# Supplements and New Media

## For the Instructor

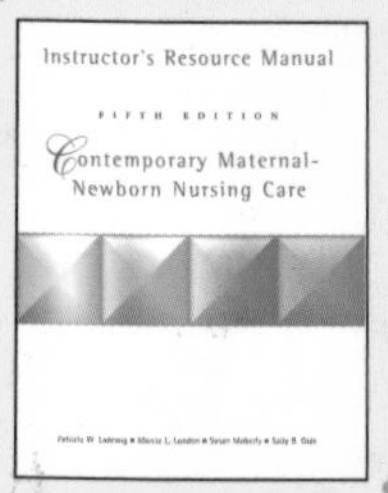

**Instructor's Resource Manual ISBN: 0-13-032505-8**

This manual contains a wealth of material to help faculty plan and manage the maternal-newborn nursing course. It includes chapter overviews, detailed lecture suggestions and outlines, learning objectives, demonstrations an activities, teaching tips, and more for each chapter. The IRM also guides faculty in how to assign and use the text-specific Companion Website, **www.prenhall.com/ladewig**, and the CD-ROM that accompany the textbook.

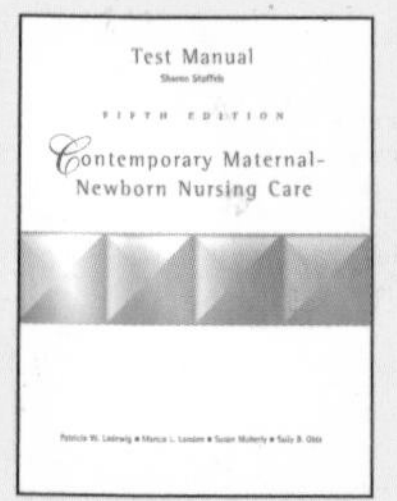

**Test Manual ISBN: 0-13-032507-4**

The printed test bank provides a thousand NCLEX-style test questions along with an answer key.

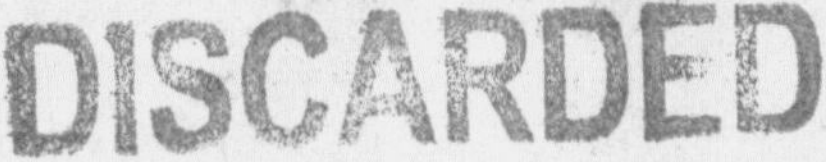


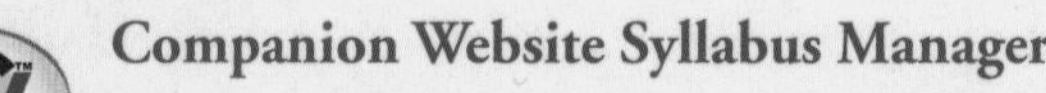

**Instructor's Resource CD-ROM with PowerPoints & Test Bank**
**ISBN: 0-13-032508-2**

This cross-platform CD-ROM provides illustrations from the new edition for use in classroom lectures. It also contains the electronic test bank. This supplement is available to faculty free upon adoption of the textbook.

**Companion Website Syllabus Manager**

Faculty adopting this textbook have ***free*** access to the online **Syllabus Manager** features of the Companion Website, **www.prenhall.com/ladewig**. It offers a whole host of features that facilitate the students' use of the Companion Website, and allows faculty to post syllabi and course information online for their students. For more information or a demonstration of **Syllabus Manager**, please contact a Prentice Hall Sales Representative.

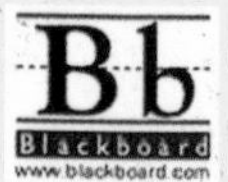


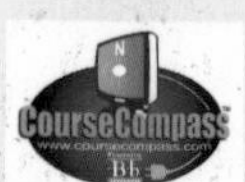


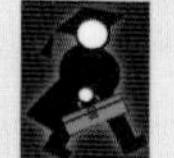

**Online Course Management Systems**

Also new to this package are online course companions available for schools using **Blackboard**, **Course Compass**, or **WebCT** course management systems. The online course management solutions feature interactive modules, electronic test bank, PowerPoint images, and an E-Book version of the textbook. For more information about adopting an online course management system to accompany **Contemporary Maternal-Newborn Nursing Care, 5th Edition** please contact your Prentice Hall Health Sales Representative or go online to **www.prenhall.com/demo**.

**Blackboard ISBN: 0-13-094248-0**
**Course Compass ISBN: 0-13-094240-5**
**WebCT ISBN: 0-13-094249-9**

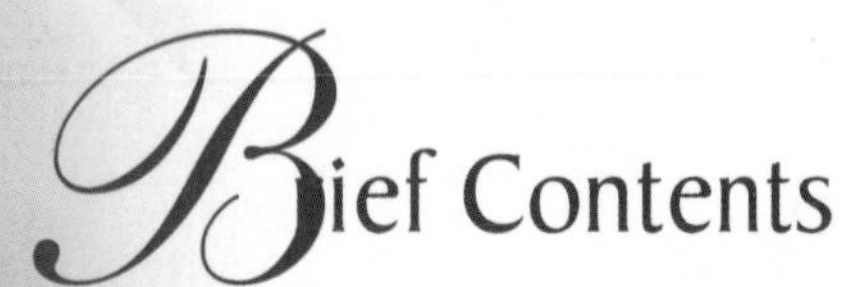

# Brief Contents

FIFTH EDITION

# Contemporary Maternal-Newborn Nursing Care

Patricia Wieland Ladewig, PhD, RN
Professor and Academic Dean
School for Health Care Professions
Regis University
Denver, Colorado

Marcia L. London, MSN, RNC, NNP
Beth-El College of Nursing and Health Sciences
University of Colorado
Colorado Springs, Colorado

Susan M. Moberly, RNC, ICCE
Labor and Delivery Nurse and Certified Childbirth Educator
Penrose Community Hospital/Centura Health
Colorado Springs, Colorado

Sally B. Olds, MS, RNC, SANE
Professor Emerita
Beth-El College of Nursing and Health Sciences
Colorado Springs, Colorado



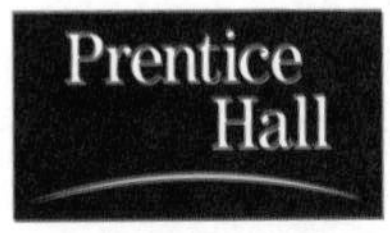


Upper Saddle River, New Jersey 07458

**Library of Congress Cataloging-in-Publication Data**

Ladewig, Patricia W.
Contemporary Maternal-Newborn Nursing Care/
Patricia Wieland, Marcia L. London, Susan M. Moberly,
Sally B. Olds.—5th ed.
p. cm.
Rev. ed. of: Maternal-Newborn Nursing Care: The
Nurse, the Family, and the Community, 4th ed. © 1998.
Includes bibliographical references and index.
ISBN: 0-8053-8051-5
1. Maternity nursing. 2. Neonatology. 3. Pediatric
nursing. I. London, Marcia L., II. Moberly, Susan M.,
III. Olds, Sally B., IV. Ladewig, Patricia W. Maternal-
Newborn Care. V. Title

2001036159

**Publisher:** Julie Alexander
**Executive Editor:** Maura Connor
**Development Editor:** Laura Bonazzoli
**Editorial Assistant:** Beth Ann Romph
**Marketing Manager:** Nicole Benson
**Director of Manufacturing and Production:**
Bruce Johnson
**Managing Editor:** Patrick Walsh
**Production Editor:** Lisa Hessel, Carlisle Publishers Services
**Production Liaison:** Cathy O'Connell
**Manufacturing Manager:** Ilene Sanford
**Media Development Editor:** Sarah Hayday
**Manager of Media Production:** Amy Peltier
**New Media Project Manager:** Stephen Hartner
**Design Director:** Cheryl Asherman
**Senior Designer:** Maria Guglielmo
**Cover Design:** Rob Richman, LaFortezza Design Group
**Interior Design:** Jennifer Bergamini, Alamini Design
**Composition:** Carlisle Communications
**Printing and Binding:** Von Hoffman

Previously published by Addison Wesley Nursing, a division of Benjamin Cummings Publishing Company Inc., under the title Maternal-Newborn Nursing Care: The Nurse, the Family, & the Community Fourth Edition.

Notice: Care has been taken to confirm the accuracy of information presented in this book. The authors, editors, and the publisher, however, cannot accept any responsibility for errors or omissions or for consequences from application of the information in this book and make no warranty, express or implied, with respect to its contents.

The authors and publisher have exerted every effort to ensure that drug selections and dosages set forth in this text are in accord with current recommendations and practice at time of publication. However, in view of ongoing research, changes in government regulations, and the constant flow of information relating to drug therapy and drug reactions, the reader is urged to check the package inserts of all drugs for any change in indications of dosage and for added warnings and precautions. This is particularly important when the recommended agent is a new and/or infrequently employed drug.

Pearson Education LTD.
Pearson Education Australia PTY, Limited
Pearson Education Singapore, Pte. Ltd.
Pearson Education North Asia Ltd.
Pearson Education Canada, Ltd.
Pearson Educación de Mexico, S.A. de C.V.
Pearson Education—Japan
Pearson Education Malaysia, Pte. Ltd.



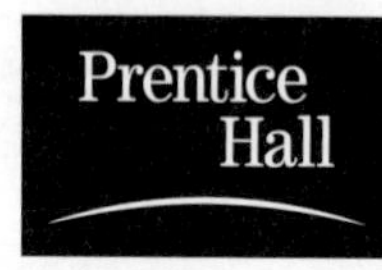


10 9 8 7 6 5 4 3 2 1
ISBN 0-8053-8051-5

# *Dedication*

Truly effective health care is not the responsibility of any one profession. It requires commitment, dedication, and collaboration on the part of many.

And so, we dedicate this book to our colleagues in health care . . .

To childbirth educators, certified nurse midwives, and physicians;
To physical therapists, medical technologists, and genetic counselors;
To dietitians, occupational therapists, and radiologic technologists;
To psychologists, social workers, and counselors;
To nurse anesthetists, paramedics, and respiratory therapists;
To audiologists, speech pathologists, and physician assistants;
To pharmacists, public health workers, and health information management professionals;
and to all those who provide care to childbearing women and their families.

Because together we touch lives,
Together we meet needs,
Together we make the world a better place
. . . one family at a time.

And, as always, we remember our beloved families —
Tim Ladewig, Ryan, and Erik
David London, Craig, and Matthew
Marty Moberly, Amanda, and Adam (AJ)
Joe Olds, Scott, Roy, Allison, and Dave

PWL MLL SMM SBO

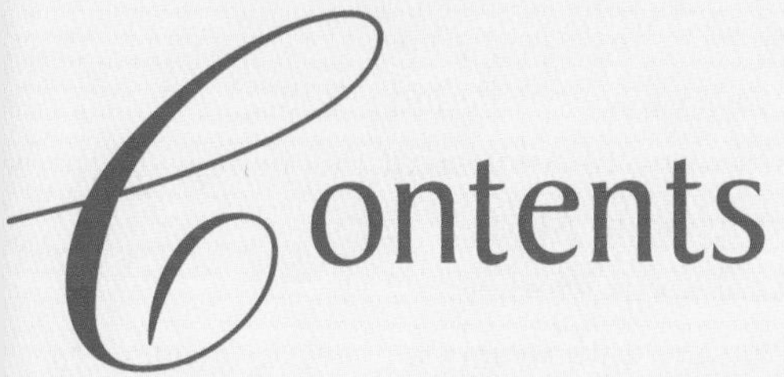

# Contents

CHAPTER **30**

## The Postpartal Family at Risk 799



## Appendixes 827

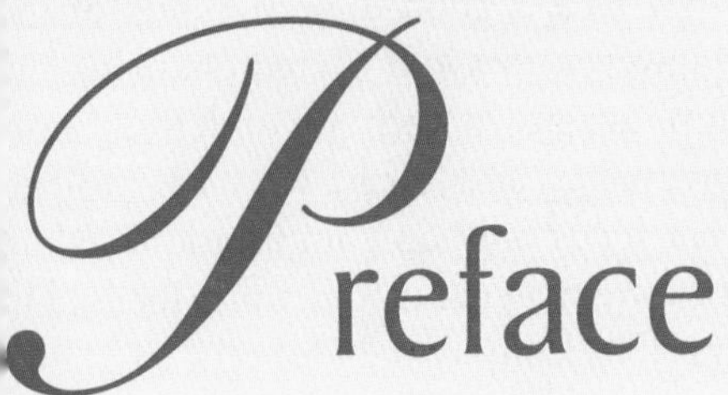

# Preface

Today, more than ever before, nurses play a central role during pregnancy and the experience of birth, and in how families feel about the experience afterward. Nevertheless, nurses working with childbearing families are challenged by a variety of forces affecting the provision of nursing care. Shortened lengths of stay, the trend toward greater use of community-based and home care, the impact of HIV/AIDS, the increased use of unlicensed assistive personnel, downsizing and mergers of health care systems, and the general aging of the population all impact the way we practice nursing today and will continue to do so in the future.

The underlying philosophy of *Contemporary Maternal-Newborn Nursing Care* (formerly *Maternal-Newborn Nursing Care: The Nurse, the Family, and the Community*) remains unchanged. We believe that pregnancy and childbirth are normal life processes and that family members are coparticipants in care. We remain committed to providing a text that is accurate and readable, a text that helps students develop the skills and abilities they need now and in the future in an ever-changing health care environment.

## Evidence-Based Practice

Health care professionals are increasingly aware of the importance of using reliable information as the basis for planning and providing effective care. This approach, referred to as *evidence-based practice,* draws on information from a variety of sources including nursing research. To help nurses become more comfortable in using evidence-based practice, we have included a brief discussion of it in chapter 1 and then provided examples of evidence-based practice as it relates to maternal-newborn nursing throughout the text. We are very proud that Lisa Sams, RN, MSN, a noted authority on the use of evidence-based practice in nursing care, developed this content for the text.

## Community-Based Nursing Care

Although pregnancy, birth, and the postpartal period cover a period of many months, in reality most women spend only two to three days (if any) in an acute care facility. Thus, by its very nature, maternal-newborn nursing is primarily community-based nursing. Moreover, because of the changes resulting from managed care, even women with high-risk pregnancies are receiving more care in their homes and in the community and are spending less time in hospital settings.

This greater emphasis on nursing care provided in community-based settings is a driving force in health care today and, consequently, forms a dominant theme through this edition. We have addressed this topic in focused, user-friendly ways. **Community-Based Nursing Care** is a special heading used throughout this text and indicated by an icon to assist students in recognizing this content. Because we consider home care to be one form of community-based care, it often has a separate heading under Community-Based Nursing Care. Even more important, a separate chapter, **Home Care of the Postpartal Family,** provides a thorough explanation of home care, both from a theoretical perspective and as a significant tool in caring for childbearing families.

## Emphasis on Client and Family Teaching

Client and family teaching remains a critical element of effective nursing care, one that we continue to emphasize and highlight in this new edition. Again, our focus is on the teaching that nurses do at all stages of pregnancy and the childbearing process—including the important postpartal teaching that is done before and after families are discharged. Throughout the text, detailed discussions of client and family teaching are summarized in **Teaching Guides** such as the one on sexual activity during pregnancy. These Teaching Guides help students plan and organize their client teaching. The tear-out **Client-Family Teaching Cards** are also handy tools for the student to use while studying or as a quick reference in the clinical setting. Two new cards for Spanish phrases and sign language have been added to the new edition of this text. In addition, a foldout, full-color **Fetal Development Chart** depicts maternal and fetal development by month and provides specific teaching guidelines for each stage of pregnancy. Students can use this chart as another study tool or as a quick clinical reference.

# Commitment to Diversity

As nurses and educators we feel a strong commitment to the importance of recognizing and honoring diversity and multiculturalism. Thus we continually strive to make our text ever more inclusive. Achieving such a goal is difficult, but we feel our success in this regard cannot be measured simply in terms of specific photos, charts, or tables. Instead, we believe that with its subtle integration of a variety of issues and scenarios affecting maternal-newborn nursing care—beyond the emphasis on ethnicity alone—our approach is more accessible overall.

# Organization: A Nursing Care Management Framework

As educators and nurses, we have organized this text to flow logically. Nurses today must be able to think critically and problem solve effectively. For these reasons, we begin with an introductory unit to set the stage by providing information about maternal-newborn nursing and important related contents. Subsequent units progress in a way that closely reflects the steps of the *nursing process.* The nurse's role is clearly delineated within this framework. Thus the units related to pregnancy, labor and birth, the newborn period, and postpartum begin with a discussion of basic theory followed by content or chapters on nursing assessment and then nursing care for essentially healthy women or infants. Within the nursing care chapters and content areas, we use the heading **Nursing Care Management** and the subheadings **Nursing Assessment and Diagnosis, Planning and Implementation,** and **Evaluation.**

Complications of a period are the last chapter or chapters in each unit, also organized using the nursing process. We believe that students can more clearly grasp the complicated content of the high-risk chapters in a given unit once they have a good understanding of the normal process. However, to avoid overemphasizing the prevalence of complications in such a wonderfully normal process as pregnancy and birth, we have avoided including units that focus only on complications. More specialized or distinctive material is sometimes focused in a single chapter, as, for example, the chapters on maternal nutrition, adolescent pregnancy, special diagnostic procedures, and newborn nutrition.

In keeping with the changing approaches to nursing care management, **Critical Pathways** are featured throughout the text. Four critical pathways—intrapartal, newborn, postpartal, and cesarean birth—are designed to help students plan and manage care within normally anticipated time frames. In addition, we provide critical pathways that address nursing care for women with complications such as pregnancy-induced hypertension and diabetes mellitus as well as for high-risk newborns. This information is designed to help students become familiar with this approach to managing care so that they are better prepared in the clinical setting.

# Notable Features

Instructors and students alike value the in-text learning aids included in our textbooks. With this edition, we have once again developed a text that is easy to learn from and easy to use as a reference. Each chapter begins with **Objectives** and a list of **Key Terms.** Page numbers are included with each key term to identify the place where the term first appears in the chapter. Each chapter ends with a chapter review that consists of a summary of **Chapter Highlights,** a list of **References,** and a *new* section entitled **Maternal-Newborn Nursing Online.** This last section encourages students to use the additional chapter-specific NCLEX review, exercises, and resources available on the accompanying free Student CD-ROM and the Companion Website at www.prenhall.com/ladewig. Finally, a **Glossary** of terms commonly used in the field of maternal-newborn nursing can be found at the back of the text.

*New* **Chapter Opening Vignettes** from nurses in a variety of maternal, newborn, and women's health roles illustrate the diversity of career options and settings available to nurses in this field and reflect the deep satisfaction that these nurses experience in their profession.

Moreover, *new* **Hints for Practice** offer hands-on suggestions and clinical tips for specific procedures and interventions.

The **Assessment Guides** incorporate physical assessment and normal findings, alterations and possible causes, and guidelines for nursing interventions. **Procedures** describe actions specific to maternal-newborn nursing care in a step-by-step fashion.

To support the development of critical thinking skills, **Critical Thinking in Practice** boxes provide brief scenarios that ask students to determine the appropriate response. Suggested answers to the scenarios are provided in Appendix I so that students will have immediate feedback on their decision-making skills.

**Community-Based Nursing Care** is a special heading and icon throughout the text that identifies specific aspects of maternal-newborn nursing care that occurs in community or home settings.

**Drug Guides** for those medications commonly used in maternal-newborn nursing are included to guide students in correctly administering the medications.

**Key Facts to Remember** provide a quick review of important content in convenient boxed format.

## Comprehensive Teaching and Learning Package

To enhance the teaching and learning process, the following supplements have been developed in close correlation with the new edition of this textbook. The full complement of supplemental teaching materials is available to all qualified instructors from your Prentice Hall Health Sales Representative.

***Student CD-ROM.*** A new addition to this package, the Student CD-ROM includes NCLEX-style multiple-choice questions that emphasize the application of nursing care. Students can test their knowledge and gain immediate feedback through rationales for right and wrong answers. The CD-ROM also provides several video clips and animations to help students understand and visualize difficult concepts in maternal-newborn nursing care. Finally, the CD-ROM allows access to the Companion Website described later in this section. This CD-ROM is packaged free with every copy of the textbook.

***Student Workbook.*** This useful workbook has been revised, streamlined, and updated in keeping with the changes made to this new edition. It provides a concise review of essential content and includes exercises and strategies to help students focus their study.

***Clinical Handbook.*** This portable handbook provides students with a succinct, quick-reference guide for use in the clinical setting. Content is organized by each stage of the childbirth process and includes normal and at-risk information. Procedures, tables, photos, and illustrations are integrated throughout.

***Instructor's Manual.*** This effective and timesaving aid has been revised and streamlined. It provides suggestions for covering important content and is organized by topics according to subject matter.

***Test Bank.*** Available in printed or electronic formats, this updated test bank helps faculty quickly and easily create numerous unique examinations. Test items follow the NCLEX format and are classified by cognitive level, nursing process step, and client need.

***Instructor's Resource CD-ROM.*** New to this package, the Instructor's Resource CD-ROM provides two resources in an electronic format. First, the CD-ROM includes the complete test bank in a PC-compatible format. Second, it includes a comprehensive collection of images from the textbook in PowerPoint format, so faculty can easily import these photographs and illustrations into their own classroom lecture presentations.

***Companion Website and Syllabus Manager®***. New to this package is a free Companion Website at www.prenhall.com/ladewig. This website serves as a text-specific, interactive online workbook to *Contemporary Maternal-Newborn Nursing Care,* 5th edition. The Companion Website includes modules for objectives, chapter outlines, key terms and definitions, discussion questions with essay responses, NCLEX review questions with automatic grading, links to other sites for student research and essay responses, and more. Instructors adopting this textbook for their courses have free access to an online Syllabus Manager with a whole host of features that facilitate the students' use of this Companion Website and allow faculty to post their syllabi online for their students. For more information or a demonstration of Syllabus Manager, please contact your Prentice Hall Health Sales Representative or go online to www.prenhall.com/demo.

***Online Course Management Systems.*** Also new to this package are online course companions available for schools using Blackboard, WebCT, or Course Compass course management systems. For more information about adopting an online course management system to accompany *Contemporary Maternal-Newborn Nursing Care,* 5th edition please contact your Prentice Hall Health Sales Representative or go online to www.prenhall.com/demo.

## Acknowledgments

With each revision, our goal remains constant—to ensure that our text reflects the most current research and the latest information about nursing. This would not be possible without the support of our colleagues in clinical practice and nursing education. Their suggestions, contributions, and words of encouragement help us achieve this goal. We recognize the intense commitment of nurses everywhere to excellence in clinical practice. And so we thank our colleagues.

We are grateful, too, to our students past, present, and future. They stimulate us with their interest; they reinvigorate us with their enthusiasm; they challenge us with their questions to make this text as clear and readable as possible. We learn so much from them.

In publishing, as in health care, quality assurance is an essential part of this process—and this is the dimension that reviewers add. Some reviewers assist us by validating the content, some by their attention to detail, and some by challenging us to examine our ways of thinking to develop a new awareness. Thus we extend a sincere thanks to all those who reviewed the manuscript for this text. Their names and affiliations are listed following this preface.

We also wish to thank the contributors to the 6th edition of our other text, *Maternal-Newborn Nursing: A Family and Community-Based Approach.* They include the following:

**Melody R. Marks Best, RN-C, MS, WHCNP, LCCE**
Colorado College
Colorado Springs, Colorado

**Deborah A. Bopp, RN, MS**
Memorial Hospital
Colorado Springs, Colorado

**Wendy Earl**
Medical Writer
San Francisco, California

**Victoria Flanagan, RN, BSN**
Dartmouth-Hitchcock Medical Center
Lebanon, New Hampshire

**Kathleen Furniss, RNC, MSN**
Associates in Woman's Health Care
Wayne, New Jersey

**Mary I. Enzman Hagedorn, RN, PhD, CNS, CPNP**
Beth El College of Nursing and Health Sciences
University of Colorado at Colorado Springs
Colorado Springs, Colorado

**Carol Ann Harrigan, RNC, MSN, NNP**
Phoenix Children's Hospital
Phoenix, Arizona

**Mary Ellen Honeyfield, RNC, MS, NNP**
Innovative Health Care, Inc.
Denver, Colorado

**Virginia Gramzow Kinnick, RN, EdD, CNM**
University of Northern Colorado
Greeley, Colorado

**Cheryl Pope Kish, RNC, MSN, EdD, WHNP**
Georgia College and Georgia State University
Milledgeville, Georgia

**Ruth Likler, RNC, BSN**
Presbyterian/St. Luke's Medical Center
Denver, Colorado

**Deborah Cooper McGee, RNC, MSN**
Regis University
St. Luke's Medical Center
Denver, Colorado

**Susan Moberly, RN, BSN, ICCE**
Centura Health/Penrose Community Birth Center
Colorado Springs, Colorado

**Patricia Moores, RN, PhD, CS**
Samuel Merritt College
Oakland, California

**Candace Polzella, RD, MSS**
The Renfrew Center
Philadelphia, Pennsylvania

**Lisa Sams, RN, MSN**
Clinician to Clinician Solutions, Inc.
Arlington, Virginia

**Lisa A. Smith-Pedersen, APRN, MSN, CNNP**
Northwestern State University of Louisiana
Louisiana State University Medical Center
Shreveport, Louisiana

**Monica Taylor, RN, MEd, LCCE**
The Toledo Hospital
Toledo, Ohio

**Candace Tulve Shoenenberger, RN, PhD, WHCNP**
Regis University
Denver, Colorado

**Mary E. English Worth, RNC, CRNP**
Pennsylvania Reproductive Associates
Philadelphia, Pennsylvania

**Sandra Worthington, RNC, MSN, CNM**
Planned Parenthood Federation of America, Inc.
New York, New York

We are especially grateful to Lisa Sams, Clinical Linkages, INC., for contributing content and boxes on evidence-based practice to this edition. She is a leader in this important, emerging focus of clinical practice and—an added plus—she is a truly delightful woman.

A project of this scope is not possible without the skill and expertise of many people. And so we extend special thanks to the following people.

First and foremost, our deepest thanks to our editor, Maura Connor, for her commitment to this book and to us as authors. She is incredibly knowledgeable about nursing education and the needs of students. As we transitioned to a new publishing company, Maura smoothed the way, helping us carry our shared vision forward in a seamless transition. She is enthusiastic, warm, and supportive, and we look forward to many years of collaboration and friendship.

Julie Alexander, our publisher, has delineated a vision for the future and a commitment to excellence for Prentice Hall Health. Her energy, responsiveness, and forward thinking are awe inspiring and challenge us to give our best. We anticipate a long and exciting relationship with this very special woman.

Special thanks to a dear friend, Laura Bonazzoli, the developmental editor for the book. Her knowledge of the book's content, her awareness of issues impacting childbearing families, and her eye for detail have helped us produce a strong, readable edition.

Beth Ann Romph, editorial assistant, kept us on track. Her kindness, patience, and unfailing efficiency coupled with her skill at handling detail were invaluable. She truly is an unsung hero. Thanks, Beth.

We also extend our deep appreciation to Lisa Hessel of Carlisle Publishers Services. She assumed the Herculean task of steering the book through all phases of production. She was effective in her role, patient and gracious in her interactions, and responsive to our needs when scheduling problems arose.

We are also grateful to Susan Brehm for her skillful copyediting. Her work improved our manuscript and helped ensure consistency.

This is a time of possibilities for nursing. The need for skilled nurses has never been higher, nor have the opportunities to make a real difference in the lives of childbearing families ever been greater. Time and again we have seen the difference a skilled nurse can make in the lives of people in need. We, like you, are committed to helping all nurses recognize and take pride in that fact. Thank you for your letters, your comments, and your suggestions. We feel embraced by your support.

PWL
MLL
SMM
SBO

# Reviewers

**Margaret Jean Auffarth, MSN**
University of Missouri, St Louis
St. Louis, MO

**Martha A. Auvenshire, RN, EdD**
California State University, Hayward
Hayward, CA

**Sandra L. Baker, RN, MSN**
Riverside Community College
Riverside, CA

**Deborah A. Bechtel-Blackwell, PhD, RNC, WHCNP, CS, ANP**
University of South Carolina, Columbia
Columbia, SC

**Karen Booth, RN, BSN, MEd, MSN**
Owens Community College
Toledo, OH

**Joyce Breed, MSN**
Bevil State Community College
Sumiton, AL

**Jacqueline A. Carrillo, RN, MSN**
Hinds Community College
Jackson, MS

**Shelly F. Conroy, BSN, MSN**
John Tyler Community College
Chester, VA

**Patricia Contrisciani, RN, BSN, MSN, EdD**
Delaware County Community College
Media, PA

**Julie Coon, RN, MSN, EdD**
Ferris State University
Big Rapids, MI

**Debra I. Craig, DNSc, CNS, RN**
Point Loma Nazarene College
San Diego, CA

**Phyllis S. Daugherty, MEd, RN**
Rowan-Cabarrus Community College
Salisbury, NC

**Kathy Deardorff, MSN, RN**
University of Texas, Tyler
Tyler, TX

**Mary Ann Duffy, RNC, BSN**
Southern Union State Community College
Valley, AL

**Eme Ekpo, PhD, PNP, WHCNP**
Adelphi University
Garden City, NY

**Judy Fillmore, BSN**
Southern Utah University
Cedar City, UT

**Janet E. Fogg, RNC, MSN**
Pennsylvania State University/Hershey Medical Center
Hershey, PA

**Roberta Gates, RN, MSN**
Darton College
Albany, GA

**S. Kim Genovese, RNC, CARN, MSN, MSA**
Purdue University
West Lafayette, IN

**Eileen Griffiths, RN, MSN**
Miami-Dade Community College
Miami, FL

**Angela Halen, RNC, MSN**
North Harris Montgomery Community College
Houston, TX

**Sally Johnson Hartman, MSN**
Indiana University Purdue University
Fort Wayne, IN

**Lori Mattrey Hoffman, PhD, RN**
DeSales University
Center Valley, PA

**Madeline Hogan, RN, MSN**
Nassau Community College
Garden City, NY

**Paulette Hopkins, RN, MSN, WHNP**
Meridian Community College
Meridian, MS

**Grace Jacobson, PhD, RNC**
Idaho State University
Pocatello, ID

**Cecilia M. Jevitt, CNM, PhD**
University of South Florida
Tampa, FL

**Linda J. Kapinos, RNC, MSN, MEd, IBCLC**
Capital Community College
Hartford, CT

**Suzanne Ketchem, RN, MSN**
University of Pittsburgh
Bradford, PA

**Jane M. Kirkpatrick, RNC, MSN**
Purdue University
West Lafayette, IN

**Janice C. Livingston, MEd, MS, ARNP**
Central Florida Community College
Ocala, FL

**Karen Lyons, RN, MS**
Oklahoma City Community College
Oklahoma City, OK

**Debbie McGregor, MSN**
Miami Dade Community College
Miami, FL

**Rhonda R. Martin, MS, RN**
University of Tulsa
Tulsa, OK

**Victoria M. Mendler, RNC, MSN, WHNP**
Macomb Community College
Clinton Township, MI

**Rita G. Mertig, BSN, MSN**
John Tyler Community College
Chester, VA

**Jan M. Nick, PhD, RNC**
Loma Linda University
Loma Linda, CA

**Jennifer Ortiz, RNC, MSN**
Suffolk Community College
Brentwood, NY

**Joanne Ottman, RN, MSN**
Naugatuck Valley Community College
Waterbury, CT

**Charlene Pope, CNM, MPH, RN, PhC**
State University of New York, Brockport
Brockport, NY

**Melissa Powell, RN, MSN**
Eastern Kentucky University
Richmond, KY

**Kristin Priddy, RN, MSN**
University of Texas, Arlington
Arlington, TX

**Kathy Records, PhD, RN**
Intercollegiate Center for Nursing Education
Spokane, WA

**Kristine Ring-Wilson, MS, RN**
Excelsior College
Albany, NY

**Carole A. Rosales, RN, MSN**
Los Angeles Valley College
Van Nuys, CA

**Constance M. Roth-Sautter, PhD, RNC**
Medical College of Ohio
Toledo, OH

**Editha C. Sanchez, RNC, MSN, MEd**
South Suburban College
South Holland, IL

**Debbie Sanders, RNC, MSN**
Pennsylvania State University/Geisinger Medical Center
Danville, PA

**Rose Schecter, PhD, RN**
Molloy College
Rockville Centre, NY

**Carol Schimer, MS, RN**
Pasco Hernando Community College
New Port Richey, FL

**Debra L. Siegel, RN, CNM, MS**
Cuyahoga Community College
Cleveland, OH

**Violetta Siguly, RN, MSN**
Miami Dade Community College
Miami, FL

**Diane Spatz, PhD, RN**
University of Pennsylvania
Philadelphia, PA

**Karen Stevens, RN, MSN**
Bowie State University
Bowie, MD

**Sharon J. Thompson, PhD, RN, MPH**
Gannon University
Erie, PA

**Mary Tobin, RN, MSN**
Kirkwood Community College
Cedar Rapids, IA

**Susanne M. Tracy, RN, MN, MA**
Rivier College/St. Joseph's Hospital
Nashua, NH

**Lois Tschetter, RN, EdD (candidate)**
South Dakota State University
Brookings, SD

**Debra J. Walden, MNSc, RNP**
Arkansas State University
State University, AK

**Kathleen A. Walsh, BSN, MSN, PhD (candidate)**
Broward Community College
Ft. Lauderdale, FL

**Linda Williams, RN, MSN**
Southwestern College
Chula Vista, CA

**Judith M. Wismont, PhD, RN**
University of Michigan, Ann Arbor
Ann Arbor, MI

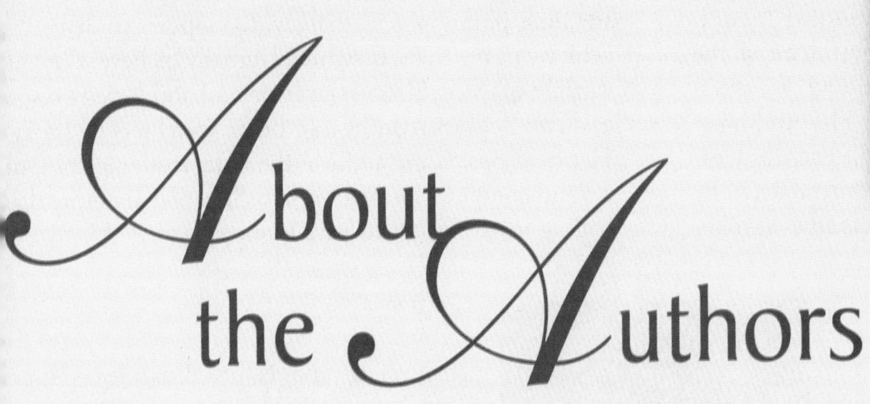

# About the Authors

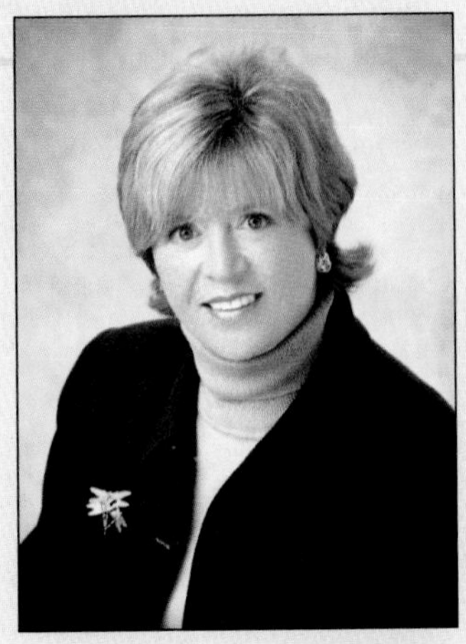

Patricia A. Wieland Ladewig

Patricia A. Wieland Ladewig received her BS from the College of Saint Teresa in Winona, Minnesota. After graduation, she worked as a pediatric nurse before joining the Air Force. After completing her tour of duty, Dr. Ladewig relocated to Florida, where she accepted a faculty position at Florida State University. There she discovered teaching as her calling. Over the years, she taught at several schools of nursing while earning her MSN in maternal-newborn nursing from Catholic University of America in Washington, DC, and her PhD in higher education administration from the University of Denver in Colorado. In addition, she became a Women's Health Nurse Practitioner and maintained a part-time clinical practice. In 1988 Dr. Ladewig became the first director of the nursing program at Regis College in Denver, and, in 1991, when the college became Regis University, she became dean of the School for Health Care Professions. Under her guidance, the Department of Nursing has added a graduate program and the School for Health Care Professions has added two departments: the Department of Physical Therapy and the Department of Health Services Administration and Management. Dr. Ladewig feels that teaching others to be excellent, caring nurses gives her the best of all worlds because it keeps her in touch with the profession she loves and enables her to help shape the future of the nursing profession. When not at work or writing textbooks, Pat and her husband, Tim, enjoy skiing, climbing Colorado's 14'ers (14,000-foot mountains, 15 of which she has climbed to date), and traveling. They are the parents of two sons, Ryan, who recently graduated with a master's degree in computer science, and Erik, a student at Regis University.

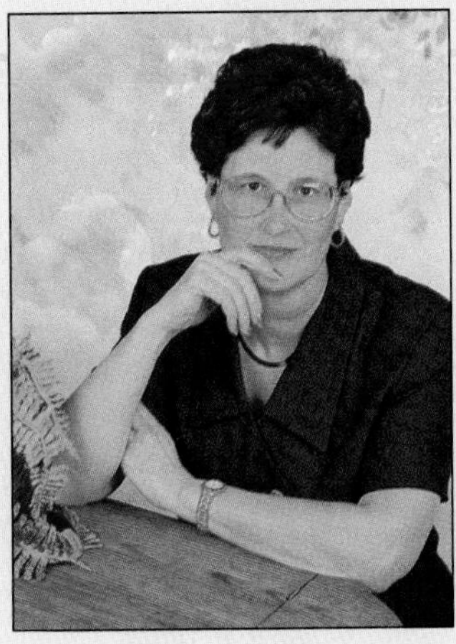

Marcia L. London

Marcia L. London has been able to combine her two greatest passions by being both a nurse caring for children and families and a teacher for almost 30 years. She received her BSN and School Nurse Certificate from Plattsburgh State University in Plattsburgh, New York. After graduation, she worked as a pediatric nurse at St. Luke's Hospital in New York City, then moved to Pittsburgh, where she began her teaching career. Mrs. London accepted a faculty position at Pittsburgh's Children's Hospital Affiliate program and received her MSN in pediatrics as a clinical nurse specialist from the University of Pittsburgh in Pennsylvania. Mrs. London began teaching at Beth-El School of Nursing and Health Science in 1974 after opening the first intensive care nursery at Memorial Hospital of Colorado Springs. She has served in many faculty positions at Beth-El, including assistant director of the School of Nursing. Mrs. London obtained her post-master's Neonatal Nurse Practitioner certificate in 1983 and subsequently developed the Neonatal Nurse Practitioner (NNP) certificate and the master's NNP program at Beth-El. She is active nationally in neonatal nursing and was involved in the development of the Neonatal Nurse Practitioner Educational program guidelines. Mrs. London is also actively involved in nurse practitioner education in general. She is involved in the revision of the Core Competency for Nurse Practitioners and

*continue*

Curriculum Guidelines for Nurse Practitioner Education, as a member of the Education Committee of the National Organization of Nurse Practitioner Faculties. Mrs. London is currently completing her PhD in higher education administration and adult studies at the University of Denver in Colorado. She feels fortunate to be involved in the education of her future colleagues and her teaching philosophy is that, with support, students ca achieve more than they may initially believe they ar capable of. Mrs. London and her husband have two son and two dogs (Samantha and Betsy, daughters by proxy Her two sons, Craig and Matthew, are studying comput ers and computer animation in college and are more tha willing to give Mom helpful hints.

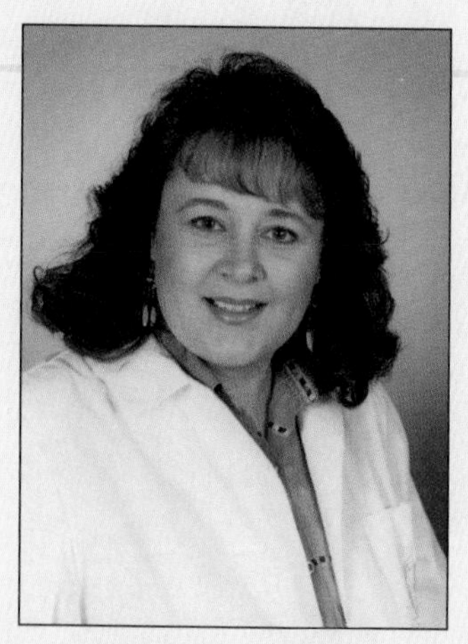

Susan M. Moberly

Susan M. Moberly is a relative newcomer to maternal-newborn nursing, but not to the vital issues of consumer advocacy, women's health, and childbearing choice. Sue began caring for expectant parents as a certified childbirth educator over 15 years ago, specializing in prenatal classes developed for those individuals with special needs and circumstances. She has taught childbirth education in many settings, both hospital and community based. In 1990 Ms. Moberly successfully completed the national certification program with the International Childbirth Education Association (ICEA), which she continues to maintain. In 1996 she graduated with her BSN from Beth-El College of Nursing and began practice as a labor and delivery nurse at Penrose Community Hospital in Colorado Springs. In 1999 Sue completed the RN certification for in-patient obstetrics.

Early in Ms. Moberly's undergraduate studies, she became convinced that the concepts of political professional development, holistic nursing practice, and career involvement *must* begin at the student level. During her time at Beth-El, Sue was a leader in both the local and state chapters of the National Student Nurse Association (NSNA), was selected as a char ter member of the then newly formed Xi-Ph chapter of Sigma Theta Tau, and was activ in the American Holistic Nurses Association In 1995 Sue Moberly was honored to b chosen as the NSNA Helene Fuld Fellow fo Colorado. She attended the Fuld Conferenc on Holistic Nursing Practice in Edinburgh Scotland, and participated in a study tour o London. Following graduation, Ms. Moberly continued her involvement with the Student Nurses Association as an adviser an served as vice president of her Sigma Theta Tau chapter fo three years. She is also an active member of the Colorad Nurses Association and AWHONN.

Currently Sue is completing final requirements for he certification in nurse-midwifery at the University of Colorado Health Sciences Center. In addition, she is trying to stay sane while working in labor and delivery, coauthoring this textbook, and raising two adolescents: he 16-year-old daughter, Amanda, and her 12-year-old son AJ. Thanks to the support of her husband, Marty, she is succeeding!

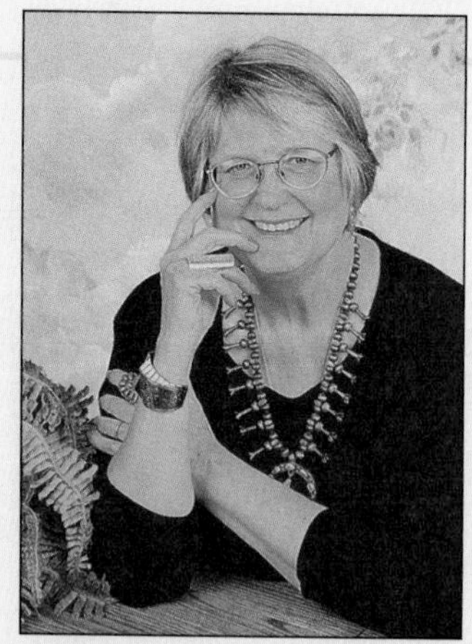

Sally B. Olds

Sally B. Olds has provided hands-on maternal-newborn nursing care and has mentored students and colleagues for more than 30 years. She received her BSN from the University of Kansas and her MS in nursing from the University of Colorado. Completing her master's degree provided Mrs. Olds with the opportunity to achieve one of her life's goals: teaching nursing students. She began teaching at the Beth-El School of Nursing and Health Science in 1975, eventually becoming the chair of the Department of Holistic Nursing, and was instrumental in developing the Clinical Nursing Specialist Program in Holistic Health for the master's program. Her teaching philosophy has been to nurture and support students as they learn, to focus on the positive aspects of learning, and to teach students the importance of respecting the client and family for whom they provide care. Mrs. Olds taught at Beth-El for over 22 years before retiring in 1997 and was named professor emerita. She became a Sexual Assault Nurse Examiner (SANE), working one-on-one with sexual assault survivors in 1996, and she continues her involvement with issues affecting women and children. Since her retirement, Mrs. Olds has had more time to spend with her husband, two grown children, and Old English sheepdog.

# A GUIDE TO
# Contemporary Maternal-Newborn Nursing Care

## FIFTH EDITION

Nurses working with childbearing families play a special role during pregnancy and birth experience. They also face a unique set of challenges, from shortened lengths of say and the impact of HIV to the increased use of unlicensed assistive personnel. The new Fifth Edition of **Contemporary Maternal-Newborn Nursing Care** (formerly *Maternal-Newborn Nursing Care, 4/e*) continues to foster the vital skills nurses need to meet these challenges—flexibility, critical thinking, and problem-solving—withing the framework of the nursing process.

The new Fifth Edition is supported by robust pedagogy and a suite of user-friendly supplements, including new CD-ROMs for both students and instructors and free Companion Website. Visit www.prenhall.com/ladewig for chapter outlines, discussion questions with essay responses, NCLEX review questions with automatic grading, links to other sites of student research and essay responses, and much more.

**Chapter Opening Vignettes** offer from the heart commentary by nurses in a variety of maternal, newborn, and women's health roles, illustrating not only the diversity of career options available, but also the deep satisfaction enjoyed by these practitioners.

**Evidence-Based Practice** boxes draw on the latest research as the basis for planning and providing effective care. The new fifth Edition introduces readers to the concept of evidence-based practice in Chapter One, with detailed examples related to maternal-newborn nursing throughout the text.

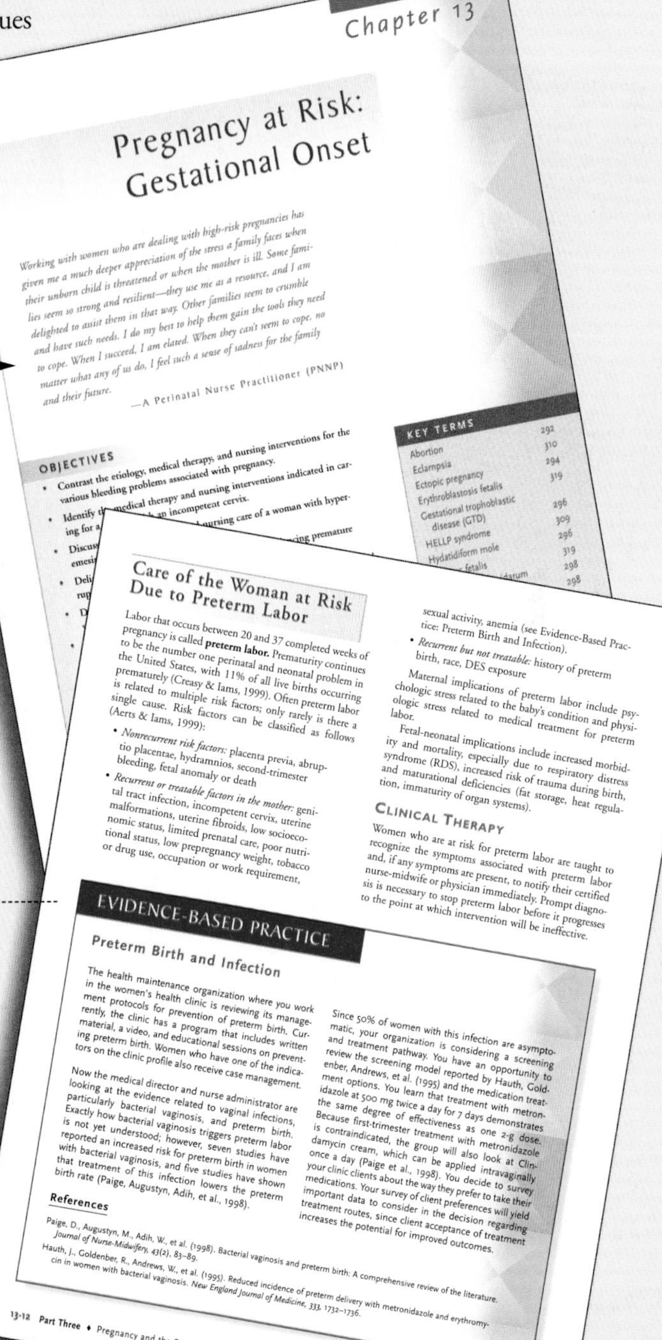

Chapter 13

Pregnancy at Risk: Gestational Onset

*Working with women who are dealing with high-risk pregnancies has given me a much deeper appreciation of the stress a family faces when their unborn child is threatened or when the mother is ill. Some families seem so strong and resilient—they use me as a resource, and I am delighted to assist them in that way. Other families seem to crumble and have such needs. I do my best to help them gain the tools they need to cope. When I succeed, I am elated. When they can't seem to cope, no matter what any of us do, I feel such a sense of sadness for the family and their future.*

—A Perinatal Nurse Practitioner (PNNP)

OBJECTIVES

- Contrast the etiology, medical therapy, and nursing interventions for the various bleeding problems associated with pregnancy.
- Identify the medical therapy and nursing interventions indicated in caring for a ... an incompetent cervix.
- Discuss ... nursing care of a woman with hyperemesis ...
- Deli... ...ing premature rup...

KEY TERMS

| | |
|---|---|
| Abortion | 292 |
| Eclampsia | 310 |
| Ectopic pregnancy | 294 |
| Erythroblastosis fetalis | 319 |
| Gestational trophoblastic disease (GTD) | 296 |
| HELLP syndrome | 309 |
| Hydatidiform mole | 296 |
| ... fetalis | 319 |
| ...darum | 298 |
| | 298 |

Care of the Woman at Risk Due to Preterm Labor

Labor that occurs between 20 and 37 completed weeks of pregnancy is called **preterm labor.** Prematurity continues to be the number one perinatal and neonatal problem in the United States, with 11% of all live births occurring prematurely (Creasy & Iams, 1999). Often preterm labor is related to multiple risk factors; only rarely is there a single cause. Risk factors can be classified as follows (Aerts & Iams, 1999):

- *Nonrecurrent risk factors:* placenta previa, abruptio placentae, hydramnios, second-trimester bleeding, fetal anomaly or death
- *Recurrent or treatable factors in the mother:* genital tract infection, incompetent cervix, uterine malformations, uterine fibroids, low socioeconomic status, limited prenatal care, poor nutritional status, low prepregnancy weight, tobacco or drug use, occupation or work requirement, sexual activity, anemia (see Evidence-Based Practice: Preterm Birth and Infection).
- *Recurrent but not treatable:* history of preterm birth, race, DES exposure

Maternal implications of preterm labor include psychologic stress related to the baby's condition and physiologic stress related to medical treatment for preterm labor.

Fetal-neonatal implications include increased morbidity and mortality, especially due to respiratory distress syndrome (RDS), increased risk of trauma during birth, and maturational deficiencies (fat storage, heat regulation, immaturity of organ systems).

CLINICAL THERAPY

Women who are at risk for preterm labor are taught to recognize the symptoms associated with preterm labor and, if any symptoms are present, to notify their certified nurse-midwife or physician immediately. Prompt diagnosis is necessary to stop preterm labor before it progresses to the point at which intervention will be ineffective.

EVIDENCE-BASED PRACTICE

Preterm Birth and Infection

The health maintenance organization where you work in the women's health clinic is reviewing its management protocols for prevention of preterm birth. Currently, the clinic has a program that includes written material, a video, and educational sessions on preventing preterm birth. Women who have one of the indicators on the clinic profile also receive case management.

Now the medical director and nurse administrator are looking at the evidence related to vaginal infections, particularly bacterial vaginosis, and preterm birth. Exactly how bacterial vaginosis triggers preterm labor is not yet understood; however, seven studies have reported an increased risk for preterm birth in women with bacterial vaginosis, and five studies have shown that treatment of this infection lowers the preterm birth rate (Paige, Augustyn, Adih, et al., 1998).

Since 50% of women with this infection are asymptomatic, your organization is considering a screening and treatment pathway. You have an opportunity to review the screening model reported by Hauth, Goldenber, Andrews, et al. (1995) and the medication treatment options. You learn that treatment with metronidazole at 500 mg twice a day for 7 days demonstrates the same degree of effectiveness as one 2-g dose. Because first-trimester treatment with metronidazole is contraindicated, the group will also look at Clindamycin cream, which can be applied intravaginally once a day (Paige et al., 1998). You decide to survey your clinic clients about the way they prefer to take their medications. Your survey of client preferences will yield important data to consider in the decision regarding treatment routes, since client acceptance of treatment increases the potential for improved outcomes.

References


Paige, D., Augustyn, M., Adih, W., et al. (1998). Bacterial vaginosis and preterm birth: A comprehensive review of the literature. *Journal of Nurse-Midwifery, 43*(2), 83–89.

Hauth, J., Goldenber, R., Andrews, W., et al. (1995). Reduced incidence of preterm delivery with metronidazole and erythromycin in women with bacterial vaginosis. *New England Journal of Medicine, 333*, 1732–1736.


13-12 Part Three ♦ Pregnancy and the Family

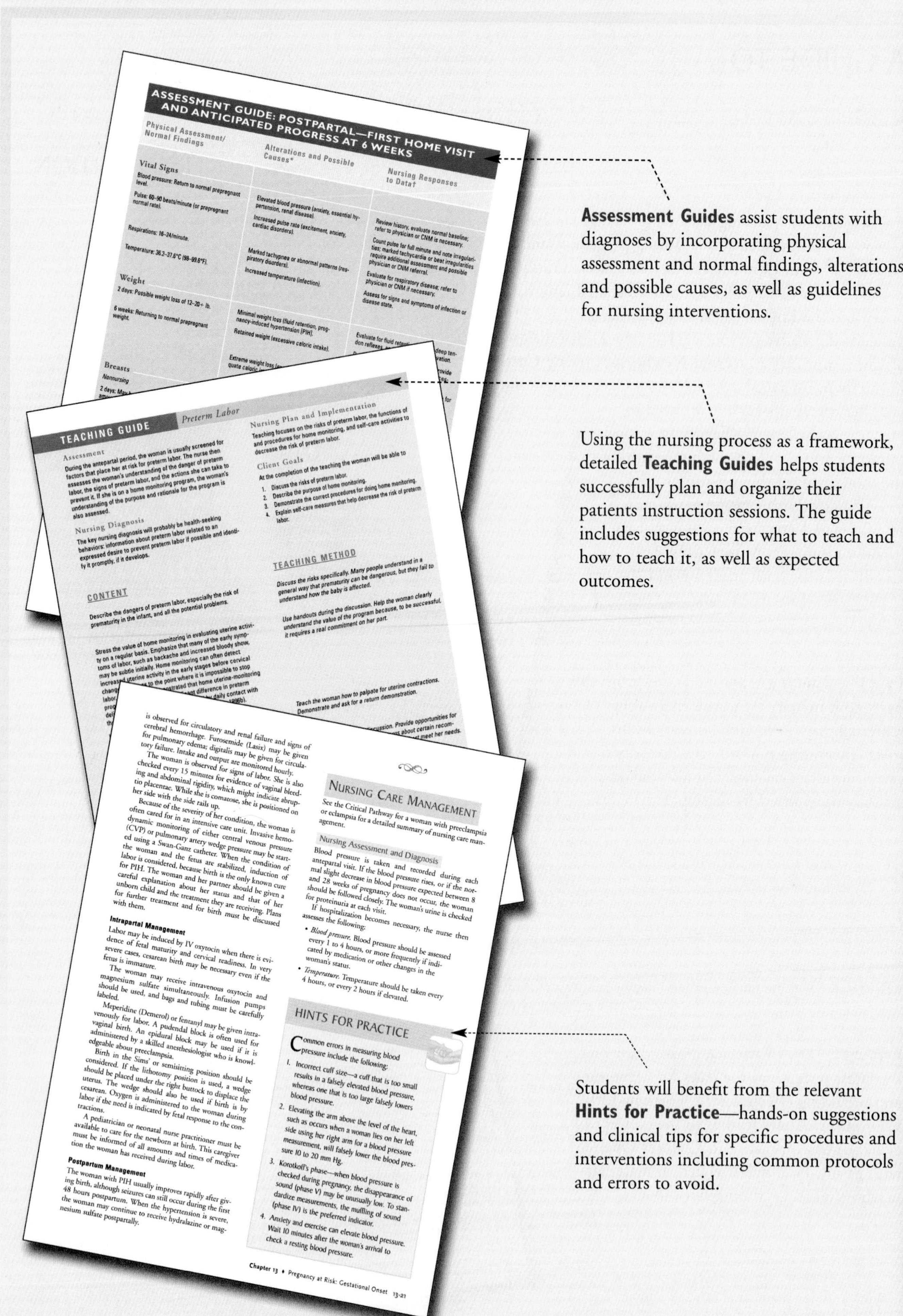

**Assessment Guides** assist students with diagnoses by incorporating physical assessment and normal findings, alterations and possible causes, as well as guidelines for nursing interventions.

Using the nursing process as a framework, detailed **Teaching Guides** helps students successfully plan and organize their patients instruction sessions. The guide includes suggestions for what to teach and how to teach it, as well as expected outcomes.

Students will benefit from the relevant **Hints for Practice**—hands-on suggestions and clinical tips for specific procedures and interventions including common protocols and errors to avoid.

Students are guided through the specific aspects of maternal-newborn nursing care that may occur in a community or home setting versus hospital-based care. Each **Community-Based Nursing Care** section offers detailed guidelines for not only physical patient care but also emotional support.

Brief yet detailed scenarios found in **Critical Thinking in Practice** prompt students to assess possible situations and offer appropriate responses. An appendix of suggested answers provide immediate feedback and reinforcement of clinical decision-making skills.

Outlining antepartal, intrapartal, and postpartal management, the **Critical Pathways** are designed to help students plan and manage care within normal anticipated time frames. With information ranging from referral sources to nursing care management and reports, Critical Pathways help students better prepare for the realities of the clinical setting.

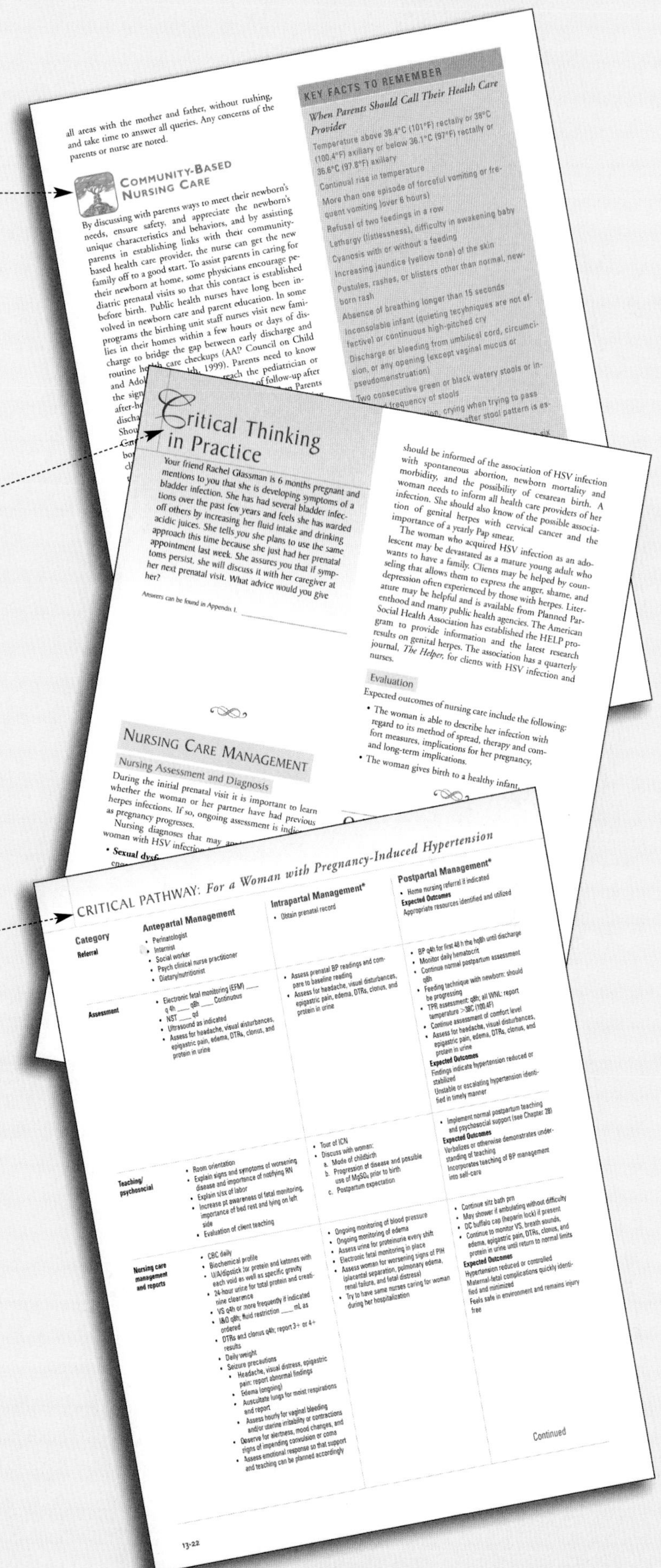

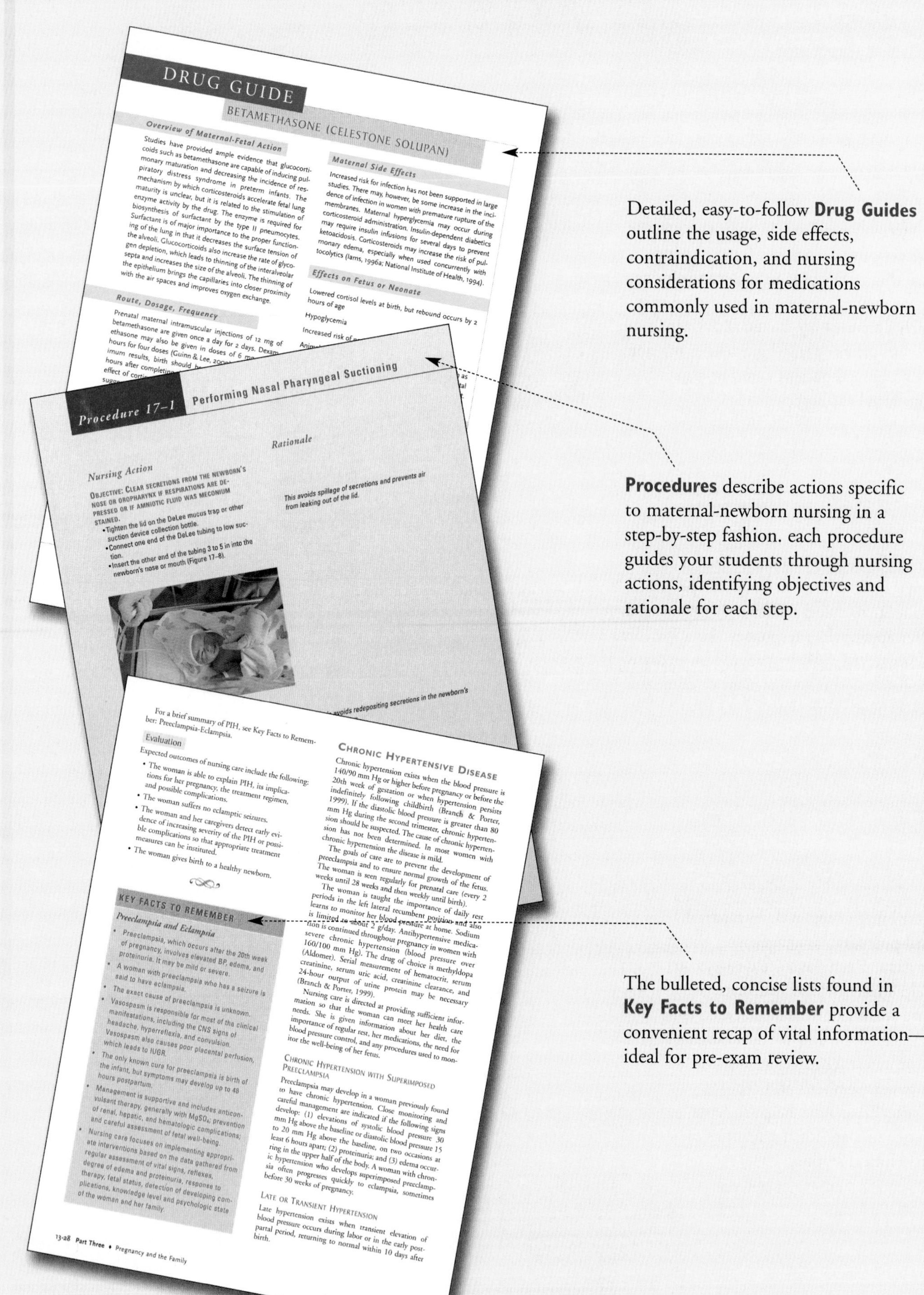

Detailed, easy-to-follow **Drug Guides** outline the usage, side effects, contraindication, and nursing considerations for medications commonly used in maternal-newborn nursing.

**Procedures** describe actions specific to maternal-newborn nursing in a step-by-step fashion. each procedure guides your students through nursing actions, identifying objectives and rationale for each step.

The bulleted, concise lists found in **Key Facts to Remember** provide a convenient recap of vital information—ideal for pre-exam review.

# Part One

# Basic Concepts

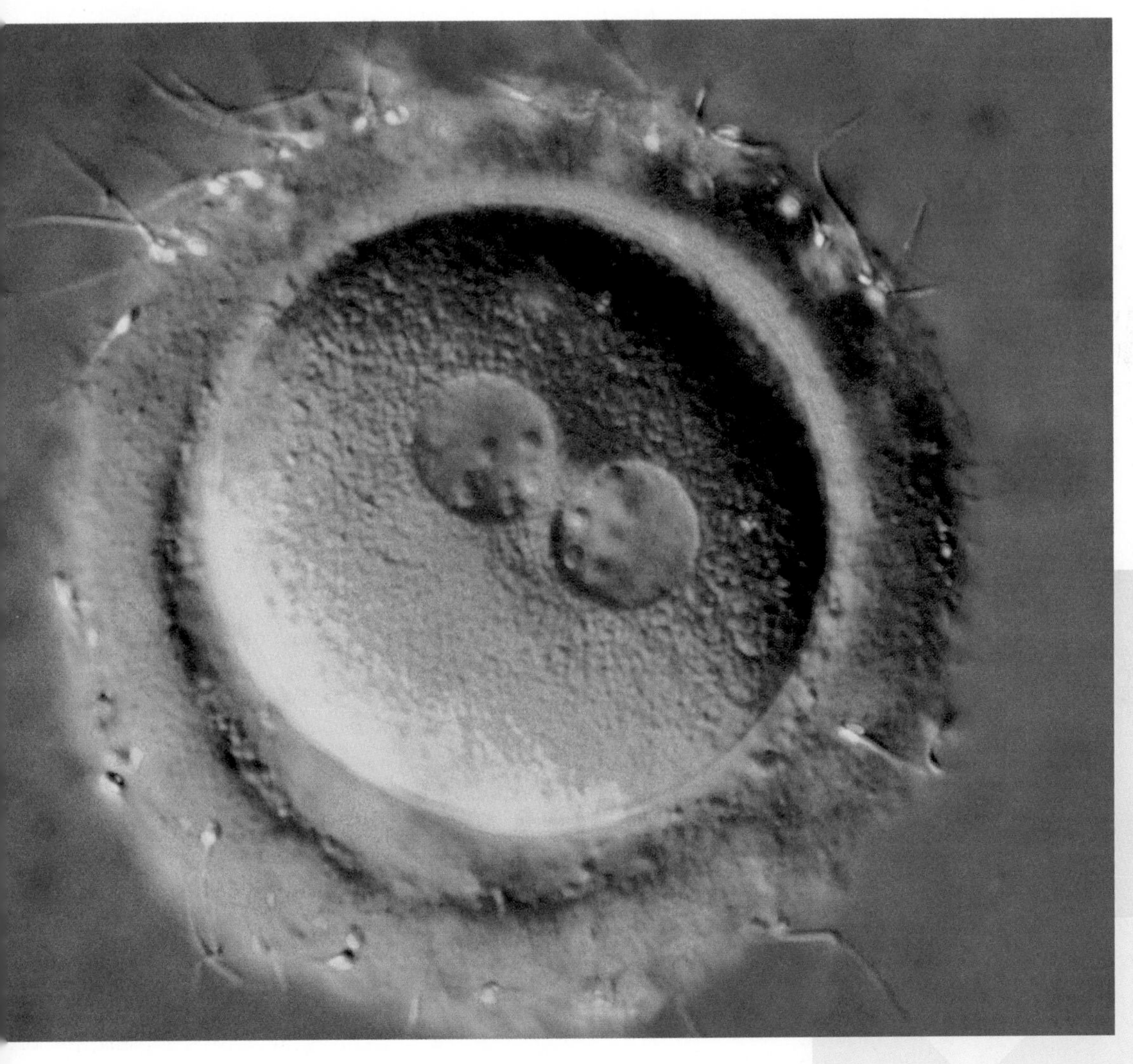

# Chapter 1

# Contemporary Maternal-Newborn Care

*The opportunities I've had as a nurse are amazing. I've been an Air Force nurse and a hospital staff nurse. I thought I could never love any type of nursing more than I loved the mother-baby unit, but then I became a nurse practitioner and found wonderful new challenges. At the same time, I became a faculty member at a local university and learned the joy of helping to shape future nurses. Now I am the dean of the program. Do you know how lucky I am? I am 54, I've been a nurse for 33 years, and I am still passionate about what I do!*

## KEY TERMS

| Term | Page |
|---|---|
| Assisted reproductive technology (ART) | 8 |
| Birth rate | 11 |
| Certified nurse-midwife (CNM) | 4 |
| Certified professional midwife (CPM) | 5 |
| Certified registered nurse (RNC) | 4 |
| Clinical nurse specialist (CNS) | 4 |
| Infant mortality rate | 11 |
| Informed consent | 6 |
| Intrauterine fetal surgery | 8 |
| Maternal mortality rate | 12 |
| Nurse practitioner (NP) | 4 |
| Professional nurse | 4 |

## OBJECTIVES

- Relate the concept of the expert nurse to nurses caring for childbearing families.
- Summarize the use of community-based nursing care in meeting the needs of childbearing families.
- Identify the nursing roles available to the maternal-newborn nurse.
- Delineate significant legal and ethical issues that influence the practice of maternal-newborn nursing.
- Describe the Human Genome Project.
- Discuss the role of evidence-based practice in improving the quality of nursing care for childbearing families.
- Contrast descriptive and inferential statistics.
- Relate the availability of statistical data to the formulation of further research questions.

he practice of most nurses is filled with special moments, shared experiences, times in which they know they have practiced the essence of nursing and, in so doing, touched a life. What is the essence of nursing? Simply stated, nurses care *for* people, care *about* people, and use their expertise to help people help themselves, as the following situation demonstrates.

> I like working with students. I enjoy their enthusiasm, the questions they ask, and the ways in which they cause me to examine my practice. I love being a nurse, I am passionate about the importance of what I do, and I want to seize every chance to influence those who will be practicing beside me someday. An incident that took place last week is a perfect example. I had a nursing student working with me in one of our birthing rooms. It was her first day caring for laboring women, and she was scared and excited at the same time. We were taking care of a healthy woman who had two boys at home and really wanted a girl. As labor progressed, the student and I worked closely together, monitoring contractions, teaching the woman and her husband, doing what we could to ease her discomfort. Sometimes the student asked how I knew when to do something—a vaginal exam, for example—and each time I'd try to think beyond "I just do" to give her some clues. During the birth the student stayed close to the mother, coaching and helping with breathing. The student felt she had an important role to play and she handled it beautifully. At the moment of birth the student and dad leaned forward, watching as the baby just slipped into the world. There wasn't a sound until the student said in a voice filled with awe, "Ooh, it's a girl!" Then we all laughed and hugged each other. What a day—using my expertise to help others and helping a future nurse recognize the importance of what we do!

All nurses who provide care and support to childbearing women and their families can make a difference. But how does this happen? How do nurses develop expertise and become skilled, caring practitioners? In her classic work, Benner (1984) suggests that, as nurses develop their skills in making clinical judgments and intervening appropriately, they progress through five levels of competence. Beginning as a novice, the new nurse progresses to advanced beginner and then to competent, proficient, and, finally, expert nurse.

The student discussed earlier was clearly a novice. Lacking in experience, the novice relies on rules to guide actions. As nurses gain experience, they begin to draw on that experience to view situations more holistically, becoming increasingly aware of subtle cues that indicate physiologic and psychologic changes. Expert nurses, like the nurse in the preceding situation, have a clear vision of what is possible in a given situation. This holistic perspective, based on a wealth of knowledge bred of experience, enables the nurse to act intuitively to provide effective care. In reality, "intuition" reflects the nurse's internalization of information. When faced with a clinical situation, nurses draw almost subconsciously on their stored knowledge and judgment.

The use of intuitive perception is especially important to the art of nursing in areas such as maternal-newborn nursing, where change occurs quickly and families look to the nurse for help and guidance. Labor nurses become attuned to a woman's progress or lack of progress, nursery nurses detect subtle changes in their small charges, and antepartal and postpartal nurses become adept at assessing and teaching. Thus skilled nursing practice depends on a solid base of knowledge and clinical expertise delivered in a caring, holistic manner.

Empowerment is an important concept for nurses today. Empowerment is both a process and an outcome. As an internal process, empowerment results as individuals develop ever-increasing awareness of competence, mastery, and control over their own lives. An empowered self develops as a result of five processes—control, competence, credibility, confidence, and comfort. For nurses, these attributes evolve as they mature in the profession (Moores, 1997).

Control develops as nurses learn to handle their own emotions and to master clinical situations by making and acting on client care decisions. Control issues are often difficult for advanced beginners (Benner, 1984), who can demonstrate only marginally acceptable performance, and they may look to expert nurses for guidance. As nurses provide good nursing care and develop a sound knowledge base, they gain competence. From this competence flows credibility as others begin to trust and believe in them. Nurses in turn become self-reliant, gaining confidence in their judgments, which is critical to feelings of empowerment. Finally a sense of comfort develops and nurses feel able to predict probable outcomes (Moores, 1997).

Empowered nurses are better able to approach client care situations effectively with full knowledge that they are legally, ethically, and morally accountable for their actions. Empowered nurses are able to interact as equals with other health care providers and collaborate with them to resolve problems and accomplish goals (Moores, 1997). When empowered nurses practice proactively, they anticipate problems before they develop and avoid undesirable client outcomes (Hagedorn, Gardner, Laux, et al., 1997). Empowered nurses share responsibility and accountability with each childbearing family, thereby helping the family become self-determining.

We believe that many nurses who work with childbearing families are experts: they are sensitive, intuitive, and technically skilled. They are empowered professionals who can collaborate effectively with others and advocate for those individuals and families who need their support. They can support the efforts of childbearing families to make decisions about their needs and desires. They can foster independence and self-reliance. Such nurses do make a difference in the quality of care that childbearing families receive.

## Nursing Roles

The depth of care provided by nurses caring for women and for childbearing families depends on the nurses' education, qualifications, and scope of practice. A **professional nurse** has graduated from an accredited basic program in nursing, has successfully completed the nursing licensure examination (NCLEX), and is currently licensed as a registered nurse (RN). RNs may be found working as labor nurses, mother-baby nurses, lactation consultants, clinic nurses, newborn nursery nurses, home health nurses, adult or newborn intensive care nurses, gynecology unit nurses, and the like. A **certified registered nurse (RNC)** has shown expertise in a field by taking a national certification exam. A **nurse practitioner (NP)** has received specialized education in a master's degree program or a certificate program and thus can function in an advanced practice role. Nurse practitioners often provide ambulatory care services to expectant families, and, in the case of *neonatal nurse practitioners (NNPs),* they care for newborns. Some NPs, such as *perinatal nurse practitioners (PNNPs),* function in acute care, high-risk settings. They focus on physical and psychosocial assessments, including history, physical examination, and certain diagnostic tests and procedures. Nurse practitioners make clinical judgments and begin appropriate treatments, seeking physician consultation when necessary. The emerging emphasis on community-based care has greatly increased opportunities for NPs.

The **clinical nurse specialist (CNS)** has a master's degree and specialized knowledge and competence in a specific clinical area. CNSs often are found on mother-baby units or in the intensive care nursery assisting staff to provide excellent, evidence-based care. The **certified nurse-midwife (CNM)** is educated in the two disciplines of nursing and midwifery and is certified by the American College of Nurse-Midwives. The CNM is prepared to manage independently the care of women at low risk for complications during pregnancy and birth and the care of healthy newborns (Figure 1–1♦).

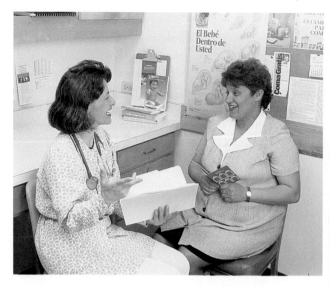

FIGURE 1–1 ♦ A certified nurse-midwife confers with her client.

## Contemporary Childbirth

Contemporary childbirth is characterized by an emphasis on the family and the family's choices about the birth experience. Today the concept of family-centered childbirth is accepted and encouraged. Fathers are active participants, not simply bystanders; siblings are encouraged to visit and meet the newest family member, and they may even attend the birth.

In addition, new definitions of family are evolving. For example, the family of a single mother may include her mother, her sister, another relative, a close friend, or the father of the child. Many cultures also recognize the importance of extended families, and several family members may provide care and support.

The family can make choices about the place of birth (hospital, birthing center, or home), the primary caregiver (physician, certified nurse-midwife, or even lay midwife), and birth-related experiences (position for birth, use of analgesia and anesthesia, and methods of childbirth preparation, for example).

In the early 1990s women who gave birth vaginally remained in the hospital for about 3 days. This provided time for nurses to assess the family's knowledge and skill and to complete essential teaching. In an effort to control costs, discharge within 12 to 24 hours after birth became the norm. This practice did not necessarily cause problems for women with supportive families, thorough prenatal preparation, and adequate resources for necessary follow-up care. However, because early discharge severely limits the time available for client teaching, women with little knowledge, experience, or support were often inadequately prepared to care for themselves and their newborn infants. Fortunately, the negative impact of this practice gained recognition nationwide and resulted in legislation that provides for a postpartum stay of up to 48 hours following a vaginal birth and up to 96 hours following a cesarean birth at the discretion of the mother and her health care provider.

Some women choose to give birth at home. Although some CNMs do home births, the majority of home births are attended by direct-entry midwives (lay midwives) who are not RNs. In the past, training as a lay midwife followed an apprenticeship model, with a more senior midwife teaching a less experienced midwife. Even today, some women gain their training in that way, but many are choosing to complete a direct-entry midwifery education program. Currently direct-entry midwives are working to be viewed as legitimate professionals. Their professional organization, the Midwives Alliance of North America (MANA), has adopted a statement of values and ethics and has assumed a leadership role in developing a certification process. Certification through the North American Registry of Midwives (NARM) is available for direct-entry midwives who meet established standards. The midwife who completes the process successfully can use the title **certified professional midwife (CPM)** (Myers-Ciecko, 1999).

Some provision for direct-entry midwifery exists in approximately 65% of the states in the United States; however, 60% of all licensed midwives practice in just four states—California, Florida, Texas, and Washington (Dower & Miller, 1999). At present, only a few managed care plans make home birth services available to their members. Time will tell whether this is an emerging trend.

## Complementary Therapies

Interest in complementary and alternative medicine (CAM) therapies continues to grow nationwide and will affect the care of childbearing families. CAM includes a wide array of therapies including, for example, acupuncture, acupressure, therapeutic touch, biofeedback, massage therapy, meditation, herbal therapies, and homeopathic remedies.

Research indicates that more than 42% of adults use some form of alternative practice and more than 46% have seen an alternative medicine practitioner. Moreover, more than 60% of those who use complementary or alternative therapies do *not* reveal this to their regular physician (Eisenberg, Davis, Ettner, et al., 1998). In response to this interest, the U.S. Congress established the National Center for Complementary and Alternative Medicine to evaluate alternative medical treatments, to support research and training in CAM, and to establish an information clearinghouse for the exchange of information about CAM with the public (Murphy, Kronenberg, & Wade, 1999).

Alternative therapies have often played a role in women's health care. For example, herbs are widely used to prevent miscarriage, to treat symptoms of menopause, and the like; homeopathic remedies are used for many reasons such as to treat musculoskeletal discomforts of pregnancy and to assist the fetus to assume a favorable position for birth; acupressure is used to reduce nausea during pregnancy; and therapeutic touch is sometimes used to decrease the discomfort of labor. It is important for nurses working with childbearing families to become knowledgeable about complementary and alternative approaches, to become familiar with those practices that have the greatest level of documented success, and to respect and support the family's right to consider alternative approaches to traditional health care.

## Community-Based Nursing Care

Primary care is the focus of much attention as caregivers search for a new, more effective direction for health care. Primary care includes a focus on health promotion, illness prevention, and individual responsibility for one's own health. These services are best provided in community-based settings. Third-party payers and managed care organizations are beginning to recognize the importance of primary care in containing costs and maintaining health. Estimates suggest that fewer than half of nurses now work in a traditional hospital setting. Community-based health care systems providing primary care and some secondary care are becoming available in schools, workplaces, homes, churches, clinics, transitional care programs, and other ambulatory settings.

The growth and diversity of managed care plans offer both opportunities and challenges for women's health care. The potential exists for managed care organizations to work with consumers to provide a model for coordinated and comprehensive well-woman care that includes improved delivery of screening and preventive services. One challenge managed care organizations will face is how to relate to essential community providers of care, such as family-planning clinics or women's health centers, that offer a unique service or serve groups of women with special needs (adolescents, disabled women, and ethnic or racial minorities).

Community-based care remains an essential element of health care for uninsured or underinsured individuals, as well as for individuals who benefit from programs such as Medicare or state-sponsored health-related programs. Whereas some of these programs, such as those offered through public health departments, are broad based, others, such as parenting classes for adolescents, are geared to the needs of a specific population.

Community-based care is also part of a trend initiated by consumers, who are asking for a "seamless" system of family-centered, comprehensive, coordinated health care, health education, and social services. This seamless system requires coordination as clients move from primary care services to acute care facilities and then back into the community. Nurses can assume this care-management role and perform an important service for individuals and families.

Maternal-child nurses are especially sensitive to these changes in health care delivery because the vast majority of health care provided to childbearing women and their families takes place outside of hospitals in clinics, offices, and community-based organizations. In addition, maternal-child nurses offer specialized services such as childbirth preparation classes and postpartal exercise classes. In essence, we are already expert at providing community-based nursing care. However, it is important that we remain knowledgeable about current practices and trends and open to new ways of meeting the needs of women and children.

### Home Care

Providing health care in the home is an especially important dimension of community-based nursing care. Shorter hospital stays end in the discharge of individuals who still require support, assistance, and teaching. Home care helps fill this gap. Conversely, home care also enables individuals to remain at home with conditions that formerly would have required hospitalization.

Nurses are the major providers of home care services. Home care nurses perform direct nursing care and also supervise unlicensed assistive personnel who provide less skilled levels of service. In a home setting, nurses use their skills in assessment, therapeutics, communication, teaching, problem solving, and organization to meet the needs of childbearing women and their families. They also play a major role in coordinating services from other providers, such as physical therapists and lactation consultants.

Postpartum and newborn home visits help ensure a satisfactory transition from the birthing center to the home. We see this trend as positive and hope that this method of meeting the needs of childbearing families will become standard practice. Chapter 29 discusses home care and provides guidance about making a home visit. Throughout the text we have also provided information on the use of home care to meet the needs of pregnant women with health problems, such as diabetes or preterm labor. We believe that home care offers nurses the opportunity to function in an autonomous role and make a significant difference for individuals and families.

## Legal Considerations

### Scope of Practice

The *scope of practice* is defined as the limits of nursing practice set forth in state statutes. Although some state practice acts continue to limit nursing practice to the traditional responsibilities of providing client care related to health maintenance and disease prevention, most state practice acts cover expanded practice roles that include collaboration with other health professionals in planning and providing care, physician-delegated diagnosis and prescriptive privilege, and the delegation of client care tasks to other specified licensed and unlicensed personnel. Specified care activities for certified nurse-midwives and women's health, perinatal, and neonatal nurse practitioners may include diagnosis and prenatal management of uncomplicated pregnancies (CNMs may also manage births) and prescribing and dispensing medications under protocols in specified circumstances. A nurse must function within the scope of practice or risk being accused of practicing medicine without a license.

### Standards of Nursing Care

*Standards of care* establish minimum criteria for competent, proficient delivery of nursing care. Such standards are designed to protect the public and are used to judge the quality of care provided. Legal interpretation of actions within standards of care is based on what a reasonably prudent nurse with similar education and experience would do in similar circumstances.

A number of different sources publish written standards of care. The American Nurses' Association (ANA) has published standards of professional practice written by the ANA Congress for Nursing Practice. The ANA Divisions of Practice have also published standards, including the standards of practice for maternal-child health. Organizations such as the Association of Women's Health, Obstetrics, and Neonatal Nurses (AWHONN), the National Association of Neonatal Nurses (NANN), and the Association of Operating Room Nurses (AORN) have developed standards for specialty practice. Agency policies, procedures, and protocols also provide appropriate guidelines for care standards. The Joint Commission on the Accreditation of Healthcare Organizations (JCAHO), a nongovernmental agency that audits the operation of hospitals and health care facilities, has also contributed to the development of nursing standards.

Some standards carry the force of law; others, although not legally binding, carry important legal significance. Any nurse who fails to meet appropriate standards of care may be subject to allegations of negligence or malpractice. However, any nurse who practices within the guidelines established by an agency, or follows local or national standards, is assured that clients are provided with competent nursing care, which, in turn, decreases the potential for litigation.

### Informed Consent

**Informed consent** is a legal concept that protects a client's right to autonomy and self-determination by specifying that no action may be taken without that person's prior understanding and freely given consent. Although this policy is usually enforced for such major procedures as surgery or regional anesthesia, it pertains to any nursing, medical, or surgical intervention. To touch a person without consent (except in an emergency) constitutes battery. Consent is not informed unless the woman understands the usual procedures, their rationales, and any associated risks. To be a truly active participant in decision making about her care, she should also understand possible alternatives.

The person who is ultimately responsible for the treatment or procedure should provide the information necessary to obtain informed consent. In most instances, this is the physician. In such cases, the nurse's role is to witness the client's signature giving consent. If the nurse determines that the client does not understand the procedure or risks, the nurse must notify the physician, who must then provide additional information to ensure that the consent is informed. Anxiety, fear, pain, and medications that alter consciousness may influence an individual's ability to give informed consent. An oral consent is legal, but written consent is easier to defend in a court of law.

Society grants parents the responsibility and authority to give consent for their minor children (generally under age 18). Special problems can occur in maternal-newborn nursing when a very young minor gives birth. It is possible, depending on state law, that the very young mother may consent to treatment for her newborn but not for herself. In most states, however, a pregnant teenager is considered an emancipated minor and may therefore give consent for herself as well.

Refusal of a treatment, medication, or procedure after appropriate information is provided also requires that a client sign a form releasing the doctor and clinical facility from liability resulting from the effects of such a refusal. Jehovah's Witnesses' refusal of blood transfusions is an example.

Nurses are responsible for educating clients about any nursing care provided. Before each nursing intervention, the maternal-newborn nurse lets the woman know what to expect, thus ensuring her cooperation and obtaining her consent. Afterward, the nurse documents the teaching and the learning outcomes in the woman's record. The importance of clear, concise, and complete nursing records cannot be overemphasized. These records are evidence that the nurse obtained consent, performed prescribed treatments, reported important observations to the appropriate staff, and adhered to acceptable standards of care.

### Right to Privacy

The *right to privacy* is the right of a person to keep her or his person and property free from public scrutiny. Maternity nurses must remember that this includes avoiding unnecessary exposure of the childbearing woman's body. To protect the woman, only those responsible for her care should examine her or discuss her case.

The right to privacy is protected by state constitutions, statutes, and common law. The ANA, National League for Nursing (NLN), and JCAHO have adopted professional standards protecting the privacy of clients. Health care agencies should also have written policies dealing with client privacy.

Laws, standards, and policies about privacy specify that information about clients' treatment, condition, and prognosis can be shared only by health professionals responsible for their care. Information considered vital statistics (name, age, occupation, and so on) may be revealed legally but is often withheld because of ethical considerations. The client should be consulted regarding what information may be released and to whom. When the client is a celebrity or is considered newsworthy, inquiries by the media are best handled by the public relations department of the agency.

## Ethical Issues

Although ethical dilemmas confront nurses in all areas of practice, those related to pregnancy, birth, and the newborn seem especially difficult to resolve.

### Maternal-Fetal Conflict

Until fairly recently, the fetus was viewed legally as a nonperson. Mother and fetus were viewed as one complex client—the pregnant woman—of which the fetus was an essential part. However, advances in technology have permitted the physician to treat the fetus and monitor fetal development. The fetus is increasingly viewed as a client separate from the mother, although treatment of the fetus necessarily involves the mother, and, thus, the medical emphasis has shifted from one of unity to one of duality (Hornstra, 1999).

Most women are strongly motivated to protect the health and well-being of their fetus. In some instances, however, women have refused interventions on behalf of the fetus, and forced interventions have occurred. These include forced cesarean birth; coercion of mothers who practice high-risk behaviors such as substance abuse to enter treatment; and, perhaps most controversial, mandating experimental in utero therapy or surgery in an attempt to correct a specific birth defect. These interventions infringe on the autonomy of the mother. They may also be detrimental to the baby if, as a result, maternal bonding is hindered, the mother is afraid to seek prenatal care, or the mother is herself harmed by the actions taken (Hornstra, 1999).

Attempts have also been made to criminalize the behavior of women who fail to follow a physician's advice or who engage in behaviors (such as substance abuse) that are considered harmful to the fetus. This raises two thorny questions: (1) What practices should be monitored? and (2) Who will determine when the behaviors pose such a risk to the fetus that the courts should intervene?

The American College of Obstetricians and Gynecologists (ACOG) Committee on Ethics (1999), the American Academy of Pediatrics Committee on Bioethics (1999), and the American Medical Association Board of Trustees (1990) all reaffirm the fundamental right of pregnant women to make informed, uncoerced decisions about medical interventions. All three groups also recognize that cases of maternal-fetal conflict involve two clients, both of whom deserve respect and treatment. All agree that such cases "are best resolved through the use of internal hospital mechanisms including counseling, the intervention of specialists, and the utilization of ethics committees . . . and that a resort to judicial intervention is rarely, if ever, appropriate" (Mitchell, 1994, p. 94).

## Abortion

Since the 1973 Supreme Court decision in *Roe v. Wade,* abortion has been legal in the United States. Abortion can be performed until the period of viability. After that time, abortion is permissible only when the life or health of the mother is threatened. Before viability, the rights of the mother are paramount; after viability, the rights of the fetus take precedence.

Personal beliefs, cultural norms, life experiences, and religious convictions shape people's attitudes about abortion. Ethicists have thoughtfully and thoroughly argued positions supporting both sides of the question. However, few issues spark the intensity of response seen when the issue of abortion is raised.

At present the decision about abortion is to be made by the woman and her physician. Nurses (and other caregivers) have the right to refuse to assist with the procedure if abortion is contrary to their moral and ethical beliefs. However, if a nurse works in an institution where abortions may be performed, the nurse may be dismissed for refusing. To avoid being placed in a situation contrary to their ethical values and beliefs, nurses should determine the practices of an institution before going to work there. A nurse who refuses to participate in an abortion because of moral or ethical beliefs has a responsibility to ensure that someone with similar qualifications is available to provide appropriate care for the client. Clients must never be abandoned, regardless of a nurse's beliefs.

## Intrauterine Fetal Surgery

**Intrauterine fetal surgery,** an example of therapeutic research, is a therapy for anatomic lesions that can be corrected surgically and are incompatible with life if not treated. The procedure involves opening the uterus during the second trimester (before viability), performing the planned surgery, and replacing the fetus in the uterus. The risks to the fetus are substantial, and the mother is committed to cesarean births for this and subsequent pregnancies (because the upper, active segment of the uterus is entered). The parents must be informed of the experimental nature of the treatment, the risks of the surgery, the commitment to cesarean birth, and alternatives to the treatment.

As in other aspects of maternity care, caregivers must respect the pregnant woman's autonomy. The procedure involves health risks to the woman, and she retains the right to refuse any surgical procedure. Health care providers must be careful that their zeal for new technology does not lead them to focus unilaterally on the fetus at the expense of the mother.

## Reproductive Assistance

**Assisted reproductive technology (ART)** is the term used to describe highly technologic approaches used to produce pregnancy. *In vitro fertilization and embryo transfer (IVF-ET),* a therapy offered to selected infertile couples, is perhaps the best-known ART technique. In this process, ovulation is induced and one or more oocytes are retrieved by transvaginal ultrasound scanning in conjunction with transvaginal aspiration. The oocytes are then fertilized with sperm from the partner or a donor. Three to four embryos are transferred to the woman's uterus when they reach the four- to eight-cell stage. *Zygote intrafallopian transfer (ZIFT)* is similar to IVF-ET, except that the developing embryo is implanted in the fallopian tube.

*Gamete intrafallopian transfer (GIFT)* is used in women with at least one functioning tube whose infertility is due to unknown causes or male factors such as low sperm count. In GIFT, multiple oocytes are retrieved by laparoscopy from the woman or a donor and transferred with sperm directly into the fallopian tubes. A resulting pregnancy is considered in vivo fertilization.

*Intracytoplasmic sperm injection (ICSI)* is a great advance in ART because it addresses male factor infertility. ICSI is a microscopic procedure designed to inject a single sperm into the outer layer of the ovum so that fertilization will occur. ICSI and other sophisticated ART efforts are resulting in significantly improved outcomes, especially in many categories of infertility that previously were considered untreatable (Hammond & Stillman, 1999).

Some legislative efforts have been made to address consumer concerns about ART. In the United States, the Federal Fertility Clinic Success Rate and Certification Act (FCSRCA) of 1992 requires standardized reporting of pregnancy success rates associated with ART programs and addresses issues related to laboratory quality. However, it does not deal with unethical practices that may occur or false reporting of success rates (Wilcox and Marks, 1996).

In Canada, the Royal Commission on New Reproductive Technologies was charged with examining the range of technologies related to reproduction. Among its most important recommendations, the commission advocated legislation to prohibit several aspects of technology, such as selling human eggs, zygotes, sperm, fetuses, or fetal tissue. It also recommended that the government establish a national regulatory body to license and regulate the provision of reproductive technology services in Canada (Baird, 1996).

*Surrogate childbearing* is another approach to infertility. Surrogate childbearing occurs when a woman agrees to become pregnant for a childless couple. She may be artificially inseminated with the male partner's sperm or a donor's sperm or may receive a gamete transfer, depending on the infertile couple's needs. If fertilization occurs, the woman carries the fetus to term and releases the infant to the couple after birth.

These methods of resolving infertility raise ethical issues about candidate selection, responsibility for a child born with a congenital defect, and religious objections to artificial conception. Other ethical questions include the following: What should be done with surplus fertilized oocytes? To whom do frozen embryos belong? Who is liable if a woman or her offspring contracts HIV from donated sperm? Should children be told about their conception?

## Embryonic Stem Cell Research

Human stem cells can be found in embryonic tissue and in the primordial germ cells of a fetus. Research has demonstrated that in tissue cultures these cells can be made to differentiate into other types of cells such as blood, nerve, or heart cells, which might then be used to treat problems such as diabetes, Parkinson and Alzheimer diseases, spinal cord injury, or metabolic disorders. The availability of specialized tissue or even organs grown from stem cells might also decrease society's dependence on donated organs for organ transplants (Ryan, 2000).

The ethical questions and dilemmas associated with embryonic stem cell research are staggering and complex. The following are two of the most pressing, initial issues to be considered (Roche & Grodin, 2000):

- What moral status should be attached to the human embryo? How should an embryo be viewed? With full status as a person? As a cluster of undifferentiated cells with no moral status? As having status somewhere in between, that is beyond mere cells and deserving of special respect?
- What sources of embryonic tissue are acceptable for research? Is it ever ethical to create embryos solely for stem cell research? Is there justification for using embryos remaining after fertility treatments?

Equally significant, advancements in stem cell research play a major role in the rapidly approaching convergence of reproductive and genetic technologies with all of their related ethical dilemmas, as the following discussion suggests.

## The Human Genome Project

*The Human Genome Project (HGP)* is an international, multidisciplinary effort to explore and map all human genetic material. In the United States, the HGP is a coordinated, national research program jointly sponsored by the U.S. Department of Energy and the National Institutes of Health (NIH). In 2000, scientists announced that they had completed a rough map of about 90% of the human genome. In 2001, it was reported that the human genome was composed of only 30,000 to 40,000 genes, far fewer than the 100,000 originally estimated. The work continues.

The HGP is also charged with analyzing the legal, ethical, and social implications arising from the availability of genetic information about individuals and identifying advanced ways of sharing the information that emerges with researchers, scientists, physicians, and others so that the data can be used for the public good (National Center for Human Genome Research, 2000).

As more genetic information becomes available, questions arise about the ethical use and protection of such information. Other emerging issues include the question of payment for genetic testing; appropriate counseling following testing; confidentiality; qualifications of individuals engaged in testing, counseling, and interventions; mandated testing; and the right to refuse to receive information about genetic findings.

## Cord Blood Banking

Cord blood, taken from a newborn's umbilical cord at birth, may play a role in combating leukemia, certain other cancers, and immune and blood system disorders. This is possible because cord blood, like bone marrow and embryonic tissue, contains regenerative stem cells, which can replace diseased cells in the affected individual. The value of bone marrow transplants is recognized, and a national registry of potential bone marrow donors exists. The process of collecting bone marrow is expensive and uncomfortable, however, and the National Marrow Donor Registry often has difficulty finding a matching bone marrow donor.

Cord blood has numerous advantages over bone marrow: (1) Collecting it involves no risk to mother or newborn. (2) Large-scale cord blood banking would promote better availability of stem cells for racial and minority groups, who are seriously underrepresented in bone marrow registries. (3) Cord blood is less likely than bone marrow to trigger a potentially fatal rejection response. (4) Cord blood works with a less-than-perfect match. (5) Cord blood is available for use more rapidly than bone marrow (Crooks, Lill, Feig, & Parkman, 1997).

Blood banks that process and store cord blood have now been established in the United States. Families can elect to register their infants' cord blood privately. The blood is collected at birth, and the family assumes all costs for analyzing, preparing, and storing the blood. The blood is quickly available for use by the donor, a sibling, or the mother. (During pregnancy mother and infant seem to become immunologically tolerant of each other.) This option is especially useful in families with a history of malignancy or genetic blood disease. Alternatively, families may elect to donate the cord blood to an established public registry for use by others.

Ethical issues associated with cord blood banking include the following (Smith & Thomson, 2000):

- Who owns the blood? The donor? The parents? Private blood banks? Society?
- How will informed consent be obtained and by whom?
- How will confidentiality be ensured? The family members must understand that if they choose to donate, the mother will be asked to provide a blood sample and a detailed history about her health and infectious disease status.
- How will obligations to notify the family and donor be addressed if testing of the blood reveals infectious diseases or genetic disorders?
- How will the harvested blood be allocated to ensure fairness and availability to individuals from all races, ethnic groups, and income levels?

### Implications for Nursing Practice

The complex ethical issues facing maternal-newborn nurses have many social, cultural, legal, and professional ramifications. Ethical decisions in maternal-child nursing are often complicated by moral obligations to more than one client. Straightforward solutions to the ethical dilemmas encountered in caring for childbearing families are often, quite simply, not available.

Nurses must learn to anticipate ethical dilemmas, clarify their own positions related to the issues, understand the legal implications of the issues, and develop appropriate strategies for ethical decision making. To accomplish these tasks, they can read about bioethical issues, participate in discussion groups, or attend courses and workshops on ethical topics pertinent to their areas of practice. Nurses also need to refine their skills in logical thinking and critical analysis.

## Evidence-Based Practice in Maternal-Newborn Nursing

Evidence-based practice is emerging as a force in health care. It provides a useful approach to problem solving/decision making and to self-directed patient-centered, lifelong learning (Sackett, Richardson, Rosenberg, et al., 1997). Evidence-based practice builds on the actions necessary to transform research findings into clinical practice by also considering other forms of evidence that can be useful in making clinical practice decisions (Goode & Piedalue, 1999). These other forms of evidence may include, for example, statistical data, quality measurements, risk management measures, and information from support services such as infection control.

As practicing clinicians, nurses need to meet two basic competencies related to evidence-based practice. Specifically, nurses need to (1) recognize which clinical practices are supported by good evidence, which practices have conflicting findings as to their effect on client outcomes, and which practices have no evidence to support their use and (2) use data in their clinical work.

Rote memorization and practicing from habit and opinion are passé, part of the industrial age. Unfortunately, some agencies and clinical units where nurses practice still operate in the old style, which often generates conflict for nurses who recognize the need for more responsible clinical practice. In truth, market pressures are forcing nurses and other health care providers to evaluate routines in order to improve efficiencies and provide better outcomes for clients.

Nurses need to know what data are being tracked where they work and how care practices and outcomes are improved as a result of this data monitoring. However, there is more to evidence-based practice than simply knowing what is being tracked and how the results are being used. Competent, effective nurses learn to question the very basis of their clinical work.

Throughout this text we have provided *snapshots* of evidence-based practice related to childbearing women and families, such as the one on page 85. We believe that these snapshots will help you understand the concept more clearly. We also expect that these examples may challenge you to question the usefulness of some of the routine care you observe in clinical practice. That is the impact of evidence-based practice—it moves clinicians beyond practices of "habit and opinion" to practices based on high-quality, current science (Gray, 1997).

## Nursing Research

Research is vital to expanding the science of nursing, fostering evidence-based practice, and improving client care. Research also plays an important role in advancing the profession of nursing. For example, nursing research can help determine the psychosocial and physical risks and benefits of both nursing and medical interventions.

The gap between research and practice is being narrowed by the publication of research findings in popular nursing journals, the establishment of departments of nursing research in hospitals, and collaborative research efforts by nurse researchers and clinical practitioners. Interdisciplinary research between nurses and other health care professionals is also becoming more common. This ever-increasing recognition of the value of nursing research is important because well-done research supports the goals of evidence-based practice.

## Critical Pathways

One result of the nursing process is the creation of critical pathways. *Critical pathways* specify essential nursing activities and provide basic guidelines about expected outcomes at specified time intervals. This enables the nurse to determine whether a client's responses meet general norms at any given time. In the text we have provided sample critical pathways for a woman experiencing a normal vaginal birth and a cesarean birth. We have also provided sample critical pathways for the healthy newborn, for a woman in the postpartal period, and for women or newborns with selected conditions or problems.

## Statistical Data and Maternal-Infant Care

Increasingly nurses are recognizing the value and usefulness of statistics. Health-related statistics provide an objective basis for projecting client needs, planning the use of resources, and determining the effectiveness of specific treatments.

There are two major types of statistics: *descriptive* and *inferential. Descriptive statistics* describe or summarize a set of data. They report the facts—what is—in a concise and easily retrievable way. An example of a descriptive statistic is the birth rate in the United States. Although these statistics support no conclusions about *why* some phenomenon has occurred, they identify certain trends and high-risk target groups and generate possible research questions. *Inferential statistics* allow the investigator to draw conclusions or inferences about what is happening between two or more variables in a population and to suggest or refute causal relationships between them.

Descriptive statistics are the starting point for the formation of research questions. Inferential statistics answer specific questions and generate theories to explain relationships between variables. Theory applied in nursing practice can help to change the specific variables that may be causing or at least contributing to certain health problems.

The following sections discuss descriptive statistics that are particularly important to maternal-newborn health care. Inferential considerations are addressed as possible research questions that may assist in identifying relevant variables.

### Birth Rate

**Birth rate** refers to the number of live births per 1000 people. In the United States, the birth rate increased to 14.6 in 1998, the first increase since 1990. Between 1990 and 1997 the birth rate fell 13%. The actual number of births in 1998 increased by 2% to 3,941,553, compared with 3,880,894 births in 1997. This overall increase was fueled primarily by increases in births among women in their 20s and 30s. One bright spot was that the teenage birth rate declined in 1998 to 51.1 births per 1000 women aged 15–19 years. This rate has decreased 18% since 1991 (Ventura, Martin, Curtin, et al., 2000).

In 1998, there were 340,891 live births in Canada, a birth rate of 11.4. The Canadian birth rate has declined steadily from a rate of 15.3 in 1990 (Statistics Canada, 2000). Table 1–1 compares the 1998 birth rates of selected countries.

Research questions that can be posed about birth rates include the following:

- Is there an association between birth rates and changing social values?
- Do the differences in birth rates among various countries reflect cultural differences? Availability of contraceptive information? Other factors?

### Infant Mortality

The **infant mortality rate** is the number of deaths of infants under 1 year of age per 1000 live births in a given population. In 1998, the infant mortality rate in the United States fell to 6.3, the lowest rate ever reported in

| TABLE 1–1 | Live Birth Rates and Infant Mortality Rates in Selected Countries, 1998 | |
|---|---|---|
| ***Country*** | ***Birth Rate*** | ***Infant Mortality Rate*** |
| Afgahnistan | 41.9 | 140.6 |
| Argentina | 19.9 | 18.4 |
| Australia | 13.2 | 5.1 |
| Canada | 11.9 | 5.5 |
| China | 15.1 | 43.3 |
| Egypt | 26.8 | 67.7 |
| Ethiopia | 44.3 | 124.6 |
| France | 11.4 | 5.6 |
| Iraq | 38.4 | 62.4 |
| Japan | 10.5 | 4.1 |
| Mexico | 25 | 24.6 |
| United Kingdom | 11.9 | 5.8 |
| United States | 14.3 | 6.3 |

*Source: 2000 World Almanac and Book of Facts.* Newark, NJ: World Almanac Books, 1999.

the U.S. (*Neonatal mortality* is the number of deaths of infants less than 28 days of age per 1000 live births, *perinatal mortality* includes both neonatal deaths and fetal deaths per 1000 live births, and *fetal death* is death in utero at 20 weeks or more gestation.) By comparison, in 1998 Canada had an infant mortality rate of 5.5 per 1000, continuing a trend of declining rates (Canadian Perinatal Surveillance System, 2000).

The U.S. infant mortality rate continues to be an area of concern because the United States has fallen to 22nd place in infant mortality rankings among industrialized nations. Health care professionals, policy makers, and the public continue to stress the need for better prenatal care, coordination of health services, and provision of comprehensive maternal-child services in the United States. In 1998, the percentage of women beginning prenatal care in the first trimester rose to 82.8%. This number has increased for 9 consecutive years (Ventura et al., 2000).

Table 1–1 identifies infant mortality rates for selected countries for 1998. As the data indicate, the range is dramatic among the countries listed. Information about birth rates and mortality rates is limited for some countries because of a lack of organized reporting mechanisms.

The information raises questions about access to health care during pregnancy and after birth and about standards of living, nutrition, and sociocultural factors. Additional factors affecting the infant mortality rate may be identified by considering the following research questions:

- What are the leading causes of infant mortality in each country?
- Why do mortality rates differ among racial groups?

### Maternal Mortality

**Maternal mortality** is the number of deaths from any cause during the pregnancy cycle (including the 42-day postpartal period) per 100,000 live births. The maternal mortality rates in both the United States and Canada have followed a similar pattern, specifically a long-term, steady decline followed by a plateau. However, the mortality rate in the United States in 1997 at 8.4 was higher than that of Canada at 5.2 (Hoyert, Danel, & Tully, 2000). Factors influencing the long-term decrease in maternal mortality include the increased use of hospitals and specialized health care personnel by maternity clients, the establishment of care centers for high-risk mothers and infants, the prevention and control of infection with antibiotics and improved techniques, the availability of blood products for transfusions, and the lowered rates of anesthesia-related deaths.

Additional factors may be identified by asking the following research questions:

- Is there a correlation between maternal mortality and age?
- Is there a correlation between maternal mortality and availability of health care? Economic status?

## Implications for Nursing Practice

Nurses can use statistics in a number of ways. For example, they can use statistical data to

- Determine populations at risk
- Assess the relationship between specific factors
- Help establish databases for specific client populations
- Determine the levels of care needed by particular client populations
- Evaluate the success of specific nursing interventions
- Determine priorities in case loads
- Estimate staffing and equipment needs of hospital units and clinics

Statistical information is available through many sources, including professional literature; state and city health departments; vital statistics sections of private, county, state, and federal agencies; special programs or agencies (such as family planning); and demographic profiles of specific geographic areas. Often the information can be found using the Internet. Nurses who use this information are better prepared to promote the health needs of maternal-newborn clients and their families.

# Chapter Review

## CHAPTER HIGHLIGHTS

- Many nurses working with childbearing families are expert practitioners who are able to serve as role models for nurses who have not yet attained the same level of competence.
- Contemporary childbirth is family centered, offers choices about birth, and recognizes the needs of siblings and other family members.
- A nurse must practice within the scope of practice or be subject to the accusation of practicing medicine without a license. The standard of care against which individual nursing practice is compared is that of a reasonably prudent nurse.
- Nursing standards provide information and guidelines for nurses in their own practice, in developing policies and protocols in health care settings, and in directing the development of quality nursing care.
- Informed consent—based on knowledge of a procedure and its benefits, risks, and alternatives—must be secured before providing treatment.
- Abortion can legally be performed until the fetus reaches the age of viability. The decision to have an abortion is made by a woman in consultation with her physician.
- *Assisted reproductive technology (ART)* is the term used to describe highly technologic approaches used to produce pregnancy, including in vitro fertilization and embryo transfer (IVF-ET), zygote intrafallopian transfer (ZIFT), and gamete intrafallopian transfer (GIFT).
- Cord blood banking provides the opportunity to have stem cells available to treat a variety of cancers and blood disorders. Its growing popularity has revealed several ethical issues.
- Evidence-based practice refers to clinical practice based on research findings and other available data. It increases nurses' accountability and results in better client outcomes.
- Nursing research plays a vital role in adding to the nursing knowledge base, expanding clinical practice, and further developing nursing theory.
- Descriptive statistics describe a set of data. Inferential statistics allow the investigator to draw conclusions about what is happening between two or more variables in a population.

## CHAPTER REFERENCES


American Academy of Pediatrics, Committee on Bioethics. (1999). Fetal therapy—Ethical considerations. *Pediatrics, 103*(5), 1061–1063.

American College of Obstetricians and Gynecologists, Committee on Ethics. (1999). *Parent choice: Maternal-fetal* (Opinion No. 214). Washington, DC: Author.

American Medical Association, Board of Trustees. (1990). Legal interventions during pregnancy. *JAMA, 264*(20), 2663–2670.

Baird, P. A. (1996). New reproductive technologies: The Canadian perspective. *Women's Health Issues, 6*(3), 156–166.

Benner, P. (1984). *From novice to expert.* Redwood City, CA: Addison-Wesley.

Canadian Perinatal Surveillance System. (2000). *Preterm birth.* [Fact sheet]. Ottawa, Ontario: Laboratory Centre for Disease Control.

Crooks, G. M., Lill, M., Feig, S., & Parkman, R. (1997). Cord blood: New source of stem cells for transplants. *Contemporary OB/GYN, 42*(8), 114–126.

Dower, C. N., & Miller, J. E. (1999). *Taskforce on midwifery. Charting a course for the 21st century: The future of midwifery.* San Francisco: Pew Health Professions Commission and the University of California–San Francisco Center for the Health Professions.

Eisenberg, D. M., Davis, R. B., Ettner, S. L., Appel, S., Wilkey, S., Van Rompey, M., & Kessler, R. C. (1998). Trends in alternative medicine use in the United States, 1990–1997. *JAMA, 280,* 1569–1575.

Goode, C., & Piedalue, F. (1999). Evidence-based clinical practice. *Journal of Nursing Administration, 29,* 15–21.

Gray, M. (1997). *Evidence based healthcare.* New York: Churchill-Livingstone.

Hagedorn, M. I. E., Gardner, S. L., Laux, M. G., & Gardner, G. L. (1997). A model for professional nursing practice. In S. L. Gardner & M. I. E. Hagedorn (Eds.), *Legal aspects of maternal-child nursing practice.* Menlo Park, CA: Addison Wesley Longman.

Hammond, C. B., & Stillman, R. J. (1999). Infertility and assisted reproduction. In J. R. Scott, P. J. DiSaia, C. B. Hammond, & W. N. Spellacy (Eds.), *Danforth's obstetrics and gynecology* (8th ed.). Philadelphia: Lippincott Williams & Wilkins.

Hornstra, D. (1999). A realistic approach to maternal-fetal conflict. *Neonatal Intensive Care, 12*(2), 24–31.

Hoyert, D. L., Danel, I., & Tully, P. (2000). Maternal mortality, United States and Canada, 1982–1997. *Birth, 27*(1), 4–11.

Hoyert, D. L., Kochanek, K. D., & Murphy, S. L. (1999). Deaths: Final data for 1997. *National Vital Statistics Reports, 47*(19), 1–112.

Mitchell, J. J. (1994). Maternal-fetal conflict: A role for the healthcare ethics committee. *Healthcare Ethics Committee Forum, 6*(2), 93.

Moores, P. (1997). Empowering women in the practice setting. In S. L. Gardner & M. I. E. Hagedorn (Eds.), *Legal aspects of maternal-child nursing practice* (pp. 9–23). Menlo Park, CA: Addison Wesley Longman.

Murphy, P. A., Kronenberg, F., & Wade, C. (1999). Complementary and alternative medicine in women's health. *Journal of Nurse-Midwifery, 44*(3), 192–200.

Myers-Ciecko, J. A. (1999). Evolution and current status of direct-entry midwifery education, regulation, and practice in the United States, with examples from Washington state. *Journal of Nurse-Midwifery, 44*(4), 384–393.

National Center for Human Genome Research. (2000). *Five-year research goals of the U.S. Human Genome Project* [On-line]. Available: http://www.ornl.gov/TechResources/Human_Genome/home.html

Roche, P. A., & Grodin, M. A. (2000). The ethical challenge of stem cell research. *Women's Health Issues, 10*(3), 136–139.

Ryan, K. J. (2000). The politics and ethics of human embryo and stem cell research. *Women's Health Issues, 10*(3), 105–110.

Sackett, D., Richardson, W., Rosenberg, W., & Haynes, R. B. (1997). *Evidence based medicine: How to practice and teach EBM.* New York: Churchill-Livingstone.

Smith, F. O., & Thomson, B. G. (2000). Umbilical cord blood collection, banking, and transplantation: Current status and issues relevant to perinatal caregivers. *Birth, 27*(2), 127–135.

Statistics Canada. (2000). *Births and birth rates, Canada, the provinces and territories.* CANSIM, Matrix 5772.

Ventura, S. J., Martin, J. A., Curtin, S. C., Mathews, T. J., & Park, M. M. (2000). Births: Final data for 1998. *National Vital Statistics Report, 48*(3), 1–105.

Wilcox, L. S., & Marks, J. S. (1996). Regulating assisted reproductive technologies: Public health, consumer protection, and public resources. *Women's Health Issues, 6*(3), 175–180.

## CONTEMPORARY MATERNAL-NEWBORN NURSING ON-LINE

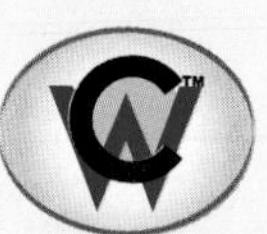

Additional interactive resources, including animations and video, for this chapter can be found on the Companion Website at http://www.prenhall.com/ladewig. Click on Chapter 1 and "Begin" to select the activities for this chapter.

For NCLEX review questions and an audio glossary, access the accompanying CD-ROM in this book.

## Chapter 2

# Reproductive Anatomy and Physiology

*I am amazed by how little many of our students know about anatomy, physiology, and reproduction. As nurses, we must use every opportunity we have to teach young people about their bodies and those of their partners. Information is the key to helping keep them safe and well!*

—University Health Clinic Nurse

## OBJECTIVES

- Identify the structures and functions of the female and male reproductive systems.
- Summarize the actions of the hormones that affect reproductive functioning.
- Identify the two phases of the ovarian cycle and the changes that occur in each phase.
- Describe the phases of the menstrual cycle, their dominant hormones, and the changes that occur in each phase.
- Discuss the significance of specific female reproductive structures during childbirth.

## KEY TERMS

| Term | Page |
|---|---|
| Ampulla | 22 |
| Areola | 27 |
| Broad ligament | 21 |
| Cardinal ligaments | 21 |
| Cervix | 21 |
| Conjugate vera | 27 |
| Corpus | 20 |
| Corpus luteum | 30 |
| Diagonal conjugate | 26 |
| Endometrium | 21 |
| Estrogens | 29 |
| Fallopian tubes | 22 |
| False pelvis | 26 |
| Female reproductive cycle (FRC) | 27 |
| Fimbriae | 22 |
| Follicle-stimulating hormone (FSH) | 29 |
| Fundus | 20 |
| Gonadotropin-releasing hormone (GnRH) | 29 |
| Graafian follicle | 30 |
| Human chorionic gonadotropin (hCG) | 31 |
| Infundibulopelvic ligament | 22 |
| Ischial spines | 24 |
| Isthmus | 22 |
| Luteinizing hormone (LH) | 29 |
| Myometrium | 20 |
| Nidation | 20 |
| Obstetric conjugate | 26 |
| Ovarian ligaments | 21 |
| Ovaries | 23 |
| Ovulation | 30 |
| Pelvic cavity | 27 |
| Pelvic diaphragm | 24 |
| Pelvic inlet | 26 |
| Pelvic outlet | 27 |
| Perimetrium | 20 |
| Perineal body | 17 |
| Progesterone | 29 |
| Prostaglandins (PGs) | 29 |
| Round ligaments | 21 |
| Sacral promontory | 24 |
| Spermatogenesis | 33 |
| Symphysis pubis | 24 |
| Testosterone | 34 |
| Transverse diameter | 27 |
| True pelvis | 26 |
| Uterosacral ligaments | 22 |
| Uterus | 19 |
| Vagina | 17 |
| Vulva | 16 |

Understanding childbearing requires more than understanding sexual intercourse or the process by which the female and male sex cells unite. The nurse must also become familiar with the structures and functions that make childbearing possible and the phenomena that initiate it. This chapter presents the anatomic, physiologic, and sexual aspects of the female and male reproductive systems. Chapter 4 discusses the psychosocial aspects of human sexuality.

The female and male reproductive organs are *homologous;* that is, they are fundamentally similar in structure and function. The primary functions of both female and male reproductive systems are to produce sex cells and transport them to locations where their union can occur. The sex cells, called *gametes,* are produced by specialized organs called *gonads.* A series of ducts and glands within both male and female reproductive systems contributes to the production and transport of the gametes.

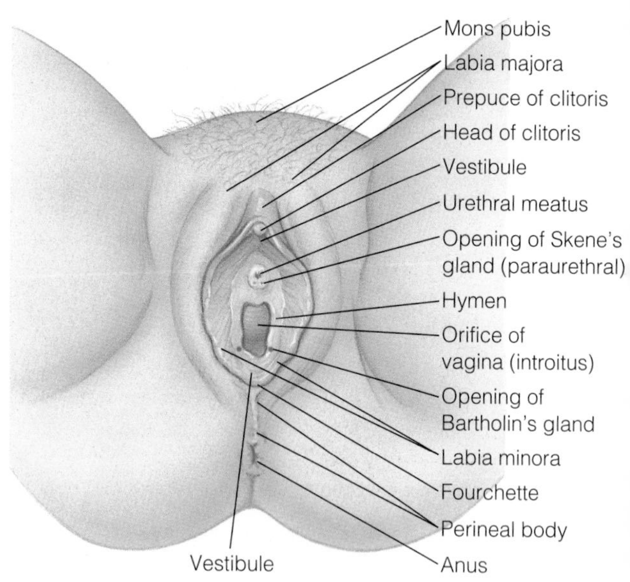


**FIGURE 2–1 ♦ Female external genitals, longitudinal view.**

## Female Reproductive System

The female reproductive system consists of the external and internal genitals and the accessory organs of the breasts. Because of its importance to childbearing, the bony pelvis is also discussed in this chapter.

### External Genitals

All the external reproductive organs except the glandular structures can be directly inspected. The size, color, and shape of these structures vary extensively among races and individuals. The female external genitals, also referred to as the **vulva,** include the following structures (Figure 2–1♦):

- Mons pubis
- Labia majora
- Labia minora
- Clitoris
- Urethral meatus and opening of the paraurethral (Skene's) glands
- Vaginal vestibule (vaginal orifice, vulvovaginal glands, hymen, and fossa navicularis)
- Perineal body

Although they are not true parts of the female reproductive system, the urethral meatus and perineal body are considered here because of their proximity and relationship to the vulva. The vulva has a generous supply of blood and nerves. As a woman ages, estrogen secretions decrease, causing the vulvar organs to atrophy and become subject to a variety of lesions.

#### Mons Pubis

The mons pubis is a softly rounded mound of subcutaneous fatty tissue beginning at the lowest portion of the anterior abdominal wall (Figure 2–1♦). Also known as the mons veneris, this structure covers the front portion of the symphysis pubis. The mons pubis is covered with pubic hair, typically with the hairline forming a transverse line across the lower abdomen. The hair is short and varies from sparse and fine in Asian women to heavy, coarse, and curly in women of African descent. The mons pubis protects the pelvic bones, especially during coitus.

#### Labia Majora

The *labia majora* are longitudinal, raised folds of pigmented skin, one on either side of the vulvar cleft. As the pair descend, they narrow and merge to form the posterior junction of the perineal skin. Their chief function is to protect the structures lying between them.

The labia majora are covered by hair follicles and sebaceous glands, with underlying adipose and muscle tissue. The dartos muscle sheet is responsible for the wrinkled appearance of the labia majora as well as for their sensitivity to heat and cold. The inner surface of the labia majora in women who have not had children is moist and looks like mucous membrane, whereas after many births it is more skinlike (Cunningham et al., 1997). With each pregnancy, the labia majora become less prominent. Because of the extensive venous network in the labia majora, varicosities may occur during pregnancy, and obstetric or sexual trauma may cause hematomas. The labia majora share an extensive lymphatic supply with the other structures of the vulva, which can facilitate the spread of cancer in the female reproductive organs.

Because of the nerves supplying the labia majora (from the first lumbar and third sacral segment of the spinal cord), certain regional anesthesia blocks will affect them and cause numbness.

### Labia Minora

The *labia minora* are soft folds of skin within the labia majora that converge near the anus, forming the *fourchette.* Each labium minus has the appearance of shiny mucous membrane, moist and devoid of hair follicles. The labia minora are rich in sebaceous glands, which lubricate and waterproof the vulvar skin and provide bactericidal secretions. Because the sebaceous glands do not open into hair follicles but open directly onto the surface of the skin, sebaceous cysts commonly occur in this area. Vulvovaginitis in this area is very irritating because the labia minora have many tactile nerve endings. The labia minora increase in size at puberty and decrease after menopause because of changes in estrogen levels.

### Clitoris

The *clitoris,* located between the labia minora, is about 5 to 6 mm long and 6 to 8 mm across. Its tissue is essentially erectile, and it is very sensitive to touch. The glans of the clitoris is partly covered by a fold of skin called the *prepuce,* or clitoral hood. This area resembles an opening to an orifice and may be confused with the urethral meatus. Accidental attempts to insert a catheter in this area produce extreme discomfort. The clitoris has rich blood and nerve supplies and exists primarily for female sexual enjoyment. In addition, it secretes *smegma,* which along with other vulval secretions has a unique odor that may be sexually stimulating to the male.

### Urethral Meatus and Paraurethral Glands

The *urethral meatus* is located 1 to 2.5 cm beneath the clitoris in the midline of the vestibule; it often appears as a puckered, slitlike opening. At times the meatus is difficult to visualize because of the presence of blind dimples or small mucosal folds. The paraurethral glands, or *Skene's glands,* open into the posterior wall of the urethra close to its opening (Figure 2–1♦). Their secretions lubricate the vaginal opening, facilitating sexual intercourse.

### Vaginal Vestibule

The vaginal vestibule is a boat-shaped depression enclosed by the labia majora and visible when they are separated. The vestibule contains the vaginal opening, or *introitus,* which is the border between the external and internal genitals.

The *hymen* is a thin, elastic collar or semicollar of tissue that surrounds the vaginal opening. The appearance changes during the woman's lifetime. The hymen is essentially avascular. For thousands of years, some societies have perpetuated the belief that the hymen covers the vaginal opening and is a sign of virginity. However, modern studies of female genital anatomy have revealed that the hymen does not completely cover the vaginal opening and can be torn through strenuous physical activity, masturbation, menstruation, or the use of tampons, thus dispelling old beliefs.

External to the hymen at the base of the vestibule are two small papular elevations containing the openings of the ducts of the *vulvovaginal (Bartholin's) glands.* They lie under the constrictor muscle of the vagina. These glands secrete a clear, thick, alkaline mucus that enhances the viability and motility of the sperm deposited in the vaginal vestibule. These gland ducts can harbor *Neisseria gonorrhea* and other bacteria, which can cause pus formation and abscesses in the Bartholin's glands.

### Perineal Body

The **perineal body** is a wedge-shaped mass of fibromuscular tissue found between the lower part of the vagina and the anus. The superficial area between the anus and the vagina is referred to as the *perineum.*

The muscles that meet at the perineal body are the external sphincter ani, both levator ani, the superficial and deep transverse perineal, and the bulbocavernosus. These muscles mingle with elastic fibers and connective tissue in an arrangement that allows a remarkable amount of stretching. During the last part of labor, the perineal body thins out until it is just a few centimeters thick. This tissue is the site of the possible episiotomy or lacerations during childbirth (see Chapter 19).

## Internal Reproductive Organs

The female internal reproductive organs are the vagina, uterus, fallopian tubes, and ovaries (Figure 2–2♦). These are target organs for estrogenic hormones, and they play a unique part in the reproductive cycle. The internal reproductive organs can be palpated during vaginal examination and assessed with various instruments.

### Vagina

The **vagina** is a muscular and membranous tube that connects the external genitals with the uterus. It extends from the vulva to the uterus. The vagina is often called the *birth canal* because it forms the lower part of the pelvis through which the fetus must pass during birth.

Because the cervix of the uterus projects into the upper part of the anterior wall of the vagina, the anterior wall is approximately 2.5 cm shorter than the posterior wall. Measurements range from 6 to 8 cm for the anterior wall and from 7 to 10 cm for the posterior wall.

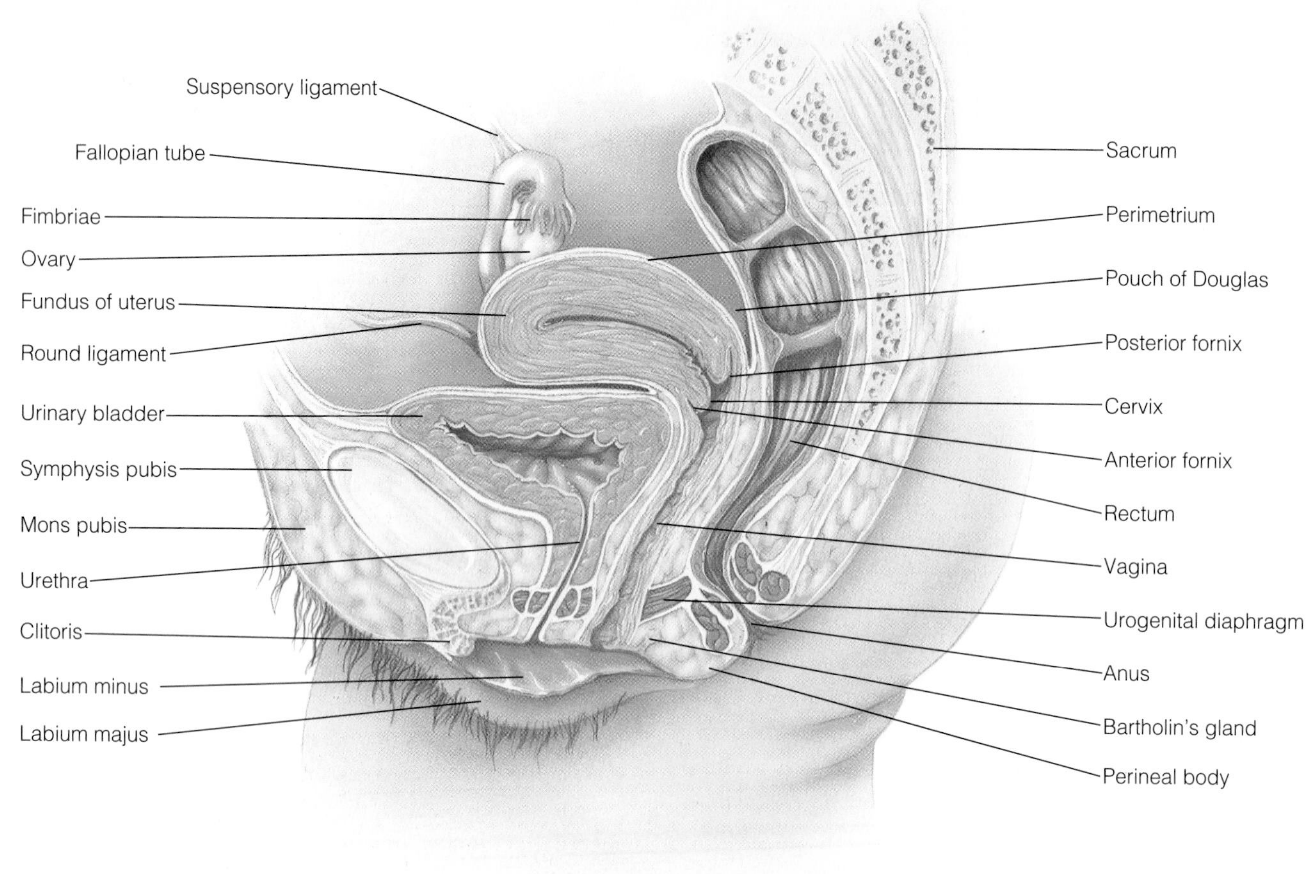


**FIGURE 2–2** ♦ Female internal reproductive organs.

In the upper part of the vagina, which is called the vaginal vault, there is a recess or hollow around the cervix. This area is called the vaginal *fornix.* Since the walls of the vaginal vault are very thin, various structures can be palpated through the walls, including the uterus, a distended bladder, the ovaries, the appendix, the cecum, the colon, and the ureters. When a woman lies on her back after intercourse, the space in the fornix permits the pooling of semen near the cervix and increases the chances of pregnancy.

The walls of the vagina are covered with ridges, or rugae, crisscrossing each other. These rugae allow the vaginal tissues to stretch enough for the fetus to pass through during childbirth.

During a woman's reproductive life, an acidic vaginal environment is normal (pH 4–5). The acidic environment is maintained by a symbiotic relationship between lactic acid–producing bacilli (Döderlein bacillus or lactobacillus) and the vaginal epithelial cells. These cells contain glycogen, which is broken down by the bacilli into lactic acid. Secretion from the vaginal epithelium provides a moist environment. The amount of glycogen is regulated by the ovarian hormones. Any interruption of this process can destroy the normal self-cleaning action of the vagina. Such interruption may be caused by antibiotic therapy, douching, or use of perineal sprays or deodorants. (For discussion of comfort issues for women, see Chapter 4.) The acidic vaginal environment is normal only during the mature reproductive years and in the first days of life when maternal hormones are operating in the infant. A relatively neutral pH of 7.5 is normal from infancy until puberty and after menopause.

The vagina's blood supplies are extensive (Figure 2–3♦). The pudendal nerve supplies what relatively little somatic innervation there is to the lower third of the vagina. Thus sensation during sexual excitement and coitus is reduced in this area, as is vaginal pain during the second stage of labor.

The vagina has three functions:

- To serve as the passage for sperm and for the fetus during birth

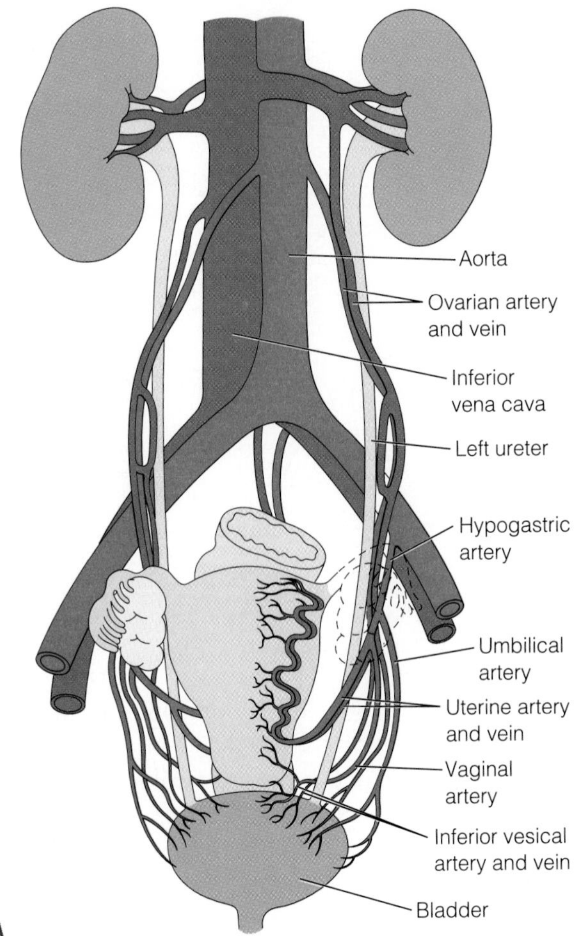


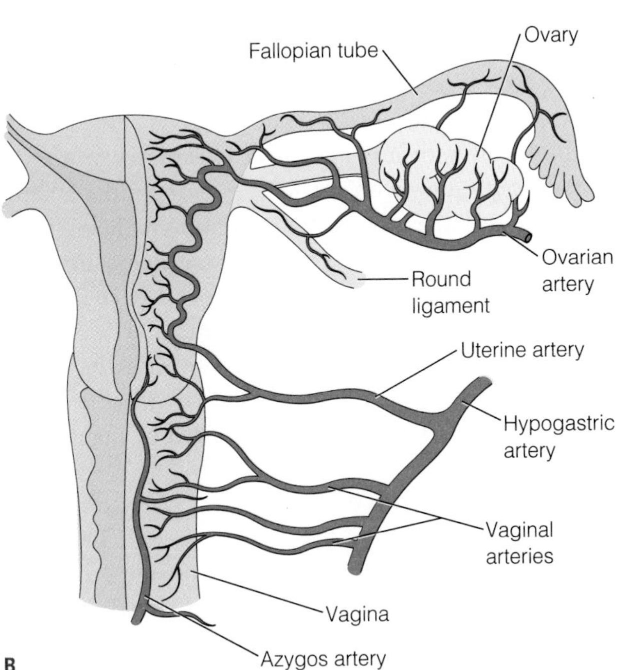


FIGURE 2–3 ♦ Blood supply to internal reproductive organs. **A**, Pelvic blood supply. **B**, Blood supply to vagina, ovaries, uterus, and fallopian tube.

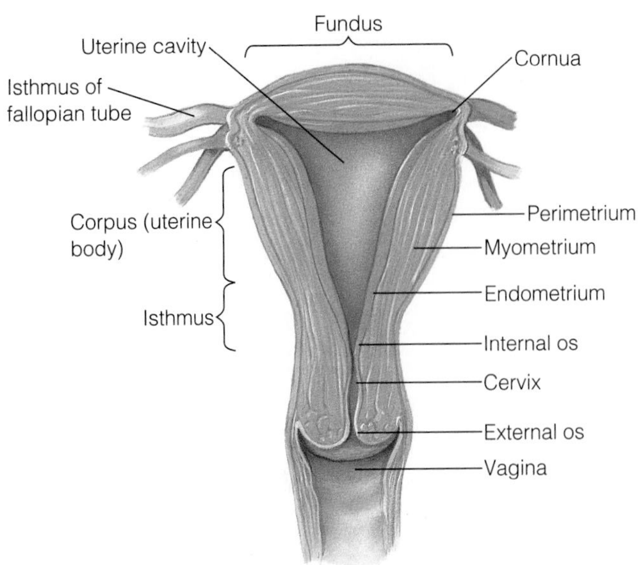


FIGURE 2–4 ♦ Structures of the uterus.

- To provide passage for the menstrual products from the uterine endometrium to the outside of the body
- To protect against trauma from sexual intercourse and infection from pathogenic organisms

## UTERUS

As the core of reproduction and hence continuation of the human race, the uterus, or womb, has been endowed with a mystical aura. Numerous customs, taboos, mores, and values have evolved about women and their reproductive function. Although scientific knowledge has replaced much of this folklore, remnants of old ideas and superstitions persist. To provide effective care, nurses must be cognizant of their own attitudes and beliefs, as well as those of their clients.

The **uterus** is a hollow, muscular, thick-walled organ shaped like an upside-down pear (Figure 2–4♦). It lies in the center of the pelvic cavity between the base of the bladder and the rectum and above the vagina. The external opening of the cervix (external os) is about the level of the ischial spines. The mature uterus weighs about 50 to 70 g and is approximately 7.5 cm long, 5 cm wide, and 1 to 2.5 cm thick (Resnik, 1999).

The position of the uterus can vary depending on a woman's posture and musculature, number of children borne, bladder and rectal fullness, and even normal respiratory patterns. Only the cervix is anchored laterally. The body of the uterus can move freely forward or backward. The axis also varies. Generally, the uterus bends forward, forming a sharp angle with the vagina. There is a bend in the area of the isthmus of the uterus; from there

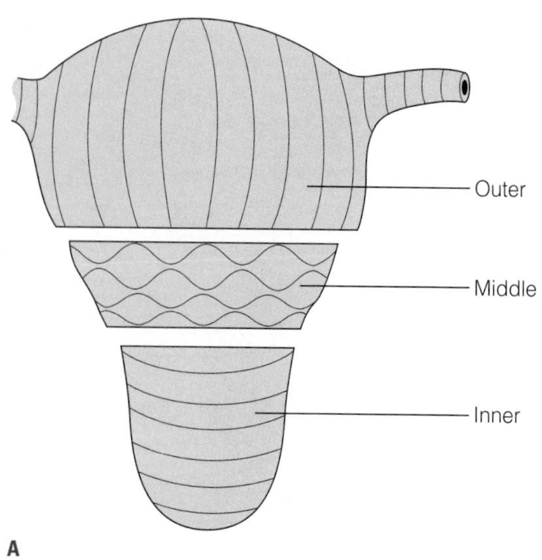


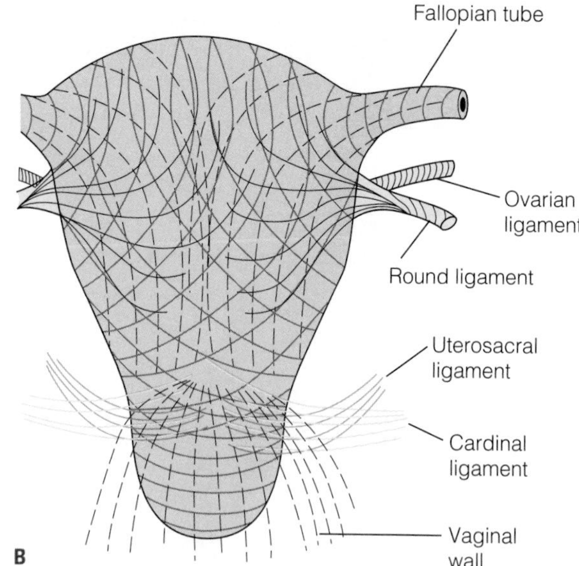


**FIGURE 2–5 ♦** Uterine muscle layers. **A,** Muscle fiber placement. **B,** Interlacing of uterine muscle layers.

the cervix points downward. The uterus is said to be anteverted when it is in this position. The anteverted position is considered normal.

The uterus is kept in place by three sets of supports. The upper supports are the broad and round ligaments. The middle supports are the cardinal, pubocervical, and uterosacral ligaments. The lower supports are those structures considered to make up the pelvic muscular floor.

The isthmus is a slight constriction in the uterus that divides it into two unequal parts. The upper two-thirds of the uterus is the **corpus,** or uterine body, composed mainly of a smooth muscle layer (myometrium). The lower third is the cervix or neck. The rounded uppermost portion of the corpus that extends above the points of attachment of the fallopian tubes is called the **fundus.** The elongated portion of the uterus where the fallopian tubes enter is called the *cornua.*

The isthmus is about 6 mm above the uterine opening of the cervix (the internal os), and it is in this area that the uterine lining changes into the mucous membrane of the cervix; it joins the corpus to the cervix. The isthmus takes on importance in pregnancy because it becomes the lower uterine segment. With the cervix, it is a passive segment and not part of the contractile uterus. At birth, this thin lower segment, situated behind the bladder, is the site for lower-segment cesarean births (see Chapter 20).

The blood and lymphatic supplies to the uterus are extensive. Innervation of the uterus is entirely by the autonomic nervous system. Even without an intact nerve supply, the uterus can contract adequately for birth; for example, hemiplegic women have adequate uterine contractions.

The function of the uterus is to provide a safe environment for fetal development. The uterine lining is cyclically prepared by steroid hormones for implantation of the embryo (**nidation**). Once the embryo is implanted, the developing fetus is protected until it is expelled.

Both the body of the uterus and the cervix are changed permanently by pregnancy. The body never returns to its prepregnant size, and the external os changes from a circular opening of about 3 mm to a transverse slit with irregular edges.

### Uterine Corpus

The uterine corpus is made up of three layers. The outermost layer is the *serosal layer,* or **perimetrium,** which is composed of peritoneum. The middle layer is the *muscular uterine* layer, or **myometrium.** This muscular uterine layer is continuous with the muscle layers of the fallopian tubes and the vagina. This continuity helps these organs present a unified reaction to various stimuli—ovulation, orgasm, or the deposit of sperm in the vagina. These muscle fibers also extend into the ovarian, round, and cardinal ligaments and minimally into the uterosacral ligaments, which helps explain the vague but disturbing pelvic "aches and pains" reported by many pregnant women.

The myometrium has three distinct layers of uterine (smooth) involuntary muscles (Figure 2–5♦). The outer layer, found mainly over the fundus, is made up of longitudinal muscles that cause cervical effacement and expel the fetus during birth. The thick middle layer is made up of interlacing muscle fibers in figure-eight patterns. These muscle fibers surround large blood vessels, and their contraction produces a hemostatic action (a tourniquet-like action on blood vessels to stop bleeding after birth). The inner muscle layer is composed of circular fibers that form sphincters at the fallopian tube attachment sites and at the internal os. The internal os sphincter inhibits the expulsion of the uterine contents during pregnancy but stretches in labor as cervical dilatation occurs. An incompetent cervical os can be caused by a torn, weak, or absent sphincter at the internal os. The sphincters at the fallopian tubes prevent menstrual blood from flowing backward into the fallopian tubes from the uterus. Although each layer of muscle has been discussed as having a unique function, the uterine musculature actually works as a whole. The uterine contractions of labor are responsible for the dilatation of the cervix and provide the major force for the passage of the fetus through the pelvis and vaginal canal at birth.

The *mucosal* layer, or **endometrium,** of the uterine corpus is the innermost layer. This single layer is composed of columnar epithelium, glands, and stroma. From menarche to menopause, the endometrium undergoes monthly degeneration and renewal in the absence of pregnancy. As it responds to the governing hormonal cycle and prostaglandin influence, the endometrium varies in thickness from 0.5 to 5 mm. The glands of the endometrium produce a thin, watery, alkaline secretion that keeps the uterine cavity moist. This endometrial milk not only helps sperm travel to the fallopian tubes but also nourishes the developing embryo before it implants in the endometrium (Chapter 3).

The blood supply to the endometrium is unique. Some of the blood vessels are not sensitive to cyclic hormonal control, whereas others are extremely sensitive to it. These differing responses allow part of the endometrium to remain intact while other endometrial tissue is shed during menstruation. When pregnancy occurs and the endometrium is not shed, the reticular stromal cells surrounding the endometrial glands become the decidual cells of pregnancy. The stromal cells are highly vascular, channeling a rich blood supply to the endometrial surface.

### Cervix

The narrow neck of the uterus is the **cervix.** It meets the body of the uterus at the internal os and descends about 2.5 cm to connect with the vagina at the external os (see Figure 2–4♦). Thus it provides a protective entrance for the body of the uterus. The cervix is divided by its line of attachment into the vaginal and supravaginal areas. The vaginal cervix projects into the vagina at an angle of from 45 to 90 degrees. The *supravaginal cervix* is surrounded by the attachments that give the uterus its main support: the uterosacral ligaments, the transverse ligaments of the cervix (Mackenrodt's ligaments), and the pubocervical ligaments.

The vaginal cervix appears pink and ends at the external os. The cervical canal appears rosy red and is lined with columnar ciliated epithelium, which contains mucus-secreting glands. Most cervical cancer begins at this *squamocolumnar junction.* The specific location of the junction varies with age and number of pregnancies. Elasticity is the chief characteristic of the cervix. Its ability to stretch is due to the high fibrous and collagenous content of the supportive tissues and also to the vast number of folds in the cervical lining.

The cervical mucus has three functions:

- To lubricate the vaginal canal
- To act as a bacteriostatic agent
- To provide an alkaline environment to shelter deposited sperm from the acidic vagina

At ovulation, cervical mucus is clearer, thinner, more profuse, and more alkaline than at other times.

### Uterine Ligaments

The uterine ligaments support and stabilize the various reproductive organs. The ligaments shown in Figure 2–6♦ are described as follows:

1. The **broad ligament** keeps the uterus centrally placed and provides stability within the pelvic cavity. It is a double layer that is continuous with the abdominal peritoneum. The broad ligament covers the uterus anteriorly and posteriorly and extends outward from the uterus to enfold the fallopian tubes. The round and ovarian ligaments are at the upper border of the broad ligament. At its lower border, it forms the cardinal ligaments. Between the folds of the broad ligament are connective tissue, involuntary muscle, blood and lymph vessels, and nerves.
2. The **round ligaments** help the broad ligament keep the uterus in place. The round ligaments arise from the sides of the uterus near the fallopian tube insertions. They extend outward between the folds of the broad ligament, passing through the inguinal ring and canals and eventually fusing with the connective tissue of the labia majora. Made up of longitudinal muscle, the round ligaments enlarge during pregnancy. During labor the round ligaments steady the uterus, pulling downward and forward so that the presenting part of the fetus is moved into the cervix.
3. The **ovarian ligaments** anchor the lower pole of the ovary to the cornua of the uterus. They are composed of muscle fibers that allow the ligaments to contract. This contractile ability influences the position of the ovary to some extent, thus helping the fimbriae of the fallopian tubes to "catch" the ovum as it is released each month.
4. The **cardinal ligaments** are the chief uterine supports and suspend the uterus from the side walls of the true pelvis. These ligaments, also known as Mackenrodt's or transverse cervical ligaments, arise

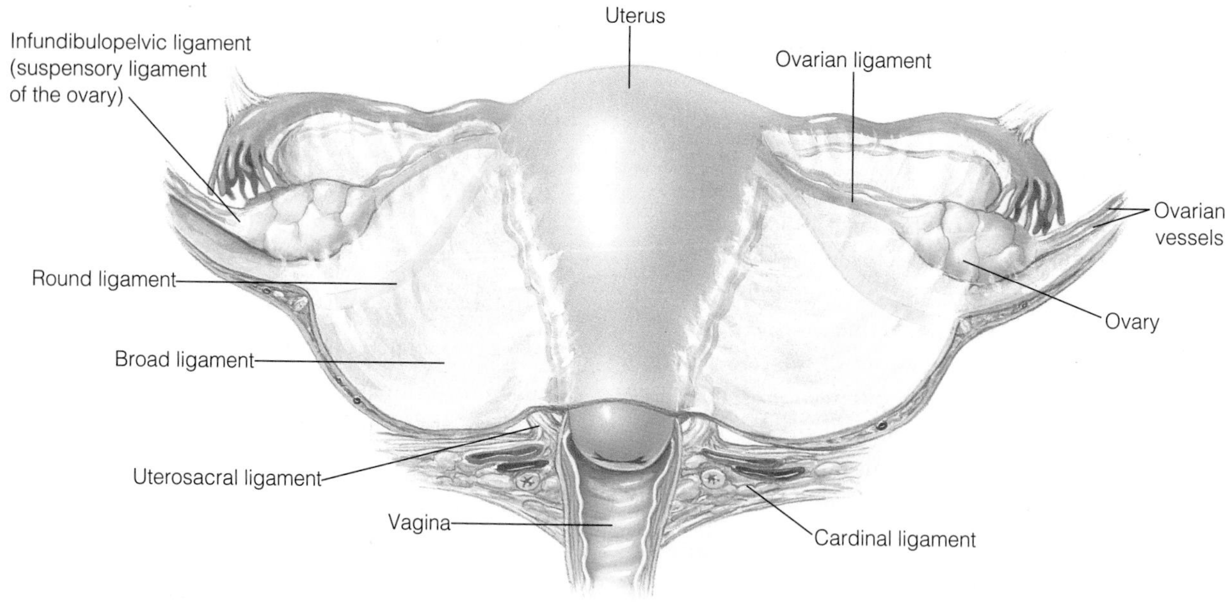


**FIGURE 2–6** ♦ Uterine ligaments.

from the sides of the pelvic walls and attach to the cervix in the upper vagina. These ligaments prevent uterine prolapse and also support the upper vagina.

5. The **infundibulopelvic ligament** suspends and supports the ovaries. Arising from the outer third of the broad ligament, the infundibulopelvic ligament contains the ovarian vessels and nerves.
6. The **uterosacral ligaments** provide support for the uterus and cervix at the level of the ischial spines. Arising on each side of the pelvis from the posterior wall of the uterus, the uterosacral ligaments sweep back around the rectum and insert on the sides of the first and second sacral vertebrae. The uterosacral ligaments contain smooth muscle fibers, connective tissue, blood and lymph vessels, and nerves. They also contain sensory nerve fibers that contribute to dysmenorrhea (painful menstruation) (see Chapter 4).

### Fallopian Tubes

The two **fallopian tubes,** also known as the *oviducts* or *uterine tubes,* arise from each side of the uterus and reach almost to the sides of the pelvis, where they turn toward the ovaries (Figure 2–7♦). Each tube is approximately 8 to 13.5 cm long. A short section of each fallopian tube is inside the uterus; its opening into the uterus is only 1 mm in diameter. The fallopian tubes link the peritoneal cavity with the uterus and vagina. This linkage increases a woman's biologic vulnerability to disease processes.

Each fallopian tube may be divided into three parts: the isthmus; the ampulla; and the infundibulum, or fimbria. The **isthmus** is straight and narrow, with a thick muscular wall and an opening (lumen) 2 to 3 mm in diameter. It is the site of tubal ligation, a surgical procedure to prevent pregnancy (see Chapter 4).

Next to the isthmus is the curved **ampulla,** which comprises the outer two-thirds of the tube. Fertilization of the secondary oocyte by a spermatozoon usually occurs here. The ampulla ends at the fimbria, which is a funnel-shaped enlargement with many projections, called **fimbriae,** reaching out to the ovary. The longest of these, the *fimbria ovarica,* is attached to the ovary to increase the chances of intercepting the ovum as it is released.

The wall of the fallopian tube is made up of four layers: peritoneal (serous), subserous (adventitial), muscular, and mucous tissues. The peritoneum covers the tubes. The subserous layer contains the blood and nerve supply, and the muscular layer is responsible for the peristaltic movement of the tube. The mucosal layer, immediately next to the muscular layer, is composed of ciliated and nonciliated cells, with the number of ciliated cells more abundant at the fimbria. Nonciliated cells secrete a protein-rich, serous fluid that nourishes the ovum. The constantly moving tubal cilia propel the ovum toward the uterus. Because the ovum is a large cell, this ciliary action is needed to assist the tube's muscular layer peristalsis. Any malformation or malfunction of the tubes can result in infertility, ectopic pregnancy, or even sterility.

A rich blood and lymphatic supply serves each fallopian tube. Thus the tubes have an unusual ability to recover from an inflammatory process (see Figure 2–3♦).

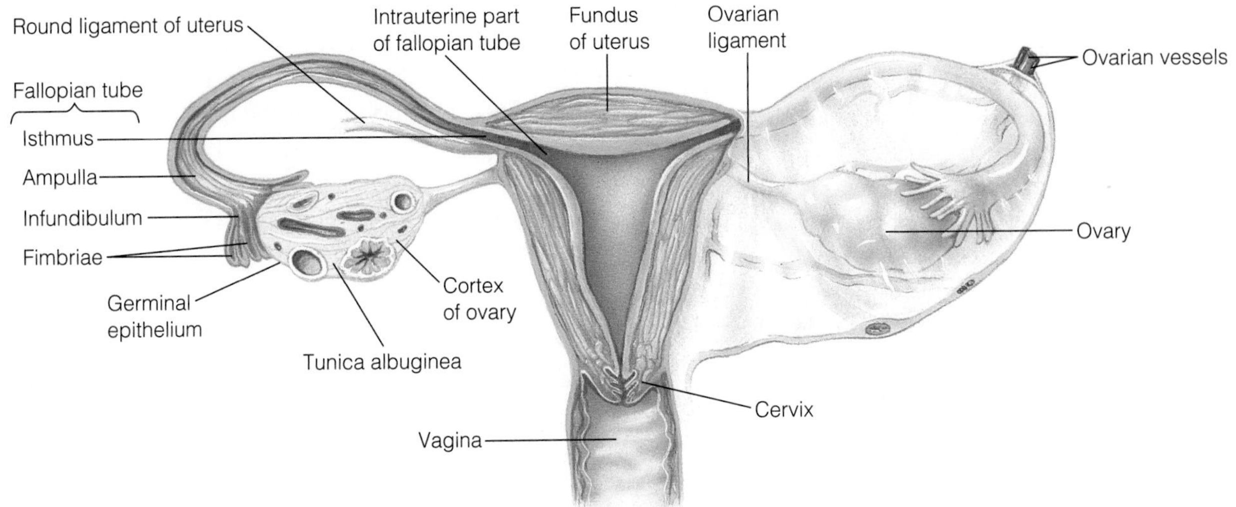


FIGURE 2–7 ♦ Fallopian tubes and ovaries.

The fallopian tubes have three functions:

- To provide transport for the ovum from the ovary to the uterus (transport time through the fallopian tubes varies from 3 to 4 days)
- To provide a site for fertilization
- To serve as a warm, moist, nourishing environment for the ovum or zygote (fertilized egg) (see Chapter 3 for further discussion)

## Ovaries

The **ovaries** are two almond-shaped structures just below the pelvic brim. One ovary is located on each side of the pelvic cavity. Their size varies among women and with the stage of the menstrual cycle. Each ovary weighs approximately 6 to 10 g and is 1.5 to 3 cm wide, 2 to 5 cm long, and 1 to 1.5 cm thick. The ovaries of girls are small, but they become larger after puberty. They also change in appearance from a dull white, smooth-surfaced organ to a pitted gray organ. The pitting is caused by scarring due to ovulation.

The ovaries are held in place by the broad, ovarian, and infundibulopelvic ligaments. There is no peritoneal covering for the ovaries. Although this lack of covering assists the mature ovum to erupt, it also allows easier spread of malignant cells from cancer of the ovaries. A single layer of cuboidal epithelial cells, called the germinal epithelium, covers the ovaries. The ovaries are composed of three layers: the tunica albuginea, the cortex, and the medulla. The *tunica albuginea* is dense and dull white and serves as a productive protective layer. The *cortex* is the main functional part because it contains ova, graafian follicles, corpora lutea, the degenerated corpora lutea (corpora albicantia), and degenerated follicles. The *medulla* is completely surrounded by the cortex and contains the nerves and the blood and lymphatic vessels.

The ovaries are the primary source of two important hormones: the estrogens and progesterone. Estrogens are associated with those characteristics contributing to femaleness, including breast alveolar lobule growth and duct development. The ovaries secrete large amounts of estrogen, while the adrenal cortex (extraglandular sites) produces minute amounts of estrogen in nonpregnant women.

*Progesterone* is often called the *hormone of pregnancy* because its effects on the uterus allow pregnancy to be maintained. The placenta is the primary source of progesterone during pregnancy. This hormone also inhibits the action of prolactin, thereby preventing lactation during pregnancy (Liu & Rebar, 1999). The interplay between the ovarian hormones and other hormones such as follicle-stimulating hormone and luteinizing hormone is responsible for the cyclic changes that allow pregnancy. The hormonal and physical changes that occur during the female reproductive cycle are discussed in depth later in this chapter.

Between the ages of 45 and 55, a woman's ovaries secrete decreasing amounts of estrogen. Eventually, ovulatory activity ceases and menopause occurs.

## Bony Pelvis

The female bony pelvis has two unique functions:

- To support and protect the pelvic contents.
- To form the relatively fixed axis of the birth passage.

Because the pelvis is so important to childbearing, its structure must be understood clearly.

## Bony Structure

The pelvis is made up of four bones: two innominate bones, the sacrum, and the coccyx. The pelvis resembles a bowl or basin; its sides are the innominate bones, and its back is the sacrum and coccyx. Lined with fibrocartilage and held tightly together by ligaments (Figure 2–8♦), the four bones join at the symphysis pubis, the two sacroiliac joints, and the sacrococcygeal joints.

The innominate bones, popularly known as the *hip bones,* are made up of three separate bones: the ilium, ischium, and pubis. These bones fuse to form a circular cavity, the *acetabulum,* which articulates with the femur.

The *ilium* is the broad, upper prominence of the hip. The *iliac crest* is the margin of the ilium. The **ischial spines,** the foremost projection nearest the groin, is the site of attachment for ligaments and muscles.

The *ischium,* the strongest bone, is under the ilium and below the acetabulum. The L-shaped ischium ends in a marked protuberance, the ischial tuberosity, on which the weight of a seated body rests. The ischial spines arise near the junction of the ilium and ischium and jut into the pelvic cavity. The shortest diameter of the pelvic cavity is between the ischial spines. The ischial spines serve as reference points during labor to evaluate the descent of the fetal head into the birth canal (see Chapter 15 and Figure 15–7♦).

The *pubis* forms the slightly bowed front portion of the innominate bone. Extending medially from the acetabulum to the midpoint of the bony pelvis, each pubis meets the other to form a joint called the **symphysis pubis.** The triangular space below this junction is known as the pubic arch. The fetal head passes under this arch during birth. The symphysis pubis is formed by heavy fibrocartilage and the superior and inferior pubic ligaments. The mobility of the inferior ligament increases during a first pregnancy and to a greater extent in subsequent pregnancies.

The sacroiliac joints also have a degree of mobility that increases near the end of pregnancy as the result of an upward, gliding movement. The pelvic outlet may be increased by 1.5 to 2 cm in the squatting, sitting, and dorsal lithotomy positions. These relaxations of the joints are induced by the hormones of pregnancy.

The *sacrum* is a wedge-shaped bone formed by the fusion of five vertebrae. On the anterior upper portion of the sacrum is a projection into the pelvic cavity known as the **sacral promontory.** This projection is another obstetric guide in determining pelvic measurements. (For a discussion of pelvic measurements, see Chapter 8.)

The small triangular bone last on the vertebral column is the *coccyx.* It articulates with the sacrum at the sacrococcygeal joint. The coccyx usually moves backward during labor to provide more room for the fetus.

## Pelvic Floor

The muscular *pelvic floor* of the bony pelvis is designed to overcome the force of gravity exerted on the pelvic organs. It acts as a buttress to the irregularly shaped pelvic outlet, thereby providing stability and support for surrounding structures.

Deep fascia, the levator ani, and coccygeal muscles form the part of the pelvic floor known as the **pelvic**

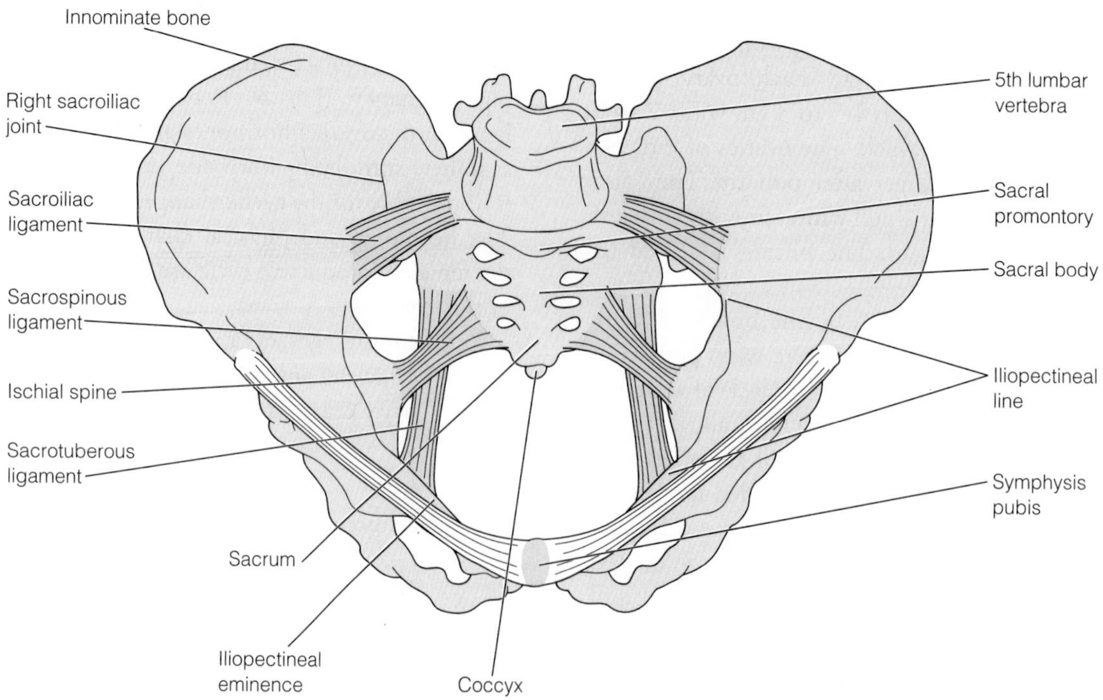


FIGURE 2–8 ♦ Pelvic bones with supporting ligaments.

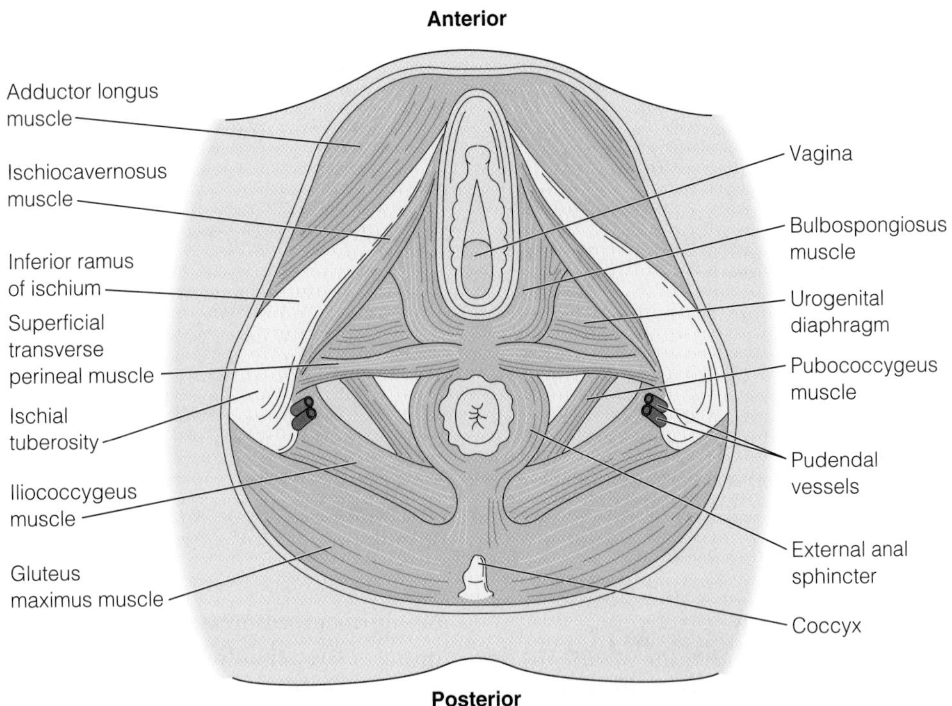


FIGURE 2–9 ♦ Muscles of the pelvic floor. (The puborectalis, pubovaginalis, and coccygeal muscles cannot be seen from this view.)

**TABLE 2–1 Muscles of the Pelvic Floor**

| *Muscle* | *Origin* | *Insertion* | *Innervation* | *Action* |
|---|---|---|---|---|
| Levator ani | Pubis, lateral pelvic wall, and ischial spine | Blends with organs in pelvic cavity | Inferior rectal, second and third sacral nerves, plus anterior rami of third and fourth sacral nerves | Supports pelvic viscera; helps form pelvic diaphragm |
| Iliococcygeus | Pelvic surface of ischial spine and pelvic fascia | Central point of perineum, coccygeal raphe, and coccyx | | Assists in supporting abdominal and pelvic viscera |
| Pubococcygeus | Pubis and pelvic fascia | Coccyx | | |
| Puborectalis | Pubis | Blends with rectum; meets similar fibers from opposite side | | Forms sling for rectum, just posterior to it; raises anus |
| Pubovaginalis | Pubis | Blends into vagina | | Supports vagina |
| Coccygeus | Ischial spine and sacrospinous ligament | Lateral border of lower sacrum and upper coccyx | Third and fourth sacral nerves | Supports pelvic viscera; helps form pelvic diaphragm; flexes and abducts coccyx |

**diaphragm.** The components of the pelvic diaphragm function as a whole, yet they are able to move over one another. This feature provides an exceptional capacity for dilatation during birth and return to prepregnancy condition following birth. Above the pelvic diaphragm is the pelvic cavity; below and behind it is the perineum.

The levator ani muscle makes up the major portion of the pelvic diaphragm and consists of four muscles: the ileococcygeus, pubococcygeus, puborectalis, and pubovaginalis. The ileococcygeal muscle, a thin muscular sheet underlying the sacrospinous ligament, helps the levator ani support the pelvic organs. Muscles of the pelvic floor are shown in Figure 2–9♦ and discussed in Table 2–1.

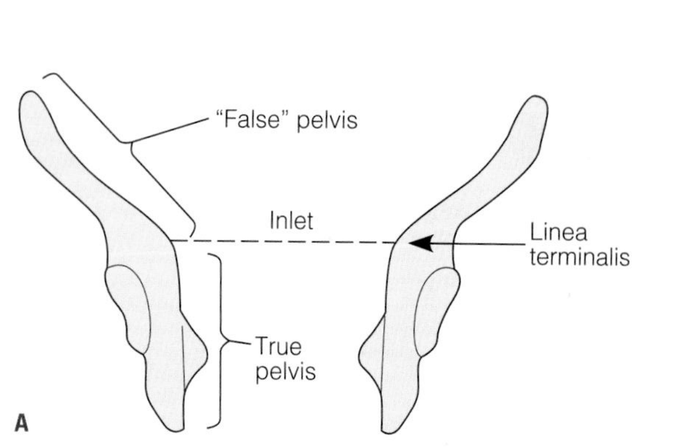


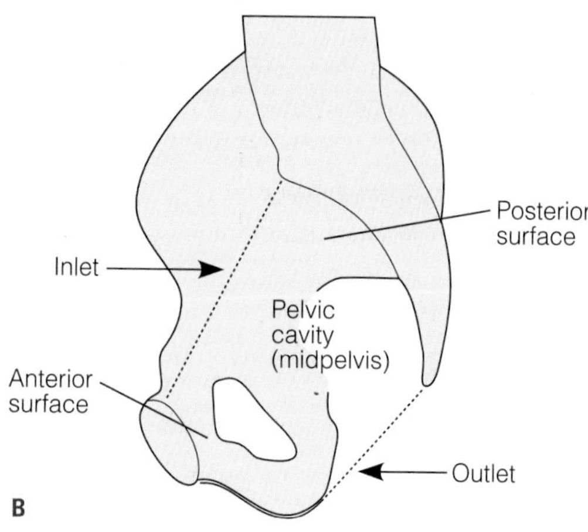


FIGURE 2–10 ♦ Female pelvis. **A**, False pelvis is shallow cavity above the inlet; true pelvis is deeper portion of cavity below the inlet. **B**, True pelvis consists of inlet, cavity (midpelvis), and outlet.

## Pelvic Division

The pelvic cavity is divided into the false pelvis and the true pelvis (Figure 2–10A♦). The **false pelvis,** the portion above the pelvic brim, or linea terminalis, serves to support the weight of the enlarged pregnant uterus and direct the presenting fetal part into the true pelvis.

The **true pelvis** is the portion that lies below the linea terminalis. The bony circumference of the true pelvis is made up of the sacrum, coccyx, and innominate bones and represents the bony limits of the birth canal. The true pelvis is of paramount importance because its size and shape must be adequate for normal fetal passage during labor and at birth.

The true pelvis consists of three parts: the inlet, the pelvic cavity, and the outlet (Figure 2–10B♦). Each part has distinct measurements that aid in evaluating the adequacy of the pelvis for childbirth. (For further discussion, see Chapter 8.)

The **pelvic inlet** is the upper border of the true pelvis. The female pelvic inlet is typically rounded. Its size and shape are determined by assessing three anteroposterior diameters. The **diagonal conjugate** extends from the subpubic angle to the middle of the sacral promontory and is typically 12.5 cm. The diagonal conjugate can be measured manually during a pelvic examination. The **obstetric conjugate** extends from the middle of the sacral promontory to an area approximately 1 cm below the pubic crest. Its length is estimated by subtracting 1.5 cm from the length of the diagonal conjugate (Figure 2–11♦). The fetus passes through the obstetric conjugate, and the

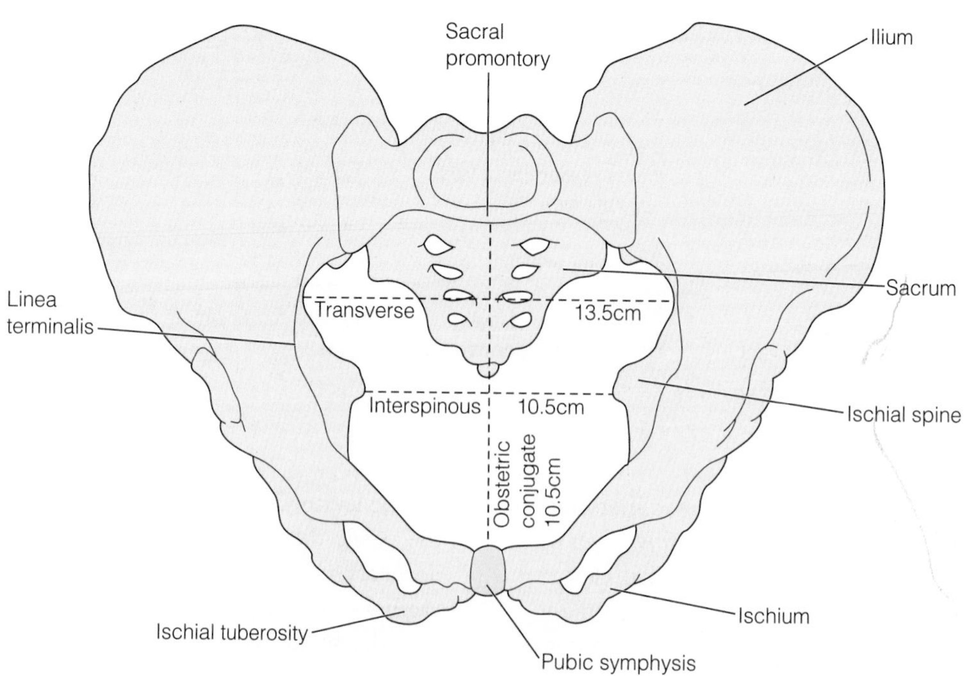


FIGURE 2–11 ♦ Pelvic planes: coronal section and diameters of the bony pelvis.

size of this diameter determines whether the fetus can move down into the birth canal in order for engagement to occur. The true (anatomic) conjugate, or **conjugate vera,** extends from the middle of the sacral promontory to the middle of the pubic crest (superior surface of the symphysis) (Di Saia, 1999). One additional measurement, the transverse diameter, helps determine the shape of the inlet. The **transverse diameter** is the largest diameter of the inlet and is measured by using the linea terminalis as the point of reference.

The **pelvic cavity** (canal) is a curved canal with a longer posterior than anterior wall. The curvature of the lumbar spine influences the shape and tilt (inclination) of the pelvic cavity (Figure 2–10B♦).

The **pelvic outlet** is at the lower border of the true pelvis. The size of the pelvic outlet can be determined by assessing the *transverse diameter,* which is also called the bi-ischial, or intertuberous, diameter. This diameter extends from the inner surface of one ischial tuberosity to the other. The pubic arch is also part of the pelvic cavity. The pubic arch has great importance because the fetus must pass under it during birth. If it is narrow, the baby's head may be pushed backward toward the coccyx, making extension of the head difficult. The shoulders of a large baby may also become wedged under the pubic arch, making birth more difficult (see Chapter 20). The clinical assessment of each of these obstetrical diameters is discussed further in Chapter 8.

### Pelvic Types

The Caldwell-Moloy classification of pelves is widely used to differentiate bony pelvic types (Caldwell & Moloy, 1933). The four basic types are *gynecoid, android, anthropoid,* and *platypelloid* (see Figure 15–1♦). Each type has a characteristic shape, and each shape has implications for labor and birth. See Chapters 8 and 15 for further discussion.

## Breasts

The *breasts,* or *mammary glands,* considered accessories of the reproductive system, are specialized sebaceous glands (Figure 2–12♦). They are conical and symmetrically placed on the sides of the chest. The greater pectoral and anterior serratus muscles underlie each breast. Suspending the breasts are fibrous tissues, called *Cooper's ligaments,* that extend from the deep fascia in the chest outward to just under the skin covering the breast. Frequently, the left breast is larger than the right. In different racial groups breasts develop at slightly different levels in the pectoral region of the chest (Rebar, 1999).

In the center of each mature breast is the *nipple,* a protrusion about 0.5 to 1.3 cm in diameter. The nipple is composed mainly of erectile tissue, which becomes more

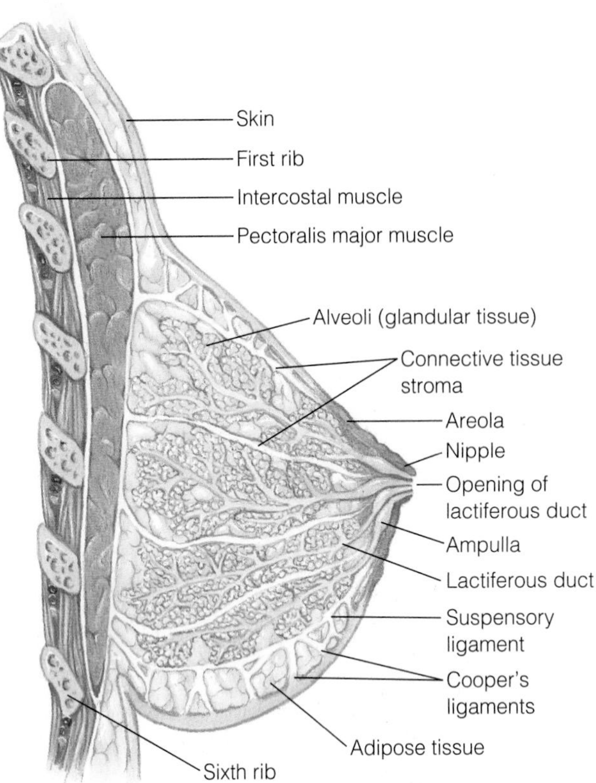


**FIGURE 2–12** ♦ Anatomy of the breast: sagittal view of left breast.

rigid and prominent during the menstrual cycle, sexual excitement, pregnancy, and lactation. The nipple is surrounded by the heavily pigmented **areola,** which is 2.5 to 10 cm in diameter. Both the nipple and the areola are roughened by small papillae called *tubercles of Montgomery.* As an infant suckles, these tubercles secrete a fatty substance that helps lubricate and protect the breasts.

The breasts are composed of glandular, fibrous, and adipose tissue. The glandular tissue is arranged in a series of 15 to 24 lobes separated by fibrous and adipose tissue. Each lobe is made up of several lobules composed of many alveoli clustered around tiny ducts. The lining of these ducts secretes the various components of milk. The ducts from several lobules merge to form the larger *lactiferous ducts,* which open on the surface of the nipple.

# The Female Reproductive Cycle

The **female reproductive cycle (FRC)** is composed of the ovarian cycle, during which ovulation occurs, and the uterine cycle, during which menstruation occurs. These two cycles take place simultaneously (Figure 2–13♦).

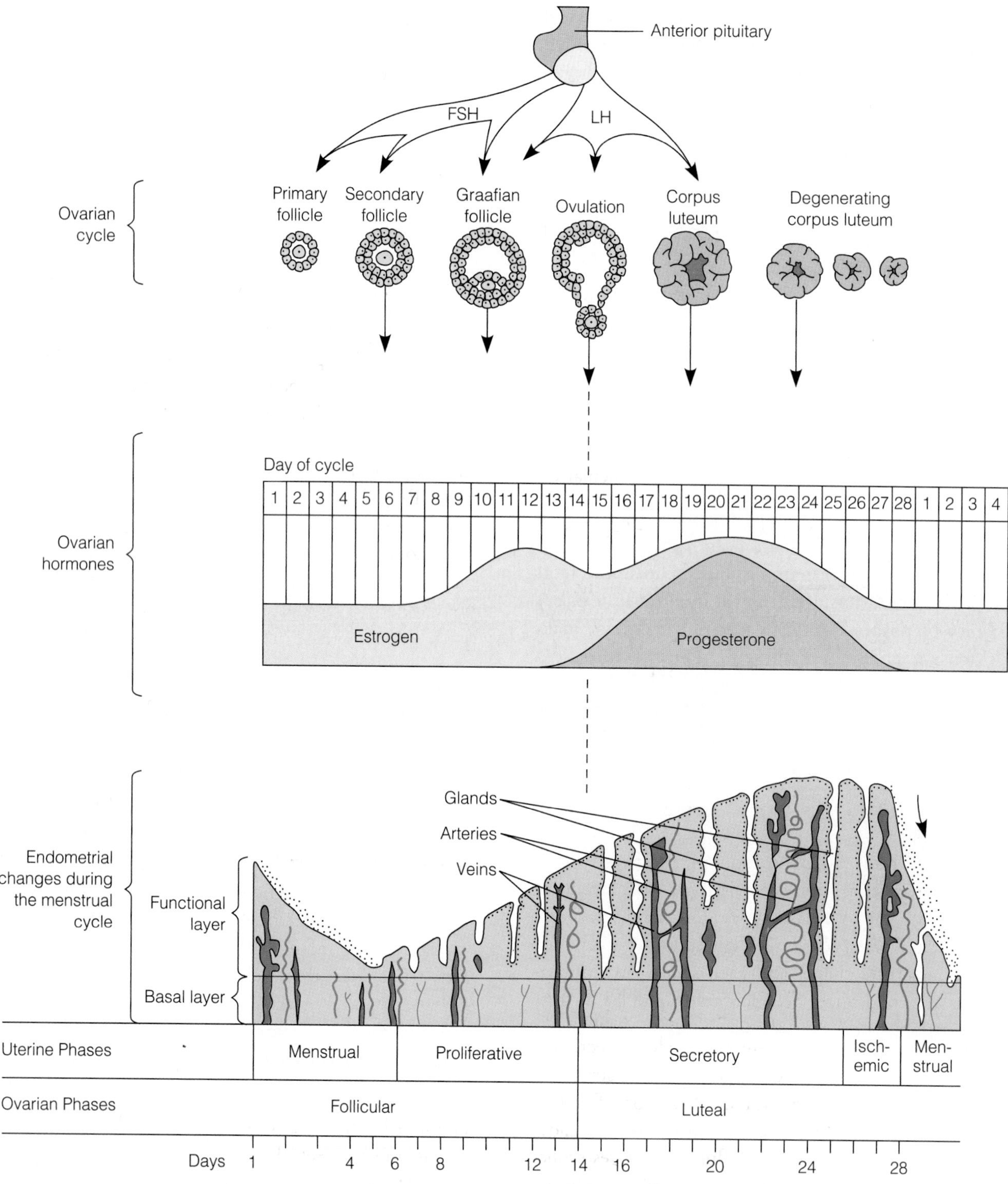


FIGURE 2–13 ♦ Female reproductive cycle: interrelationships of hormones with the four phases of the uterine cycle and the two phases of the ovarian cycle in an ideal 28-day cycle.

## Effects of Female Hormones

After menarche, a female undergoes a cyclic pattern of ovulation and menstruation (if pregnancy does not occur) for a period of 30 to 40 years. This cycle is an orderly process under neurohormonal control. Each month one oocyte matures, ruptures from the ovary, and enters the fallopian tube. The ovary, vagina, uterus, and fallopian tubes are major target organs for female hormones.

The ovaries produce mature gametes and secrete hormones. Ovarian hormones include the estrogens, progesterone, and testosterone. The ovary is sensitive to the follicle-stimulating hormone (FSH) and luteinizing hormone (LH). The uterus is sensitive to estrogen and progesterone. The relative proportion of these hormones to each other controls the events of both ovarian and menstrual cycles.

### Estrogens

**Estrogens** are secreted in large amounts by the ovaries in nonpregnant women. The major estrogenic effects are due primarily to three classical estrogens: estrone, β-estradiol, and estriol. The major estrogen is β-estradiol.

Estrogens control the development of the female secondary sex characteristics: breast development, widening of the hips, and deposits of tissue (fat) in the buttocks and mons pubis. Estrogens also assist in the maturation of the ovarian follicles and cause the endometrial mucosa to proliferate following menstruation. The amount of estrogens is greatest during the proliferative (follicular or estrogenic) phase of the menstrual cycle. Estrogens also cause the uterus to increase in size and weight because of increased glycogen, amino acids, electrolytes, and water. Blood supply is expanded as well. Under the influence of estrogens, myometrial contractility increases in both the uterus and the fallopian tubes, and uterine sensitivity to oxytocin increases. Estrogens inhibit FSH production and stimulate LH production.

Estrogens have effects on many hormones and other carrier proteins, such as contributing to the increased amount of protein-bound iodine in pregnant women and women who use oral contraceptives containing estrogen. Estrogens may increase libidinal feelings in humans. They decrease the excitability of the hypothalamus, which may cause an increase in sexual desire.

### Progesterone

**Progesterone** is secreted by the corpus luteum and is found in greatest amounts during the secretory (luteal or progestational) phase of the menstrual cycle. It decreases uterine motility and contractility caused by estrogens, thereby preparing the uterus for implantation after the ovum is fertilized. The endometrial mucosa is in a ready state as a result of estrogenic influence. Progesterone causes the uterine endometrium to further increase its supply of glycogen, arterial blood, secretory glands, amino acids, and water. Under the influence of progesterone, the vaginal epithelium proliferates and the cervix secretes thick, viscous mucus. Breast glandular tissue increases in size and complexity. Progesterone also prepares the breasts for lactation.

The temperature rise of about 0.3 to 0.6°C (0.5 to 1.0°F) that accompanies ovulation and persists throughout the secretory phase of the menstrual cycle is due to progesterone.

### Prostaglandins

**Prostaglandins (PGs)** are oxygenated fatty acids that are produced by the cells of the endometrium and are also classified as hormones. Prostaglandins have varied action in the body depending on the different type of PGs. Generally PGEs relax smooth muscles and are potent vasodilators; PGFs are potent vasoconstrictors and increase the contractility of muscles and arteries. Although their primary actions seem antagonistic, their basic regulatory functions in cells are achieved through an intricate pattern of reciprocal events. The discussion here sums up their role in ovulation and menstruation.

Prostaglandin production increases during follicular maturation, is dependent on gonadotropins, and is essential to ovulation. Extrusion of the ovum, resulting from the increased contractility of the smooth muscle in the theca layer of the mature follicle, is thought to be caused by $PGF_{2\alpha}$. Significant amounts of PGs are found in and around the follicle at the time of ovulation.

Although the exact mechanism by which the corpus luteum degenerates in the absence of pregnancy remains obscure, $PGF_{2\alpha}$ is thought to induce progesterone withdrawal, the lowest point of which coincides with the onset of menses.

During the late secretory phase, the level of $PGF_{2\alpha}$ is higher than that of PGE (Clark & Myatt, 1999). This event increases vasoconstriction and contractility of the myometrium, which contributes to the ischemia preceding menstruation. A high concentration of PGs may also account for the vasoconstriction of the endometrium venous lacunae, allowing for platelet aggregation at vascular rupture points and thereby preventing rapid blood loss during menstruation. The menstrual flow's high concentration of PGs may also facilitate the process of tissue digestion, which allows for an orderly shedding of the endometrium during menstruation.

## Neurohumoral Basis of the Female Reproductive Cycle

The female reproductive cycle is controlled by complex interactions between the nervous and endocrine systems and their target tissues. These interactions involve the hypothalamus, anterior pituitary, and ovaries.

The hypothalamus secretes **gonadotropin-releasing hormone (GnRH)** to the pituitary gland in response to signals received from the central nervous system. This releasing hormone is often called both luteinizing hormone–releasing hormone (LHRH) and follicle-stimulating hormone–releasing hormone (FSHRH).

In response to GnRH, the anterior pituitary secretes the gonadotropic hormones **follicle-stimulating hormone (FSH)** and **luteinizing hormone (LH).** FSH is primarily responsible for the maturation of the ovarian follicle. As the follicle matures, it secretes increasing amounts of estrogen, which enhance the development of the follicle (Ferin, 1998). (This estrogen is also responsible for the building or proliferation phase of the endometrium after it is shed during menstruation.)

Final maturation of the follicle cannot come about without the action of LH. The anterior pituitary's production of LH increases 6- to 10-fold as the follicle matures. The peak production of LH can precede ovulation by as much as 36 hours (Couchman & Hammond, 1999).

The LH is also responsible for the "luteinizing" of the theca and granulosa cells of the ruptured follicle. As a result, estrogen production is reduced and progesterone secretion continues. Thus estrogen levels fall a day before ovulation; tiny amounts of progesterone are in evidence. **Ovulation** takes place following the very rapid growth of the follicle, as the sustained high level of estrogen diminishes and progesterone secretion begins.

The ruptured follicle undergoes rapid change, complete luteinization is accomplished, and the mass of cells becomes the **corpus luteum.** The lutein cells secrete large amounts of progesterone with smaller amounts of estrogen. (Concurrently, the excessive amounts of progesterone are responsible for the secretory phase of the uterine cycle.) Seven or eight days following ovulation, the corpus luteum begins to involute, losing its secretory function. The production of both progesterone and estrogen is severely diminished. The anterior pituitary responds with increasingly large amounts of FSH; a few days later LH production begins. As a result, new follicles become responsive to another ovarian cycle and begin maturing.

## Ovarian Cycle

The ovarian cycle has two phases: the *follicular phase* (days 1–14) and the *luteal phase* (days 15–28 in a 28-day cycle). Figure 2–14♦ depicts the changes that the follicle undergoes during the ovarian cycle. In women whose menstrual cycles vary, usually only the length of the follicular phase varies, because the luteal phase is of fixed length. During the follicular phase, the immature follicle matures as a result of FSH. Within the follicle, the oocyte grows. A mature **graafian follicle** appears on about the 14th day under dual control of FSH and LH. It is a large structure, measuring about 5 to 10 mm. The mature follicle produces increasing amounts of estrogen. In the mature graafian follicle, the cells surrounding the antral cavity are granulosa cells. The oocyte is surrounded by fluid and enclosed in a thick elastic capsule called the zona pellucida.

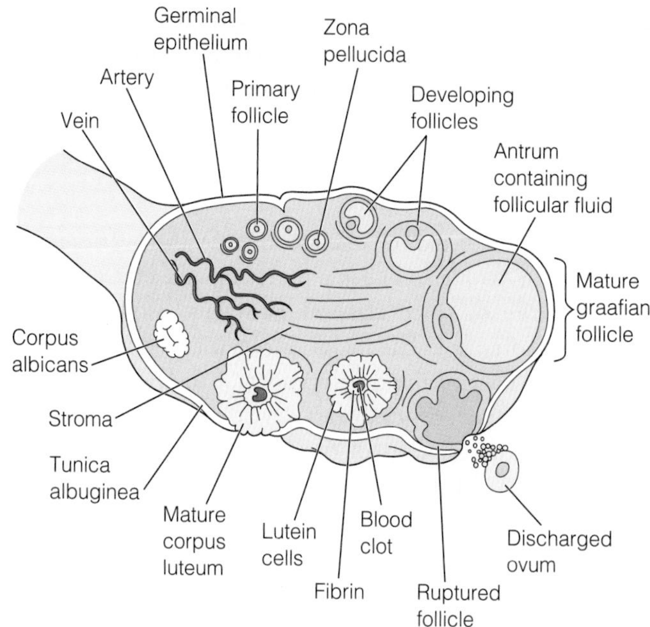


**FIGURE 2–14 ♦** Various stages of development of the ovarian follicles.

Just before ovulation, the mature oocyte completes its first meiotic division (see Chapter 3 for a description of meiosis). As a result of this division, two cells are formed: a small cell, called a *polar body,* and a larger cell, called the *secondary oocyte.* The secondary oocyte matures into the ovum (see Figure 3–2♦).

As the graafian follicle matures and enlarges, it comes close to the surface of the ovary. The ovary surface forms a blisterlike protrusion 10 to 15 mm in diameter, and the follicle walls become thin. The secondary oocyte, polar body, and follicular fluid are pushed out. The ovum is discharged near the fimbria of the fallopian tube and is pulled into the tube to begin its journey toward the uterus.

Occasionally, ovulation is accompanied by midcycle pain known as *mittelschmerz.* This pain may be caused by a thick tunica albuginea or by a local peritoneal reaction to the expelling of the follicular contents. Vaginal discharge may increase during ovulation, and a small amount of blood (midcycle spotting) may be discharged as well.

The body temperature increases about 0.3 to 0.6°C (0.5–1.0°F) 24 to 48 hours after the time of ovulation. It remains elevated until the day before menstruation begins. There may be an accompanying sharp basal body temperature drop before the increase. These temperature changes are useful clinically to determine the approximate time ovulation occurs.

Generally the ovum takes several minutes to travel through the ruptured follicle to the fallopian tube opening. The contractions of the tube's smooth muscle and its ciliary action propel the ovum through the tube. The ovum remains in the ampulla, where, if it is fertilized, cleavage can begin. The ovum is thought to be fertile for only 6 to 24 hours. It reaches the uterus 72 to 96 hours after its release from the ovary.

The luteal phase begins when the ovum leaves its follicle. Under the influence of LH, the corpus luteum develops from the ruptured follicle. Within 2 or 3 days, the corpus luteum becomes yellowish and spherical and increases in vascularity. If the ovum is fertilized and implants in the endometrium, the fertilized egg begins to secrete **human chorionic gonadotropin (hCG),** which is needed to maintain the corpus luteum. If fertilization does not occur, within about a week after ovulation the corpus luteum begins to degenerate, eventually becoming a connective tissue scar called the *corpus albicans.* With degeneration comes a decrease in estrogen and progesterone. This allows for an increase in LH and FSH, which trigger the hypothalamus. Approximately 14 days after ovulation (in a 28-day cycle), in the absence of pregnancy, menstruation begins.

### Uterine (Menstrual) Cycle

*Menstruation* is cyclic uterine bleeding in response to cyclic hormonal changes. Menstruation occurs when the ovum is not fertilized and begins about 14 days after ovulation in a 28-day cycle. The menstrual discharge, also referred to as the *menses,* or *menstrual flow,* is composed of blood mixed with fluid, cervical and vaginal secretions, bacteria, mucus, leukocytes, and other cellular debris. The menstrual discharge is dark red and has a distinctive odor.

Menstrual parameters vary greatly among individuals. Generally, menstruation occurs every 28 days, plus or minus 5 to 10 days. Emotional and physical factors such as illness, excessive fatigue, stress or anxiety, and vigorous exercise programs can alter the cycle interval. Certain environmental factors such as temperature and altitude may also affect the cycle. The duration of menses is from 2 to 8 days, with the blood loss averaging 30 mL and the loss of iron averaging 0.5 to 1 mg daily.

The uterine (menstrual) cycle has four phases: menstrual, proliferative, secretory, and ischemic. Menstruation occurs during the *menstrual phase.* Some endometrial areas are shed, while others remain. Some of the remaining tips of the endometrial glands begin to regenerate. The endometrium is in a resting state following menstruation. Estrogen levels are low, and the endometrium is 1 to 2 mm deep. During this part of the cycle, the cervical mucosa is scanty, viscous, and opaque.

The *proliferative phase* begins when the endometrial glands enlarge, becoming twisted and longer in response to increasing amounts of estrogen. The blood vessels become prominent and dilated, and the endometrium increases in thickness six- to eightfold. This gradual process reaches its peak just before ovulation. The cervical mucosa becomes thin, clear, watery, and more alkaline, making the mucosa more favorable to spermatozoa. As ovulation nears, the cervical mucosa shows increased elasticity, called *spinnbarkheit.* At ovulation, the mucus will stretch more than 5 cm. The cervical mucosa pH increases from below 7.0 to 7.5 at the time of ovulation. On microscopic examination, the mucosa shows a characteristic ferning pattern (see Figure 5–3♦). This fern pattern is a useful aid in assessing ovulation time.

The *secretory phase* follows ovulation. The endometrium, under estrogenic influence, undergoes slight cellular growth. Progesterone, however, causes such marked swelling and growth that the epithelium is warped into folds. The amount of tissue glycogen increases. The glandular epithelial cells begin to fill with cellular debris, become twisted, and dilate. The glands secrete small quantities of endometrial fluid in preparation for a fertilized ovum. The vascularity of the entire uterus increases greatly, providing a nourishing bed for implantation. If implantation occurs, the endometrium, under the influence of progesterone, continues to develop and become even thicker (see Chapter 3 for a discussion of implantation).

If fertilization does not occur, the *ischemic phase* begins. The corpus luteum begins to degenerate, and as a result both estrogen and progesterone levels fall. Areas of necrosis appear under the epithelial lining. Extensive vascular changes also occur. Small blood vessels rupture, and the spiral arteries constrict and retract, causing a deficiency of blood in the endometrium, which becomes pale. This ischemic phase is characterized by the escape of blood into the stromal cells of the uterus. The menstrual flow begins, thus beginning the menstrual cycle again. After menstruation the basal layer remains, so that the tips of the glands can regenerate the new functional endometrial layer. For further discussion, see Key Facts to Remember: Summary of Female Reproductive Cycle.

## Male Reproductive System

The primary reproductive functions of the male genitals are to produce and transport sex cells (sperm) through and eventually out of the male genital tract and into the female genital tract. The external and internal genitals of the male reproductive system are shown in Figure 2–15♦.

### External Genitals

The two external reproductive organs are the penis and scrotum. The *penis* is an elongated, cylindrical structure consisting of a body, called the *shaft,* and a

## KEY FACTS TO REMEMBER

### *Summary of Female Reproductive Cycle*

**Ovarian Cycle**

*Follicular phase* (days 1–14): Primordial follicle matures under influence of FSH and LH up to the time of ovulation.

*Luteal phase* (days 15–28): Ovum leaves follicle; corpus luteum develops under LH influence and produces high levels of progesterone and low levels of estrogen.

**Uterine (Menstrual) Cycle**

*Menstrual phase* (days 1–6): Estrogen levels are low, cervical mucus is scant, viscous, and opaque.

*Proliferative phase* (days 7–14): Estrogen peaks just prior to ovulation. Cervical mucus at ovulation is clear, thin, watery, alkaline, and more favorable to sperm; shows ferning pattern; and has spinnbarkheit greater than 5 cm. Just before ovulation, body temperature may drop slightly, then at ovulation body temperature rises sharply and remains elevated under the influence of progesterone.

*Secretory phase* (days 15–26): Estrogen drops sharply, and progesterone dominates.

*Ischemic phase* (days 27–28): Both estrogen and progesterone levels drop.

cone-shaped end, called the *glans.* The penis lies in front of the scrotum.

The shaft of the penis is made up of three longitudinal columns of erectile tissue: the paired *corpora cavernosa* and the *corpus spongiosum.* These columns are covered by dense fibrous connective tissue and then enclosed by elastic tissue. The penis is covered by a thin outer layer of skin.

The corpus spongiosum contains the urethra and becomes the glans at the distal end of the penis. The urethra widens within the glans and ends in a slitlike opening, located in the tip of the glans, called the *urethral meatus.* A circular fold of skin arises just behind the glans and covers it. Known as the *prepuce,* or *foreskin,* it may be removed by the surgical procedure of circumcision (see Chapter 23). If the corpus spongiosum does not surround the urethra completely, the urethral meatus may occur on the ventral aspect of the penile shaft (hypospadias) or on the dorsal aspect (epispadias).

Sexual stimulation causes the penis to elongate, thicken, and stiffen, a process called *erection.* The penis becomes erect when its blood vessels become engorged, a consequence of parasympathetic nerve stimulation. If sexual stimulation is intense enough, the forceful and sudden expulsion of semen occurs through the rhythmic contractions of the penile muscles. This phenomenon is called *ejaculation.*

The penis serves both the urinary and the reproductive systems. Urine is expelled through the urethral meatus. The reproductive function of the penis is to deposit sperm in the vagina so that fertilization of the ovum can occur.

The *scrotum* is a pouchlike structure that hangs in front of the anus and behind the penis. Composed of skin and the *dartos muscle,* the scrotum shows increased pigmentation and scattered hairs. The sebaceous glands open directly onto the scrotal surface; their secretion has

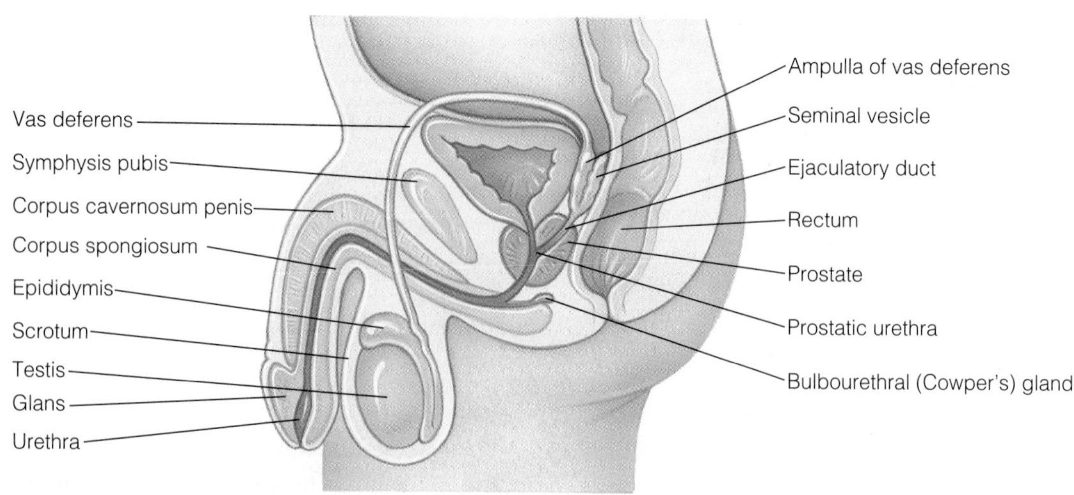


FIGURE 2–15 ♦ Male reproductive system, sagittal view.

a distinctive odor. Contraction of the dartos and cremasteric muscles shortens the scrotum and draws it closer to the body, thus wrinkling its outer surface. The degree of wrinkling is greatest in young men and at cold temperatures and is least in older men and at warm temperatures.

Inside the scrotum are two lateral compartments. Each compartment contains a testis with its related structures. Because the left spermatic cord grows longer, the left testis and its scrotal sac hang lower than on the right. A ridge (raphe) on the external scrotal surface marks the position of the medial septum.

The function of the scrotum is to protect the testes and the sperm by maintaining a temperature lower than that of the body. Spermatogenesis cannot occur if the testes fail to descend and thus remain at body temperature. Because it is sensitive to touch, pressure, temperature, and pain, the scrotum defends against potential harm to the testes.

## Internal Reproductive Organs

The male internal reproductive organs include the gonads (testes or testicles), a system of ducts (epididymides, vas deferens, ejaculatory duct, and urethra), and accessory glands (seminal vesicles, prostate gland, bulbourethral glands, and urethral glands). See Key Facts to Remember: Summary of Male Reproductive Organ Functions.

### Testes

The *testes* are a pair of oval, compound glandular organs contained in the scrotum. In the sexually mature male, they are the site of spermatozoa production and the secretion of several male sex hormones.

Each testis is 4 to 6 cm long, 2 to 3 cm wide, and 3 to 4 cm thick and weighs about 10 to 15 g. Each is covered by an outer serous membrane and an inner capsule that is tough, white, and fibrous. The connective tissue sends projections inward to form septa, dividing the testis into 250 to 400 lobules. Each lobule contains one to three tightly packed, convoluted *seminiferous tubules* containing sperm cells in all stages of development.

The seminiferous tubules are surrounded by loose connective tissue that houses abundant blood and lymph vessels and *interstitial (Leydig's) cells.* The interstitial cells produce testosterone, the primary male sex hormone. The tubules also contain *Sertoli's cells,* which nourish and protect the spermatocytes. The seminiferous tubules come together to form 20 to 30 straight tubules, which in turn form an anastomotic network of thin-walled spaces, the *rete testis.* The rete testis forms 10 to 15 efferent ducts that empty into the duct of the epididymis.

Most of the cells lining the seminiferous tubules undergo **spermatogenesis,** a process of maturation in which spermatocytes become spermatozoa. (Chapter 3 further discusses the process of spermatogenesis.) Sperm production varies among and within the tubules, with cells in different areas of the same tubule undergoing different stages of spermatogenesis. The sperm are eventually released from the tubules into the epididymis, where they continue to mature.

Like the female reproductive cycle, the process of spermatogenesis and other functions of the testes are the result of complex neural and hormonal controls. The hypothalamus secretes releasing factors that stimulate the anterior pituitary to release the gonadotropins—FSH and LH. These hormones cause the testes to produce testosterone, which maintains spermatogenesis, increases

**KEY FACTS TO REMEMBER**

***Summary of Male Reproductive Organ Functions***

The testes house seminiferous tubules and gonads.

- Seminiferous tubules contain sperm cells in various stages of development and undergoing meiosis.
- Sertoli's cells nourish and protect spermatocytes (phase between spermatids and spermatozoa).
- Leydig's cells are the main source of testosterone.
- Epididymides provide an area for maturation of sperm and a reservoir for mature spermatozoa.
- The vas deferens connects the epididymis with the prostate gland, then connects with ducts from the seminal vesicle to become an ejaculatory duct.
- Ejaculatory ducts provide a passageway for semen and seminal fluid into the urethra.
- Seminal vesicles secrete yellowish fluid rich in fructose, prostaglandins, and fibrinogen. This provides nutrition that increases motility and fertilizing ability of sperm. Prostaglandins also aid fertilization by making the cervical mucus more receptive to sperm.
- The prostate gland secretes thin, alkaline fluid containing calcium, citric acid, and other substances. Alkalinity counteracts acidity of ductus and seminal vesicle secretions.
- Bulbourethral (Cowper's) glands secrete alkaline, viscous fluid into semen, aiding in neutralization of acidic vaginal secretions.

sperm production by the seminiferous tubules, and stimulates production of seminal fluid.

**Testosterone** is the most prevalent and potent of the testicular hormones. It is also responsible for the development of secondary male characteristics and certain behavioral patterns. The effects of testosterone include structural and functional development of the male genital tract, emission and ejaculation of seminal fluid, distribution of body hair, promotion of growth and strength of long bones, increased muscle mass, and enlargement of the vocal cords. The action of testosterone on the central nervous system is thought to produce aggressiveness and sexual drive. The action of testosterone is constant, not cyclic like that of the female hormones. Its production is not limited to a certain number of years, but it is thought to decrease with age.

The testes have two primary functions:

- To serve as the site of spermatogenesis
- To produce testosterone

### Epididymis

The *epididymis* (plural, *epididymides*) is a duct about 5.6 m long, although it is convoluted into a compact structure about 3.75 cm long. An epididymis lies behind each testis. It arises from the top of the testis, courses downward, and then passes upward, where it becomes the vas deferens.

The epididymis provides a reservoir where maturing spermatozoa can survive for a long period. When discharged from the seminiferous tubules into the epididymis, the sperm are immotile and incapable of fertilizing an ovum. The spermatozoa remain in the epididymis for 2 to 10 days. As the sperm move along the tortuous course of the epididymis they become both motile and fertile.

### Vas Deferens and Ejaculatory Ducts

The *vas deferens,* also known as the *ductus deferens,* is about 40 cm long and connects the epididymis with the prostate. One vas deferens arises from the posterior border of each testis. It joins the spermatic cord and weaves over and between several pelvic structures until it meets the vas deferens from the opposite side. Each vas deferens terminus expands to form the *terminal ampulla.* It then unites with the seminal vesicle duct (a gland) to form the ejaculatory duct, which enters the prostate gland and ends in the prostatic urethra. The ejaculatory ducts serve as passageways for semen and fluid secreted by the seminal vesicles. The main function of the vas deferens is to rapidly squeeze the sperm from their storage sites (the epididymis and distal part of the vas deferens) into the urethra.

### Urethra

The male urethra is the passageway for both urine and semen. The urethra begins in the bladder and passes through the prostate gland, where it is called the *prostatic urethra.* The urethra emerges from the prostate gland to become the *membranous urethra.* It terminates in the penis, where it is called the *penile urethra.* In the penile urethra, goblet secretory cells are present, and smooth muscle is replaced by erectile tissue.

### Accessory Glands

The male accessory glands secrete a unique and essential component of the total seminal fluid in an ordered sequence.

The *seminal vesicles* are two glands composed of many lobes. Each vesicle is about 7.5 cm long. They are situated between the bladder and the rectum, immediately above the base of the prostate. The epithelium lining the seminal vesicles secretes an alkaline, viscid, clear fluid rich in high-energy fructose, prostaglandins, fibrinogen, and amino acids. During ejaculation, this fluid mixes with the sperm in the ejaculatory ducts. This fluid helps provide an environment favorable to sperm motility and metabolism (Aumüller & Riva, 1992).

The *prostate gland* encircles the upper part of the urethra and lies below the neck of the bladder. Made up of several lobes, it measures about 4 cm in diameter and weighs 20 to 30 g. The prostate is made up of both glandular and muscular tissue. It secretes a thin, milky, alkaline fluid containing high levels of zinc, calcium, citric acid, and acid phosphatase. This fluid protects the sperm from the acidic environment of the vagina and the male urethra, which could be spermicidal.

The *bulbourethral (Cowper's) glands* are a pair of small, round structures on either side of the membranous urethra. The glands secrete a clear, thick, alkaline fluid rich in mucoproteins that becomes part of the semen. This secretion also lubricates the penile urethra during sexual excitement and neutralizes the acid in the male urethra and vagina, thereby enhancing sperm motility.

The *urethral (Littré's) glands* are tiny mucus-secreting glands found throughout the membranous lining of the penile urethra. Their secretions add to those of the bulbourethral glands.

## SEMEN

The male ejaculate, *semen* or *seminal fluid,* is made up of spermatozoa and the secretions of all the accessory glands. The seminal fluid transports viable and motile sperm to the female reproductive tract. Effective transportation of sperm requires adequate nutrients, an adequate pH (about 7.5), a specific concentration of sperm to fluid, and an optimal osmolarity.

A spermatozoon is made up of a *head* and a *tail.* The tail is divided into the middle piece and end piece (Figure 2–16♦). The head's main components are the *acrosome* and *nucleus.* The head carries the male's haploid number of chromosomes (23), and it is the part that enters the ovum at fertilization (see Chapter 3). The tail, or flagellum, is divided into the middle and end piece and is specialized for motility.

Sperm may be stored in the male genital system for up to 42 days, depending primarily on the frequency of ejaculations. The average volume of ejaculate following abstinence for several days is 2 to 5 mL but may vary from 1 to 10 mL. Repeated ejaculation results in decreased volume. Once ejaculated, sperm can live only two or three days in the female genital tract.

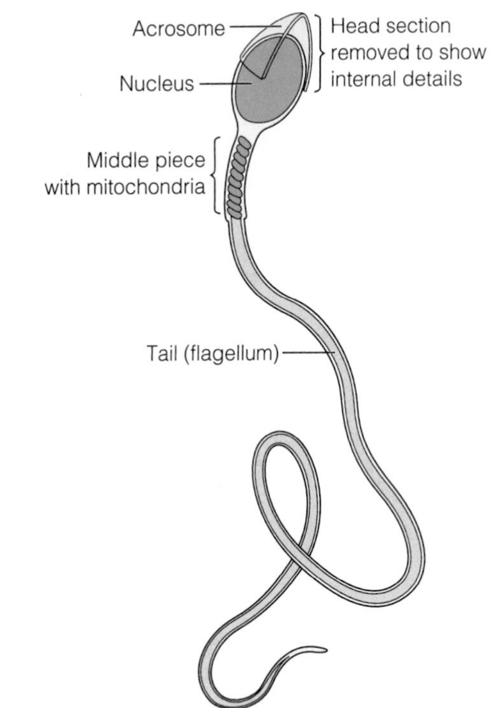


**FIGURE 2–16** ♦ Schematic representation of a mature spermatozoon.

# Chapter Review

## CHAPTER HIGHLIGHTS

- Reproductive activities require a complex interaction between the reproductive structures, the central nervous system, and such endocrine glands as the pituitary, hypothalamus, testes, and ovaries.
- The female reproductive system consists of the ovaries, where female germ cells and female sex hormones are formed; the fallopian tubes, which capture the ovum and allow transport to the uterus; the uterus, which is the implantation site for the fertilized ovum (blastocyst); the cervix, which is a protective portal for the body of the uterus and the connection between the vagina and the uterus; and the vagina, which is the passageway from the external genitals to the uterus and provides for discharge of menstrual products out of the body.
- The female reproductive cycle is composed of the ovarian cycle, during which ovulation occurs, and the uterine cycle, during which menstruation occurs. These two cycles take place simultaneously and are under neurohumoral control.
- The ovarian cycle has two phases: the follicular phase and the luteal phase. During the follicular phase, the primordial follicle matures under the influence of FSH and LH until ovulation occurs. The luteal phase begins when the ovum leaves the follicle and the corpus luteum develops under the influence of LH. The corpus luteum produces high levels of progesterone and low levels of estrogen.

- The uterine (menstrual) cycle has four phases: menstrual, proliferative, secretory, and ischemic. Menstruation is the actual shedding of the endometrial lining, when estrogen levels are low. The proliferative phase begins when the endometrial glands begin to enlarge under the influence of estrogen and cervical mucosal changes occur; the changes peak at ovulation. The secretory phase follows ovulation, and, influenced primarily by progesterone, the uterus increases its vascularity to make ready for possible implantation. The ischemic phase is characterized by degeneration of the corpus luteum, decreases in both estrogen and progesterone levels, constriction of the spiral arteries, and escape of blood into the stromal cells of the endometrium.
- The male reproductive system consists of the testes, where male germ cells and male sex hormones are formed; a series of continuous ducts through which spermatozoa are transported outside the body; accessory glands that produce secretions important to sperm nutrition, survival, and transport; and the penis, which serves as the reproductive organ of intercourse.

## CHAPTER REFERENCES


Aumüller, G., & Riva, A. (1992). Morphology and functions of the human seminal vesicle. *Andrologia, 24* (4):183–196.

Caldwell, W. E., & Moloy, H. C. (1933). Anatomical variations in the female pelvis and their effect on labor with a suggested classification [Historical article]. *American Journal of Obstetrics and Gynecology, 26,* 479–505.

Clark, K. E., & Myatt, L. (1999). Prostaglandins and the reproductive cycle. In J. J. Sciarri & T. J. Watkins (Eds.), *Gynecology and obstetrics* (Vol. 5, chap. 42, pp. 1–18). Hagerstown, MD: Harper & Row.

Couchman, G. M., & Hammond, C. B. (1999). Clinical anatomy of the female. In J. R. Scott, P. J. Di Saia, C. B. Hammond, & W. N. Spellacy (Eds.), *Danforth's obstetrics and gynecology* (8th ed., pp. 19–28). Philadelphia: Lippincott.

Cunningham, F. G., MacDonald, P. C., Gant, N. F., Leveno, K. J., Gilstrap, L. C., Hankins, G. D. V., & Clark, S. L. (1997). *Williams obstetrics* (20th ed.). Stamford, CT: Appleton & Lange.

Di Saia, P. J. (1999). Clinical anatomy of the female. In J. R. Scott, P. J. Di Saia, C. B. Hammond, & W. N. Spellacy (Eds.), *Danforth's obstetrics and gynecology* (8th ed., pp. 47–64). Philadelphia: Lippincott.

Ferin, M. (1998). The hypothalmus-hypophyseal-ovarian axis and the menstrual cycle. In J. J. Sciarri & T. J. Watkins (Eds.). *Gynecology and obstetrics* (Vol. 5, chap. 6, pp. 1–15). Hagerstown, MD: Harper & Row.

Liu, J. H., & Rebar, R. W. (1999). Endocrinology of pregnancy. In R. W. Creasy & R. Resnik (Eds.), *Maternal-fetal medicine: Principles and practice* (4th ed., pp. 379–391). Philadelphia: Saunders.

Rebar, R. W. (1999). The breast and the physiology of lactation. In R. W. Creasy & R. Resnik (Eds.), *Maternal-fetal medicine: Principles and practice* (4th ed., pp. 106–121). Philadelphia: Saunders.

Resnik, R. (1999). Anatomic alterations in the reproductive tract. In R. K. Creasy & R. Resnik (Eds.), *Maternal-fetal medicine: Principles and practice* (4th ed., pp. 90–94). Philadelphia: Saunders.


## CONTEMPORARY MATERNAL-NEWBORN NURSING ON-LINE

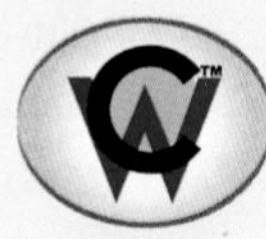

Additional interactive resources, including animations and video, for this chapter can be found on the Companion Website at http://www.prenhall.com/ladewig. Click on Chapter 2 and "Begin" to select the activities for this chapter.

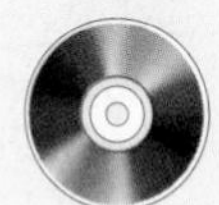

For NCLEX review questions and an audio glossary, access the accompanying CD-ROM in this book.

## Chapter 3

# Conception and Fetal Development

*I love teaching the course content on conception and fetal development. Each time, I am struck anew by the absolute magic of human reproduction.*

—Department of Nursing Faculty Member

## OBJECTIVES

- Explain the difference between meiotic cellular division and mitotic cellular division.
- Compare the processes by which ova and sperm are produced.
- Describe the components of the process of fertilization.
- Identify the differing processes by which fraternal (dizygotic) and identical (monozygotic) twins are formed.
- Describe in order of increasing complexity the structures that form during the cellular multiplication and differentiation stages of intrauterine development.
- Describe the development, structure, and functions of the placenta and umbilical cord during intrauterine life.
- Summarize the significant changes in growth and development of the fetus in utero at 4, 6, 12, 16, 20, 24, 28, 36, and 40 weeks' gestation.
- Identify the vulnerable periods during which malformations of the various organ systems may occur and describe the resulting congenital malformations.

## KEY TERMS

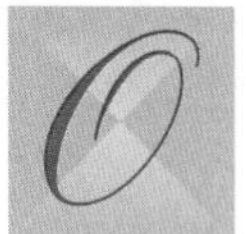

Our bodies are very similar, in both structure and function. Even our chromosomes are made of the same biochemical substances. What, then, makes each of us unique? The answer lies in the physiologic mechanisms of heredity, the processes of cellular division, and the environmental factors that influence our development from the moment we are conceived. This chapter explores the processes involved in conception and fetal development—the basis of human uniqueness.

## Cellular Division

Each human begins life as a single cell (fertilized ovum, or zygote). This single cell reproduces itself, and in turn each resulting cell also reproduces itself in a continuing process. The new cells are similar to the cells from which they came. Cells are reproduced by either mitosis or meiosis, two different but related processes. **Mitosis** produces exact copies of the original cell, making growth and development possible, and in mature individuals it is the process by which our body cells continue to divide and replace themselves. **Meiosis** is a process of cell division leading to the development of eggs and sperm needed to produce a new organism.

### Mitosis

During mitosis, the cell undergoes several changes ending in cell division. As the last phase of cell division nears completion, a furrow develops in the cell cytoplasm, which divides it into two *daughter cells,* each with its own nucleus. Daughter cells have the same **diploid number of chromosomes** (46) and same genetic makeup as the cell from which they came. After a cell with 46 chromosomes goes through mitosis, the result is two identical cells, each with 46 chromosomes.

### Meiosis

Meiosis is a special type of cell division by which diploid cells give rise to sperm and ova. Meiosis consists of two successive cell divisions. In the first division, the chromosomes replicate, doubling the structure of each of the 46 chromosomes. Next, a pairing takes place between homologous chromosomes (Sadler, 1995). Instead of separating immediately, as in mitosis, the chromosomes become closely intertwined. At each point of contact, there is a physical exchange of genetic material between the chromatids (the arms of the chromosomes). New combinations are provided by the newly formed chromosomes; these combinations account for the wide variation of traits in people (eg, hair or eye color). The chromosome pairs then separate, and the members of the pair move to opposite sides of the cell. The cell divides, forming two daughter cells, each with 23 double-structured chromosomes—the same amount of deoxyribonucleic acid (DNA) as a normal somatic cell. In the second division, the chromatids of each chromosome separate and move to opposite poles of each of the daughter cells. Cell division occurs, resulting in the formation of four cells, each containing 23 single chromosomes (the **haploid number of chromosomes**). These daughter cells contain only half the DNA of a normal somatic cell. See Key Facts to Remember: Comparison of Meiosis and Mitosis.

Mutations may occur during the second meiotic division, if two of the chromatids do not move apart rapidly enough when the cell divides. The still-paired chromatids are carried into one of the daughter cells and eventually form an extra chromosome. This condition, *autosomal nondisjunction* (chromosomal mutation), is harmful to the offspring if fertilization occurs.

Another type of chromosomal mutation can occur if chromosomes break during meiosis. If the broken segment is lost, the result is a shorter chromosome; this situation is known as *deletion.* If the broken segment becomes attached to another chromosome, a harmful mutation called a *translocation* is the result. The effects of translocation and autosomal nondisjunction are described in Chapter 5.

Meiosis occurs during *gametogenesis,* the process by which germ cells, or **gametes,** are produced. The gametes must have a haploid number (23) of chromosomes so that when the female gamete (egg or ovum) and the male gamete (sperm or spermatozoon) unite to form the *zygote* (fertilized ovum), the normal human diploid number of chromosomes (46) is reestablished.

#### Oogenesis

*Oogenesis* is the process by which the female gametes, or ova, are produced. The ovaries begin to develop early in the fetal life of the female. All the ova that the female will produce are formed by the sixth month of fetal life. The ovary gives rise to oogonial cells, which develop into *oocytes.* Meiosis begins in all oocytes before the female fetus is born but stops before the first division is complete and remains in this arrested phase until puberty. During puberty, the mature primary oocyte proceeds (by oogenesis) through the first meiotic division in the graafian follicle of the ovary.

The first meiotic division produces two cells of unequal size with different amounts of cytoplasm but with the same number of chromosomes. These two cells are the *secondary oocyte* and a minute *polar body.* Both the secondary oocyte and the polar body contain 22 double-structured autosomal chromosomes and one double-structured sex chromosome (X). At the time of ovulation, a second meiotic division begins immediately and pro-

## KEY FACTS TO REMEMBER

### *Comparison of Meiosis and Mitosis*

*Meiosis*

**Purpose**

Produce reproductive cells (gametes). Reduction of chromosome number by half (from diploid [46] to haploid [23]), so that when fertilization occurs the normal diploid number is restored. Introduces genetic variability.

**Cell division**

Two-stage reduction.

**Number of daughter cells**

Four daughter cells, each containing one-half the number of chromosomes as the mother cell, or 23 chromosomes. Nonidentical to original cell.

*Mitosis*

**Purpose**

Produce cells for growth and tissue repair. Cell division characteristic of all somatic cells.

**Cell division**

One-stage cell division.

**Number of daughter cells**

Two daughter cells identical to the mother cell, each with the diploid number (46 chromosomes).

ceeds as the oocyte moves down the fallopian tube. Division is again not equal, and the secondary oocyte moves into the metaphase stage of cell division, where its meiotic division is arrested.

When the secondary oocyte completes the second meiotic division after fertilization, the result is a mature ovum with the haploid number of chromosomes and virtually all the cytoplasm. In addition, the second polar body (also haploid) forms at this time. The first polar body has also divided in two, producing two additional polar bodies. Thus, at the completion of meiosis, four haploid cells have been produced: the three polar bodies, which eventually disintegrate, and one ovum (Sadler, 1995) (Figure 3–1♦).

#### SPERMATOGENESIS

During puberty, the germinal epithelium in the seminiferous tubules of the testes begins the process of spermatogenesis, which produces the male gamete (sperm). The diploid spermatogonium replicates before it enters the first meiotic division, during which it is called the primary spermatocyte. During this first meiotic division, the spermatogonium forms two cells called secondary spermatocytes, each of which contains 22 double-structured autosomal chromosomes and either a double-structured X sex chromosome or a double-structured Y sex chromosome. During the second meiotic division, they divide to form four spermatids, each with the haploid number of chromosomes. The spermatids undergo a series of changes during which they lose most of their cytoplasm and become sperm (spermatozoa) (Figure 3–1♦).

# The Process of Fertilization

**Fertilization** is the process by which a sperm fuses with an ovum to form a new diploid cell, or zygote. Following are the events that lead to fertilization.

## PREPARATION FOR FERTILIZATION

The process of fertilization takes place in the ampulla (outer third) of the fallopian tube. During ovulation, high estrogen levels increase peristalsis within the fallopian tubes, which helps move the ovum through the tube toward the uterus. The ovum has no inherent power of movement. The high estrogen levels also cause a thinning of the cervical mucus, facilitating movement of the sperm through the cervix, into the uterus, and up the fallopian tube.

The ovum's cell membrane is surrounded by two layers of tissue. The layer closest to the cell membrane is called the *zona pellucida.* It is a clear, noncellular layer whose thickness influences the fertilization rate. Surrounding the zona pellucida is a ring of elongated cells, called the *corona radiata* because they radiate from the ovum like the gaseous corona around the sun. These cells are held together by hyaluronic acid.

The mature ovum and spermatozoa have only a brief time to unite. Ova are considered fertile for about 12 to 24 hours after ovulation. Sperm can survive in the female reproductive tract for 48 to 72 hours but are believed to be healthy and highly fertile for only about 24 hours (De Jonge, 2000).

In a single ejaculation, the male deposits approximately 200 to 500 million spermatozoa in the vagina, of which only hundreds of sperm actually reach the ampulla (Brannigan & Lipshultz, 2000). The spermatozoa propel themselves up the female tract by the flagellar movement of their tails. Transit time from the cervix into the fallopian tube can be as short as 5 minutes but usually takes an average of 4 to 6 hours after ejaculation

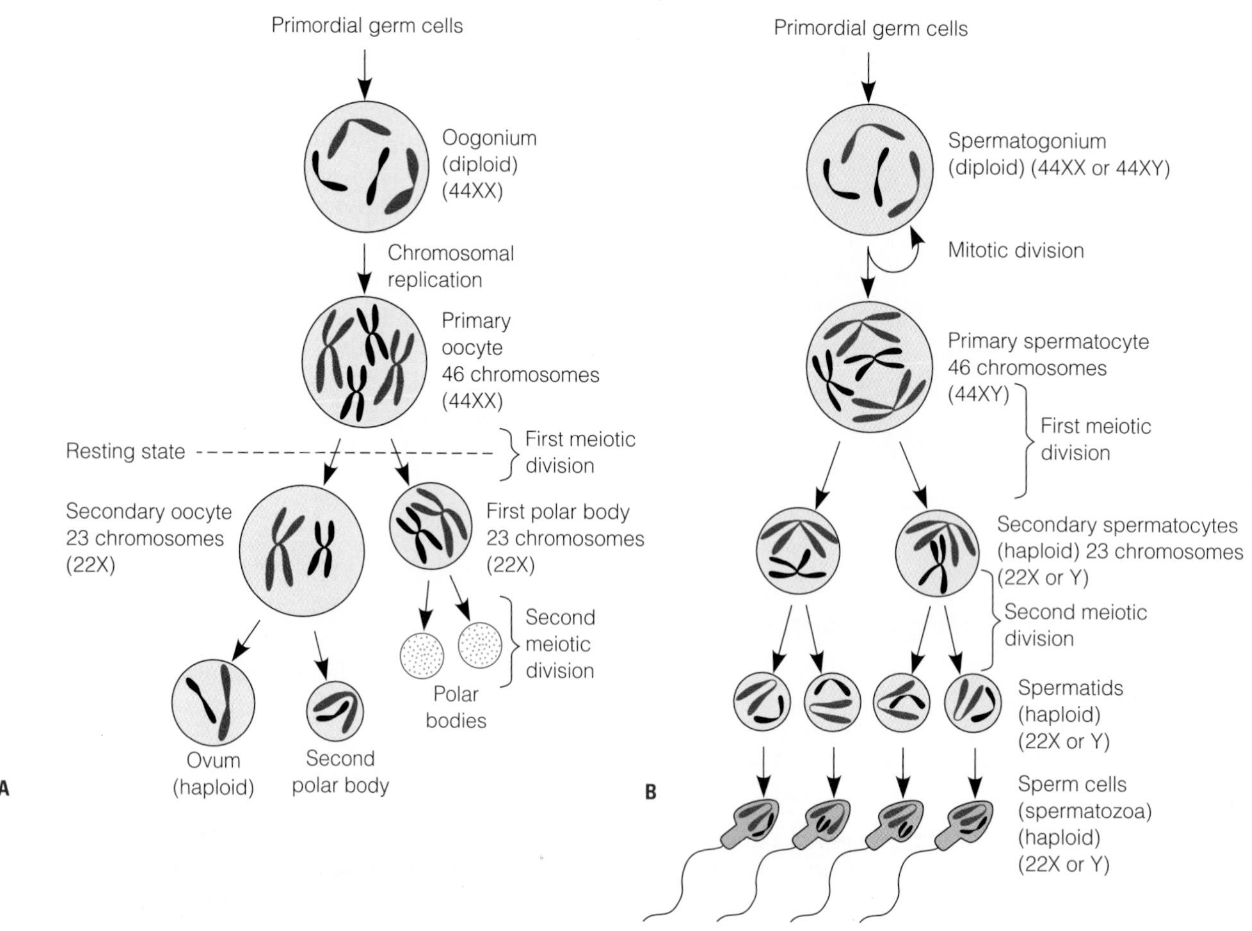


**FIGURE 3–1 ♦** Gametogenesis involves meiosis within the ovary and testis. **A,** During meiosis each oogonium produces a single haploid ovum once some cytoplasm moves into the polar bodies. **B,** Each spermatogonium produces four haploid spermatozoa.

(Brannigan & Lipshultz, 2000). Prostaglandins in the semen may increase uterine smooth muscle contractions, which help transport the sperm. The fallopian tubes have a dual ciliary action that facilitates movement of the ovum toward the uterus and movement of the sperm from the uterus toward the ovary.

The sperm's nucleus, which contains its genetic material, is compacted into the head of the sperm and covered by a protective cap called an acrosome, which is in turn covered by a plasma membrane. The sperm must undergo two processes before fertilization can occur: capacitation and the acrosomal reaction. **Capacitation** is the removal of the plasma membrane overlying the spermatozoa's acrosomal area and the loss of seminal plasma lipids, proteins, and the glycoprotein coat. If the sperm plasma membrane is not removed, the sperm will not be able to fertilize the ovum (Brannigan & Lipshultz, 2000). Capacitation occurs in the female reproductive tract (aided by uterine enzymes) and is thought to take about 7 hours.

The **acrosomal reaction** follows capacitation. The acrosomes of the sperms surrounding the ovum release their enzymes (hyaluronidase, a protease called acrosin, and corona-dispersing enzymes) and thus break down the hyaluronic acid in the ovum's corona radiata (Brannigan & Lipshultz, 2000). Hundreds of acrosomes must rupture before enough hyaluronic acid is cleared for a single sperm to penetrate the ovum's zona pellucida successfully. At the moment of penetration, a cellular change occurs in the ovum that renders it impenetrable by other sperm (Figure 3–2♦).

## The Moment of Fertilization

After the sperm enters the ovum, a chemical signal prompts the secondary oocyte to complete the second meiotic division, forming the nucleus of the ovum and ejecting the second polar body. Then the nuclei of the ovum and sperm swell and approach each other. The true moment of fertilization occurs as the nuclei unite. Their individual nuclear membranes disappear, and their chromosomes pair up to produce the diploid **zygote.** Since each nucleus contains a haploid number of chromosomes (23), this union restores the diploid number (46). The zygote contains a new combination of genetic material that results in an individual different from either parent and anyone else.

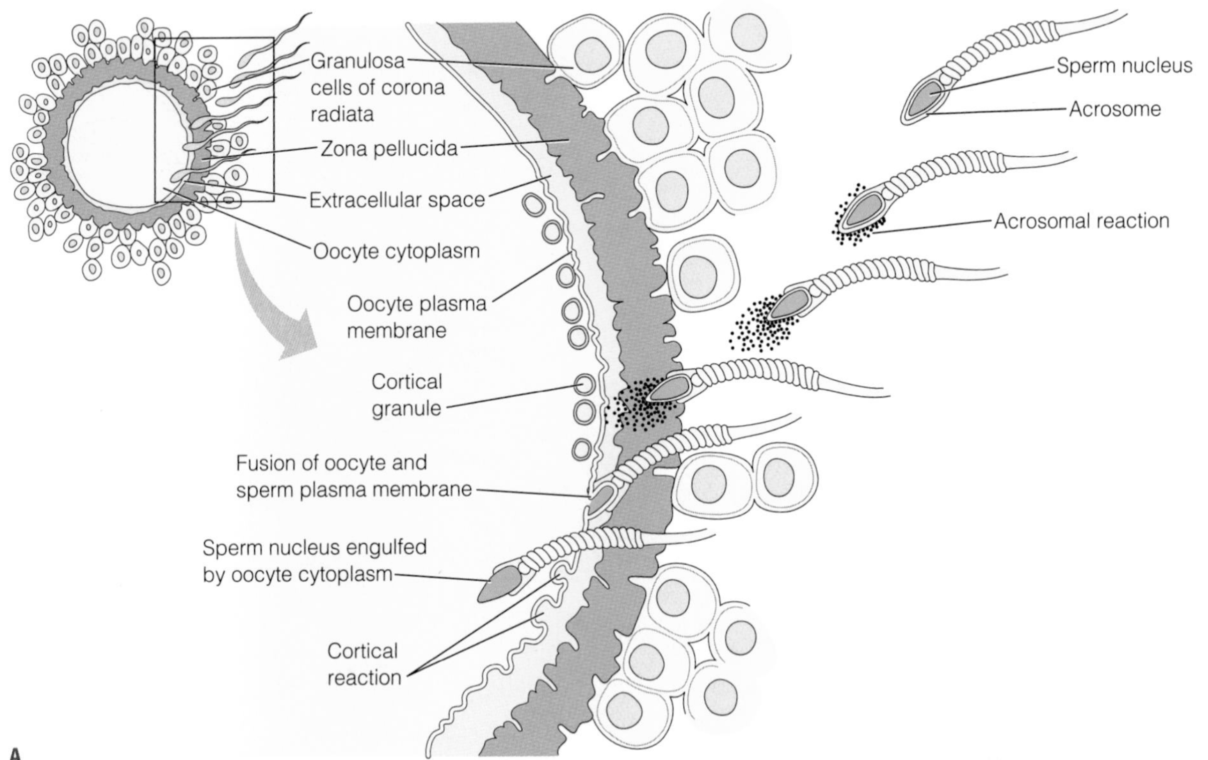


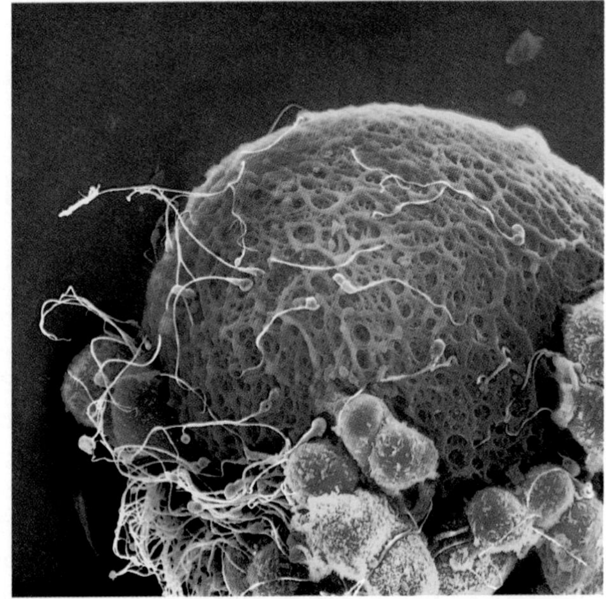


FIGURE 3–2 ♦ Sperm penetration of an ovum. **A**, The sequential steps of oocyte penetration by a sperm are depicted moving from top to bottom. **B**, Scanning electron micrograph of a human sperm surrounding a human ovum (750×). The smaller spherical cells are granulosa cells of the corona radiata. *Source:* Scanning electron micrograph from Nilsson, L. (1990). *A child is born.* New York: Dell Publishing.

It is also at the moment of fertilization that the sex of the zygote is determined. As discussed in Chapter 5, the two chromosomes (the sex chromosomes) of the 23rd pair—either XX or XY—determine the sex of an individual. X chromosomes are larger and bear more genes than Y chromosomes. Females have two X chromosomes, and males have an X and a Y chromosome. Whereas the mature ovum produced by oogenesis can have only one type of sex chromosome—an X—spermatogenesis produces two sperm with an X chromosome and two sperm with a Y chromosome. When each gamete contributes an X chromosome, the resulting zygote is female. When the ovum contributes an X and the sperm contributes a Y chromosome, the resulting zygote is male. Certain traits are termed sex linked because they are controlled by the genes on the X sex chromosome. Two examples of sex-linked traits are color blindness and hemophilia.

## Twins

Twins normally occur in approximately 1 in 80 pregnancies, and triplets occur in 1 in 8000 pregnancies (Spellacy, 1999). Twins have been reported to occur more often among black women than among white women and more often among white women than among women of Asian origin (Benirschke, 1999a). Among all groups, as parity (having given birth to a viable infant) increases, so does the chance for multiple births.

Twins may be either fraternal or identical. If they are fraternal, they are dizygotic, which means they arise from two separate ova fertilized by two separate spermatozoa (Figure 3–3♦). There are two placentas, two chorions, and two amnions; however, the placentas sometimes fuse and appear to be one. Despite their birth relationship, fraternal twins are no more similar to each other than they would be to siblings born singly. They may be of the same or different sex.

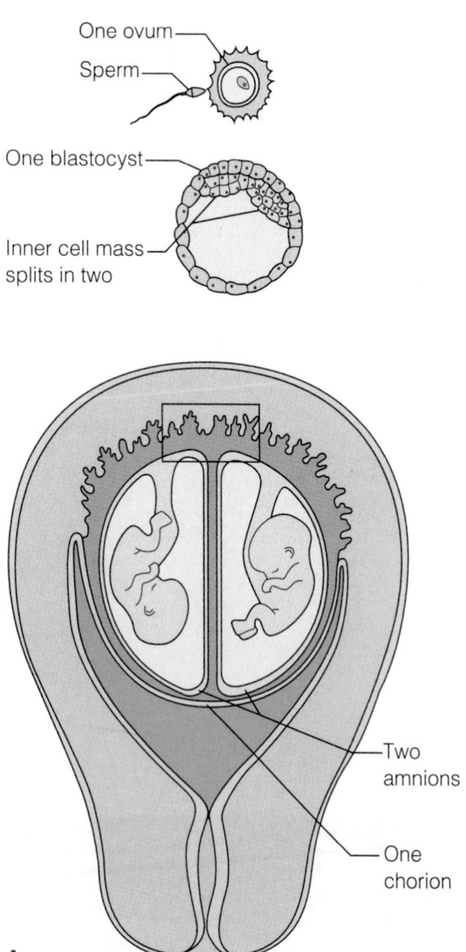


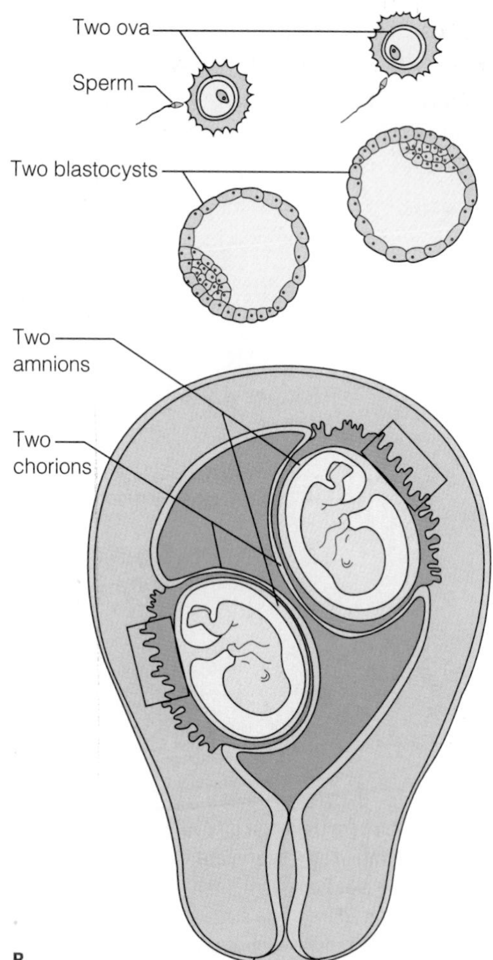


**FIGURE 3–3** ♦ **A,** Formation of identical twins. **B,** Formation of fraternal twins (Note separate placentas.)

The likelihood of dizygotic twinning increases with maternal age up to about age 35 and then decreases abruptly. The chance of dizygotic twins increases with parity, in conceptions that occur in the first 3 months of marriage, and also with coital frequency. The chance of dizygotic twinning decreases during periods of malnutrition and during winter and spring for women living in the northern hemisphere. Studies indicate that dizygotic twins occur in certain families, perhaps because of genetic factors that result in elevated serum gonadotropin levels and thus double ovulation (Spellacy, 1999).

Identical, or monozygotic, twins develop from a single fertilized ovum. They are of the same sex and have the same genotype (appearance). Identical twins usually have a common placenta (Figure 3–3♦). Monozygosity is not affected by environment, race, physical characteristics, or fertility.

Monozygotic twins originate from division of the fertilized ovum at different stages of early development, after the zygote consists of thousands of cells. Complete separation of the cellular mass into two parts is necessary for twin formation. The number of amnions and chorions present depends on the timing of the division:

1. If division occurs within 3 days of fertilization (before the inner cell mass and chorion are formed), two embryos, two amnions, and two chorions will develop. This dichorionic-diamniotic situation occurs about 20% to 30% of the time, and there may be two distinct placentas or a single fused placenta.
2. If division occurs about 5 days after fertilization (when the inner cell mass is formed and the chorion cells have differentiated but those of the amnion have not), two embryos develop with separate amnion sacs. These sacs will eventually be covered by a common chorion; thus there will be a monochorionic-diamniotic placenta.
3. If the amnion has already developed, approximately 7 to 13 days after fertilization, division results in two embryos with a common amnion sac and a common chorion (a monochorionic-monoamniotic placenta). This type occurs about 1% of the time (Spellacy, 1999).

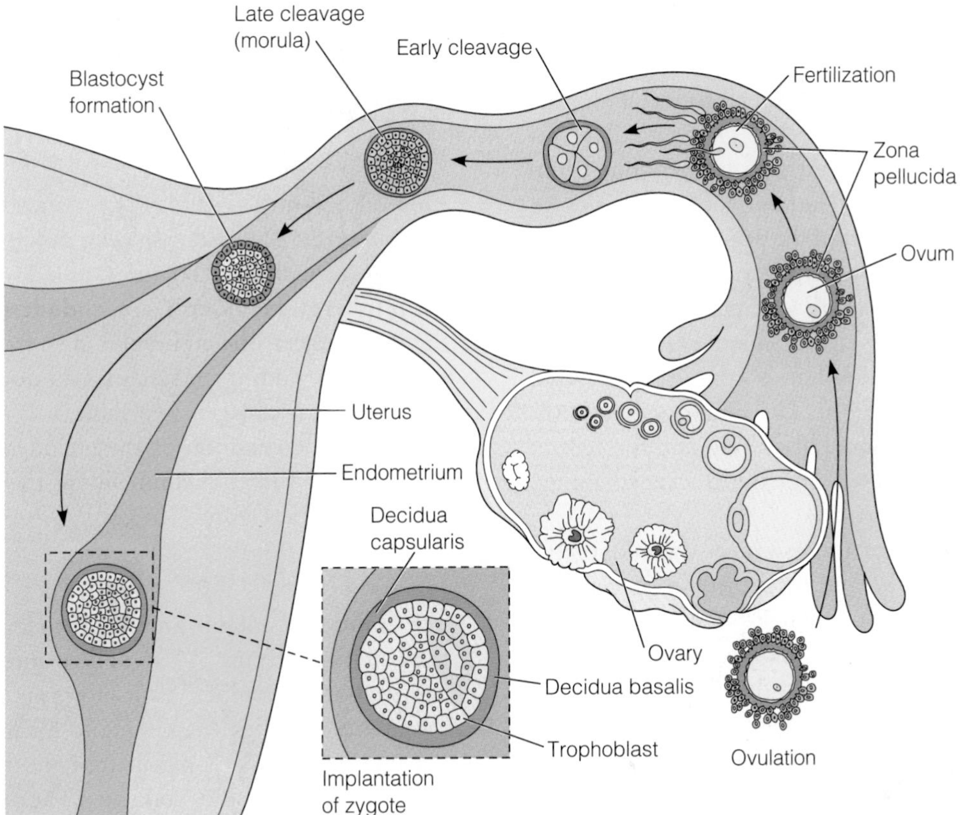


FIGURE 3–4 ♦ During ovulation, the ovum leaves the ovary and enters the fallopian tube. Fertilization generally occurs in the outer third of the fallopian tube. Subsequent changes in the fertilized ovum from conception to implantation are depicted.

Monozygotic twinning is considered a random event and occurs in approximately 3.5 per 1000 live births (Spellacy, 1999). The survival rate of monozygotic twins is 10% lower than that of dizygotic twins, and congenital anomalies are more prevalent. Both twins may have the same malformation.

# Preembryonic Development

The first 14 days of development, starting the day the ovum is fertilized (conception), are called the preembryonic stage, or the stage of the ovum (Craven & Ward, 1999). Development after fertilization can be divided into two phases: cellular multiplication and cellular (embryonic membrane) differentiation. This stage is characterized by rapid cellular multiplication and differentiation and the establishment of the embryonic membranes and primary germ layers. These phases and the process of implantation (nidation), which occurs between them, are discussed next.

## Cellular Multiplication

Cellular multiplication begins as the zygote moves through the fallopian tube toward the cavity of the uterus. This transport takes 3 days or more and is accomplished mainly by a very weak fluid current in the fallopian tube resulting from the beating action of the ciliated epithelium that lines the tube.

The zygote now enters a period of rapid mitotic divisions called **cleavage,** during which it divides into two cells, four cells, eight cells, and so on. These cells, called *blastomeres,* are so small that the developing cell mass is only slightly larger than the original zygote. The blastomeres are held together by the zona pellucida, which is under the corona radiata. The blastomeres eventually form a solid ball of 12 to 16 cells called the **morula.** As the morula enters the uterus, its intracellular fluid increases, and a cavity begins to form within it. The inner solid mass of cells is called the **blastocyst.** The outer layer of cells that surrounds the cavity and replaces the zona pellucida is the **trophoblast.** Eventually, the trophoblast develops into one of the embryonic membranes, the chorion. The blastocyst develops into a double layer of cells called the embryonic disc, from which the embryo will develop, and the other embryonic membrane (the amnion). The journey of the fertilized ovum to its destination in the uterus is illustrated in Figure 3–4♦.

## Implantation (Nidation)

While floating in the uterine cavity, the blastocyst is nourished by the uterine glands, which secrete a mixture of lipids, mucopolysaccharides, and glycogen. The trophoblast attaches itself to the surface of the endometrium for further nourishment. The most frequent site of attachment is the upper part of the posterior uterine wall. Between days 7 and 10 after fertilization, the zona pellucida disappears and the blastocyst implants itself by burrowing into the uterine lining. It penetrates down toward the maternal capillaries until it is completely covered (Ahokas & McKinney, 2000). The lining of the uterus thickens below the implanted blastocyst, and the cells of the trophoblast grow down into the thickened lining, forming processes called *villi.*

Under the influence of progesterone, the endometrium increases in thickness and vascularity in preparation for implantation and nutrition of the ovum. After implantation, the endometrium is called the *decidua.* The portion of the decidua that covers the blastocyst is called the **decidua capsularis,** the portion directly under the implanted blastocyst is the **decidua basalis,** and the portion that lines the rest of the uterine cavity is the **decidua vera (parietalis)** (Ahokas & McKinney, 2000). The maternal part of the placenta develops from the decidua basalis, which contains large numbers of blood vessels (see magnified insert in Figure 3–4♦). The chorionic villi in contact with the decidua basalis will form the fetal portion of the placenta.

## Cellular Differentiation

### Primary Germ Layers

About the 10th to 14th day after conception, the homogeneous mass of blastocyst cells differentiates into the primary germ layers (Figure 3–5♦). These three layers, the **ectoderm, mesoderm,** and **endoderm,** are formed at the same time as the embryonic membranes, and all tissues, organs, and organ systems will develop from these primary germ cell layers (see Table 3–1, on page 45). For example, differentiation of the endoderm results in the formation of the epithelium lining the respiratory and digestive tracts (Figure 3–6♦).

### Embryonic Membranes

The **embryonic membranes** begin to form at the time of implantation (Figure 3–7♦). These membranes protect and support the embryo as it grows and develops inside the uterus. The first membrane to form is the **chorion,** the outermost embryonic membrane that encloses the amnion, embryo, and yolk sac. The chorion, a thick membrane that develops from the trophoblast, has many fingerlike projections called *chorionic villi* on its surface. These chorionic villi can be used for early genetic testing of the embryo at 8 to 10 weeks' gestation by chorionic

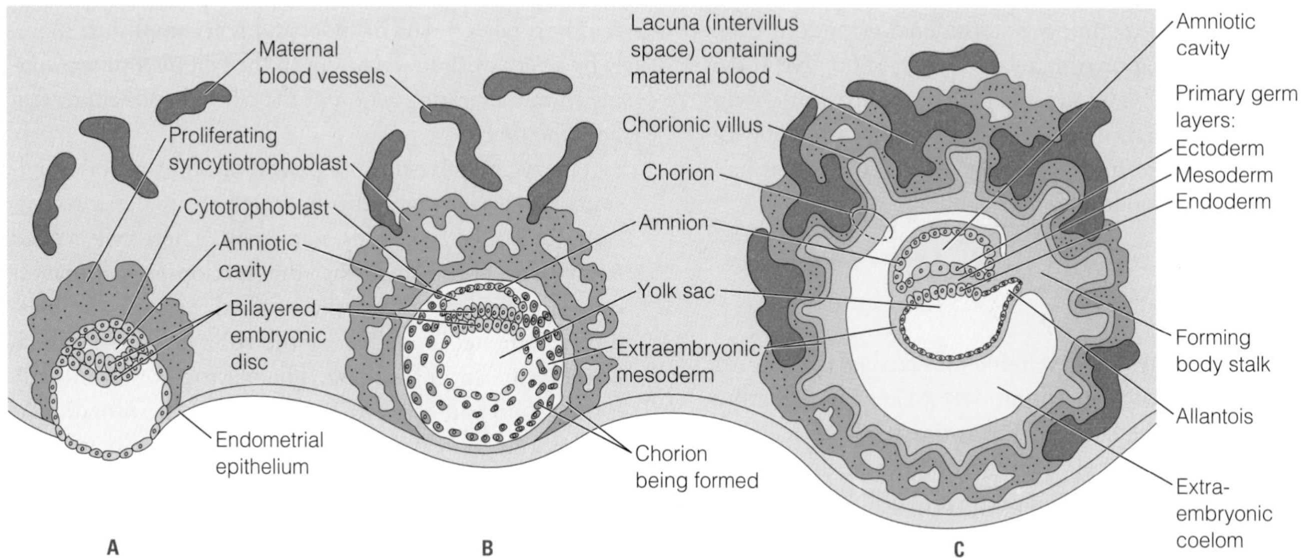


FIGURE 3–5 ♦ Formation of primary germ layers. **A**, Implantation of a 7½-day blastocyst in which the cells of the embryonic disc are separated from the amnion by a fluid-filled space. The erosion of the endometrium by the syncytiotrophoblast is ongoing. **B**, Implantation is completed by day 9, and extraembryonic mesoderm is beginning to form a discrete layer beneath the cytotrophoblast. **C**, By day 16 the embryo shows all three germ layers, a yolk sac, and an allantois (an outpouching of the yolk sac that forms the structural basis of the body stalk, or umbilical cord). The cytotrophoblast and associated mesoderm have become the chorion, and chorionic villi are developing. *Source:* Adapted from Marieb, E. N. (1998). *Human anatomy and physiology* (4th ed., p. 1088). Redwood City, CA: Benjamin/Cummings.

| TABLE 3–1 Derivation of Body Structures from Primary Cell Layers | | |
|---|---|---|
| *Ectoderm* | *Mesoderm* | *Endoderm* |
| Epidermis | Dermis | Respiratory tract epithelium |
| Sweat glands | Wall of digestive tract | Epithelium (except nasal), including pharynx, tongue, tonsils, thyroid, parathyroid, thymus, and tympanic cavity |
| Sebaceous glands | Kidneys and ureter (suprarenal cortex) | Lining of digestive tract |
| Nails | Reproductive organs (gonads, genital ducts) | Primary tissue of liver and pancreas |
| Hair follicles | Connective tissue (cartilage, bone, joint cavities) | Urethra and associated glands |
| Lens of eye | Skeleton | Urinary bladder (except trigone) |
| Sensory epithelium of internal and external ear, nasal cavity, sinuses, mouth, and anal canal | Muscles (all types) | Vagina (parts) |
| Central and peripheral nervous systems | Cardiovascular system (heart, arteries, veins, blood, bone marrow) | |
| Nasal cavity | Pleura | |
| Oral glands and tooth enamel | Lymphatic tissue and cells | |
| Pituitary gland | Spleen | |
| Mammary glands | | |

villi sampling (see Chapter 19). The villi begin to degenerate, except for those just under the embryo, which grow and branch into depressions in the uterine wall, forming the fetal portion of the placenta. By the fourth month of pregnancy, the surface of the chorion is smooth except at the place of attachment to the uterine wall.

The second membrane, the **amnion,** originates from the ectoderm, a primary germ layer, during the early stages of embryonic development. The amnion is a thin protective membrane that contains amniotic fluid. The space between the membrane and the embryo is the amniotic cavity. This cavity surrounds the embryo and yolk sac, except where the developing embryo (germ-layer disc) attaches to the trophoblast via the umbilical cord. As the embryo grows, the amnion expands until it comes in contact with the chorion. These two slightly adherent fetal membranes form the fluid-filled amniotic sac, or **bag of waters (BOW),** that protects the floating embryo.

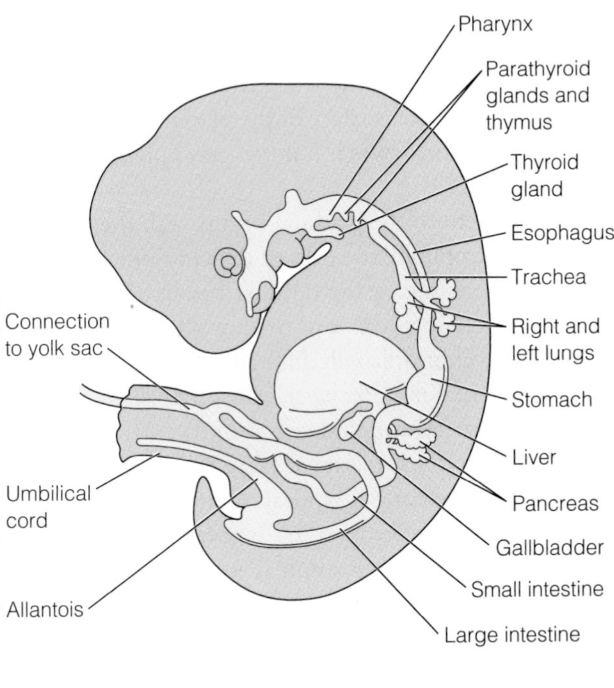


FIGURE 3–6 ♦ Endoderm differentiates to form the epithelial lining of the digestive and respiratory tracts and associated glands. *Source:* Adapted from Marieb, E. N. (1998). *Human anatomy and physiology* (4th ed., p. 1092). Redwood City, CA: Benjamin/Cummings.

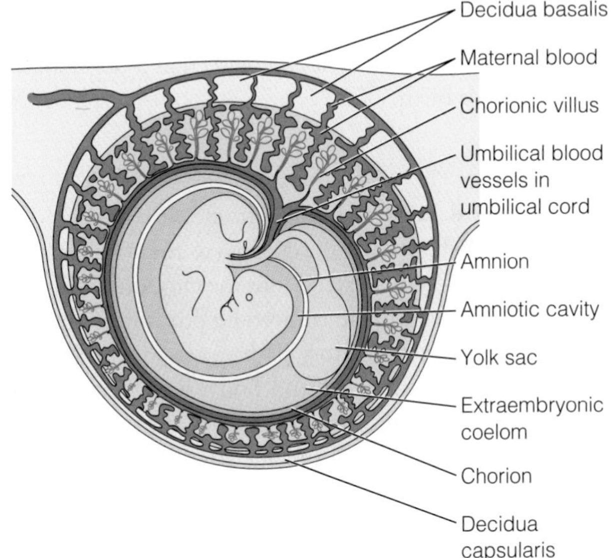


FIGURE 3–7 ♦ Early development of primary embryonic membranes. At 4½ weeks, the decidua capsularis (placental portion enclosing the embryo on the uterine surface) and decidua basalis (placental portion encompassing the elaborate chorionic villi and maternal endometrium) are well formed. The chorionic villi lie in blood-filled intervillous spaces within the endometrium. The amnion and yolk sac are well developed. *Source:* Adapted from Marieb, E. N. (1998). *Human anatomy and physiology* (4th ed., p. 1088). Redwood City, CA: Benjamin/Cummings.

### Amniotic Fluid

**Amniotic fluid** functions as a cushion to protect against mechanical injury. It also helps control the embryo's temperature, permits symmetrical external growth of the embryo, prevents adherence of the amnion, and allows freedom of movement so that the embryo-fetus can change position, thus aiding in musculoskeletal development. The amount of amniotic fluid at 10 weeks is about 30 mL, and it increases to 350 mL at 20 weeks. After 20 weeks, the volume ranges from 700 to 1000 mL. The amniotic fluid volume is constantly changing as the fluid moves back and forth across the placental membrane. As the pregnancy continues, the fetus contributes to the volume of amniotic fluid by excreting urine. The fetus swallows up to 600 mL every 24 hours, and about 400 mL of amniotic fluid flows out of the fetal lungs each day (Gilbert & Brace, 1993). See Chapter 19 for an in-depth discussion of alterations in amniotic fluid volume.

Amniotic fluid is slightly alkaline and contains albumin, uric acid, creatinine, lecithin, sphingomyelin, bilirubin, vernix, leukocytes, epithelial cells, enzymes, and fine hair called lanugo.

### Yolk Sac

In humans, the yolk sac is small and functions early in embryonic life. It develops as a second cavity in the blastocyst on about day 8 or 9 after conception. It forms primitive red blood cells during the first 6 weeks of development, until the embryo's liver takes over the process. As the embryo develops, the yolk sac is incorporated into the umbilical cord, where it can be seen as a degenerated structure after birth.

### Umbilical Cord

The **umbilical cord** is formed from the amnion. The *body stalk,* which attaches the embryo to the yolk sac, contains blood vessels that extend into the chorionic villi. The body stalk fuses with the embryonic portion of the placenta to provide a circulatory pathway from the chorionic villi to the embryo. As the body stalk elongates to become the umbilical cord, the vessels in the cord decrease to one large vein and two smaller arteries. About 1% of umbilical cords have only two vessels, an artery and a vein; this condition may be associated with congenital malformations primarily of the renal, gastrointestinal, and cardiovascular systems. A specialized connective tissue known as **Wharton's jelly** surrounds the blood vessels in the umbilical cord. This tissue, plus the high blood volume pulsating through the vessels, prevents compression of the umbilical cord in utero. At term (38 to 42 weeks' gestation), the average cord is 2 cm (0.8 in) across and about 55 cm (22 in) long. The cord can attach itself to the placenta in various sites. Central insertion into the placenta is considered normal. (See Chapter 19 for a discussion of the various attachment sites.)

Umbilical cords appear twisted or spiraled. This is most likely caused by fetal movement (Benirschke, 1999b). A true knot in the umbilical cord rarely occurs; if it does, the cord is usually long. More common are so-called false knots, caused by the folding of cord vessels. A nuchal cord is said to exist when the umbilical cord encircles the fetal neck.

## Development and Functions of the Placenta

The **placenta** is the means of metabolic and nutrient exchange between the embryonic and maternal circulations. Placental development and circulation do not begin until the third week of embryonic development. The placenta develops at the site where the embryo attaches to the uterine wall. Expansion of the placenta continues until about the 20th week, when it covers approximately one-half of the internal surface of the uterus. After 20 weeks' gestation, the placenta becomes thicker but not wider. At 40 weeks' gestation, the placenta is about 15 to 20 cm (5.9 to 7.9 in) in diameter and 2.5 to 3.0 cm (1.0 to 1.2 in) in thickness. At that time, it weighs about 400 to 600 g (14 to 21 oz).

The placenta has two parts: the maternal and fetal portions. The maternal portion consists of the decidua basalis and its circulation. Its surface is red and fleshlike. The fetal portion consists of the chorionic villi and their circulation. The fetal surface of the placenta is covered by the amnion, which gives it a shiny, gray appearance (Figures 3–8 and 3–9♦).

Development of the placenta begins with the chorionic villi. The trophoblastic cells of the chorionic villi form spaces in the tissue of the decidua basalis. These spaces fill with maternal blood, and the chorionic villi grow into them. As the chorionic villi differentiate, two trophoblastic layers appear: an outer layer, called the *syncytium* (consisting of syncytiotrophoblasts), and an inner layer, known as the *cytotrophoblast* (Figure 3–5♦). The cytotrophoblast thins out and disappears about the fifth month, leaving only a single layer of syncytium covering the chorionic villi. The syncytium is in direct contact with the maternal blood in the intervillous spaces. It is the functional layer of the placenta and secretes the placental hormones of pregnancy.

A third, inner layer of connective mesoderm develops in the chorionic villi, forming *anchoring villi.* These anchoring villi eventually form the septa (partitions) of the placenta. The septa divide the mature placenta into 15 to 20 segments called **cotyledons** (subdivisions of the

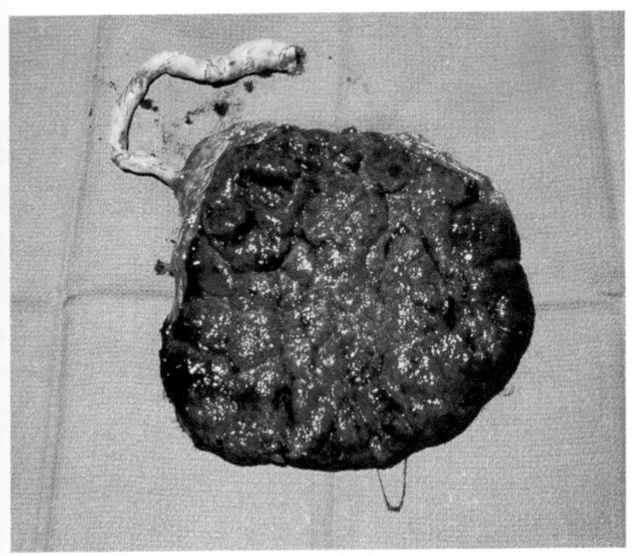

FIGURE 3–8 ♦ Maternal side of placenta.

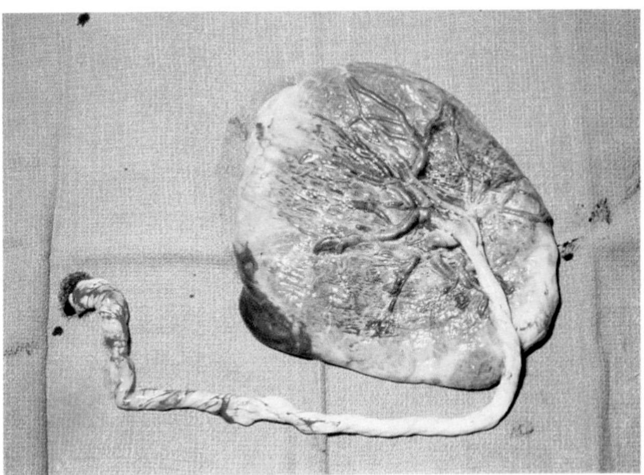

FIGURE 3–9 ♦ Fetal side of placenta.

placenta made up of anchoring villi and decidual tissue). In each cotyledon, the *branching villi* form a highly complex vascular system that allows compartmentalization of the utero placental circulation. The exchange of gases and nutrients takes place across these vascular systems.

Exchange of substances across the placenta is minimal during the first 3 to 5 months of development because of limited permeability. The villous membrane is initially too thick. As the villous membrane thins, placental permeability increases until about the last month of pregnancy, when permeability begins to decrease as the placenta ages.

In the fully developed placenta, fetal blood in the villi and maternal blood in the intervillous spaces are separated by three to four thin layers of tissue.

## Placental Circulation

After implantation of the blastocyst, the cells distinguish themselves into fetal cells and trophoblastic cells. The proliferating trophoblast successfully invades the decidua basalis of the endometrium, first opening the uterine capillaries and later opening the larger uterine vessels. The chorionic villi are an outgrowth of the blastocystic tissue. As these villi continue to grow and divide, the fetal vessels begin to form. The intervillous spaces in the decidua basalis develop as the endometrial spiral arteries are opened.

By the fourth week, the placenta has begun to function as a means of metabolic exchange between embryo and mother. The completion of the maternal-placental-fetal circulation occurs about 17 days after conception, when the embryonic heart begins functioning (Benirschke, 1999b). By 14 weeks, the placenta is a discrete organ. It has grown in thickness as a result of growth in the length and size of the chorionic villi and accompanying expansion of the intervillous space.

In the fully developed placenta's umbilical cord, fetal blood flows through the two umbilical arteries to the capillaries of the villi, becomes oxygen enriched, and then flows back through the umbilical vein into the fetus (Figure 3–10♦). Late in pregnancy, a soft blowing sound (*funic souffle*) can be heard over the area of the umbilical cord. The sound is synchronous with the fetal heartbeat and fetal blood flow through the umbilical arteries.

Maternal blood, rich in oxygen and nutrients, spurts from the spiral uterine arteries into the intervillous spaces. These spurts are produced by the maternal blood pressure. The blood is directed toward the chorionic plate, and as the spurt loses pressure, it becomes lateral (spreads out). Fresh blood enters continuously and exerts pressure on the contents of the intervillous spaces, pushing blood toward the exits in the basal plate. The blood then drains through the uterine and other pelvic veins. A *uterine souffle,* timed precisely with the mother's pulse, is also heard just above the mother's symphysis pubis during the last months of pregnancy. This souffle is caused by the augmented blood flow entering the dilated uterine arteries.

Braxton Hicks contractions (see Chapter 15) are believed to facilitate placental circulation by enhancing the movement of blood from the center of the cotyledon through the intervillous space. Placental blood flow is enhanced when the woman is lying on her left side because the vena cava is not compromised.

## Placental Functions

Placental exchange functions occur only in those fetal vessels that are in intimate contact with the covering syncytial membrane. The syncytium villi have brush borders containing many microvilli, which greatly increase the exchange rate between maternal and fetal circulation (Benirschke, 1999b).

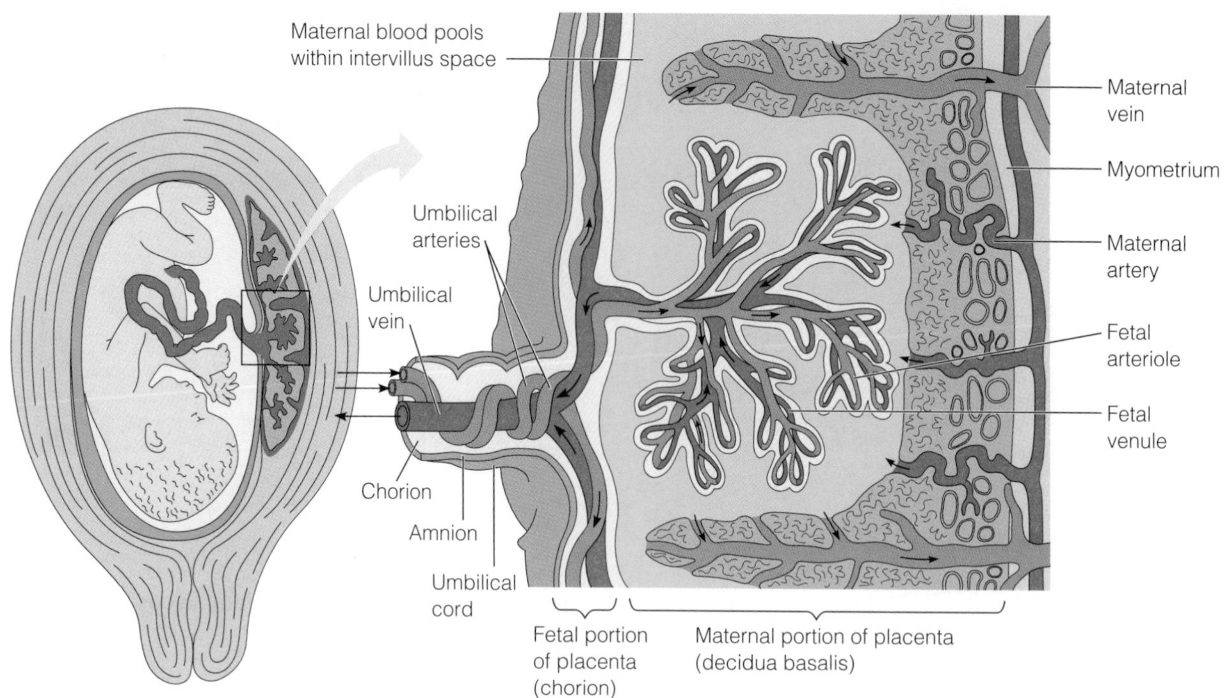


FIGURE 3–10 ♦ Vascular arrangement of the placenta. Arrows indicate the direction of blood flow. Maternal blood flows through the uterine arteries to the intervillous spaces of the placenta and returns through the uterine veins to maternal circulation. Fetal blood flows through the umbilical arteries into the villous capillaries of the placenta and returns through the umbilical vein to the fetal circulation.

The placental functions, many of which begin soon after implantation, include fetal respiration, nutrition, and excretion. To carry out these functions, the placenta is involved in metabolic and transfer activities. In addition, it has endocrine functions and special immunologic properties.

## Metabolic Activities

The placenta continuously produces glycogen, cholesterol, and fatty acids for fetal use and hormone production. The placenta also produces numerous enzymes required for fetoplacental transfer, breaks down certain substances such as epinephrine and histamine, and stores glycogen and iron.

## Transport Function

The placental membranes actively control the transfer of a wide range of substances by five major mechanisms:

1. *Simple diffusion* moves substances from an area of higher concentration to an area of lower concentration. Substances that move across the placenta by simple diffusion include water, oxygen, carbon dioxide, electrolytes (sodium and chloride), anesthetic gases, and drugs. Insulin and steroid hormones originating from the adrenals and thyroid hormones also cross the placenta, but at a very slow rate. The rate of oxygen transfer across the placental membrane is greater than that allowed by simple diffusion, indicating that oxygen is also transferred by some type of facilitated diffusion transport. Unfortunately many substances of abuse, such as cocaine, cross the placenta via simple diffusion.
2. *Facilitated transport* involves a carrier system to move molecules from an area of greater concentration to an area of lower concentration at a more rapid rate than by simple diffusion. Molecules such as glucose, galactose, and some oxygen are transported by this method. The glucose level in the fetal blood ordinarily is approximately 20% to 30% lower than the glucose level in the maternal blood, because the fetus is metabolizing glucose rapidly. This lower level, in turn, causes rapid transport of additional glucose from the maternal blood into the fetal blood.
3. *Active transport* can work against a concentration gradient and allows molecules to move from areas of lower concentration to areas of higher concentration. Amino acids, calcium, iron, iodine, water-soluble vitamins, and glucose are transferred across the placenta in this way (Ahokas & McKinney, 2000).
4. *Pinocytosis* is important for transferring large molecules such as albumin and gamma globulin. Materials are engulfed by ameba-like cells, forming plasma droplets.
5. *Hydrostatic* and *osmotic pressures* allow the bulk flow of water and some solutes.

Other modes of transfer also exist. For example, fetal red blood cells pass into the maternal circulation through breaks in the placental membrane, particularly during labor and birth. Certain cells, such as maternal leukocytes, and microorganisms, such as viruses (eg, the human immunodeficiency virus [HIV], which causes acquired immunodeficiency syndrome [AIDS]) and the bacterium *Treponema pallidum,* which causes syphilis, can also cross the placental membrane under their own power (Moore, Persaud, & Shiota, 2000). Some bacteria and protozoa infect the placenta by causing lesions and then entering the fetal blood system.

Reduction of the placental surface area, as with abruptio placentae (partial or complete premature separation of an abnormally implanted placenta), lessens the area that is functional for exchange. Placental diffusion distance also affects exchange. In conditions such as diabetes and placental infection, edema of the villi increases the diffusion distance, thus increasing the distance the substance has to be transferred. Blood flow alteration changes the transfer rate of substances. Decreased blood flow in the intervillous space is seen in labor and with certain maternal diseases such as hypertension. Mild fetal hypoxia increases the umbilical blood flow, but severe hypoxia results in decreased blood flow.

As the maternal blood picks up fetal waste products and carbon dioxide, it drains back into the maternal circulation through the veins in the basal plate. Fetal blood is hypoxic by comparison; it therefore attracts oxygen from the mother's blood. Affinity for oxygen increases as the fetal blood gives up its carbon dioxide, which also decreases its acidity.

### Endocrine Functions

The placenta produces hormones that are vital to the survival of the fetus. These include human chorionic gonadotropin (hCG); human placental lactogen (hPL); and two steroid hormones, estrogen and progesterone.

The hormone hCG is similar to luteinizing hormone (LH) and prevents the normal involution of the corpus luteum at the end of the menstrual cycle. If the corpus luteum stops functioning before the 11th week of pregnancy, spontaneous abortion occurs. The hCG also causes the corpus luteum to secrete increased amounts of estrogen and progesterone.

After the 11th week, the placenta produces enough progesterone and estrogen to maintain pregnancy. In the male fetus, hCG also exerts an interstitial cell-stimulating effect on the testes, resulting in the production of testosterone. This small secretion of testosterone during embryonic development is the factor that causes male sex organs to grow. Human chorionic gonadotropin may play a role in the trophoblast's immunologic capabilities (ability to exempt the placenta and embryo from rejection by the mother's system). Human chorionic gonadotropin is used as a basis for pregnancy tests (see Chapter 7).

Human chorionic gonadotropin is present in maternal blood serum as early as 10 days after fertilization, just as soon as implantation has occurred, and is detectable in maternal urine at the time of missed menses. It reaches its maximum level at 45 to 60 days' gestation and then begins to decrease as placental hormone production increases (Ahokas & McKinney, 2000).

*Progesterone* is a hormone essential for pregnancy. It increases the secretions of the fallopian tubes and uterus to provide appropriate nutritive matter for the developing morula and blastocyst. It also appears to aid in ovum transport through the fallopian tube (Ahokas & McKinney, 2000). Progesterone causes decidual cells to develop in the uterine endometrium, and it must be present in high levels for implantation to occur. Progesterone also decreases the contractility of the uterus, thus preventing uterine contractions from causing spontaneous abortion.

Prior to stimulation by hCG, the production of progesterone by the corpus luteum reaches a peak about 7 to 10 days after ovulation. Implantation occurs at about the same time as this peak. At 16 days after ovulation, progesterone reaches a level between 25 and 50 mg/day and continues to rise slowly in subsequent weeks (Cunningham et al., 1997). After 10 weeks, the placenta (specifically, the syncytiotrophoblast) takes over the production of progesterone and secretes it in tremendous quantities, reaching levels of more than 250 mg/day late in pregnancy.

By 7 weeks, the placenta produces more than 50% of the estrogens in the maternal circulation. *Estrogens* serve mainly a proliferative function, causing enlargement of the uterus, breasts, and breast glandular tissue. Estrogens also have a significant role in increasing vascularity and vasodilation, particularly in the villous capillaries toward the end of pregnancy. Placental estrogens increase markedly toward the end of pregnancy, to as much as 30 times the daily production in the middle of a normal monthly menstrual cycle. The primary estrogen secreted by the placenta is different from that secreted by the ovaries. The placenta secretes mainly *estriol,* whereas the ovaries secrete primarily *estradiol.* The placenta cannot synthesize estriol by itself. Essential precursors are provided by the fetal adrenal glands and are transported to the placenta for the final conversion to estriol.

The hormone *human placental lactogen (hPL),* also referred to as human chorionic somatomammotropin (hCS), is similar to human pituitary growth hormone; hPL stimulates certain changes in the mother's metabolic processes. These changes ensure that more protein, glucose, and minerals are available for the fetus. Secretion of hPL can be detected by about 4 weeks after conception.

### Immunologic Properties

The placenta and embryo are transplants of living tissue within the same species and are therefore considered *homografts.* Unlike other homografts, the placenta and embryo appear exempt from immunologic reaction by the host. Most recent data suggest that there is a suppression of cellular immunity by the placental hormones (progesterone and hCG) during pregnancy. One theory suggests that trophoblastic tissue is immunologically inert. It may contain a cell coating that masks transplantation antigens, repels sensitized lymphocytes, and protects against antibody formation.

## Fetal Circulatory System

The circulatory system of the fetus has several unique features that, by maintaining the blood flow to the placenta, provide the fetus with oxygen and nutrients while removing carbon dioxide and other waste products.

Most of the blood supply bypasses the fetal lungs, since they do not carry out respiratory gas exchange. The placenta assumes the function of the fetal lungs by supplying oxygen and allowing the fetus to excrete carbon dioxide into the maternal bloodstream. Figure 3–11♦ shows the fetal circulatory system. The blood from the placenta flows through the umbilical vein, which enters the abdominal wall of the fetus at the site that, after birth, is the umbilicus (belly button). It divides into two branches, one of which circulates a small amount of blood through the fetal liver and empties into the inferior vena cava through the hepatic vein. The second and larger branch, called the **ductus venosus,** empties directly into the fetal vena cava. This blood then enters the right atrium, passes through the **foramen ovale** into the left atrium, and pours into the left ventricle, which pumps it into the aorta. Some blood returning from the head and upper extremities by way of the superior vena cava is emptied into the right atrium and passes through the tricuspid valve into the right ventricle. This blood is pumped into the pulmonary artery, and a small amount passes to the lungs for nourishment only. The larger portion of blood passes from the pulmonary artery through the **ductus arteriosus** into the descending aorta, bypassing the lungs. Finally, blood returns to the placenta through the two umbilical arteries, and the process is repeated.

The fetus obtains oxygen via diffusion from the maternal circulation because of the gradient difference of $PO_2$ of 50 mm Hg in maternal blood in the placenta to 30 mm Hg $PO_2$ in the fetus. At term the fetus receives oxygen from the mother's circulation at a rate of 20 to 30 mL per minute (Sadler, 1995). Fetal hemoglobin facilitates obtaining oxygen from the maternal circulation, because it carries as much as 20% to 30% more oxygen than adult hemoglobin. For further discussion, see Chapter 21.

Fetal circulation delivers the highest available oxygen concentration to the head, neck, brain, and heart (coronary circulation) and a lesser amount of oxygenated blood to the abdominal organs and the lower body. This circulatory pattern leads to cephalocaudal (head-to-tail) development in the fetus.

# Embryonic and Fetal Development

Pregnancy is calculated to last an average of 10 lunar months: 40 weeks, or 280 days. This period of 280 days is calculated from the onset of the last normal menstrual period to the time of birth. Estimated date of birth (EDB) is usually calculated by this method. The postfertilization age, or postconception age, of the fetus is calculated to be *about* 2 weeks less, or 266 days (38 weeks) after fertilization. This latter measurement is more accurate because it measures time from the fertilization of the ovum, or conception. The basic events of organ development in the embryo and fetus are outlined in Table 3–2. The time periods in the table are postfertilization or **postconception age periods.** For detailed discussion of the development of each body system, see Chapter 21.

Human development follows three stages. The preembryonic stage, as we have seen, consists of the first 14 days of development after the ovum is fertilized; the embryonic stage covers the period from day 15 until approximately the end of the eighth week, and the fetal stage extends from the end of the eighth week until birth.

## Embryonic Stage

The stage of the **embryo** starts on day 15 (the beginning of the third week after conception) and continues until approximately the eighth week, or until the embryo reaches a *crown-to-rump* (*C–R*) length of 3 cm (1.2 in). This length is usually reached about 56 days after fertilization (the end of the eighth gestational week). During the embryonic stage, tissues differentiate into essential organs and the main external features develop (See Figure 3–12♦, on page 54). The embryo is the most vulnerable to teratogens during this period.

### Third Week

In the third week, the embryonic disk becomes elongated and pear shaped, with a broad cephalic end and a narrow caudal end. The ectoderm has formed a long cylindrical tube for brain and spinal cord development. The gastrointestinal tract, created from the endoderm, appears as another tubelike structure communicating

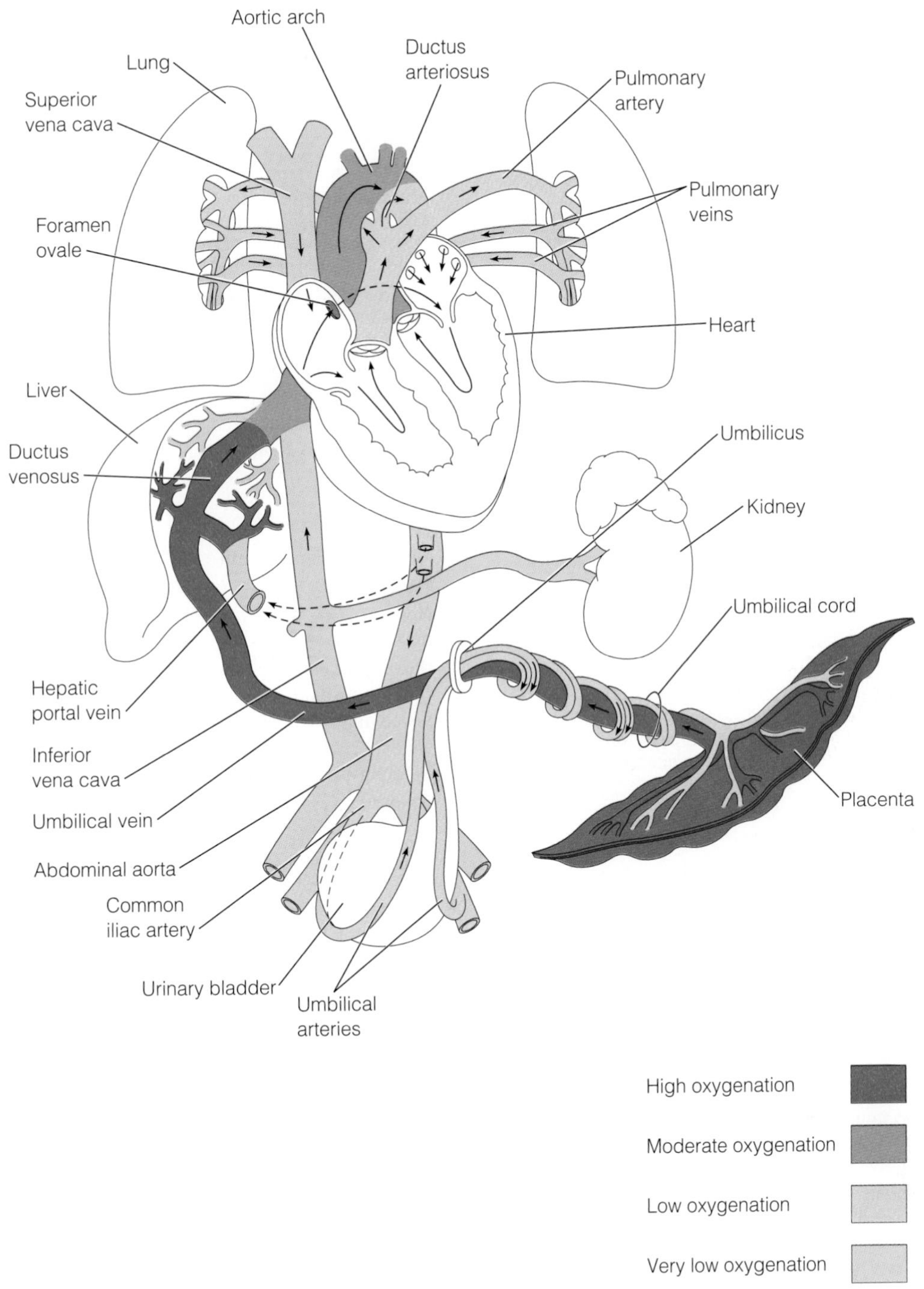


**FIGURE 3–11** ♦ Fetal circulation. Blood leaves the placenta and enters the fetus through the umbilical vein. After circulating through the fetus, the blood returns to the placenta through the umbilical arteries. The ductus venosus, the foramen ovale, and the ductus arteriosus allow the blood to bypass the fetal liver and lungs.

with the yolk sac. The most advanced organ is the heart. At 3 weeks, a single tubular heart forms just outside the body cavity of the embryo.

### Fourth to Fifth Week

During days 21 to 32, *somites* (a series of mesodermal blocks) form on either side of the embryo's midline. The vertebrae that form the spinal column will develop from these somites. Prior to 28 days, arm and leg buds are not visible, but the tail bud is present. The pharyngeal arches—which will form the lower jaw, hyoid bone, and larynx—develop at this time. The pharyngeal pouches appear now; these pouches will form the eustachian tube and cavity of the middle ear, the tonsils, and the parathyroid and thymus glands. The primordia of the ear and eye are also present. By the end of 28 days, the tubular heart

## TABLE 3–2 Summary of Organ System Development

### AGE: 2–3 WEEKS

**Length:** 2 mm C–R (crown to rump)

**Nervous system:** Groove forms along middle back as cells thicken; neural tube forms from closure to neural groove.

**Cardiovascular system:** Beginning of blood circulation; tubular heart begins to form during third week.

**Gastrointestinal system:** Liver begins to function.

**Genitourinary system:** Formation of kidneys beginning.

**Respiratory system:** Nasal pits forming.

**Endocrine system:** Thyroid tissue appears.

**Eyes:** Optic cup and lens pit have formed; pigment in eyes.

**Ear:** Auditory pit is now enclosed structure.

### AGE: 4 WEEKS

**Length:** 4–6 mm C–R

**Weight:** 0.4 g

**Nervous system:** Anterior portion of neural tube closes to form brain; closure of posterior end forms spinal cord.

**Musculoskeletal system:** Noticeable limb buds.

**Cardiovascular system:** Tubular heart beats at 28 days, and primitive red blood cells circulate through fetus and chorionic villi.

**Gastrointestinal system:** Mouth: formation of oral cavity; primitive jaws present; esophagotracheal septum begins division of esophagus and trachea. Digestive tract: stomach forms; esophagus and intestine become tubular; ducts of pancreas and liver forming.

### AGE: 5 WEEKS

**Length:** 8 mm C–R

**Weight:** Only 0.5% of total body weight is fat (to 20 weeks).

**Nervous system:** Brain has differentiated and cranial nerves are present.

**Musculoskeletal system:** Developing muscles have innervation.

**Cardiovascular system:** Atrial division has occurred.

### AGE: 6 WEEKS

**Length:** 12 mm C–R

**Musculoskeletal system:** Bone rudiments present; primitive skeletal shape forming; muscle mass begins to develop; ossification of skull and jaws begins.

**Cardiovascular system:** Chambers present in heart; groups of blood cells can be identified.

**Gastrointestinal system:** Oral and nasal cavities and upper lip formed; liver begins to form red blood cells.

**Respiratory system:** Trachea, bronchi, and lung buds present.

**Ear:** Formation of external, middle, and inner ear continues.

**Sexual development:** Embryonic sex glands appear.

### AGE: 7 WEEKS

**Length:** 18 mm C–R

**Cardiovascular system:** Fetal heartbeats can be detected.

**Gastrointestinal system:** Mouth: tongue separates; palate folds. Digestive tract: stomach attains final form.

**Genitourinary system:** Separation of bladder and urethra from rectum.

**Respiratory system:** Diaphragm separates abdominal and thoracic cavities.

**Eyes:** Optic nerve formed; eyelids appear, thickening of lens.

**Sexual development:** Differentiation of sex glands into ovaries and testes begins.

### AGE: 8 WEEKS

**Length:** 2.5–3 cm C–R

**Weight:** 2 g

**Musculoskeletal system:** Digits formed; further differentiation of cells in primitive skeleton; cartilaginous bones show first signs of ossification; development of muscles in trunk, limbs, and head; some movement of fetus now possible.

**Cardiovascular system:** Development of heart essentially complete; fetal circulation follows two circuits—four extraembryonic and two intraembryonic.

**Gastrointestinal system:** Mouth: completion of lip fusion. Digestive tract: rotation in midgut; anal membrane has perforated.

**Ear:** External, middle, and inner ear assuming final forms.

**Sexual development:** Male and female external genitals appear similar until end of ninth week.

### AGE: 10 WEEKS

**Length:** 5–6 cm C–H (crown to heel)

**Weight:** 14 g

**Nervous system:** Neurons appear at caudal end of spinal cord; basic divisions of brain present.

**Musculoskeletal system:** Fingers and toes begin nail growth.

**Gastrointestinal system:** Mouth: separation of lips from jaw; fusion of palate folds. Digestive tract: developing intestines enclosed in abdomen.

**Genitourinary system:** Bladder sac formed.

**Endocrine system:** Islets of Langerhans differentiated.

**Eyes:** Eyelids fused closed; development of lacrimal duct.

**Sexual development:** Males: production of testosterone and physical characteristics between 8 and 12 weeks.

### AGE: 12 WEEKS

**Length:** 8 cm C–R; 11.5 cm C–H

**Weight:** 45 g

**Musculoskeletal system:** Clear outlining of miniature bones (12–20 weeks); process of ossification is established throughout fetal body; appearance of involuntary muscles in viscera.

**Gastrointestinal system:** Mouth: completion of palate. Digestive tract: appearance of muscles in gut; bile secretion begins; liver is major producer of red blood cells.

**Respiratory system:** Lungs acquire definitive shape.

**Skin:** Pink and delicate.

**Endocrine system:** Hormonal secretion from thyroid; insulin present in pancreas.

**Immunologic system:** Appearance of lymphoid tissue in fetal thymus gland.

### AGE: 16 WEEKS

**Length:** 13.5 cm C–R; 15 cm C–H

**Weight:** 200 g

**Musculoskeletal system:** Teeth beginning to form hard tissue that will become central incisors.

**Gastrointestinal system:** Mouth: differentiation of hard and soft palate. Digestive tract: development of gastric and intestinal glands; intestines begin to collect meconium.

**Genitourinary system:** Kidneys assume typical shape and organization.

**Skin:** Appearance of scalp hair; lanugo present on body; transparent skin with visible blood vessels; sweat glands developing.

**Eye, ear, and nose:** Formed.

**Sexual development:** Sex determination possible.

## TABLE 3–2 Summary of Organ System Development *continued*

### AGE: 18 WEEKS

**Musculoskeletal system:** Teeth beginning to form hard tissue (enamel and dentine) that will become lateral incisors.

**Cardiovascular system:** Fetal heart tones audible with fetoscope at 16–20 weeks.

### AGE: 20 WEEKS

**Length:** 19 cm C–R; 25 cm C– H

**Weight:** 435 g (6% of total body weight is fat)

**Nervous system:** Myelination of spinal cord begins.

**Musculoskeletal system:** Teeth beginning to form hard tissue that will become canine and first molar. Lower limbs are of final relative proportions.

**Gastrointestinal system:** Fetus actively sucks and swallows amniotic fluid; peristaltic movements begin.

**Skin:** Lanugo covers entire body; brown fat begins to form; vernix caseosa begins to form.

**Immunologic system:** Detectable levels of fetal antibodies (IgG type).

**Blood formation:** Iron is stored and bone marrow is increasingly important.

### AGE: 24 WEEKS

**Length:** 23 cm C–R; 28 cm C–H

**Weight:** 780 g

**Nervous system:** Brain looks like mature brain.

**Musculoskeletal system:** Teeth are beginning to form hard tissue that will become the second molars.

**Respiratory system:** Respiratory movements may occur (24–40 weeks). Nostrils reopen. Alveoli appear in lungs and begin production of surfactant; gas exchange possible.

**Skin:** Reddish and wrinkled, vernix caseosa present.

**Immunologic system:** IgG levels reach maternal levels.

**Eyes:** Structurally complete.

### AGE: 28 WEEKS

**Length:** 27 cm C–R; 35 C–H

**Weight:** 1200–1250 g

**Nervous system:** Begins regulation of some body functions.

**Skin:** Adipose tissue accumulates rapidly; nails appear; eyebrows and eyelashes present.

**Eyes:** Eyelids open (28–32 weeks).

**Sexual development:** Males: testes descend into inguinal canal and upper scrotum.

### AGE: 32 WEEKS

**Length:** 31 cm C–R; 38–43 cm C–H

**Weight:** 2000 g

**Nervous system:** More reflexes present.

### AGE: 36 WEEKS

**Length:** 35 cm C–R; 42–48 cm C–H

**Weight:** 2500–2750 g

**Musculoskeletal system:** Distal femoral ossification centers present.

**Skin:** Pale; body rounded, lanugo disappearing, hair fuzzy or woolly; few sole creases; sebaceous glands active and helping to produce vernix caseosa (36–40 weeks).

**Ears:** Earlobes soft with little cartilage.

**Sexual development:** Males; scrotum small and few rugae present; descent of testes into upper scrotum to stay (36–40 weeks). Females: labia majora and minora equally prominent.

### AGE: 38–40 WEEKS

**Length:** 40 cm C–R; 48–52 C–H

**Weight:** 3200+ g (16% of total body weight is fat)

**Respiratory system:** At 38 weeks, lecithin-sphingomyelin (L/S) ratio approaches 2:1 (indicates decreased risk of respiratory distress from inadequate surfactant production if born now).

**Skin:** Smooth and pink; vernix present in skin folds; moderate to profuse silky hair; lanugo on shoulders and upper back; nails extend over tips or digits; creases cover sole.

**Ears:** Earlobes firmer due to increased cartilage.

**Sexual development:** Males: rugous scrotum. Females: labia majora well developed and minora small or completely covered.

*Note:* Age refers to postfertilization or postconception age.

*Sources:* Sadler, T. W. (1995). *Langman's medical embryology* (7th ed). Baltimore: Williams & Wilkins; and Moore, K. L. & Persaud, T. V. N. (1998). *The developing human: Clinically oriented embryology* (6th ed). Philadelphia: Saunders.

is beating at a regular rhythm and pushing its own primitive blood cells through the main blood vessels.

During the fifth week, the optic cups and lens vessels of the eye form and the nasal pits develop. Partitioning in the heart occurs with the dividing of the atrium. The embryo has a marked C-shaped body, accentuated by the rudimentary tail and the large head folded over a protuberant trunk (Figure 3–13♦). By day 35, the arm and leg buds are well developed, with paddle-shaped hand and foot plates. The heart, circulatory system, and brain show the most advanced development. The brain has differentiated into five areas, and 10 pairs of cranial nerves are recognizable.

### Sixth to Seventh Week

At 6 weeks the head structures are more highly developed and the trunk is straighter than in earlier stages. The upper and lower jaws are recognizable, and the external nares are well formed. The trachea has developed, and its caudal end is bifurcated for beginning lung formation. The upper lip has formed, and the palate is developing. The ears are developing rapidly. The arms have begun to extend ventrally across the chest, and both arms and legs have digits, although they may still be webbed. There is a slight elbow bend in the arms, which are more advanced in development than the legs. Beginning at this stage, the

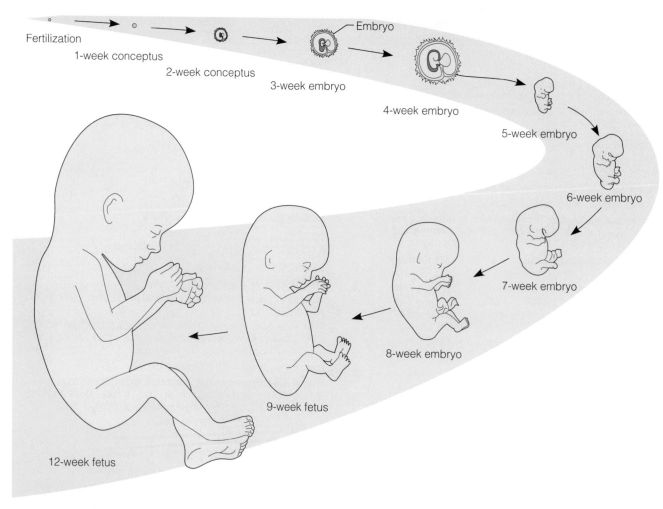

Fertilization
1-week conceptus
2-week conceptus
Embryo
3-week embryo
4-week embryo
5-week embryo
6-week embryo
7-week embryo
8-week embryo
9-week fetus
12-week fetus

FIGURE 3–12 ♦ The actual size of a human conceptus from fertilization to the early fetal stage. The embryonic stage begins in the third week after fertilization; the fetal stage begins in the ninth week. Source: Adapted from Marieb, E. N. (1998). *Human anatomy and physiology* (4th ed., p. 1079). Redwood City, CA: Benjamin/Cummings.

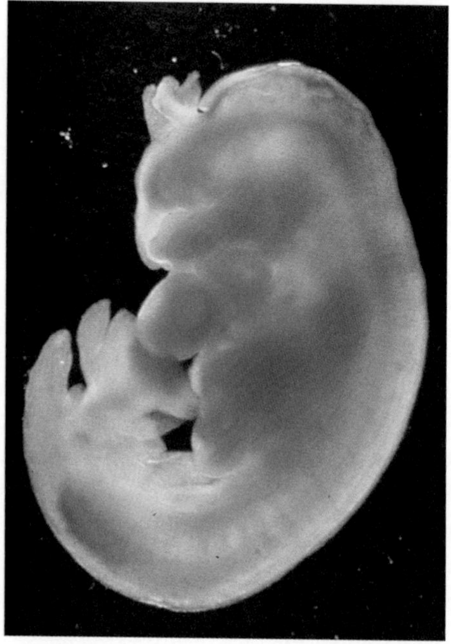

FIGURE 3–13 ♦ The embryo at 5 weeks. The embryo has a marked C-shaped body and a rudimentary tail.

prominent tail will recede. The heart now has most of its definitive characteristics, and fetal circulation begins to be established. The liver starts to produce blood cells. At 7 weeks the head of the embryo is rounded and nearly erect (Figure 3–14♦). The eyes have shifted and are closer together, and the eyelids are beginning to form. Prior to this time the rectal and urogenital passages formed one tube that ended in a blind pouch; they now separate into two tubular structures. The intestines enter the extraembryonic coelom in the area of the umbilical cord (called umbilical herniation) (Moore, Persaud, & Shiota, 2000). At this point the beginnings of all essential external and internal structures are present.

### Eighth Week

At 8 weeks the embryo is approximately 3 cm (1.2 in) long C–R and clearly resembles a human being. Facial features continue to develop. The eyelids begin to fuse. Auricles of the external ears begin to assume their final shape, but they are still set low (Moore, Persaud, &

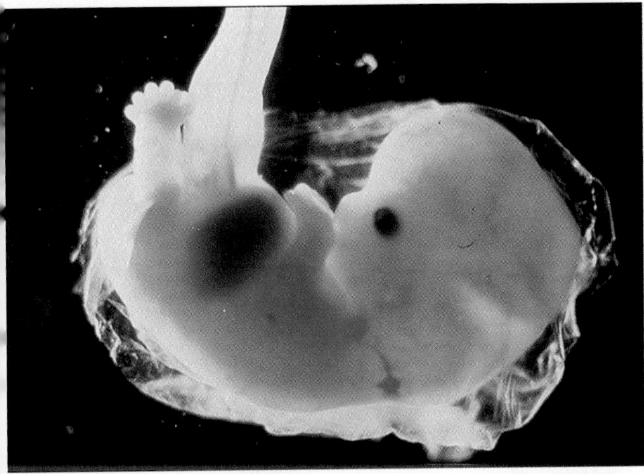

FIGURE 3–14 ♦ The embryo at 7 weeks. The head is rounded and nearly erect. The eyes have shifted forward and closer together, and the eyelids begin to form.

Shiota, 2000). External genitals appear, but the embryo's sex is not clearly discernible, and the rectal passage opens with the perforation of the anal membrane. The circulatory system through the umbilical cord is well established. Long bones are beginning to form, and the large muscles are now capable of contracting.

## Fetal Stage

By the end of the eighth week, the embryo is sufficiently developed to be called a **fetus.** Every organ system and external structure that will be found in the full-term newborn is present. The remainder of gestation is devoted to refining structures and perfecting function.

### Ninth to Twelfth Week

By the end of the ninth week the fetus reaches a C–R length of 5 cm (2 in) and weighs about 14 g. The head is large and comprises almost half of the fetus's entire size (Figure 3–15♦). At 12 weeks, the fetus reaches 8 cm (3.2 in) C–R and weighs about 45 g (1.6 oz). The face is well formed, with the nose protruding, the chin small and receding, and the ear acquiring a more adult shape. The eyelids close at about the 10th week and will not reopen until about the 28th week. Some reflex movement of the lips suggestive of the sucking reflex has been observed at 3 months. Tooth buds now appear for all 20 of the child's first teeth (baby teeth). The limbs are long and slender, with well-formed digits. The fetus can curl the fingers toward the palm and begins to make a tiny fist. The legs are still shorter and less developed than the arms. The urogenital tract completes its development, well-differentiated genitals appear, and the kidneys begin to produce urine. Red blood cells are produced primarily by the liver. Fetal heart rates can be ascertained by electronic devices between 8 and 12 weeks. The rate is 120 to 160 beats per minute.

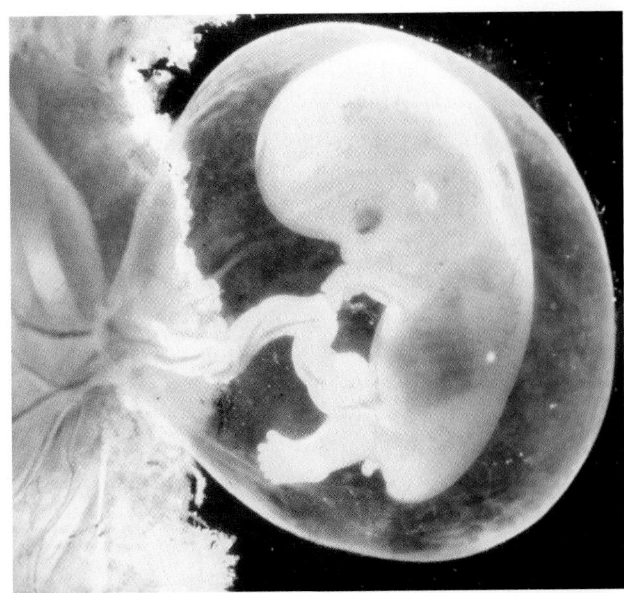

FIGURE 3–15 ♦ The fetus at 9 weeks. Every organ system and external structure is present. *Source:* Nilsson, L. (1990). *A child is born.* New York: Dell Publishing.

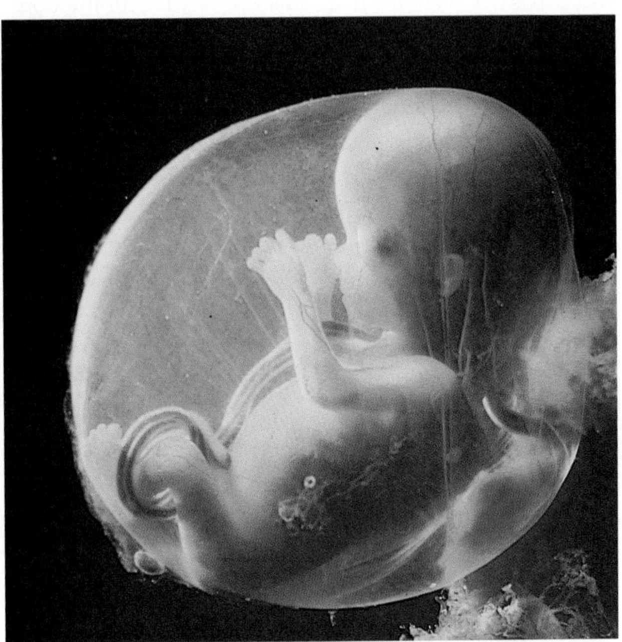

FIGURE 3–16 ♦ The fetus at 14 weeks. During this period of rapid growth the skin is so transparent that blood vessels are visible beneath it. More muscle tissue and body skeleton have developed, and they hold the fetus more erect. *Source:* Nilsson, L. (1990). *A child is born.* New York: Dell Publishing.

Between 13 and 16 weeks is a period of rapid growth. **Lanugo,** or fine hair, begins to develop, especially on the head. The skin is so transparent that blood vessels are clearly visible beneath it. More muscle tissue and body skeleton have developed and hold the fetus more erect (Figure 3–16♦). Active movements are present; the fetus stretches and exercises its arms and legs. It makes sucking motions, swallows amniotic fluid, and produces meconium in the intestinal tract.

### Twentieth Week

The fetus doubles its C–R length and now measures 19 cm (8 in) long. Fetal weight is between 435 and 465 g (15.2 and 16.3 oz). Lanugo covers the entire body and is especially prominent on the shoulders. Subcutaneous deposits of brown fat, which has a rich blood supply, make the skin less transparent. Nipples now appear over the mammary glands. The head is covered with fine, woolly hair, and the eyebrows and eyelashes are beginning to form. Nails are present on both fingers and toes. Muscles are well developed, and the fetus is active (Figure 3–17♦). The mother feels fetal movement, known as quickening. The fetal heartbeat is audible through a fetoscope. Quickening and fetal heartbeat can help in validating the estimated date of birth.

### Twenty-Fourth Week

The fetus at 24 weeks reaches a crown-to-heel (C–H) length of 28 cm (11.2 in). It weighs about 780 g (1 lb, 10 oz). The hair on the head is growing long, and eyebrows and eyelashes have formed. The eye is structurally complete and will soon open. The fetus has a reflex hand grip (grasp reflex) and, by the end of 6 months, a startle reflex. Skin covering the body is reddish and wrinkled, with little subcutaneous fat. Skin on the hands and feet has thickened, with skin ridges on palms and soles forming distinct foot- and fingerprints. The skin over the entire body is covered with **vernix caseosa,** a protective cheeselike, fatty substance secreted by the sebaceous glands. The alveoli in the lungs are just beginning to form.

### Twenty-Fifth to Twenty-Eighth Week

At 6 months the fetal skin is still red, wrinkled, and covered with vernix caseosa. During this time the brain is developing rapidly, and the nervous system is complete enough to provide some degree of regulation of body functions. The eyelids open and close under neural control. In the male fetus, the testes begin to descend into the scrotal sac. Respiratory and circulatory systems have developed; even though the lungs are still physiologically immature, they are sufficiently developed to provide gas exchange. A fetus born at this time will require immediate and prolonged intensive care to survive and then to decrease the risk of major handicap. The fetus at 28 weeks is about 35 to 38 cm (14 to 15 in) long C–H and weighs 1200 to 1250 g (2 lb, 10.5 oz to 2 lb, 12 oz).

### Twenty-Ninth to Thirty-Second Week

At 30 weeks the pupillary light reflex is present (Moore, Persaud, & Shiota, 2000). The fetus is gaining weight from an increase in body muscle and fat and weighs about 2000 g (4 lb, 6.5 oz), with a C–H length of about 38 to 43 cm (15 to 17 in), by 32 weeks of age. The central nervous system (CNS) has matured enough to direct

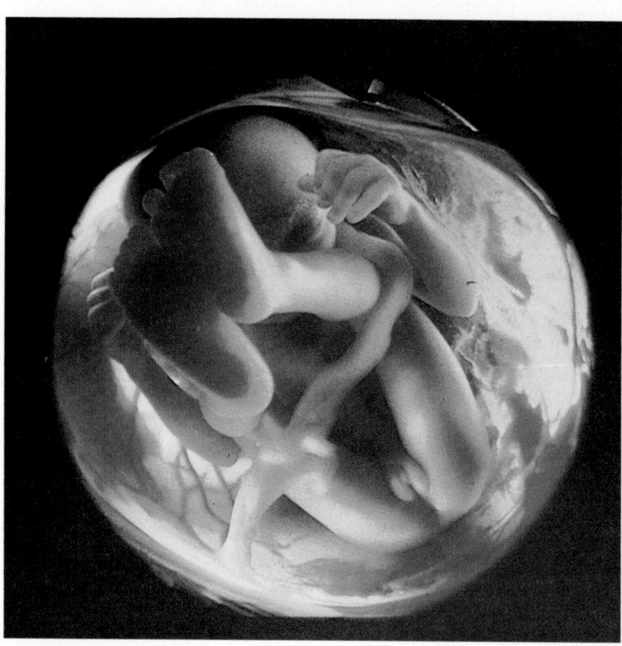

FIGURE 3–17 ♦ The fetus at 20 weeks. The fetus now weighs 435 to 465 g and measures about 19 cm. Subcutaneous deposits of brown fat make the skin a little less transparent. "Woolly" hair covers the head, and nails have developed on the fingers and toes. *Source:* Nilsson, L. (1990). *A child is born.* New York: Dell Publishing.

rhythmic breathing movements and partially control body temperature. However, the lungs are not yet fully mature. Bones are fully developed but soft and flexible. The fetus begins storing iron, calcium, and phosphorus. In males the testicles may be located in the scrotal sac but are often still high in the inguinal canals.

### Thirty-Sixth Week

The fetus begins to get plump, and less wrinkled skin covers the deposits of subcutaneous fat. Lanugo begins to disappear, and the nails reach the edge of the fingertips. By 35 weeks of age the fetus has a firm grasp and exhibits spontaneous orientation to light. By 36 weeks of age the weight is usually 2500 to 2750 g (5 lb, 12 oz to 6 lb, 11.5 oz), and the C–H length of the fetus is about 42 to 48 cm (16 to 19 in). An infant born at this time has a good chance of surviving but may require some special care, especially if there is intrauterine growth retardation.

### Thirty-Eighth to Fortieth Week

The fetus is considered full term 38 weeks after conception. The C–H length varies from 48 to 52 cm (19 to 21 in), with males usually longer than females. Generally males also weigh more than females. The weight at term is about 3000 to 3600 g (6 lb, 10 oz to 7 lb, 15 oz). The skin is pink and has a smooth, polished look. The only lanugo left is on the upper arms and shoulders. The hair on the head is no longer woolly but is coarse and about 1 in long. Vernix caseosa is present, with heavier deposits remaining in the creases and folds of the skin. The body and extremities are plump, with good skin turgor, and the fingernails extend beyond the fingertips. The chest is prominent but still a little smaller than the head, and mammary glands protrude in both sexes. The testes are in the scrotum or palpable in the inguinal canals.

As the fetus enlarges, amniotic fluid diminishes to about 500 mL or less, and the fetal body mass fills the uterine cavity. The fetus assumes what is called its position of comfort, or lie. The head is generally pointed downward, following the shape of the uterus (and possibly because the head is heavier than the feet). The extremities, and often the head, are well flexed. After 5 months, feeding patterns, sleeping patterns, and activity patterns become established, so at term the fetus has its own body rhythms and individual style of response.

Key Facts to Remember (Fetal Development: What Parents Want to Know), lists some important developmental milestones.

## Factors Influencing Embryonic and Fetal Development

Factors that may affect embryonic development include the quality of the sperm or ovum from which the zygote was formed, the genetic code established at fertilization, and the adequacy of the intrauterine environment. If the environment is unsuitable before cellular differentiation occurs, all the cells of the zygote are affected. The cells may die, which causes spontaneous abortion, or growth may be slowed, depending on the severity of the situation. When differentiation is complete and the fetal membranes have formed, an injurious agent has the greatest effect on those cells undergoing the most rapid growth. Thus the time of injury is critical in the development of anomalies.

Because organs are formed primarily during embryonic development, the growing organism is considered most vulnerable to noxious agents during the first months of pregnancy; therefore it is important to know the gestational age of the embryo or fetus to determine the potential effects of teratogens. Any agent, such as a drug, virus, or radiation, that can cause development of abnormal structures in an embryo is called a *teratogen.* Chapter 7 discusses the effects of specific teratogenic agents on the developing fetus.

Adequacy of the maternal environment is also important during the periods of rapid embryonic and fetal development. Maternal nutrition can affect brain development. The period of maximum brain growth and myelination begins with the fifth lunar month before birth and continues during the first 6 months after birth, when there is a twofold increase in myelination. From 6 months to 2 years of age there is about a 50% further increase in myelination (Volpe, 2000). Amino acids, glucose, and fatty acids are considered to be the primary dietary factors in brain growth. A subtle type of damage that affects the associative capacity of the brain, possibly leading to learning disabilities, may be caused by nutritional deficiency at this stage. Maternal nutrition may also predispose offspring to the development of adult coronary heart disease, hypertension, and diabetes in babies who were small or disproportionate at birth. (Maternal nutrition is discussed in depth in Chapter 11.)

Another prenatal influence on the intrauterine environment is maternal hyperthermia associated with sauna or hot tub use. Studies of the effects of maternal hyperthermia during the first trimester have raised concern about possible CNS defects and failure of neural tube closure. Maternal substance abuse also affects the intrauterine environment and is discussed in Chapters 12 and 13.

### KEY FACTS TO REMEMBER

*Fetal Development: What Parents Want to Know*

| | |
|---|---|
| 4 weeks: | The fetal heart begins to beat. |
| 8 weeks: | All body organs are formed. |
| 8–12 weeks: | Fetal heart rate can be heard by ultrasound Doppler device. |
| 16 weeks: | Baby's sex can be seen.<br>Although thin, the fetus looks like a baby. |
| 20 weeks: | Heartbeat can be heard with fetoscope.<br>Mother feels movement (quickening).<br>Baby develops a regular schedule of sleeping, sucking, and kicking.<br>Hands can grasp.<br>Baby assumes a favorite position in utero.<br>Vernix (lanolin-like covering) protects the body, and lanugo (fine hair) keeps oil on skin.<br>Head hair, eyebrows, and eyelashes present. |
| 24 weeks: | Weighs 1 lb, 10 oz.<br>Activity is increasing.<br>Fetal respiratory movements begin. |
| 28 weeks: | Eyes begin to open and close.<br>Baby can breathe at this time.<br>Surfactant needed for breathing at birth is formed.<br>Baby is two-thirds its final size. |
| 32 weeks: | Baby has fingernails and toenails.<br>Subcutaneous fat is being laid down.<br>Baby appears less red and wrinkled. |
| 38–40 weeks: | Baby fills total uterus.<br>Baby gets antibodies from mother. |

# Chapter Review

## CHAPTER HIGHLIGHTS

- Humans have 46 chromosomes, which are divided into 23 pairs—22 pairs of autosomes and 1 pair of sex chromosomes.
- Mitosis is the process by which additional somatic (body) cells are formed. It provides growth and development of the organisms and replacement of body cells.
- Meiosis is the process by which new organisms are formed. It occurs during gametogenesis (oogenesis and spermatogenesis) and consists of two successive cell divisions (reduction division), which produce a gamete with 23 chromosomes (22 autosomal chromosomes and 1 sex chromosome), the haploid number of chromosomes.
- Gametes must have a haploid number of chromosomes (23) so that when the female gamete (ovum) and the male gamete (spermatozoon) unite (fertilization) to form the zygote, the normal human diploid number of chromosomes (46) is reestablished.
- An ovum is considered fertile for about 24 hours after ovulation, and the sperm is capable of fertilizing the ovum for only about 24 hours after it is deposited in the female reproductive tract.
- Fertilization usually takes place in the ampulla (outer third) of the fallopian tube.
- Both capacitation and acrosomal reaction must occur for the sperm to fertilize the ovum. Capacitation is the removal of the plasma membrane, which exposes the acrosomal covering of the sperm head. Acrosomal reaction is the deposit of hyaluronidase in the corona radiata, which allows the sperm head to penetrate the ovum.
- Sex chromosomes are referred to as X and Y. Females have two X chromosomes, and males have an X and a Y chromosome. Y chromosomes are carried only by the sperm. To produce a male child, the mother contributes an X chromosome and the father contributes a Y chromosome.
- Twins are either monozygotic (identical) or dizygotic (fraternal). Dizygotic twins arise from two separate ova fertilized by two separate spermatozoa. Monozygotic twins develop from a single ovum fertilized by a single spermatozoon.
- Preembryonic development first proceeds via cellular multiplication in which the zygote undergoes rapid mitotic division called cleavage. As a result of cleavage, the zygote divides and multiplies into cell groupings called blastomeres, which are held together by the zona pellucida. The blastomeres eventually become a solid ball of cells called the morula. When a cavity forms in the morula cell mass, the inner solid cell mass is called the blastocyst.
- Implantation usually occurs in the upper part of the posterior uterine wall when the blastocyst burrows into the uterine lining.
- After implantation, the endometrium is called the decidua. Decidua capsularis is the portion that covers the blastocyst. Decidua basalis is the portion that is directly under the blastocyst. Decidua vera is the portion that lines the rest of the uterine cavity.
- Primary germ layers will give rise to all tissues, organs, and organ systems. The three primary germ cell layers are ectoderm, endoderm, and mesoderm.
- Embryonic membranes are called the amnion and the chorion. The amnion is formed from the ectoderm and is a thin protective membrane that contains the amniotic fluid and the embryo. The chorion is a thick membrane that develops from the trophoblast and encloses the amnion, embryo, and yolk sac.
- Amniotic fluid cushions the fetus against mechanical injury, controls the embryo's temperature, allows symmetrical external growth, prevents adherence to the amnion, and permits freedom of movement.

- The umbilical cord contains two umbilical arteries, which carry deoxygenated blood from the fetus to the placenta, and one umbilical vein, which carries oxygenated blood from the placenta to the fetus. The umbilical cord normally has a central insertion into the placenta. Wharton's jelly, a specialized connective tissue, helps prevent compression of the umbilical cord in utero.
- The placenta develops from the chorionic villi and decidua basalis and has two parts: The maternal portion, consisting of the decidua basalis, is red and fresh looking; the fetal portion, consisting of chorionic villi, is covered by the amnion and appears shiny and gray. The placenta is made up of 15 to 20 segments called cotyledons.
- The placenta serves endocrine (production of hPL, hCG, estrogen, and progesterone), metabolic, and immunologic functions. It acts as the fetus's respiratory organ, is an organ of excretion, and aids in the exchange of nutrients.
- Fetal circulation is a specially designed circulatory system that provides for oxygenation of the fetus while bypassing the fetal lungs.
- Stages of fetal development include the pre-embryonic stage (the first 14 days of human development starting at the time of fertilization), the embryonic stage (from day 15 after fertilization, or the beginning of the third week, until approximately 8 weeks), and the fetal stage (from 8 weeks until birth, at approximately 40 weeks after the last normal menstrual period).
- Significant events that occur during the embryonic stage include the fetal heart beginning to beat at 4 weeks and the establishment of fetal circulation at 6 weeks.
- The fetal stage is devoted to refining structures and perfecting function. Some significant developments during the fetal stage are as follows:
- At 8 to 12 weeks, all organ systems are formed and simply require maturation.
- At 16 weeks, the sex can be determined visually.
- At 20 weeks, the fetal heartbeat can be auscultated by a fetoscope, and the mother can feel movement (quickening).
- At 24 weeks, vernix caseosa covers the entire body.
- At 26 to 28 weeks, the eyes reopen.
- At 32 weeks, skin appears less wrinkled and red, since subcutaneous fat has been laid down.
- At 36 weeks, fingernails reach the ends of fingers.
- At 40 weeks, vernix caseosa is apparent only in the creases and folds of the skin, and lanugo remains on upper arms and shoulders only.
- The embryo is particularly vulnerable to teratogenesis during the first 8 weeks of cell differentiation and organ system development.

## CHAPTER REFERENCES


Ahokas, R. A., & McKinney, E. T. (2000). Development and physiology of the placenta and membranes. In J. J. Sciarra & T. J. Watkins (Eds.), *Gynecology and obstetrics* (Vol. 2, chap. 11, pp. 1–21). Philadelphia: Lippincott Williams & Wilkins.

Benirschke, K. (1999a). Multiple gestation: Incidence, etiology, and inheritance. In R. K. Creasy & R. Resnik (Eds.), *Maternal-fetal medicine* (4th ed., pp. 585–597). Philadelphia: Saunders.

Benirschke, K. (1999b). Normal development. In R. K. Creasy & R. Resnik (Eds.), *Maternal-fetal medicine* (4th ed., pp. 63–71). Philadelphia: Saunders.

Brannigan, R. E., & Lipshultz, L. I. (2000). Sperm transport and capacitation. In J. J. Sciarra & T. J. Watkins (Eds.), *Gynecology and obstetrics* (Vol. 1, chap. 45, pp. 1–9). Philadelphia: Lippincott Williams & Wilkins.

Craven, C., & Ward, K. (1999). Embryology, fetus, and placenta: Normal and abnormal. In J. R. Scott, P. J. Di Saia, C. B. Hammond, & W. N. Spellacy (Eds.), *Danforth's obstetrics and gynecology* (8th ed., pp. 29–46). Philadelphia: Lippincott Williams & Wilkins.

Cunningham, F. G., MacDonald, P. C., Gant, N. G., Leveno, K. J., Gilstrapp, L. C., III, Hankins, G. D. V., & Clark, S. L. (1997). *Williams' obstetrics* (20th ed.). Stamford, CT: Appleton & Lange.

De Jonge, C. J. (2000). Egg transport and fertilization. In J. J. Sciarra & T. J. Watkins (Eds.), *Gynecology and obstetrics* (Vol. 1, chap. 46, pp. 1–7). Philadelphia: Lippincott Williams & Wilkins.

Gilbert, W. M., & Brace, R. A. (1993). Amniotic fluid volume and normal flows to and from the amniotic cavity. *Seminars in Perinatology, 17*(3), 150–157.

Moore, K. L., Persaud, T. V. N., & Shiota, K. (2000). *Color Atlas of Clinical embryology* (2nd ed.). Philadelphia: Saunders.

Sadler, T. W. (1995). *Langman's medical embryology* (7th ed.). Baltimore: Williams & Wilkins.

Spellacy, W. N. (1999). Multiple pregnancies. In J. R. Scott, P. J. Di Saia, C. B. Hammond, & W. N. Spellacy (Eds.), *Danforth's obstetrics and gynecology* (8th ed., pp. 293–300). Philadelphia: Lippincott Williams & Wilkins.

Volpe, J. J. (2000). *Neurology of the newborn* (4th ed.). Philadelphia: Saunders.

## CONTEMPORARY MATERNAL-NEWBORN NURSING ON-LINE

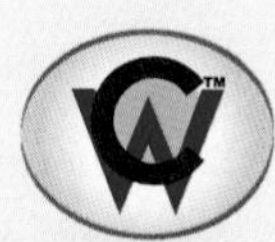

Additional interactive resources, including animations and video, for this chapter can be found on the Companion Website at http://www.prenhall.com/ladewig. Click on Chapter 3 and "Begin" to select the activities for this chapter.

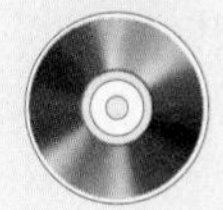

For NCLEX review questions and an audio glossary, access the accompanying CD-ROM in this book.

# Part Two

# Women: The Reproductive Years

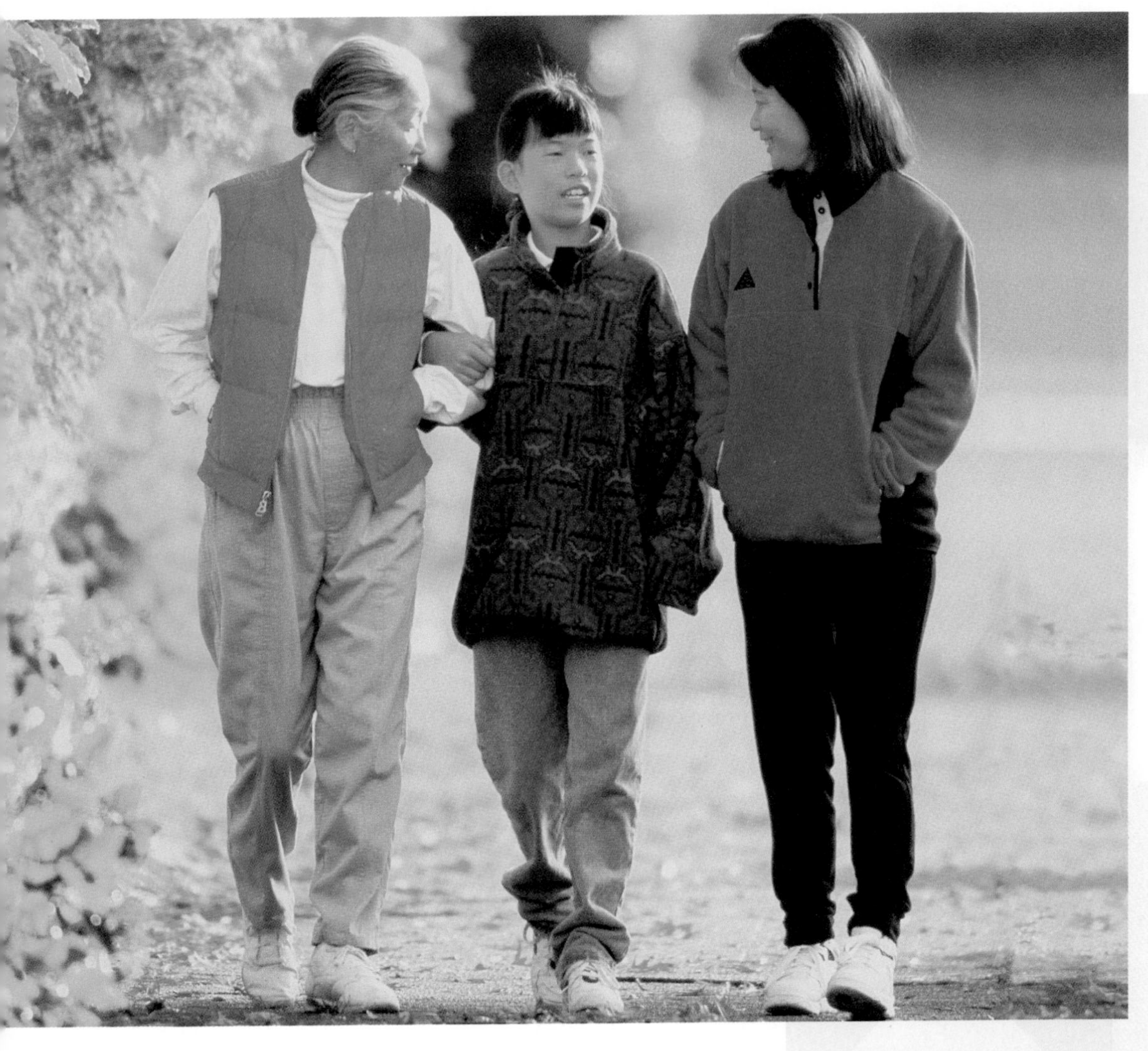

Chapter 4

# Women's Health Care

*I have started caring for the teenage daughters of many of my longtime clients. Making each teen's first pelvic exam a positive experience has become something of a mission for me. Every time I complete an exam and the young woman says, "That was easy. Why do women make such a fuss about a pelvic?" I want to jump up and shout, "Yes!" Attitudes are changed one person at a time.*

—A Women's Health Nurse Practitioner

## KEY TERMS



## OBJECTIVES

- Summarize information that women may need to implement effective self-care measures for dealing with menstruation.
- Compare the advantages, disadvantages, and effectiveness of the various methods of contraception.
- Delineate basic gynecologic screening procedures indicated for well women.
- Discuss the physical and psychologic aspects of menopause.
- Delineate the nurse's role in working with women who are the victims of violence through female partner abuse and rape.
- Contrast the common benign breast disorders.
- Discuss the signs and symptoms, medical therapy, and implications for fertility of endometriosis.
- Identify the risk factors, treatment options, and nursing interventions for a woman with toxic shock syndrome.
- Compare vulvovaginal candidiasis and bacterial vaginosis.
- Describe the common sexually transmitted infections.
- Summarize the health teaching a nurse needs to provide to a woman with a sexually transmitted infection.
- Relate the implications of pelvic inflammatory disease (PID) for future fertility to its pathology, signs and symptoms, and treatment.
- Identify the implications of an abnormal finding during a pelvic examination.
- Contrast cystitis and pyelonephritis.

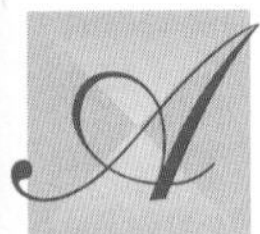

A woman's health care needs change throughout her lifetime. As a young girl she needs health teaching about menstruation, sexuality, and personal responsibility. As a teen she needs information about reproductive choices and safe sexual activity. During this time she should also be introduced to the importance of health care practices such as breast self-examination and regular Pap smears. The mature woman may need to be reminded of these self-care issues and prepared for physical changes that accompany childbirth and aging. By educating women about their bodies, their health care choices, and their right to be knowledgeable consumers, nurses can help women assume responsibility for the health care they receive.

The contemporary woman is likely to encounter various major or minor gynecologic or urinary problems during her lifetime. The nurse can assist a woman in this situation by providing accurate, sensitive, and supportive health education and counseling. To meet the woman's needs, the nurse must have up-to-date information about health care practices and available diagnostic and treatment options.

This chapter provides information about selected aspects of women's health care with an emphasis on conditions typically addressed in a community-based setting.

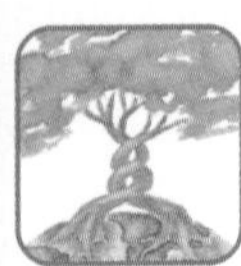

## Community-Based Nursing Care

*Women's health* refers to a holistic view of women and their health-related needs within the context of their everyday lives. It is based on the awareness that a woman's physical, mental, and spiritual status are interdependent and affect her state of health or illness. The woman's view of her situation, her assessment of her needs, her values, and her beliefs are valid and important factors to be incorporated into any health care intervention.

Nurses can work with women to provide health teaching and information about self-care practices in schools, during routine examinations in a clinic or office, at senior centers, at meetings of volunteer organizations, through classes offered by local agencies or schools, or in the home. This community-based focus is the key to providing effective nursing care to women of all ages.

In reality, the vast majority of women's health care is provided outside of acute care settings. Nurses oriented to community-based care are especially effective in recognizing the autonomy of each individual and in dealing with clients holistically. This holistic approach is important in addressing not only physical problems but also major health issues such as violence against women, which may go undetected unless care providers are alert for signs of it.

## The Nurse's Role in Addressing Issues of Sexuality

Because sexuality and its reproductive implications are such an intrinsic and emotion-laden part of life, people have many concerns, problems, and questions about sex roles, behaviors, education, inhibitions, morality, and related areas such as family planning. The reproductive implications of sexual intercourse must also be considered. Some people desire pregnancy; others wish to avoid it. Health factors are another consideration. The increase in the incidence of sexually transmitted infections, especially human immunodeficiency virus, acquired immunodeficiency syndrome (HIV/AIDS), and herpes, has caused many people to modify their sexual practices and activities. Women frequently ask questions or voice concerns about these issues to the nurse in a clinic or ambulatory setting. Thus the nurse may need to assume the role of counselor on sexual and reproductive matters.

Nurses who assume this role must be secure about their own sexuality. They must also recognize their own feelings, values, and attitudes about sexuality so they can be more sensitive and objective when they encounter the values and beliefs of others. Nurses need to have accurate, up-to-date information about topics related to sexuality, sexual practices, and common gynecologic problems. They also need to know about the structures and functions of female and male reproductive systems. In addition, when a woman is accompanied by her partner, it is important that the nurse be sensitive to the dynamics of the relationship between the partners.

Continuing education for the practicing nurse and appropriate courses in undergraduate and graduate nursing education programs can help nurses achieve the requisite knowledge about aspects of sexuality. These courses can help nurses learn about sexual values, attitudes, alternative lifestyles, cultural factors, and misconceptions and myths about sex and reproduction.

## Taking a Sexual History

Nurses are often responsible for taking a woman's initial history, including her gynecologic and sexual history. To be effective, the nurse must have good communication skills and should conduct the interview in a quiet, private place free of distractions.

Opening the discussion with a brief explanation of the purpose of such questions is often helpful. For example, the nurse might say, "As your nurse I'm interested in all aspects of your well-being. Often women have concerns or questions about sexual matters, especially when they are pregnant (or starting to be sexually active). I will be asking you some questions about your sexual history as part of your general health history."

It may be helpful to use direct eye contact as much as possible unless the nurse knows it is culturally unacceptable to the woman. The nurse should do little, if any, writing during the interview, especially if the woman seems ill at ease or is discussing very personal issues. Open-ended questions are often useful in eliciting information. For example, "What, if anything, would you change about your sex life?" will elicit more information than "Are you happy with your sex life now?" The nurse needs to clarify terminology and proceed from easier topics to those that are more difficult to discuss. Throughout the interview the nurse should be alert to body language and nonverbal cues. It is important that the nurse not assume that the client is heterosexual. Some women are open about lesbian relationships; others are more reserved until they develop a sense of trust in their caregivers.

After completing the sexual history, the nurse assesses the information obtained. If there is a problem that requires further medical tests and assessments, the nurse will refer the woman to a nurse practitioner, certified nurse-midwife, physician, or counselor as necessary. In many instances the nurse alone will be able to develop a nursing diagnosis and then plan and implement therapy. For example, if the nurse determines that a woman who is interested in conceiving a child does not have a clear understanding of when she ovulates, the nurse may formulate the following nursing diagnosis: Health-seeking behaviors: information about ovulation related to an expressed desire to time intercourse to enhance the possibility of conception. The nurse can then evaluate the woman's knowledge through discussion and review and work with the woman to provide necessary information. The nurse might also suggest that the woman keep a menstrual calendar and monitor basal body temperatures to identify the time of ovulation.

The nurse must be realistic in making assessments and planning interventions. It requires insight and skill to recognize when a woman's problem requires interventions that are beyond a nurse's preparation and ability. In such situations, the nurse must make appropriate referrals.

# Menstruation

Girls today begin to learn about puberty and menstruation at a surprisingly young age. Unfortunately the source of their "education" is sometimes their peers or the media; thus the information is often incomplete, inaccurate, and sensationalized. Nurses who work with young girls and adolescents recognize this and are working hard to provide accurate health teaching and to correct misinformation about menarche (the onset of menses) and the menstrual cycle.

Cultural, religious, and personal attitudes about menstruation are part of the menstrual experience and often reflect negative attitudes toward women. In the past, many myths surrounded menstruation. Women were often isolated or restricted to the company of other women during their monthly flow because they were considered "unclean." Currently there are fewer customs associated with menstruation, although many women hide the fact of menstruation entirely. Sexual intercourse during menses is a common practice and is not generally contraindicated. For most couples, the decision is one of personal preference. (The physiology of menstruation is discussed in Chapter 2.)

## Counseling the Premenstrual Girl about Menarche

Many young women find it embarrassing or stressful to discuss the menstrual experience, both because of the many taboos associated with the subject and because of their immaturity. However, the most critical factor in successful adaptation to menarche is the adolescent's level of preparedness. Information should be given to premenstrual girls over time rather than all at once. This allows them to absorb information and develop questions.

The following basic information is helpful for young clients:

- *Cycle length.* Cycle length is determined from the first day of one menses to the first day of the next menses. Initially a female's cycle length is about 29 days, but the normal length may vary from 21 to 35 days. As a woman matures, cycle length often shortens to a median of 25+ days just before menopause. Cycle length often varies by a day or two from one cycle to the next, although greater normal variations may also occur.
- *Amount of flow.* The average flow is approximately 30 mL per period. Usually women characterize the amount of flow in terms of the number of pads or tampons used. Flow often is heavier at first and lighter toward the end of the period.
- *Length of menses.* Menses usually lasts from 2 to 8 days, although this may vary.

The nurse should make it clear that variations in age at menarche, length of cycle, and duration of menses are normal because girls may worry if their experience varies from that of their peers. It also is helpful to acknowledge the negative aspects of menstruation (messiness and embarrassment) while stressing its positive role as a symbol of maturity and womanhood.

## Educational Topics

The nurse's primary role is to provide accurate information and assist in clarifying misconceptions, so that girls will develop positive self-images and progress smoothly through this phase of maturation.

### Pads and Tampons

Since early times women have made pads and tampons from cloth or rags, which required washing but were reusable. Commercial tampons were introduced in the 1930s.

Today adhesive-stripped minipads and maxipads and flushable tampons are readily available. However, the deodorants and increased absorbency that manufacturers have added to both sanitary napkins and tampons may prove harmful. The chemical used to deodorize can create a rash on the vulva and damage the tender mucous lining of the vagina. Excessive or inappropriate use of tampons can produce dryness or even small sores or ulcers in the vagina.

Because the use of superabsorbent tampons has been linked to the development of toxic shock syndrome (TSS) (page 93), women should avoid using them. They should use regular-absorbency tampons only for heavy menstrual flow (during the first 2 or 3 days of the period), not during the whole period, and change them every 3 to 6 hours. Because *Staphylococcus aureus,* the causative organism of TSS, is frequently found on the hands, a woman should wash her hands before inserting a fresh tampon and should avoiding touching the tip of the tampon when unwrapping it or before insertion.

In the absence of a heavy menstrual flow, tampons absorb moisture, leaving the vaginal walls dry and subject to injury. The absorbency of regular tampons varies. If the tampon is hard to pull out or shreds when removed, or if the vagina becomes dry, the tampon is probably too absorbent. If a woman is worried about accidental spotting, she can check the diagrams on the packages of regular tampons; those that expand in width are better able to prevent leakage without being too absorbent.

A woman may want to use tampons only during the day and switch to napkins at night to avoid vaginal irritation. She should avoid using tampons on the last, spotty days of the period and should never use them for midcycle spotting or leukorrhea. If a woman experiences vaginal irritation, itching, or soreness or notices an unusual odor while using tampons, she should stop using them or change brands or absorbencies to see if that helps.

The choice of sanitary protection—whether napkins or tampons—must meet the individual's needs and feel comfortable.

### Vaginal Spray, Douching, and Cleansing

Vaginal sprays are unnecessary and can cause infections, itching, burning, vaginal discharge, rashes, and other problems. If a woman chooses to use a spray, she needs to know that these sprays are for external use only and should never be applied to irritated or itching skin or used with sanitary napkins.

Although douching is sometimes used to treat vaginal infections, douching as a hygiene practice is unnecessary, since the vagina cleanses itself. Douching washes away the natural mucus and upsets the vaginal ecology, which can make the vagina more susceptible to infection. Douching with perfumed douches can cause allergic reactions, and too frequent use of an undiluted or strong douche solution can cause irritation or even tissue damage. Propelling water up the vagina may also erode the antibacterial cervical plug and force bacteria and germs from the vagina into the uterus. Women should avoid douching during menstruation because the cervix is dilated to permit the downward flow of menstrual fluids from the uterine lining. Douching may force tissue back up into the uterine cavity, which could contribute to endometriosis.

The mucous secretions that continually bathe the vagina are odor-free while they are in the vagina; odor develops only when they mingle with perspiration and are exposed to the air. Keeping one's skin clean and free of bacteria with plain soap and water is the most effective method of controlling odor. A soapy finger or soft washcloth should be used to wash gently between the vulvar folds. Bathing is as important during menses as at any other time. A long, leisurely soak in a warm tub promotes menstrual blood flow and relieves cramps by relaxing the muscles.

Keeping the vulva fresh throughout the day means keeping it dry and clean. A woman can ensure adequate ventilation by wearing cotton panties and clothes loose enough to permit the vaginal area to breathe. After using the toilet, a woman should always wipe herself from front to back and, if necessary, follow up with a moistened paper towel or toilet paper. If an unusual odor persists despite these efforts, it may be a sign that something is awry. Certain conditions such as vaginitis produce a foul-smelling discharge.

## Associated Menstrual Conditions

A variety of menstrual irregularities have been identified. An abnormally short duration of menstrual flow is termed *hypomenorrhea;* an abnormally long one is called *hypermenorrhea.* Excessive, profuse flow is called *menorrhagia,* and bleeding between periods is known as *metrorrhagia.* Infrequent and too frequent menses are termed *oligomenorrhea* and *polymenorrhea,* respectively. An *anovulatory cycle* is one in which ovulation does not occur. Such irregularities should be investigated to rule out any disease process.

### Amenorrhea

**Amenorrhea,** the absence of menses, is classified as primary or secondary. Primary amenorrhea is said to occur if menstruation has not been established by 18 years of age. Secondary amenorrhea is said to occur when an established menses (of longer than 3 months) ceases.

Primary amenorrhea necessitates a thorough assessment of the young woman to determine its cause. Possible causes include congenital obstructions, congenital absence of the uterus, testicular feminization (external genitals appear female but uterus and ovaries are absent and testes are present), or absence or imbalance of hormones. Success of treatment depends on the causative factors. Many causes are not correctable.

Secondary amenorrhea is caused most frequently by pregnancy. Additional causes include lactation, hormonal imbalances, poor nutrition (anorexia nervosa, obesity, and fad dieting), ovarian lesions, strenuous exercise (associated with long-distance runners, dancers, and other athletes with low body fat ratios), debilitating systemic diseases, stress of high intensity and/or long duration, stressful life events, a change in season or climate, use of oral contraceptives, use of the phenothiazine and chlorpromazine group of tranquilizers, and syndromes such as Cushing and Sheehan. Treatment is dictated by the causative factors. The nurse can explain that once the underlying condition has been corrected—for example, when sufficient body weight is gained—menses will resume. Female athletes and women who participate in strenuous exercise routines may be advised to increase their caloric intake or reduce their exercise levels for a month or two to see whether a normal cycle ensues. If it does not, medical referral is indicated.

### Dysmenorrhea

**Dysmenorrhea,** or painful menstruation, occurs at, or a day before, the onset of menstruation and disappears by the end of menses. Dysmenorrhea is classified as primary or secondary. Primary dysmenorrhea is defined as cramps without underlying disease. Prostaglandins $F_2$ and $F_{2\alpha}$, which are produced by the uterus in higher concentrations during menses, are the primary cause. They increase uterine contractility and decrease uterine artery blood flow, causing ischemia. The end result is the painful sensation of cramps. Dysmenorrhea typically disappears after a first pregnancy and does not occur if cycles are anovulatory. Treatment of primary dysmenorrhea incudes oral contraceptives (which block ovulation), prostaglandin inhibitors (such as ibuprofen, aspirin, and naproxen), and self-care measures such as regular exercise, rest, heat, and good nutrition. Biofeedback has also been used with some success.

Secondary dysmenorrhea is associated with pathology of the reproductive tract and usually appears after menstruation has been established. Conditions that most frequently cause secondary dysmenorrhea include endometriosis; residual pelvic inflammatory disease (PID); anatomic anomalies such as cervical stenosis, imperforate hymen, and uterine displacement; ovarian cysts; and the presence of an intrauterine device. Because primary and secondary dysmenorrhea may coexist, accurate differential diagnosis is essential for appropriate treatment.

Some nutritionists suggest that vitamins B and E help relieve the discomforts associated with menstruation. Vitamin $B_6$ may help relieve the premenstrual bloating and irritability some women experience. Vitamin E, a mild prostaglandin inhibitor, may help decrease menstrual discomfort. Avoiding salt can decrease discomfort from fluid retention.

Heat is soothing and promotes increased blood flow. Any source of warmth, from sipping herbal tea to soaking in a hot tub or using a heating pad, may be helpful during painful periods. Massage can also soothe aching back muscles and promote relaxation and blood flow.

Daily exercise can ease menstrual discomfort and help prevent cramps and other menstrual complaints. Aerobic exercises such as jogging, cycling, swimming, and fast-paced walking are especially helpful. Persistent discomfort should be medically evaluated.

### Premenstrual Syndrome

**Premenstrual syndrome (PMS)** refers to a symptom complex associated with the luteal phase of the menstrual cycle (2 weeks prior to the onset of menses). Women over 30 years of age are the most likely to have PMS. The symptoms must, by definition, occur between ovulation and the onset of menses. They repeat at the same stage of each menstrual cycle and include some or all of the following:

- Psychologic: irritability, lethargy, depression, low morale, anxiety, sleep disorders, crying spells, and hostility
- Neurologic: classic migraine, vertigo, and syncope
- Respiratory: rhinitis, hoarseness, and occasionally asthma
- Gastrointestinal: nausea, vomiting, constipation, abdominal bloating, and craving for sweets
- Urinary: retention and oliguria
- Dermatologic: acne
- Mammary: swelling and tenderness

## Critical Thinking in Practice

Rita Cooper is a 16-year-old, vivacious teenager who comes to the clinic because of irregular menses. She is captain of the cheerleading squad at the local high school and believes that her periods are "really messed up" and interfering with her cheering activities. She wants to get her periods regulated and asks for birth control pills.

As you take Rita's menstrual history, you find that her menarche was at age 12 and that her periods occur every 24 to 34 days. She usually has cramps, and the flow, which she describes as heavy, lasts 4 to 5 days. She uses an average of five tampons per day. What should you advise Rita about her menstrual cycle?

Answers can be found in Appendix I.

Most women experience only some of these symptoms. The symptoms usually are most pronounced 2 or 3 days before the onset of menstruation and subside as menstrual flow begins, with or without treatment. *Premenstrual dysphoric disorder (PMDD)* is a diagnosis that may be applied to a subgroup of women with PMS whose symptoms are primarily mood related and severe (Endicott, Bardack, Grady-Weliky, et al., 2000).

The exact cause of PMS is unknown, although a variety of theories have been put forth to explain it. These include, for example, hormone imbalance, nutritional deficiency, prostaglandin excess, and endorphin deficiency.

## Nursing Care Management

The nurse can help the woman identify specific symptoms and develop healthy behavior. After assessment, counseling for PMS may include advising the woman to restrict her intake of foods containing methylxanthines such as chocolate, cola, and coffee; restrict her intake of alcohol, nicotine, red meat, and foods containing salt and sugar; increase her intake of complex carbohydrates and protein; and increase the frequency of meals. For women whose primary symptoms are psychologic, supplementation with B complex vitamins, especially $B_6$, may decrease anxiety and depression. However, treatment trials do not demonstrate a consistent effect, and megadoses of $B_6$ are associated with peripheral neurologic changes (Moline & Zendell, 2000). Vitamin E supplements may help reduce breast tenderness, and a program of aerobic exercise such as fast walking, jogging, and aerobic dancing is generally beneficial. In addition to vitamin supplements, pharmacologic treatments for PMS include progesterone suppositories, diuretics, psychotropic drugs (such as tricyclic antidepressants and selective serotonin reuptake inhibitors), and prostaglandin inhibitors. All have been effective in some women and not in others. For women who are not planning a pregnancy, low-dose oral contraceptives, which suppress ovulation, are often helpful.

An empathic relationship with a health care professional to whom the woman feels free to voice concerns is highly beneficial. The nurse can encourage the woman to keep a diary to help identify life events associated with PMS. Self-care groups and self-help literature both help women feel they have control over their bodies. Some women elect to use complementary therapies such as homeopathic remedies or herbs. Thus it is helpful for the nurse to have a general familiarity with commonly used remedies. It is important that women using such alternatives seek advice from knowledgeable, experienced homeopaths or herbalists.

# Contraception

The decision to use a method of contraception may be made individually by a woman (or, in the case of vasectomy, by a man) or jointly by a couple. The decision may be motivated by a desire to avoid pregnancy, to gain control over the number of children conceived, or to determine the spacing of future children. In choosing a specific method, consistency of use outweighs the absolute reliability of the given method.

Decisions about contraception should be made voluntarily, with full knowledge of advantages, disadvantages, effectiveness, side effects, contraindications, and long-term effects. Many outside factors influence this choice, including cultural practices, religious beliefs, attitudes and personal preferences, cost, effectiveness, misinformation, practicality of method, and self-esteem. Different methods of contraception may be appropriate at different times for couples.

### Fertility Awareness Methods

**Fertility awareness methods,** also known as *natural family planning,* are based on an understanding of the changes that occur throughout a woman's ovulatory cycle. All these methods require periods of abstinence and recording of certain events throughout the cycle; cooperation of the partners is important.

Fertility awareness methods are free, safe, and acceptable to many whose religious beliefs prohibit other methods. They provide an increased awareness of the body, involve no artificial substances or devices, encourage a couple to communicate about sexual activity and family planning, and are useful in helping a couple plan a pregnancy.

On the other hand, these methods require extensive initial counseling to be used effectively. They may interfere with sexual spontaneity; they require extensive maintenance of records for several cycles before beginning to use them; they may be difficult or impossible for women with irregular cycles to use; and, although theoretically they should be very reliable, in practice they may not be as reliable in preventing pregnancy as other methods.

The *basal body temperature (BBT)* method to detect ovulation requires that a woman take her BBT every morning upon awakening (before any activity) and record the readings on a temperature graph. To do this, she uses a basal body temperature thermometer, which shows tenths of a degree rather than the two-tenths shown on standard thermometers. She may also use tympanic thermometry (an "ear thermometer"). After 3 to 4 months of recording temperatures, a woman with regular cycles should be able to predict when ovulation will occur. The method is based on the fact that the temperature sometimes drops just before ovulation and almost always rises and remains elevated for several days after. The temperature rise occurs in response to the increased progesterone levels that occur in the second half of the cycle. Figure 4–1♦ shows a sample BBT chart. To avoid conception, the couple abstains from intercourse on the day of the temperature rise and for 3 days after. Because the temperature rise does not occur until after ovulation, a woman who had intercourse just before the rise is at risk of pregnancy. To decrease this risk, some couples abstain from intercourse for several days before the *anticipated* time of ovulation and then for 3 days after.

The *calendar,* or *rhythm, method* is based on the assumptions that ovulation tends to occur 14 days (plus or minus 2 days) before the start of the next menstrual period, sperm are viable for 48 to 72 hours, and the ovum is viable for 24 hours (Hatcher et al., 1998). To use this method, the woman must record her menstrual cycles for 6 to 8 months to identify the shortest and longest cycles. The first day of menstruation is the first day of the cycle. The fertile phase is calculated from 18 days before the end of the shortest recorded cycle through 11 days from the end of the longest recorded cycle (Hatcher et al., 1998). For example, if a woman's cycle lasts from 24 to 28 days, the fertile phase would be calculated as day 6 through day 17. Once this information is obtained, the woman can identify the fertile and infertile phases of her cycle. For effective use of this method, she must abstain from intercourse during the fertile phase. The calendar method is the least reliable of the fertility awareness methods and has largely been replaced by other, more scientific approaches.

The *cervical mucus method,* sometimes called the *ovulation method* or the *Billings method,* involves the assessment of cervical mucus changes that occur during the menstrual cycle. The amount and character of cervical mucus change because of the influence of estrogen and progesterone. At the time of ovulation the mucus (estrogen-dominant mucus) is clearer, more stretchable (a quality called *spinnbarkeit*), and more permeable to sperm. It also shows a characteristic fern pattern when placed on a glass slide and allowed to dry (see Figure 5–3♦). During the luteal phase, the cervical mucus is thick and sticky (progesterone-dominant mucus) and forms a network that traps sperm, making their passage more difficult.

To use the cervical mucus method, the woman abstains from intercourse for the first menstrual cycle. Cervical

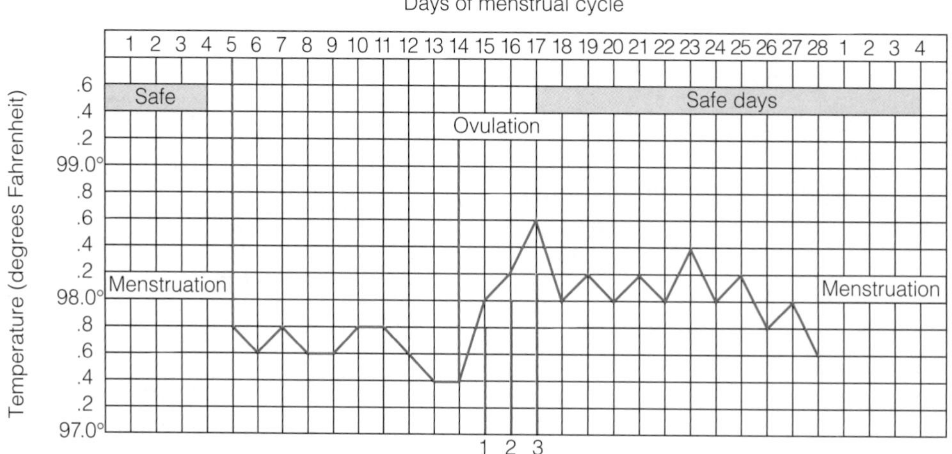


**FIGURE 4–1 ♦ Sample basal body temperature chart.** Source: Crooks, R., & Baur, K. (1993) *Our sexuality* (5th ed.). Monterey, CA: Brooks/Cole.

mucus is assessed daily for amount, feeling of slipperiness or wetness, color, clearness, and spinnbarkheit, as the woman becomes familiar with varying characteristics.

The peak day of wetness and clear, stretchable mucus is assumed to be the time of ovulation. To use this method correctly, the woman should abstain from intercourse from the time she first notices that the mucus is becoming clear, more elastic, and slippery until 4 days after the last wet mucus (ovulation) day. Because this method evaluates the effects of hormonal changes, it can be used by women with irregular cycles.

The *symptothermal method* consists of various assessments made and recorded by the couple. These include information regarding cycle days, coitus, cervical mucus changes, and secondary signs such as increased libido, abdominal bloating, mittelschmerz (midcycle abdominal pain), and basal body temperature. Through the various assessments, the couple learns to recognize signs that indicate ovulation. This combined approach tends to improve the effectiveness of fertility awareness as a method of birth control.

## Situational Contraceptives

*Abstinence* can be considered a method of contraception, and, partly because of changing values and the increased risk of infection with intercourse, it is gaining increased acceptance.

**Coitus interruptus,** or *withdrawal,* is one of the oldest and least reliable methods of contraception. This method requires that the male withdraw from the female's vagina when he feels that ejaculation is impending. He then ejaculates away from the external genitalia of the woman. Failure tends to occur for two reasons: (1) this method demands great self-control on the part of the man, who must withdraw just as he feels the urge for deeper penetration with impending orgasm, and (2) some preejaculatory fluid, which can contain sperm, may escape from the penis during the excitement phase prior to ejaculation. The fact that the quantity of sperm in this preejaculatory fluid is increased after a recent ejaculation is especially significant for couples who engage in repeated episodes of intercourse within a short period of time. Couples who use this method should be aware of postcoital contraceptive options in case the man fails to withdraw in time.

*Douching after intercourse* is an ineffective method of contraception and is not recommended. It may actually facilitate conception by pushing sperm farther up the birth canal.

## Spermicides

**Spermicides,** available as creams, jellies, foams, vaginal film, and suppositories, are inserted into the vagina before intercourse. They destroy sperm or neutralize vaginal secretions and thereby immobilize sperm. Spermicides that effervesce in a moist environment offer more rapid protection, and coitus may take place immediately after they are inserted. Suppositories may require up to 30 minutes to dissolve and will not offer protection until they do so. The nurse instructs the woman to insert these spermicide preparations high in the vagina and maintain a supine position.

Spermicides are minimally effective when used alone, but their effectiveness increases in conjunction with a diaphragm or condom. The major advantages of spermicides are their wide availability and low toxicity. They are readily available over the counter without prescription. In addition, they provide significant protection from gonorrhea and chlamydia (Hatcher et al., 1998).

Skin irritation and allergic reactions to spermicides are the primary disadvantages. Although some studies have suggested that the use of spermicides at the time of conception or early in pregnancy may be associated with an increased risk of congenital anomalies, recent studies have shown no increased incidence (Hatcher et al., 1998).

## Mechanical Contraceptives

Mechanical contraceptive methods either prevent the transport of sperm to the ovum or prevent implantation of the zygote.

### Male and Female Condoms

The male **condom** offers a viable means of contraception when used consistently and properly (Figure 4–2♦). Acceptance has been increasing as a growing number of men are assuming responsibility for regulation of fertility. The condom is applied to the erect penis, rolled from the tip to the end of the shaft, before vulvar or vaginal contact. A small space must be left at the end of the condom to allow for collection of the ejaculate, so that the condom will not break at the time of ejaculation. If the condom or vagina is dry, water-soluble lubricants, such as K-Y jelly, should be used to prevent irritation and possible condom breakage.

Care must be taken in removing the condom after intercourse. For optimal effectiveness, the man should withdraw his penis from the vagina while it is still erect and hold the condom rim to prevent spillage. If after ejaculation the penis becomes flaccid while still in the vagina, the male should hold onto the edge of the condom while withdrawing to avoid spilling the semen and to prevent the condom from slipping off.

The effectiveness of male condoms is largely determined by their use. The condom is small, disposable, and inexpensive; it has no side effects, requires no medical examination or supervision, and offers visual evidence of effectiveness. Most condoms are made of latex, although

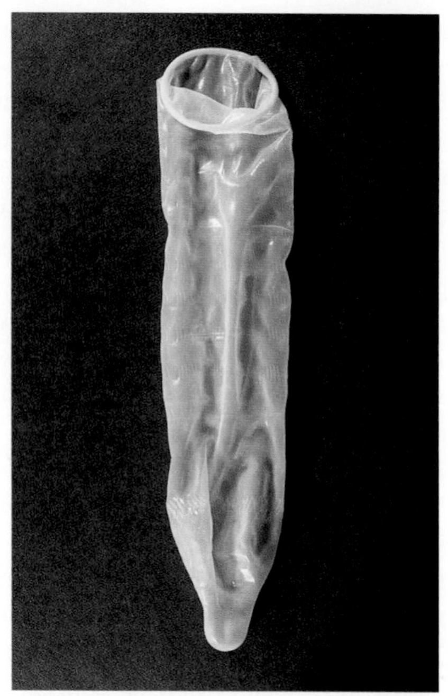
A

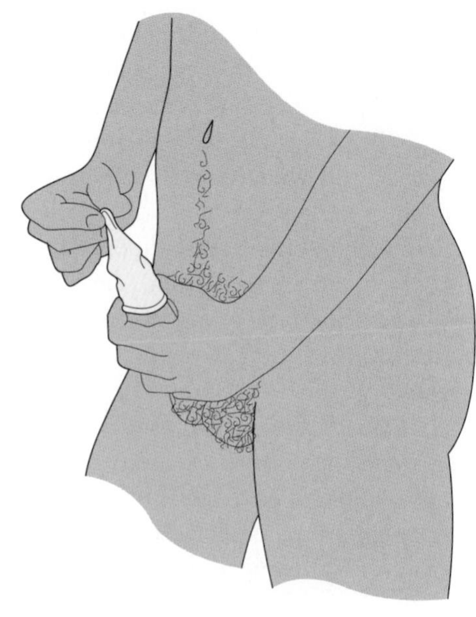
B

FIGURE 4–2 ♦ **A**, Unrolled condom with reservoir tip. **B**, Correct use of a condom.

polyurethane and silicone rubber condoms are available for individuals allergic to latex. All condoms except natural "skin" condoms, made from lamb's intestines, offer protection against both pregnancy and sexually transmitted infections (STIs). Breakage, displacement, perineal or vaginal irritation, and dulled sensation are possible disadvantages.

The male condom is becoming increasingly popular because of the protection it offers from infections. For women, sexually transmitted infection increases the risk of PID and resultant infertility. Many women are beginning to insist that their sexual partners use condoms, and many women carry condoms with them.

The *Reality female condom* (Figure 4–3♦) is a thin polyurethane sheath with a flexible ring at each end. The inner ring, at the closed end of the condom, serves as the means of insertion and fits over the cervix like a diaphragm. The second ring remains outside the vagina and covers a portion of the woman's perineum. It also covers the base of the man's penis during intercourse. Available over the counter and designed for onetime use, the condom may be inserted up to 8 hours before intercourse. The inner sheath is prelubricated but does not contain spermicide and is not designed to be used with a male condom. Data on its effectiveness against pregnancy are still limited, although the female condom has been compared favorably to other barrier methods. Because it also covers a portion of the vulva, it probably provides better protection than other methods against some pathogens. High cost, noisiness during intercourse, and the cumbersome feel of the device make acceptability a problem for some couples.

### Diaphragm and Cervical Cap

The **diaphragm** (Figure 4–4♦) is used with spermicidal cream or jelly and offers a good level of protection from conception. The woman must be fitted with a diaphragm and instructed in its use by trained personnel. The diaphragm should be rechecked for correct size after each childbirth and whenever a woman has gained or lost 15 lbs or more.

The diaphragm must be inserted before intercourse, with approximately 1 teaspoonful (or 1.5 in from the tube) of spermicidal jelly placed around its rim and in the cup. This chemical barrier supplements the mechanical barrier of the diaphragm. The diaphragm is inserted through the vagina and covers the cervix. The last step in insertion is to push the edge of the diaphragm under the symphysis pubis, which may result in a "popping" sensation. When fitted properly and correctly in place, the diaphragm should not cause discomfort to the woman or her partner. Correct placement of the diaphragm can be checked by touching the cervix with a fingertip through the cup. The cervix feels like a small, firm, rounded structure and has a consistency similar to that of the tip of the nose. The center of the diaphragm should be over the cervix. If more than 4 hours elapse between insertion of the diaphragm and intercourse, additional spermicidal cream should be used. It is necessary to leave the diaphragm in place for at least 6 hours after coitus. If intercourse is desired again within the 6 hours, another type of contraception must be used or additional spermicidal jelly placed in the vagina with an applicator, taking care not to disturb the placement of

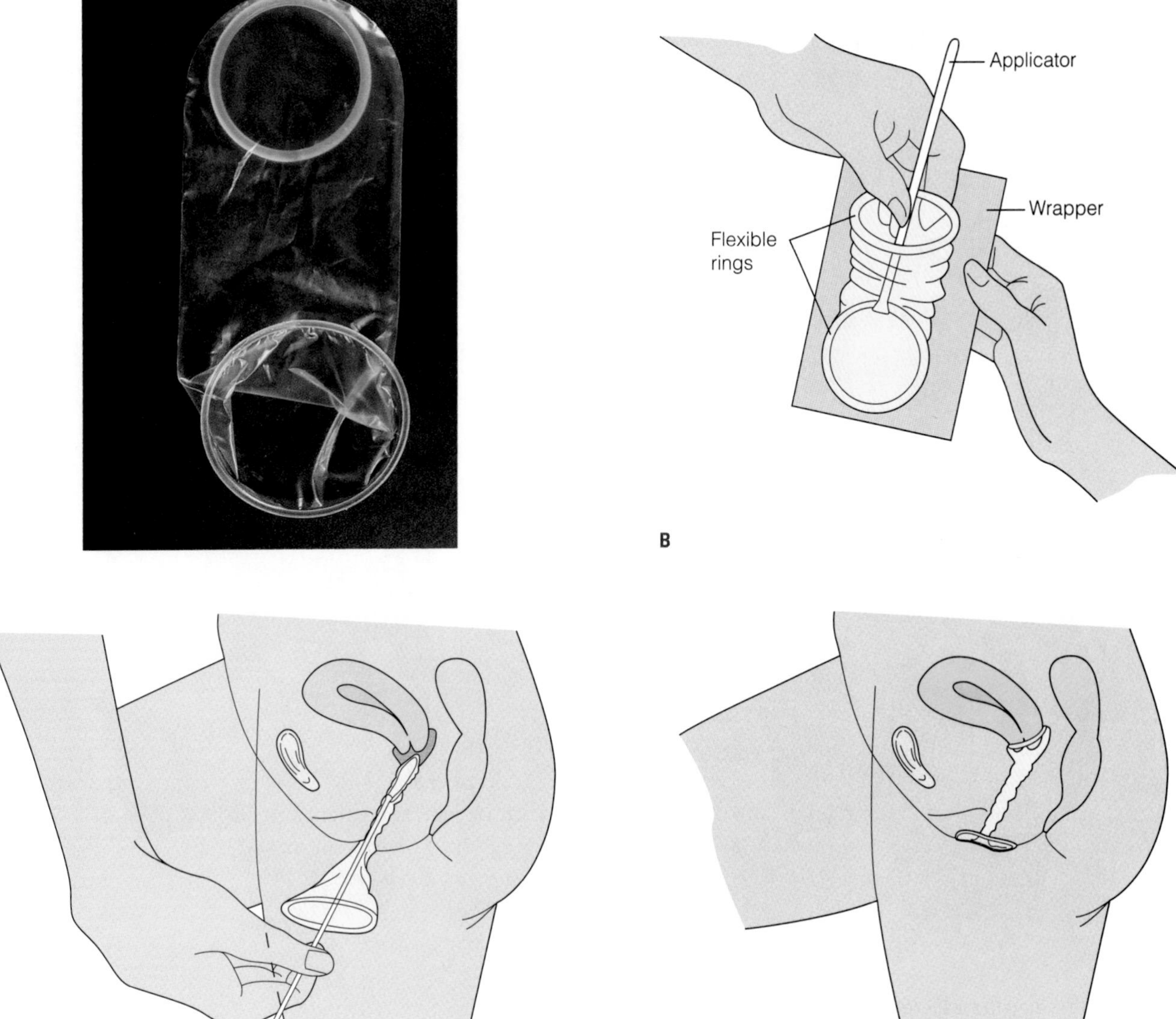


FIGURE 4–3 ♦ **A,** The female condom. To insert the condom: **B,** Remove condom and applicator from wrapper by pulling up on the ring. **C,** Insert condom slowly by gently pushing the applicator toward the small of the back. **D,** When properly inserted, the outer ring should rest on the folds of skin around the vaginal opening, and the inner ring (closed end) should fit loosely against the cervix. Source: Crooks, R., & Baur, K. (1993). *Our sexuality* (5th ed.). Monterey, CA: Brooks/Cole.

the diaphragm. Periodically the diaphragm should be held up to the light and inspected for tears or holes.

Some couples feel that the use of a diaphragm interferes with the spontaneity of intercourse. The nurse can suggest that the partner insert the diaphragm as part of foreplay. The woman can then easily verify the placement herself.

Diaphragms are an excellent contraceptive method for women who are lactating, who cannot or do not wish to use the pill (oral contraceptives), who are smokers over age 35, or who wish to avoid the increased risk of PID associated with intrauterine devices.

Women who object to manipulating their genitals to insert the diaphragm, check its placement, and remove it may find this method unsatisfactory. It is not recommended for women with a history of urinary tract infection, because pressure from the diaphragm on the urethra may interfere with complete bladder emptying and lead to recurrent urinary tract infections (UTIs). Women with a history of toxic shock syndrome should not use diaphragms or any of the barrier methods because they are left in place for prolonged periods. For the same reason, the diaphragm should not be used during a menstrual period or if a woman has abnormal vaginal discharge.

The **cervical cap** (Figure 4–5♦) is a cup-shaped device, used with spermicidal cream or jelly, that fits snugly over the cervix and is held in place by suction. Effectiveness rates and method of insertion are similar to those for the diaphragm. Unlike the diaphragm, however, the cap may be left in place for up to 48 hours, and it does not require

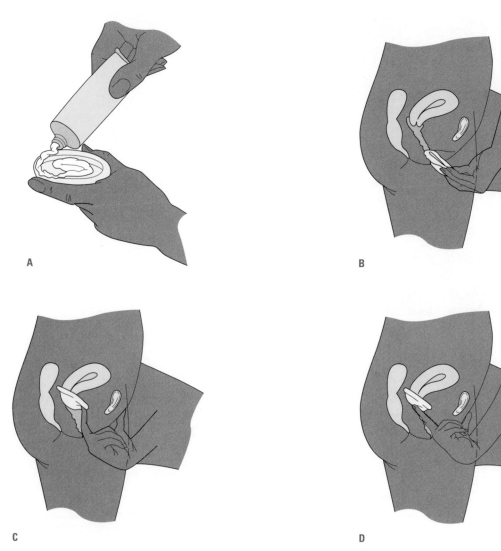

FIGURE 4–4 ♦ Inserting the diaphragm. A, Apply jelly to the rim and center of the diaphragm. B, Insert the diaphragm. C, Push the rim of the diaphragm under the symphysis pubis. D, Check placement of the diaphragm. Cervix should be felt through the diaphragm.

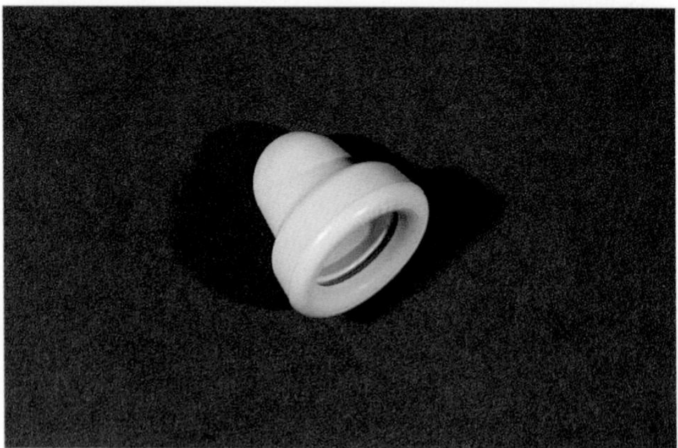

FIGURE 4–5 ♦ A cervical cap.

additional spermicide for repeated intercourse (Hatcher et al., 1998). Advantages, disadvantages, and contraindications are similar to those associated with the diaphragm. The cervical cap may be more difficult to fit because of limited size options. It also tends to be more difficult for women to insert and remove.

### Intrauterine Devices

The **intrauterine device (IUD)** is designed to be inserted into the uterus by a qualified health care provider and left in place for an extended period, providing continuous contraceptive protection. The exact mechanism of IUD action is not clearly understood. Traditionally the IUD was believed to act by preventing the implantation of a fertilized ovum. Thus the IUD was considered an abortifacient (abortion-causing) method. Current evidence on the new generation of IUDs suggests that they truly are contraceptives; they act by altering or inhibiting sperm migration and ovum transport in some way (Chez & Strathman, 1999). The IUD is also known to have local inflammatory effects on the endometrium (Hatcher et al., 1998).

Advantages of the IUD include high rate of effectiveness, continuous contraceptive protection, no coitus-related

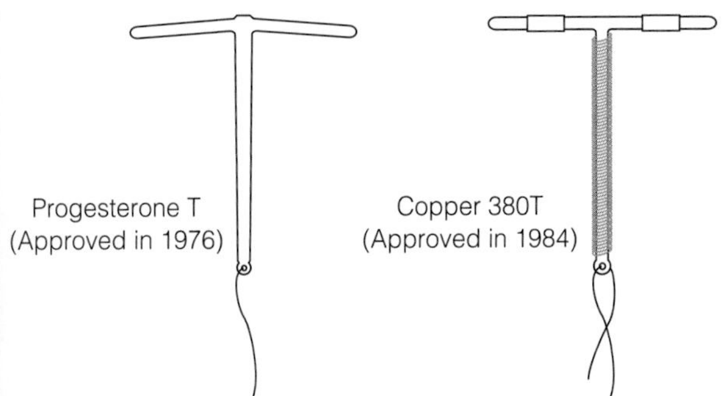


FIGURE 4–6 ♦ Two types of IUDs.

activity, and relative inexpensiveness over time. Possible adverse reactions to the IUD include discomfort to the wearer, increased bleeding during menses, PID, perforation of the uterus, intermenstrual bleeding, dysmenorrhea, and expulsion of the device.

Two IUDs are currently available in the United States (Figure 4–6♦). The progesterone T (Progestasert) must be changed annually and should be used only by women with an allergy to copper. The copper T380A (ParaGard) is highly effective and can be left in place for up to 10 years. The IUD is recommended only for women who have at least one child and are in a monogamous relationship, because these women have the lowest risk of developing a pelvic infection. It is not recommended for women with multiple sexual contacts, because they are at higher risk for sexually transmitted infections (STIs).

The IUD is inserted into the uterus with its string or tail protruding through the cervix into the vagina. It may be inserted during a menstrual period or during the 4- to 6-week postpartum check. After insertion, the clinician instructs the woman to check for the presence of the string once a week for the first month and then after each menses. She is told that she may have some cramping or bleeding intermittently for 2 to 6 weeks and that her first few menses may be irregular. Follow-up examination is suggested 4 to 8 weeks after insertion.

Women with IUDs should contact their health care providers if they are exposed to a STI or if they develop the following warning signs: late period, abnormal spotting or bleeding, pain with intercourse, abdominal pain, abnormal discharge, signs of infection (fever, chills, and malaise), or missing string. If the woman becomes pregnant with an IUD in place, the device is generally removed if the string is visible.

## ORAL CONTRACEPTIVES

**Oral contraceptives (OCs),** also called *birth control pills,* are typically a combination of the hormones estrogen and progesterone. OCs work by inhibiting the release of an ovum and by maintaining cervical mucus that is hostile to sperm. Many OCs are available. The pill is taken daily for 21 days, typically beginning on the Sunday after the first day of the menstrual cycle. In most cases menses occurs 1 to 4 days after the last pill is taken. Seven days after taking her last pill, the woman restarts the pill. Thus the woman always begins the pill on the same day. Some companies offer a 28-day pack with seven "blank" pills so that the woman never stops taking a pill. The pill should be taken at approximately the same time each day—usually upon arising or before retiring in the evening.

**TABLE 4–1 Side Effects Associated with Oral Contraceptives**

| *Estrogen Effects* | *Progestin Effects* |
|---|---|
| Alterations in lipid metabolism | Acne, oily skin |
| Breast tenderness, engorgement; increased breast size | Breast tenderness; increased breast size |
| Cerebrovascular accident | Decreased libido |
| Changes in carbohydrate metabolism | Decreased high-density lipoprotein (HDL) cholesterol levels |
| Chloasma | Depression |
| Fluid retention; cyclic weight gain | Fatigue |
| Headache | Hirsutism |
| Hepatic adenomas | Increased appetite; weight gain |
| Hypertension | Increased low-density lipoprotein |
| Leukorrhea, cervical erosion, ectopia | (LDL) cholesterol levels |
| Nausea | Oligomenorrhea, amenorrhea |
| Nervousness, irritability | Pruritus |
| Telangiectasia | Sebaceous cysts |
| Thromboembolic complications—thrombophlebitis, pulmonary embolism | |

Although they are highly effective, OCs may produce side effects ranging from breakthrough bleeding to thrombus formation. Side effects from OCs may be either progesterone or estrogen related (Table 4–1). The use of low-dose (35 μg or less estrogen) preparations has reduced many of the side effects; the newer 20-μg pills appear to provide comparable cycle control and have even fewer side effects (Rosenberg, Meyers, & Roy, 1999).

Contraindications to the use of oral contraceptives include pregnancy, previous history of thrombophlebitis or thromboembolic disease, acute or chronic liver disease of cholestatic type with abnormal function, presence of estrogen-dependent carcinomas, undiagnosed uterine bleeding, heavy smoking, hypertension, diabetes, and hyperlipidemia. In addition, women with the following

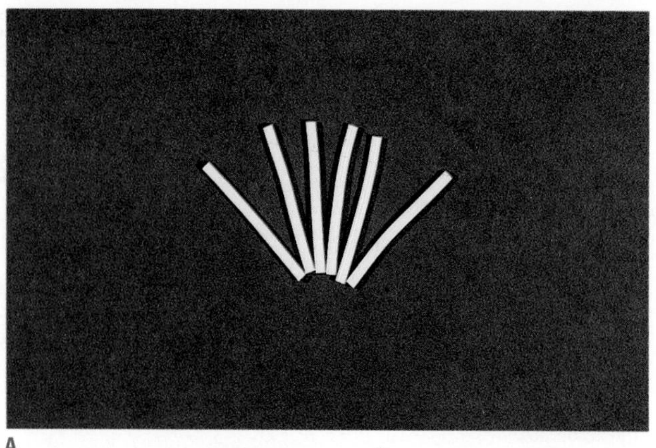

A

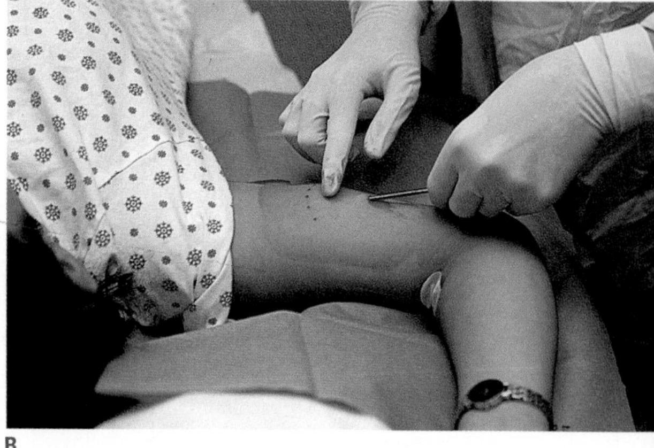

B

FIGURE 4–7 ♦ A, The Norplant system. B, Norplant, a long-acting progestin contraceptive, is implanted in a woman's upper arm.

conditions who use oral contraceptives need to be examined every 3 months: migraine headaches, epilepsy, depression, oligomenorrhea, and amenorrhea. Women who choose this method of contraception should be fully advised of its potential side effects.

OCs also have some important noncontraceptive benefits. Many women experience relief of uncomfortable menstrual symptoms. Cramps are lessened, flow is decreased, and cycle regularity is increased. Mittelschmerz is eliminated, and the incidence of functional ovarian cysts is decreased. There is also a substantial reduction in the incidence of ectopic pregnancy, ovarian cancer, endometrial cancer, iron deficiency anemia, benign breast disease, and hospitalization for pelvic inflammatory disease (Wallach & Grimes, 2000). OCs are considered a fine solution to the physiologic problems some women experience during the perimenopause, and their use in nonsmoking women ages 40 to 45 has quadrupled since 1990 (Speroff, 1998).

The woman using oral contraceptives should contact her health care provider if she becomes depressed, becomes jaundiced, develops a breast lump, or experiences any of the following warning signs: severe abdominal pain, severe chest pain or shortness of breath, severe headaches, dizziness, changes in vision (vision loss or blurring), speech problems, or severe leg pain.

Another OC is the progesterone-only pill, also called the minipill. It is used primarily by women who have a contraindication to the estrogen component of the combination preparation, such as history of thrombophlebitis, but are strongly motivated to use this form of contraception. The major problems with this preparation are amenorrhea or irregular spotting and bleeding patterns.

## Long-Acting Progestin Contraceptives

**Subdermal implants (Norplant)** consist of six silastic capsules containing levonorgestrel, a progestin, which are implanted in the woman's arm. They are effective for up to 5 years (Figure 4–7♦). Norplant prevents ovulation in most women. It also stimulates the production of thick cervical mucus, which inhibits sperm penetration. Norplant provides effective continuous contraception removed from the act of coitus. Possible side effects include spotting, irregular bleeding or amenorrhea, an increased incidence of ovarian cysts, weight gain, headaches, fluid retention, acne, mood changes, and depression. Women should be advised that the implant may be visible, especially in very slender users, and that it requires a minor surgical procedure to insert and remove the implants. A biodegradable form of implant, which is currently under development, would eliminate the need for surgical removal.

Depot-medroxyprogesterone acetate (DMPA) **(Depo-Provera),** another long-acting progestin, provides highly effective birth control for 3 months when given as a single injection of 150 mg. DMPA, which acts primarily by suppressing ovulation, is safe, convenient, private, and relatively inexpensive. It also separates birth control from the act of coitus. It can safely be given to nursing mothers because it contains no estrogen. DMPA provides levels of progesterone high enough to block the LH surge, thereby suppressing ovulation. It also thickens the cervical mucus to block sperm penetration. Side effects include menstrual irregularities, headache, weight gain, breast tenderness, and depression. Return of fertility may be delayed for an average of 9 months (Kaunitz & Jordon, 1997).

In 2000, a monthly contraceptive IM injection was approved by the FDA. The medication, Lunelle, is a combination of medroxyprogesterone acetate (MPA) and estradiol cypionate ($E_2C$). Lunelle is a highly effective contraceptive that has a side effect pattern similar to that of OCs (Shulman, 2000).

## Emergency Postcoital Contraception

Emergency **postcoital contraception** is indicated when a woman is worried about pregnancy because of unprotected intercourse or possible contraceptive failure (eg, broken condom, slipped diaphragm, or too long a time between DMPA injections). The most commonly prescribed emergency postcoital contraceptive is levonorgestrel and ethinyl estradiol (Ovral), a combination oral contraceptive containing 50 μg estrogen. Though sometimes called the "morning-after pill," the phrase is misleading because the woman actually takes two pills as soon after intercourse as possible and two more 12 hours later. This regimen must be started within 72 hours after unprotected intercourse. In addition, a progestin-only (levonorgestrel) emergency contraceptive pill called Plan-B is also available. One pill is taken following the same schedule as Ovral. The Plan-B regimen is more effective than other emergency contraceptives and has a much lower incidence of associated nausea and vomiting (Trussell, Ellertson, Stewart, et al., 2000).

## Operative Sterilization

Before sterilization is performed on either partner, the physician provides a thorough explanation of the procedure to both. Each needs to understand that sterilization is not a decision to be taken lightly or entered into when psychologic stresses, such as separation or divorce, exist. Even though both male and female procedures are theoretically reversible, the permanency of the procedure should be stressed and understood.

Male sterilization is achieved through a relatively minor procedure called a **vasectomy.** This procedure involves surgically severing the vas deferens in both sides of the scrotum. It takes about 4 to 6 weeks and 6 to 36 ejaculations to clear the remaining sperm from the vas deferens. During that period, the couple is advised to use another method of birth control and to bring in two or three semen samples for a sperm count. The man is rechecked at 6 and 12 months to ensure that fertility has not been restored by recanalization. Side effects of a vasectomy include pain, infection, hematoma, sperm granulomas, and spontaneous reanastomosis (reconnecting).

Vasectomies can sometimes be reversed by using microsurgery techniques. Restored fertility, as measured by subsequent pregnancy, ranges from 30% to 76%, depending primarily on the length of time between vasectomy and reversal (Pollack & Barone, 2000).

Female sterilization is most frequently accomplished by **tubal ligation.** The tubes are located through a small subumbilical incision or by minilaparotomy techniques and are crushed, ligated, electrocoagulated, or banded or plugged (in the newer, reversible procedures). Tubal ligation may be done at any time. However, the postpartal period is an ideal time to perform a tubal ligation because the tubes are somewhat enlarged and easily located.

Complications of female sterilization procedures include coagulation burns on the bowel, bowel perforation, pain, infection, hemorrhage, and adverse anesthesia effects. Reversal of a tubal ligation depends on the type of procedure performed. With microsurgical techniques, a pregnancy rate of 44% to 81% is possible (DeLeon & Peters, 2000).

## Male Contraception

The vasectomy and the condom, discussed previously, are currently the only forms of male contraception available in the United States. Hormonal contraception for men has yet to be developed, although studies are under way.

# Nursing Care Management

In most cases, the nurse who provides information and guidance about contraceptive methods works with the woman partner, because most contraceptive methods are female oriented. Since a man can purchase condoms without seeing a health care provider, only with vasectomy does a man require counseling and interaction with a nurse. The nurse can play an important role in helping a woman choose a method of contraception that is acceptable to her and to her partner.

In addition to completing a history and assessing for any contraindications to specific methods, the nurse can spend time with a woman learning about her lifestyle, personal attitudes about particular contraceptive methods, religious beliefs, personal biases, and plans for future childbearing, before helping the woman select a particular contraceptive method. Once the method is chosen, the nurse can help the woman learn to use it effectively. Table 4–2 summarizes factors to consider in choosing an appropriate method of contraception.

The nurse also reviews any possible side effects and warning signs related to the method chosen and counsels the woman about what action to take if she suspects she is pregnant. In many cases the nurse is involved in telephone counseling of women who call with questions and concerns about contraception. Thus it is vital that the nurse be knowledgeable about this topic and have resources available to find answers to less common questions.

The Teaching Guide: Using a Method of Contraception provides guidelines for helping women use a method of contraception effectively.

## TEACHING GUIDE *Using a Method of Contraception*

### Assessment

The nurse determines the woman's general knowledge about contraceptive methods, identifies the methods the woman has used previously (if any), identifies contraindications or risk factors for any methods, discusses the woman's personal preferences and biases about various methods, and discusses her commitment (and her partner's commitment if appropriate) to a chosen method.

### Nursing Diagnosis

The key nursing diagnosis will probably be health-seeking behaviors: information on contraception related to an expressed desire to practice family planning.

### Nursing Plan and Implementation

The teaching plan focuses on confirming that a chosen method of contraception is a good choice for the woman. The nurse then helps the woman learn the method so that she can use it effectively.

### Client Goals

At the completion of the teaching, the woman will be able to

1. Confirm for herself that the chosen method of contraception is appropriate for her.
2. List the advantages, disadvantages, and risks of the chosen method.
3. Describe (or demonstrate) the correct procedure for using the chosen method.
4. Cite warning signs that should be reported to the caregiver.

## *Teaching Plan*

| CONTENT | TEACHING METHOD |
|---|---|
| Discuss the factors that a woman should consider in choosing a method of contraception (Table 4–2). Stress that the different methods may be appropriate at different times in the woman's life. Review the woman's reasons for selecting a particular method and confirm any contraindications to specific methods. | Contraception is a personal decision, so the discussion should take place in a private area free of interruptions.<br>Create a supportive, warm, and comfortable atmosphere by attitude and communication style—both verbal and nonverbal.<br>Provide accurate information in an open, nonjudgmental way. |
| Discuss the advantages, disadvantages, and risks of the chosen method. | Focus on open discussion. It may help to have written information about the method chosen. If a signed permit is required (as with sterilization or IUD insertion), the physician should also discuss the advantages, disadvantages, and risks. |
| Describe the correct procedure for using a method. Go through step-by-step. Periodically stop and have the woman review the information. If a technique is to be learned (as with inserting a diaphragm or charting basal body temperature), demonstrate and then have the woman do a return demonstration as appropriate. (*Note:* If certain aspects are beyond the nurse's level of expertise, the nurse can review the content and confirm that the woman has the opportunity to do a return demonstration. For example, an office nurse who does not do cervical cap fittings may cover information on its use, have the woman try inserting the cap herself, and then have the placement checked by the nurse practitioner or physician.) | Learning is best accomplished when material is broken down into smaller steps.<br>Have a model or chart available to enable the woman to visualize what is being described. Have a sample of the chosen method available: a package of oral contraceptives, an open IUD, or a symptothermal chart. |
| Provide information on what the woman should do if unusual circumstances arise (she forgets a pill or misses a morning temperature).<br>Stress warning signs that require immediate action on the part of the woman and explain why these signs indicate a risk. Carefully delineate the actions the woman should take. | Provide a written handout identifying the warning signs of her chosen method and listing the actions a woman should take. The handout should also cover actions the woman should take if an unusual situation develops. For example, what should she do if she vomits or has diarrhea while taking oral contraceptives?<br>Arrange to talk with the woman again soon, either on the phone or at a return visit, to determine if she has any questions about the method and to ensure that no problems have arisen. |

### EVALUATION

Evaluate the woman's learning by asking her to describe the method she has chosen, its contradictions and warning signs, and the procedure for using it correctly. In some cases, a return demonstration is useful.

**TABLE 4–2 Factors to Consider in Choosing a Method of Contraception**

| | |
|---|---|
| Effectiveness of method in preventing pregnancy<br>Safety of the method:<br>Are there inherent risks?<br>Does it offer protection against STIs or other conditions?<br>Client's age and future childbearing plans<br>Any contraindications in client's health history<br>Religious or moral factors influencing choice | Personal preferences, biases<br>Lifestyle:<br>How frequently does client have intercourse?<br>Does she have multiple partners?<br>Does she have ready access to medical care in the event of complications?<br>Is cost a factor?<br>Partner's support and willingness to cooperate<br>Personal motivation to use method |

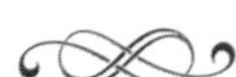

### Clinical Interruption of Pregnancy

Although abortion was legalized in the United States in 1973, the associated controversy over moral and legal issues continues. This controversy is as readily apparent in the medical and nursing professions as in other groups.

Many women are strongly opposed to abortion for religious, ethical, or personal reasons. Other women feel that access to a safe, legal abortion is every woman's right. A number of physical and psychosocial factors influence a woman's decision to seek an abortion. The presence of a disease or health state that jeopardizes the mother's life and serious, life-threatening fetal problems are frequently suggested as indications for abortion. In other instances, the timing or circumstance of the pregnancy creates an inordinate stress on the woman and she chooses an abortion. Some of these situations may involve contraceptive failure, rape, or incest.

Abortion in the first trimester is technically easier and safer than abortion in the second trimester. It may be performed by dilatation and curettage (D&C), minisuction, or vacuum curettage. The major risks include perforation of the uterus, laceration of the cervix, systemic reaction to the anesthetic agent, hemorrhage, and infection. Second trimester abortion may be done using dilatation and extraction (D&E), hypertonic saline, systemic prostaglandins, and intrauterine prostaglandins.

In 2000 the FDA approved mifepristone (Mifeprex), originally called RU 486, for use to induce abortion medically during the first 7 weeks of pregnancy (up to 49 days following conception). Mifepristone blocks the action of progesterone, thereby altering the endometrium. After the length of the woman's gestation is confirmed, she takes a dose of mifepristone. Two days later she returns to her caregiver and takes a dose of the prostaglandin misoprostel, which induces contractions that expel the embryo/fetus. About 12 days after taking the misoprostel, the woman is seen a third time to confirm that the abortion was successful.

### Nursing Care Management

Important aspects of nursing care for a woman who chooses to have an abortion include providing information about the methods of abortion and associated risks; counseling regarding available alternatives to abortion and their implications; encouraging verbalization by the woman; providing support before, during, and after the procedure; monitoring vital signs, intake, and output; providing for physical comfort and privacy throughout the procedure; and health teaching about self-care, the importance of the postabortion checkup, and contraception review.

## Recommended Gynecologic Screening Procedures

The accepted standard of care for women today involves the regular completion of a variety of screening procedures designed to detect potential problems early to permit the most effective treatment. This section focuses on some of the most commonly used screening procedures: breast self-examination and breast examination by a trained health care provider, mammography, Pap smear, and pelvic examination.

### Breast Examination

Like the uterus, the breast undergoes regular cyclical changes in response to hormonal stimulation. Each month, in rhythm with the cycle of ovulation, the breasts become engorged with fluid in anticipation of pregnancy, and the woman may experience sensations of tenderness, lumpiness, or pain. If conception does not occur, the accumulated fluid drains away via the lymphatic network. *Mastodynia* (premenstrual swelling and tenderness of the breasts) is common. It usually lasts for 3 to 4 days before the onset of menses, but the symptoms may persist throughout the month.

After menopause, adipose breast tissue atrophies and is replaced by connective tissue. Elasticity is lost, and the breasts may droop and become pendulous. The recurring breast engorgement associated with ovulation ceases. If estrogen replacement therapy is used to counteract other symptoms of menopause, breast engorgement may resume.

Monthly **breast self-examination (BSE)** is the best method for detecting breast masses early. A woman who knows the texture and feel of her own breasts is far more likely to detect changes that develop. Thus it is important for a woman to develop the habit of doing routine BSE as early as possible, preferably as an adolescent. Women at high risk for breast cancer are especially encouraged to be attentive to the importance of early detection through routine BSE.

In the course of a routine physical examination or during an initial visit to the caregiver, the woman should be taught BSE technique and its importance as a monthly practice. The effectiveness of BSE is determined by the woman's ability to perform the procedure correctly.

Breast self-examination should be performed on a regular monthly basis about 1 week after each menstrual period, when the breasts are typically not tender or swollen. After menopause, BSE should be performed on the same day each month (chosen by the woman for ease of remembrance).

Breast self-examination is most effective when it uses a dual approach incorporating both inspection and palpation. See the Teaching Guide: Teaching Breast Self-Examination.

Clinical breast examination by a trained health care provider, such as a physician, nurse-practitioner, or nurse-midwife, is an essential element of a routine gynecologic examination. Experience in differentiating among benign, suspicious, and worrisome breast changes enables the caregiver to reassure the woman if the findings are normal or move forward with additional diagnostic procedures or referral if the findings are suspicious or worrisome.

## Mammography

A **mammogram** is a soft tissue x-ray of the breast without the injection of a contrast medium. It can detect lesions in the breast before they can be felt and has gained wide acceptance as an effective screening tool for breast cancer. Currently the American Cancer Society, the American Medical Association, and the American College of Radiology recommend that all women age 40 and over have an annual mammogram. The National Cancer Institute recommends mammograms every 1 to 2 years for women ages 40 to 49 and annually for all women ages 50 and older.

## Pap Smear and Pelvic Examination

The Papanicolaou test (**Pap smear**) has played an important role in decreasing the incidence of death from cervical cancer. In countries without routine cervical screening, cervical cancer is the first or second leading cause of cancer-related deaths among women. By contrast, in the United States, cervical cancer is ranked 11th as a cancer-related cause of death (Cox, 1999). The purpose of the Pap smear is to detect cellular abnormalities by obtaining a smear containing cells from the cervix and the endocervical canal. Precancerous and cancerous conditions, as well as atypical findings and inflammatory changes, can be identified by microscopic examination of a Pap smear slide. A newer test, the *ThinPrep Pap test,* is proving even more effective than the traditional Pap smear in detecting abnormalities. In this test, no slide is prepared. Instead, the cervical cells, which are gathered in the same way as for the Pap smear, are transferred directly to a vial of preservative fluid, thereby preserving the entire specimen.

Women should be advised to avoid douching, intercourse, female hygiene products, and spermicidal agents immediately before a specimen is obtained for screening. Specimens should not be obtained during menstruation or when visible cervicitis exists.

Women who have reached the age of 18 and women, regardless of age, who are or have been sexually active should have a pelvic examination and Pap smear annually.

The pelvic examination enables the health care provider to assess a variety of factors about the woman's vagina, uterus, ovaries, and lower abdominal area. It is often performed after the Pap smear but may also be performed without a Pap for diagnostic purposes. Women sometimes perceive the pelvic exam as uncomfortable and embarrassing. The negative feelings may cause women to delay having yearly gynecologic examinations, and this avoidance may pose a threat to life and health.

Text continues on page 81.

### HINTS FOR PRACTICE

Whenever you teach about pelvic examination and Pap smear, be certain that the woman understands that she should not douche for at least 24 hours beforehand. Douching can interfere with the accuracy of the Pap smear. Occasionally a caregiver will specifically request that a woman use a douche before a Pap smear; douching should only be done in this circumstance.

## TEACHING GUIDE *Teaching Breast Self-Examination*

### Assessment

The nurse determines the woman's general knowledge about breast self-examination (BSE), identifies previous experience with BSE, identifies risk factors for breast cancer, determines the woman's general knowledge about breast cancer, identifies barriers to BSE, and discusses her commitment to practice BSE.

### Nursing Diagnosis

The key nursing diagnosis will probably be health-seeking behavior: information on BSE related to an expressed need to take action to detect breast abnormalities.

### Nursing Plan and Implementation

The teaching plan focuses on assisting the woman to learn BSE so that she can use it effectively.

### Client Goals

At the completion of the teaching, the woman will be able to

1. Discuss her risk of breast cancer.
2. Describe the use of BSE in breast cancer detection.
3. Demonstrate the correct procedure for BSE.
4. List warning signs of breast cancer to be reported to the caregiver.
5. Incorporate monthly BSE into her personal routine.

## *Teaching Plan*

| CONTENT | TEACHING METHOD |
|---|---|
| Discuss the risk factors associated with breast cancer. | Breast cancer should be discussed in a private area free of interruptions. The room needs to have a mirror; bed, couch, or examining table; pillows; a patient gown; and a private area for the woman to disrobe. |
| Stress the unique risk factors associated with the woman's personal history and lifestyle. | Create a supportive, warm, and comfortable atmosphere by attitude and communication style—both verbal and nonverbal. A discussion of breast cancer may bring forth many emotions in the woman, including grief for previous breast cancer–related losses. |
| Discuss the use of BSE in breast cancer detection. | Focus on open discussion. A brochure with statistics and illustrations may be useful. Stress the positive outcomes of early detection to counterbalance fears. |

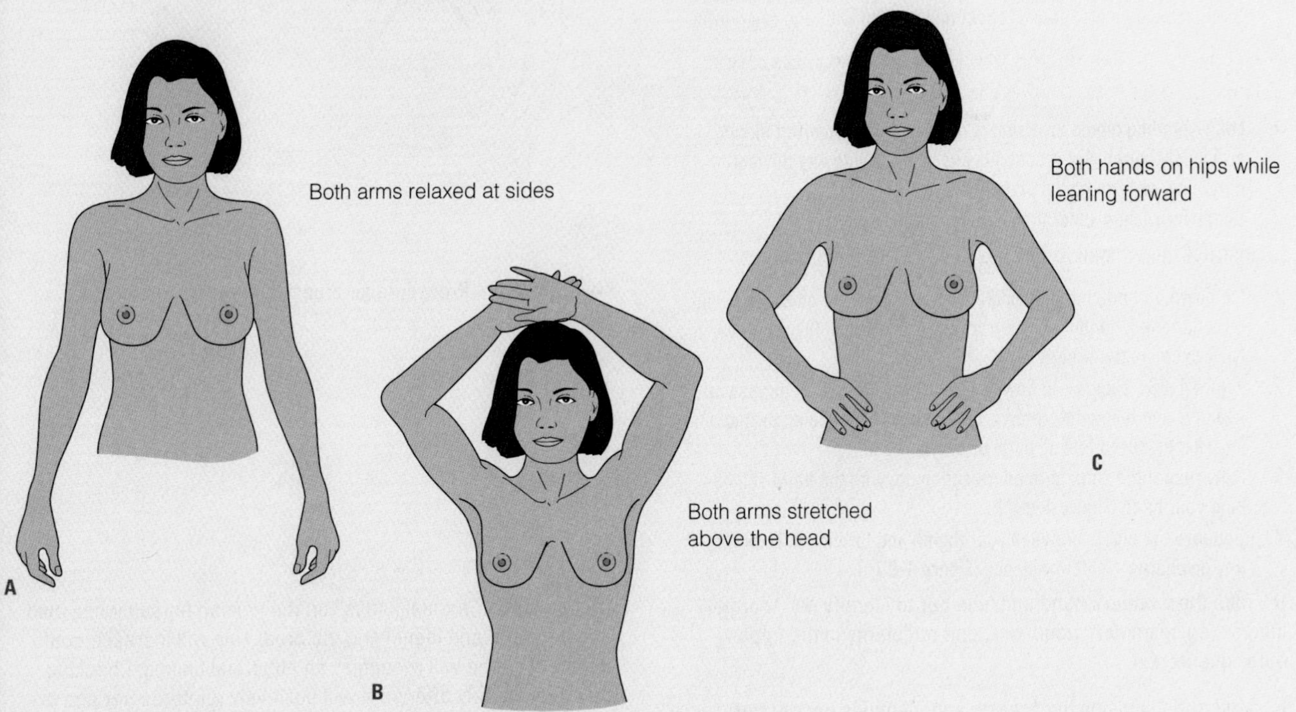


FIGURE 4–8 ♦ Positions for inspection of the breasts.

Describe and demonstrate the correct procedure for BSE.

A. Instruct the woman to inspect her breasts by standing or sitting in front of a mirror. She needs to inspect her breasts in three positions: with both arms relaxed down at her sides, both arms stretched straight over her head, and both hands placed on her hips while leaning forward (Figure 4–8♦).

B. Advise the woman to look at her breasts individually and in comparison with one another. Note and record the following characteristics for each position:

### Size and Symmetry of the Breasts

1. Breasts may vary, but the variations should remain constant during rest or movement—note abnormal contours.
2. Some size difference between the breasts is normal.

### Shape and Direction of the Breasts

1. The shape of the breasts can be rounded or pendulous with some variation between breasts.
2. The breasts should be pointing slightly laterally.

### Color, Thickening, Edema, and Venous Patterns

1. Check for redness or inflammation.
2. A blue hue with a marked venous pattern that is focal or unilateral may indicate an area of increased blood supply due to tumor. Symmetric venous patterns are normal.
3. Skin edema observed as thickened skin with enlarged pores ("orange peel") may indicate blocked lymphatic drainage due to tumor.

### Surface of the Breasts

1. Skin dimpling, puckering, or retraction (pulling) when the woman presses her hands together or against her hips suggests malignancy.
2. Striae (stretch marks) red at onset and whitish with age are normal.

### Nipple Size and Shape, Direction, Rashes, Ulcerations, and Discharge

1. Long-standing nipple inversion is normal, but an inverted nipple previously capable of erection is suspicious. Note any deviation, flattening, or broadening of the nipples.
2. Check for rashes, ulcerations, or discharge.

C. Instruct the woman to palpate (feel) her breasts as follows:

1. Lie down. Put one hand behind your head. With the other hand, fingers flattened, gently feel your breast. Press lightly (Figure 4–9A♦). Now examine the breast.
2. Figure 4–9B♦ shows you how to check each breast. Begin as you see in B and follow the arrows, feeling gently for a lump or thickening. Remember to feel all parts of each breast.
3. Now repeat the same procedure sitting up, with the hand still behind your head (Figure 4–9C♦).
4. Squeeze the nipple between your thumb and forefinger. Look for any discharge—clear or bloody (Figure 4–9D♦).

D. Take the woman's hand and help her to identify her "normal lumps" (eg, mammary ridge, ribs, and nodularity in the upper outer quadrants).

E. After she examines her breasts and identifies her normal lumps, instruct her to palpate her breasts once more to identify any areas that she may have questions about. If questions arise,

Learning is best accomplished when material is broken down into smaller steps and presented with multiple approaches. Prior to asking the woman to perform BSE, use a model or a chart to demonstrate the procedure. Then have the woman perform BSE. Be very supportive and give a lot of positive feedback because some women may be embarrassed. Demonstrate a nonjudgmental, accepting attitude.

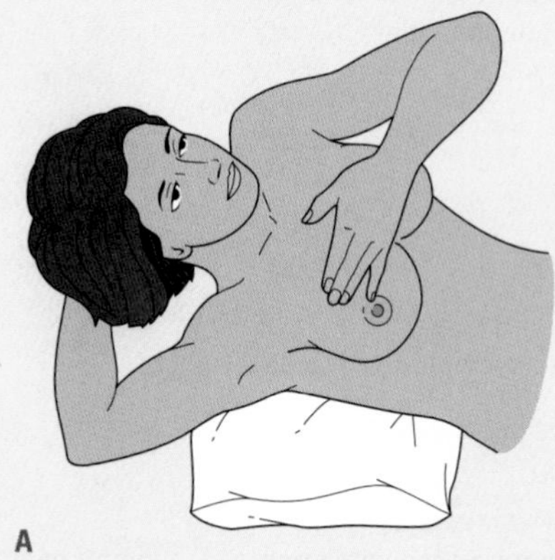

With one hand behind your head, flatten your fingers and press lightly on your breast, feeling gently for a lump or thickening.
A


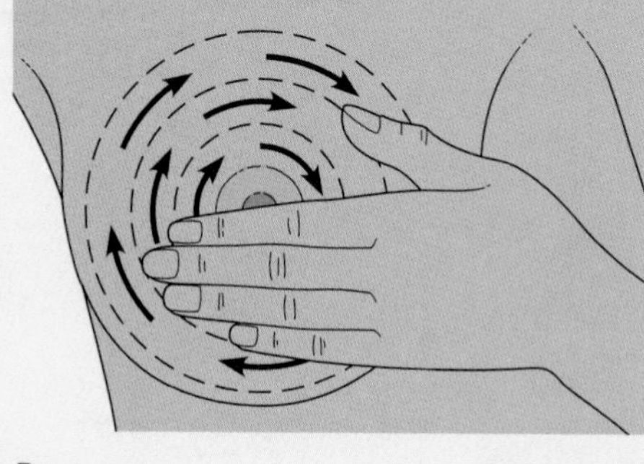

Check each breast in a circular manner, feeling all parts of the breast.
B


FIGURE 4–9 ♦ Procedure for breast self-examination.

Demonstrate "normal lumps" on the woman herself while guiding her hand and identifying the area. This will increase confidence that she will recognize an abnormal finding. Checking her immediately afterward will positively reinforce her and diminish the fear associated with BSE.

the nurse should palpate the area and attempt to identify whether it is normal.

F. If a breast model is available, instruct the woman to palpate it and identify the lumps.

G. Provide information on the warning signs of breast cancer and what she should do if she identifies any of these signs during BSE.

Provide a written handout on the warning signs of breast cancer. The handout should also cover actions that the woman should take if a warning sign is discovered. Stress the positive effects of early detection.

## TIMING

Instruct the woman to perform BSE on a monthly basis. Be specific based on whether she is premenopausal, pregnant, postmenopausal, or postmenopausal receiving hormone replacement therapy.

Provide the woman with a reminder symbol for monthly BSE. The American Cancer Society provides such items to hang in the shower, place on a refrigerator, and so forth. Praise her commitment to do monthly BSE. Give the woman a follow-up telephone number (eg, American Cancer Society) to use if she needs additional information or has questions.

## EVALUATION

Evaluate the woman's learning through discussion and return demonstration. Learning has occurred if the woman performs BSE correctly and can identify timing, normal and abnormal findings, and follow-up activities.

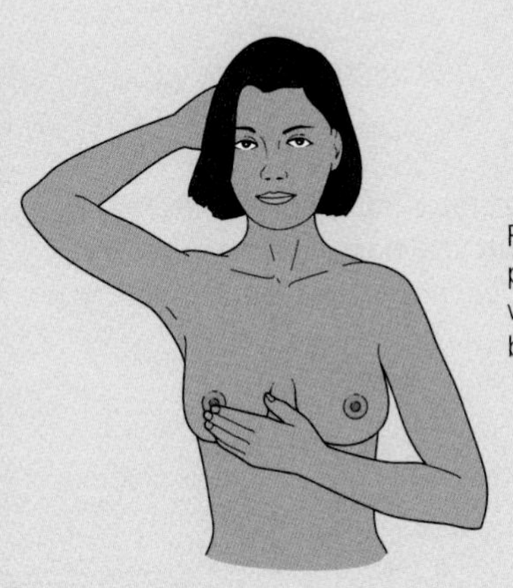
Repeat the same procedure sitting up with your hand still behind your head.
C

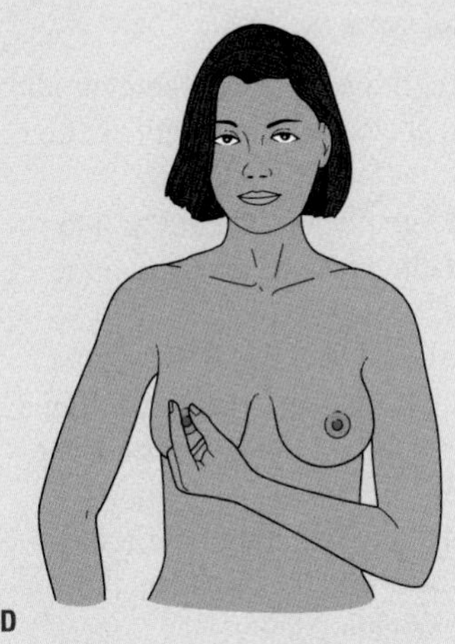
Squeeze your nipple between your thumb and forefinger; look for any clear or bloody discharge.
D

**FIGURE 4–9** ♦ Procedure for breast self-examination (*continued*).

Source: American Cancer Society. (1973). Breast self-examination and the nurse, No. 3408 PE. New York: Author.

To make the pelvic examination less threatening, and thus improve health-seeking behavior, more health care providers are performing what is called an educational pelvic examination. This includes offering the woman a mirror to watch the procedure, pointing out anatomic parts to her, and positioning and draping her to allow eye-to-eye contact with the practitioner. The woman is encouraged to participate by asking questions and giving feedback.

Nurse practitioners, certified nurse-midwives, and physicians all perform pelvic examinations. Nurses assist the practitioner and the woman during the examination. Procedure 4–1 provides information on assisting with a pelvic examination.

# Menopause

**Menopause,** the time when menses cease, is a time of transition for a woman, marking the end of her reproductive abilities. *Climacteric,* or *change of life* (often used synonymously with menopause), refers to the host of psychologic and physical alterations that occur around the time of menopause.

# *Procedure 4–1* Assisting with a Pelvic Examination

| *Nursing Action* | *Rationale* |
|---|---|
| **Objective: Provide a warm environment.**<br>Turn on overhead heat lights, if available, or turn up the thermostat. | *Warm environment promotes comfort.* |
| **Objective: Assemble and prepare the equipment.** | |
| • Prepare and arrange the following items so that they are easily accessible: | *Equipment organization facilitates the examination.* |
| a. Vaginal specula of various sizes, warmed with water or on a heating pad prior to insertion<br>b. Gloves<br>c. Water-soluble lubricant<br>d. Materials for Pap smear and cultures<br>e. Good light source | *A warmed speculum assists in lubrication and facilitates initial insertion when culture and smears are taken.* |
| • Do not use lubricant on the speculum before insertion. | *Use of lubricant may alter findings or cultures.* |
| **Objective: Prepare the woman.** | |
| • Explain the procedure. If the woman has never had a pelvic examination, show her the equipment and explain the procedure before examination. | *Explanation of the procedure decreases anxiety.* |
| • Instruct the woman to empty her bladder and to remove clothing below the waist. She may want to leave her shoes on. | *An empty bladder promotes comfort during internal examination. Some women feel more comfortable with shoes on, rather than supporting their weight with bare heels against cold stirrups.* |
| • Give the woman a disposable drape or sheet to place on her lap. Encourage her to sit on the end of the examining table with the drape across her lap. | |
| • Position the woman in the lithotomy position with her thighs flexed and adducted. Place her feet in the stirrups. Her buttocks should extend slightly beyond the end of the examining table. | |
| • Drape the woman with the sheet, leaving a flap so the perineum can be exposed. | |
| **Objective: Provide support to the woman as the physician or nurse practitioner performs the examination.** | |
| • Explain each part of the examination as it is performed: inspection of external genitals, vagina, and cervix; bimanual examination of internal organs. | *Explanations promote relaxation.* |
| • Instruct the woman to relax and breathe slowly. | |
| • Advise the woman when the speculum is about to be inserted and ask her to bear down. | *When the speculum is inserted, the woman may feel intravaginal pressure. Bearing down helps open the vaginal orifice and relaxes the perineal muscles.* |
| • Lubricate the examiner's finger prior to bimanual examination. | *Lubrication decreases friction and eases insertion.* |

## *Procedure 4–1* Assisting with a Pelvic Examination

*continued*

| *Nursing Action* | *Rationale* |
|---|---|
| **OBJECTIVE: PROVIDE FOR THE WOMAN'S COMFORT AT THE END OF THE EXAMINATION.** | |
| • Move to the end of the examination table and face the woman's perineum. Cover the woman with the drape. Apply gentle pressure to the woman's knees and encourage her to move toward the head of the table. Offer your hand to the woman, remove her heels from the stirrups, and assist her to a sitting position. Be sure that she is not dizzy and that she is sitting or standing safely before you leave the room. | *The supine position may cause postural hypotension.* |
| • Provide tissues to wipe lubricant from the perineum.<br>• Provide privacy while the woman dresses. | *Upon assuming a sitting position, vaginal secretions along with lubricant may be discharged.* |

Today the average age at menopause is 51.4 years, and the average life span of a woman in the United States is over 80 years. Thus the average woman will live one-third of her life after menopause (Hammond, 1999). A woman's psychologic adaptation to menopause and the climacteric is multifactorial. She is influenced by her own expectations and knowledge, physical well-being, family views, marital stability, and sociocultural expectations. As the number of women reaching menopause increases, the negative emotional connotations society once attached to menopause are diminishing, enabling menopausal women to cope more effectively and even encouraging them to view menopause as a time of personal growth.

The physical characteristics of menopause are linked to the shift from a cyclic to a noncyclic hormonal pattern. Menopause usually occurs between 45 and 52 years of age. The age at onset may be influenced by nutritional, cultural, or genetic factors. The physiologic mechanisms initiating its onset are not precisely known. The onset of menopause occurs when estrogen levels become so low that menstruation stops.

Generally ovulation ceases 1 to 2 years before menopause, but individual variations exist. Atrophy of the ovaries occurs gradually. FSH levels rise, and less estrogen is produced. Menopausal symptoms include atrophic changes in the vagina, vulva, and urethra and in the trigonal area of the bladder.

Many menopausal women experience a vasomotor disturbance commonly known as *hot flashes,* a feeling of heat arising from the chest and spreading to the neck and face. The hot flashes are often accompanied by sweating and sleep disturbances. These episodes may occur as often as 20 to 30 times a day and generally last 3 to 5 minutes. Some women also experience dizzy spells, palpitations, and weakness. Many women find their own most effective ways to deal with the hot flashes. Some report that using a fan or drinking a cool liquid helps relieve distress; others seek relief through hormone replacement therapy. In addition, many women use complementary therapies (see later discussion).

The uterine endometrium and myometrium atrophy, as do the cervical glands. The uterine cavity constricts. The fallopian tubes and ovaries atrophy extensively. The vaginal mucosa becomes smooth and thin, and the rugae disappear, leading to loss of elasticity. As a result, intercourse can be painful, but this problem may be overcome by using lubricating gel. Dryness of the mucous membrane can lead to burning and itching. The vaginal pH level increases as the number of Döderlein's bacilli decreases.

Postmenopausal women can still be multiorgasmic. Some women find that their sexual interest and activity improve as the need for contraception disappears and personal growth and awareness increase. Other women experience a decrease in libido at this time. Vulvar atrophy occurs late, and the pubic hair thins, turns gray or white, and may ultimately disappear. The labia shrivel and lose their heightened pigmentation. Pelvic fascia and muscles atrophy, resulting in decreased pelvic support. The breasts become pendulous and decrease in size and firmness.

Long-range physical changes may include **osteoporosis,** a decrease in the bony skeletal mass. This change is thought to be associated with lowered estrogen and androgen levels, lack of physical exercise, and a chronic low intake of calcium. Moreover, the estrogen deprivation that occurs in menopausal women may significantly increase their risk of coronary heart disease. Loss of protein from the skin and supportive tissues causes wrinkling. Postmenopausal women frequently gain weight, which may be due to excessive caloric intake or to lower caloric need with the same level of intake.

## Clinical Therapy

### Hormone Replacement Therapy

**Hormone replacement therapy (HRT),** usually involving estrogen with or without a progestin, had been controversial for years, but currently the American College of Obstetricians and Gynecologists recommends HRT in menopause. Estrogen replacement is helpful in stopping hot flashes and night sweats and in reversing atrophic vaginal changes. Perhaps most significantly, HRT may reduce the incidence of coronary artery disease, the leading cause of death in postmenopausal women. Other benefits of HRT include prevention and treatment of bone loss associated with osteoporosis, improved bladder and vaginal tone, and improved quality of life. It may also improve memory and offer protection against Alzheimer's disease, colon cancer, and macular degeneration (the leading cause of legal blindness in the United States) (Hammond, 1999). Whether HRT increases the incidence of breast cancer is debated, but research suggests that there is an increased risk of breast cancer in women who use HRT that includes progesterone for extended periods of time (Schairer, Lubin, Troisi, et al., 2000).

When estrogen is given alone, it can produce endometrial hyperplasia and increase the risk of endometrial cancer. Thus, in women who still have a uterus, estrogen is opposed by giving a progestin, often Provera, for a portion of the cycle. HRT may be given continuously or sequentially. The continuous approach involves the daily administration of 0.625 mg estrogen with 2.5 mg progestin. This regimen is associated with less vaginal bleeding and is sufficient to prevent endometrial hyperplasia and osteoporosis; it also retains most of estrogen's beneficial effects on the cardiovascular system (Speroff, 1999). With the sequential approach, estrogen is given the first 25 days of the month, with 5 to 10 mg progestin added during the last 12 days of the estrogen administration (days 14 to 25). Although most women prefer to take estrogen orally, some choose the transdermal estrogen skin patch. Estrogen may also be given by injection. For women experiencing decreased libido, combination estrogen-testosterone preparations are available.

A thorough history, physical examination including Pap smear, and baseline mammogram are indicated before starting HRT. An initial endometrial biopsy is indicated for women with an increased risk of endometrial cancer; biopsy is also indicated if excessive, unexpected, or prolonged vaginal bleeding occurs. Women taking estrogen should be advised to stop immediately if they develop headaches, visual changes, signs of thrombophlebitis, or chest pain.

### Alternative and Complementary Therapies

For women who do not wish to take HRT or who have medical contraindications to it, a variety of approaches have been proposed as alternative or complementary treatment or preventive measures for the discomforts of the perimenopausal and postmenopausal years. These include diet and nutrition, specifically a high-fiber, low-fat diet with supplements of vitamins D and E. Phytoestrogens (substances with estrogen properties), found in a number of foods, especially soy products, can play a significant role in reducing menopausal symptoms. About 10% of women have tried herbal remedies such as long quai and black cohosh, which have been used in traditional Chinese medicine for years but have not yet been well studied (Nachtigall, 2000). Weight-bearing exercises such as walking, jogging, tennis, and low-impact aerobics help increase bone mass and decrease the risk of osteoporosis. Exercise also improves cholesterol profiles and contributes to overall health. Stress management and relaxation techniques such as biofeedback, meditation, yoga, visualization, and massage may provide a sense of well-being. Some women also use homeopathic remedies for symptom relief (Lindsay, 1999).

### Prevention and Treatment of Osteoporosis

Osteoporosis is more common in women who are middle-aged or older. The following risk factors are also associated with osteoporosis:

- White or Asian heritage
- Small-boned and thin
- Family history of osteoporosis
- Lack of regular exercise
- Nulliparous
- Early onset of menopause
- Consistently low intake of calcium
- Cigarette smoking
- Moderate to heavy alcohol intake

Pre- or postmenopausal women with four or more risk factors for osteoporosis should have their bone mass measured. Women's height should be measured at each visit, because a loss of height is often an early sign that vertebrae are being compressed because of reduced bone

## EVIDENCE-BASED PRACTICE

### Osteoporosis

You are scheduled to spend a day in the women's clinic of a local retirement center working with a nurse who does health teaching with the clinic's clients. Your instructor recommends that you be prepared to discuss osteoporosis, nutrition, and bone density testing and refers you to the National Guideline Clearinghouse at www.guideline.gov. The guideline she suggests is titled *Physician's Guide to Prevention and Treatment of Osteoporosis.* This guideline seems daunting when you read that it was developed as a collaborative effort by 10 specialty organizations. However, when you begin the review, you find it clear and easy to use.

The guideline recommends that women consume at least 1200 mg/day of dietary calcium. A supplemental capsule may be necessary if this intake is not achievable with dairy products and the appropriate vegetables. Studies show that this simple intervention can reduce the rate of osteoporosis-related fractures by 10%. When combined with vitamin D (400 to 800 IU/day recommended as a supplement for women at risk of deficiency) a single study shows a 25% decrease in fractures of the hip and 15% decrease in other fractures. This will be important information to include in the education sessions.

The clinic also offers referrals for bone mineral density testing, but you do not know who should be tested. This guideline tells you that women under age 65 who have risk factors besides menopause should be tested. After age 65 all women should be tested regardless of risk factors. You also learn that there are several ways bone mineral density testing can be done using technologies such as single photon absorptimometry, quantitative computed tomography, and ultrasound densitometry.

In addition, the guideline offers detailed information on hormone replacement therapy and other interventions that have been studied for their effectiveness in treating osteoporosis. You pay heed to an especially strong statement in the guidelines. It advises caregivers to urge every postmenopausal woman to consider her risk of osteoporosis. "Osteoporosis is a 'silent risk' factor for fracture just as hypertension is for stroke."

You feel more confident about having current and accurate information for the women you will see at the clinic. You recognize that your instructor guided you to a solid resource that offers a systematic review of the evidence so that your practice is grounded by accurate, up-to-date information.

*Source:* National Osteoporosis Foundation. (1999). *Physician's guide to prevention and treatment of osteoporosis* [Online]. Washington, DC: Author. Available: www.guideline.gov

mass. A variety of conditions, including malabsorption syndrome, cancer, cirrhosis of the liver, chronic use of cortisone, and rheumatoid arthritis, can cause secondary arthritis, which resembles osteoporosis. If these secondary causes have been eliminated, treatment for osteoporosis is initiated.

Prevention of osteoporosis is a primary goal of care. Women are advised to maintain an adequate calcium intake. Women over age 50 should have a daily calcium intake of 1200 mg. Most women require supplements to achieve this level. They should also have a daily vitamin D intake of 400 to 800 IU. Women are also advised to participate regularly in exercise, to consume only modest quantities of alcohol and caffeine, and to stop smoking. Alcohol and smoking have a negative effect on the rate of bone resorption.

The effectiveness of estrogen in preventing osteoporosis is well documented. Women with no contraindications to estrogen who are showing evidence of bone loss are good candidates for HRT. For women who are unable or unwilling to take estrogen, other medications available to treat or help prevent osteoporosis include the following (National Institutes of Health, 2000):

- Alendronate (Fosamax), etidronate (Didronel), and risedronate (Actonel): calcium regulators that act by inhibiting bone resorption and increasing bone mass
- Raloxifene (Evista): one of a new class of drugs called selective estrogen receptor modulators that preserve the beneficial effects of estrogen, including its protection against osteoporosis, but do not stimulate uterine or breast tissue
- Intranasal calcitonin: a calcium regulator that may inhibit bone loss; its value is less clear than that of the other medications listed.

## Nursing Care Management

Most menopausal women deal well with this developmental phase of life, although some women may need counseling to adjust successfully. Reaction to menopause is determined to a large extent by the life the woman has lived, by the security she has in her feminine identity, and by her feelings of self-worth and self-esteem.

Nurses and other health care professionals can help the menopausal woman achieve high-level functioning at this time in her life. Of paramount importance is the nurse's ability to understand and provide support for the woman's views and feelings. Whether the woman expresses relief and delight or tearfulness and fear, the nurse needs to use an empathic approach in counseling, health teaching, and providing physical care.

Nurses should explore the question of the woman's comfort during sexual intercourse. In counseling, the nurse may say, "After menopause many women notice that their vagina seems dryer and intercourse can be uncomfortable. Have you noticed any changes?" This gives the woman information and may open discussion. The nurse can then go on to explain that dryness and shrinking of the vagina can be addressed by use of a water-soluble jelly. Use of estrogen, orally or in vaginal creams, may also be indicated. Increased frequency of intercourse will maintain some elasticity in the vagina. When assessing the menopausal woman, the nurse should address the question of sexual activity openly but tactfully, because the woman may have been socialized to be reticent in discussing sex.

The crucial need of women in the perimenopausal period of life is for adequate information about the changes taking place in their bodies and their lives. Supplying that information provides both a challenge and an opportunity for nurses.

# Violence Against Women

Violence against women has reached epidemic proportions in society today. Violence affects women of all ages, races, ethnic backgrounds, socioeconomic levels, educational levels, and walks of life. Two of the most common forms of violence are intimate partner abuse and rape. Society not only accepts these forms of violence against women but also shifts the blame for the violence to the women themselves by asking questions such as "How did she make him so mad?" "Why does she stay?" "What was she doing out so late?" and "Why did she dress that way?"

Violence against women is a major health concern, one that costs the health care system millions of dollars and thousands of lives. In response to this epidemic health care providers are becoming more knowledgeable about actions they should take to provide effective care.

## Female Partner Abuse

*Intimate partner abuse* can be defined as collective methods used to exert power and control by one individual over another in an adult domestic or intimate relationship. Gay men, heterosexual women, and lesbian women batter, but most abusers are male, and the overwhelming majority of victims are women (Gantt & Bickford, 1999). Consequently, we use the term **female partner abuse** in discussing this serious health problem.

Female partner abuse is the most common form of violence in the United States but the least reported serious crime. Research suggests that 18% to 25% of women treated in emergency departments and almost one-fourth of women seeking prenatal care are victims of violence (Valente, 2000). Worldwide, as many as one in three women will be the victim of violence or sexual coercion at some point in her life (State of the World Population, 2000).

The woman may or may not be married to her abuser. She may be living with, dating, or divorced from him. Female partner abuse takes many forms, including verbal attacks, insults, intimidation, threats, emotional abuse, social isolation, economic deprivation, intellectual derision, ridicule, stalking, and physical attacks and injury. Physical battering includes slapping, kicking, shoving, punching, forms of torture, attacks with objects or weapons, and sexual assault. Women who are physically abused can also suffer psychologic and emotional abuse.

### Cycle of Violence

In an effort to explain the experience of battered women, Walker (1984) developed the theory of the *cycle of violence.* Battering takes place in a cyclic fashion through three phases:

1. In the *tension-building phase,* the batterer demonstrates power and control. This phase is characterized by anger, arguing, blaming the woman for external problems, and possibly minor battering incidents. The woman may blame herself and believe she can prevent the escalation of the batterer's anger by her own actions.
2. The *acute battering incident* is typically triggered by some external event or internal state of the batterer. It is an episode of acute violence distinguished by lack of control, lack of predictability, and major destructiveness. The cycle of violence

can be interrupted before the acute battering incident if proper interventions take place.

3. The *tranquil, loving phase* is sometimes termed the honeymoon period. This phase may be characterized by extremely kind and loving behavior on the part of the batterer as he tries to make up with the woman, or it may simply be manifested as an absence of tension and violence. Without intervention, this phase will end and the cycle of violence will continue. Over time the violence increases in severity and frequency.

### Characteristics of Battered Women

Battered women often hold traditional views of sex roles. Many were raised to be submissive, passive, and dependent and to seek approval from male figures. Some battered women were exposed to violence between their parents, whereas others first experienced it from their partners. Many battered women do not work outside the home. As part of the manipulation of batterers, they are isolated from family and friends and totally dependent on their partners for their financial and emotional needs.

Battered women may attribute their beatings to some personal shortcoming or inadequacy. Many believe their batterers' insults and accusations that they are bad wives or partners and negligent mothers. As these women become more isolated, they find it harder to judge who is right. Eventually they fully believe in their inadequacy, and their low self-esteem reinforces their belief that they deserve to be beaten. Battered women often feel a pervasive sense of guilt, fear, and depression. Their sense of hopelessness and helplessness reduces their problem-solving ability. Some women develop a pattern of behavior termed *learned helplessness,* in which the unknown becomes terrifying. Learned helplessness often plays a role in a woman's decision to stay in a known, though abusive, situation rather than leave and face the unknown. Some researchers suggest that a theory of survivorship better describes the behavior of many women who experience abuse. These women actively seek help and have found creative ways to survive in a relationship when help is not forthcoming (Poirier, 1997).

### Characteristics of Batterers

Batterers come from all backgrounds, professions, religious groups, and socioeconomic levels. Batterers often have feelings of insecurity, socioeconomic inferiority, powerlessness, and helplessness that conflict with their assumptions of male supremacy. Emotionally immature and aggressive men have a tendency to express these overwhelming feelings of inadequacy through violence. Many batterers feel undeserving of their partners, yet they blame and punish the very women they value.

Battered women often describe their husbands or partners as lacking respect toward women in general, having come from homes where they witnessed abuse of their mothers or were themselves abused as children, and having a hidden rage that erupts occasionally. Batterers accept traditional macho values, yet when they are not angry or aggressive, they appear childlike, dependent, seductive, manipulative, and in need of nurturing. They may be well respected in the community. This dual personality of batterers reflects the conflict between their belief that they must live up to their macho image and their feelings of inadequacy in the role of husband or provider. Combined with low frustration tolerance and poor impulse control, their pervasive sense of powerlessness leads them to strike out at life's inequities by abusing women.

## Nursing Care Management

Nurses in many different health care settings often come in contact with abused women but fail to recognize them, especially if their bruises are not visible. Women who are at high risk of battering often have a history of alcohol or drug abuse, child abuse, or abuse in the previous or present relationship. Other possible signs of abuse include expressions of helplessness and powerlessness; low self-esteem revealed by the woman's dress, appearance, and the way she relates to health care providers; signs of depression evidenced by fatigue, hopelessness, and somatic problems such as headache, insomnia, chest pain, back pain, or pelvic pain; and possible suicide attempts. In addition, the abused woman may have a history of missed or frequently changed appointments, perhaps because she had signs of abuse that kept her from coming in or her partner prevented it.

Because female partner abuse is so prevalent, many caregivers now advocate *universal screening of all female clients at every health encounter.* Screening should be done privately, with only the caregiver and client present, in a safe and quiet place. Specific language leads to higher disclosure rates. Possible screening questions include the following (American College of Obstetricians and Gynecologists [ACOG], 1999a):

1. Has your partner or anyone close to you ever threatened to hurt you?
2. During the past year, have you been kicked, hit, choked, or hurt physically?
3. Has your partner or anyone else ever forced you to have sex?

During the screening the nurse should assure the woman that her privacy will be respected. It is essential that the nurse remain nonjudgmental; create a warm, caring climate conducive to sharing; and demonstrate a willingness to talk about violence. A battered woman often interprets the nurse's willingness to discuss violence as permission for her to discuss it as well.

When a woman seeks care for an injury, the nurse should be alert to the following cues of abuse:

- Hesitation in providing detailed information about the injury and how it occurred
- Inappropriate affect for the situation
- Delayed reporting of symptoms
- Pattern of injury consistent with abuse, including multiple injury sites involving bruises, abrasions, and contusions to the head (eyes and back of the neck), throat, chest, abdomen, or genitals
- Inappropriate explanation for the injuries
- Lack of eye contact
- Signs of increased anxiety in the presence of the possible batterer, who frequently does much of the talking

When a battered woman comes in for treatment, she needs to feel safe physically and secure in talking about her injuries and problems. If a man is with her, the nurse should ask or tell him to remain in the waiting room while the woman is examined. A battered woman also needs to reestablish a feeling of control over her world. She needs to regain a sense of predictability by knowing what to expect and how she can interact. The nurse should provide sufficient information about what to expect in terms the woman can understand.

In providing care the nurse needs to let the woman work through her story, problems, and situation at her own pace. The nurse should reassure the woman that she is believed and not considered crazy. The nurse should anticipate the woman's ambivalence (due to her fear and possible love-hate relationship with her batterer) but also respect the woman's capacity to change and grow when she is ready. The woman may require assistance in identifying specific problems and in developing realistic ideas for reducing or eliminating those problems. In all interactions the nurse should stress that no one should be abused and that the abuse is not the woman's fault.

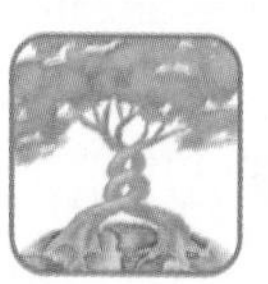

## Community-Based Nursing Care

The nurse should inform any woman suspected of being in an abusive situation of the services available in the health care agency and the community. A battered woman may need the following:

- Medical treatment for injuries
- Temporary shelter to provide a safe environment for her and her children
- Counseling to raise her self-esteem and help her understand the dynamics of family violence
- Legal assistance for a restraining order, protection, and/or prosecution
- Financial assistance to obtain shelter, food, and clothing
- Job training or employment counseling
- An ongoing support group with counseling

If the woman returns to an abusive situation, the nurse should encourage her to develop an exit plan for herself and her children, if any. As part of the plan, she should pack a change of clothing for herself and her children, including toiletries and an extra set of car and house keys. She should store these items away from the house with a friend or relative. If possible she should have money, identification papers (driver's license, social security card, and birth certificates for herself and her children), checkbook, savings account information, other financial information (such as mortgage papers, automobile papers, and pay stubs), court papers or orders, and information about the children to help her enroll them in school. She should also plan where she will go, regardless of the time of day. The nurse should ensure that the woman has a planned escape route and emergency telephone numbers she can call, including local police, a phone hotline, and a women's shelter if one is available in the community.

Working with battered women is challenging, and many health care providers feel frustrated and impotent when the women repeatedly return to their abusive situations without developing sufficient ego strength or coping abilities. On average, women leave their battering situation seven times before they stay away permanently. Nurses must realize that they cannot rescue battered women; battered women must decide on their own how to handle their situations. Effective nurses provide battered women with information that empowers them in decision making and supports their decisions, knowing that incremental assistance over the years may be the only alternative until the battered women are ready to explore other options.

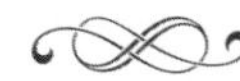

## Sexual Assault and Rape

In its broadest sense, **sexual assault** is involuntary sexual contact with another person. The National Crime Victimization Survey defines rape as follows: "**Rape** is forced sexual intercourse and includes both psychological coercion as well as physical force. Forced sexual intercourse means vaginal, anal, or oral penetration by the offender(s)." The person who commits a sexual assault may be an acquaintance, spouse, other relative, employer, or stranger. Sexual assault is an act of violence expressed sexually—most commonly, a man's aggression and rage acted out against a woman.

Sexual assault is one of the most underreported violent crimes in the United States. The National Center for the Prevention and Control of Rape estimates that one out of three women will be sexually assaulted at some time in her life. Estimates suggest that 1.3 rapes occur every minute in the United States (Haddix-Hill, 1997).

No woman of any age or ethnicity is immune, but statistics indicate that young, unmarried women, women who are unemployed or have a low family income, and students have the highest incidence of sexual assault or attempted assault. Adolescent survivors of sexual assault are often reluctant to report the assault because of embarrassment, feelings of guilt, fear of retribution, lack of knowledge of their legal rights, concerns about confidentiality, lack of funds, and limited access to health care. Young adolescents may also avoid disclosing an assault to authorities because they may be worried about revealing the circumstances, especially if they involved risk-taking behaviors such as underage drinking, drug use, accepting a ride from a stranger, or socializing with older men (Holmes, 1998).

Like their victims, the assailants come from all ethnic backgrounds and walks of life. More than half are under age 25, and three out of five are married and leading "normal" sex lives. Why do men rape? Of the many theories put forth, none provides a completely satisfactory explanation.

So few assailants are actually caught and convicted that a clear characteristic of the assailant has not been developed. However, rapists tend to be emotionally weak and insecure and may have difficulty maintaining interpersonal relationships. Many assailants also have trouble dealing with the stresses of daily life. Such men may become angry and overcome by feelings of powerlessness. They then commit a sexual assault as an expression of power or anger.

One type of sexual assault, *date rape* (a form of acquaintance rape), is an increasing problem on high school and college campuses. In some cases an assailant uses alcohol or other drugs to sedate his intended victim. One drug, flunitrazepam (Rohypnol) has gained notoriety as a date rape drug because it frequently produces amnesia in its victims. In date rape situations, the male is usually determined to have sex and will do whatever he feels necessary if denied. Thus in date rape the primary motivation is sexual gratification (Crooks & Baur, 1998), but it is still expressed as violence against the woman.

## Responses to Sexual Assault

Sexual assault is a situational crisis. It is a traumatic event that the victim cannot be prepared to handle because it is unforeseen. Following the assault, the victim generally experiences a cluster of symptoms, described by Burgess and Holmstrom (1979) as the *rape trauma syndrome,* that last far beyond the rape itself. These phases are described in Table 4–3. Although the phases of response are listed individually, they often overlap, and individual responses and their duration may vary. Recently a fourth phase—integration and recovery—has been suggested (Holmes, 1998).

Research also suggests that survivors of sexual assault may exhibit high levels of posttraumatic stress disorder, the same disorder that developed in many of the veterans of the Vietnam War. Posttraumatic stress disorder is marked by varying degrees of intensity. Assault victims with this disorder often require lengthy, intensive therapy to regain a sense of trust and feeling of personal control.

## Care of the Sexual Assault Survivor

Survivors of sexual assault often enter the health care system by way of the emergency room. Thus the emergency room nurse is often the first person to counsel them. Because the values, attitudes, and beliefs of the caregiver will necessarily affect the competence and focus of the care, it is essential that nurses clearly understand their feelings about sexual assault and assault survivors and resolve any conflicts that may exist. In many communities, specially trained sexual assault nurse examiner (SANE) nurses coordinate the care of survivors of sexual assault, gather necessary forensic evidence, and are then available as expert witnesses when assailants are tried for the crime.

The first priority in caring for a survivor of a sexual assault is to create a safe, secure milieu. Admission information is gathered in a quiet, private room. The woman should be reassured that she is safe and not alone. The nurse assesses the survivor's appearance, demeanor, and ways of communicating for the purpose of planning care. Initially, the woman is evaluated to determine the need for emergency care. Obtaining a careful, detailed history is essential. After the woman has received any necessary emergency care, a forensic chart and kit are completed.

The woman is given a thorough explanation of the procedures to be carried out and signs a consent form for the forensic examination and collection of materials. Sexual assault kits contain all the necessary supplies for collecting and labeling evidence. The woman's clothing is collected and bagged, swabs of stains and secretions are taken, hair samples and any fingernail scrapings are collected, blood samples are drawn, tissue swabs are obtained, and photographs are taken. Vaginal and rectal examinations are performed, along with a complete physical examination for

| TABLE 4–3 Phases of Recovery Following Sexual Assault | |
|---|---|
| ***Phase*** | ***Response*** |
| Acute Phase (Disorganization) | Fear, shock, disbelief, desire for revenge, anger, anxiety, guilt, denial, embarrassment, humiliation, helplessness, dependence, self-blame, wide variety of physical reactions, lost or distorted coping mechanisms |
| Outward Adjustment Phase (Denial) | Survivor appears outwardly composed, denying and repressing feelings (eg, she returns to work, buys a weapon); refuses to discuss the assault; denies need for counseling |
| Reorganization | Survivor makes many life adjustments, such as moving to a new residence or changing her phone number; uses emotional distancing; may engage in risky sexual behaviors; may experience sexual dysfunction, phobias, flashbacks, sleep disorders, nightmares, anxiety; has a strong urge to talk about or resolve feelings; may seek counseling or remain silent |
| Integration and Recovery | Time of resolution; survivor begins to feel safe and be comfortable trusting others; places blame on assailant; may become an advocate for others |

trauma. The woman is offered prophylactic treatment for sexually transmitted infections. The woman is also questioned about her menstrual cycle and contraceptive practices. If she could become pregnant as a result of the rape, she is offered postcoital contraceptive therapy.

Throughout the experience the nurse acts as the sexual assault survivor's advocate, providing support without usurping decision making. The nurse need not agree with all the survivor's decisions but should respect and defend her right to make them.

The family members and friends on whom the survivor calls will also need nursing care. Like those of the survivor, the reactions of the family will depend on the values to which they ascribe. Many families or mates blame the survivor for the assault and feel angry with her for not having been more careful. They may also incorrectly view the assault as a sexual act rather than an act of violence. They may feel personally wronged and see the survivor as devalued or unclean. Their reactions may compound the survivor's crisis. By spending some time with family members before their first interaction with the survivor, the nurse can perhaps reduce their anxiety and absorb some of their frustrations, sparing the woman further trauma.

Sexual assault counseling, provided by qualified nurses or other counselors, is a valuable tool in helping the survivor come to terms with her assault and its impact on her life. In counseling the woman is encouraged to explore and identify her feelings and determine appropriate actions to resolve her problems and concerns. It is important for the counselor to avoid reinforcing the prevalent myth that the assault was somehow the woman's fault. The fault lies with the assailant. The counselor also plays an important role in emphasizing that the loss of control the woman experienced during the rape was temporary and that the woman can regain a feeling of control over life.

### Prosecution of the Assailant

Legally, sexual assault is considered a crime against the state, and prosecution of the assailant is a community responsibility. The survivor, however, must begin the process by reporting the assault and pressing charges against her assailant. In the past, the police and the judicial system were notoriously insensitive in dealing with survivors. However, many communities now have classes designed to help officers work effectively with sexual assault survivors or have special teams to carry out this important task.

Many women who have sought to use the judicial process have had such a traumatic experience that they refer to it as a second assault. The woman may be asked repeatedly to describe the experience in intimate detail, and her reputation and testimony will be attacked by the defense attorney. In addition, publicity may intensify her feelings of humiliation, and, if her assailant is released on bail or found not guilty, she may fear retaliation.

The nurse acting as a counselor needs to be aware of the judicial sequence to anticipate rising tension and frustration in the survivor and her support system. She will need consistent, effective support at this crucial time.

## Care of the Woman with a Benign Disorder of the Breast

Throughout her lifetime a woman may experience a variety of breast disorders. Some, like mastitis, are acute disorders, whereas others, such as fibrocystic breast disease, are chronic. This section deals with some of the common breast disorders a woman may encounter. For information on breast cancer, readers should refer to a medical-surgical nursing textbook.

### Fibrocystic Breast Disease

**Fibrocystic breast disease,** the most common of the benign breast disorders, is most prevalent in women 30 to 50 years of age. Only women with fibrocystic breast disease who show certain histologic changes (usually found incidentally when a biopsy is done) have an increased risk of developing cancer. Fibrosis is a thickening of the normal breast tissue. Cyst formation that may accompany fibrosis is considered a later change in the condition. Fibrocystic breast disease is probably caused by an imbalance in estrogen and progesterone that distorts the normal changes of the menstrual cycle. The symptoms often increase as the woman approaches menopause and generally decrease after menopause. However, if a postmenopausal woman is treated with hormone replacement therapy, the cyclic breast changes may resume.

The woman often reports pain, tenderness, and swelling that occur cyclically and are most pronounced just before menses. Physical examination may reveal only mild signs of irregularity, or the breasts may feel dense, with areas of irregularity and nodularity. Women often refer to this irregularity as "lumpiness." Some women may also have expressible nipple discharge. Although unilateral discharge and serosanguineous discharge are the most worrisome findings, all breast discharge should be investigated further.

If the woman has a large, fluid-filled cyst, she may experience a localized painful area as the capsule containing the accumulated fluid distends coincident with her cycle. However, if small cysts form, the woman may experience not a solitary tender lump but a diffuse tenderness. A cyst may often be differentiated from a malignancy because a cyst is more mobile and tender and is not associated with skin retraction (pulling) in the surrounding tissue.

Mammography, sonography, palpation, and fine-needle aspiration are used to confirm fibrocystic breast disease. Often, fine-needle aspiration is the treatment as well, affording relief from the tenderness or pain. Treatment of palpable cysts is conservative; invasive procedures such as biopsy are used only if the diagnosis is questionable.

Women with mild symptoms may benefit from restricting sodium intake and taking a mild diuretic during the week before the onset of menses. This counteracts fluid retention, relieves pressure in the breast, and helps decrease the pain. In other cases, a mild analgesic is necessary. Other treatment approaches include the use of thiamine and vitamin E. In severe cases, the hormone inhibitor danazol is the drug of choice.

Some researchers suggest that methylxanthines (found in caffeine products, such as coffee, tea, colas, and chocolate, and in some medications) may contribute to the development of fibrocystic breast changes and that limiting intake of these substances will help decrease fibrocystic changes. Other research fails to demonstrate a clear association between methylxanthines and fibrocystic breast changes. Additional medical therapies that are helpful in varying degrees include oral contraceptives, progestins, and bromocriptine. All work on the principle of estrogen suppression and progesterone stimulation or augmentation.

### Other Benign Breast Disorders

*Fibroadenoma* is a common benign tumor seen in women in their teens and early twenties. It has not been significantly associated with breast cancer. Fibroadenomas are freely movable, solid tumors that are well defined, sharply delineated, and rounded, with a rubbery texture. They are asymptomatic and nontender.

If there are any disquieting features to the appearance of a lump, fine-needle biopsy or excision of the mass may be indicated. Caution is exercised when deciding on biopsy because excision of the mass in a young girl may interfere with normal breast development. Watchful observation and possible surgical excision are the only treatments for fibroadenomas. Surgery is often deferred. When advisable, surgical removal of the fibroadenoma concludes its treatment.

*Intraductal papillomas,* most often occurring during the menopausal years, are tumors growing in the terminal portion of a duct or, sometimes, throughout the duct system within a section of the breast. They are typically benign but have the potential to become malignant. Although relatively uncommon, they are the most frequent cause of nipple discharge in women who are not pregnant or lactating.

The majority of papillomas present as solitary nodules. These small, ball-like lesions may be detected on mammography but often are nonpalpable. The presence of a papilloma is often frightening to the woman, because her primary symptom is a discharge from the nipple that may be serosanguineous or brownish green due to old blood. The location of the papilloma within the duct system and its pattern of growth determine whether nipple discharge will be present.

If the woman reports a nipple discharge, the breast should be milked to obtain fluid. The fluid obtained is sent for a Pap smear. The diagnosis is confirmed if papilloma cells are present. The lesion must be excised and histologically examined because of the difficulty in differentiating between a benign papilloma and a papillary carcinoma. Treatment for benign intraductal papilloma is excision with follow-up care.

*Duct ectasis* (comedomastitis), an inflammation of the ducts behind the nipple, commonly occurs during or near the onset of menopause and is not associated with malignancy. The condition typically occurs in women who have borne and nursed children. It is characterized by a thick, sticky nipple discharge and by burning pain, pruritus, and inflammation. Nipple retraction may also be noted, especially in postmenopausal women. Treatment is conservative, with drug therapy aimed at symptomatic relief. The major central ducts of the breast occasionally have to be excised.

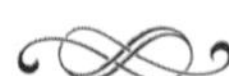

## Nursing Care Management

### Nursing Assessment and Diagnosis

During the period of diagnosis of any breast disorder, the woman may be anxious about a possible change in body image or a diagnosis of cancer. The nurse can use therapeutic communication to assess the significance the woman places on her breasts; her current emotional status, coping mechanisms used during periods of stress, and knowledge and beliefs about cancer; and other variables that may influence her coping and adjustment.

Nursing diagnoses that may apply to a woman with a benign disorder of the breast include the following:

- ***Knowledge deficit*** related to a lack of information about the diagnostic procedures
- ***Anxiety*** related to threat to body image

### Nursing Plan and Implementation

During the prediagnosis period the nurse should clarify misconceptions and encourage the woman to express her anxiety. Once a diagnosis is made, the nurse should ensure that the woman clearly understands her condition, its association to breast malignancy, and the treatment options.

The nurse can also point out that frequent professional breast examinations and regular mammograms are tools that help detect any abnormalities and that the woman who practices monthly BSE, follows her caregiver's advice, and is examined regularly has taken positive action to protect her health.

### Evaluation

Expected outcomes of nursing care include the following:

- The woman is able to discuss her fears, concerns, and questions during the period of diagnosis.
- The diagnosis is made quickly and accurately.

## Care of the Woman with Endometriosis

**Endometriosis,** a condition characterized by the presence of endometrial tissue outside the endometrial cavity, occurs in about 5% to 10% of premenopausal women (Esposito, Tureck, & Mastroianni, 1999). Endometriosis has been found almost everywhere in the body, including the vagina, lungs, cervix, central nervous system, and gastrointestinal tract. The most common location, however, is the pelvis. This tissue responds to the hormonal changes of the menstrual cycle and bleeds in a cyclic fashion. The bleeding results in inflammation, scarring of the peritoneum, and formation of adhesions.

Endometriosis may occur at any age after puberty, although it is most common in women between ages 30 and 40. The exact cause of endometriosis is unknown. Leading theories include retrograde menstrual flow and inflammation of the endometrium, hereditary tendency, and a possible immunologic defect.

The most common symptom of endometriosis is pelvic pain, which is often dull or cramping. Usually the pain is related to menstruation and is thought to be dysmenorrhea by the affected woman. **Dyspareunia** (painful intercourse) and abnormal uterine bleeding are other common signs. The condition is often diagnosed when the woman seeks evaluation for infertility. Bimanual examination may reveal a fixed, tender, retroverted uterus and palpable nodules in the cul-de-sac. Diagnosis is confirmed by laparoscopy. However, to avoid the need for diagnostic surgery, in some cases medical therapy may be instituted based on signs and symptoms and careful pretreatment evaluation (ACOG, 1999b).

Treatment may be medical, surgical, or a combination of the two. During a laporoscopic examination to confirm the diagnosis, any visible implants of endometrial tissue are removed using excision, endocoagulation, electrocautery, or laser vaporization (ACOG, 1999b). Surgery is very effective in relieving pain symptoms, at least for a period of time. In women with minimal disease and symptoms, treatment includes observation, analgesics, and nonsteroidal antiinflammatory drugs

(NSAIDs). If the woman does not currently desire pregnancy, she may be started on a combined oral contraceptive (OC). OCs create a pseudopregnancy state with decreased menstrual bleeding. If OCs do not relieve symptoms, therapy with medroxyprogesterone acetate (MPA), danazol, or a GnRH agonist may be indicated.

MPA causes endometrial tissue to atropy, thereby decreasing symptoms. It may be administered in oral form daily or given intramuscularly every 1 to 3 months. Side effects include weight gain, bloating, acne, headaches, emotional liability, and irregular bleeding (Propst & Laufer, 1999).

Danazol is a testosterone derivative that suppresses GnRH and has high-androgen and low-estrogen effects that inhibit the growth of the endometrium. It suppresses ovulation and causes amenorrhea. Danazol has some significant side effects, however, including hirsutism, vaginal bleeding, acne, oily skin, weight gain, reduced libido, voice changes and hoarseness, clitoral enlargement, and decreased breast size.

Gonadotropin-releasing hormone (GnRH) agonists such as nafarelin acetate (given as a metered nasal spray twice daily) and leuprolide acetate (Lupron) (given once a month as an intramuscular injection) are gaining popularity because many women tolerate them better than danazol and their results in treating endometriosis are comparable. GnRH agonists suppress the menstrual cycle through estrogen antagonism. This may result in the hypoestrogen side effects of hot flashes, vaginal dryness, decreased libido, and loss of bone density (Kim & Adamson, 2000).

In more advanced cases, surgery may be done to remove implants and break up adhesions. If severe dyspareunia or dysmenorrhea are symptoms, the surgeon may perform a presacral neurectomy. In advanced cases in which childbearing is not an issue, treatment may be a hysterectomy with bilateral salpingo-oophorectomy.

## Nursing Care Management

### Nursing Assessment and Diagnosis

The nurse should be aware of the common symptoms of endometriosis and elicit an accurate history if a woman mentions these symptoms. If a woman is being treated for endometriosis, the nurse should assess the woman's understanding of the condition, its implications, and the treatment alternatives.

Nursing diagnoses that may apply to a woman with endometriosis include the following:

- ***Pain*** related to peritoneal irritation secondary to endometriosis
- ***Ineffective individual coping*** related to depression secondary to infertility

### Nursing Plan and Implementation

The nurse can be available to explain the condition, its symptoms, treatment alternatives, and prognosis. The nurse can help the woman evaluate treatment options and make appropriate choices. If medication is begun, the nurse can review the dosage, schedule, possible side effects, and any warning signs. A woman with endometriosis is often advised to avoid delaying pregnancy because of the risk of infertility. The woman may wish to discuss the implications of this decision on her life choices, relationship with her partner, and personal preferences. The nurse can be a nonjudgmental listener and help the woman consider her options.

### Evaluation

Expected outcomes of nursing care include the following:

- The woman is able to discuss her condition, its implications for fertility, and her treatment options.
- After considering the alternatives, the woman chooses appropriate treatment options.

## Care of the Woman with Toxic Shock Syndrome

Although **toxic shock syndrome (TSS)** has been reported in children, postmenopausal women, and men, it is primarily a disease of women in their reproductive years, especially women at or near menses or during the postpartum period. The causative organism is a strain of *Staphylococcus aureus.* As discussed earlier, the use of superabsorbent tampons was once related to an increased incidence of TSS. That incidence has declined, probably because of changes in tampon design and changes in menses hygiene practices. Occluding the cervical os with a contraceptive device such as a diaphragm or cervical cap during menses may also increase the risk of TSS (McGregor, 2000).

Early diagnosis and treatment are important in preventing a fatal outcome. The most common signs of TSS include fever (often greater than 38.9°C [102°F]); desquamation of the skin, especially the palms and soles, which usually occurs 1 to 2 weeks after the onset of symptoms; rash; hypotension; and dizziness. Systemic symptoms often include vomiting, diarrhea, severe myalgia, and inflamed mucous membranes (oropharyngeal, conjunctival, or vaginal). Disorders of the central nervous system, including alterations in consciousness, disorientation, and coma, may also occur. Laboratory findings reveal elevated blood urea nitrogen (BUN), creatinine, serum glutamic-oxaloacetic transaminase (SGOT), serum glutamic-pyruvic transaminase (SGPT), and total bilirubin levels, while platelets are often less than 100,000/mm$^3$.

Women with TSS are generally hospitalized and given supportive therapy, including intravenous fluids to maintain blood pressure. Severe cases may require renal dialysis, administration of vasopressors, and intubation. Broad-spectrum antibiotic therapy (including antistaphylococcal agents) is initiated immediately until septisemia is excluded as a diagnosis; antibiotic therapy also reduces the risk of recurrence (McGregor, 2000).

## Nursing Care Management

Nurses play a major role in helping educate women about ways to prevent the development of TSS. Women should understand the importance of avoiding prolonged use of tampons. They should change tampons every 3 to 6 hours and avoid using superabsorbent tampons. Some women may choose to use other products, such as sanitary napkins or minipads. Women who choose to continue using tampons may reduce their risk of TSS by alternating them with napkins and avoiding overnight use of tampons.

Postpartal women should avoid the use of tampons for 6 to 8 weeks after childbirth. Women with a history of TSS should never use tampons. Women who use diaphragms or cervical caps should not leave them in place for prolonged periods and should not use them during the postpartum period or when they are menstruating. Nurses can also help make women aware of the signs and symptoms of TSS so that they will seek treatment promptly if symptoms occur.

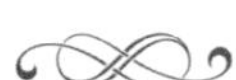

# Care of the Woman with Vulvovaginal Candidiasis

Vulvovaginal candidiasis (VVC), also called moniliasis or yeast infection, is the most common form of vaginitis affecting the vagina and vulva. Recurrences are frequent for some women. Factors that contribute to the occurrence of this infection are use of oral contraceptives, use of antibiotics, frequent douching, pregnancy, diabetes mellitus, and use of immunosuppressants. *Candida albicans* is responsible for most vaginal yeast infections.

The woman with VVC often complains of thick, curdy vaginal discharge, severe itching, dysuria, and dyspareunia. A male sexual partner may experience a rash or excoriation of the skin of the penis and possibly pruritus. The male may be symptomatic and the female asymptomatic.

On physical examination, the woman's labia may be swollen and excoriated if pruritus has been severe. A speculum examination reveals thick, white, tenacious cheeselike patches adhering to the vaginal mucosa. Diagnosis is confirmed by microscopic examination of the vaginal discharge; hyphae and spores are usually seen on a wet-mount preparation (Figure 4–10♦).

Medical treatment of VVC includes intravaginal insertion of miconazole, tioconazole, butoconazole, terconazole, clotrimazole, or nystatin suppositories or cream at bedtime for 3 days to 1 week (Centers for Disease Control and Prevention [CDC], 1998). If the vulva is also infected, the cream is applied topically. VVC may also be treated with a single oral dose of 150 mg fluconazole, but fluconazole has been associated with liver toxicity and its use should be reserved for special situations such as recalcitrant infection (Cullins, Dominguez, Guberski, et al., 1999). Some of the topical medications are available over the counter. They are indicated for women with a history of yeast infections who clearly recognize the symptoms.

Topical miconazole usually eliminates the yeast infection from the male. However, the CDC states that treatment of the male partner is not necessary unless candidal balanitis (inflammation of the glans penis) is present or chronicity is a problem (CDC, 1998).

If a woman experiences frequent recurrences of VVC, she should be tested for an elevated blood glucose level to determine whether a diabetic or prediabetic condition is present. Women at high risk for HIV infection should be

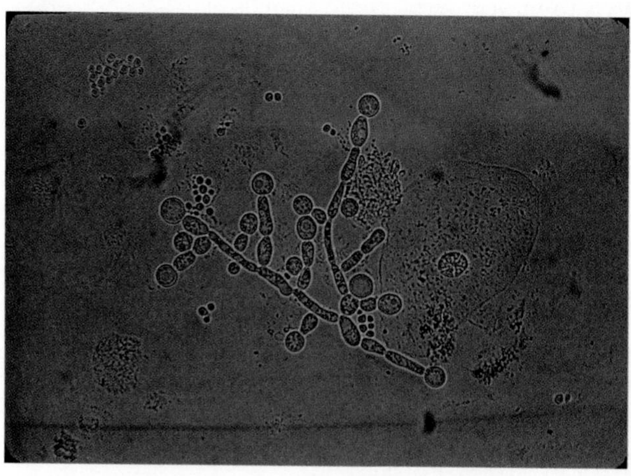

FIGURE 4–10 ♦ The hyphae and spores of *Candida albicans*.
*Source:* Courtesy Centers for Disease Control and Prevention.

tested for the virus. Pregnant women are treated the same as nonpregnant women (CDC, 1998). Infection at the time of birth may cause thrush (a mouth infection) in the newborn.

## Nursing Care Management

### Nursing Assessment and Diagnosis

The nurse should suspect VVC if a woman complains of intense vulvar itching and a curdy, white discharge. Because pregnant women with diabetes mellitus are especially susceptible to this infection, the nurse should be alert for symptoms in these women. In some areas nurses are trained to do speculum examinations and wet-mount preparations and can confirm the diagnosis themselves. In most cases, however, the nurse who suspects a vaginal infection reports it to the woman's health care provider. See Key Facts to Remember: Vaginitis.

Nursing diagnoses that might apply to the woman with VVC include the following:

- ***Risk for impaired skin integrity*** related to scratching secondary to discomfort of the infection
- ***Knowledge deficit*** related to lack of information about ways of preventing the development of VVC

### Nursing Plan and Implementation

If the woman is experiencing discomfort because of pruritus, the nurse can recommend gentle bathing of the vulva with a weak sodium bicarbonate solution. If a topical treatment is being used, the woman will need to bathe the area before applying the medication.

The nurse also discusses with the woman the factors that contribute to the development of VVC and suggests ways to prevent recurrences, such as wearing cotton underwear and avoiding vaginal powders or sprays that may irritate the vulva. Some women report that the addition of yogurt to the diet or the use of activated culture of plain yogurt as a vaginal douche helps prevent recurrence by maintaining high levels of lactobacilli.

### Evaluation

Expected outcomes of nursing care include the following:

- The woman's symptoms are relieved, and the infection is cured.
- The woman is able to identify self-care measures to prevent further episodes of VVC.

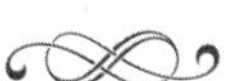

**KEY FACTS TO REMEMBER**

*Vaginitis*

To distinguish among the common types of vaginitis and their treatments , it is useful to remember the following:

**Vulvovaginal candidiasis (moniliasis)**

Cause: *Candida albicans*

Appearance of discharge: Thick, curdy, like cottage cheese

Diagnostic test: Slide of vaginal discharge (treated with potassium hydroxide [KOH]) shows characteristic hyphae and spores

Treatment: Clotrimazole vaginal cream or suppositories

**Bacterial vaginosis (Gardnerella vaginalis vaginitis)**

Cause: *Gardnerella vaginalis*

Appearance of discharge: Gray, milky

Diagnostic test: Slide of vaginal discharge shows characteristic "clue" cells

Treatment: Metronidazole

**Trichomoniasis**

Cause: *Trichomonas vaginalis*

Appearance of discharge: Greenish white and frothy

Diagnostic test: Saline slide of vaginal discharge shows motile flagellated organisms

Treatment: Metronidazole

# Care of the Woman with a Sexually Transmitted Infection

The occurrence of **sexually transmitted infection (STI)**, or *sexually transmitted disease (STD),* has increased over the past few decades. In fact, vaginitis and STIs are the most common reasons for outpatient, community-based treatment of women.

## Bacterial Vaginosis

*Bacterial vaginosis (BV),* a sexually associated condition, was formerly referred to as nonspecific vaginitis or *Gardnerella vaginalis* vaginitis. It is an alteration of normal

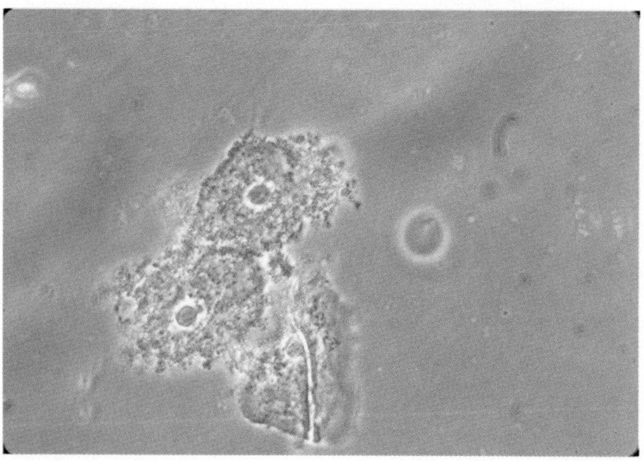

FIGURE 4–11 ♦ Depiction of the clue cells characteristically seen in bacterial vaginosis.

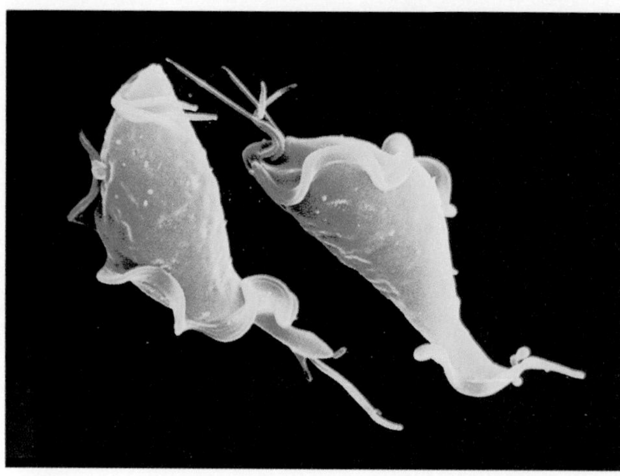

FIGURE 4–12 ♦ Microscopic appearance of *Trichomonas vaginalis.*

vaginal bacterial flora that results in the loss of hydrogen peroxide producing lactobacilli, which are normally the main vaginal flora. With the loss of this natural defense, bacteria such as *Gardnerella,* mycoplasmas, and anaerobes overgrow in large numbers, causing vaginitis (Thomason & Scaglione, 1999). The cause of this overgrowth is not clear, although tissue trauma and sexual intercourse are sometimes identified as contributing factors.

The infected woman often notices an excessive amount of thin, watery, yellow-gray vaginal discharge with a foul odor described as "fishy." The characteristic "clue" cell is seen on a wet-mount preparation (Figure 4–11♦). The vaginal pH is usually greater than 4.5.

The nonpregnant woman is generally treated with metronidazole (Flagyl) or clindamycin (Cleocin) orally or as a vaginal cream. Because of its potential teratogenic effects, metronidazole is avoided during the first trimester of pregnancy; one full applicator of clindamycin is inserted intravaginally at bedtime instead. During the second and third trimesters, oral metronidazole or clindamycin or vaginal metronidazole gel can be used (CDC, 1998). BV during pregnancy may be a factor in premature rupture of the membranes and preterm birth. Treatment of sexual partners is only recommended in cases of recurrent BV (Thomason & Scaglione, 1999).

## Trichomoniasis

*Trichomonas vaginalis* is a microscopic motile protozoan that thrives in an alkaline environment. Most infections are acquired through sexual intimacy. Transmission by shared bath facilities, wet towels, or wet swimsuits may also be possible (CDC, 1998).

Symptoms of trichomoniasis include a yellow-green, frothy, odorous discharge frequently accompanied by inflammation of the vagina and cervix, dysuria, and dyspareunia. Visualization of *T. vaginalis* under the microscope on a wet-mount preparation of vaginal discharge confirms the diagnosis (Figure 4–12♦).

Treatment for trichomoniasis is metronidazole (Flagyl) administered in a single 2-g dose for both male and female sexual partners; a 7-day regimen is also available (Eschenbach, 2000). Partners should avoid intercourse until both are cured (see Key Facts to Remember: Vaginitis).

The woman should be informed that metronidazole is contraindicated in the first trimester of pregnancy because of possible teratogenic effects on the fetus. However, no other adequate treatment exists. For women with severe symptoms after the first trimester, treatment with 2 g metronidazole in a single dose may be considered (Eschenbach, 2000). The woman and her partner should be cautioned to avoid alcohol while taking metronidazole; the combination has an effect similar to that of alcohol and Antabuse—abdominal pain, flushing, and tremors.

## Chlamydial Infection

*Chlamydial infection,* caused by *Chlamydia trachomatis,* is the most common STI in the United States. The organism is an intracellular bacterium with several different immunotypes. Immunotypes of chlamydia are responsible for lymphogranuloma venereum and trachoma, which is the world's leading cause of preventable blindness.

Chlamydia is a major cause of nongonococcal urethritis (NGU) in men. In women it can cause infections similar to those that occur with gonorrhea. It can infect the fallopian tubes, cervix, urethra, and Bartholin's glands. Pelvic inflammatory disease, infertility, and ectopic pregnancy are associated with chlamydia. The newborn of a woman with untreated chlamydia is at risk of developing ophthalmia neonatorum, which responds to erythromycin ophthalmic ointment but not to silver nitrate eye prophylaxis at birth. The newborn may also develop chlamydia pneumonia.

Symptoms of chlamydia include a thin or purulent discharge, burning and frequency of urination, and lower abdominal pain. Women, however, are often asymptomatic. Diagnosis is often made after treatment of a male partner for NGU or in a symptomatic woman with a negative gonorrhea culture. Laboratory detection is now simpler, due to the use of new deoxyribonucleic acid (DNA) methods (ligase chain reaction [LCR] and polymerase chain reaction [PCR]). These DNA amplification tests are over 95% sensitive to *C. trachomatis* and, because they can be done on a woman's first-voided urine of the day, are noninvasive (Hammerschlag, 1999).

The recommended treatment is azithromycin or doxycycline. Sexual partners should also be treated, and couples should abstain from intercourse for 7 days, the course of therapy. Pregnant women should be treated with erythromycin ethylsuccinate or amoxicillin, although neither is highly effective (CDC, 1998).

## GONORRHEA

*Gonorrhea* is an infection caused by the bacteria *Neisseria gonorrhoeae.* If a nonpregnant woman contracts the disease, she is at risk of developing pelvic inflammatory disease. If a woman becomes infected after the third month of pregnancy, the mucous plug in the cervix will prevent the infection from ascending, and it will remain localized in the urethra, cervix, and Bartholin's glands until the membranes rupture. Then it can spread upward.

The majority of women with gonorrhea are asymptomatic. Thus it is accepted practice to screen for this infection by doing a cervical culture during the initial prenatal examination. For women at high risk, the culture may be repeated during the last month of pregnancy. Cultures of the urethra, throat, and rectum may also be required for diagnosis, depending on the body orifices used for intercourse.

The most common symptoms of gonorrheal infection include a purulent, greenish yellow vaginal discharge, dysuria, and urinary frequency. Some women also develop inflammation and swelling of the vulva. The cervix may appear swollen and eroded and may secrete a foul-smelling discharge in which gonococci are present.

Treatment consists of antibiotic therapy with ceftriaxone intramuscularly and doxycycline or azithromycin administered orally. This combined approach provides dual treatment for gonorrhea and chlamydia because the two infections often occur together. Additional treatment may be required if the cultures remain positive 7 to 14 days after completion of treatment. All sexual partners must also be treated or the woman may become reinfected. Pregnant women should be treated with ceftriaxone intramuscularly or cefixime orally. This treatment is combined with erythromycin or amoxicillin to address the risk of coinfection with chlamydia (CDC, 1998).

Women should be informed of the need for reculture to verify cure and the need for abstinence or condom use until cure is confirmed. Both sexual partners should be treated if either has a positive test for gonorrhea.

## HERPES GENITALIS

*Herpes* infections are caused by the herpes simplex virus (HSV). Two types of herpes infections can occur: HSV-1 (the cold sore) typically occurs above the waist and is not sexually transmitted; HSV-2 is usually associated with genital infections. The clinical symptoms and treatment of both types are the same. At least 45 million people in the United States have been diagnosed with genital HSV-2 infection (CDC, 1998).

The primary episode of herpes genitalis is characterized by the development of single or multiple blisterlike vesicles, which usually occur in the genital area and sometimes affect the vaginal walls, cervix, urethra, and anus. The vesicles may appear within a few hours to 20 days after exposure and rupture spontaneously to form very painful, open, ulcerated lesions. Inflammation and pain secondary to the presence of herpes lesions can cause difficult urination and urinary retention. Inguinal lymph node enlargement may be present. Flulike symptoms and genital pruritus or tingling also may be noticed. Primary episodes usually last the longest and are the most severe. Lesions heal spontaneously in 2 to 4 weeks.

After the lesions heal, the virus enters a dormant phase, residing in the nerve ganglia of the affected area. Some individuals never have a recurrence, whereas others have regular recurrences. Recurrences are usually less severe than the initial episode and seem to be triggered by emotional stress, menstruation, ovulation, pregnancy, frequent or vigorous intercourse, poor health status or a generally run-down physical condition, tight clothing, or overheating. Diagnosis is made on the basis of the clinical appearance of the lesions, Pap smear or culture of the lesions, and sometimes blood testing for antibodies.

No known cure for herpes exists. Prescriptive treatment is available to provide relief from pain and prevent complications from secondary infection. The recommended treatment of the first clinical episode of genital herpes is oral acyclovir, valacyclovir, or famciclovir. These same medications, in somewhat different dosages, are also recommended for recurrent herpes infection and for daily suppression therapy for people who have frequent recurrences. Therapy should be started during the prodromal period for the greatest benefit (CDC, 1998).

Self-help suggestions include cleansing with povidone-iodine (Betadine) solution to prevent secondary infection and with Burow's solution to relieve discomfort. Use of vitamin C or lysine is frequently suggested to prevent recurrence, although studies have not documented the effectiveness of these supplements. Keeping the genital area clean and dry, wearing loose clothing, and wearing cotton underwear or none at all will promote healing. Primary and recurrent lesions will heal without prescriptive therapies.

If herpes is present in the genital tract of a woman during childbirth, it can have a devastating, even fatal, effect on the newborn. For further discussion, see Chapter 13.

## Syphilis

*Syphilis* is a chronic infection caused by the spirochete *Treponema pallidum.* Syphilis can be acquired congenitally through transplacental inoculation and can result from maternal exposure to infected exudate during sexual contact or from contact with open wounds or infected blood. The incubation period varies from 10 to 90 days, and even though no symptoms or lesions are noted during this time, the woman's blood contains spirochetes and is infectious.

Syphilis is divided into early and late stages. During the early stage (primary), a chancre appears at the site where the *T. pallidum* organism entered the body. Symptoms include slight fever, loss of weight, and malaise. The chancre persists for about 4 weeks and then disappears. In 6 weeks to 6 months, secondary symptoms appear. Skin eruptions called condylomata lata, which resemble wartlike plaques and are highly infectious, may appear on the vulva. Other secondary symptoms are acute arthritis, enlargement of the liver and spleen, nontender enlarged lymph nodes, iritis, and a chronic sore throat with hoarseness. When infected in utero, the newborn exhibits secondary-stage symptoms of syphilis. Transplacentally transmitted syphilis may cause intrauterine growth restriction, preterm birth, and stillbirth.

As a result of the disease's impact on the fetus in utero, serologic testing of every pregnant woman is recommended; some state laws require it. Testing is done at the initial prenatal screening and repeated in the third trimester. Blood studies may be negative if blood is drawn too early in the pregnancy.

Diagnosis is made by dark-field examination for spirochetes. Blood tests such as the venereal disease research laboratory (VDRL) test, rapid plasma reagin (RPR) test, or the more specific fluorescent treponemal antibody-absorption (FTA-ABS) test are commonly done.

For pregnant and nonpregnant women with syphilis of less than a year's duration, the CDC (1998) recommends 2.4 million units of benzathine penicillin G administered intramuscularly. If syphilis is of long (more than a year) duration, 2.4 million units of benzathine penicillin G is given intramuscularly once a week for 3 weeks. If a woman is allergic to penicillin and nonpregnant, doxycycline can be given. The pregnant woman who is allergic to penicillin should be desensitized to penicillin (CDC, 1998). Maternal serologic testing may remain positive for 8 months, and the newborn may have a positive test for 3 months.

## Condylomata Acuminata (Venereal Warts)

The infection *condylomata acuminata,* also called *venereal warts,* is a relatively common sexually transmitted condition caused by the human papillomavirus (HPV). Because of the increasing evidence of a link between HPV and cervical cancer, the condition is receiving increasing attention.

Often a woman seeks medical care after noticing single or multiple soft, grayish pink, cauliflower-like lesions in her genital area (Figure 4–13♦). The moist, warm environment of the genital area is conducive to the growth of the warts, which may be present on the vulva, vagina, cervix, and anus. The incubation period following exposure is 3 weeks to 3 years.

Because condylomata sometimes resemble other lesions and malignant transformation is possible, all atypical, pigmented, and persistent warts should be biopsied and treatment should be instituted promptly. The CDC does not specify a treatment of choice for genital warts but recommends that treatment be determined based on client preference, available resources, and experience of the health care provider. Client-applied therapies include podofilox solution or gel or imiquimod cream. Provider-administered therapies include cryotherapy with liquid nitrogen or cryoprobe; topical podophyllin; trichloroacetic acid (TCA); bichloroacetic acid (BCA); intralesional interferon; surgical removal by tangential scissor excision, shave excision, or curettage; or laser surgery

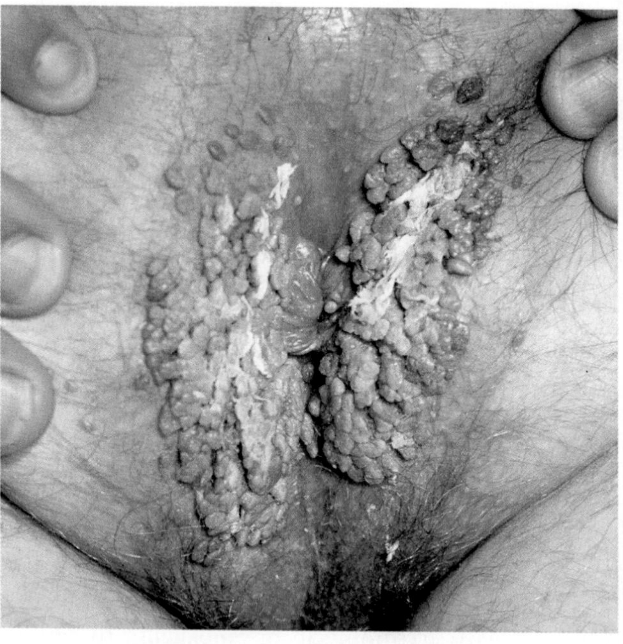

**FIGURE 4–13** ♦ Condylomata acuminata on the vulva.

(CDC, 1998). Imiquimod, podophyllin, and podofilox are not used during pregnancy because they are thought to be teratogenic and in large doses have been associated with fetal death.

Women with HPV infections should have frequent Pap smears to monitor cervical cellular changes. Sex partners are probably infected but do not require treatment unless large lesions are present. The use of male or female condoms may reduce the risk of transmitting the virus to an uninfected partner.

## Acquired Immunodeficiency Syndrome

*Acquired immunodeficiency syndrome (AIDS)* is a fatal disorder caused by the human immunodeficiency virus (HIV). Medical-surgical texts more fully describe care of patients with HIV and AIDS. However, because the diagnosis of HIV/AIDS or the presence of the HIV antibody has profound implications for a fetus if the woman is pregnant, AIDS is discussed in more detail in Chapter 12.

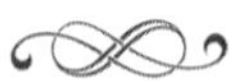

# Nursing Care Management

## Nursing Assessment and Diagnosis

Nurses working with women must become adept at taking a thorough history and identifying women at risk for STIs. Risk factors include multiple sexual partners, a partner's involvement with other partners, high-risk sexual behaviors such as intercourse without barrier contraception or anal intercourse, partners with high-risk behaviors, treatment with antibiotics while taking oral contraceptives, and young age at onset of sexual activity. Nurses should be alert for signs and symptoms of STIs and be familiar with diagnostic procedures if an STI is suspected.

Although each STI has certain distinctive characteristics, the following complaints suggest the possibility of infection and warrant further investigation:

- Presence of a sore or lesion on the vulva
- Increased vaginal discharge or malodorous vaginal discharge
- Burning with urination
- Dyspareunia
- Bleeding after intercourse
- Pelvic pain

In many instances the woman is asymptomatic but may report symptoms in her partner, especially painful urination or urethral discharge. It is often helpful to ask the woman whether her partner is experiencing any symptoms.

Nursing diagnoses that may apply when a woman has an STI include the following:

- ***Altered family processes*** related to the effects of a diagnosis of STI on the couple's relationship
- ***Knowledge deficit*** related to lack of information about the long-term effects of the diagnosis on childbearing status

## Nursing Plan and Implementation

In a supportive, nonjudgmental way the nurse provides the woman who has an STI with information about the infection, methods of transmission, implications for pregnancy or future fertility, and the importance of thorough treatment. If treatment of her partner is indicated, the woman must understand that it is necessary to prevent a cycle of reinfection. She should also understand the need to abstain from sexual activity, if necessary, during treatment.

Some STIs such as trichomoniasis or chlamydia may cause a woman concern but, once diagnosed, are rather simply treated. Other STIs may also be fairly simple to treat medically but may carry a stigma and be emotionally devastating for the woman. Thus the nurse should stress prevention with all women and encourage them to require partners, especially new partners, to use condoms.

The nurse can be especially helpful in encouraging the woman to explore her feelings about the diagnosis. She may experience anger or feel betrayed by a partner, she may feel guilt or see her diagnosis as a form of punishment, or she may feel concern about the long-term implications for future childbearing or ongoing intimate relationships. She may experience a myriad of emotions that she never expected. Opportunities to discuss her feelings in a nonjudgmental environment can be very helpful. The nurse can offer suggestions about support groups, if indicated, and assist the woman in planning for future sexual activity.

More subtly, the nurse's attitude of acceptance and matter-of-factness conveys to the woman that she is still an acceptable person who happens to have an infection. See Key Facts to Remember: Information about Sexually Transmitted Infections.

## Evaluation

Expected outcomes of nursing care include the following:

- The infection is identified and cured, if possible; if not, supportive therapy is provided.

## KEY FACTS TO REMEMBER

### *Information about Sexually Transmitted Infections*

- The risk of contracting a sexually transmitted infection increases with the number of sexual partners. Because of the extended periods of time between infection with HIV and evidence of infection, intercourse with an individual exposes a woman or man to all the other sex partners of that individual for the past 5 or more years.
- The condom is the best contraceptive method currently available (other than abstinence) for protection from sexually transmitted infections.
- Other contraceptive methods such as the diaphragm, cervical cap, and spermicides also offer some protection against sexually transmitted infections.
- A person diagnosed with a sexually transmitted infection has a responsibility to notify any sexual partners so they can obtain treatment.
- Absence of symptoms or disappearance of symptoms does not mean that treatment is unnecessary if a person suspects a sexually transmitted infection. She or he should be seen for evaluation and treatment. All prescribed medications should be taken completely.
- The presence of a genital infection may lead to an abnormal Pap smear. Women with certain infections should have more frequent Pap tests according to a schedule recommended by their caregiver.

- The woman and her partner can describe the infection, its method of transmission, its implications, and the therapy.
- The woman copes successfully with the impact of the diagnosis on her self-concept.

# Care of the Woman with Pelvic Inflammatory Disease

**Pelvic inflammatory disease (PID)** occurs in approximately 1% of women between ages 15 and 39, although sexually active young women between 15 and 24 have the highest infection rate (Eschenbach, 1999). The disease is more common in women who have had multiple sexual partners, a history of PID, early onset of sexual activity, a recent gynecologic procedure, or an intrauterine device. It usually produces a tubal infection (salpingitis) that may or may not be accompanied by a pelvic abscess. However, perhaps the greatest problem of PID is postinfection tubal damage, which is closely associated with infertility.

The organisms most frequently identified with PID include *Chlamydia trachomatis* and *Neisseria gonorrhoeae.* Bacterial vaginosis may facilitate the ascending spread of pathogens.

Symptoms of PID include bilateral sharp, cramping pain in the lower quadrants, fever, chills, purulent vaginal discharge, irregular bleeding, malaise, nausea, and vomiting. However, it is also possible to be asymptomatic and have normal laboratory values.

Diagnosis consists of a clinical examination to define symptoms, plus blood tests, a gonorrhea culture, and a LCR or PCR test for chlamydia. Physical examination usually reveals direct abdominal tenderness with palpation, adnexal tenderness, and cervical and uterine tenderness with movement (chandelier sign). A palpable mass is evaluated with ultrasound. Fluid may be aspirated via needle from the cul-de-sac of Douglas through the posterior vaginal fornix. Purulent fluid suggests an intraabdominal infection. Laparoscopy may be used to confirm the diagnosis and to enable the examiner to obtain cultures from the fallopian tubes and directly from the fluid of the cul-de-sac (Wölner-Hanssen, 1999).

Except in mild cases, the woman is hospitalized and treated with intravenous administration of cefoxitan sodium, cefotetan disodium, or clindamycin plus gentamicin. Outpatient therapy usually includes antibiotics such as cefoxitan, ceftriaxone, doxycycline, and clindamycin used singly or in combination. Ofloxacin (Floxin) is also available for women with PID caused by chlamydia or gonorrhea. Ofloxacin, taken twice daily for 10 to 14 days, has a 98% cure rate ("A Simpler Cure," 1997). In addition, supportive therapy is often indicated for severe symptoms. The sexual partner should also be treated. If the woman has an IUD, it is generally removed 24 to 48 hours after antibiotic therapy is started.

## Nursing Care Management

### Nursing Assessment and Diagnosis

The nurse is alert to factors in a woman's history that put her at risk for PID. Even though fewer types of IUDs are available, many women still have them, and the nurse should question the woman about possible symptoms, such as aching pain in the lower abdomen, foul-smelling discharge, malaise, and the like. The woman who is acutely ill will have obvious symptoms, but a low-grade infection is more difficult to detect.

Nursing diagnoses that may apply to a woman with PID include the following:

- ***Pain*** related to peritoneal irritation
- ***Knowledge deficit*** related to a lack of information about the possible effects of PID on fertility

### Nursing Plan and Implementation

The nurse plays a vital role in helping to prevent or detect PID. Accordingly, the nurse spends time discussing risk factors related to this infection. The woman who uses an IUD for contraception and has multiple sexual partners needs to understand clearly the risk she faces. The nurse discusses signs and symptoms of PID and stresses the importance of early detection.

The woman who develops PID should be counseled on the importance of completing her antibiotic treatment and of returning for follow-up evaluation. She should also understand the possibility of decreased fertility following the infection.

### Evaluation

Expected outcomes of nursing care include the following:

- The woman describes her condition, her therapy, and the possible long-term implications of PID on her fertility.
- The woman completes her course of therapy and the PID is cured.

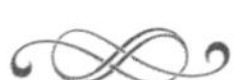

# Care of the Woman with an Abnormal Finding during Pelvic Examination

## Abnormal Pap Smear Results

The Bethesda system (Table 4–4) has become the most widely used system in the United States for reporting Pap smear results. The system provides a uniform format and classification of terminology based on current understanding of cervical disease. Early detection of abnormalities allows early changes to be treated before cells reach the precancerous or cancerous stage.

Notification of an abnormal Pap smear usually causes anxiety for a woman, so it is important that she be told in a caring way. Research indicates that the concerns of women with an abnormal Pap test focused on not understanding the results and meaning of the findings, worry about cancer, and concerns about fertility (Lauver, Baggot, & Kruse, 1999). Thus, the woman needs accurate, complete information about the meaning of the results and the next steps to be taken. She should also be given time to ask questions and express her concerns.

Diagnostic or therapeutic procedures employed in cases of abnormalities include repetition of the Pap test using the ThinPrep method rather than a smear, Pap tests at shorter intervals, colposcopy and endocervical biopsy, cryotherapy, laser conization, or large loop excision of the transformation zone (LLETZ). Management is based on the specific report.

**Colposcopy** has evolved as an appropriate second step in many cases of abnormal Pap. The examination, typically done in an office or clinic, permits more detailed visualization of the cervix in bright light, using a microscope with 6× to 40× magnification. The cervix can be visualized directly and again following application of 3% acetic acid. The acetic acid causes abnormal epithelium to assume a characteristic white appearance. The colposcope can be used to localize and obtain a directed biopsy.

Women who had first coitus at an early age or have a history of, or a sex partner with a history of, multiple sexual partners, exposure to sexually transmitted infections, immunosuppressive therapy, or antenatal exposure to diethylstilbestrol (DES) have an increased risk of abnormal cell changes and cervical cancer.

## Ovarian Masses

Between 70% and 80% of ovarian masses are benign. More than 50% are functional cysts, occurring most commonly in women 20 to 40 years of age. Functional cysts are rare in women who take oral contraceptives.

Ovarian cysts usually represent physiologic variations in the menstrual cycle. Dermoid cysts (cystic teratomas) comprise 10% of all benign ovarian masses. Cartilage, bone, teeth, skin, or hair can be observed in these cysts. Endometriomas, or "chocolate cysts," are another common type of ovarian mass.

No relationship exists between ovarian masses and ovarian cancer. However, ovarian cancer is the most fatal of all cancers in women because it is difficult to diagnose and often has spread throughout the pelvis before it is detected.

A woman with an ovarian mass may be asymptomatic; the mass may be noted on a routine pelvic examination. She may experience a sensation of fullness or cramping in the lower abdomen (often unilateral), dyspareunia, irregular bleeding, or delayed menstruation.

**TABLE 4–4 The Bethesda System for Classifying Pap Smears**

**ADEQUACY OF THE SPECIMEN**
Satisfactory for evaluation
Satisfactory for evaluation but limited by . . . (specify reason)
Unsatisfactory for evaluation

**GENERAL CATEGORIZATION (OPTIONAL)**
Within normal limits
Benign cellular changes (See descriptive diagnoses.)
Epithelial cell abnormality (See descriptive diagnoses.)

**DESCRIPTIVE DIAGNOSES**
Benign cellular changes
- Infection
  - *Trichomonas vaginalis*
  - Fungal organisms morphologically consistent with *Candida* spp.
  - Predominance of coccobacilli consistent with shift in vaginal flora
  - Bacteria morphologically consistent with *Actinomyces* spp.
  - Cellular changes associated with herpes simplex virus
  - Other

Reactive changes
- Reactive cellular changes associated with
  - Inflammation (includes typical repair)
  - Atrophy with inflammation (atrophic vaginitis)
  - Radiation
  - Intrauterine contraceptive device (IUD)
  - Other

Reactive changes *continued*
- Epithelial cell abnormalities
  - Squamous cell
  - Atypical squamous cells of undetermined significance (ASCUS): Qualify*
  - Low-grade squamous intraepithelial lesion (SIL) encompassing HPV† mild dysplasia/CIN 1
  - High-grade squamous intraepithelial lesion encompassing: Moderate and severe dysplasia, CIS/CIN 2 and CIN 3
  - Squamous cell carcinoma
- Glandular cell
  - Endometrial cells, cytologically benign, in a postmenopausal woman
  - Atypical glandular cells of undetermined significance: Qualify*
  - Endocervical adenocarcinoma
  - Endometrial adenocarcinoma
  - Extrauterine adenocarcinoma
  - Adenocarcinoma, not otherwise specified
- Other malignant neoplasms: Specify
  - Hormonal evaluation (applies to vaginal smears only)
  - Hormonal pattern compatible with age and history
  - Hormonal pattern incompatible with age and history: Specify
  - Hormonal evaluation not possible due to: Specify

*Atypical squamous or glandular cells of undetermined significance should be futher qualified as to whether a reactive or a premalignant/malignant process is favored.
†Cellular changes of human papillomavirus (HPV)—previous. termed koilocytosis, koilocytotic atypia, or condylomatous atypia—are included in the category of low-grade squamous intraepithelial lesion.

Diagnosis is made on the basis of a palpable mass with or without tenderness and other related symptoms. Radiography or ultrasonography may be used to assist in the diagnosis.

The woman is frequently kept under observation for a month or two because most cysts will resolve on their own and are harmless. Oral contraceptives may be prescribed for 1 to 2 months to suppress ovarian function. If this regimen is effective, a repeat pelvic examination should be normal. If the mass is still present after 60 days of observation and oral contraceptive therapy, a diagnostic laparoscopy or laparotomy may be considered. Tubal or ovarian lesions, ectopic pregnancy, cancer, infection, or appendicitis also must be ruled out before a diagnosis can be confirmed.

Surgery is not always necessary but will be considered if the mass is larger than 6 to 7 cm in circumference; if the woman is over 40 years of age with an adnexal mass, a persistent mass, or continuous pain; or if the woman is taking oral contraceptives. Surgical exploration is also indicated when a palpable mass is found in an infant, a young girl, or a postmenopausal woman.

Women who are taking oral contraceptives should be informed of their preventive effect against ovarian masses. Women may need clear explanations about why the initial therapy is observation. A discussion of the origin and resolution of ovarian cysts may clarify this treatment plan. If a surgical treatment removes or impairs the function of one ovary, the woman needs to be assured that the remaining ovary can be expected to take over ovarian functioning and that pregnancy is still possible.

## Uterine Masses

Fibroid tumors, or leiomyomas, are among the most common benign disease entities in women and are the most common reason for gynecologic surgery. Between 20% and 50% of women develop leiomyomas by age 40. The potential for cancer is minimal. Leiomyomas are more common in women of African heritage.

Fibroid tumors develop when smooth muscle cells are present in whorls and arise from uterine muscles and connective tissue. The size varies from 1 to 2 cm to the size of a 10-week fetus. Frequently the woman is asymptomatic.

Lower abdominal pain, fullness or pressure, menorrhagia, metrorrhagia, or increased dysmenorrhea may occur, particularly with large leiomyomas. Ultrasonography revealing masses or nodules can assist and confirm the diagnosis. Leiomyoma is also considered a possible diagnosis when masses or nodules involving the uterus are palpated on a pelvic examination.

The majority of these masses require no treatment and will shrink after menopause. Close observation for symptoms or an increase in size of the uterus or the masses is the only management most women will require. Routine pelvic examinations every 3 to 6 months are recommended unless new symptoms appear.

If a woman notices symptoms, or pelvic examination reveals that the mass is increasing in size, surgery (myomectomy, D&C, or hysterectomy) will be recommended. The choice of surgery depends on the age and reproductive status of the woman and the significance of the noted changes. There are no medications or therapies to prevent fibroids.

Endometrial cancer, most commonly a disease of postmenopausal women, has a high rate of cure if detected early. The hallmark sign is vaginal bleeding in postmenopausal women not treated with hormone replacement therapy. Diagnosis is made by endometrial biopsy or posthysterectomy pathology examination of the uterus. The treatment is total abdominal hysterectomy and bilateral salpingo-oophorectomy. Radiation therapy may also be indicated, depending on the stage of the cancer.

## Nursing Care Management

Pelvic examinations and Pap smears are not done by nurses except those with special training. In most cases, nursing assessment is directed toward an evaluation of the woman's understanding of the findings and their implications and her psychosocial response.

The woman needs accurate information on etiology, symptomatology, and treatment options. She should be encouraged to report symptoms and keep appointments for follow-up examination and evaluation. The woman needs realistic reassurance if her condition is benign; she may require counseling and effective emotional support if a malignancy is likely. If the management plan includes surgery, she may need the nurse's support in obtaining a second opinion and making her decision.

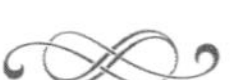

# Care of the Woman with a Urinary Tract Infection

A *urinary tract infection (UTI)* may be life threatening or a mere inconvenience. Bacteria usually enter the urinary tract by way of the urethra. The organisms are capable of migrating against the downward flow of urine. The shortness of the female urethra facilitates the passage of bacteria into the bladder. Other conditions that are associated with bacterial entry are relative incompetence of the urinary sphincter, frequent enuresis (bed-wetting) before adolescence, and urinary catheterization. Wiping from back to front after urination may transfer bacteria from the anorectal area to the urethra.

Voluntarily suppressing the desire to urinate is a predisposing factor. Retention overdistends the bladder and can lead to an infection. There also seems to be a relationship between recurring UTI and sexual intercourse. General poor health or lowered resistance to infection can increase a woman's susceptibility to UTI.

*Asymptomatic bacteriuria (ASB)* (bacteria in the urine actively multiplying without accompanying clinical symptoms) constitutes about 6% to 8% of UTIs. This condition becomes especially significant if the woman is pregnant. About 30% to 40% of pregnant women with untreated ASB will go on to develop cystitis or pyelonephritis (Lentz, 2000). Asymptomatic bacteriuria is almost always caused by a single organism, typically *Escherichia coli.* Other commonly found causative organisms include *Klebsiella* and *Proteus.* If more than one type of bacteria is cultured, the possibility of urine-culture contamination must be considered.

A woman who has had a UTI is susceptible to recurrent infection. If a pregnant woman develops an acute UTI, especially with a high temperature, amniotic fluid infection may develop and retard the growth of the placenta.

### Lower Urinary Tract Infection (Cystitis)

Because urinary tract infections are ascending, it is important to recognize and diagnose a lower UTI early to avoid the sequelae associated with upper UTI.

Symptoms of frequency, pyuria, and dysuria without bacteriuria may indicate urethritis caused by *Chlamydia trachomatis;* it has become a common pathogen in the genitourinary system.

When cystitis develops, the initial symptom is often dysuria, specifically at the end of urination. Urgency and frequency also occur. Cystitis is usually accompanied by a low-grade fever (38.3°C [101°F] or lower), and hematuria is occasionally seen. Urine specimens usually contain an abnormal number of leukocytes and bacteria. Diagnosis is made with a urine culture.

Treatment depends on the causative organism. Oral trimethoprim-sulfamethoxazole, fluoroquinolones, and fomycin tromethamine are frequently used in single-dose, 3-day, and 7-day regimens. (For treatment options during pregnancy, see Table 13–3.) Phenazopyridine (Pyridium), a bladder analgesic, may also be prescribed to treat the dysuria.

# Nursing Care Management

## Nursing Assessment and Diagnosis

During each visit the nurse notes any complaints from the woman of pain on urination or other urinary difficulties. If any concerns arise, the nurse obtains a clean-catch urine specimen from the woman.

Nursing diagnoses that may apply to a woman with a lower UTI include the following:

- ***Pain*** related to dysuria secondary to the UTI
- ***Knowledge deficit*** related to a lack of information about self-care measures to help prevent recurrence of UTI

## Nursing Plan and Implementation

The nurse should make sure the woman is aware of good hygiene practices, since most bacteria enter through the urethra after having spread from the anal area. See Key Facts to Remember: Information for Women about Ways to Avoid Cystitis. The nurse should also reinforce instructions or answer questions regarding the prescribed antibiotic, the amount of liquids to take, and the reasons for these treatments. Cystitis usually responds rapidly to treatment, but follow-up urinary cultures are important.

## Evaluation

Expected outcomes of nursing care include the following:

- The woman implements self-care measures to help prevent cystitis as part of her personal routine.
- The woman can identify the signs, symptoms, therapy, and possible complications of cystitis.
- The woman's infection is cured.

### KEY FACTS TO REMEMBER

*Information for Women about Ways to Avoid Cystitis*

- If you use a diaphragm for contraception, try changing methods or using another size of diaphragm.
- Avoid bladder irritants such as alcohol, caffeine products, and carbonated beverages.
- Increase fluid intake, especially water, to a minimum of six to eight glasses per day.
- Make regular urination a habit; avoid long waits.
- Practice good genital hygiene, including wiping from front to back after urination and bowel movements.
- Be aware that vigorous or frequent sexual activity may contribute to urinary tract infection.
- Urinate before and after intercourse to empty the bladder and cleanse the urethra.
- Complete medication regimens even if symptoms decrease.
- Do not use medication left over from previous infections.
- Drink cranberry juice to acidify the urine. This has been found to relieve symptoms in some cases.

## Upper Urinary Tract Infection (Pyelonephritis)

*Pyelonephritis* (inflammatory disease of the kidneys) is less common but more serious than cystitis and is often preceded by lower UTI. It is more common during the latter part of pregnancy or early postpartum and poses a serious threat to maternal and fetal well-being. Women with symptoms of pyelonephritis during pregnancy have an increased risk of preterm birth and of intrauterine growth restriction.

Acute pyelonephritis has a sudden onset, with chills, high temperature of 39.6°C to 40.6°C (103°F to 105°F), and flank pain (either unilateral or bilateral). The right side is almost always involved if the woman is pregnant because the large bulk of intestines to the left pushes the uterus to the right, putting pressure on the right ureter and kidney. Nausea, vomiting, and general malaise may ensue. With accompanying cystitis, the woman may experience frequency, urgency, and burning with urination.

Edema of the renal parenchyma or ureteritis with blockage and swelling of the ureter may lead to temporary suppression of urinary output. This is accompanied by severe colicky (spastic, intense) pain, vomiting, dehydration, and ileus of the large bowel. Women with acute pyelonephritis generally have increased diastolic blood pressure, positive fluorescent antibody titer (FA test), low creatinine clearance, significant bacteremia in urine culture, pyuria, and presence of white blood cell casts.

Often the woman is hospitalized and started on intravenous antibiotics. In the case of obstructive pyelonephritis, a blood culture is necessary. The woman is kept on bed rest. After the sensitivity report is received, the antibiotic is changed as necessary. If signs of urinary obstruction occur or continue, the ureter may be catheterized to establish adequate drainage.

With appropriate drug therapy, the woman's temperature should return to normal. The pain subsides and the urine shows no bacteria within 2 to 3 days. Follow-up urinary cultures are needed to determine that the infection has been eliminated completely.

## Nursing Care Management

### Nursing Assessment and Diagnosis

During a woman's visit, the nurse obtains a sexual and medical history to identify whether she is at risk for UTI. A clean-catch urine specimen is evaluated for evidence of ASB.

Nursing diagnoses that may apply to a woman with an upper UTI include the following:

- ***Knowledge deficit*** related to lack of information about the disease and its treatment
- ***Fear*** related to the possible long-term effects of the disease

### Nursing Plan and Implementation

The nurse provides the woman with information to help her recognize the signs of UTI, so she can contact her caregiver as soon as possible. The nurse also discusses hygiene practices, the advantages of wearing cotton underwear, and the need to void frequently to prevent urinary stasis.

The nurse stresses the importance of maintaining a good fluid intake. Drinking cranberry juice daily and taking 500 mg of vitamin C help acidify the urine and may help prevent recurrence of infection. Women with a history of UTI find it helpful to drink a glass of fluid before sexual intercourse and to void afterward.

### Evaluation

Expected outcomes of nursing care include the following:

- The woman completes her prescribed course of antibiotic therapy.
- The woman's infection is cured.
- The woman incorporates preventive self-care measures into her daily regimen.

## Pelvic Relaxation

A *cystocele* is the downward displacement of the bladder, which appears as a bulge in the anterior vaginal wall. Arbitrary classifications of mild to severe are frequently given. Genetic predisposition, childbearing, obesity, and increased age are factors that may contribute to cystocele.

Symptoms of stress incontinence are most common, including loss of urine with coughing, sneezing, laughing, or sudden exertion. Vaginal fullness, a bulging out of the vaginal wall, or a dragging sensation may also be noticeable.

If pelvic relaxation is mild, Kegel exercises are helpful in restoring tone. The exercises involve contraction and relaxation of the pubococcygeal muscle (see Chapter 9). Women have found these exercises helpful before and after childbirth in maintaining vaginal muscle tone. Estrogen may improve the condition of vaginal mucous membranes, especially in menopausal women. Vaginal pessaries or rings may be used if surgery is undesirable or impossible or until surgery can be scheduled. Surgery may be considered for cystoceles considered moderate to severe.

The nurse may instruct the woman in the use of Kegel exercises. Information on causes and contributing factors and discussion of possible alternative therapies will greatly assist the woman.

# Chapter Review

## CHAPTER HIGHLIGHTS

- Nurses should provide girls and women with clear information about menstrual issues, such as use of tampons (deodorant and absorbency); vaginal spray and douching practices; and self-care comfort measures during menstruation, such as nutrition, exercise, and use of heat and massage.
- Dysmenorrhea usually begins at, or a day before, onset of menses and disappears by the end of menstruation. Therapy with hormones such as oral contraceptives or the use of nonsteroidal antiinflammatory drugs or prostaglandin inhibitors is useful. Self-care measures include improved nutrition, exercise, applications of heat, and extra rest.
- Premenstrual syndrome occurs most often in women over age 30, and symptoms occur 2 to 3 days before onset of menstruation and subside as menstruation starts, with or without treatment. Medical management usually includes progesterone agonists and prostaglandin inhibitors. Self-care measures include improved nutrition (vitamin B complex and E supplementation and avoidance of methylxanthines found in chocolate and caffeine), a program of aerobic exercise, and participation in self-care support groups.
- Fertility awareness methods are natural, noninvasive methods of contraception often used by people whose religious beliefs prevent their using other methods.
- Mechanical contraceptives such as the diaphragm, cervical cap, and condom act as barriers to prevent the transport of sperm. These methods are used in conjunction with a spermicide.
- The intrauterine device (IUD) is a mechanical contraceptive. Although its exact method of action is not clearly understood, research suggests it acts by immobilizing sperm or by impeding the progress of sperm from the cervix to the fallopian tubes. The IUD may also act by speeding the movement of the ovum through the fallopian tube. In addition, the IUD has a local inflammatory effect.
- Oral contraceptives (the pill) are combinations of estrogen and progesterone. When taken correctly, they are the most effective of the reversible methods of fertility control.
- Spermicides are far less effective in preventing pregnancy when they are not used with a barrier method.
- Permanent sterilization is accomplished by tubal ligation for women and vasectomy for men. Although theoretically reversible, clients are advised that the method should be considered irreversible.
- Recommendations about the frequency of screening mammograms vary somewhat. Currently the American Medical Association, the American Cancer Society, and the American College of Radiology all recommend annual mammography in women beginning at age 40.
- Menopause is a physiologic, maturational change in a woman's life. Physiologic changes include the cessation of menses and decrease in circulating hormones. Hormonal changes sometimes bring unsettling emotional responses. The most common physiologic symptoms are hot flashes, palpitations, dizziness, and increased perspiration at night. The woman's anatomy also undergoes changes, such as atrophy of the vagina, reduction in size and pigmentation of the labia, and myometrial atrophy. Osteoporosis becomes an increasing concern.
- Current management of menopause centers around hormone replacement therapy and client health care education.
- Battering occurs in a cyclic pattern called the "cycle of violence" and increases in frequency and severity over time.
- Nurses are in an excellent position to intervene and assist battered women by recognizing their cues, diagnosing their problems appropriately, and understanding the complex dynamics of the battering family. Nurses provide information about available community resources, medical attention, and community support.

- Sexual assault is a form of violence acted out sexually. Most sexual assaults are expressions of anger or power.
- Following sexual assault the survivor usually experiences an assortment of symptoms known as the rape trauma syndrome.
- In fibrocystic breast disease the cysts tend to be round, mobile, and well delineated. The woman generally experiences increased discomfort premenstrually. Because of the increased risk of breast cancer, women with fibrocystic breast disease should understand the importance of monthly breast self-examination.
- Endometriosis is a condition in which endometrial tissue occurs outside the endometrial cavity. This tissue bleeds in a cyclic fashion in response to the menstrual cycle. The bleeding leads to inflammation, scarring, and adhesions. The primary symptoms include dysmenorrhea, dyspareunia, and infertility.
- Treatment of endometriosis may be medical, surgical, or a combination. For the woman not desiring pregnancy at present, oral contraceptives are used.
- Toxic shock syndrome, caused by a toxin of *Staphylococcus aureus,* is most common in women of childbearing age. There is an increased incidence in women who use tampons or barrier methods of contraception, such as the diaphragm and cervical cap.
- Vulvovaginal candidiasis (moniliasis), a vaginal infection caused by *Candida albicans,* is most common in women who use oral contraceptives, are on antibiotics, are currently pregnant, or have diabetes mellitus. It is generally treated with intravaginal suppositories or, in certain cases, with oral medication.
- Bacterial vaginosis, a common vaginal infection, is diagnosed by its characteristic fishy odor and by the presence of "clue" cells on a vaginal smear. It is treated with metronidazole unless the woman is in the first trimester of pregnancy.
- Chlamydial infection is difficult to detect in a woman but may result in pelvic inflammatory disease (PID) and infertility. It is treated with antibiotic therapy.
- Gonorrhea, a common sexually transmitted infection, may be asymptomatic in women initially but may cause PID if not diagnosed early. The treatment of choice is penicillin.
- Herpes genitalis, caused by the herpes simplex virus, is a recurrent infection with no known cure. Acyclovir (Zovirax), valacyclovir, or famciclovir may reduce the symptoms and decrease the length of viral shedding.
- Syphilis, caused by *Treponema pallidum,* is a sexually transmitted infection that is treatable if diagnosed. The characteristic lesion is the chancre. Syphilis can also be transmitted in utero to the fetus of an infected woman. The treatment of choice is penicillin.
- Condylomata accuminata (venereal warts) are transmitted by the human papillomavirus. Treatment is indicated, because research suggests a possible link with abnormal cervical changes. The treatment chosen depends on the size and location of the warts.
- Pelvic inflammatory disease may be life threatening and may lead to infertility.
- Women with an abnormal finding on a pelvic examination need a careful explanation of the finding and techniques of diagnosis and emotional support during the diagnostic period.
- The classic symptoms of a lower urinary tract infection (UTI) are dysuria, urgency, frequency, and sometimes hematuria.
- An upper UTI is a serious infection that can permanently damage the kidneys if untreated. Generally the woman is acutely ill and requires supportive therapy as well as antibiotics.
- A cystocele is a downward displacement of the bladder into the vagina. Often it is accompanied by stress incontinence. Kegel exercises may help restore tone in mild cases.

# CHAPTER REFERENCES


American College of Obstetricians and Gynecologists. (1999a). *Domestic violence* (ACOG Educational Bulletin No. 257). Washington, DC: Author.

American College of Obstetricians and Gynecologists. (1999b). *Medical management of endometriosis* (ACOG Practice Bulletin No. 11). Washington, DC: Author.

A simpler cure for pelvic infections. (1997, April). *Health,* p. 18.

Burgess, A. W., & Holmstrom, L. L. (1979). *Rape: Crisis and recovery.* Englewood Cliffs, NJ: Prentice-Hall.

Centers for Disease Control and Prevention. (1998). 1998 sexually transmitted disease treatment guidelines. *Mortality and Morbidity Weekly Report, 47*(RR-1), 1–116.

Chez, R. A., & Strathman, I. (1999). Contraception and sterilization. In J. R. Scott, P. J. DiSaia, C. B. Hammond, & W. N. Spellacy (Eds). *Danforth's Obstetrics and Gynecology* (8th ed.). Philadelphia: Lippincott Williams & Wilkins, pp. 553–566.

Cox, J. T. (1999). New primary cervical screening technologies. *The Female Patient, 24*(10), 37–56.

Crooks, R., & Baur, K. (1998). *Our sexuality* (7th ed.). Monterey, CA: Brooks/Cole.

Cullins, V. E., Dominguez, L., Guberski, T., Secor, R. M., & Wysocki, S. J. (1999). Treating vaginitis. *The Nurse Practitioner, 24*(10), 46–60.

DeLeon, F. D., & Peters, A. J. (2000). Reversal of female sterilization. In J. J. Sciarra (Ed.), *Gynecology and obstetrics* (Vol. 6). Chapter 46. Philadelphia: Lippincott Williams & Wilkins , pp. 1–6.

Endicott, J., Bardack, L., Grady-Weliky, T. A., Ling, F. W., & Schmidt, P. J. (2000). An update on premenstrual dysphoric disorder. *The Female Patient, 25*(2), 45–56.

Eschenbach, D. A. (1999). Pelvic infections and sexually transmitted diseases. In J. R. Scott, P. J. DiSaia, C. B. Hammond, & W. N. Spellacy (Eds.), *Danforth's obstetrics and gynecology* (8th ed.). Philadelphia: Lippincott Williams & Wilkins, pp. 579–600.

Eschenbach, D. A. (2000). Infectious vaginitis. In J. J. Sciarra (Ed.), *Gynecology and obstetrics* (Vol. 1). Chapter 40. Philadelphia: Lippincott Williams & Wilkins, pp. 1–17.

Esposito, M. A., Tureck, R. W., & Mastroianni, L. (1999). Understanding endometriosis. *The Female Patient, 24*(6), 79–85.

Gantt, L., & Bickford, A. (1999). Screening for domestic violence. *AWHONN Lifelines, 3*(2), 36–42.

Haddix-Hill, K. (1997). The violence of rape. *Critical Care Nursing Clinics of North America, 9*(2), 167–174.

Hammerschlag, M. R. (1999). New diagnostic methods for chlamydial infection in women. *Medscape Women's Health, 4*(5), 1–7.

Hammond, C. B. (1999). *Confronting aging and disease: The role of HRT.* Symposium conducted at the annual meeting of the American College of Obstetricians and Gynecologists, Philadelphia, PA.

Hatcher, R. A., Trussell, J., Stewart, F., Cates, W., Jr., Stewart, G. K., Guest, F., & Kowal, D. (1998). *Contraceptive technology* (17th ed.). New York: Ardent Media.

Holmes, M. M. (1998). The clinical management of rape in adolescents. *Contemporary OB/GYN, 43*(5), 62–78.

Kaunitz, A., & Jordon, C. (1997). Two long acting hormonal contraceptive options. *Contemporary Nurse Practitioner, 2*(2), 10–12.

Kim, A. H., & Adamson, G. D. (2000). Endometriosis. In J. J. Sciarra (Ed.), *Gynecology and obstetrics* (Vol. 1) Chapter 20. Philadelphia: Lippincott Williams & Wilkins, pp. 1–22.

Lauver, D. R., Baggot, A., & Kruse, K. (1999). Women's experiences in coping with abnormal Papanicolaou results and follow-up colposcopy. *Journal of Obstetric, Gynecologic, and Neonatal Nursing, 28*(3), 283–290.

Lentz, G. M. (2000). Urinary tract infections in obstetrics and gynecology. In J. J. Sciarra (Ed.), *Gynecology and obstetrics* (Vol. 2.). Philadelphia: Lippincott Williams & Wilkins.

Lindsay, S. H. (1999). Menopause, naturally. *AWHONN Lifelines, 3*(5), 32–38.

McGregor, J. A. (2000). Toxic shock syndrome. In J. J. Sciarra (Ed.), *Gynecology and obstetrics* (Vol. 1). Chapter 43. Philadelphia: Lippincott Williams & Wilkins, pp. 1–9.

Moline, M. L., & Zendell, S. M. (2000 Mar). Evaluating and managing premenstrual syndrome. *Medscape Women's Health, 5*(2), 1–3.

Nachtigall, L. E. (2000 June). Assessing alternative approaches to menopause. *Supplement to Contemporary OB/GYN,* 3–10.

National Institutes of Health. (2000, March 27–29). Osteoporosis prevention, diagnosis, and therapy. *NIH Consensus Statement Online, 17*(2):1–34.

Poirier, L. (1997). The importance of screening for domestic violence in all women. *The Nurse Practitioner, 22*(5), 105–115.

Pollack, A. E., & Barone, M. A. (2000). Reversing vasectomy. In J. J. Sciarra (Ed.), *Gynecology and obstetrics* (Vol. 6). Chapter 48. Philadelphia: Lippincott Williams & Wilkins, pp. 1–5.

Propst, A. M., & Laufer, M. R. (1999). Diagnosing and treating adolescent endometriosis. *Contemporary OB/GYN, 44*(12), 52–59.

Rosenberg, M. J., Meyers, A., & Roy, V. (1999). Efficacy, cycle control, and side effects of low- and lower-dose oral contraceptives: A randomized trial of 20 micrograms and 35 micrograms estrogen preparations. *Contraception, 60*(6), 321–329.

Schairer, C., Lubin, J., Troisi, R., Sturgeon, S., Brinton, L., & Hoover, R. (2000). Menopausal estrogen and estrogen-progestin replacement therapy and breast cancer risk. *JAMA, 283,* 485–491.

Shulman, L. P. (2000). Monthly contraceptive injection. *The Female Patient, 25*(11), 14–20.

Speroff, L. (May 15, 1998). A quarter century of contraception: Remarkable advances, increasing success. *Contemporary OB/GYN, 43*(S), 13–26.

Speroff, L. (1999, November). Hormone therapy and heart health in postmenopausal women. *Contemporary OB/GYN, 44* Suppl., 4–26.

State of the World Population (2000). Ending Violence Against Women and Girls. *United Nations Population Fund.* New York, NY: http:/www.unfpa.org/5wp 2000

Thomason, J. L., & Scaglione, N. J. (1999). Bacterial vaginosis. *Contemporary OB/GYN, 44*(6), 15–24.

Trussell, J., Ellertson, C., Stewart, F., et al. (2000). Emergency contraception: A cost-effective approach to preventing unwanted pregnancy. *Office of Population Research, Medscape/Women's Health.*

Valente, S. M. (2000). Evaluating and managing intimate partner violence. *The Nurse Practitioner, 25*(5), 18–33.

Walker, L. (1984). *The battered woman syndrome.* New York: Springer.

Wallach, M., & Grimes, D. A. (2000). Modern oral contraception: Update from the Contraception Report. Totowa, N.J.: Emron.

Wölner-Hanssen, P. (1999). Pelvic inflammatory disease: Diagnosis. *Contemporary OB/GYN, 44*(8), 108–116.

## CONTEMPORARY MATERNAL-NEWBORN NURSING ON-LINE

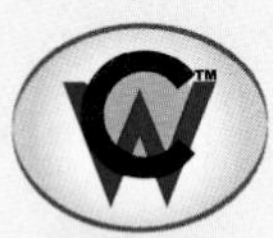

Additional interactive resources, including animations and video, for this chapter can be found on the Companion Website at http://www.prenhall.com/ladewig. Click on Chapter 4 and "Begin" to select the activities for this chapter.

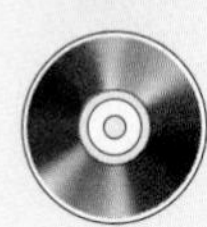

For NCLEX review questions and an audio glossary, access the accompanying CD-ROM in this book.

# Chapter 5

# Families with Special Reproductive Concerns

*When I first began working in genetics I focused primarily on the science of it, on the odds, on the disorders. Now I recognize the courage of those with known genetic disorders who must decide whether to risk childbirth, the commitment of those who care for and love children with profound disabilities, and the constant sorrow of those who lose a child because of a previously undetected genetic problem. This work is about people—not genes, not DNA, but people.*

—A Nurse Genetic Counselor

## KEY TERMS

| Term | Page |
|---|---|
| Autosomes | 125 |
| Basal body temperature (BBT) | 114 |
| Chromosomes | 125 |
| Endometrial biopsy | 117 |
| Ferning capacity | 118 |
| Genotype | 128 |
| Hysterosalpingography (HSG) | 119 |
| Infertility | 111 |
| In vitro fertilization (IVF) | 122 |
| Karyotype | 125 |
| Laparoscopy | 119 |
| Mendelian (single-gene) inheritance | 128 |
| Monosomies | 126 |
| Mosaicism | 126 |
| Non-Mendelian (multifactorial) inheritance | 128 |
| Pedigree | 128 |
| Phenotype | 128 |
| Postcoital test or Huhner test | 119 |
| Sex chromosomes | 128 |
| Spinnbarkheit | 117 |
| Subfertility | 111 |
| Therapeutic insemination | 121 |
| Transvaginal ultrasound | 117 |
| Trisomies | 125 |
| Tubal embryo transfer (TET) | 122 |

## OBJECTIVES

- Identify the essential components of fertility.
- Describe the elements of the preliminary investigation of infertility.
- Summarize the indications for the tests and associated treatments, including assisted reproductive technologies, that are done in an infertility workup.
- Identify the physiologic and psychologic effects of infertility on a couple.
- Describe the nurse's role as counselor, educator, and advocate for couples during infertility evaluation and treatment.
- Discuss the indications for preconceptual chromosomal analysis and prenatal testing.
- Identify the characteristics of autosomal dominant, autosomal recessive, and X-linked (sex-linked) recessive disorders.
- Compare prenatal and postnatal diagnostic procedures used to determine the presence of genetic disorders.
- Explore the emotional impact on a couple undergoing genetic testing or coping with the birth of a baby with a genetic disorder and explain the nurse's role in genetic counseling.

ost couples who want children are able to conceive them with little trouble. Pregnancy and childbirth usually take their normal course, and a healthy baby is born without problems. But some less fortunate couples are unable to fulfill their dream of having the desired baby because of infertility or genetic problems.

This chapter explores two particularly troubling reproductive problems: the inability to conceive and the risk of bearing babies with genetic abnormalities.

# Infertility

**Infertility** is defined as lack of conception despite unprotected sexual intercourse for at least 12 months (Bopp & Seifer, 2000). Infertility has a profound emotional, psychologic, and economic impact on both the affected couples and society. Approximately 10% to 15% of couples in their reproductive years are infertile (Speroff, Glass, & Kase, 1999). *Sterility* is the term applied when there is an absolute factor preventing reproduction. **Subfertility** is used to describe a couple that has difficulty conceiving because both partners have reduced fertility (Hatcher, Stewart, Trussell, et al., 1998).

*Primary infertility* identifies women who have never conceived, whereas *secondary infertility* indicates those who have been pregnant in the past but have not conceived during one or more years of unprotected intercourse (Hatcher et al., 1998).

Public perception is that the incidence of infertility is increasing, but in fact there has been no significant change in the proportion of infertile couples in the United States (Speroff et al., 1999). What has changed is the composition of the infertile population; the infertility diagnosis has increased in the age group 25 to 44 because of delayed childbearing and the entry of the baby boom cohort into this age range in Western society (Bopp & Seifer, 2000). The perception that infertility is on the rise may be related to the following factors:

- The deferring of pregnancy and then the desire to have a family within a short time frame
- The increase in assisted reproduction techniques
- The increase in availability and use of infertility services
- The increase in insurance coverage of some ethnic groups for diagnosis of and treatment for infertility
- The increased number of childless women over age 35 seeking medical attention for infertility
- The increased acceptance of infertility as a problem

## Essential Components of Fertility

Understanding the elements essential for normal fertility can help the nurse identify the many factors that may cause infertility. The following components must be present for normal fertility:

- Female partner
  - The cervical mucus must be favorable to ensure survival of spermatozoa and facilitate passage to the upper genital tract.
  - The fallopian tubes must be patent and have normal fimbria with peristaltic movements toward the uterus to facilitate transport and interaction of ovum and sperm.
  - The ovaries must produce and release normal ova in a regular, cyclic fashion.
  - There must be no obstruction between the ovaries and the uterus.
  - The endometrium must be in a physiologic state to allow implantation of the blastocyst and to sustain normal growth.
  - Adequate reproductive hormones must be present.
- Male partner
  - The testes must produce spermatozoa of normal quality, quantity, and motility.
  - The male genital tract must not be obstructed.
  - The male genital tract secretions must be normal.
  - Ejaculated spermatozoa must be deposited in the female vaginal tract in such a manner that they reach the cervix.

These normal findings are correlated with possible causes of deviation in Table 5–1.

With intricacies of timing and environment playing such a crucial role, it is an impressive natural phenomenon that the majority of couples in the United States are able to conceive. The remaining couples suffer infertility due to a male factor (35%), a female factor (50%), or either an unknown cause (unexplained infertility) or a problem with both partners (15%) (Speroff et al., 1999). In 35% of infertile couples, multiple causes are present. Professional intervention can help approximately 65% of infertile couples achieve pregnancy.

Couples should be referred for infertility evaluation if they have been unable to conceive after at least 1 year of attempting to achieve pregnancy. If the woman is over age 35, it may be appropriate to refer the couple after only 6 to 9 months of unprotected intercourse without conception. At age 25, when couples are the most fertile, the average length of time needed to achieve conception is 5.3 months. In about 20% of

**TABLE 5–1 Possible Causes of Infertility**

| *Necessary Norms* | *Deviations from Normal* |
|---|---|
| **FEMALE** | |
| Favorable cervical mucus | Cervicitis, cervical stenosis, use of coital lubricants, antisperm antibodies (immunologic response) |
| Clear passage between cervix and tubes | Myomas, adhesions, adenomyosis, polyps, endometritis, cervical stenosis, endometriosis, congenital anomalies (eg, septate uterus, diethylstilbestrol (DES) exposure) |
| Patent tubes with normal motility | Pelvic inflammatory disease, peritubal adhesions, endometriosis, intrauterine device, salpingitis (eg, chlamydia, recurrent sexually transmitted infections), neoplasm, ectopic pregnancy, tubal ligation |
| Ovulation and release of ova | Primary ovarian failure, polycystic ovarian disease, hypothyroidism, pituitary tumor, lactation, periovarian adhesions, endometriosis, premature ovarian failure, hyperprolactinemia, Turner syndrome |
| No obstruction between ovary and tubes | Adhesions, endometriosis, pelvic inflammatory disease |
| Endometrial preparation | Anovulation, luteal phase defect, malformation, uterine infection, Asherman's syndrome |
| **MALE** | |
| Normal semen analysis | Abnormalities of sperm or semen, polyspermia, congenital defect in testicular development, mumps after adolescence, cryptorchidism, infections, gonadal exposure to x-rays, chemotherapy, smoking, alcohol abuse, malnutrition, chronic or acute metabolic disease, medications (eg, morphine, ASA, ibuprofen), cocaine, marijuana use, constrictive underclothing, heat |
| Unobstructed genital tract | Infections, tumors, congenital anomalies, vasectomy, strictures, trauma, varicocele |
| Normal genital tract secretions | Infections, autoimmunity to semen, tumors |
| Ejaculate deposited at the cervix | Premature ejaculation, impotence, hypospadias, retrograde ejaculation (eg, diabetic), neurologic cord lesions, obesity (inhibiting adequate penetration) |

cases, conception occurs within the first month of unprotected intercourse (Speroff et al., 1999).

## Preliminary Investigation

Extensive testing for infertility is avoided until data confirm that the timing of intercourse and length of coital exposure have been adequate. The nurse provides information about the most fertile times to have intercourse during the menstrual cycle. Teaching the couple the signs and timing of ovulation and most effective times for intercourse within the cycle may solve the problem (see Table 5–2). Primary assessment, including a comprehensive history and physical examination for any obvious causes of infertility, is done before a costly, time-consuming, and emotionally trying investigation is initiated. During the first visit for the preliminary investigation, the nurse explains the basic infertility workup. The basic investigation for the couple depends on the individuals' history and usually includes assessment of ovarian function, cervical mucosal adequacy and receptivity to sperm, sperm adequacy, tubal patency, and the general condition of the pelvic organs (Bradshaw, 1998). Since about 35% of infertility is related to a male factor, a semen analysis should be one of the first diagnostic tests done before moving on to more invasive diagnostic procedures involving the woman.

**TABLE 5–2 Fertility Awareness**

Avoid douching and artificial lubricants. Prevent alteration of pH of vagina and introduction of spermicidal agents.

Promote retention of sperm. The male superior position with female remaining recumbent for at least 1 hour after intercourse maximizes the number of sperm reaching the cervix.

Avoid leakage of sperm. Elevate the woman's hips with a pillow after intercourse. Avoid getting up to urinate for 1 hour after intercourse.

Maximize the potential for fertilization. Have intercourse one to three times per week at intervals no less than 48 hours.

Avoid emphasizing conception during sexual encounters to decrease anxiety and potential sexual dysfunction.

Maintain adequate nutrition and reduce stress. Using stress-reduction techniques and good nutritional habits increases sperm production.

Explore other methods to increase fertility awareness, such as home assessment of cervical mucus and basal body temperature (BBT) recordings.

Seek counsel and advice from valued friend or family member.

Consider incorporating culturally appropriate methods to enhance fertility.

The mutual desire to have children is a cornerstone of many marriages. A fertility problem is a deeply personal, emotion-laden area in a couple's life. The self-esteem of one or both partners may be threatened if the inability to conceive is perceived as a lack of virility or femininity (Leon, 2000). The nurse can provide comfort to couples by offering a sympathetic ear, a nonjudgmental approach, and appropriate information and instructions throughout the diagnostic and therapeutic process. Because counseling includes discussion of very personal matters, nurses who are comfortable with their own sexuality are able to establish rapport and elicit relevant information from couples with fertility problems.

The first interview should involve both partners and include a comprehensive history and physical examination. Table 5–3 lists the items in a complete infertility physical workup and laboratory evaluation for both partners. Figure 5–1♦ outlines the historical database, diagnostic tests usually performed, and health care interventions used in cases of infertility.

**TABLE 5–3 Initial Infertility Physical Workup and Laboratory Evaluations**

| *Female* | *Male* |
|---|---|
| **PHYSICAL EXAMINATION** | **PHYSICAL EXAMINATION** |
| Assessment of height, weight, blood pressure, temperature, and general health status | General health (assessment of height, weight, blood pressure) |
| Endocrine evaluation of thyroid for exophthalmos, lid lag, tremor, or palpable gland | Endocrine evaluation (eg, presence of gynecomastia) |
| Optic fundi evaluation for presence of increased intracranial pressure, especially in oligomenorrheal or amenorrheal women (possible pituitary tumor) | Visual fields evaluation for bitemporal hemianopia |
| Reproductive features (including breast and external genital area) | Abnormal hair patterns |
| Physical ability to tolerate pregnancy | |
| **PELVIC EXAMINATION** | **UROLOGIC EXAMINATION** |
| Papanicolaou smear | Presence or absence of phimosis |
| Culture for gonorrhea if indicated and possibly chlamydia or mycoplasma culture (opinions vary) | Location of urethral meatus |
| Signs of vaginal infections (Chapter 4) | Size and consistency of each testis, vas deferens, and epididymis |
| Shape of escutcheon (eg, does pubic hair distribution resemble that of a male?) | Presence of varicocele |
| Size of clitoris (enlargement caused by endocrine disorders) | |
| Evaluation of cervix: old lacerations, tears, erosion, polyps, condition and shape of os, signs of infections, cervical mucus (evaluate for estrogen effect of spinnbarkheit and cervical ferning) | **RECTAL EXAMINATION** |
| **BIMANUAL EXAMINATION** | Size and consistency of prostate, with microscopic evaluation of prostate fluid for signs of infection |
| Size, shape, position, and motility of uterus | Size and consistency of seminal vesicles |
| Presence of congenital anomalies | **LABORATORY EXAMINATION** |
| Presence of endometriosis | Complete blood count |
| Evaluation of adnexa: ovarian size, cysts, fixations, or tumors | Sedimentation rate, if indicated |
| **RECTOVAGINAL EXAMINATION** | Serology |
| Presence of retroflexed or retroverted uterus | Urinalysis |
| Presence of rectouterine pouch masses | Rh factor and blood grouping |
| Presence of possible endometriosis | Semen analysis |
| **LABORATORY EXAMINATION** | If indicated, testicular biopsy, buccal smear |
| Complete blood count | Hormonal assays, FSH, LH, prolactin |
| Sedimentation rate, if indicated | |
| Serology | |
| Urinalysis | |
| Rh factor and blood grouping | |
| If indicated, thyroid function tests, prolactin levels, glucose tolerance test, hormonal assays including estradiol, LH, progesterone, FSH, dehydroepiandrosterone (DHEA), androstendione, testosterone, 17 $\alpha$-hydroxy progesterone (17-OHP). | |

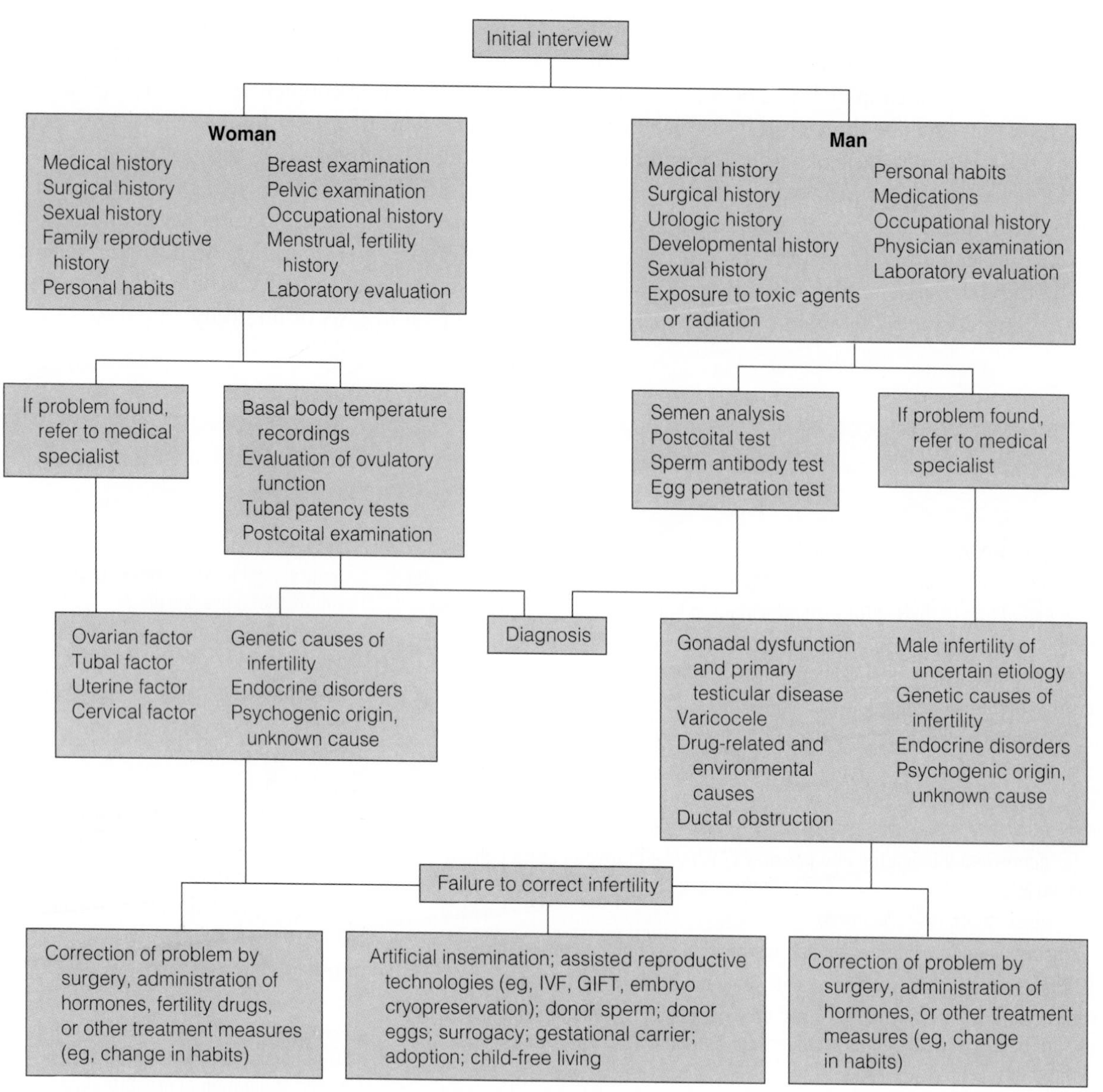


**FIGURE 5–1** ♦ Flow chart for management of the infertile couple.

## Tests for Infertility

Because of the high incidence of multifactorial infertility, a thorough female evaluation includes assessment of ovulatory function, as well as structure and function of the cervix, uterus, fallopian tubes, and ovaries. See Chapter 3 for an in-depth discussion of the fertility cycle. If the man's history indicates the need, he may be referred to a urologist and further testing. Evaluation of the man may include at least two semen analyses to confirm or rule out a seminal deficiency. Tests such as the hamster sperm penetration assay, (SPA), acrosome reaction assay, sperm density evaluation, and semen immunobead testing for the presence of antisperm antibody (immunologic infertility) may be performed, but their usefulness is controversial.

### Assessment of the Woman

**Evaluation of Ovulatory Factors** Ovulation problems account for approximately 15% of infertility causes (Speroff et al., 1999). For a review of female reproductive cycle characteristics, see Chapter 2.

One basic test of ovulatory function is the **basal body temperature (BBT)** recording, which aids in identification of follicular and luteal phase abnormalities. At the initial visit, the nurse instructs the woman in the technique of recording BBT on a special form. The woman is instructed to begin a new chart on the first day of every monthly cycle. The temperature can be taken with a standard oral or rectal thermometer calibrated by tenths of a degree, making slight temperature changes readily apparent (Carcio, 1998). A special kind of thermometer (BBT) may be used to measure temperatures only between 35°C and 37.8°C (96°F and 100°F). The woman should take the BBT every morning before getting out of bed (after 6 to 8 hours of uninterrupted sleep) (Moghissi, 1998). In addition to the traditional glass and mercury thermometer, tympanic thermometry, which provides a reading in

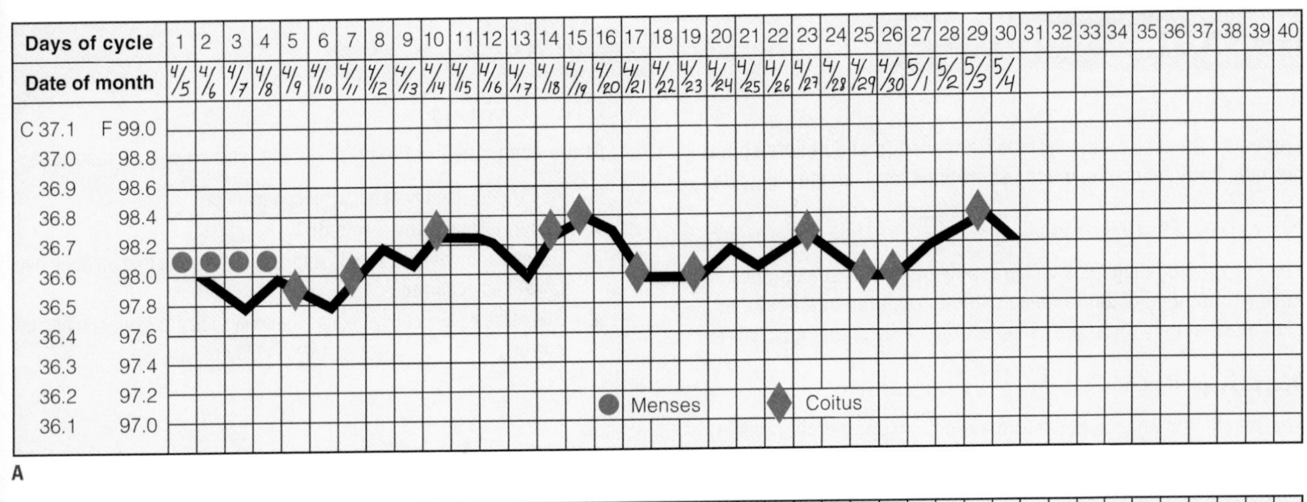


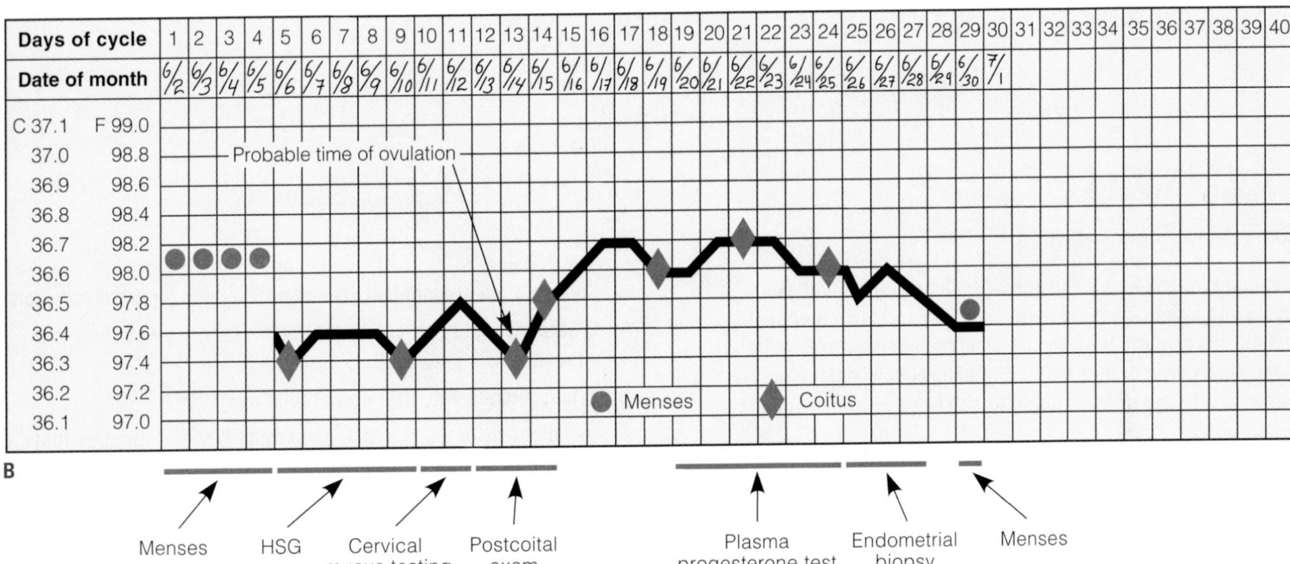


**FIGURE 5–2** ♦ **A,** A monophasic, anovulatory basal body temperature (BBT) chart. **B,** A biphasic BBT chart illustrating probable time of ovulation, the different types of testing, and the time in the cycle that each would be performed.

only a few seconds, may also be a valid method. In addition, computerized or digitalized BBT devices ("the Rabbit," Fertil-A-Chron) are being developed to identify the fertile period more accurately at home.

The woman records daily variations on the temperature graph. The temperature graph shows a typical biphasic pattern during ovulatory cycles, whereas in anovulatory cycles it remains monophasic. The woman uses the readings on the temperature graph to detect ovulation and timing of intercourse (Figure 5–2♦).

Basal temperature for females in the preovulatory phase is usually below 36.7°C (98°F). As ovulation approaches, production of estrogen increases. At its peak estrogen may cause a slight drop, then a rise, in the basal temperature. The slight drop in temperature before ovulation is often difficult to capture on the BBT chart (Carcio, 1998). Prior to ovulation, there is a surge of luteinizing hormone (LH), which stimulates production of progesterone, causing a 0.3°C to 0.6°C (0.5°F to 1.0°F) rise in basal temperature. These changes in the basal temperature create the typical biphasic pattern. Figure 5–2B♦ shows a biphasic ovulatory BBT chart. Progesterone is thermogenic (produces heat); therefore it maintains the temperature increase during the second half of the menstrual cycle (luteal phase). Temperature elevation does not predict the day of ovulation, but it does provide supportive evidence of ovulation about a day after it has occurred. Actual release of the ovum probably occurs 24 to 36 hours before the first temperature elevation (Carcio, 1998; Speroff et al., 1999).

Based on serial BBT charts, the clinician might recommend sexual intercourse every other day beginning 3 to 4 days prior to and continuing for 2 to 3 days after the expected time of ovulation. See Teaching Guide: Methods of Determining Ovulation, on pages 116 and 117.

## TEACHING GUIDE *Methods of Determining Ovulation*

### Assessment

The nurse focuses on the woman's knowledge and beliefs about her own body functions, mucus secretions, and menstrual cycle.

### Nursing Diagnosis

The key nursing diagnosis will probably be health-seeking behaviors: methods of determining ovulation related to a desire to plan a pregnancy (or to practice natural family planning)

### Nursing Plan and Implementation

The teaching plan includes information on expected changes in cervical mucus and body temperature related to menstrual cycle, how to recognize that ovulation has occurred, and self-care methods for determining fertility days.

### Client Goals

At the completion of the teaching the woman will be able to

1. Accurately identify cervical mucus changes
2. Accurately take and record BBT
3. Discuss the changes in BBT and cervical mucus that indicate ovulation has occurred
4. Summarize physical symptoms that may indicate ovulation has occurred.

## *Teaching Plan*

| CONTENT | TEACHING METHOD |
|---|---|
| **Basal Body Temperature (BBT) Method** | |
| Describe the expected findings with an ovulatory (biphasic) cycle and stress the need to monitor BBT for 3 to 4 months to establish a pattern. BBT can be used to time intercourse if pregnancy is desired or as a method of natural family planning. Describe the timing of intercourse to achieve or avoid pregnancy. | Choose a private location, free of distractions for the discussion.<br>Create a supportive, comfortable atmosphere by attitude and communication style.<br>*Briefly* explain why BBT can predict ovulation.<br>Use pictures or graphs to demonstrate the BBT changes that indicate ovulatory and anovulatory cycles. |
| Describe the procedure for measuring BBT:<br>• Using a BBT thermometer, the woman chooses one site (oral, vaginal, or rectal), which she uses consistently.<br>• The woman takes her temperature for 5 minutes every day before arising and before starting any activity, including smoking.<br>• The result is then recorded immediately on a BBT chart, and the temperature dots for each day are connected to form a graph.<br>• She then shakes the thermometer down in preparation for use the next day. | Learning is best accomplished when content is broken down into smaller steps.<br>Show the woman the BBT thermometer and demonstrate its use. *Note:* A tympanic (ear) electric thermometer may also be used.<br>Provide a blank chart. Ask the woman to chart 3 days' findings using temperature results you identify. |
| Explain that certain situations can disturb body temperature such as large alcohol intake, sleeplessness, fever, warm climate, jet lag, shift work, or the use of an electric blanket. | Provide a handout summarizing the procedure.<br>Provide frequent opportunities for questions and discussion. |
| **Cervical Mucus Method** | |
| Explain that cervical mucus changes throughout a woman's menstrual cycle and that the quality of the mucus can be used to predict ovulation. Describe the various characteristics of the cervical mucus throughout the menstrual cycle. Stress that it may take several cycles for the woman to become familiar with the pattern. | Discuss the characteristics of the mucus and the rationale for the changes.<br>Explore the woman's feelings about using the procedure. |
| Describe the procedure for assessing cervical mucus changes:<br>• Every day when she uses the bathroom the woman checks her vagina, either by dabbing the vaginal opening with toilet paper or by putting a finger in the opening. | Show pictures of the mucus changes including spinnbarkheit of different degrees of elasticity.<br>Encourage the woman to ask questions. |

## TEACHING GUIDE *Methods of Determining Ovulation continued*

- She notes the wetness (presence of mucus), collects some mucus, determines its color and consistency, and records her findings on a chart.
- She washes her hands before and after the procedure.

Stress that the presence and consistency of the mucus are altered by vaginal infection, vaginal medications, spermicides, lubricants, douching, sexual arousal, and semen.

Provide a written handout describing the process and findings so that the woman has information readily available.

### EVALUATION

Evaluate the learning by providing time for discussion, questions, and practice using the charts and thermometer. Ask the woman to describe the selected procedure in her own words.

Hormonal assessments of ovulatory function fall into the following categories:

1. *Gonadotropin levels (FSH, LH).* Baseline hormonal assessment of (FSH) and LH provides valuable information about normal ovulatory function. Measured on cycle day 3, FSH is the single most valuable test of ovarian reserve and function. FSH should always be measured, particularly in women over age 35, to predict the potential for successful treatment with ovulation-induction treatment cycles. LH levels may be measured early in the cycle to rule out androgen excess disorders, which disrupt normal follicular development and oocyte maturation. Daily sampling of LH at midcycle can detect the LH surge. The day of the LH surge is believed to be the day of maximum fertility. Urine LH ovulation prediction kits are also available for home use to better time postcoital testing, insemination, and coitus (Moghissi, 1998).
2. *Progesterone assays.* Progesterone levels furnish the best evidence of ovulation and corpus luteum functioning. Serum levels begin to rise with the LH surge and peak about 8 days later. A level of 5 ng/mL 3 days after the LH surge confirms ovulation (Moghissi, 1998). On day 21 (7 days postovulation) a level of 10 ng/mL or higher indicates an adequate luteal phase.

Hormonal assessment may also be conducted for prolactin, thyroid-stimulating hormone, and androgen (testosterone, dehydroepiandrosterone (DHEAS), and androstenedione) levels.

**Endometrial biopsy** provides information about the effects of progesterone produced by the corpus luteum after ovulation and endometrial receptivity. The biopsy is performed not earlier than 10 to 12 days after ovulation and involves removing a sample of endometrium with a small pipette attached to suction (Speroff et al., 1999). The woman should be informed that some pelvic discomfort, cramping, and vaginal spotting are normal during and following the procedure. The onset of menses following biopsy should be disclosed for accurate interpretation of the biopsy report.

A dysfunction may exist if the endometrial lining does not show the expected amount of secretory tissue for that day of the woman's menstrual cycle. Endometrial biopsies and serum progesterone assay may both be necessary to confirm luteal phase dysfunction.

**Transvaginal ultrasound** is an invaluable adjunct in infertility diagnosis and treatment. Transvaginal ultrasound is the method of choice for follicular monitoring of women undergoing induction cycles, for timing ovulation for insemination and intercourse, for retrieving oocytes for in vitro fertilization, and for monitoring early pregnancy. The use of a transvaginal color-flow Doppler to investigate uterine blood flow may in the future help the endocrinologist evaluate the adequacy of the developing follicle, further assess oocyte maturity and endometrial development and patterns, and improve the diagnosis of luteal phase defects (Moghissi, 1998).

**Evaluation of Cervical Factors** The mucous cells of the endocervix consist predominantly of water. As ovulation approaches, the ovary increases its secretion of estrogen and produces changes in the cervical mucus. The amount of mucus increases 10-fold, and the water content rises significantly.

At ovulation, mucus elasticity **(spinnbarkheit)** increases and viscosity decreases. Excellent spinnbarkheit exists when the mucus can be stretched 8 to 10 cm or longer (Speroff et al., 1999). Mucus elasticity is determined by using two glass slides (Figure 5–3A♦) or by

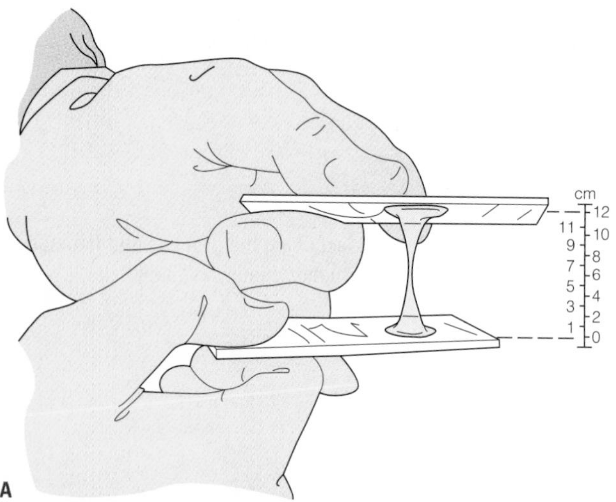


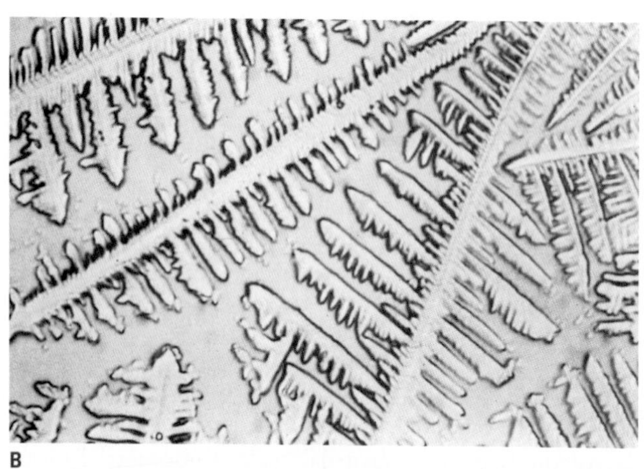


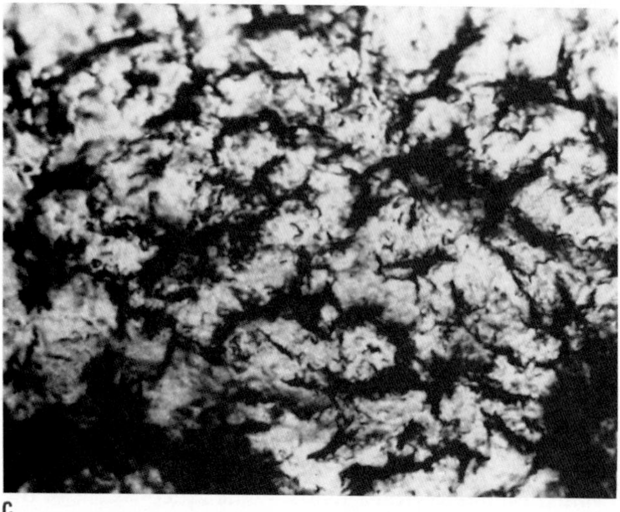


FIGURE 5–3 ♦ **A,** Spinnbarkheit (elasticity). **B,** Ferning pattern. **C,** Lack of ferning. *Source:* Speroff, L., et al. (1994). *Clinical gynecologic endocrinology and infertility* (5th ed., p. 818). Baltimore: Williams & Wilkins.

grasping some mucus at the external os and stretching it through the vagina toward the introitus. (See Teaching Guide: Methods of Determining Ovulation.)

The **ferning capacity** (crystallization) (Figure 5–3B♦) of the cervical mucus also increases as ovulation approaches.

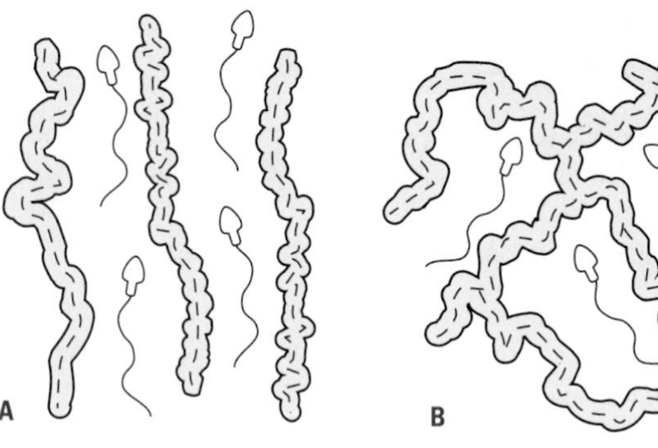


FIGURE 5–4 ♦ Sperm passage through cervical mucus. **A,** Appearance at the time of ovulation with channels favoring efficient sperm penetration and migration upward. **B,** Unfavorable mazelike configuration found at other times during the menstrual cycle. *Source:* Corson, S. (1990). *Conquering infertility* (p. 16). New York: Prentice-Hall.

Ferning is caused by decreased levels of salt and water interacting with the glycoproteins in the mucus during the ovulatory period and is thus an indirect indication of estrogen production. To test for ferning, mucus is obtained from the cervical os, spread on a glass slide, allowed to air dry, and examined under the microscope. Within 24 to 48 hours postovulation, rising levels of progesterone markedly decrease the quantity of cervical mucus and increase its viscosity and cellularity. The resulting absence of spinnbarkheit and ferning capacity decreases sperm survival.

To be receptive to sperm, cervical mucus must be thin, clear, watery, profuse, alkaline, and acellular. As shown in Figure 5–4♦, the mazelike microscopic mucoid strands align in a parallel manner to allow for easy sperm passage. The mucus is termed inhospitable if these changes do not occur.

Cervical mucus inhospitable to sperm survival can have several causes, some of which are treatable. For example, estrogen secretion may be inadequate for development of receptive mucus. Cervical infection, another cause of mucosal hostility to sperm, can be treated, depending on the type of infection. Cone biopsy, electrocautery, or cryosurgery of the cervix may remove large numbers of mucus-producing glands, creating a "dry cervix" that decreases sperm survival. Finally, treatment with clomiphene citrate may have harmful effects on cervical mucus due to its antiestrogenic properties. Therefore, therapy with supplemental estrogen for approximately 6 days before expected ovulation encourages the formation of suitable spinnbarkheit (Speroff et al., 1999). However, intrauterine insemination (IUI) is more often the most appropriate therapy to overcome these obstacles. Profuse mucus is necessary for a hospitable sperm environment.

The cervix can also be the site of secretory immunologic reactions in which antisperm antibodies are produced, causing agglutination or immobilization of sperm. The most widely used serum-sperm bioassay to detect specific classes of antibodies in serum and seminal fluid is immunobead testing by radio immunoassay. The treatment for antisperm antibodies may include IUI of the man's washed sperm to bypass the cervical factor.

The **postcoital test,** (PCT), also called the **Huhner test,** is performed 1 or 2 days before the expected date of ovulation as determined by previous BBT charts, the length of prior cycles, or a urinary LH kit. This examination evaluates the cervical mucus, sperm motility, sperm-mucus interaction, and the sperm's ability to negotiate the cervical mucus barrier (Speroff et al., 1999). The couple can have intercourse up to 12 hours before the examination. If the results are abnormal, the test should be repeated at the optimal time of 2 to 3 hours after intercourse. A small plastic catheter aspirates mucus from the internal and external os. The mucus is measured and examined microscopically for signs of infection, spinnbarkheit, ferning, number and motility of active spermatozoa per high-power field (HPF) and number of sperm with poor or no motility. The focus of the postcoital exam on the timing of intercourse may promote sexual difficulties in some infertile couples.

#### Evaluation of Uterine Structures and Tubal Patency

Tubal patency tests are usually done after BBT evaluation, semen analysis, and other less invasive tests. Tubal patency and uterine structure are usually evaluated by hysterosalpingography. Other invasive tests of tubular function are laparoscopy and hysteroscopy. Hysteroscopy may be performed earlier in the evaluation if the woman's history suggests possible tubal or adhesive disease or uterine abnormalities.

**Hysterosalpingography (HSG)** or hysterogram involves an instillation of a radiopaque substance into the uterine cavity. As the substance fills the uterus and fallopian tubes and spills into the peritoneal cavity, it is viewed with x-ray techniques. This procedure can reveal tubal patency and any distortions of the uterine cavity. In addition, the oil-based dye and injection pressure used in HSG may have a therapeutic effect. This effect may be caused by the flushing of debris, breaking of adhesions, or induction of peristalsis by the instillation (Carcio, 1998).

The HSG should be performed in the proliferative phase of the cycle to avoid interrupting an early pregnancy. This timing also avoids the lush secretory changes in the endometrium that occur after ovulation, which may prevent the passage of the dye through the tubes and present a false picture of cornual obstruction. HSG causes moderate discomfort. The pain is referred from the peritoneum (which is irritated by the subdiaphragmatic collection of gas) to the shoulder. The cramping may be decreased if the radiopaque dye is warmed to body temperature before instillation. Women can take an over-the-counter (OTC) prostaglandin synthesis inhibitor (such as ibuprofen) 30 minutes before the procedure to decrease the pain, cramping, and discomfort. HSG can also cause recurrence of pelvic inflammatory disease, so prophylactic antibiotics are recommended to prevent infection that could be triggered by the procedure (Speroff et al., 1999).

*Hysteroscopy* allows the physician to further evaluate any areas of suspicion within the uterine cavity or fallopian tubes revealed by the HSG. It is often done in conjunction with a laparoscopy, but it can be done independently and does not require general anesthesia. A fiber-optic instrument is inserted into the uterus for further evaluation of polyps, fibroids, or structural variations (Speroff et al., 1999).

**Laparoscopy** enables direct visualization of the pelvic organs and is usually done 6 to 8 months after the HSG unless symptoms suggest the need for earlier evaluation. Diagnostic laparoscopy is an outpatient procedure requiring the use of general anesthesia. Generally, a three-puncture approach is used, entry is made through the umbilical area, and supporting instruments are inserted in two suprapubic incisions. The peritoneal cavity is distended with carbon dioxide gas so that the pelvic organs can be directly visualized with a fiber-optic instrument. Tubular patency can be assessed by instillation of dye into the uterine cavity through the cervix. The pelvis is evaluated for endometriosis, adhesions, organ fixations, pelvic inflammatory disease, tumors, and cysts. The intraperitoneal gas is usually manually expressed at the end of the procedure. In routine preanesthesia instructions, the woman is told that she may have some discomfort from organ displacement and shoulder and chest pain caused by gas in the abdomen. She should be informed that she can resume normal activities as tolerated after 24 hours. Using postoperative pain medication and assuming a supine position may help relieve discomfort caused by any remaining gas.

### Assessment of the Man

A semen analysis is the single most important initial diagnostic study of the man; it should be done early in the couple's evaluation, before invasive testing of the woman. Although a postcoital test can provide information about sperm viability, it does not provide sufficient information about normal seminal parameters. To obtain adequate results, the specimen is collected after 2 to 3 days of abstinence, usually by masturbation to avoid contamination or loss of any ejaculate. If the man has difficulty producing sperm by masturbation, special medical-grade condoms are available to collect the sperm during intercourse. Neither regular nor nonlatex condoms should be used, because they contain spermicidal agents and sperm can be lost in the condom. Most lubricants also are spermicidal and should not be used unless approved by the andrology laboratory. Both seasonal and incidental variability may be seen in count and motility in successive semen analyses from the same individual. Thus, a repeat semen analysis may be required to assess the man's fertility potential adequately; a minimum of two separate analyses is recommended for confirmation. In cases in which a known testicular insult has occurred (infection, high fevers, or surgery), a repeat analysis may not be done for at least 2.5 months to allow for new sperm maturation.

Sperm analysis provides information about sperm motility and morphology and a determination of the absolute number of spermatozoa present (Table 5–4). Although low numbers and motility may indicate compromised fertility, other parameters, such as morphology, motion patterns, and progression, are important prognostic indicators. Values previously thought to indicate subfertility may in fact be compatible with normal fertility when morphology, motion patterns and progression factors are considered. An infertile specimen is one that has fewer than 20 million sperm per milliliter, less than 50% motility at 6 hours, or less than 30% normal sperm forms (Damani & Shaban, 1999). Some studies have indicated that the quality of sperm decreases with increased age (Speroff et al., 1999).

Spermatozoa have been shown to possess intrinsic antigens that can provoke male immunologic infertility. Immunologic infertility is especially apparent following vasectomy reversals or genital trauma, such as testicular torsion, in which autoimmunity to sperm (the man produces antibodies to his sperm) develops. Research now indicates that it is the actual presence of antibodies on the spermatozoal surface (not just the presence of antibodies in the serum) that affects sperm function and thus leads to subfertility. Treatment for antisperm antibodies is directed toward preventing the formation of antibodies or arresting the underlying mechanism that compromises sperm function. Different therapies that have been used, such as immunosuppression with corticosteriods and intrauterine insemination, have not proved effective. The treatment of choice for clinically significant antisperm antibodies is in vitro fertilization (IVF) or intrauterine insemination (IUI) (Damani & Shaban, 1999).

**TABLE 5–4 Normal Semen Analysis**

| *Factor* | *Value* |
|---|---|
| Volume | >2 mL |
| pH | 7.0 to 8.0 |
| Total sperm count | > 20 million/mL |
| Liquefaction | Complete in 1 hour |
| Motility | 50% or greater forward progression |
| Normal forms | 30% or greater |
| Round cells | < 5 million/mL |
| White cells | < 1 million/mL |

*Source:* World Health Organization. (1993). *The WHO laboratory manual for the examination of human semen and sperm-cervical mucus interaction* (3rd ed.). Geneva: Author.

# Methods of Infertility Management

## Pharmacological Methods

If an ovulation defect is detected during the fertility testing, the treatment depends on the specific cause. If a woman has normal ovaries, a normal prolactin level, and an intact pituitary gland, *clomiphene citrate* (Clomid or Serophene) is often used. This medication induces ovulation in 80% of women by actions at both the hypothalamic and ovarian levels; 40% of these women will become pregnant. Approximately 5% of women develop multiple-gestation pregnancies, almost exclusively twins.

Clomiphene citrate works by increasing the secretion of LH and FSH, which stimulates follicle growth. The woman usually takes 50 to 150 mg/day orally for 5 days beginning anywhere from cycle day 3 to cycle day 5 after last menses (Miller & Soules, 1998; Leibowitz & Hoffman, 2000). The woman usually starts with 50 mg/day and increases the dose by 50 mg/day to a maximum of 200 to 250 mg/day. The clinician may need to give estrogen simultaneously if the amount of cervical mucus decreases.

The woman is informed that if ovulation occurs, it is expected 5 to 10 days after the last dose. The presence of ovulation and evaluation of the response to therapy are assessed by BBT or urinary LH kit for in-home use, ultrasound evaluation, and possibly progesterone assays in conjunction with an endometrial biopsy.

After the first treatment cycle, a pelvic exam is done to rule out ovarian enlargement and hyperstimulation syndrome. Ovarian enlargement and abdominal discomfort (bloating) may result from follicular growth and formation of multiple corpora lutea. Persistence of ovarian cysts is a contraindication for further clomiphene citrate administration. Other side effects include hot flashes, abdominal distention, bloating, breast discomfort, nausea and vomiting, vision problems (such as visual spots), headache, and dryness or loss of hair (Carcio, 1998; Leibowitz & Hoffman, 2000). Supplemental low-dose estrogen may be given to ensure appropriate quality and quantity of cervical mucus.

The nurse ensures that the couple has been advised to have sexual intercourse every other day for 1 week beginning 5 days after the last day of medication. The nurse also reminds the couple that if the woman does not have a period she must be checked for the possibility of pregnancy before another trial of clomiphene citrate is started.

The woman can assess the presence of ovulation and possible response to clomiphene citrate therapy by doing BBT and urinary LH tests. The woman should be knowledgeable about side effects and call her health care provider if they occur. When visual disturbances (flashes, blurring, or spots) occur, bright lighting should be avoided. This side effect disappears within a few days or weeks after discontinuation of therapy (Speroff et al., 1999). The occurrence of hot flashes may be due to the antiestrogenic properties of clomiphene citrate. The woman can obtain some relief by increasing intake of fluids and using fans.

Therapy using *human menopausal gonadotropins (hMG),* which include *menotropins* (Pergonal®, Hemegon™, and Repronex) and *urofollitropin* (Fertinex), is indicated as a first line of therapy for anovulatory infertile women with low to normal levels of gonadotropins (FSH and LH) and as a second line of therapy in women who fail to ovulate or conceive with clomiphene citrate therapy and in women undergoing assisted reproduction to induce superovulation. Menotropin is a combination of FSH and LH obtained from postmenopausal women's urine. Gonadotropin therapy requires close observation by use of serum estradiol levels and ultrasound. Monitoring of follicle development is necessary to minimize the risk of multiple pregnancy and to avoid ovarian hyperstimulation syndrome. The daily dose of medication given is titrated based on serum estradiol and ultrasound findings. When follicle maturation has occurred, hCG may be administered by intramuscular injection to stimulate ovulation. The couple is advised to have intercourse 24 to 36 hours after hCG administration and for the next 2 days. Women who elect to have hMG medication usually have passed through all other forms of management without conceiving. Strong emotional support and thorough education are needed because of the numerous office visits and injections. Often the male partner is instructed, with return demonstration, to administer the daily injections (Leibowitz & Hoffman, 2000).

High prolactin levels may impair the glandular production of FSH and LH or block their action on the ovaries. When hyperprolactinemia accompanies anovulation, the infertility may be treated with *bromocriptine* (Parlodel). This medication acts directly on the prolactin-secreting cells in the anterior pituitary. It inhibits the pituitary's secretion of prolactin, thus preventing suppression of the pulsatile secretion of FSH and LH. Thus normal menstrual cycles are restored and ovulation is induced by allowing FSH and LH production. If treatment is successful, the tests of ovulatory function will indicate that ovulation is occurring with a normal luteal phase. Bromocriptine should be discontinued if pregnancy is suspected or at the anticipated time of ovulation because of its possible teratogenic effects. Side effects include nausea, diarrhea, dizziness, headache, and fatigue. To minimize side effects for women who are extremely sensitive, treatment may be initiated with a dose of 1.25 mg, slowly building tolerance toward the usual dose of 2.5 mg given twice daily. An intravaginal preparation may also be used to decrease the occurrence of side effects (Carcio, 1998).

When endometriosis is determined to be the cause of infertility, *danazol* (Danocrine®) may be given to suppress ovulation and menstruation and to effect atrophy of the ectopic endometrial tissue. Temporary suppression has been shown to result in healing of the endometriosis. The treatment regimen may last for 6 to 12 months or longer, depending on the severity of the disease. Other pharmacological treatments involve use of oral contraceptives or oral medroxyprogesterone acetate and gonadotropin-releasing hormone (GnRH) agonists (Yuen, 1999; Leibowitz & Hoffman, 2000). The management and care of endometriosis is further discussed in Chapter 4.

Treatment of luteal phase defects may include the use of progesterone to augment luteal phase progesterone levels. Ovulation-induction agents, such as clomiphene citrate or menotropins, may be used to augment proliferative phase FSH production in the developing follicle. It is also common to use progesterone supplementation in conjunction with these ovulation-induction agents if the drug alone does not correct the luteal phase. Occasionally hCG therapy may be used in the luteal phase to stimulate corpus luteum production of progesterone.

### Therapeutic Insemination

**Therapeutic insemination** has replaced the previously used term *artificial insemination* and involves the depositing of semen at the cervical os or in the uterus by mechanical means. *Therapeutic donor insemination (TDI)* is the current term for use of donor semen, and *therapeutic husband insemination (THI)* is the current term for use of the husband's semen. Therapeutic husband insemination is used in cases of inadequate volumes of sperm, decreased motility, and anatomic defects accompanied by inadequate deposition or penetration of semen, or retrograde ejaculation (Sigman, 1999). It is also indicated in cases of unexplained infertility and some cases of female factor infertility, such as scant or inhospitable mucus, persistent cervicitis, or cervical stenosis. Because the seminal fluid contains high levels of prostaglandins, intrauterine insemination prevents the violent reaction of nausea, severe cramps, abdominal pain, and diarrhea that can result from the absorption of prostaglandins by the uterine lining (Sigman, 1999). Sperm preparation for IUI involves washing sperm from the seminal plasma.

Therapeutic donor insemination is considered in cases of azoospermia (absence of sperm), severe oligo- or asthenospermia, inherited male sex-linked disorders, and autosomal dominant disorders. Some states have specified the parental rights of single women and donors, but most are silent on this issue (Speroff et al., 1999).

Therapeutic donor insemination has become more complicated and expensive in the past decade because of the need for strict screening and processing procedures. Guidelines established by the American Fertility Society (1994) include mandatory medical (genetic) and infectious disease screening of both donor and recipient, the need for informed consent from all parties, the need to limit the number of pregnancies per donor, and the need for accurate means of record keeping. Finally, because of the risk of transmitting infectious diseases, donated sperm must be frozen and quarantined for 6 months from the time of acquisition, and the donor must be retested before sperm can be released for use.

Numerous factors need to be evaluated before TDI is performed. Has every possible effort been made to diagnose and treat the cause of the male infertility? Do tests indicate normal fertility and sperm-ovum transport in the woman? Has the couple had an opportunity to discuss this option with an infertility counselor to explore the issues of secrecy, disclosure, and potential feelings of loss the couple (particularly the male partner) may feel about not having a genetic child? Are there any religious constraints? After making the decision, the couple should allow themselves time to further assess their concerns and explore their feelings individually and together to ensure that this option is acceptable to both.

*Intrauterine insemination (IUI),* with or without ovulation induction therapy, is an option for many couples before more aggressive treatments such as in vitro fertilization (IVF) and gamete intrafallopian transfer (GIFT) are employed.

## In Vitro Fertilization

The **in vitro fertilization (IVF)** procedure is selectively used in cases in which infertility has resulted from tubal factors, mucus abnormalities, male infertility, unexplained infertility, male and female immunologic infertility, and cervical factors. In IVF a woman's eggs are collected from her ovaries, fertilized in the laboratory, and placed into her uterus after normal embryo development has begun. If the procedure is successful, the embryo continues to develop in the uterus, and pregnancy proceeds naturally.

The potential for a successful pregnancy with IVF is maximized when three to four embryos (rather than one) are placed in the uterus. For this reason, fertility drugs are used to induce ovulation prior to the process. Follicular development and oocyte maturity are monitored frequently with ultrasound and hormonal assays. Monitoring usually begins around cycle day 5, and medications are titrated according to individual response. When follicles appear mature, hCG is given to stimulate final egg maturation and control the induction of ovulation. Egg retrieval is performed approximately 35 hours later. Once the eggs are fertilized and progress to the embryo stage, the embryos are placed in the uterus. After the procedure, the woman is advised to engage in only minimal activity for 12 to 24 hours, and progesterone supplementation is prescribed.

Success with IVF depends on many factors, but especially the woman's age and the specific indication. Women have a good chance of achieving pregnancy with an average of three cycles of IVF. Many couples find the emotional, physical, and financial costs of going beyond three cycles too great (Speroff et al., 1999). Clinical delivery rates reported by the Society of Assisted Reproductive Technology (SART) in 1996 were 26.0% per embryo transfer for women regardless of age or indication (American Society for Reproductive Medicine, 1999). The increase in maternal and neonatal morbidity associated with IVF because of the rates of multiple gestation remains an issue. Differences in successful IVF may exist between various ethnic groups (Sharara & McClamrock, 2000).

## Other Assisted Reproductive Techniques (ART)

*Gamete intrafallopian transfer (GIFT)* involves the retrieval of oocytes by laparoscopy; immediate placement of the oocytes in a catheter with washed, motile sperm; and placement of the gametes into the fimbriated end of the fallopian tube. Fertilization occurs in the fallopian tube as with normal conception (in vivo) rather than in the laboratory (in vitro). From the GIFT technology evolved procedures such as *zygote intrafallopian transfer (ZIFT) and* ***tubal embryo transfer (TET).*** In these procedures eggs are retrieved and incubated with the man's sperm. However, the eggs are transferred back to the woman's body at a much earlier stage of cell division than in IVF and, as in GIFT, are placed in the fallopian tube or tubes and not the uterus. In TET the placement is done at the embryo stage. These procedures allow fertilization to be documented, which is not possible with GIFT, and the pregnancy rate is theoretically increased when the fertilized ovum is placed in the fallopian tube. IVF success rates approximate those that have been achieved with the GIFT procedure, and IVF is a much less invasive and costly procedure. For these reasons, GIFT and other tubal procedures have lost some acceptance and IVF techniques are more often employed. However, GIFT may be more acceptable to adherents of some religions, since fertilization does not occur outside the woman's body. Other technologies involve oocyte donation and cryopreservation of the embryo (Kingsberg, Applegarth, & Janata, 2000).

Several new reproductive technologies are available to assist families with genetic problems or infertile women who are unable to carry a pregnancy. The diagnosis of genetic disorders via blastomere analysis before implantation provides couples with the option of foregoing the attempt to establish a pregnancy and thereby avoiding a difficult decision about terminating an affected pregnancy (Verp, 1999a). Assisted embryo hatching is a micromanipulation procedure that has proved to be an effective adjunct therapy in IVF. In vitro fertilization using a gestational carrier allows infertile women who are genetically sound but unable to carry a pregnancy to exercise the option of having their own biologic child (Pergament & Fiddler, 2000).

**TABLE 5–5 Tasks of the Infertile Couple**

| *Tasks* | *Nursing Interventions* |
|---|---|
| Recognize how infertility affects their lives and express feelings (may be negative toward self or mate) | Supportive: help to understand and facilitate free expression of feelings |
| Grieve the loss of potential offspring | Help to recognize feelings |
| Evaluate reasons for wanting a child | Help to understand motives |
| Decide about management | Identify alternatives; faciliate partner communication |

*Source:* Sawatzky, M. (1981). Tasks of the infertile couple. *Journal of Obstetric, Gynecologic, and Neonatal Nursing,* 10, 132.

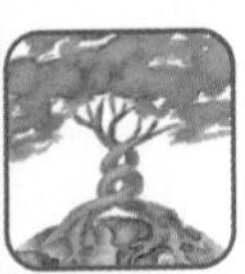

## Community-Based Nursing Care

Infertility therapy taxes a couple's financial, physical, and emotional resources. Treatment can be costly, and often insurance coverage is limited. Years of effort and numerous evaluations and examinations may take place before conception occurs, if it occurs at all. In a society that values children and considers them to be the natural result of marriage, infertile couples face a myriad of tensions and discrimination. Clinic nurses need to be constantly aware of the emotional needs of the couple confronting infertility evaluation and treatment. Often an intact marriage will become stressed with intrusive infertility procedures and treatments. Constant attention to temperature charts and instructions about their sex life from a person outside the relationship naturally affect the spontaneity of a couple's interactions. Tests and treatments may heighten feelings of frustration or anger between partners. The need to share this intimate area of a relationship, especially when one or the other is identified as "the cause" of infertility, may precipitate feelings of guilt or shame. The nurse's role can be summarized as that of counselor, educator, and advocate. Tasks of the infertile couple and appropriate nursing interventions are summarized in Table 5–5. Throughout the evaluation process nurses play a key role in lessening the stress these couples must endure by providing resources and accurate information about what is entailed in treatment and what physical, emotional, and financial demands they can anticipate throughout the process (Glover, Hunter, Richards, et al., 2000).

The nurse's ability to assess and respond to emotional and educational needs is essential to give infertile couples a sense of control (Carcio, 1998; Klock & Greenfield, 2000). An assessment tool such as an infertility questionnaire (Table 5–6) may be helpful. Extensive and repeated explanations and written instruction may be necessary because the couple's anxiety often overwhelms their ability to retain all the information given. It is important to use a nursing framework that recognizes the multidimensional needs of the infertile individual or couple within physical, social, psychologic, spiritual, and environmental contexts.

Infertility may be perceived as a loss by one or both partners. Affected individuals have described this loss as loss of their relationship with spouse, family, or friends; their health; their status or prestige; their self-esteem and self-confidence; their security; and the potential child. One such loss may lead to depression, but in many cases the crisis of infertility evokes feelings of all these losses (Bradshaw, 1998). Each couple passes through several stages of feelings, not unlike those identified by Kübler-Ross: surprise, denial, anger, isolation, guilt, grief, and resolution. The impact of these feelings on the couple and how fast they move into resolution, if ever, may depend on the cause and on the duration of treatment. Each partner may progress through the stages at different rates (Sandelowski, 1994). Nonjudgmental acceptance and a professional, caring attitude on the nurse's part can go far in dissipating the negative emotions the couple may experience while going through these stages.

This is also a time when the nurse may assess the couple's relationship: Are they able and willing to communicate verbally and share feelings? Are they mutually supportive? The answers to such questions may help the nurse to identify areas of strength and weakness and to construct an appropriate plan of care. Referral to mental health professionals is helpful when the emotional issues become too disruptive in the couple's relationship or life. The couple should be aware of infertility support and education organizations such as RESOLVE, which may help meet some of their needs and validate their feelings. Finally, individual or group counseling with other infertile couples may help the couple resolve feelings brought about by their own difficult situation.

## TABLE 5–6 Infertility Questionnaire

**SELF-IMAGE**

1. I feel bad about my body because of our inability to have a child.
2. Since our infertility, I feel I can do anything as well as I used to.
3. I feel as attractive as before our infertility.
4. I feel less masculine/feminine because of our inability to have a child.
5. Compared with others, I feel I am a worthwhile person.
6. Lately, I feel I am sexually attractive to my wife/husband.
7. I feel I will be incomplete as a man/woman if we cannot have a child.
8. Having an infertility problem makes me feel physically incompetent.

**GUILT/BLAME**

1. I feel guilty about somehow causing our infertility.
2. I wonder if our infertility problem is due to something I did in the past.
3. My spouse makes me feel guilty about our problem.
4. There are times when I blame my spouse for our infertility.
5. I feel I am being punished because of our infertility.

**SEXUALITY**

1. Lately I feel I am able to respond to my spouse sexually.
2. I feel sex is a duty, not a pleasure.
3. Since our infertility problem, I enjoy sexual relations with my spouse.
4. We have sexual relations for the purpose of trying to conceive.
5. Sometimes I feel like a "sex machine," programmed to have sex during the fertile period.
6. Impaired fertility has helped our sexual relationship.
7. Our inability to have a child has increased my desire for sexual relations.
8. Our inability to have a child has decreased my desire for sexual relations.

*Note:* The questionnaire is scored on a Likert scale, with responses ranging from "strongly agree" to "strongly disagree." Each question is scored separately, and the mean score is determined for each section (Self-Image, Guilt/Blame, and Sexuality). The total mean score is then divided by 3. A final mean score of greater than 3 indicates distress.

*Source:* Bernstein, J. (1985). Assessment of psychological dysfunction associated with infertility. *Journal of Obstetric, Gynecologic, and Neonatal Nursing, 14* (Suppl.), 63.

### ADOPTION

Infertile couples consider various alternatives for resolving their infertility; adoption is one option that will be considered at several points during the treatment process. The adoption of an infant can be a difficult and frustrating experience for all persons involved. As couples begin to consider adoption, an important aspect of this exploration is the reading of magazines and informational books on adoption, attending adoption support groups and conferences, and meeting with adoptive parents to discuss their experiences with adoption (Carcio, 1998). Some couples seek international adoption or consider adopting older children, children with handicaps, or children of mixed parentage because the adoption process in such cases is quicker and more children are available. Nurses in the community can assist couples considering adoption by providing information on community resources for adoption and support through the adoption process. Couples also need support if they choose to remain childless.

### PREGNANCY AFTER INFERTILITY

The feeling of being infertile does not necessarily disappear with pregnancy. Although there may be initial ecstacy, couples may face a whole new arena of fear and anxiety, and the parents-to-be often do not know where they "fit in." They may feel a great sense of isolation because those who have had no trouble conceiving cannot relate to the physical and emotional pain they endured to achieve the pregnancy. Contact with their past support system composed of other infertile couples may vanish when peers learn they have resolved their infertility problems. Although the desperation to become pregnant may have superseded the couple's ability to acknowledge their concerns about undergoing various treatments or procedures, questions about the repeated cycle of fertility drugs or the achievement of pregnancy through IVF technology or cryopreservation may now arise. The expectant couple may be very concerned about the potential of these treatments to adversely affect the fetus (Buitendijk, 1999). Couples may need reassurance throughout the pregnancy to allay these anxieties. The nurse can assist couples who conceive after infertility by acknowledging their past experiences of infertility treatment; validating their fears and anxieties as they face childbirth classes, birth, and parenting issues; and providing support and education about what to anticipate physically and emotionally throughout the pregnancy.

## Genetic Disorders

Even when conception has been achieved, families can have special reproductive concerns. The desired and expected outcome of any pregnancy is the birth of a healthy, "perfect" baby. Parents experience grief, fear, and anger when they discover that their baby has been born with a defect or a genetic disease. Such an abnormality may be evident at birth or may not appear for some time. The baby may have inherited a disorder from one parent, creating guilt and strife within the family.

Regardless of the type or scope of the problem, parents will have many questions: "What did I do?" "What caused it?" "Will it happen again?" The nurse must anticipate the couple's questions and concerns and guide, direct, and support the family (Olsen, 1994). To do so, the nurse must have a basic knowledge of genetics and genetic counseling. Many congenital malformations and diseases are genetic or have a strong genetic component. Others are not genetic at all. Professional nurses can help expedite this process if they understand the principles involved and can direct the family to the appropriate resources.

## Chromosomes and Chromosomal Analysis

All hereditary material is carried on tightly coiled strands of (DNA) known as **chromosomes.** Chromosomes carry the genes, the smallest units of inheritance.

All *somatic (body) cells* contain 46 chromosomes, which is the *diploid* number; the sperm and egg contain 23 chromosomes, or the *haploid* number (see Chapter 3). There are 23 pairs of homologous chromosomes (a matched pair of chromosomes, one inherited from each parent); 22 of the pairs are **autosomes** (nonsex chromosomes), and one pair is made up of the sex chromosomes, X and Y. A normal female has a 46,XX chromosome constitution; a normal male has a 46,XY chromosome constitution (Figures 5–5 and 5–6♦). The **karyotype,** or pictorial analysis of these chromosomes, is usually obtained from specially treated and stained peripheral blood lymphocytes. Placental tissue taken from a site near the insertion of the cord and deep enough to include chorion can also be sent for karyotyping.

Chromosomal abnormalities can occur in either the autosomes or the sex chromosomes and can be divided into two categories: abnormalities of number and abnormalities of structure. Even small alterations in chromosomes can cause problems, especially those associated with slow growth and development or with mental retardation. The child need not have obvious major congenital malformations to be affected. Some of these abnormalities can be passed on to other offspring. Thus, in some cases, chromosomal analysis is appropriate even if clinical manifestations are mild. Whatever the case, too much or too little genetic material usually produces adverse effects on a child's growth and development.

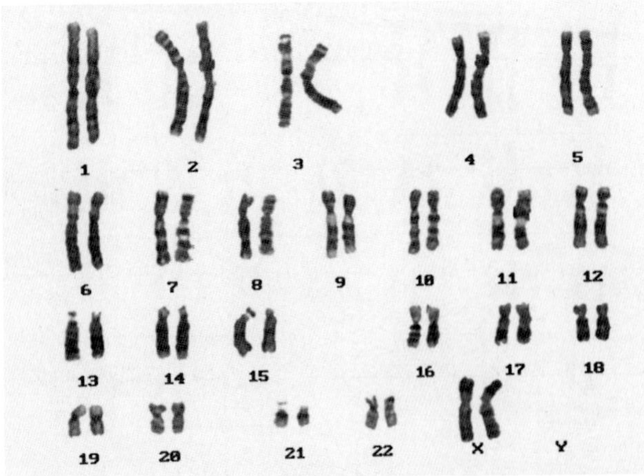


FIGURE 5–5 ♦ Normal female karyotype. *Source:* Courtesy David Peakman, Reproductive Genetics Center, Denver, CO.

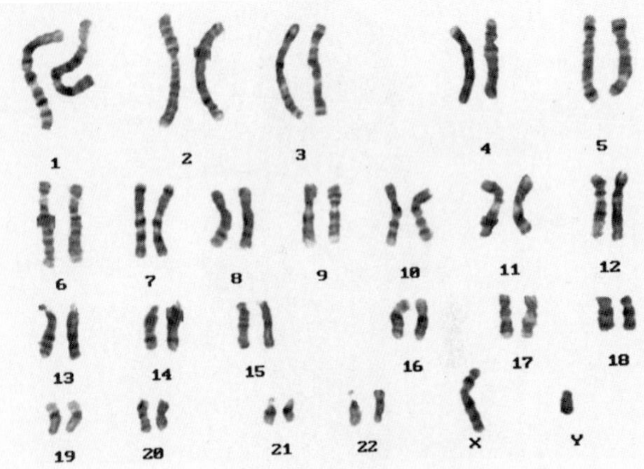


FIGURE 5–6 ♦ Normal male karyotype. *Source:* Courtesy David Peakman, Reproductive Genetics Center, Denver, CO.

## Autosomal Abnormalities

*Abnormalities of chromosome number* are most commonly seen as trisomies, monosomies, and mosaicism. In all three cases, the abnormality is most often caused by nondisjunction. Nondisjunction occurs when paired chromosomes fail to separate during cell division. If nondisjunction occurs in either the sperm or the egg before fertilization, the resulting zygote (fertilized egg) will have an abnormal chromosome makeup in all of the cells (trisomy or monosomy). If nondisjunction occurs after fertilization, the developing zygote will have cells with two or more different chromosome makeups, evolving into two or more different cell lines (mosaicism).

**Trisomies** are the product of the union of a normal gamete (egg or sperm) with a gamete that contains an extra chromosome. The individual will have 47 chromosomes and is trisomic (has three copies of the same chromosome) for whichever chromosome is extra. Down syndrome (formerly called mongolism) is the most common trisomy abnormality seen in children (see Figure 5–7♦). The presence of the extra chromosome 21 produces distinctive clinical features (see Table 5–7 on page 127 and Figure 5–8♦). With the advent of modern surgical techniques and antibiotics, children with Down's syndrome are now living into their fifth and sixth decades.

Two other common trisomies are trisomy 18 and trisomy 13 (see Table 5–7 on page 127 and Figures 5–9 and 5–10♦). The prognosis for both trisomy 13 and 18 is extremely poor. Most children (70%) die within the first 3 months of life secondary to complications related

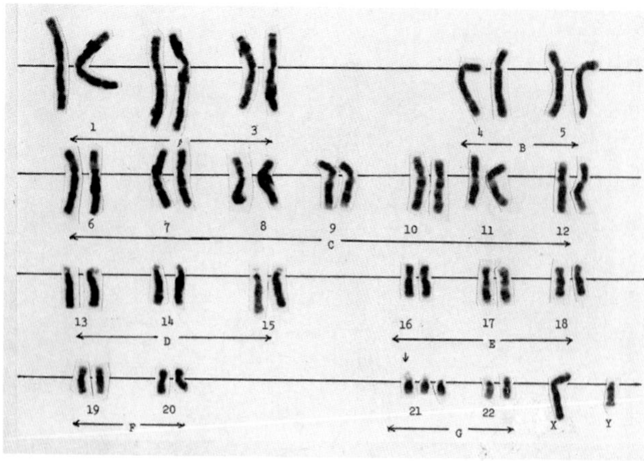


**FIGURE 5–7 ♦** Karyotype of a male who has trisomy 21, Down syndrome. Note the extra 21 chromosome. *Source:* Courtesy Dr. Arthur Robinson, National Jewish Hospital and Research Center, Denver, CO.

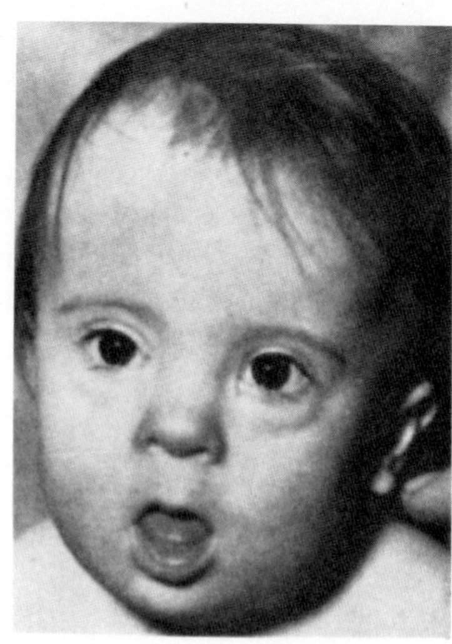

**FIGURE 5–8 ♦** A child with Down syndrome. *Source:* Jones, K. L. (1988). *Smith's recognizable patterns of human malformations* (4th ed.). Philadelphia: Saunders.

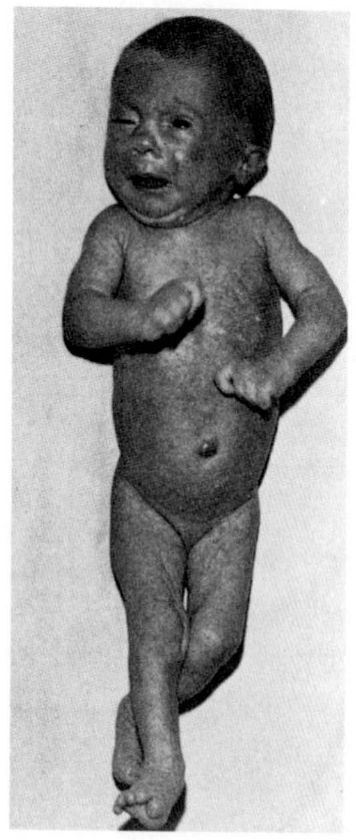

**FIGURE 5–9 ♦** Infant with trisomy 18. *Source:* Jones, K. L. (1988). *Smith's recognizable patterns of human malformations* (4th ed.). Philadelphia: Saunders.

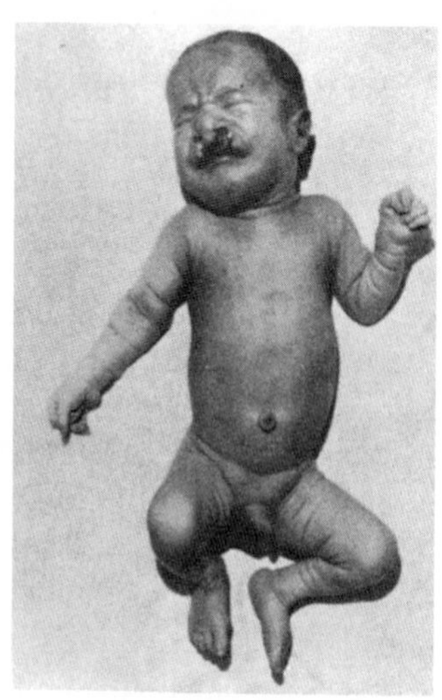

**FIGURE 5–10 ♦** Infant with trisomy 13. *Source:* Jones, K. L. (1988). *Smith's recognizable patterns of human malformations* (4th ed.). Philadelphia: Saunders.

to respiratory and cardiac abnormalities. However, 10% survive the first year of life; therefore, the family needs to plan for the possibility of long-term care of a severely affected infant and for family support.

**Monosomies** occur when a normal gamete unites with a gamete that is missing a chromosome. In this case, the individual has only 45 chromosomes and is said to be monosomic. Monosomy of an entire autosomal chromosome is incompatible with life.

**Mosaicism** occurs after fertilization and results in an individual who has two different cell lines, each with a different chromosomal number. Mosaicism tends to be more common in the sex chromosomes than in the autosomes; when it occurs in the autosomes it is most common in those with Down syndrome. An individual with many classic signs of Down syndrome but with normal or near-normal intelligence should be investigated for the possibility of mosaicism.

*Abnormalities of chromosome structure* involve only parts of the chromosome and occur in two forms: translocation and deletions or additions. Some children born with Down syndrome have an abnormal rearrangement of chromosomal material known as a *translocation.* Clinically, the two types of Down syndrome are indistinguishable. What is of major importance to the family is that the two different types have significantly different risks of recurrence. The only way to distinguish the two types of Down syndrome is to do a chromosome analysis. Risk of trisomy is 1 in 700 live births; in contrast, the risk is 1 in 1500 live births with a balanced translocation.

## TABLE 5–7 Chromosomal Syndromes

| ALTERED CHROMOSOME | CHARACTERISTICS |
|---|---|
| **ALTERED CHROMOSOME: 21**<br>Genetic defect: trisomy 21 (Down syndrome) (secondary nondisjunction or 14/21 unbalanced translocation)<br>Incidence: average 1 in 700 live births, incidence variable with age of woman **(Figure 5–8♦)** | CNS: mental retardation; hypotonia at birth<br>Head: flattened occiput; depressed nasal bridge; mongoloid slant of eyes; epicanthal folds; white specking of the iris (Brushfield spots); protrusion of the tongue; high, arched palate; low-set ears<br>Hands: broad, short fingers; abnormalities of finger and foot; dermal ridge patterns (dermatoglyphics); transverse palmar crease (simian line)<br>Other: congenital heart disease |
| **ALTERED CHROMOSOME: 18**<br>Genetic defect: trisomy 18<br>Incidence: 1 in 3000 live births **(Figure 5–9♦)** | CNS: mental retardation; severe hypotonia<br>Head: prominent occiput; low-set ears; corneal opacities; ptosis (drooping eyelids)<br>Hands: third and fourth fingers overlapped by second and fifth fingers; abnormal dermatoglyphics; syndactyly (webbing of fingers)<br>Other: congenital heart defects; renal abnormalities; single umbilical artery; gastrointestinal tract abnormalities; rocker-bottom feet; cryptorchidism; various malformations of other organs |
| **ALTERED CHROMOSOME: 13**<br>Genetic defect: trisomy 13<br>Incidence: 1 in 5000 live births **(Figure 5–10♦)** | CNS: mental retardation; severe hypotonia; seizures<br>Head: microcephaly; microphthalmia and/or coloboma (keyhole-shaped pupil); malformed ears; aplasia of external auditory canal; micrognathia (abnormally small lower jaw); cleft lip and palate<br>Hands: polydactyly (extra digits); abnormal posturing of fingers; abnormal dermatoglyphics<br>Other: congenital heart defects; hemangiomas; gastrointestinal tract defects; various malformations of other organs |
| **ALTERED CHROMOSOME: 5P**<br>Genetic defect: deletion of short arm of chromosome 5 (cri du chat, or cat cry syndrome)<br>Incidence: 1 in 20,000 live births | CNS: severe mental retardation; a catlike cry in infancy<br>Head: microcephaly; hypertelorism (widely spaced eyes); epicanthal folds; low-set ears<br>Other: failure to thrive; various organ malformations |
| **ALTERED CHROMOSOME: XO (SEX CHROMOSOME)**<br>Genetic defect: only one X chromosome in female (Turner syndrome)<br>Incidence: 1 in 300–7000 live female births **(Figure 5–11♦)** | CNS: no intellectual impairment; some perceptual difficulties<br>Head: low hairline; webbed neck<br>Trunk: short stature; cubitus valgus (increased carrying angle of arm); excessive nevi (congenital discoloration of skin due to pigmentation); broad, shieldlike chest with widely spaced nipples; puffy feet; no toenails<br>Other: fibrous streaks in ovaries; underdeveloped secondary sex characteristics; primary amenorrhea; usually infertile; renal anomalies; coarctation of the aorta |
| **ALTERED CHROMOSOME: XXY (SEX CHROMOSOME)**<br>Genetic defect: extra X chromosome in male (Klinefelter syndrome)<br>Incidence: 1 in 1000 live male births, approximately 1%–2% of institutionalized males | CNS: mild mental retardation<br>Trunk: occasional gynecomastia (abnormally large male breasts); eunuchoid body proportions (lack of male muscular and sexual development)<br>Other: small, soft testes; underdeveloped secondary sex characteristics; usually sterile |

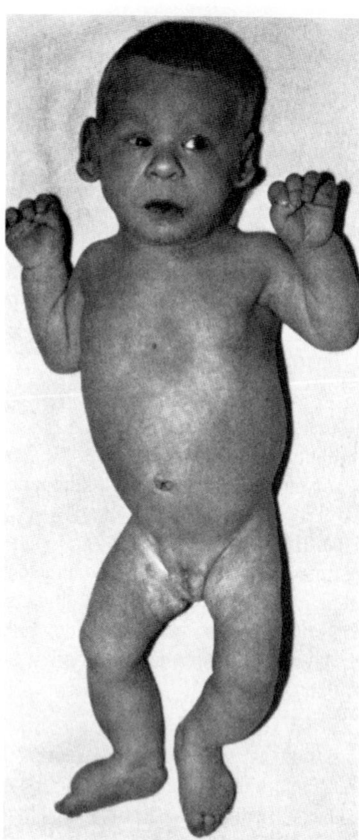

**FIGURE 5–11** ♦ Infant with Turner syndrome at 1 month of age. Note prominent ears. *Source:* Lemli, L., & Smith, D. W. (1963). The XO syndrome: A study of the differentiated phenotype in 25 patients. *Journal of Pediatrics, 63,* 577.

The translocation occurs when the carrier parent has 45 chromosomes, usually with one chromosome fused to another. A common translocation is one in which the parent has one normal 14, one normal 21, and one 14/21 chromosome. Since all the chromosomal material is present and functioning normally, the parent is clinically normal. This individual is known as a *balanced translocation carrier.* When a person who is a balanced translocation carrier has a child with a partner who has a structurally normal chromosome constitution, the child can have a normal number of chromosomes, be a carrier, or have an extra chromosome 21. Such a child has an *unbalanced translocation* and has Down syndrome.

Structure abnormality is also caused by *additions* or *deletions* of chromosomal material. Any portion of a chromosome may be lost or added, generally leading to some adverse effect. Depending on how much chromosomal material is involved, the clinical effects may be mild or severe. Many types of additions and deletions have been described, such as the deletion of the short arm of chromosome 5 (cri du chat, or cat cry, syndrome) or the deletion of the long arm of chromosome 18 (see Table 5–7).

## Sex Chromosome Abnormalities

To better understand abnormalities of the **sex chromosomes,** the nurse should know that in a female, at an early embryonic stage, one of the two normal X chromosomes becomes inactive. The inactive X chromosome forms a dark staining area known as the *Barr body.* The normal female has one Barr body, since one of her two X chromosomes has been inactivated. The normal male has no Barr bodies because he has only one X chromosome.

The most common sex chromosome abnormalities are Turner syndrome in females (45,XO with no Barr bodies present; see Figure 5–11♦) and Klinefelter syndrome in males (47,XXY with one Barr body present). See Table 5–7 for clinical descriptions of these abnormalities.

## Modes of Inheritance

Many inherited diseases are produced by an abnormality in a single gene or pair of genes. In such instances, the chromosomes are grossly normal. The defect is at the gene level. Some of these gene defects can be detected by technologies such as DNA and biochemical assays.

The two major categories of inheritance are **Mendelian (single-gene) inheritance** and **non-Mendelian (multifactorial) inheritance.** Each single-gene trait is determined by a pair of genes working together. These genes are responsible for the observable expression of the traits (eg, blue eyes, fair skin), referred to as the **phenotype.** The total genetic makeup of an individual is referred to as the **genotype** (pattern of the genes on the chromosomes).

One of the genes for a trait is inherited from the mother, the other from the father. An individual who has two identical genes at a given locus is considered to be *homozygous* for that trait. An individual is considered to be *heterozygous* for a particular trait when he or she has two different *alleles* (alternate forms of the same gene) at a given locus on a pair of homologous chromosomes.

The best-known modes of single-gene inheritance are autosomal dominant, autosomal recessive, and X-linked (sex-linked) recessive. There is also an X-linked dominant mode of inheritance, which is less common, and the now identified mode of inheritance, fragile X syndrome.

### Autosomal Dominant Inheritance

An individual is said to have an autosomal dominant inherited disorder if the disease trait is heterozygous—that is, the abnormal gene overshadows the normal gene of the pair to produce the trait. It is essential to remember that in autosomal dominant inheritance

1. An affected individual generally has an affected parent. Thus the family **pedigree** (graphic representation of a family tree) usually shows multiple generations with the disorder.

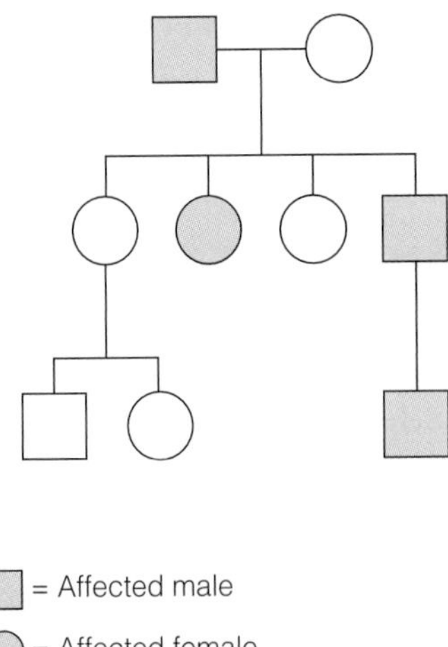


**FIGURE 5–12** ♦ Autosomal dominant pedigree. One parent is affected. Statistically, 50% of offspring will be affected, regardless of sex.

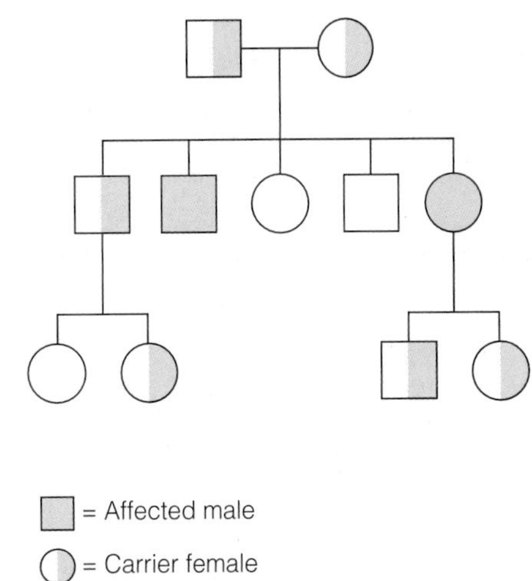


**FIGURE 5–13** ♦ Autosomal recessive pedigree. Both parents are carriers. Statistically, 25% of offspring are affected, regardless of sex.

2. An affected individual has a 50% chance of passing on the abnormal gene to each of his or her children (Figure 5–12♦).
3. Males and females are equally affected, and a father can pass the abnormal gene on to his son. This is an important principle when distinguishing autosomal dominant disorders from X-linked disorders.
4. Autosomal dominant inherited disorders have varying degrees of presentation. This is an important factor when counseling families concerning autosomal dominant disorders. A parent with a mild form of the disease may have a child with a more severe form.

Some common autosomal dominant inherited disorders are Huntington's disease, polycystic kidney disease, neurofibromatosis (von Recklinghausen disease), and achondroplastic dwarfism.

## Autosomal Recessive Inheritance

In an autosomal recessive inherited disorder, the individual must have two abnormal genes to be affected. The notion of a *carrier state* is appropriate here. A carrier is an individual who is heterozygous for the abnormal gene and clinically normal. It is not until two individuals mate and pass on the same abnormal gene that affected children may appear. It is essential to remember that in autosomal recessive inheritance

1. An affected individual may have clinically normal parents, but both parents are carriers of the abnormal gene (Figure 5–13♦).
2. With two carrier parents there is a 25% chance that the abnormal gene will be passed on to any of their offspring. Each pregnancy has a 25% chance of resulting in an affected child.
3. If a child of two carrier parents is clinically normal, there is a 50% chance that he or she is a carrier of the gene.
4. Both males and females are equally affected.
5. There is an increased history of consanguineous matings (mating of close relatives).

Some common autosomal recessive inherited disorders are cystic fibrosis, phenylketonuria, (PKU), galactosemia, sickle-cell anemia, Tay-Sachs disease, and most metabolic disorders.

## X-Linked Recessive Inheritance

X-linked, or sex-linked, disorders are those for which the abnormal gene is carried on the X chromosome. Thus an X-linked disorder is manifested in a male who carries the abnormal gene on his X chromosome. His mother is considered to be a carrier when the normal gene on one X chromosome overshadows the abnormal gene on the other X chromosome. It is essential to remember that in X-linked recessive inheritance

1. There is no male-to-male transmission. Affected males are related through the female line (see Figure 5–14♦).
2. There is a 50% chance that a carrier mother will pass the abnormal gene to each of her sons, who will thus be affected. There is a 50% chance that a carrier mother will pass the normal gene to each of her sons, who will thus be unaffected. Finally, there is a 50% chance that a carrier mother will pass the abnormal gene to each of her daughters, who will become carriers.
3. Fathers affected with an X-linked disorder cannot pass the disorder to their sons, but all their daughters become carriers of the disorder.

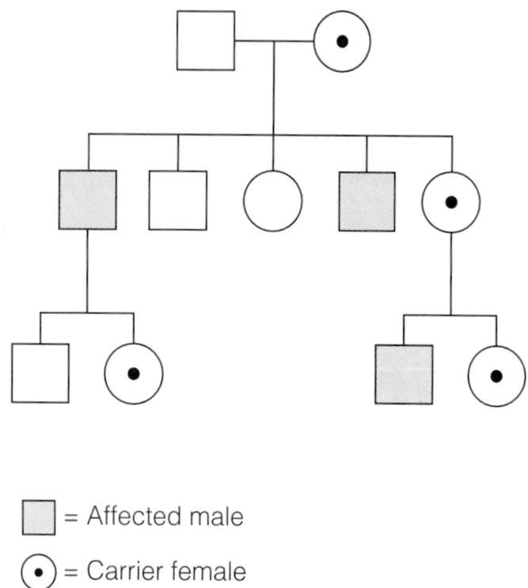


**FIGURE 5–14** ♦ X-linked recessive pedigree. The mother is the carrier. Statistically, 50% of male offspring are affected, and 50% of female offspring are carriers.

Common X-linked recessive disorders are hemophilia, Duchenne muscular dystrophy, and color blindness.

### X-Linked Dominant Inheritance

X-linked dominant disorders are extremely rare, the most common being vitamin D–resistant rickets. When X-linked dominance does occur, the pattern is similar to that of X-linked recessive inheritance except that heterozygous females are affected. It is essential to remember that in X-linked dominant inheritance there is no male-to-male transmission. Affected fathers will have affected daughters but no affected sons.

### Fragile X Syndrome

Fragile X syndrome is a common inherited form of mental retardation second only to Down syndrome among all causes of moderate mental retardation in males (Hogge & Lanasa, 1999). Fragile X syndrome is a central nervous system disorder linked to a "fragile" site on the X chromosome. It is characterized by moderate mental retardation, large protuberant ears, and large testes after puberty. The carrier females do not have the abnormal features, but about one-third are mildly mentally retarded.

### Multifactorial Inheritance

Many common congenital malformations, such as cleft palate, heart defects, spina bifida, dislocated hips, clubfoot, and pyloric stenosis, are caused by an interaction of many genes and environmental factors. They are, therefore, multifactorial in origin. It is essential to remember that in multifactorial inheritance

1. The malformations may vary from mild to severe. For example, spina bifida may range in severity from mild (spina bifida occulta) to more severe (myelomeningocele). It is believed that the more severe the defect, the greater the number of genes present for that defect.
2. There is often a sex bias. For example, pyloric stenosis is more common in males, whereas cleft palate is more common among females. When a member of the less commonly affected sex shows the condition, a greater number of genes must usually be present to cause the defect.
3. In the presence of environmental influences (such as seasonal changes, altitude, irradiation, chemicals in the environment, or exposure to toxic substances), fewer genes are needed to manifest the disease in the offspring.
4. In contrast to single-gene disorders, there is an additive effect in multifactorial inheritance. The more family members who have the defect, the greater the risk that the next pregnancy will also be affected.

Although most congenital malformations are multifactorial traits, a careful family history should always be taken, since cleft lip and palate, certain congenital heart defects, and other malformations occasionally can be inherited as autosomal dominant or recessive traits. Other disorders thought to be within the multifactorial inheritance group are diabetes, hypertension, some heart diseases, and mental illness.

## Prenatal Diagnostic Tests

Parent-child and family-planning counseling have become a major responsibility of professional nurses. To be effective counselors, nurses must have the most up-to-date information about prenatal diagnosis. It is essential that couples be completely informed about the known and potential risks of each of the genetic diagnostic procedures. Nurses must recognize the emotional impact on the family of a decision to have or not have a genetic diagnostic procedure.

The ability to diagnose certain genetic diseases has enormous implications for the practice of preventive health care. Several methods are available for prenatal diagnosis, although some are still being used on an experimental basis.

### Genetic Ultrasound

Ultrasound may be used to assess the fetus for genetic or congenital problems. With ultrasound, one can visualize the fetal head for fetal abnormalities in size, shape, and structure (for a detailed discussion of ultrasound technology, see Chapter 14). Craniospinal defects (anencephaly, microcephaly, hydrocephalus), thoracic malformations (diaphragmatic hernia), gastrointestinal malformations (omphalocele, gastroschisis), renal malformations (dysplasia or obstruction), and skeletal malformations (caudal regression, conjoined twins) are only some of the disorders that have been diagnosed in utero by ultrasound.

Screening by ultrasound for congenital anomalies is best done at 18 to 20 weeks, when fetal structures have developed completely. There is no information documenting harm to the fetus or long-term effects from exposure to ultrasound. However, complete safety is not guaranteed; therefore, the practitioner and the parents must evaluate the risks against the benefits on an individual basis.

### Genetic Amniocentesis

The major method of prenatal diagnosis is genetic amniocentesis (Figure 5–15♦). The procedure is described in Chapter 14. The indications for genetic amniocentesis include the following:

1. *Maternal age 35 or older.* Women age 35 or older are at greater risk for having children with chromosomal abnormalities (see Chapter 10 for further discussion). Chromosomal abnormalities due to maternal age include trisomy 21, trisomy 13, trisomy 18, XXX, or XXY. The risk of having a live-born infant with a chromosome problem is 1 in 200 for a 35-year-old woman; the risk for trisomy 21 is 1 in 400 (Hook, Cross, & Jackson, 1988). At age 45, the risks are 1 in 20 and 1 in 40, respectively.
2. *Previous child born with a chromosomal abnormality.* Young couples who have had a child with a trisomy 21, 18, or 13 have an approximately 1% to 2% risk of a future child having a chromosomal abnormality.
3. *Parent carrying a chromosomal abnormality (balanced translocation).* A woman who carries a balanced 14/21 translocation has a risk of approximately 10% to 15% that her children will be affected with the unbalanced translocation of Down syndrome; if the father is the carrier, there is a 2% to 5% risk.
4. *Mother carrying an X-linked disease.* In families in which the woman is a known or possible carrier of an X-linked disorder such as hemophilia or Duchenne muscular dystrophy, genetic amniocentesis, chorionic villus sampling (CVS), or percutaneous umbilical blood sampling (PUBS) may be options. For a known female carrier, the risk of an affected male fetus is 50%. Now DNA testing may make it possible to identify affected males from nonaffected males in some disorders. In disorders in which female carriers can be distinguished from noncarriers, only the carrier females would be offered prenatal diagnosis.
5. *Parents carrying an inborn error of metabolism that can be diagnosed in utero.* Metabolic disorders detectable in utero include argininosuccinicaciduria, cystinosis, Fabry disease, galactosemia, Gaucher disease, homocystinuria, Hunter syndrome, Hurler syndrome, Krabbe's disease, Lesch-Nyhan syndrome, maple syrup urine disease, metachromatic leukodystrophy, methylmalonic aciduria, Niemann-Pick disease, Pompe disease, Sanfilippo syndrome, and Tay-Sachs disease.
6. *Both parents carrying an autosomal recessive disease.* When both parents are carriers of an autosomal recessive disease, there is a 25% risk for each pregnancy that the fetus will be affected. Diagnosis is made by testing the cultured amniotic fluid cells (enzyme level, substrate level, product level, or DNA) or the fluid itself. Autosomal recessive diseases identified by amniocentesis are hemoglobinopathies such as sickle-cell anemia, thalassemia, and cystic fibrosis.
7. *Family history of neural tube defects.* Genetic amniocentesis is available to couples who have had a child with neural tube defects or who have a family history of these conditions, which include anencephaly, spina bifida, and myelomeningocele. Neural tube defects are usually multifactorial traits.

### Percutaneous Umbilical Blood Sampling (PUBS) and Chorionic Villus Sampling (CVS)

Percutaneous umbilical blood sampling is a technique used for obtaining blood that allows for rapid chromosome diagnosis, genetic studies, or transfusion for Rh isoimmunization or hydrops. Chorionic villus sampling is used in selected regional centers, and its diagnostic capability is similar to that of amniocentesis. Its advantage is that diagnostic information is available at 8 to 10 weeks' gestation and that products of conception are tested directly. For further discussion, see Chapter 14.

### Alpha-Fetoprotein (AFP)

The maternal circulation or amniotic fluid is tested for alpha-fetoprotein (AFP). The maternal serum AFP (MSAFP) level is elevated in cases of infants with open neural tube defects, anencephaly, omphalocele, and gastroschisis; fetal death; vaginal bleeding; or multiple gestations (Rose & Mennuti, 2000). A woman with a family history of neural tube defects should consult her prenatal care provider for recommended folic acid dosages. Low MSAFP level has been associated with Down syndrome. MSAFP testing is done at 15 to 22 weeks' gestation (Scioscia, 1999). Ultrasound and amniocentesis are offered to patients with low or high MSAFP levels. Inaccurate dating is the most common cause for abnormal AFP; therefore, ultrasound dating is very important (Rose & Mennuti, 2000). With high MSAFP levels, normal amniotic fluid AFP, and normal

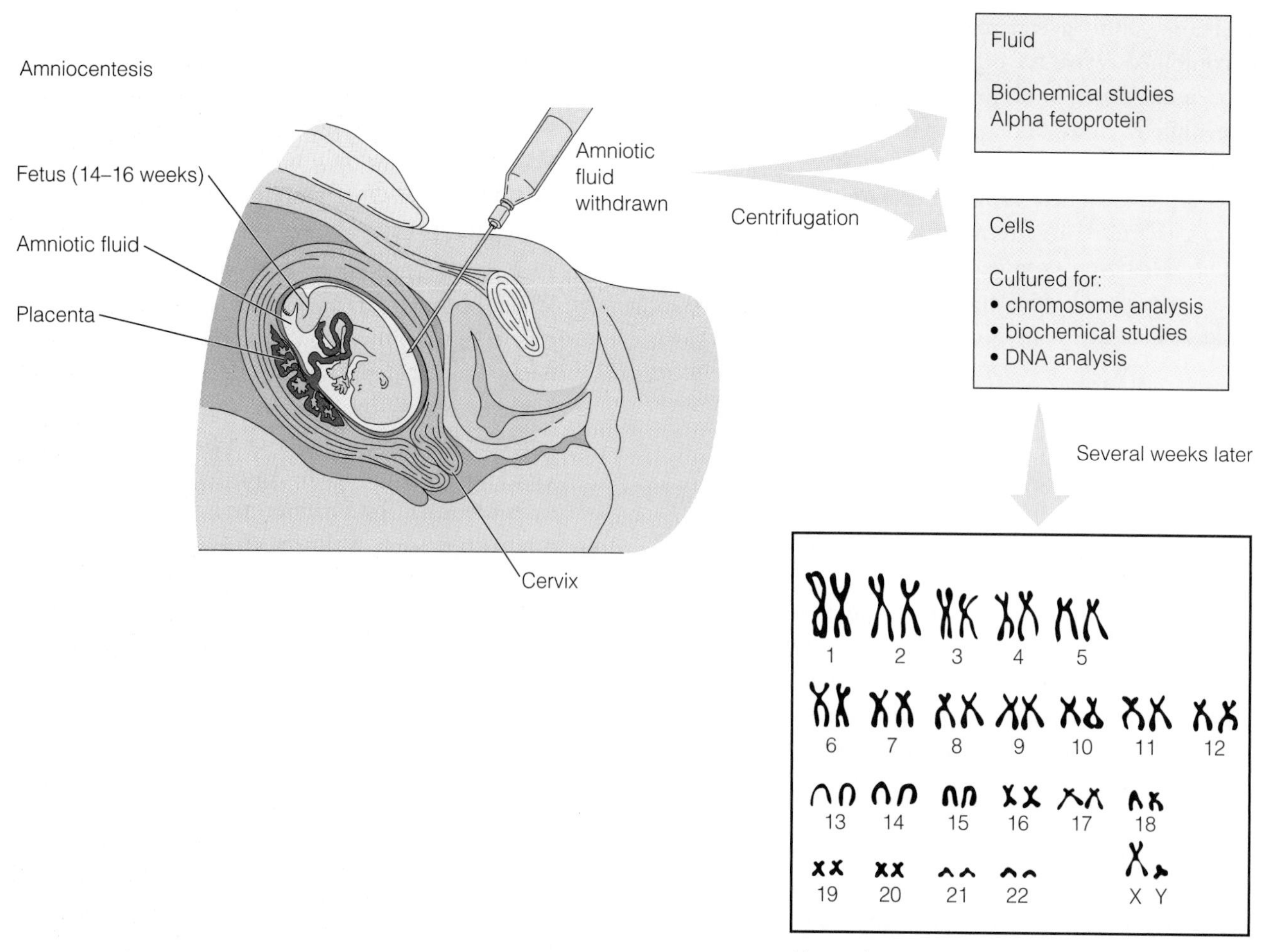


**FIGURE 5–15** ♦ Genetic amniocentesis for prenatal diagnosis is done at 14 to 16 weeks' gestation.

ultrasound, there is an increased risk for preterm labor, perinatal death, and intrauterine growth retardation.

## Implications of Prenatal Diagnostic Testing

It is imperative that counseling precede any procedure for prenatal diagnosis. Many questions and points must be considered if the family is to reach a satisfactory decision. See Table 5–8 and Key Facts to Remember: Couples Who May Benefit from Prenatal Diagnosis.

With the advent of diagnostic techniques such as amniocentesis and chorionic villus sampling, couples at risk who would not otherwise have additional children can decide to conceive. Following prenatal diagnosis, a couple can decide not to have a child with a genetic disease. For many couples, prenatal diagnosis is not a solution, however, since the only method of preventing a genetic disease is preventing the birth by terminating the pregnancy. The decision about whether to use prenatal diagnosis can only be made by the family. Even when termination is not an option, prenatal diagnosis can give parents an opportunity to prepare for the birth of a child with special needs, contact the families of children with similar problems, or access support services before the birth.

Every pregnancy has a 3% to 4% risk of resulting in an infant with a birth defect. When an abnormality is detected or suspected before birth, an attempt is made to determine the diagnosis by assessing the family health history (via the pedigree) and the pregnancy history and by evaluating the fetal anomaly or anomalies via ultrasound. Health care professionals can then present the parents with options. A family with a baby who has a lethal anomaly, such as trisomy 13 or 18, may wish to consider nonaggressive intervention. Many disorders can be diagnosed prenatally; the list has grown and continues to grow almost daily. Nurses should consult experts on a specific disorder before giving information to couples or discussing options.

Treatment of prenatally diagnosed disorders may begin during the pregnancy, thus possibly preventing irreversible damage. For example, a mother carrying a fetus with galactosemia may follow a galactose-free diet. In

| TABLE 5–8 Genetic Screening Recommendations for Various Ethnic and Age Groups | | | |
|---|---|---|---|
| *Background of Population at Risk* | *Disorder* | *Screening Test* | *Definitive Test* |
| Ashkenazic Jewish | Tay-Sachs disease | Decreased serum hexosaminidase-A | CVS* or amniocentesis for hexosaminidase-A assay |
| African; Hispanic from Caribean, Central America, or South America | Sickle-cell anemia | Presence of sickle-cell hemoglobin; confirmatory hemoglobin electrophoresis | CVS or amniocentesis for genotype determination; direct molecular studies |
| Greek, Italian | beta-thalassemia | Mean corpuscular volume < 80%; confirmatory hemoglobin electrophoresis | CVS or amniocentesis for genotype determiniation (direct molecular studies or indirect RFLP† analysis) |
| Southeast Asian (Vietnamese, Loatian, Cambodian), Philippine | alpa-thalassemia | Mean corpuscular volume < 80%; confirmatory hemoglobin electrophoresis | CVS or amniocentesis for genotype determination (direct molecular studies) |
| Women over age 35 (all ethnic groups) | Chromosomal trisomies | None | CVS or amniocentesis for cytogenetic analysis |
| Women of any age (all ethnic groups; particularly suggested for women from British Isles, Ireland) | Neural tube defects and selected other anomlies | Maternal serum alphafetoprotein (MSAFP) | Amniocentesis for amniotic fluid, alpha-fetoprotein, and acetylcholinesterase assays |

*Chronic villus sampling.
†Restriction fragment length polymorphism.

**KEY FACTS TO REMEMBER**

*Couples Who May Benefit from Prenatal Diagnosis*

Women age 35 or over at time of birth

Couples with a balanced translocation (chromosomal abnormality)

Mother carrying X-linked disease (eg, hemophilia)

Couples with a previous child with chromosomal abnormality

Couples in which either partner or a previous child is affected with a diagnosable metabolic disorder

Couples in which both partners are carriers for a diagnosable metabolic or autosomal recessive disorder

Family or personal history of neural tube defects

Ethnic groups at increased risk for specific disorders (Table 5–8)

Couples with history of two or more first-trimester spontaneous abortions

Women with an abnormal maternal serum alpha-fetoprotein (MSAFP or AFP3) test

light of the philosophy of preventive health care, information that can be obtained prenatally should be made available to all couples who are expecting a baby or who are contemplating pregnancy.

## Postnatal Diagnosis

Questions concerning genetic disorders (cause, treatment, and prognosis) are most often first discussed in the newborn nursery or during the infant's first few months of life. When a child is born with anomalies, has a stormy newborn period, or does not progress as expected, a genetic evaluation may be warranted. An accurate diagnosis and an optimal treatment plan incorporate the following:

- Complete detailed history to determine whether the problem is prenatal (congenital), postnatal, or familial in origin.
- Thorough physical examination, including dermatoglyphics analysis (Figure 5–16♦).
- Laboratory analysis, which includes chromosome analysis; enzyme assay for inborn errors of metabolism (see Chapter 25 for further discussion of these tests); DNA studies (both direct and by linkage); and antibody titers for infectious teratogens, such as toxoplasmosis, rubella, cytomegalovirus, and herpesvirus (TORCH syndrome) (see Chapter 13).

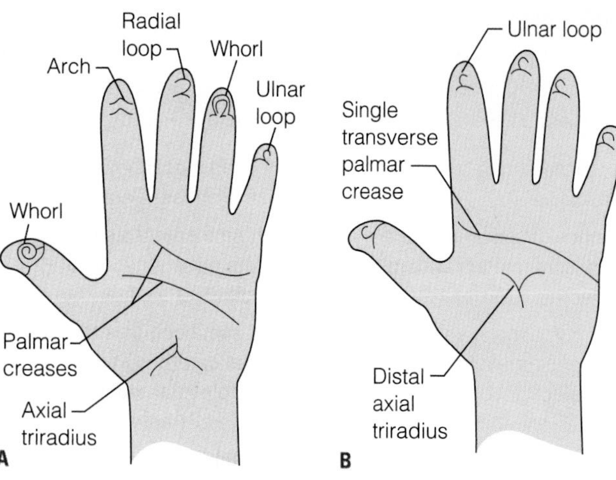


FIGURE 5–16 ♦ Dermatoglyphic patterns of the hands in **A**, a normal individual, and **B**, a child with Down syndrome. Note the single transverse palmar crease, distally placed axial triradius, and increased number of ulnar loops.

To make an accurate diagnosis, the geneticist consults with other specialists and reviews the current literature. This permits the geneticist to evaluate all the available information before arriving at a diagnosis and plan of action.

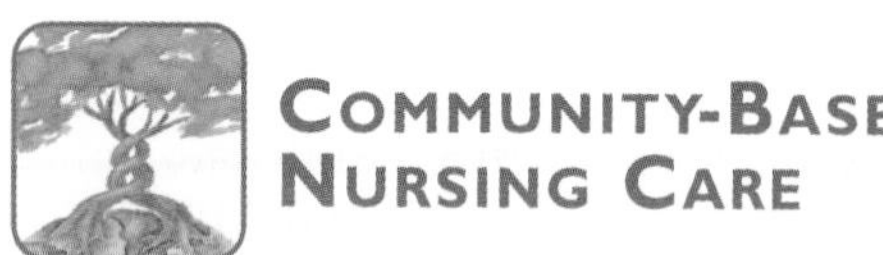

## Community-Based Nursing Care

*Genetic counseling* is a communication process in which a genetic counselor provides a family with the most complete and accurate information about the occurrence or the risk of recurrence of a genetic disease in that family (Verp, 1999b).

In retrospective genetic counseling, time is a crucial factor. One cannot expect a couple who has just learned that their child has a birth defect or Down syndrome to take in any information concerning future risks. However, the couple should never be "put off" from genetic counseling for so long that they conceive another affected child because of lack of information. The perinatal nursing team nurse frequently has the first contact with the family who have a newborn with a congenital abnormality. At the birth of an affected child, the nurse can inform the parents that genetic counseling is available before they attempt to have another child. Genetic counseling is an appropriate course of action for any family wondering "Will it happen again?" The nursery nurse frequently has the first contact with the family that has a newborn with a congenital anomaly. The family nurse practitioner or family-planning nurse is in an excellent position to reach at-risk families before the birth of another baby with a congenital problem.

Genetic counseling referral is advised for any of the following categories:

1. *Congenital abnormalities, including mental retardation.* Any couple who has a child or a relative with a congenital malformation may be at increased risk and should be so informed. If mental retardation of unidentified cause has occurred in a family, there may be an increased risk of recurrence. In many cases, the genetic counselor will identify the cause of a malformation as a teratogen (see Chapter 9). The family should be aware of teratogenic substances so they can avoid exposure during any subsequent pregnancy.
2. *Familial disorders.* Families should be told that certain diseases may have a genetic component and that the risk of their occurrence in a particular family may be higher than that in the general population. Such disorders as diabetes, heart disease, cancer, and mental illness fall into this category.
3. *Known inherited diseases.* Families may know that a disease is inherited but not know the mechanism or the specific risk for them. An important point to remember is that family members who are not at risk for passing on a disorder should be as well informed as family members who are at risk.
4. *Metabolic disorders.* Any family at risk for having a child with a metabolic disorder or biochemical defect should be referred. Because most inborn errors of metabolism are inherited in an autosomal recessive manner, a family may not be identified as being at risk until the birth of an affected child. Carriers of the sickle-cell trait can be identified before they conceive a child, and the risk of having an affected child can be determined. Prenatal diagnosis of an affected fetus is available on an experimental basis only.
5. *Chromosomal abnormalities.* As discussed previously, any couple who has had a child with a chromosomal abnormality may be at increased risk of having another child similarly affected. This group includes families in which there is concern about a possible translocation.

After a couple has been referred to the genetics clinic, they are sent a form requesting information on the health status of various family members. At this time, the nurse can help by discussing the form with the couple or clarifying the information needed to complete it.

A pedigree and history facilitate identification of other family members who might also be at risk for the same disorder (Figure 5–17♦). The couple being counseled may wish to notify relatives at risk so that they, too, can begin genetic counseling. When done correctly, the family history and pedigree can be powerful tools for determining a family's risk.

The counselor gathers additional information about the pregnancy, the affected child's growth and development, and the family's understanding of the problem.

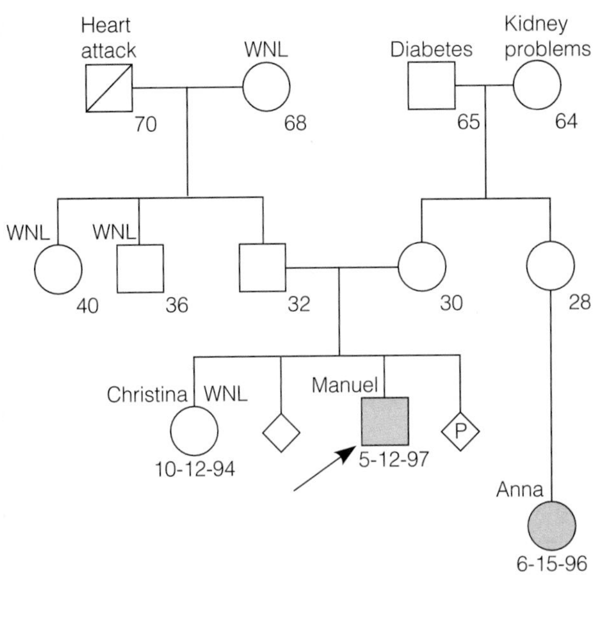


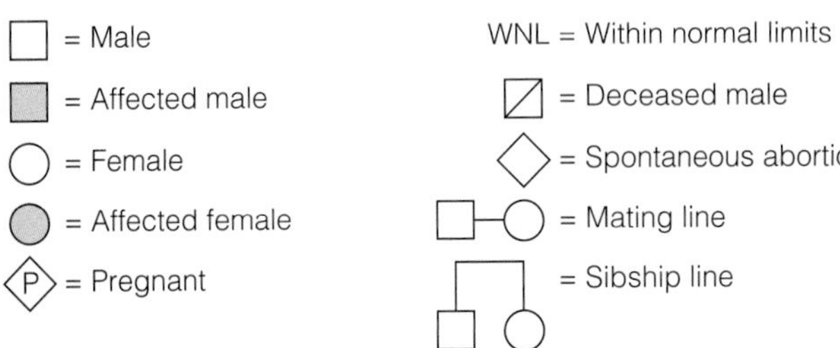


**FIGURE 5–17** ♦ Screening pedigree. Arrow indicates the nearest family member affected with the disorder being investigated. Basic data have been recorded. Numbers refer to the ages of the family members.

Generally the child undergoes a physical examination. Other family members may also be examined. If laboratory tests such as chromosomal analyses, metabolic studies, or viral titers are indicated, they are performed at this time. The genetic counselor may then give the parents some preliminary information based on the data at hand.

Finally, the nurse should elicit information concerning ethnic background, family origin, and religion. Many genetic disorders are more common among certain ethnic groups or more commonly found in particular geographic areas. For example, compared with individuals of other ethnic backgrounds, families from the British Isles are at higher risk for neural tube defects, Ashkenazic Jews (from eastern Europe) are at higher risk for Tay-Sachs disease, people of African descent are at higher risk for sickle-cell anemia, and people of Mediterranean heritage are at higher risk for thalassemias.

## Follow-Up Counseling

When all the data have been carefully examined and analyzed, the couple returns for a follow-up visit. At this time, the genetic counselor gives the parents all the information available, including the medical facts, diagnosis, probable course of the disorder, and any available management; the inheritance pattern for this particular family and the risk of recurrence; and the options or alternatives for dealing with the risk of recurrence. The remainder of the counseling session is spent discussing the course of action that seems appropriate to the family in view of the risk and family goals. Among the options or alternatives are prenatal diagnosis, early detection and treatment, and, in some cases, adoption, artificial insemination, and delayed childbearing.

The couple may consider therapeutic donor insemination, discussed earlier in this chapter. This alternative is appropriate, for example, if the male partner has an autosomal dominant disorders; TDI would decrease to zero the risk of having an affected child (if the sperm donor is not at risk) because the child would not inherit any genes from the affected parent. If the man has an X-linked disorder and does not wish to continue the gene in the family (all his daughters would be carriers), TDI is an alternative to terminating all pregnancies with a female fetus. If the man is a carrier for a balanced translocation and if termination of pregnancy is against family ethics, TDI is the most appropriate alternative. If both parents are carriers of an autosomal recessive disorders. TDI lowers the risk to a very low level or to zero if a carrier test is available. Finally, TDI may be appropriate if the couple is at high risk for a multifactorial disorder.

Couples who are young and at risk may decide to delay childbearing for a few years. These couples may find in a few years that prenatal diagnosis is available or that a disease can be detected and treated early to prevent irreversible damage.

The family may return to the genetic counselor a number of times to ask questions and express concerns. It is most desirable for the nurse working with the family to attend many or all of these counseling sessions. Because the nurse has already established a rapport with the couple, she or he can act as a liaison between the family and the genetic counselor. Hearing directly what the genetic counselor says helps the nurse clarify the issues for the family, which in turn helps them formulate questions.

When the parents have completed the counseling sessions, the counselor sends them and their certified nurse-midwife or physician a letter detailing the contents of the sessions. The parents keep this document for reference. See Key Facts to Remember: Nursing Responsibilities in Genetic Counseling.

A nurse with the appropriate knowledge of genetics is in an ideal position to help couples review what has been discussed during the counseling sessions and to answer any additional questions they might have. As families return to daily living, the nurse can provide helpful information on the day-to-day aspects of caring for a child, answer questions as they arise, support parents in their decisions, and refer families to other health and community agencies (Mackta & Weiss, 1994).

## KEY FACTS TO REMEMBER

### *Nursing Responsibilities in Genetic Counseling*

Identify families at risk for genetic problems.

Determine how the genetic problem is perceived and what information is desired before proceeding.

Assist families in acquiring accurate information about the specific problem.

Act as liaison between family and genetic counselor.

Assist the family in understanding and dealing with information received.

Provide information on support groups.

Aid families in coping with this crisis.

Provide information about known genetic factors.

Assure continuity of nursing care to the family.

If the couple is considering having more children, or if siblings want information about their affected brother or sister, the nurse should recommend that the family return for another follow-up visit with the genetic counselor. Appropriate options can again be defined and discussed, and any new information can be given to the family. Many genetic centers have found the public health nurse to be the ideal health professional to provide such follow-up care.

Nurses must be careful not to assume a diagnosis, determine carrier status or recurrence risks, or provide genetic counseling without adequate information and training. Inadequate, inappropriate, or inaccurate information may be misleading or harmful. Health care professionals need to learn the appropriate referral systems and options for care in their region.

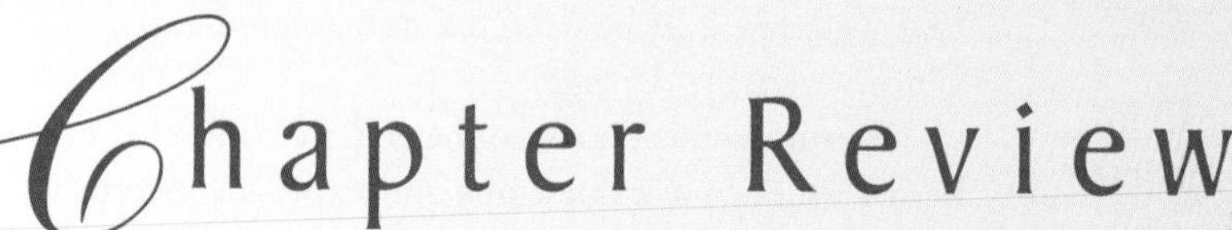

# Chapter Review

## CHAPTER HIGHLIGHTS

- A couple is considered infertile when they do not conceive after 1 year of unprotected coitus.
- About 10% to 15% of couples in the United States are infertile.
- A thorough history and physical exam of both partners are essential as a basis for infertility investigation.
- General fertility investigations include evaluation of ovarian function, cervical mucus adequacy and receptivity to sperm, sperm number and function, tubal patency, general condition of the pelvic organs, and certain laboratory tests.
- Among cases of infertility, 35% involve male factors, 50% involve female factors, and 15% have no identifiable cause; and 35% have multifactorial causes.
- Medications may be prescribed to induce ovulation, facilitate cervical mucus formation, reduce antibody concentration, increase sperm count and motility, and suppress endometriosis.
- The emotional aspects of infertility may be even more difficult for the couple than the testing and therapy.
- The nurse needs to be prepared to dispel myths and provide accurate information about infertility.

- The nurse assesses coping responses and initiates counseling referrals as indicated.
- In autosomal dominant inherited disorders, an affected parent has a 50% chance of having an affected child. Such disorders equally affect males and females. The characteristic presentation varies in each individual with the gene. Some of the common autosomal dominant inherited disorders are Huntington disease, polycystic kidney disease, and neurofibromatosis (von Recklinghausen disease).
- Autosomal recessive inherited disorders are characterized by both parents being carriers; each offspring having a 25% chance of having the disease, a 25% chance of not being affected, and a 50% chance of being a carrier; and males and females being equally affected. Some common autosomal recessive inherited disorders are cystic fibrosis, phenylketonuria, galactosemia, sickle-cell anemia, Tay-Sachs disease, and most metabolic disorders.
- X-linked recessive disorders are characterized by no male-to-male transmission, effects limited to males, a 50% chance that a carrier mother will pass the abnormal gene to her son, a 50% chance that a carrier mother will not transmit the abnormal gene to her son; a 50% chance that the daughter of a carrier mother will be a carrier, and a 100% chance that daughters of affected fathers will be carriers. Common X-linked recessive disorders are hemophilia, color blindness, and Duchenne muscular dystrophy.
- Multifactorial inheritance disorders include cleft lip and palate, spina bifida, dislocated hips, clubfoot, and pyloric stenosis.
- Some genetic conditions that can currently be diagnosed prenatally are craniospinal defects, renal malformations, hemophilia, fragile X syndrome, thalassemia, cystic fibrosis, many inborn errors of metabolism such as Tay-Sachs disease, and neural tube defects. This list expands daily as new technology allows for the detection of more conditions.
- The chief tools of prenatal diagnosis are ultrasound, serum alpha-fetoprotein testing, amniocentesis, chorionic villus sampling, and percutaneous umbilical blood sampling.
- Based on sound knowledge about common genetic problems, the nurse should prepare the family for counseling and act as a resource person during and after the counseling sessions.

## CHAPTER REFERENCES


American Fertility Society. (1994). *Infertility: Questions and answers.* Washington, DC: Author.

American Society for Reproductive Medicine. (1999). Assisted reproductive technology in the United States: 1996 results generated from the American Society for Reproductive Medicine/Society for Assisted Reproductive Technology Registry. *Fertility and Sterility 7*(5), 798–807.

Bernstein, J. (1985). Assessment of psychological dysfunction associated with infertility. *Journal of Obstetrics, Gynecologic, and Neonatal Nursing 14*(Suppl.), 63.

Bopp, B. L., & Seifer, D. B. (2000). Age and reproduction. In J. J. Sciarri & T. J. Watkins (Eds.), *Gynecology and obstetrics* (Vol. 5, chap. 72, pp. 1–26). Philadelphia: Lippincott Williams & Wilkins.

Bradshaw, K. D. (1998). Evaluation and management of the infertile couple. In J. J. Sciarri & T. J. Watkins (Eds.), *Gynecology and obstetrics* (Vol. 5, chap. 50, pp. 1–15). Hagerstown, MD: Harper & Row.

Buitendijk, S. E. (1999). Children after in vitro fertilization. *International Journal of Technology Assessment in Health Care, 15*(1), 52–65.

Carcio, H. A. (1998). *Management of the infertile woman.* Philadelphia: Lippincott-Raven.

Damani, M. N., & Shaban, S. F. (1999). Medical treatment of male infertility. In J. J. Sciarri & T. J. Watkins (Eds.), *Gynecology and obstetrics* (Vol. 5, chap. 65, pp. 1–20). Hagerstown, MD: Harper & Row.

Glover, L., Hunter, M., Richards, J. M., Katz, M., & Abel, P. D. (2000). Development of the fertility adjustment scale. *Fertility and Sterility 72*(4), 623–628.

Hatcher, R. A., Stewart, F., Trussell, J., Kowal, D., Guest, F., Stewart, G. K., Gates, W., & Policat, M. (1998). *Contraceptive technology* (17th ed.). New York: Ardent Media.

Hogge, W. A., & Lanasa, M. C. (1999). Molecular and Mendelian disorders. In J. J. Sciarri & T. J. Watkins (Eds.), *Gynecology and obstetrics* (Vol. 5, chap. 115, pp. 1–13). Hagerstown, MD: Harper & Row.

Hook, E. B., Cross, P. K., & Jackson, L., (1988). Maternal age-specific rates of 47,121 and other cytogenetic abnormalities diagnosed in the first trimester of pregnancy in chorionic villus biopsy specimens: Comparison with rates expected from observations at amniocentesis. *American Journal of Human Genetics,* 42, 797.

Leibowitz, D., & Hoffman, D. (2000). Fertility drug therapies: Past, present, and future. *Journal of Obstetric, Gynecologic, and Neonatal Nursing,* 29(2), 201–210.

Leon, I. G. (2000). Psychology of reproduction: Pregnancy, parenthood, and parental ties. In J. J. Sciarri & T. J. Watkins (Eds.), *Gynecology and obstetrics* (Vol. 6, chap. 62, pp. 1–29). Philadelphia: Lippincott Williams & Wilkins.

Kingsberg, S. A., Applegarth, L. D., & Janata, J. W. (2000). Embryo donation programs and policies in North America: Survey results and implications for health and mental health professionals. *Fertility and Sterility, 73*(2), 215–220.

Klock, S. C. & Greenfeld, D. A. (2000). Psychological status of in vitro fertilization patients during pregnancy: a longitudinal study. *Fertility and Sterility,* 73(6), 1159–1164.

Mackta, J., & Weiss, J. O. (1994). The role of genetic support groups. *Journal of Obstetric, Gynecologic, and Neonatal Nursing, 23*(6), 519–523.

Miller, P. B., & Soules, M. R. (1998). Luteal phase deficiency: Pathophysiology, diagnosis, and treatment. In J. J. Sciarri & T. J. Watkins (Eds.), *Gynecology and obstetrics* (Vol. 5, chap. 56, pp. 1–29). Hagerstown, MD: Harper & Row.

Moghissi, K. S. (1998). How to document ovulation. In J. J. Sciarri & T. J. Watkins (Eds.), *Gynecology and obstetrics* (Vol. 5, chap. 54, pp. 1–14). Hagerstown, MD: Harper & Row.

Olsen, D. G. (1994). Parental adjustment to a child with a genetic disease: One parent's reflections. *Journal of Obstetric, Gynecologic, and Neonatal Nursing, 23*(6), 516–518.

Pergament, E., & Fiddler, M. (2000). Indications and patient selection for preimplantation-related chromosome abnormalities. In J. J. Sciarri & T. J. Watkins (Eds.), *Gynecology and obstetrics* (Vol. 5, chap. 107, pp. 1–7). Philadelphia: Lippincott Williams & Wilkins.

Rose, N. C., & Mennuti, M. T. (2000). Alphafetoprotein and neural tube defects. In J. J. Sciarri & T. J. Watkins (Eds.), *Gynecology and obstetrics* (Vol. 3, chap. 116, pp. 1–14). Philadelphia: Lippincott Williams & Wilkins.

Sandelowski, M. (1994). On infertility. *Journal of Obstetric, Gynecologic, and Neonatal Nursing, 23*(9), 749–752.

Sawatzky, M. (1981). Tasks of the infertile couple. *Journal of Obstetric, Gynecologic, and Neonatal Nursing, 10,* 132–133.

Scioscia, A. L. (1999). Prenatal genetic diagnosis. In R. K. Creasy & R. Resnik (Eds.), *Maternal-fetal medicine* (4th ed., pp. 40–62). Philadelphia: Saunders.

Sharara, F. I. & McClamrock, H. D. (2000). Differences in in vitro fertilization (IVF) outcome between white and black women in an inner-city, university-based IVF program. *Fertility and Sterility, 73*(6), 1170–1173.

Sigman, M. (1999). Therapeutic insemination. In J. J. Sciarri & T. J. Watkins (Eds.), *Gynecology and obstetrics* (Vol. 5, chap. 67, pp. 1–21) Hagerstown, MD: Harper & Row.

Speroff, L., Glass, R. H., & Kase, N. G. (1999). *Clinical gynecologic endocrinology and infertility* (6th ed.). Philadelphia: Lippincott Williams & Wilkins.

Verp, M. S. (1999a). Antenatal diagnosis of chromosomal abnormalities. In J. J. Sciarri & T. J. Watkins (Eds.), *Gynecology and obstetrics* (Vol. 3, chap. 113, pp. 1–17). Hagerstown, MD: Harper & Row.

Verp, M. S. (1999b). Genetic counseling. In J. J. Sciarri & T. J. Watkins (Eds.), *Gynecology and obstetrics* (Vol. 3, chap. 111, pp. 1–13). Hagerstown, MD: Harper & Row.

World Health Organization. (1992). *WHO manual for the examination of human semen and sperm–cervical mucus interaction.* Cambridge, UK: Cambridge University Press.

Yuen, B. H. (1999). New methods for induction of ovulation. In J. J. Sciarri & T. J. Watkins (Eds.), *Gynecology and obstetrics* (Vol. 5, chap. 70, pp. 1–13). Hagerstown, MD: Harper & Row.

## CONTEMPORARY MATERNAL-NEWBORN NURSING ON-LINE

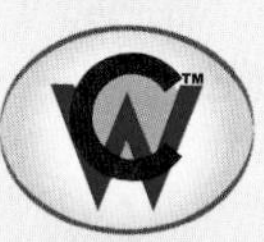

Additional interactive resources, including animations and video, for this chapter can be found on the Companion Website at http://www.prenhall.com/ladewig. Click on Chapter 5 and "Begin" to select the activities for this chapter.

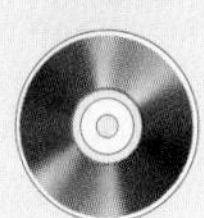

For NCLEX review questions and an audio glossary, access the accompanying CD-ROM in this book.

Chapter 6

# Preparation for Parenthood

*One of the most important things I can do for couples is to help them expand their awareness—awareness of the inherent "rightness" and naturalness of the birth process, awareness of the multitude of options that are available to them, awareness of the health care environment, awareness that control is an illusion, and awareness of the intuitions and strengths that they already possess.*

—A Childbirth Educator (CBE) and Nurse

## OBJECTIVES

- Provide a rationale for preconception counseling.
- Delineate the various issues related to pregnancy, labor, and birth that require decision making by the parents.
- Discuss the basic goals of childbirth education.
- Describe the types of antepartal education programs available to expectant couples and their families.
- Describe the childbirth educator's role in decreasing pregnant women's anxiety.
- Compare methods of childbirth preparation.
- Identify a variety of ways in which the nurse conveys respect for client individuality in preparing for childbirth.

## KEY TERMS

| Term | Page |
|---|---|
| Abdominal effleurage | 145 |
| Birth preference plan | 141 |
| Doula | 144 |
| La Leche League | 145 |
| Lamaze classes | 147 |
| Prenatal education | 145 |

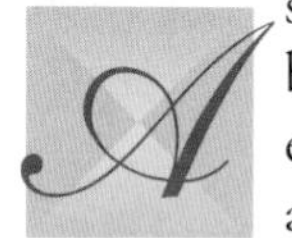s pregnancy progresses, expectant parents begin to look forward to their birth experience and the challenges of parenthood. In addition to gathering information about the pregnancy, there are many decisions and plans to be made. Where will the birth be? Who do they wish to be present? What steps can they take to prepare themselves for this wonderful occasion? How do they approach their new roles as parents?

Today's professional nurse can assist a pregnant woman or expectant couple, if the father is involved, to make the choices that are part of pregnancy and birth. The nurse can help them select a health care provider, find prenatal classes that meet their needs, and make informed choices based on accurate and adequate information. Even more important, as the parents work through these decisions, the nurse is able to affirm their decision-making abilities and the taking on of the parenting role. For first-time parents, the decisions may seem numerous and complicated, and the nurse has a unique opportunity to help them establish a pattern of decision making that will serve them well in their years as parents.

## Preconception Counseling

One of the first questions a couple should ask before conception is whether they wish to have children. This decision involves consideration of each person's goals, expectations of the relationship, and desire to be a parent. Sometimes one individual wishes to have a child, but the other does not. In such situations, an open discussion is essential to reach a mutually acceptable decision.

Couples who wish to have children face a decision about the timing of pregnancy. At what point in their lives do they believe it would be best to become parents? Pregnancy is a life-changing event and comes as a surprise even when the decision about timing is made.

For couples who have religious beliefs that do not support contraception or who feel that fertility planning is unnatural, planning the timing of the pregnancy is unacceptable and irrelevant. These couples can still take steps to ensure that they are in the best possible physical and mental health when pregnancy occurs.

### Preconception Health Measures

The nurse begins by teaching the couple about known or suspected health risks. The nurse advises the woman to cease smoking if possible or to limit her cigarette intake to less than half a pack per day. Because of the hazards of secondhand smoke, it is helpful if her partner refrains from smoking around her. Although the effects of caffeine are less clearly understood, the woman is advised to avoid or limit her intake of caffeine. Alcohol, social drugs, and street drugs pose a real threat to the fetus. A woman who uses any prescription or over-the-counter medications needs to discuss the implications of their use with her health care provider. It is best to avoid using any medication if possible. Because of the possible teratogenic effects of environmental hazards, the nurse urges the couple contemplating pregnancy to determine whether they are exposed to any environmental hazards at work or in their community.

#### Physical Examination

It is advisable for both partners to have a physical examination to identify any health problems so that they can be corrected if possible. These problems might include medical conditions such as high blood pressure or obesity; problems that pose a threat to fertility, such as certain sexually transmitted infections; or conditions that keep the individual from achieving optimal health, such as anemia or colitis. If the family history indicates previous genetic disorders, or if the couple is planning pregnancy when the woman is over age 35, the health care provider may suggest that the couple consider genetic counseling. In addition to the history and physical exam, the woman may have a variety of laboratory tests. (See Assessment Guide: Initial Prenatal Assessment, in Chapter 8). Prior to conception the woman is also advised to have a dental examination and any necessary dental work to avoid exposure to x-rays and the risk of infection while she is pregnant.

#### Nutrition

Prior to conception it is advisable for the woman to be at an average weight for her body build and height. The woman is advised to follow a nutritious diet that contains ample quantities of all the essential nutrients. Some nutritionists advocate emphasizing the following nutrients: calcium, protein, iron, B complex vitamins, vitamin C, folic acid, and magnesium. Intake of vitamins in greater than the recommended dietary allowance (RDA) can cause severe fetal problems and should be avoided. (See Chapter 11 for further discussion of nutrition.)

#### Exercise

A woman is advised to continue her present pattern of exercise or to establish a regular exercise plan beginning at least 3 months before she attempts to become pregnant. An exercise routine that she enjoys and maintains will provide the best results. Exercise that includes some aerobic conditioning and some general muscle toning will improve the woman's circulation and genral health. Once an exercise program is well established, the woman is generally encouraged to continue t during pregnancy.

### Contraception

A woman who takes oral contraceptives is advised to stop taking the pill and have two or three normal menses before attempting to conceive. This wait period allows the natural hormonal cycle to return and facilitates dating the subsequent pregnancy. A woman using an intrauterine device is advised to have it removed and wait 1 month before attempting to conceive. During the waiting period, she can use barrier methods of contraception (condoms, diaphragm, or cervical cap with spermicides).

### Conception

Most preconception recommendations focus on helping the couple attain their best possible health state so that they do not enter pregnancy with unnecessary risks. Conception is a personal and emotional experience, and even if a couple is prepared, they may feel some ambivalence. Ambivalence is a normal response, but they may require reassurance that this feeling will pass. A couple may get so caught up in preparation and in their efforts to "do things right" that they lose sight of the pleasure they derive from each other and their lives together and cease to value the joy of spontaneity in their relationship. It is often helpful for the health care provider to remind an overly zealous couple to take pleasure in the present moment.

## Childbearing Decisions

Once the couple has achieved conception, they should begin exploring their options for a health care provider and birth setting, as well as labor support and sibling preparation, if appropriate.

### Care Provider

One of the first decisions facing expectant parents is the selection of a health care provider. The nurse assists them by explaining the various options and outlining what can be expected from each. A thorough understanding of the differences of education preparation, skill level, general philosophy, and characteristics of practice of certified nurse-midwives, obstetricians, family practice physicians, and lay midwives is essential. For instance, research shows that as many as 40% of adults use some form of complementary or alternative medicine (Allaire, Moos, & Wells, 2000). To determine whether a particular practice is safe during pregnancy, an open avenue for communication must exist between the expectant parent and the primary care provider. In addition to concerns about philosophy, the nurse should encourage expectant parents to investigate the care provider's credentials, education and training, fee schedule, and availability to new clients; this information is often obtained by telephoning the provider's office. The nurse can also help the expectant parents develop a list of questions for their first visit to a care provider to help determine compatibility. Some questions could include the following:

- Who is in practice with you, or who covers for you when you are unavailable?
- How do your partners' philosophies compare with yours?
- How do you feel about my partner, other support person, or other children coming to the prenatal visits?
- What are your feelings about _____ (fill in special desires for the birth event, such as different positions assumed during labor, episiotomy, induction of labor, other people present during the birth, breastfeeding immediately after the birth, no separation of infant and parents following birth, and so on)?
- If a cesarean birth is necessary, could my partner be present?
- Are you familiar with _____ (fill in complementary or alternative forms of health care that may be used currently)? How will this practice impact my plan of care?

Choosing a care provider is just one of the decisions pregnant women and couples make. A method that has assisted many couples in making these choices is called a **birth preference plan.** By writing down preferences, prospective parents identify aspects of the childbearing experience that are most important to them. (A sample birth preference sheet is presented in Figure 6–1♦.) Used as a tool for communication among the expectant parents, the health care provider, and the health care professionals at the birth setting, the written plan identifies options that are available as well as those that are not (England & Horowitz, 1998).

The preference sheet or plan also helps pregnant women and couples set priorities. Using the plan, they identify areas that they want to incorporate into their own birth experience. They can then discuss the document at a visit with their certified nurse-midwife or other care provider and use it to compare their wishes with the philosophy and beliefs of the provider. They can also take the birth plan to the birth setting and use it as a basis for communicating their needs during the childbirth experience.

| Choice | I would like to have Yes | No | Available Yes | No |
|---|---|---|---|---|
| Care provider: | | | | |
| Certified nurse-midwife | | | | |
| Obstetrician | | | | |
| Lay midwife | | | | |
| Birth setting | | | | |
| Hospital: | | | | |
| Birthing room | | | | |
| Delivery room | | | | |
| Birth center | | | | |
| Home | | | | |
| Partner present | | | | |
| Doula present | | | | |
| During labor and birth | | | | |
| During cesarean | | | | |
| During whole postpartum period | | | | |
| During labor: | | | | |
| Ambulate as desired | | | | |
| Shower if desired | | | | |
| Wear own clothes | | | | |
| Use whirlpool | | | | |
| Use rocking chair | | | | |
| Have enema | | | | |
| Water birth | | | | |
| Intermittent electronic fetal monitor | | | | |
| Membranes: | | | | |
| Rupture naturally | | | | |
| Amniotomy if needed | | | | |
| Labor stimulation if needed | | | | |
| Medication: | | | | |
| Identify type desired | | | | |
| Food and fluids or ice as desired | | | | |
| Music during labor and birth | | | | |
| Massage | | | | |
| Therapeutic touch | | | | |
| Position during birth: | | | | |
| On side | | | | |
| Hands and knees | | | | |
| Kneeling | | | | |
| Squatting | | | | |
| Birthing chair | | | | |
| Birthing bed | | | | |
| Other: | | | | |
| Family present (sibs) | | | | |
| Filming of birth/videotaping | | | | |
| Leboyer | | | | |
| Episiotomy | | | | |
| Partner to cut umbilical cord | | | | |
| Hold baby immediately after birth | | | | |
| Breastfeed immediately after birth | | | | |
| No separation after birth | | | | |
| Save the placenta | | | | |
| Collect cord blood | | | | |
| Newborn care: | | | | |
| Eye treatment for the baby | | | | |
| Vitamin K injection | | | | |
| Breastfeeding | | | | |
| Formula feeding | | | | |
| Glucose water | | | | |
| Circumcision | | | | |
| Postpartum care: | | | | |
| Rooming-in | | | | |
| Short stay (48° after vaginal birth) | | | | |
| Sibling visitation | | | | |
| Infant care classes | | | | |
| Self-care classes | | | | |
| Home visits following discharge | | | | |
| Home doula | | | | |
| Other: | | | | |

FIGURE 6–1 ♦ Birth preference sheet. The column on the left lists various choices that the couple may consider during their childbirth experience. Once the couple has considered each of the choices, they may mark the "yes" or "no" space in the middle columns. The right columns are used to note the availability of some of the choices For instance, the couple may want to use hydrotherapy (whirlpool) during labor, but the birthing settings in their community do not have whirlpool tubs available. All choices need to be made in the context of what is available in the couple's community.

Expectant parents also need to discuss the qualities they want in a care provider for the newborn. They may want to visit several before the birth to select someone who will meet their needs and those of their child.

Pregnant women and couples will make many more choices. Some are explored in Table 6–1. Although most birth experiences are very close to the desired experience at times expectations cannot be met. Expectations may not be met because of the unavailability of some choices in the community, limitations set by insurance providers, or unexpected problems during pregnancy or birth. It is important for nurses to help expectant parents keep sight of what is realistic for their situation while also acting as an advocate for them.

## Birth Setting

The nurse can help expectant parents choose a birth setting by suggesting they tour facilities and talk with nurses there and talk with friends or acquaintances who are recent parents. However, it is important to note that the birth setting may be largely determined by the choice of health care provider. Questions that expectant parents may ask of new parents include the following:

- What kind of care and support did you receive during labor?
- If the setting has both labor and delivery rooms and birthing rooms, was a birthing room available when you wanted it?
- Were you encouraged to be mobile during labor or to do what you wanted to do (walking, sitting in a rocking chair, sitting in a whirlpool bath, standing in a shower, and so on)? If not, were there reasonable circumstances that prevented you from doing so?
- Were you encouraged to be actively involved in your plan of care and kept well informed of progress or proposed changes?
- Was your labor partner or coach treated well?
- Were your birth preferences respected? Did you share them with the facility before the birth? If something did not work, why do you think there were problems?

**TABLE 6–1 Benefits and Risks of Some Consumer Decisions during Pregnancy, Labor, and Birth**

| *Issue* | *Benefits* | *Risks* |
|---|---|---|
| Breastfeeding | No additional expense<br>Contains maternal antibodies<br>Decreases incidence of infant otitis media, vomiting, and diarrhea<br>Easier to digest than formula<br>Immediately after birth, promotes uterine contractions and decreases incidence of postpartum hemorrhage | Transmission of pollutants to newborn<br>Irregular ovulation and menses can cause false sense of security and nonuse of contraceptives<br>Increased nutritional requirement in mother |
| Enema | May facilitate labor<br>Increases space for infant in pelvis<br>May increase strength of contractions<br>May prevent contamination of sterile field | Increases discomfort and anxiety |
| Ambulation during labor | Comfort for laboring woman<br>May assist in labor progression by<br>a. Stimulating contractions<br>b. Allowing gravity to help descent of fetus<br>c. Giving sense of independence and control | Cord prolapse will rupture membranes unless engagement has occurred<br>Birth of infant in undesirable situations |
| Electronic fetal monitoring | Helps evaluate fetal well-being<br>Helps identify fetal stress<br>Useful in diagnostic testing<br>Helps evaluate labor progress | Supine postural hypotension<br>Intrauterine perforation (with internal uterine pressure device)<br>Infection (with internal monitoring)<br>Decreases personal interaction with mother because of attention paid to the machine<br>Mother is unable to ambulate or change her position freely |
| Whirlpool (jet hydrotherapy) | Increased relaxation<br>Decreased anxiety<br>Stimulation of labor<br>Nonmedicated pain relief<br>Slight decrease in B/P<br>Increased diuresis | May slow contractions if used before active labor is established<br>Possible risk of infection if membranes are ruptured<br>Slight increase in maternal temperature and heart rate and fetal heart rate during whirlpool and/or in first 30 minutes after being in tub. |
| Analgesia | Maternal relaxation facilitates labor | All drugs reach the fetus in varying degrees and with varying effects<br>May slow contractions if used before active labor is established |
| Episiotomy | May facilitate birth in emergency situations | Increased pain after birth and for several weeks following birth<br>Infection<br>Increased frequency of 3rd- and 4th-degree lacerations (Wolcott & Conry, 2000) |

- During labor, did the nurse offer or suggest a variety of comfort measures?
- How were medications handled during labor? Were you comfortable with this arrangement?
- Were siblings welcomed in the birth setting? After the birth?
- Was the nursing staff helpful after the baby was born? Did you receive self-care and infant care information? Did you have a choice about what information was provided?

The nurse can encourage expectant parents to consider options early in the pregnancy to allow time to talk with their health care provider and other parents and to tour the facilities.

## Labor Support

Another important choice the expectant family faces is how active a support role the father or other partner wants to take during labor and birth. Although many partners are comfortable acting as the primary physical and emotional support for the laboring woman, some partners are not. Studies have found that many men are discouraged when the comfort measures they learned in childbirth classes do not seem to work in labor, and they are left with a negative feeling about the experience (Chapman, 2000). Over the past decade a variety of options for labor support have emerged as families and health care providers have come to understand and respect individual needs (Simkin, 1999). Some possible choices include asking a friend or family member to attend the birth and help with comfort needs, contacting a local childbirth advocate group for a volunteer referral, or hiring a specialized childbirth support person, known as a doula.

The role of the **doula** is to attend to the needs of the childbearing family. Specially trained to assist with births and provide support to new parents and family members, the doula is an adjunct to the health care team. In a managed care environment in which nursing staff are often stretched thin, a doula can be an asset to the nurse by attending to the many comfort needs of the laboring mother and her family (England & Horowitz, 1998; Simkin, 1999).

## Sibling Preparation for Birth

Some expectant parents may wish to have their other children present at the birth. Children who will attend a birth can be prepared through books, audiovisual materials, models, discussion, and sibling classes. Nurses can assist parents with sibling preparation by helping them understand the stresses a child may experience. For example, the child may become frightened if the laboring mom is irritable and visibly showing discomfort, feel left out when there is a new child to love, or feel disappointed if a brother is born when a sister was expected.

It is highly recommended that a sibling have his or her own support person whose sole responsibility is tending to the child's needs. The support person needs to be familiar to the child; warm, sensitive, and flexible; knowledgeable about the birth process; and comfortable with sexuality and birth. This person must be prepared to interpret what is happening for the child and to intervene when necessary. For example, the support person needs to be prepared to remove the child from the birthing room at the child's request or if the situation warrants that action.

Siblings should be given the option of relating to the birth in whatever manner they choose, as long as it is not disruptive. They should understand that they may stay or leave the room as they choose. The nurse may elicit from the children exactly what they expect from the experience and ensure that they feel free to ask questions and express feelings.

In general, siblings who are present at birth tend to have feelings of interest and the desire to nurture "our" baby, as opposed to jealousy and rivalry directed at "Mom's" baby. The mother does not disappear mysteriously into the hospital and return with a demanding outsider. Instead, the family attending the birth together finds a new opportunity for closeness and growth by sharing in the birth of a new member.

### KEY FACTS TO REMEMBER

*Possible Content of Classes for Childbirth Preparation*

**Early Classes (First Trimester)**

Early gestational changes

Self-care during pregnancy

Fetal development, environmental dangers for the fetus

Sexuality in pregnancy

Birth settings and types of care providers

Nutrition, rest, and exercise suggestions

Relief measures for common discomforts of pregnancy

Psychologic changes in pregnancy

Information for getting pregnancy off to a good start

**Later Classes (Second and Third Trimesters)**

Preparation for birth process

Postpartum self-care

Birth choices (e.g., episiotomy, medications, fetal monitoring, enema)

Relaxation techniques

Breathing techniques

Infant stimulation or infant massage

Newborn safety issues, such as car seats

**Adolescent Preparation Classes**

How to be a good parent

Newborn care

Health dangers for the baby

Healthy diet during pregnancy

How to recognize when baby is ill

Baby care: physical and emotional

**Breastfeeding Programs**

Advantages and disadvantages

Techniques of breastfeeding

Methods of breast milk storage

Involvement of fathers in feeding process

# Classes for Family Members during Pregnancy

**Prenatal education** programs provide important opportunities to share information about pregnancy and childbirth and to enhance the parents' decision-making skills. The content of each class is generally directed by the overall goals of the program. For example, in classes that aim to provide preconceptual information, preparations for becoming pregnant are the major topics. Other classes may be directed toward childbirth choices available today, preparation of the mother and her partner for pregnancy and birth, preparation for a vaginal birth after a (previous) cesarean (VBAC) birth, and preparation for the birth by specific people such as grandparents or siblings. The nurse who knows the types of prenatal programs available in the community can direct expectant parents to programs that meet their special needs and learning goals. See Key Facts to Remember: Possible Content of Classes for Childbirth Preparation.

From the expectant parents' point of view, class content is best presented in chronology with the pregnancy. It is important to begin the classes by finding out what each parent wants to learn and including a discussion of related choices. Whereas both parents may expect to learn breathing and relaxation techniques and infant care, fathers usually expect facts and mothers expect coping strategies. Prenatal classes are often divided into early and late classes.

## Early Classes: First Trimester

Early prenatal classes often include prepregnant women and couples as well as those in early pregnancy. The classes cover early gestational changes; self-care during pregnancy; fetal development and environmental dangers for the fetus; sexuality in pregnancy; birth settings and types of care providers; nutrition, rest, and exercise suggestions; common discomforts of pregnancy and relief measures; psychologic changes in pregnancy for the woman and man; methods of coping with stress; and the benefits of following a healthful lifestyle. Early classes provide information about factors that place the woman at risk for preterm labor and about how to recognize symptoms of preterm labor. Early classes should also present information about breastfeeding and bottle-feeding. The majority of women (50 to 80%) have made their infant feeding decision before the sixth month of pregnancy.

## Later Classes: Second and Third Trimesters

The later classes focus on preparation for the birth, including birth choices (episiotomy, medications, fetal monitoring, epidural, and so forth), postpartum self-care, infant care and feeding, and newborn safety issues. Since many expectant parents purchase a car seat before the birth of their child, later classes should also include information about the importance of car seats, how they work, and how to select an approved car seat.

Childbirth preparation classes are an ideal time to incorporate infant stimulation concepts. These concepts aid in the development of parenting skills and enhance prenatal and neonatal bonding. Tactile, vestibular, and auditory stimulation can be explained. Information regarding tactile stimulation can be presented while discussing maternal anatomy and physiology. As the uterine wall thins during the pregnancy, the mother and father are better able to feel the baby, and the fetus can sense the parents' stroking and patting through the abdominal wall. **Abdominal effleurage** (a light stroking movement made over the abdominal wall with the fingertips) can be used to provide tactile stimulation to the fetus.

Vestibular stimulation through movement of the fetus is provided while the expectant woman does the pelvic-tilt exercise. Rocking in a rocking chair is also a comfortable way to provide both relaxation for the expectant woman and vestibular stimulation for the fetus. Auditory stimulation can be provided by playing music. Classical music (such as works by Vivaldi, Bach, Beethoven, and Mozart) is found to stimulate the fetus.

## Adolescent Parenting Classes

Adolescents have special learning needs during pregnancy. Areas of concern for teens focus on how to be a good parent, how to care for the new baby, health dangers to the baby, and healthful foods to eat during pregnancy. Teens also have information needs about how to recognize when the baby is sick, protect the baby from accidents, and make the baby feel happy and loved. Expectant teens are often eager to hear more about the birth process (especially ways to cope with pain during the birth process), the personal health of the mother, the discomforts and life changes that accompany pregnancy, and sexuality.

## Breastfeeding Programs

Programs offering information on breastfeeding are increasing. For many years, a primary source of information has been a nonprofit organization that promotes breastfeeding, called **La Leche League.** Information can also be obtained from certified lactation educators, clinical lactation consultants, birthing centers, hospitals, and health clinics. Expectant parents learn positioning and techniques of breastfeeding, advantages and disadvantages, and methods of breast pumping and milk storage. The father's support and encouragement of the mother is vital, so it is important to include him in the educational programs and decision making. Some fathers may feel ambivalent or resentful about breastfeeding and need opportunities in the prenatal period for discussion and sharing of feelings and experiences.

### Sibling Preparation: Adjustment to a Newborn

The birth of a new sibling is a significant event in a child's life. Positive adjustment can be enhanced by attendance at sibling preparation classes (see Figure 6–2♦). The classes usually focus on reducing anxiety in the child, providing opportunities for the child to express feelings and concerns, and encouraging realistic expectations of the newborn. Parents learn strategies to help prepare the child for the birth and to assist the child in coping with a new family member.

Sibling preparation can be addressed through a formal class or in a less formal way by providing a booklet for parents that addresses issues affecting both parents and children.

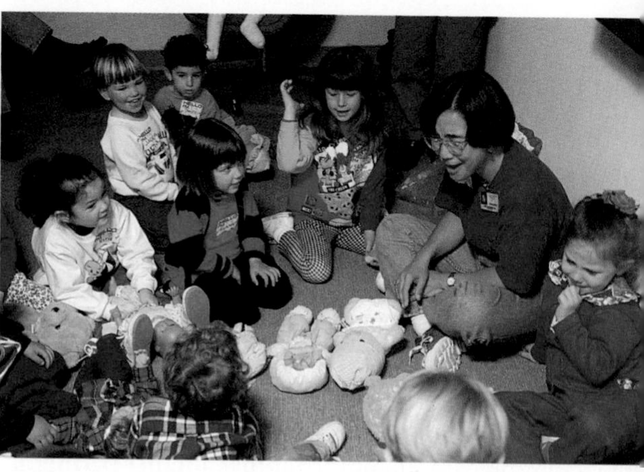

FIGURE 6–2 ♦ It is especially important that siblings be well prepared when they are going to be present for the birth. However, all siblings can benefit from information about birth and the new baby ahead of time.

### Classes for Grandparents

Grandparents are an important source of support and information for prospective and new parents. They are now often included in the birthing process. Prenatal programs for grandparents can be an important source of information about current beliefs and practices in childbearing. The most useful content may include changes in birthing and parenting practices and helpful tips for being a supportive grandparent. Grandparents who will be integral members of the labor and birth team need information about that role.

## Education of the Family Having Cesarean Birth

Cesarean birth is an alternative method of birth. However, because the need for a cesarean birth is rarely known in advance, specific classes covering this alternative are uncommon. Since one out of every four or five births is by cesarean, preparation for this possibility should be an integral part of every childbirth education curriculum.

### Preparation for Cesarean Birth

Cesarean birth class content should cover what the parents can expect to happen during a cesarean birth, what they might feel, and what choices are available to them. All pregnant women and couples should be encouraged to discuss with their certified nurse-midwife or physician the progression of events if a cesarean birth becomes necessary. They can also discuss their needs and preferences regarding the following:

- Choice of anesthetic
- Father (or significant other) being present during the birth
- Immediate initial contact with their newborn

### Preparation for Repeat Cesarean Birth

When expectant parents are anticipating a repeat cesarean birth, they have time to plan and prepare. Many birthing units provide preparation classes for repeat cesarean birth. Parents who have had previous negative experiences need an opportunity to describe what contributed to their feelings. They should be encouraged to identify what they would like to change and to list interventions that would make the experience more positive. Those who have had positive experiences require reassurance that their needs and desires will be met in a similar manner. In addition, all parents are encouraged to air any fears or anxieties.

A specific concern of the woman facing a repeat cesarean is anticipation of pain. She needs reassurance that subsequent cesarean births are often less painful than the first. In addition, planned cesarean births involve less fatigue than unplanned procedures because they are not preceded by a long, strenuous labor. Providing this information will help the woman cope more effectively with stressful stimuli, including pain. The nurse can remind the client that she has already had experience with how to reduce, cope with, and alleviate discomfort during the first few days following surgery.

## Preparation for Parents Desiring Vaginal Birth after Cesarean Birth (VBAC)

Parents who have had a cesarean birth and are now anticipating a vaginal birth have unique needs. Because they may have unresolved questions and concerns about the last birth, it is helpful to begin the series of classes with an informational session. During this session, couples can ask questions, share experiences, and begin to form bonds with each other. The nurse can supply information regarding the criteria necessary to attempt a trial of labor and identify decisions to be made regarding the birth experience. Some childbirth educators suggest that parents prepare two birth preference plans: one for vaginal birth and one for cesarean birth. Preparation of the birth plans seems to give parents some sense of control over the birth experience and tends to increase the positive aspects of the experience.

After an informational session, the classes may be divided according to the needs of the expectant parents. Those with recent childbirth experiences may need only refresher classes, whereas others may need complete training. Some parents may choose to attend regular classes after participating in the informational session.

## Childbirth Preparation Methods

Childbirth preparation classes are usually taught by *certified childbirth educators* (CBE or CCE). Various types of childbirth preparation are available. Vital to each method is the educational component, which helps alleviate fear. The classes vary in coverage of subjects related to the maternity cycle, but all teach relaxation and coping techniques, as well as what to expect during labor and birth. Most classes also feature exercises to relax and condition muscles and breathing exercises for use in labor. The greatest differences among the methods lie in the theories of why they work and in the specific comfort techniques and breathing patterns they teach.

Childbirth preparation offers several advantages. Most important is that the baby's health will be optimized by judicious use of analgesics and anesthetics. Another advantage is the satisfaction of the parents, for whom childbirth becomes a shared and profound emotional experience. In addition, each method has been shown to shorten labor. All nurses should know how these techniques differ, so that they can support each birth experience effectively.

### Programs for Preparation

Some antepartal classes, specifically oriented to preparation for labor and birth, have a name associated with a theory of pain reduction in childbirth. The most common methods of this type are the Lamaze (psychoprophylactic), Kitzinger (sensory-memory), and Bradley (partner-coached childbirth). Each of these programs is designed to provide the woman or couple with self-help measures so that the pregnancy and birth are healthy and happy events (Haire, 1999). See Table 6–2 for differentiating characteristics of each method.

The *psychoprophylactic method* is the childbirth preparation method generally called **Lamaze classes.** *Psychoprophylactic* means "mind prevention." Dr. Fernand Lamaze, a French obstetrician, introduced this method of childbirth preparation to the Western world. In 1960 proponents of the method formed a nonprofit group called the American Society for Psychoprophylaxis in Obstetrics (ASPO). This organization offers a standardized training and certification for childbirth educators, and has helped establish many programs throughout the United States. Lamaze has become one of the most familiar types of childbirth education.

Another prominent organization that provides educational resources and certification for educators is the International Childbirth Education Association (ICEA). Also formed in 1960, this organization does not advocate a particular method of childbirth preparation but rather promotes a philosophy of "freedom of choice based on knowledge of alternatives" (ICEA, 2000). Many expectant parents find this approach consistent with their own desires to experience birth as informed

TABLE 6–2 Summary of Selected Childbirth Preparation Methods

| *Method* | *Characteristics* | *Breathing Technique* |
|---|---|---|
| Lamaze | See narrative discussion in text. | Uses patterned breathing. |
| Bradley | Frequently referred to as partner- or husband-coached natural childbirth. Uses various exercises and slow, controlled abdominal breathing to accomplish relaxation. | Uses primarily abdominal breathing. |
| Kitzinger | Uses sensory memory to help the woman understand and work with her body in preparation for birth. Incorporates the Stanislavsky method of acting as a way to teach relaxation. | Uses chest breathing in conjunction with abdominal relaxation. |

health care consumers. ICEA educators often teach a combination of techniques designed to meet individual needs.

## Body-Conditioning Exercises

Some body-conditioning exercises, such as the pelvic tilt, pelvic rock, and Kegel exercises, are taught in childbirth preparation classes. Other exercises strengthen the abdominal muscles for the expulsive phase of labor. (See Chapter 8 for a description of recommended exercises.)

## Relaxation Exercises

Relaxation during labor allows the woman to conserve energy and allows the uterine muscles to work more efficiently. Without practice it is very difficult to relax the whole body in the midst of intense uterine contractions. However, *progressive relaxation* exercises such as those taught to induce sleep can be helpful during labor. Instructions for one relaxation exercise follow:

- Lie down on your back or side. (Lying on the left side is best for pregnant women.)
- Tighten your muscles in both feet. Hold the tightness for a few seconds and then relax the muscles completely, letting all the tension drain out.
- Tighten your lower legs, hold for a few seconds, and then relax the muscles, letting all the tension drain out.
- Continue tensing and relaxing parts of your body, moving up the body as you do so.

Another relaxation technique, called *touch relaxation,* is based on interaction between the woman and her partner (See an example in Table 6–3).

An additional exercise specific to Lamaze is *disassociation relaxation.* The woman is taught to become familiar with the sensation of contracting and relaxing the voluntary muscle groups throughout her body. She then learns to contract a specific muscle group and relax the rest of her body. The exercise conditions the woman to relax uninvolved muscles while the uterus contracts, creating an active relaxation pattern.

The relaxation techniques described are most effective if the woman practices them regularly both alone and with the participation of her support person. During a practice session, the partner can begin by checking the woman's neck, shoulders, arms, and legs for relaxation. As tense areas are found, the helper encourages the woman to relax those particular body parts. By gentle touch and verbal cues the woman learns to respond to her own perceptions of tense muscles and also to the suggestion from others. The exercises are usually practiced each day so that they become comfortable and easy to do.

### TABLE 6–3 Touch Relaxation

Touch relaxation technique often combines patterned abdominal breathing with focused relaxation, It may be used to achieve relaxation of specific body parts or for general body relaxation.

Goals: The woman learns to release tension in the areas that her partner touches. The partner learns to watch his or her partner carefully and becomes attuned to tense, tightened muscles.

Technique

- The partner gently touches the woman's brow.
- The woman uses abdominal breathing. As she breathes in through her nose, her abdomen rises, and as she breathes out through her mouth, her abdomen falls. As each breath is released, she lets all tightness and tension flow out with the breath.
- The partner continues to lightly touch her brow until relaxation is felt. The partner may want to provide quiet encouragement such as, "You are doing fine, you are releasing the tension in your forehead." After at least five breaths, the partner may now touch the woman's shoulders and repeat the pattern described earlier.
- The partner moves on to the arms, chest, abdomen, thighs, and calves. The last aspect is to breathe in, let the whole body relax and go limp, and slowly release the breath. It will be helpful at the end of each labor contraction to let the body go limp and release all tension.
- As the couple practices, it is important for the woman to relax each part of her body. When she is in labor it will not be possible to go through the whole body; however, the woman can indicate what would be most helpful (e.g., touch her shoulder during each contraction). The partner can also be alert for signs of muscle tension and tightening. As the partner and woman practice touch relaxation, they may want to make the situation more realistic. They could decide that uterine contractions are occurring every 5 minutes and are lasting for 30 seconds. A clock will help the partner keep track of time. The partner can indicate that a contraction is beginning and suggest the woman begin her breathing. To help her focus the partner may touch her shoulder or hand. In some instances, it is helpful for the partner to breathe along with the woman. Each couple can determine what works best for them.

Relaxation may also be promoted by cutaneous stimulation. One type commonly used prior to the transitional phase of labor is known as abdominal effleurage (Figure 6–3♦). This light abdominal stroking is used effectively to relieve mild to moderate pain but is not useful for relieving intense pain. Deep pressure over the sacrum is effective for relieving back pain. In addition to the measures just described, the nurse can promote relaxation by encouraging and supporting the expectant mother's breathing techniques.

## Breathing Techniques

Breathing techniques are a key element of most childbirth preparation programs. They help keep the mother and her unborn baby adequately oxygenated and help the

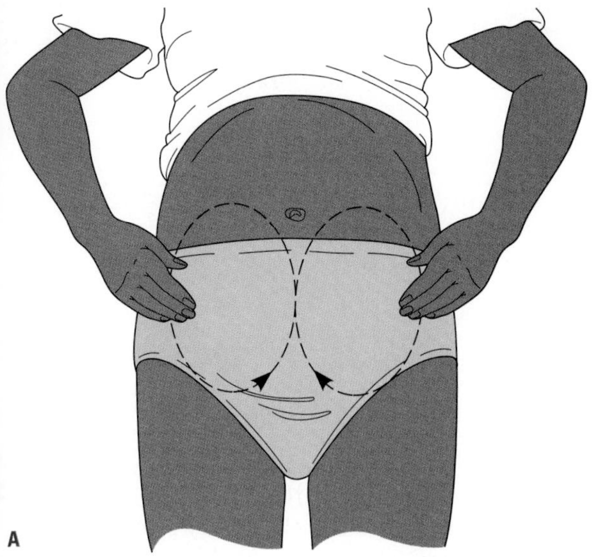


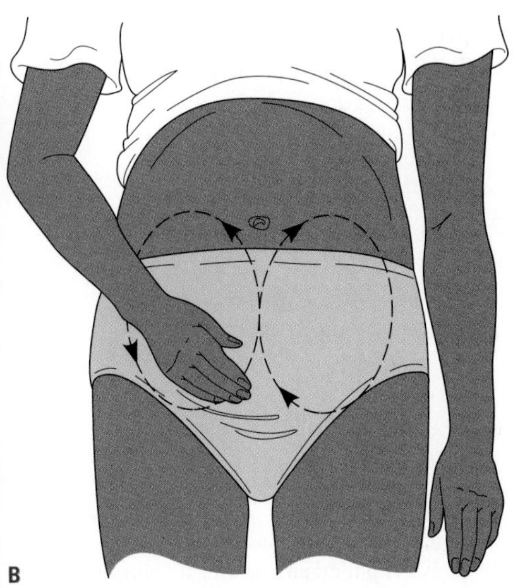


FIGURE 6–3 ♦ Effleurage is light stroking of the abdomen with the fingertips. **A,** Starting at the symphysis, the woman lightly moves her fingertips up and around in a circular pattern. **B,** An alternative approach involves using one hand in a figure-eight pattern. This light stroking can also be done by the support person.

## KEY FACTS TO REMEMBER

### *Goals of Breathing Techniques*

- Provide adequate oxygenation of mother and baby, open maternal airways, and avoid inefficient use of muscles
- Increase physical and mental relaxation
- Decrease pain and anxiety
- Provide a means of focusing attention
- Control inadequate ventilation patterns that are related to pain and stress

## HINTS FOR PRACTICE

Call the birthing facilities in your community and inquire about what choices are available in each facility.

mother relax and focus her attention appropriately. Breathing techniques are best taught during the final trimester of pregnancy, when the expectant mother's attention is focused on the birth experience. The nurse then supports the mother's use of breathing techniques during labor. See Key Facts to Remember: Goals of Breathing Techniques. Breathing techniques are described in detail in Chapter 17.

# Preparation for Childbirth That Supports Individuality

Nurses involved in childbirth education need to include the concept of individuality when providing information to expectant parents about the process of childbirth. Controversy exists over the use of prescribed breathing techniques in childbirth. The current focus in childbirth education is to encourage women to incorporate their own natural responses into coping with the pain of labor and birth. Self-care activities that may be used include the following:

- Vocalization or "sounding" to relieve tension in pregnancy and labor
- Massage (light touch) to facilitate relaxation
- Use of warm water for showers or bathing during labor
- Visualization (imagery)
- Relaxing music and subdued lighting

Nurses should encourage expectant mothers and couples to make the birth a personal experience. Women might choose to bring items from home that help create a more personal birthing space to enhance relaxation and comfort. These items might include warm socks, extra pillows, bath powder, lotion, or a favorite blanket. She may wish to bring photos of special people or places. Many expectant parents enjoy listening to tapes of favorite music or watching favorite home videos. Such personalization of the birth experience may give expectant parents feelings of increased serenity and empowerment (England & Horowitz, 1998).

# Chapter Review

## CHAPTER HIGHLIGHTS

- Preconception counseling may help couples make decisions regarding childbearing.
- Prenatal classes may be offered early and late in the pregnancy. Expectant parents tend to want information in chronological sequence with the pregnancy.
- Adolescents have special learning needs related to pregnancy, the birthing process, and newborn care.
- Breastfeeding programs are offered in the prenatal period.
- Siblings are often included in the whole birthing process, and special classes are available for them.
- Grandparents have unique needs for information.
- Information regarding cesarean birth is beneficial in prenatal classes.
- Prenatal education programs vary in their goals, content, and method of teaching, but all seek to enhance knowledge and decrease anxiety.
- Lamaze is a psychoprophylactic method of preparing for labor and birth. The classes include information on toning exercises, relaxation exercises and techniques, and breathing methods for labor.
- Childbirth education groups, such as ICEA and ASPO, provide consumer health information and certification for teaching prenatal classes.
- Childbirth classes must meet the individual needs of families and their members.

## CHAPTER REFERENCES


Allaire, A. D., Moos, M. K., & Wells, S. R. (2000). Complementary and alternative medicine in pregnancy: A survey of North Carolina certified nurse-midwives. *Obstetrics and Gynecology, 95*(1), 19–23.

Chapman, L. L. (2000). Expectant fathers and labor epidurals. *American Journal of Maternal-Child Nursing, 25*(3), 133–138.

England, P., & Horowitz, R. (1998). *Birthing from within.* Albuquerque, NM: Pantera Press.

Haire, D. (1999). The history of childbirth education. *International Journal of Childbirth Education, 14*(4), 26.

International Childbirth Education Association. (2000). ICEA philosophy statement. *International Journal of Childbirth Education, 15*(1).

Simkin, P. (1999). Labor support: Where has it been and where is it going? *International Journal of Childbirth Education, 14*(4), 22.

Wolcott, H. D. & Conry, J. A. (2000). Normal labor. In A. T. Evans & K. R. Niswander's (Eds.) *Manual of Obstetrics,* (6th ed.), pp. 392–424. Philadelphia, PA: Lippincott, Williams & White.


## CONTEMPORARY MATERNAL-NEWBORN NURSING ON-LINE

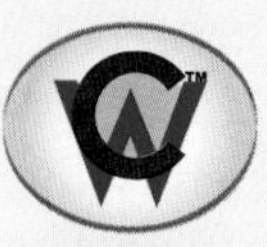

Additional interactive resources, including animations and video, for this chapter can be found on the Companion Website at http://www.prenhall.com/ladewig. Click on Chapter 6 and "Begin" to select the activities for this chapter.

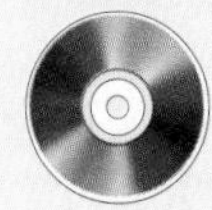

For NCLEX review questions and an audio glossary, access the accompanying CD-ROM in this book.

# Part Three

# Pregnancy and the Family

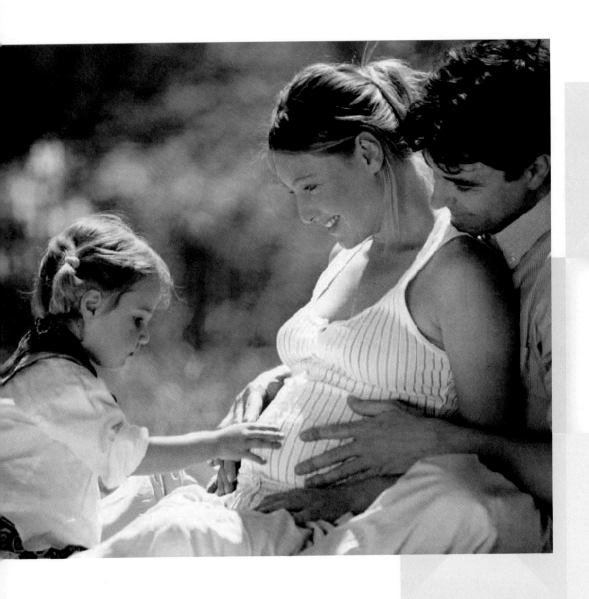

Chapter 7

# Physical and Psychologic Changes of Pregnancy

*In my experience, few women are ever really prepared for all the changes they experience during pregnancy, especially a first pregnancy. That is why early prenatal care is important. Yes, starting care early gives us a better chance to identify risk factors, but it also enables us to do a better job of prenatal education. I am constantly amazed by what a difference it makes for a woman when she has a good idea of what to expect and why.*

—A Nurse Working with an Obstetrician in Private Practice

## KEY TERMS

| | |
|---|---|
| Ballottement | 160 |
| Braxton Hicks contractions | 153 |
| Chadwick's sign | 153 |
| Chloasma | 155 |
| Couvade | 165 |
| Diastasis recti | 156 |
| Goodell's sign | 153 |
| Hegar's sign | 159 |
| Linea nigra | 155 |
| McDonald's sign | 159 |
| Morning sickness | 158 |
| Physiologic anemia of pregnancy | 154 |
| Quickening | 158 |
| Striae | 154 |
| Supine hypotensive syndrome (vena caval syndrome, aortocaval compression) | 154 |

## OBJECTIVES

- Identify the anatomic and physiologic changes that occur during pregnancy.
- Relate these anatomic and physiologic changes to the signs and symptoms that develop in the woman.
- Compare subjective (presumptive), objective (probable), and diagnostic (positive) changes of pregnancy.
- Contrast the various types of pregnancy tests.
- Discuss the emotional and psychologic changes that commonly occur in a woman, her partner, and her family during pregnancy.
- Summarize cultural factors that may influence a family's response to pregnancy.

No matter how much we learn about pregnancy and the changes that occur in the woman and the developing fetus, we never cease to be amazed. First, it is nothing short of a miracle that the union of two microscopic entities—an ovum and a sperm—can produce a living being. Second, the woman's body must undergo extraordinary physical changes to maintain a pregnancy.

Pregnancy is divided into three trimesters, each a 3-month period. Each trimester brings predictable changes for both the mother and fetus. This chapter describes the physical and psychologic changes caused by pregnancy. It also presents the various cultural factors that can affect a pregnant woman's well-being. Subsequent chapters build on this information in describing effective approaches to planning and providing care.

# Anatomy and Physiology of Pregnancy

## Reproductive System

### Uterus

The changes in the uterus during pregnancy are amazing. Before pregnancy, the uterus is a small, semisolid, pear-shaped organ measuring approximately 7.5 × 5 × 2.5 cm and weighing about 60 g (2 oz). At the end of pregnancy it measures about 28 × 24 × 21 cm and weighs approximately 1000 g; its capacity has also increased from about 10 mL to 5000 mL (5 L) or more.

The enlargement of the uterus is primarily due to the enlargement (hypertrophy) of the preexisting myometrial cells as a result of the stimulating influence of estrogen and the distention caused by the growing fetus. Only a limited increase in cell number (hyperplasia) occurs. The fibrous tissue between the muscle bands increases markedly, which adds to the strength and elasticity of the muscle wall. The enlarging uterus, developing placenta, and growing fetus require additional blood flow to the uterus. By the end of pregnancy, one-sixth of the total maternal blood volume is contained within the vascular system of the uterus.

**Braxton Hicks contractions,** which are irregular, generally painless contractions of the uterus, occur intermittently throughout pregnancy. They may be felt through the abdominal wall beginning about the fourth month of pregnancy. In later months, these contractions become uncomfortable and may be confused with true labor contractions.

### Cervix

Estrogen stimulates the glandular tissue of the cervix, which increases in cell number and becomes hyperactive.

> **HINTS FOR PRACTICE**
>
> Beginning early in pregnancy, have the woman feel her uterus periodically so that she becomes familiar with the size and the way it feels. As her pregnancy progresses she then will be more likely to identify Braxton Hicks contractions and preterm labor, if it occurs.

The endocervical glands secrete a thick, sticky mucus that accumulates and forms a plug, which seals the endocervical canal and prevents the ascent of organisms into the uterus. This mucous plug is expelled when cervical dilatation begins. The hyperactivity of the glandular tissue also increases the normal physiologic mucorrhea, at times resulting in profuse discharge. Increased cervical vascularity also causes both the softening of the cervix (**Goodell's sign**) and its bluish discoloration (**Chadwick's sign**).

### Ovaries

The ovaries stop producing ova during pregnancy, but the corpus luteum continues to produce hormones until about weeks 10 to 12. The progesterone it secretes until about the seventh week of pregnancy maintains the endometrium until the placenta assumes the task. The corpus luteum then begins to regress and is almost completely obliterated by the middle of pregnancy.

### Vagina

Estrogen causes a thickening of the vaginal mucosa, a loosening of the connective tissue, and an increase in vaginal secretions. These secretions are thick, white, and acidic (pH 3.5 to 6.0). The acid pH helps prevent bacterial infection but favors the growth of yeast organisms. Thus the pregnant woman is more susceptible to monilial infection than usual.

The supportive connective tissue of the vagina loosens throughout pregnancy. By the end of pregnancy, the vagina and perineal body are sufficiently relaxed to permit passage of the infant. Because blood flow to the vagina is increased, the vagina may show the same blue-purple color (Chadwick's sign) as the cervix.

### Breasts

Estrogen and progesterone cause many changes in the mammary glands. The breasts enlarge and become more nodular as the glands increase in size and number in preparation for lactation. Superficial veins become more prominent, the nipples become more erectile, and the areolas darken. Montgomery's follicles (sebaceous glands) enlarge, and **striae** (reddish stretch marks that slowly turn silver after childbirth) may develop.

Colostrum, an antibody-rich yellow secretion, may leak or be expressed from the breasts during the last trimester. Colostrum gradually converts to mature milk during the first few days after childbirth.

## Respiratory System

Many respiratory changes occur to meet the increased oxygen requirements of a pregnant woman. The volume of air breathed each minute increases 30% to 40%. In addition, progesterone decreases airway resistance, permitting a 15% to 20% increase in oxygen consumption, as well as increases in carbon dioxide production and in the respiratory functional reserve.

As the uterus enlarges, it presses upward and elevates the diaphragm. The subcostal angle increases, so that the rib cage flares. The anteroposterior diameter increases, and the chest circumference expands by as much as 6 cm; as a result, there is no significant loss of intrathoracic volume. Breathing changes from abdominal to thoracic as pregnancy progresses, and descent of the diaphragm on inspiration becomes less possible. Some hyperventilation and difficulty in breathing may occur.

Nasal stuffiness and epistaxis (nosebleeds) may also occur because of estrogen-induced edema and vascular congestion of the nasal mucosa.

## Cardiovascular System

Blood volume progressively increases beginning in the first trimester, increases rapidly in the second trimester, and slows in the third. It peaks in the middle of the third trimester, at about 45% above nonpregnant levels. This increase is due to increases in both erythrocytes and plasma.

During pregnancy, blood flow increases to organ systems with an increased workload. Thus blood flow increases to the uterus and kidneys, while hepatic and cerebral flow remains unchanged. Cardiac output begins to increase early in pregnancy and remains elevated throughout gestation.

The pulse may increase by as many as 10 to 15 beats per minute at term. The blood pressure decreases slightly, reaching its lowest point during the second trimester. It gradually increases to near prepregnant levels by the end of the third trimester.

The enlarging uterus puts pressure on pelvic and femoral vessels, interfering with returning blood flow and causing stasis of blood in the lower extremities. This condition may lead to dependent edema and varicosity of the veins in the legs, vulva, and rectum (hemorrhoids) in late

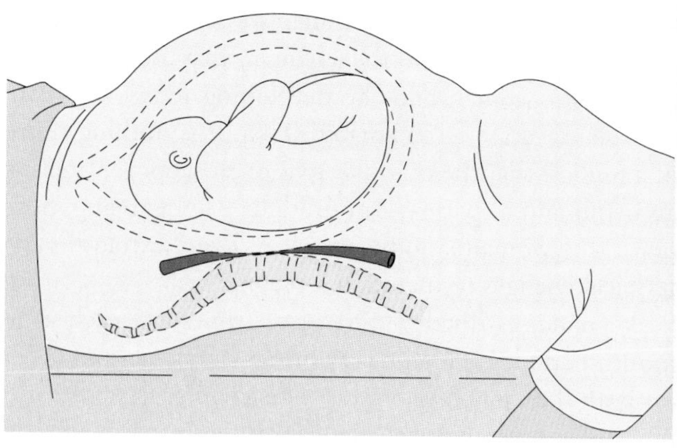

FIGURE 7–1 ♦ Vena caval syndrome. The gravid uterus compresses the vena cava when the woman is supine. This reduces the blood flow returning to the heart and may cause maternal hypotension.

pregnancy. This increased blood volume in the lower legs may also make the pregnant woman prone to postural hypotension.

When the pregnant woman lies supine, the enlarging uterus may press on the vena cava, thus reducing blood flow to the right atrium, lowering blood pressure, and causing dizziness, pallor, and clamminess. Research indicates that the enlarging uterus may also press on the aorta and its collateral circulation (Cunningham, MacDonald, Gant, et al., 1997). This condition is called **supine hypotensive syndrome.** It may also be referred to as **vena caval syndrome** or **aortocaval compression** (Figure 7–1♦). It can be corrected by having the woman lie on her left side or by placing a pillow or wedge under her right hip.

The total erythrocyte (red blood cell) volume increases by about 30% in women who receive iron supplementation (but only about 18% without iron supplementation) (Cruikshank, Wigton, & Hays, 1996). This increase in erythrocytes is necessary to transport the additional oxygen required during pregnancy. However, the increase in plasma volume during pregnancy averages about 50%. Because the plasma volume increase (50%) is greater than the erythrocyte increase (30%), the hematocrit, which measures the concentration of red blood cells in the plasma, decreases by an average of about 7% during pregnancy. This decrease is referred to as the **physiologic anemia of pregnancy** (pseudoanemia).

Iron is necessary for hemoglobin formation, and hemoglobin is the oxygen-carrying component of erythrocytes. Thus the increase in erythrocyte levels results in an increased need for iron by the pregnant woman. Even though the gastrointestinal absorption of iron is moderately increased during pregnancy, it is usually necessary to add supplemental iron to the diet to meet the expanded red blood cell and fetal needs.

Leukocyte production increases slightly to an average of 5000 to 12,000/mm$^3$; a few women develop levels as high as 15,000/mm³. During labor and the early postpartum period, these levels may reach 25,000/mm³ or higher (Cunningham, et al., 1997).

Both the fibrin and plasma fibrinogen levels increase during pregnancy. Although the blood-clotting time of the pregnant woman does not differ significantly from that of the nonpregnant woman, clotting factors VII, VIII, IX, and X increase; thus pregnancy is a somewhat hypercoagulable state. These changes, coupled with venous stasis in late pregnancy, increase the pregnant woman's risk of developing venous thrombosis.

## Gastrointestinal System

Nausea and vomiting are common during the first trimester because of elevated human chorionic gonadotropin levels and changed carbohydrate metabolism. Gum tissue may soften and bleed easily. The secretion of saliva may increase and even become excessive (ptyalism).

Elevated progesterone levels cause smooth muscle relaxation, resulting in delayed gastric emptying and decreased peristalsis. As a result, the pregnant woman may complain of bloating and constipation. These symptoms are aggravated as the enlarging uterus displaces the stomach upward and the intestines laterally and posteriorly. The cardiac sphincter also relaxes, and heartburn (pyrosis) may occur due to reflux of acidic secretions into the lower esophagus. Hemorrhoids frequently develop in late pregnancy from constipation and from pressure on vessels below the level of the uterus.

Only minor liver changes occur with pregnancy. Plasma albumin concentrations and serum cholinesterase activity decrease with normal pregnancy, as with certain liver diseases.

The emptying time of the gallbladder is prolonged during pregnancy as a result of smooth muscle relaxation from progesterone. This, coupled with the elevated levels of cholesterol in the bile, can predispose the woman to gallstone formation.

## Urinary Tract

During the first trimester, the enlarging uterus is still a pelvic organ and presses against the bladder, producing urinary frequency. This symptom decreases during the second trimester, when the uterus becomes an abdominal organ and pressure against the bladder lessens. Frequency reappears during the third trimester, when the presenting part descends into the pelvis and again presses on the bladder, reducing bladder capacity, contributing to hyperemia, and irritating the bladder.

The ureters (especially the right ureter) elongate and dilate above the pelvic brim. The glomerular filtration rate (GFR) rises by as much as 50% beginning in the second trimester and remains elevated until birth. To compensate for this increase, renal tubular reabsorption also increases. However, glycosuria is sometimes seen during pregnancy because of the kidneys' inability to reabsorb all the glucose filtered by the glomeruli. Glycosuria may be normal or may indicate gestational diabetes, so it always warrants further testing.

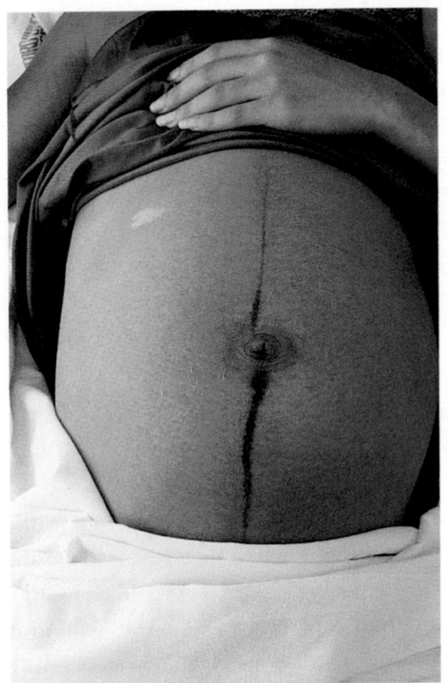

**FIGURE 7–2** ♦ Linea nigra.

## Skin and Hair

Changes in skin pigmentation commonly occur during pregnancy. They are thought to be stimulated by increased estrogen, progesterone, and α-melanocytic-stimulating hormone levels (Cruikshank, Wigton, Hays, et al., 1996). Pigmentation of the skin increases primarily in areas that are already hyperpigmented: the areola, the nipples, the vulva, and the perianal area. The skin in the middle of the abdomen may develop a pigmented line, the **linea nigra,** which usually extends from the umbilicus or above to the pubic area (Figure 7–2♦). Facial **chloasma** (also known as the "mask of pregnancy"), a darkening of the skin over the forehead and around the eyes, may develop. Chloasma is more prominent in dark-haired women and is aggravated by exposure to the sun. Fortunately, chloasma fades or becomes less prominent soon after childbirth when the hormonal influence of pregnancy subsides. In addition, the sweat and sebaceous glands are often hyperactive during pregnancy.

Striae, or stretch marks, are reddish, wavy streaks that may appear on the abdomen, thighs, buttocks, and breasts. They result from reduced connective tissue strength due to elevated adrenal steroid levels.

*Vascular spider nevi,* small, bright-red elevations of the skin radiating from a central body, may develop on the chest, neck, face, arms, and legs. They may be caused by increased subcutaneous blood flow in response to elevated estrogen levels.

The rate of hair growth may decrease during pregnancy; the number of hair follicles in the resting or dormant phase also decreases. After birth, the number of hair follicles in the resting phase increases sharply and the woman may notice increased hair shedding for 1 to 4 months. Practically all hair is replaced within 6 to 12 months, however (Cunningham, et al., 1997).

## Musculoskeletal System

No demonstrable changes occur in the teeth of pregnant women. The dental caries that sometimes accompany pregnancy are probably caused by inadequate oral hygiene and dental care, especially if the woman has problems with bleeding gums or nausea and vomiting.

The joints of the pelvis relax somewhat because of hormonal influences. The result is often a waddling gait. As the pregnant woman's center of gravity gradually changes, the lumbar spinal curve becomes accentuated, and her posture changes (Figure 7–3♦). This posture change compensates for the increased weight of the uterus anteriorly and frequently results in low backache.

Pressure of the enlarging uterus on the abdominal muscles may cause the rectus abdominis muscle to separate, producing **diastasis recti.** If the separation is severe and muscle tone is not regained postpartally, subsequent pregnancies will not have adequate support and the woman's abdomen may appear pendulous.

## Eyes

During pregnancy, intraocular pressure decreases, probably because of increased vitreous outflow, and the cornea thickens slightly because of fluid retention. As a result, some pregnant women experience difficulty wearing previously comfortable contact lenses (Cunningham, et al., 1997). These changes usually disappear by 6 weeks postpartum.

## Metabolism

Most metabolic functions increase during pregnancy because of the increased demands of the growing fetus and its support system. The expectant mother must meet both her own tissue replacement needs and those of her unborn child. Her body must also anticipate the needs of labor and lactation. For a detailed discussion of nutrient, vitamin, and mineral metabolism, see Chapter 11.

### Weight Gain

The recommended weight gain for women of normal weight before pregnancy is 25 to 35 lb (11.4 to 15.9 kg), whereas for women who were overweight, the recommended gain is 15 to 25 lb (6.8 to 11.4 kg). Underweight women are advised to gain the weight needed to reach their ideal weight plus 25 to 35 lb (11.4 to 15.9 kg) (Mattson & Smith, 2000). The average pattern of weight gain is 3.5 to 5 lb (1.6 to 2.3 kg) during the first trimester and 12 to 15 lb (5.5 to 6.8 kg) during each of the last two trimesters. Adequate nutrition and weight gain are important during pregnancy (see discussion in Chapter 11).

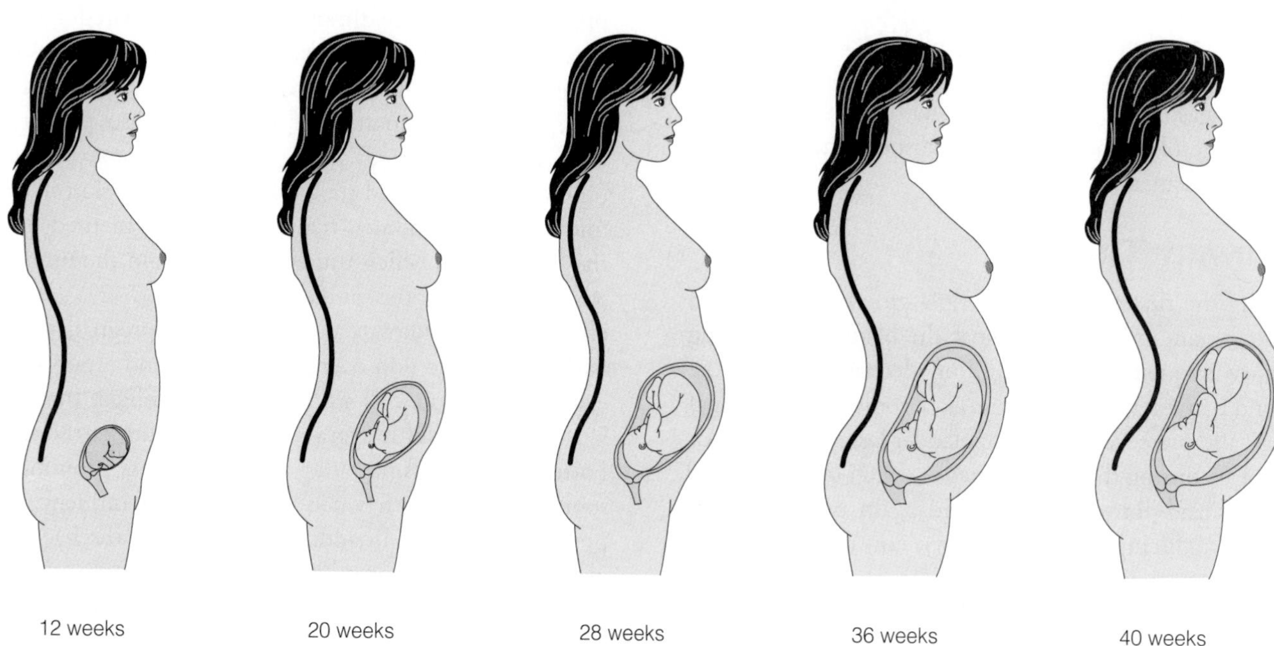


**FIGURE 7–3 ♦** Postural changes during pregnancy. Note the increasing lordosis of the lumbosacral spine and the increasing curvature of the thoracic area.

### Water Metabolism

Increased water retention, a basic alteration of pregnancy, is caused by several interrelated factors. The increased level of steroid sex hormones affects sodium and fluid retention. The lowered serum protein also influences fluid balance, as do increased intracapillary pressure and permeability. The extra water is needed for the fetus, placenta, and amniotic fluid and the mother's increased blood volume, interstitial fluids, and enlarged organs.

### Nutrient Metabolism

The fetus makes its greatest protein and fat demands during the second half of pregnancy, doubling in weight during the last 6 to 8 weeks. Protein (contributing nitrogen) must be stored during pregnancy to maintain a constant level within the breast milk and to avoid depletion of maternal tissues. Carbohydrate needs also increase, especially during the second and third trimesters.

Fats are more completely absorbed during pregnancy, and the level of free fatty acids increases in response to human placental lactogen. The levels of lipoproteins and cholesterol also increase. Because of these changes, increased levels of dietary fat or reduced carbohydrate production may lead to ketonuria in the pregnant woman.

## Endocrine System

### Thyroid

The thyroid gland often enlarges slightly during pregnancy because of increased vascularity and hyperplasia of glandular tissue. Its capacity to bind thyroxine is greater, resulting in an increase in serum protein-bound iodine. These changes are due to higher blood levels of estrogen during pregnancy.

The basal metabolic rate increases by as much as 25% during pregnancy. However, within a few weeks after birth all thyroid function returns to normal limits.

### Pituitary

Pregnancy is made possible by the hypothalamic stimulation of the anterior pituitary gland, which in turn produces follicle-stimulating hormone (FSH), which stimulates ovum growth, and luteinizing hormone (LH), which brings about ovulation. Stimulation of the pituitary also prolongs the ovary's corpus luteal phase, which maintains the endometrium in case conception occurs. Prolactin, another anterior pituitary hormone, is responsible for initial lactation.

The posterior portion of the pituitary secretes vasopressin (antidiuretic hormone) and oxytocin. Vasopressin causes vasoconstriction, which results in increased blood pressure; it also helps regulate water balance. Oxytocin promotes uterine contractility and stimulates ejection of milk from the breasts (the letdown reflex) in the postpartum period.

### Adrenals

No significant increase in the weight of the adrenal glands occurs during pregnancy. Circulating cortisol, which regulates carbohydrate and protein metabolism, increases in response to increased estrogen levels. Cortisol blood levels return to normal within 1 to 6 weeks postpartum.

The adrenals secrete increased levels of aldosterone by the early part of the second trimester. This increase in aldosterone in a normal pregnancy may be the body's protective response to the increased sodium excretion associated with progesterone (Cunningham, et al., 1997).

### Pancreas

The pregnant woman has increased insulin needs, and the pancreatic islets of Langerhans, which secrete insulin, are stressed to meet this increased demand. Any marginal pancreatic function quickly becomes apparent, and the woman may show signs of gestational diabetes.

### Hormones in Pregnancy

#### Human Chorionic Gonadotropin (hCG)

The trophoblast secretes human chorionic gonadotropin (hCG) in early pregnancy. This hormone stimulates progesterone and estrogen production by the corpus luteum to maintain the pregnancy until the placenta is developed sufficiently to assume that function.

#### Human Placental Lactogen (hPL)

Also called human chorionic somatomammotropin, human placental lactogen (hPL) is produced by the syncytiotrophoblast. Human placental lactogen is an antagonist of insulin; it increases the amount of circulating free fatty acids for maternal metabolic needs and decreases maternal metabolism of glucose to favor fetal growth.

#### Estrogen

Estrogen, secreted originally by the corpus luteum, is produced primarily by the placenta as early as the seventh week of pregnancy. Estrogen stimulates uterine development to provide a suitable environment for the fetus. It also helps develop the ductal system of the breasts in preparation for lactation.

#### Progesterone

Progesterone, also produced initially by the corpus luteum and then by the placenta, plays the greatest role in maintaining pregnancy. It maintains the endometrium and inhibits spontaneous uterine contractility, thus preventing early spontaneous abortion. Progesterone also helps develop the acini and lobules of the breasts in preparation for lactation.

#### Relaxin

Relaxin is detectable in the serum of a pregnant woman by the time of the first missed menstrual period. Relaxin inhibits uterine activity, diminishes the strength of uterine contractions, aids in the softening of the cervix, and has the long-term effect of remodeling collagen. Its primary source is the corpus luteum, but small amounts are believed to be produced by the placenta and uterine decidua (Buster & Carson, 1996).

### Prostaglandins in Pregnancy

Prostaglandins (PGs) are lipid substances that can arise from most body tissues but occur in high concentrations in the female reproductive tract and are present in the decidua during pregnancy. The exact functions of PGs during pregnancy are still unknown, although it has been proposed that they are responsible for maintaining reduced placental vascular resistance. Decreased prostaglandin levels may contribute to pregnancy-induced hypertension (PIH). Prostaglandins are also believed to play a role in the complex biochemistry that initiates labor.

## Signs of Pregnancy

Many of the changes women experience during pregnancy are used to diagnose the pregnancy itself. They are called the subjective, or presumptive, changes; the objective, or probable, changes; and the diagnostic, or positive, changes of pregnancy. The guidelines for differentiating among these three are identified in Key Facts to Remember: Differentiating the Signs of Pregnancy.

### Subjective (Presumptive) Changes

The subjective changes of pregnancy are the symptoms the woman experiences and reports. Because they can be caused by other conditions, they cannot be considered proof of pregnancy (Table 7–1). The following subjective signs can be diagnostic clues when other signs and symptoms of pregnancy are also present.

*Amenorrhea,* or the absence of menses, is the earliest symptom of pregnancy. The missing of more than one menstrual period, especially in a woman whose cycle is ordinarily regular, is an especially useful diagnostic clue.

*Nausea and vomiting in pregnancy (NVP)* occur frequently during the first trimester. Because these symptoms often occur in the early part of the day, they are commonly referred to as **morning sickness.** In reality, the symptoms may occur at any time and can range from a mere distaste for food to severe vomiting. Research suggests that women who experience NVP have a decreased incidence of spontaneous abortion and perinatal mortality (Cruikshank et al., 1996).

*Excessive fatigue* may be noted within a few weeks after the first missed menstrual period and may persist throughout the first trimester.

*Urinary frequency* is experienced during the first trimester as the enlarging uterus presses on the bladder.

*Changes in the breasts* are frequently noted in early pregnancy. These changes include tenderness and tingling sensations, increased pigmentation of the areola and nipple, and changes in Montgomery's glands. The veins also become more visible and form a bluish pattern beneath the skin.

**Quickening,** or the mother's perception of fetal movement, occurs about 18 to 20 weeks after the last menstrual period in a woman pregnant for the first time but may occur as early as 16 weeks in a woman who has been preg-

**KEY FACTS TO REMEMBER**

*Differentiating the Signs of Pregnancy*

These guidelines help differentiate among the presumptive, probable, and positive changes of pregnancy.

**Subjective (Presumptive) Changes**

- Symptoms the woman experiences and reports
- May have causes other than pregnancy

**Objective (Probable) Changes**

- Signs perceived by the examiner
- May have causes other than pregnancy

**Diagnostic (Positive) Changes**

- Signs perceived by the examiner
- Can be caused only by pregnancy

**HINTS FOR PRACTICE**

Some women suggest that it is easiest to imagine the fluttering associated with quickening by letting the outer tips of the eyelashes brush a finger and then imagining that same sensation deep inside the abdomen.

**TABLE 7–1 Differential Diagnosis of Pregnancy: Subjective Changes**

| *Subjective Changes* | *Possible Alternative Causes* |
|---|---|
| Amenorrhea | Endocrine factors; early menopause; lactation; thyroid, pituitary, adrenal, ovarian dysfunction |
| | Metabolic factors: malnutrition, anemia, climatic changes, diabetes mellitus, degenerative disorders, long-distance running |
| | Psychologic factors: emotional shock, fear of pregnancy or sexually transmitted infection, intense desire for pregnancy (pseudocyesis), stress |
| | Obliteration of endometrial cavity by infection or curettage |
| | Systemic disease (acute or chronic), such as tuberculosis or malignancy |
| Nausea and vomiting | Gastrointestinal disorders |
| | Acute infections such as encephalitis |
| | Emotional disorders such as pseudocyesis or anorexia nervosa |
| Urinary frequency | Urinary tract infection |
| | Cystocele |
| | Pelvic tumors |
| | Urethral diverticula |
| | Emotional tension |
| Breast tenderness | Premenstrual tension |
| | Chronic cystic mastitis |
| | Pseudocyesis |
| | Hyperestrinism |
| Quickening | Increased peristalsis |
| | Flatus ("gas") |
| | Abdominal muscle contractions<br>Shifting of abdominal contents |

nant before. Quickening is a fluttering sensation in the abdomen that gradually increases in intensity and frequency.

## Objective (Probable) Changes

An examiner can perceive the objective changes that occur in pregnancy. Since these changes can also have other causes, they do not confirm pregnancy (Table 7–2).

*Changes in the pelvic organs*—the only physical changes detectable during the first 3 months of pregnancy—are caused by increased vascular congestion. These changes are noted on pelvic examination. There is a softening of the cervix called Goodell's sign. Chadwick's sign is a bluish, purple, or deep-red discoloration of the mucous membranes of the cervix, vagina, and vulva (some sources consider this a presumptive sign). **Hegar's sign** is a softening of the isthmus of the uterus, the area between the cervix and the body of the uterus (Figure 7–4♦). **McDonald's sign** is an ease in flexing the body of the uterus against the cervix.

General enlargement and softening of the body of the uterus can be noted after the eighth week of pregnancy. The fundus of the uterus is palpable just above the symphysis pubis at about 10 to 12 weeks' gestation and at the level of the umbilicus at 20 to 22 weeks' gestation (Figure 7–5♦).

**TABLE 7–2 Differential Diagnosis of Pregnancy: Objective Changes**

| *Objective Changes* | *Possible Alternative Causes* |
|---|---|
| Changes in pelvic organs | Increased vascular congestion |
| Goodell's sign | Estrogen-progestin oral contraceptives |
| Chadwick's sign | Vulvar, vaginal, cervical hyperemia |
| Hegar's sign | Excessively soft walls of nonpregnant uterus |
| Uterine enlargement | Uterine tumors |
| Braun von Fernwald's sign | Uterine tumors |
| Piskacek's sign | Uterine tumors |
| Enlargement of abdomen | Obesity, ascites, pelvic tumors |
| Braxton Hicks contractions | Hematometra, pedunculated, submucous, and soft myomas |
| Uterine souffle | Large uterine myomas, large ovarian tumors, or any condition with greatly increased uterine blood flow |
| Pigmentation of skin | Estrogen-progestin oral contraceptives |
| Chloasma | Melanocyte hormonal stimulation |
| Linea nigra | |
| Nipples and areola | |
| Abdominal striae | Obesity, pelvic tumor |
| Ballottement | Uterine tumors or polyps, ascites |
| Pregnancy tests | Increased pituitary gonadotropins at menopause, choriocarcinoma, hydatidiform mole |
| Palpation for fetal outline | Uterine myomas |

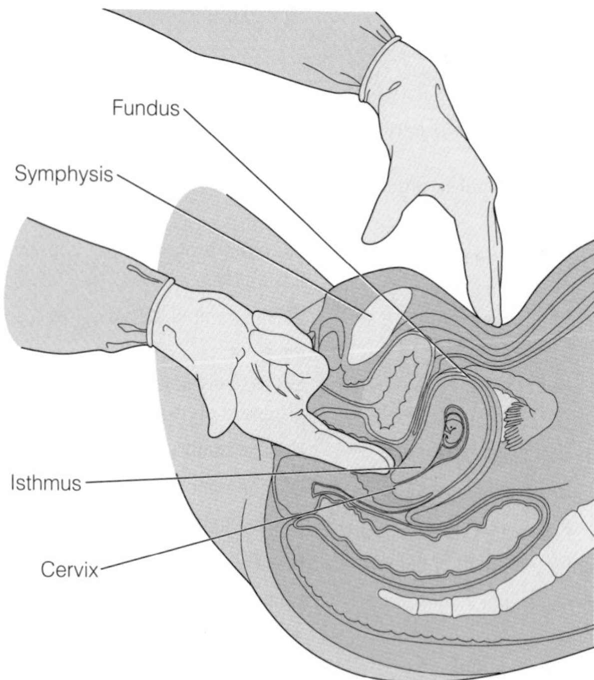


FIGURE 7–4 ♦ Hegar's sign, a softening of the isthmus of the uterus, can be determined by the examiner during a vaginal examination.

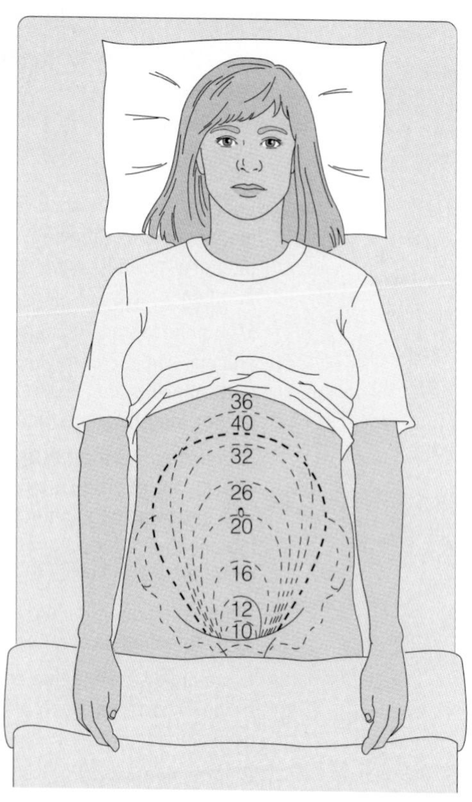


FIGURE 7–5 ♦ Approximate height of the fundus at various weeks of pregnancy.

*Enlargement of the abdomen* during the childbearing years is usually regarded as evidence of pregnancy, especially if it is continuous and accompanied by amenorrhea.

*Braxton Hicks contractions* can be palpated most commonly after the 28th week. As the woman approaches the end of pregnancy, these contractions may become uncomfortable. They are then often called false labor.

*Uterine souffle* may be heard when the examiner auscultates the abdomen over the uterus. It is a soft, blowing sound that occurs at the same rate as the maternal pulse and is caused by the increased uterine blood flow and blood pulsating through the placenta. It is sometimes confused with the *funic souffle,* a soft, blowing sound of blood pulsating through the umbilical cord. The funic souffle occurs at the same rate as the fetal heart rate.

*Changes in pigmentation of the skin* are common in pregnancy. The nipples and areola may darken, and the linea nigra may develop. Facial chloasma may become noticeable, and striae may appear.

The *fetal outline* may be identified by palpation in many pregnant women after 24 weeks' gestation. **Ballottement** is the passive fetal movement elicited when the examiner inserts two gloved fingers into the vagina and pushes against the cervix. This action pushes the fetal body up, and, as it falls back, the examiner feels a rebound.

*Pregnancy tests* detect the presence of hCG in the maternal blood or urine. These are not considered a positive sign of pregnancy because other conditions can cause elevated hCG levels.

## Clinical Pregnancy Tests

A variety of assay techniques are available to detect hCG during early pregnancy.

- *Hemagglutination-inhibition test* (Pregnosticon R), an immunoassay, is based on the fact that no clumping of cells occurs when the urine of a pregnant woman is added to the hCG-sensitized red blood cells of sheep.
- *Latex agglutination test* (Gravindex and Pregnosticon Slide tests), also an immunoassay, is based on the fact that latex particle agglutination is inhibited in the presence of urine containing hCG.

The two tests just described are done on the first early morning urine specimen of the woman because it is adequately concentrated. The tests become positive within 10 to 14 days after the first missed period.

Several pregnancy tests are done on maternal serum, including the following:

- *β-subunit radioimmunoassay* (RIA) uses an antiserum with specificity for the β-subunit of hCG in maternal blood. This very accurate pregnancy test becomes positive a few days after presumed implantation, thereby permitting early diagnosis of pregnancy. This test is also used in the diagnosis of ectopic pregnancy or trophoblastic disease. However, because it requires several hours to perform and has only limited sensitivity, it is being replaced by other, technically simpler tests such as the immunoradiometric assay (Buster & Carson, 1996).

- *Immunoradiometric assay* (IRMA) (Neocept, Pregnosis) uses a radioactive antibody to identify the presence of hCG in the serum. This test can detect very low concentrations of hCG and requires only about 30 minutes to perform.
- *Enzyme-linked immunosorbent assay* (ELISA) (Model Sensichrome, Quest Confidot) does not use radioisotopes but a substance that results in a color change after binding. The test is sensitive, quick, and can detect hCG levels as early as 7 to 9 days after ovulation and conception, which is 5 days before the first missed period (Buster & Carson, 1996).
- *Fluoroimmunoassay* (FIA) (Opus hCG, Stratus hCG) uses an antibody tagged with a fluorescent label to detect serum hCG. The test, which takes about 2 to 3 hours to perform, is extremely sensitive and is used primarily to identify and follow hCG concentrations.
- *Radioreceptor assay* (Biocept-G) uses the principle of high-affinity receptors to detect pregnancy. It is a sensitive test and can be performed in 1 hour, but because it fails to distinguish between hCG and LH, cross reactions may occur and it has generally been replaced by more effective tests.

#### Over-the-Counter Pregnancy Tests

Home pregnancy tests are available over the counter at a reasonable cost. These enzyme immunoassay tests, performed on urine, are quite sensitive and detect even low levels of hCG.

Home pregnancy test instructions are quite explicit and should be followed carefully for optimal results. Best results are obtained with a first morning urine specimen, although some of the tests can be used on any voided specimen. Furthermore, because the newer kits require only a short wait (usually 3 to 5 minutes), the margin for error is very small. Most of the current kits can detect a pregnancy as early as the first day of the missed period, but to avoid false-negative results, women should be encouraged to wait 6 to 9 days after a missed period before using the test.

### Diagnostic (Positive) Changes

The positive signs of pregnancy are completely objective, cannot be confused with a pathologic state, and offer conclusive proof of pregnancy.

The *fetal heartbeat* can be detected with a fetoscope by weeks 17 to 20 of pregnancy. The electronic Doppler device allows the examiner to detect the fetal heartbeat as early as weeks 10 to 12.

*Fetal movement* is actively palpable by a trained examiner after about the 20th week of pregnancy.

*Visualization of the fetus* by ultrasound examination confirms a pregnancy. The gestational sac can be observed by 4 to 5 weeks' gestation (2 to 3 weeks after conception). Fetal parts and fetal movement can be seen as early as 8 weeks' gestation. More recently ultrasound using a vaginal probe has been used to detect a gestational sac as early as 10 days after implantation (Cunningham, et al., 1997).

## Psychologic Response of the Expectant Family to Pregnancy

Pregnancy is a developmental challenge, a turning point in a family's life, and thus it is accompanied by stress and anxiety, whether the pregnancy is desired or not. Pregnancy confirms the biologic capability to reproduce. It is an affirmation of sexuality. For beginning families, pregnancy is the transition period from childlessness to parenthood. If the pregnancy results in the birth of a child, the couple enters a new, irreversible stage of their life together.

The expectant couple may be unaware of the physical, emotional, and cognitive changes of pregnancy and may anticipate no problems from such a normal event. Thus they may be confused and distressed by new feelings and behaviors that are essentially normal.

If the expectant woman is married or has a stable partner, she no longer is only a mate but must also assume the role of mother. Her partner will soon be a father. In essence, parenthood brings significant role changes for the couple. Career goals and mobility may be affected, and the couple's relationship takes on a different meaning to them and their families and community. Routines and family dynamics are altered with each pregnancy, requiring readjustment and realignment.

As pregnancy progresses, the couple must face the anxieties of labor and birth and must also deal with fears that the baby may be ill or disfigured. Classes in prepared childbirth can help the couple overcome concerns based on misinformation or lack of information.

If the pregnant woman has no stable partner, she must deal alone with the role changes, fears, and adjustments of pregnancy or seek support from family or friends. She also faces the reality of planning for the future as a single parent. Even if the pregnant woman plans to relinquish her infant, she must still deal with the adjustments of pregnancy. This adjustment can be especially difficult without a good support system.

In most pregnancies, finances are an important consideration. Traditional lore relegates to the father the role of primary breadwinner, and indeed finances are often a very real concern for fathers. However, in today's society even pregnant women with stable partners recognize the financial impact of a child and may feel concern about financial issues. For the single mother, finances may be a major source of concern.

Decisions about financial matters need to be made at this time. Will the woman work during her pregnancy and return to work after her child is born? If so, who will provide child care? Couples may also need to decide about the division of domestic tasks. Any differences of opinion must be discussed openly and resolved so that the family can meet the needs of its members.

Pregnancy can be viewed as a developmental stage with its own distinct developmental tasks. For a couple, it can be a time of support or conflict, depending on the amount of adjustment each is willing to make to maintain the family's equilibrium.

During a first pregnancy, the couple plans together for the child's arrival, collecting information on how to be parents. At the same time, each continues to participate in some separate activities with friends or family members. The availability of social support is an important factor in psychosocial well-being during pregnancy. The social network is often a major source of advice for the pregnant woman. However, both sound and unsound information may be conveyed.

During pregnancy, the expectant mother and father both face significant changes and must deal with major psychosocial adjustments (Table 7–3). Other family members, especially other children of the woman or couple and the grandparents-to-be, must also adjust to the pregnancy.

For some, pregnancy is more than a developmental stage; it is a crisis. *Crisis* can be defined as a disturbance or conflict in which the individual cannot maintain a state of equilibrium. Pregnancy can be considered a *maturational crisis,* since it is a common event in the normal growth and development of the family. During such a crisis, the individual or family is in disequilibrium. Egos weaken, usual defense mechanisms are not effective, unresolved material from the past reappears, and relationships shift. The period of disequilibrium and disorganization is marked by unsuccessful attempts to solve the perceived problems. If the crisis is not resolved, it will result in maladaptive behaviors in one or more family members and possible disintegration of the family. Families that are able to resolve a maturational crisis will return successfully to normal functioning and can even strengthen the bonds in the family relationship.

## The Mother

Pregnancy is a condition that alters body image and also necessitates a reordering of social relationships and changes in roles of family members. The way each woman meets the stresses of pregnancy is influenced by her emotional makeup, her sociologic and cultural background, and her acceptance or rejection of the pregnancy. However, many women manifest similar psychologic and emotional responses during pregnancy, including ambivalence, acceptance, introversion, mood swings, and changes in body image.

A woman's attitude toward her pregnancy can be a significant factor in its outcome. Even if the pregnancy is planned, there is an element of surprise at first. Many women commonly experience feelings of ambivalence during early pregnancy. This ambivalence may be related to feelings that the timing is somehow wrong; worries about the need to modify existing relationships or career plans; fears about assuming a new role; unresolved emotional conflicts with the woman's own mother; and fears about pregnancy, labor, and birth. These feelings may be more pronounced if the pregnancy is unplanned or unwanted. Indirect expressions of ambivalence include complaints about considerable physical discomfort, prolonged or frequent depression, significant dissatisfaction with changing body shape, excessive mood swings, and difficulty in accepting the life changes resulting from the pregnancy (Lederman, 1996).

Women who view their pregnancy as unwanted are more likely to delay prenatal care and to experience complications. Research indicates that the support and opinion of the woman's current partner, even if he is not the father of the child, has a major impact on pregnancy wantedness. Financial and emotional support from the partner are essential to the woman's positive attitude (Kroelinger & Oths, 2000). Involving the partner in the prenatal care may help promote a supportive attitude.

Conflicts about adapting to pregnancy are no more pronounced for older pregnant women (age 35 and over) than for younger ones. Moreover, older pregnant women tend to be less concerned about the normal physical changes of pregnancy and are confident about handling issues that arise during pregnancy and parenting. This difference may result because mature pregnant women have more experience with problem solving. However, mature pregnant women may have fewer pregnant peers and thus may have fewer people with whom to share concerns and expectations (Stark, 1997).

Pregnancy produces marked changes in a woman's body within a relatively short period of time. Pregnant women experience changes in body image because of physical alterations and may feel a loss of control over their bodies during pregnancy and later during childbirth.

**TABLE 7–3 Parental Reactions to Pregnancy**

| *First Trimester* | *Second Trimester* | *Third Trimester* |
|---|---|---|
| **MOTHER'S REACTIONS** | **MOTHER'S REACTIONS** | **MOTHER'S REACTIONS** |
| Informs father secretively or openly<br>Feels ambivalent toward pregnancy, anxious about labor and responsibility of child<br>Is aware of physical changes, daydreams of possible miscarriage<br>Develops special feelings for and renewed interest in her own mother, with formation of a personal identity | Remains regressive and introspective, projects all problems with authority figures onto partner, may become angry as if lack of interest is sign of weakness in him<br>Continues to deal with feelings as a mother and looks for furniture as something concrete<br>May have other extreme of anxiety and wait until ninth month to look for furniture and clothes for baby<br>Feels movement and is aware of fetus and incorporates it into herself<br>Dreams that partner will be killed, telephones him often for reassurance<br>Experiences more distinct physical changes; sexual desires may increase or decrease | Experiences more anxiety and tension, with physical awkwardness<br>Feels much discomfort and insomnia from physical condition<br>Prepares for birth, assembles layette, picks out names<br>Dreams often about misplacing baby or not being able to give birth, fears birth of deformed baby<br>Feels ecstasy and excitement, has spurt of energy during last month |
| **FATHER'S REACTIONS** | **FATHER'S REACTIONS** | **FATHER'S REACTIONS** |
| Differ according to age, parity, desire for child, economic stability<br>Acceptance of pregnant woman's attitude or complete rejection and lack of communication<br>Is aware of his own sexual feelings, may develop more or less sexual arousal<br>Accepts, rejects, or resents mother-in-law<br>May develop new hobby outside of family as sign of stress | If he can cope, will give her extra attention she needs; if he cannot cope, will develop a new time-consuming interest outside of home<br>May develop a creative feeling and a "closeness to nature"<br>May become involved in pregnancy and buy or make furniture<br>Feels for movement of baby, listens to heartbeat, or remains aloof, with no physical contact<br>May have fears and fantasies about himself being pregnant, may become uneasy with this feminine aspect in himself<br>May react negatively if partner is too demanding, may become jealous of physician and of physician's importance to partner and her pregnancy | Adapts to alternative methods of sexual contact<br>Becomes concerned over financial responsibility<br>May show new sense of tenderness and concern, treats partner like doll<br>Daydreams about child as if older and not newborn, dreams of losing partner<br>Renewed sexual attraction to partner<br>Feels he is ultimately responsible for whatever happens |

Research suggests that these feelings may be reflected in the theme, "I want my body back" (Cline, Martin, & Deyo, 1998). These perceptions are related to a certain extent to personality factors, social network responses, and attitudes toward pregnancy. Although changes in body image are normal, they can be very stressful for the woman. Explanation and discussion of the changes may help both the woman and her partner deal with the stress associated with this aspect of pregnancy.

Fantasies about the unborn child are common among pregnant women. However, the themes of the fantasies (baby's appearance, gender, traits, impact on parents, and so forth) vary by trimester and also differ between women pregnant for the first time and women who already have children (Sorenson & Schuelke, 1999).

### First Trimester

During the first trimester, feelings of disbelief and ambivalence are paramount. The woman's baby does not seem real, and she focuses on herself and her pregnancy. She may experience one or more of the early symptoms of pregnancy, such as breast tenderness or morning sickness, which are unsettling and at times unpleasant.

During the first trimester, the expectant mother begins to exhibit some characteristic behavioral changes. She may become increasingly introspective and passive. She may be emotionally labile, with characteristic mood swings from joy to despair. She may fantasize about a miscarriage and feel guilt because of these fantasies. She may worry that these thoughts will harm the baby in some way.

### Second Trimester

During the second trimester, quickening occurs. This perception of fetal movement helps the woman think of her baby as a separate person, and she generally becomes excited about the pregnancy even if earlier she was not. The woman becomes increasingly introspective as she evaluates her life, her plans, and her child's future. This introspection helps the woman prepare for her new mothering role. Emotional lability, which may be unsettling to her partner, persists. In some instances, the partner may react by withdrawing. This withdrawal is especially distressing to the woman, because she needs increased love and affection. Once the couple understands that these behaviors are characteristic of pregnancy, it is easier for the couple to deal with them effectively, although they may be sources of stress to some extent throughout pregnancy.

As pregnancy becomes more noticeable, the woman's body image changes. She may feel great pride, embarrassment, or concern. Generally women feel best during the second trimester, which is a relatively tranquil time.

### Third Trimester

In the third trimester, the woman feels both pride about her pregnancy and anxiety about labor and birth. Physical discomforts increase, and the woman is eager for the pregnancy to end. She experiences increased fatigue, her body movements are more awkward, and her interest in sexual activity may decrease. During this time, the woman tends to be concerned about the health and safety of her unborn child and may worry that she will not cope well during childbirth. Toward the end of this period, there is often a surge of energy as the woman prepares a "nest" for the infant. Many women report bursts of energy, during which they vigorously clean and organize their homes.

### Psychological Tasks of the Mother

Rubin (1984) has identified four major tasks that the pregnant woman undertakes to maintain her intactness and that of her family and at the same time incorporate her new child into the family system. These tasks form the foundation for a mutually gratifying relationship with her infant.

1. *Ensuring safe passage through pregnancy, labor, and birth.* The pregnant woman feels concern for both her unborn child and herself. She looks for competent maternity care to provide a sense of control. She may seek information from literature, observation of other pregnant women and new mothers, and discussion with others. She also attempts to ensure safe passage by engaging in self-care activities related to diet, exercise, alcohol consumption, and so forth (Patterson, Freese, & Goldenberg, 1990). In the third trimester she becomes more aware of external threats in the environment—a toy on the stairs, the awkwardness of an escalator—that pose a threat to her well-being. She may worry if her partner is late or if she is home alone. Sleep becomes more difficult and she longs for birth even though it, too, is frightening.
2. *Seeking acceptance of this child by others.* The birth of a child alters a woman's primary support group (her family) and her secondary affiliative groups. The woman slowly and subtly alters her network to meet the needs of her pregnancy. In this adjustment the woman's partner is the most important figure. The partner's support and acceptance help form a maternal identity. If there are other children in the home, the mother also works to ensure their acceptance of the coming child. Acceptance of the anticipated change is sometimes stressful, and the woman may work to maintain some special time with her partner or older children. The woman without a partner looks to others such as a family member or friend for this support.
3. *Seeking commitment and acceptance of herself as mother to the infant (binding-in).* During the first trimester the child remains a rather abstract concept. With quickening, however, the child begins to become a real person, and the mother begins to develop bonds of attachment. The mother experiences the movement of the child within her in an intimate, exclusive way, and out of this experience bonds of love form. The mother develops a fantasy image of her ideal child. This binding-in process, characterized by its strong emotional component, motivates the pregnant woman to become competent in her role and provides satisfaction for her in the role of mother (Mercer, 1995). This possessive love increases her maternal commitment to protect her fetus now and her child after he or she is born.
4. *Learning to give of oneself on behalf of one's child.* Childbirth involves many acts of giving. The man "gives" a child to the woman; she in turn "gives" a child to him. Life is given to an infant; a sibling is given to older children of the family. The woman begins to develop a capacity for self-denial and learns to delay immediate personal gratification to meet the needs of another. Baby showers and gifts

are acts of giving that increase the mother's self-esteem and help her recognize the separateness and needs of the coming baby.

Accomplishment of these tasks helps the expectant woman develop her self-concept as mother. The expectant woman who was well nurtured by her own mother may view her mother as a role model and emulate her; the woman who views her mother as a "poor mother" may worry that she will make similar mistakes (Lederman, 1996). A woman's self-concept as a mother expands with actual experience and continues to grow through subsequent childbearing and child rearing. Occasionally a woman fails to accept the mother role, instead playing the role of baby-sitter or older sister to her child.

## The Father

For the expectant father, pregnancy is a psychologically stressful time because he, too, must make the transition from nonparent to parent or from parent of one or more to parent of two or more. Research suggests that expectant fathers who have more self-actualizing behaviors, exercise regularly, use more stress management techniques, and have good interpersonal support tend to find pregnancy less stressful and feel more confident about parenting (Walker, Fleschler, & Heaman, 1998).

Initially, expectant fathers may feel pride in their virility, which pregnancy confirms, but also have many of the same ambivalent feelings expectant mothers have. The extent of ambivalence depends on many factors, including the father's relationship with his partner, his previous experience with pregnancy, his age, his economic stability, and whether the pregnancy was planned.

In adjusting to his role, the expectant father must first deal with the reality of the pregnancy and then struggle to gain recognition as a parent from his partner, family, friends, coworkers, and society—and from his baby as well. The expectant mother can help her partner be a participant and not merely a helpmate to her if she has a definite sense of the experience as *their* pregnancy and *their* infant and not *her* pregnancy and *her* infant (Jordan, 1990).

The expectant father must establish a fatherhood role, just as the woman develops a motherhood role. Fathers who are most successful at this task generally like children, are excited about the prospect of fatherhood, are eager to nurture a child, and have confidence in their ability to be a parent. They also share the experiences of pregnancy and birth with their partners (Lederman, 1996). See Table 7–3.

### First Trimester

After the initial excitement attending the announcement of the pregnancy, an expectant father may begin to feel left out. He may be confused by his partner's mood changes. He might resent the attention she receives and her need to modify their relationship as she experiences fatigue and possibly a decreased interest in sex. In addition, he might be concerned about what kind of father he will be. During this time his child is a "potential" baby. Fathers often picture interacting with a child of 5 or 6 years, not a newborn. The pregnancy itself may seem unreal until the woman shows more physical signs.

### Second Trimester

The father's role in the pregnancy is still vague in the second trimester, but his involvement may increase as he watches and feels fetal movement and listens to the fetal heartbeat during a prenatal visit. Like expectant mothers, expectant fathers need to confront and resolve some of their conflicts about the fathering they received. A father needs to sort out which behaviors of his own father he wants to imitate and which he wants to avoid.

Evidence suggests that the father-to-be's anxiety is lessened if both parents agree on the paternal role the man is to assume. For example, if both see his role as that of breadwinner, the man's stress is low. However, if the man views his role as that of breadwinner and the woman expects him to be actively involved in child care, his stress increases. Thus the ability of the couple to negotiate a mutually agreeable role for the man may provide a significant coping mechanism for expectant fathers (Diemer, 1997).

As the woman's appearance begins to change, her partner may have several reactions. Her changed appearance may decrease his sexual interest, or it may have the opposite effect. Because of the variety of emotions both partners may feel, continued communication and acceptance are important.

### Third Trimester

If the couple's relationship has grown through effective communication of their concerns and feelings, the third trimester is often a rewarding time. They may attend childbirth classes and make concrete preparations for the arrival of the baby. If the father has developed a detached attitude about the pregnancy, however, it is unlikely he will become a willing participant, even though his role becomes more obvious.

Concerns and fears may recur. The father may worry about hurting the unborn baby during intercourse or become concerned about labor and birth. Also, he may wonder what kind of parents he and his partner will be.

### Couvade

**Couvade** has traditionally referred to the observance of certain rituals and taboos by the male to signify the transition to fatherhood. This observance affirms his psychosocial and biophysical relationship to the woman and child. Some taboos restrict his actions. For example, in some cultures the man may be forbidden to eat certain foods or carry certain weapons before and immediately after the birth. More recently, the term has been used to describe the unintentional development of physical symptoms such as fatigue, increased appetite, difficulty sleeping, depression, headache, or backache by the partner of a pregnant woman. Men who demonstrate couvade syndrome may tend to have a higher degree of paternal role preparation and be involved in more activities related to this preparation.

## SIBLINGS

Bringing a new baby home often marks the beginning of sibling rivalry. The siblings view the baby as a threat to the security of their relationships with their parents. Parents who recognize this potential problem early in pregnancy and begin constructive actions can minimize the problem of sibling rivalry.

Preparation of the young child begins several weeks before the anticipated birth. Because they do not have a clear concept of time, young children should not be told too early about the pregnancy. From the toddler's point of view, several weeks is an extremely long time. The mother may let the child feel the baby moving in her uterus, explaining that the uterus is "a special place where babies grow." The child can help the parents put the baby clothes in drawers or prepare the nursery.

The concept of consistency is important in dealing with young children. They need reassurance that certain people, special things, and familiar places will continue to exist after the new baby arrives. The crib is often an important though transient object in a child's life. If it is to be given to the new baby, the parents should thoughtfully help the older child adjust to this change. Any move from crib to bed or from one room to another should precede the baby's birth by at least several weeks. If the new baby will share a room with siblings, the parents must also discuss this situation with the older child or children.

Some parents advocate cosleeping (one or both parents sleeping with their baby or young child), and so the crib is less an issue. Cosleeping, common in many non-Western cultures, is attracting more support in the United States (Small, 1998). Opinion varies sharply about the advantages and risks of the practice. Parents who choose to cosleep must make decisions about the sleeping arrangements of other siblings following the birth of the baby.

If the child is ready, toilet training is most effective several months before or after the baby's arrival. It is not unusual for an older, toilet-trained child to regress to wetting or soiling because of the attention the newborn gets for such behavior. The older, weaned child may want to nurse or drink from the bottle again after the baby arrives. If the new mother anticipates these behaviors, they will be less frustrating during her early postpartum days.

Pregnant women may find it helpful to bring their children on a prenatal visit to the certified nurse-midwife or physician to give them an opportunity to listen to the fetal heartbeat. Such a visit helps make the baby more real to the children; they may also become involved in the prenatal care.

If siblings are school-age children, pregnancy should be viewed as a family affair. Teaching should be suitable to the child's level of understanding and may be supplemented with appropriate books. Taking part in family discussions, attending sibling preparation classes, feeling fetal movement, and listening to the fetal heartbeat help the school-age child take part in the experience of pregnancy and not feel like an outsider.

Older children or adolescents may appear to have sophisticated knowledge but may have many misconceptions about pregnancy and birth. The parents should make opportunities to discuss their concerns and involve the children in preparations for the new baby.

Even after birth, siblings need to feel that they are taking part. Having siblings visit their mother and the new baby at the hospital or birthing center will help. After the baby comes home, siblings can share in "showing off" the new baby.

Sibling preparation is essential, but other factors are equally important. These factors include how much parental attention the new arrival receives, how much attention the older child receives after the baby comes home, and how well the parents handle regressive or aggressive behavior.

## GRANDPARENTS

The first relatives told about a pregnancy are usually the grandparents. Often, the expectant grandparents become increasingly supportive of the couple, even if conflicts previously existed. But it can be difficult for even sensitive grandparents to know how deeply to become involved in the childrearing process.

Because grandparenting can occur over a wide expanse of years, people's response to this role can vary considerably. Younger grandparents leading active lives may not demonstrate as much interest as the young couple would like. In other cases, expectant grandparents may give advice and gifts unsparingly. For grandparents, conflict may be related to the expectant couple's need to feel in control of their lives, or it may stem from events signaling changing roles in the grandparents' own lives (eg, retirement, financial concerns, menopause, or death of a friend). Some parents of expectant couples may already be grandparents with a developed style of grandparenting. This influences their response to the pregnancy.

Because childbearing and childrearing practices have changed, family cohesiveness is promoted by effective communication and frank discussion between young couples and interested grandparents about the changes and the reasons for them. Clarifying the role of the helping grandparent ensures a comfortable situation for all.

Classes for grandparents may provide information about changes in birth and parenting practices. These classes help familiarize grandparents with new parents' needs and may offer suggestions for ways in which the grandparents can support the childbearing couple.

# Cultural Values and Reproductive Behavior

A universal tendency exists to create ceremonial rituals or rites around important life events. Thus pregnancy, childbirth, marriage, and death are often tied to ritual. The rituals and customs of a group are a reflection of the group's values. Thus the identification of cultural values is useful in predicting reactions to pregnancy. An understanding of male and female roles, family lifestyles, religious values, or the meaning of children in a culture may explain reactions of joy or shame.

Health values and beliefs are also important in understanding reactions and behavior. Certain behaviors can be expected if a culture views pregnancy as a sickness, whereas other behaviors can be expected if the culture views pregnancy as a natural occurrence. Prenatal care may not be a priority for women who view pregnancy as a natural phenomenon or for women challenged by financial constraints.

Generalization about cultural characteristics or values is difficult because not every individual in a culture may display these characteristics. Just as variations are seen between cultures, variations are also seen within cultures. For example, because of their exposure to the American culture, a third-generation Cambodian-American family might have very different values and beliefs from those of a Cambodian family that has recently immigrated to America. For this reason, the nurse needs to supplement a general knowledge of cultural values and practices with a complete assessment of the individual's values and practices.

The meaning assigned to childbearing may vary from culture to culture. For example, most Native American groups generally view pregnancy as a natural condition, and children are desired. In some cultures, a woman who gives birth, especially to a son, achieves higher status. This is true in traditional Chinese families, for example. Similarly, in the western United States, people of the Mormon faith view motherhood as the most important aspect of a woman's life, comparable to the male role of priesthood (Conley, 1990). In traditional Mexican-American families, having children may be seen as proving the male's manliness, or *machismo,* a desired trait among many Mexican-American men.

## Health Beliefs

Although many cultures view pregnancy as a natural occurrence, it may also be seen as a time of increased vulnerability. In Orthodox Judaism, for example, it is a man's responsibility to procreate, but it is a woman's right, not her obligation, to do so. This is because, according to Orthodox Jewish law, the health of the mother, both physically and mentally, is of primary concern, and she should never be obliged to do something that threatens her life (Bodo & Gibson, 1999a).

Individuals of many cultures take certain protective precautions based on their beliefs. For example, many Southeast Asian women fear that they will have a complicated labor and birth if they sit in a doorway or on a step. Thus they tend to avoid areas near doors in waiting rooms and examining rooms (Mattson, 1995). In the Mexican-American culture, the concept of *mal aire,* or bad air, is sometimes related to evil spirits. It is thought that air, especially night air, may enter the body and cause harm. For many Vietnamese women, lifting the arms above the head is believed to increase the risk of preterm birth. Vietnamese women also are discouraged from sitting or lying down for lengthy periods because doing so might permit the baby to become too large (Bodo & Gibson, 1999b).

Most taboos stemming from the belief in evil spirits are grounded in fear of injuring the unborn child. Taboos also arise from the belief that a pregnant woman has evil powers. As a result, pregnant women are sometimes prohibited from taking part in certain activities with other people.

The equilibrium model of health is based on the concept of balance between light and dark, heat and cold. Some Eastern philosophies focus on the notion of yin and yang. Yin represents the female, passive principle—darkness, cold, wetness—whereas yang is the masculine, active principle—light, heat, and dryness. When the two are combined, they are all that can be. The hot-cold classification is seen in cultures in Latin America, the Near East, and Asia.

Mexican-Americans may consider illness to be an excess of either hot or cold. To restore health, imbalances are often corrected by the proper use of foods, medications, or herbs. These substances are also classified as hot or cold. For example, an illness attributed to an excess of cold will be treated only with hot foods or medications. The classification of foods is not always consistent, but it conforms to a general structure of traditional knowledge. Certain foods, spices, herbs, and medications are perceived to cool or heat the body. These perceptions do not necessarily correspond to the actual temperature; some hot dishes are said to have a cooling quality.

Southeast Asians believe it is important to keep the woman "warm" after birth, because blood, which is considered "hot," has been lost, and the woman is at risk of becoming "cold." Therefore they avoid cold drinks and foods following birth (Mattson, 1995). In contrast, many women in India consider pregnancy a "hot" period and eat "cool" foods to balance the hot state (Choudhry, 1997).

The concepts of hot and cold are not as important in Native American or African-American beliefs. There are some similarities, however, in all of these groups because of their emphasis on a balance in nature.

## Health Practices

Health care practices during pregnancy are influenced by numerous factors, such as the prevalence of traditional home remedies and folk beliefs, the importance of indigenous healers, and the influence of professional health care workers. In an urban setting, the age, length of time in the city, marital status, and strength of the family may affect these patterns. Socioeconomic status is also important, since modern medical services are more accessible to those who can afford them.

An awareness of alternative health sources is crucial for health professionals, since these practices affect health outcomes. For example, in the traditional Mexican-American culture, mothers are often influenced by *familism,* a close-knit, interdependent network of nuclear and extended family members who are connected for the good of the family. Familism is also reflected in a high regard for parental roles, and young mothers will seek and follow the advice of their mothers or older women in the childbearing period (Lederman & Miller, 1998).

Indigenous healers are also important to specific cultures. In the Mexican-American culture, the healer is called a *curandero* or *curandera.* In some Native American tribes, the medicine man or woman may fulfill the healing role. Herbalists are often found in Asian cultures, and faith healers, root doctors, and spiritualists are sometimes consulted by members of some African cultures.

### KEY FACTS TO REMEMBER

*Providing Effective Prenatal Care to Families of Different Cultures*

Nurses who are interacting with expectant families from a different culture or ethnic group can provide more effective, culturally sensitive nursing care by

- Critically examining their own cultural beliefs
- Identifying personal biases, attitudes, stereotypes, and prejudices
- Making a conscious commitment to respect the values and beliefs of others
- Using sensitive, current language when describing others' cultures
- Learning the rituals, customs, and practices of the major cultural and ethnic groups with whom they have contact
- Including cultural assessment and assessment of the family's expectations of the health care system as a routine part of prenatal nursing care
- Incorporating the family's cultural practices into prenatal care as much as possible
- Fostering an attitude of respect for and cooperation with alternative healers and caregivers whenever possible
- Providing for the services of an interpreter if language barriers exist
- Learning the language (or at least several key phrases) of at least one of the cultural groups with whom they interact
- Recognizing that ultimately it is the woman's right to make her own health care choices
- Evaluating whether the client's health care beliefs have any potential negative consequences for her health

## Cultural Factors and Nursing Care

Health care providers are often unaware of the cultural characteristics they themselves demonstrate. Without cultural awareness, caregivers tend to project their own cultural responses onto foreign-born clients; clients from different socioeconomic, religious, or educational groups; or clients from different regions of the country. This projection leads caregivers to assume that the clients are demonstrating a specific behavior for the same reason that they themselves would. Moreover, health care providers often fail to realize that medicine has its own culture, which has been dominated historically by traditional middle-class values and beliefs (American College of Obstetricians and Gynecologists [ACOG], 1998).

*Ethnocentrism* is the conviction that the values and beliefs of one's own cultural group are the best or only acceptable ones. It is characterized by an inability to understand the beliefs and worldview of another culture. To a certain extent, all of us are guilty of ethnocentrism, at least some of the time. Thus the nurse who values stoicism during labor may be uncomfortable with the more vocal response of some Latin American women. Another nurse may be disconcerted by a Southeast Asian woman who believes that pain is something to be endured rather than alleviated and who is intent on maintaining self-control in labor (Mattson, 1995).

Health care providers sometimes believe that if members of other cultures do not share Western values and beliefs, they should adopt them. For example, a nurse who believes strongly in equality of the sexes may find it difficult to remain silent if a woman from a Middle Eastern culture defers to her husband in decision making. It is important to remember that pressure to defy cultural values and beliefs can be stressful and anxiety provoking for these women.

To address issues of cultural diversity in the provision of health care, emphasis is being placed on developing *cultural competency*—that is, the skills and knowledge necessary to appreciate, respect, and work with individuals from different cultures. It requires self-awareness, awareness and understanding of cultural differences, and the ability to adapt clinical skills and practices as needed (Beckman & Dysart, 2000).

Cultural assessment is an important aspect of prenatal care. Health care professionals are becoming increasingly aware that they must address cultural needs in the prenatal assessment to provide culturally sensitive health care during pregnancy. The nurse needs to identify the prospective parents' main beliefs, values, and behaviors related to pregnancy and childbearing. This includes information about ethnic background, amount of affiliation with the ethnic group, patterns of decision making, religious preference, language, communication style, and common etiquette practices. The nurse can also explore the woman's (or family's) expectations of the health care system.

In planning care, the nurse considers the extent to which the woman's personal values, beliefs, and customs are in accord with the values, beliefs, and customs of the woman's identified cultural group, the nurse providing care, and the health care agency. If discrepancies exist, the nurse then considers whether the woman's system is supportive, neutral, or harmful in relation to possible interventions. If the woman's system is supportive or neutral, it should be incorporated into the plan. For example, individual food practices or methods of pain expression may differ from those of the nurse or agency but would not necessarily pose a risk to the woman. On the other hand, certain cultural practices might pose a threat to her health. For example, some Filipinas will not take any medication during pregnancy. The health care provider may consider a certain medication essential to the woman's well-being. In this case, the woman's cultural belief may be detrimental to her own health. The nurse and client must carefully discuss the reasons for her refusal. After discussing and understanding the reasons, the nurse faces three possible outcomes: (1) identifying ways to persuade the woman to accept the proposed medication, (2) accepting the woman's decision to refuse the medication, or (3) explaining alternate therapies that might be acceptable to the woman in light of her cultural beliefs.

Key Facts to Remember: Providing Effective Prenatal Care to Families of Different Cultures summarizes the key actions a nurse can take to become more culturally aware.

# Chapter Review

## CHAPTER HIGHLIGHTS

- Virtually all systems of a woman's body are altered in some way during pregnancy.
- Blood pressure decreases slightly during pregnancy. It reaches its lowest point in the second trimester and gradually increases to near normal levels in the third trimester.
- The enlarging uterus may cause pressure on the vena cava when the woman lies supine, causing supine hyotensive syndrome.

- A physiologic anemia may occur during pregnancy because the total plasma volume increases more than the total number of erythrocytes. This difference produces a drop in the hematocrit.
- The glomerular filtration rate increases somewhat during pregnancy. Glycosuria may be caused by the body's inability to reabsorb all the glucose filtered by the glomeruli.
- Changes in the skin include the development of chloasma; linea nigra; darkened nipples, areola, and vulva; striae; and spider nevi.
- Insulin needs increase during pregnancy. A woman with a latent deficiency state may respond to the increased stress on the islets of Langerhans by developing gestational diabetes.
- The subjective (presumptive) signs of pregnancy are symptoms experienced and reported by the woman, such as amenorrhea, nausea and vomiting, fatigue, urinary frequency, breast changes, and quickening.
- The objective (probable) signs of pregnancy can be perceived by the examiner but may be caused by conditions other than pregnancy.
- The diagnostic (positive) signs of pregnancy can be perceived by the examiner and can be caused only by pregnancy.
- During pregnancy, the expectant mother may experience ambivalence, acceptance, introversion, emotional lability, and changes in body image.
- Rubin (1984) has identified four developmental tasks for the pregnant woman: (1) ensuring safe passage through pregnancy, labor, and birth; (2) seeking acceptance of this child by others; (3) seeking commitment and acceptance of herself as mother to the infant; and (4) learning to give of oneself on behalf of one's child.
- The father faces a series of adjustments as he accepts his new role. The father must deal with the reality of pregnancy, gain recognition as a parent, and confront and resolve any personal conflicts about the fathering he himself received.
- Siblings of all ages require assistance in dealing with the birth of a new baby.
- Cultural values, beliefs, and behaviors influence a family's response to childbearing and the health care system.
- Ethnocentrism is the belief that one's own cultural beliefs, values, and practices are the best ones—indeed, the only ones worth considering. To combat ethnocentrism, health care providers need to develop cultural competency.
- A cultural assessment does not have to be exhaustive, but it should focus on factors that will influence the practices of the childbearing family with regard to health needs.

## CHAPTER REFERENCES


American College of Obstetricians and Gynecologists. (1998). *Cultural competency in health care* (Opinion No. 201). Washington, DC: Author.

Beckman, C. R. B., & Dysart, D. (2000). The challenge of multicultural medical care. *Contemporary OB/GYN, 45*(12), 12–33.

Bodo, K., & Gibson, N. (1999a). Childbirth customs in Orthodox Jewish traditions. *Canadian Family Physician, 45,* 682–686.

Bodo, K., & Gibson, N. (1999b). Childbirth customs in Vietnamese traditions. *Canadian Family Physician, 45,* 690–697.

Buster, J. E., & Carson, S. A. (1996). Endocrinology and diagnosis of pregnancy. In S. G. Gabbe, J. R. Niebyl, & J. L. Simpson (Eds.), *Obstetrics: Normal and problem pregnancies* (3rd ed.). New York: Churchill-Livingstone.

Choudhry, U. K. (1997). Traditional practices of women from India: Pregnancy, childbirth, and newborn care. *Journal of Obstetric, Gynecologic, and Neonatal Nursing, 26*(5), 533–539.

Cline, C. R., Martin, D. P., & Deyo, R. A. (1998). Health consequences of pregnancy and childbirth as perceived by women and clinicians. *Obstetrics and Gynecology, 92*(5), 842–848.

Conley, L. J. (1990). Childbearing and childrearing practices in Mormonism. *Neonatal Network, 9*(3), 41–48.

Cruikshank, D. P., Wigton, T. R., & Hays, P. M. (1996). Maternal physiology in pregnancy. In S. G. Gabbe, J. R. Niebyl, & J. L. Simpson (Eds.), *Obstetrics: Normal and problem pregnancies* (3rd ed.). New York: Churchill-Livingstone.

Cunningham, F. G., MacDonald, P. C., Gant, N. F., Leveno, K. J., Gilstrap, L. C., III, Hankins, G. D. V., & Clark, S. L. (1997). *Williams obstetrics* (20th ed.). Stamford, CT: Appleton & Lange.

Diemer, G. A. (1997). Expectant fathers: Influence of perinatal education on stress, coping, and spousal relations. *Research in Nursing and Health, 20*(4), 281–293.

Jordan, P. L. (1990). Laboring for relevance: Expectant and new fatherhood. *Nursing Research, 39*(1), 11–16.

Kroelinger, C. D., & Oths, K. S. (2000). Partner support and pregnancy wantedness. *Birth, 27*(2), 112–119.

Lederman, R. P. (1996). *Psychosocial adaptation in pregnancy* (2nd ed.). New York: Springer.

Lederman, R., & Miller, D. S. (1998). Adaptations to pregnancy in three different ethnic groups: Latin-American, African-American, and Anglo-American. *Canadian Journal of Nursing Research, 30*(3), 37–51.

Mattson, S. (1995). Culturally sensitive perinatal care for Southeast Asians. *Journal of Obstetric, Gynecologic, and Neonatal Nursing, 24*(4), 335–341.

Mattson, S., & Smith, J. E. (2000). *Core curriculum for maternal-newborn nursing* (2nd ed.). Philadelphia: Saunders.

Mercer, R. T. (1995). *Becoming a mother.* New York: Springer.

Patterson, E. T., Freese, M. P., & Goldenberg, R. L. (1990). Seeking safe passage: Utilizing health care during pregnancy. *Image, 22*(1), 27–31.

Rubin, R. (1984). *Maternal identity and the maternal experience.* New York: Springer.

Small, M. F. (1998, November). Sleep with me: A trans-cultural look at the power and protection of sharing a bed. *Mothering,* pp. 62–64.

Sorenson, D. S., & Schuelke, P. (1999). Fantasies of the unborn among pregnant women. *Maternal-child nursing 24*(2), 92–97.

Stark, M. A. (1997). Psychosocial adjustment during pregnancy: The experience of mature gravidas. *Journal of Obstetric, Gynecologic, and Neonatal Nursing, 26*(2), 206–211.

Walker, L. O., Fleschler, R. G., & Heaman, M. (1998). Is a healthy lifestyle related to stress, parenting confidence, and health symptoms among new fathers? *Canadian Journal of Nursing Research, 30*(3), 21–36.

## CONTEMPORARY MATERNAL-NEWBORN NURSING ON-LINE

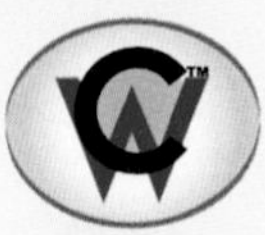

Additional interactive resources, including animations and video, for this chapter can be found on the Companion Website at http://www.prenhall.com/ladewig. Click on Chapter 7 and "Begin" to select the activities for this chapter.

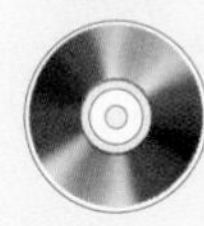

For NCLEX review questions and an audio glossary, access the accompanying CD-ROM in this book.

Chapter 8

# Antepartal Nursing Assessment

*When I work the prenatal clinic I constantly remind myself to look past stereotypes about people of different cultures and ethnic groups to see each woman and family as unique. It has helped me tremendously to do some reading about various cultural groups and their common practices—that way I don't make glaring mistakes during my initial contact with a family. However, I have found it most useful simply to ask people about their preferences in a respectful, accepting way. Almost always they tell me gladly because their childbearing experience is important to them and they sense that I am sincere.*

—A Nurse Working in a Large County Health Department

## KEY TERMS



## OBJECTIVES

- Summarize the essential components of a prenatal history.
- Define common obstetric terminology found in the history of maternity clients.
- Identify factors related to the father's health that are generally recorded on the prenatal record.
- Describe areas that should be evaluated as part of the initial assessment of psychosocial and cultural factors related to a woman's pregnancy.
- Describe the normal physiologic changes one would expect to find when performing a physical assessment of a pregnant woman.
- Compare the methods most commonly used to determine the estimated date of birth.
- Develop an outline of the essential measurements that can be determined by clinical pelvimetry.
- Delineate the possible causes of the danger signs of pregnancy.
- Relate the components of the subsequent prenatal history and assessment to the progress of pregnancy.

he registered nurse caring for a woman who is pregnant establishes an environment of comfort and open communication with each antepartal visit. The nurse conveys interest in the woman as an individual and discusses the woman's concerns and desires. This nurse can also complete many areas of prenatal assessment. Advanced practice nurses such as certified nurse-midwives (CNMs) and certified women's health nurse practitioners have the education and skill to perform full and complete antepartal assessments.

This chapter focuses on the prenatal assessments completed initially and at subsequent visits to provide optimum care for the childbearing family.

# Initial Client History

The course of a pregnancy depends on a number of factors, including the woman's prepregnancy health, presence of disease states, emotional status, and past health care. A thorough history is useful in determining the status of a woman's prepregnancy health.

## Definition of Terms

The following terms are used in recording the history of maternity clients:

**Gestation:** the number of weeks since the first day of the last menstrual period.
**Abortion:** birth that occurs before the end of 20 weeks' gestation.
**Term:** the normal duration of pregnancy (38 to 42 weeks' gestation).
**Antepartum:** time between conception and the onset of labor; usually used to describe the period during which a woman is pregnant; used interchangeably with *prenatal.*
**Intrapartum:** time from the onset of true labor until the birth of the infant and placenta.
**Postpartum:** time from birth until the woman's body returns to an essentially prepregnant condition.
**Preterm or premature labor:** labor that occurs after 20 weeks' but before completion of 37 weeks' gestation.
**Postterm labor:** labor that occurs after 42 weeks' gestation.
**Gravida:** any pregnancy, regardless of duration, including present pregnancy.
**Nulligravida:** a woman who has never been pregnant.
**Primigravida:** a woman who is pregnant for the first time.
**Multigravida:** a woman who is in her second or any subsequent pregnancy.
**Para:** birth after 20 weeks' gestation regardless of whether the infant is born alive or dead.
**Nullipara:** a woman who has had no births at more than 20 weeks' gestation.
**Primipara:** a woman who has had one birth at more than 20 weeks' gestation, regardless of whether the infant was born alive or dead.
**Multipara:** a woman who has had two or more births at more than 20 weeks' gestation.
**Stillbirth:** an infant born dead after 20 weeks' gestation.

The terms *gravida* and *para* are used in relation to pregnancies, not to the number of fetuses. Thus twins, triplets, and so forth count as *one* pregnancy and *one* birth.

The following examples illustrate how these terms are applied in clinical situations:

1. Jean Sanchez has one child born at 38 weeks' gestation and is pregnant for the second time. At her initial prenatal visit, the nurse indicates her obstetric history as "gravida 2 para 1 ab 0." Jean Sanchez's present pregnancy terminates at 16 weeks' gestation. She is now "gravida 2 para 1 ab 1."
2. Liz Buehl is pregnant for the fourth time. At home she has a child who was born at 35 weeks' gestation. One pregnancy ended at 10 weeks' gestation, and she gave birth to another infant stillborn at term. At her antepartal assessment the nurse records her obstetric history as "gravida 4 para 2 ab 1."

To provide more comprehensive data, a more detailed approach is used in some settings. Using the detailed system, *gravida* keeps the same meaning, but the meaning of *para* changes because the detailed system counts *each infant born* rather than the number of pregnancies carried to viability (Varney, 1997). Thus, for example, twins count as *one* pregnancy but *two* babies.

A useful acronym for remembering the system is TPAL:

**T:** number of *term* infants born—that is, the number of infants born after 37 weeks' gestation or more
**P:** number of *preterm* infants born—that is, the number of infants born after 20 weeks' but before the completion of 37 weeks' gestation
**A:** number of pregnancies ending in either spontaneous or therapeutic *abortion*
**L:** number of currently *living* children

Using this approach, the nurse would have initially described Jean Sanchez (see the first example) as "gravida 2 para 1001." Following Jean's spontaneous abortion she would be "gravida 2 para 1011." Liz Buehl would be described as "gravida 4 para 1111." (Figure 8–1♦ illustrates this method.)

| Name | Gravida | Term | Preterm | Abort | Living Child |
|---|---|---|---|---|---|
| Jean Sanchez | 2 | 1 | 0 | 0 | 1 |
| Liz Buehl | 4 | 1 | 1 | 1 | 1 |

FIGURE 8–1 ♦ The TPAL approach provides detailed information about the woman's pregnancy history.

## Critical Thinking in Practice

Karen Blade, a 23-year-old, GIPO, is 10 weeks pregnant when she sees the certified nurse-midwife (CNM) for her first prenatal exam. She has been experiencing some mild nausea and fatigue but otherwise is feeling well. She asks the CNM about continuing with her routine exercises (walking 3 miles a day and lifting light weights). She also asks about using the heated pool and a hot tub. What should she be told?

Answers can be found in Appendix I.

### Client Profile

The history is essentially a screening tool that identifies factors that may place the mother or fetus at risk during the pregnancy. The following information is obtained for each pregnant woman at the first prenatal assessment:

1. Current pregnancy
   - First day of last normal menstrual period (LMP)
   - Presence of cramping, bleeding, or spotting since LMP
   - Woman's opinion about the time when conception occurred and when infant is due
   - Woman's attitude toward pregnancy (Is this pregnancy planned? Wanted?)
   - Results of pregnancy tests, if completed
   - Any discomforts since LMP such as nausea, vomiting, urinary frequency, fatigue, or breast tenderness
2. Past pregnancies
   - Number of pregnancies
   - Number of abortions, spontaneous or induced
   - Number of living children
   - History of previous pregnancies, length of pregnancy, length of labor and birth, type of birth (vaginal, forceps or vacuum-assisted birth, or cesarean), type of anesthesia used ,(if any), woman's perception of the experience, and complications (antepartal, intrapartal, and postpartal)
   - Neonatal status of previous children: Apgar scores, birth weights, general development, complications, and feeding patterns
   - Loss of a child (miscarriage, elective or medically indicated abortion, stillbirth, neonatal death, relinquishment, or death after the neonatal period). What was the experience like for her? What coping skills helped? How did her partner, if involved, respond?
   - If Rh negative, was medication received after birth to prevent sensitization?
   - Prenatal education classes, and resources (books)
3. Gynecologic history
   - Date of last Pap smear; any history of abnormal Pap smear
   - Previous infections: vaginal, cervical, or sexually transmitted
   - Previous surgery
   - Age at menarche
   - Regularity, frequency, and duration of menstrual flow
   - History of dysmenorrhea
   - Sexual history
   - Contraceptive history (If birth control pills were used, did pregnancy occur immediately following cessation of pills? If not, how long after?)
4. Current medical history
   - Weight
   - Blood type and Rh factor, if known
   - General health including nutrition, normal dietary practices, and regular exercise program (type, frequency, and duration)
   - Any medications presently being taken (including nonprescription, homeopathic, or herbal medications) or taken since the onset of pregnancy
   - Previous or present use of alcohol, tobacco, or caffeine (Ask specifically about the amounts of alcohol, cigarettes, and caffeine [specify coffee, tea, colas, or chocolate] consumed each day.)
   - Illicit drug use or abuse (Ask about specific drugs such as cocaine, crack, and marijuana.)
   - Drug allergies and other allergies
   - Potential teratogenic insults to this pregnancy such as viral infections, medications, x-ray examinations, surgery, or cats in the home (possible source of toxoplasmosis)
   - Presence of disease conditions such as diabetes, hypertension, cardiovascular disease, renal problems, or thyroid disorder
   - Record of immunizations (especially rubella)
   - Presence of any abnormal symptoms
5. Past medical history
   - Childhood diseases
   - Past treatment for any disease condition (Any hospitalizations? History of hepatitis? Rheumatic fever? Pyelonephritis?)

- Surgical procedures
- Presence of bleeding disorders or tendencies (Has she received blood transfusions?)

6. Family medical history
   - Presence of diabetes, cardiovascular disease, cancer, hypertension, hematologic disorders, tuberculosis, or preeclampsia-eclampsia (pregnancy-induced hypertension [PIH])
   - Occurrence of multiple births
   - History of congenital diseases or deformities
   - Occurrence of cesarean births and cause, if known
7. Religious, spiritual, and cultural history
   - Does the woman wish to specify a religious preference on her chart? Does she have any religious beliefs or practices that might influence her health care or that of her child, such as prohibition against receiving blood products, dietary considerations, or circumcision rites?
   - What practices are important to maintain her spiritual well-being?
   - Might practices in her culture or that of her partner influence her care or that of her child?
8. Occupational history
   - Occupation
   - Physical demands (Does she stand all day, or are there opportunities to sit and elevate her legs? Any heavy lifting?)
   - Exposure to chemicals or other harmful substances
   - Opportunity for regular meals and breaks for nutritious snacks
   - Provision for maternity or family leave
9. Partner's history
   - Presence of genetic conditions or diseases
   - Age
   - Significant health problems
   - Previous or present alcohol intake, drug use, or tobacco use
   - Blood type and Rh factor
   - Occupation
   - Educational level; methods by which he learns best
   - Attitude toward the pregnancy
10. Personal information about the woman
    - Age
    - Educational level; methods by which she learns best
    - Race or ethnic group (to identify need for prenatal genetic screening and racially or ethnically related risk factors)
    - Housing; stability of living conditions
    - Economic level
    - Acceptance of pregnancy
    - Any history of emotional or physical deprivation or abuse of herself or children or any abuse in her current relationship (Ask specifically whether she has been hit, slapped, kicked, or hurt within the past year or since she has been pregnant. Ask whether she is afraid of her partner or anyone else. If yes, of whom is she afraid?)
    - History of emotional problems
    - Support systems
    - Personal preferences about the birth (expectations of both the woman and her partner, presence of others, and so on) (See Chapter 6.)
    - Plans for care of child following birth
    - Feeding preference for the baby (Breast or bottle?)

## Obtaining Data

A questionnaire is used in many instances to obtain information. The woman should complete the questionnaire in a quiet place with a minimum of distractions. The nurse can obtain further information in an interview, which allows the pregnant woman to clarify her responses to questions and gives the nurse and client the opportunity to begin developing rapport.

The expectant father can be encouraged to attend the prenatal examinations. He is often able to contribute to the history and may use the opportunity to ask questions or express concerns that are important to him.

## High-Risk Screening

**Risk factors** are any findings that suggest the pregnancy may have a negative outcome, for either the woman or her unborn child. Screening for risk factors is an important part of the prenatal assessment. Many risk factors can be identified during the initial assessment; others may be detected during subsequent prenatal visits. It is important to identify high-risk pregnancies early so that appropriate interventions can be started promptly. Not all risk factors threaten a pregnancy equally; thus many agencies use a scoring sheet to determine the degree of risk. Information must be updated throughout pregnancy as necessary. Any pregnancy may begin as low risk and change to high risk because of complications.

Table 8–1 identifies the major risk factors currently recognized. The table also identifies maternal and fetal or newborn implications if the risk is present in the pregnancy.

**TABLE 8–1 Prenatal High-Risk Factors**

| *Factor* | *Maternal Implications* | *Fetal or Neonatal Implications* |
|---|---|---|
| **SOCIAL AND PERSONAL** | | |
| Low income level and/or low educational level | Poor antenatal care<br>Poor nutrition<br>↑ risk of preeclampsia | Low birth weight<br>Intrauterine growth restriction (IUGR) |
| Poor diet | Inadequate nutrition<br>↑ risk anemia<br>↑ risk preecalmpsia | Fetal malnutrition<br>Prematurity |
| Living at high altitude | ↑ hemoglobin | Prematurity<br>IUGR<br>↑ hemoglobin (polycythemin) |
| Multiparity >3 | ↑ risk antepartum or postpartum hemorrhage | Anemia<br>Fetal death |
| Weight <45.5 kg (100 lb) | Poor nutrition<br>Cephalopelvic disproportion<br>Prolonged labor | IUGR<br>Hypoxia associated with difficult labor and birth |
| Weight >91 kg (200 lb) | ↑ risk hypertension<br>↑ risk cephalopelvic disproportion<br>↑ risk diabetes | ↓ fetal nutrition<br>↑ risk macrosomia |
| Age < 16 | Poor nutrition<br>Poor antenatal care<br>↑ risk preeclampsia<br>↑ risk cephalopelvic disproportion | Low birth weight<br>↑ fetal demise |
| Age > 35 | ↑ risk preeclampsia<br>↑ risk cesarean birth | ↑ risk congenital anomalies<br>↑ chromosomal aberrations |
| Smoking one pack/day or more | ↑ risk hypertension<br>↑ risk cancer | ↓ placental perfusion →↓ $O_2$ and nutrients available<br>Low birth weight<br>IUGR<br>Preterm birth |
| Use of addicting drugs | ↑ risk poor nutrition<br>↑ risk of infection with IV drugs<br>↑ risk HIV, hepatitis C | ↑ risk congenital anomalies<br>↑ risk low birth weight<br>Neonatal withdrawal<br>Lower serum bilirubin |
| Excessive alcohol consumption | ↑ risk poor nutrition<br>Possible hepatic effects with long-term consumption | ↑ risk fetal alcohol syndrome |
| **PREEXISTING MEDICAL DISORDERS** | | |
| Diabetes mellitus | ↑ risk preeclampsia, hypertension<br>Episodes of hypoglycemia and hyperglycemia<br>↑ risk cesarean birth | Low birth weight<br>Macrosomia<br>Neonatal hypoglycemia<br>↑ risk congenital anomalies<br>↑ risk respiratory distress syndrome |
| Cardiac disease | Cardiac decompensation<br>Further strain on mother's body<br>↑ maternal death rate | ↑ risk fetal demise<br>↑ prenatal mortality |
| Anemia: hemoglobin <9 g/dL (white)<br><29% hematocrit (white)<br><8.2 g/dL hemoglobin (black)<br><26% hematocrit (black) | Iron-deficiency anemia<br>Low energy level<br>Decreased oxygen-carrying capacity | Fetal death<br>Prematurity<br>Low birth weight |
| Hypertension | ↑ vasospasm<br>↑ risk central nervous system irritability<br>→ convulsions<br>↑ risk cerebrovascular accident<br>↑ risk renal damage | ↓ placental perfusion<br>→ low birth weight<br>Preterm birth |

TABLE 8–1 Prenatal High-Risk Factors *continued*

| *Factor* | *Maternal Implications* | *Fetal or Neonatal Implications* |
|---|---|---|
| **PREEXISTING MEDICAL DISORDERS** ***continued*** | | |
| Thyroid disorder | ↑ infertility | ↑ spontaneous abortion |
| Hypothyroidism | ↓ basal metabolic rate, goiter, myxedema | ↑ risk congenital goiter |
| Hyperthyroidism | ↑ risk postpartum hemorrhage<br>↑ risk preeclampsia<br>Danger of thyroid storm | Mental retardation → cretinism<br>↑ incidence congenital anamolies<br>↑ incidence preterm birth<br>↑ tendency to thyrotoxicosis |
| Renal disease (moderate to severe) | ↑ risk renal failure | ↑ risk IUGR<br>↑ risk preterm birth |
| Diethylstilbestrol (DES) exposure | ↑ infertility, spontaneous abortion<br>↑ cervical incompetence | ↑ spontaneous abortion<br>↑ risk preterm birth |
| **OBSTETRIC CONSIDERATIONS** | | |
| *Previous Pregnancy* | | |
| Stillborn | ↑ emotional or psychologic distress | ↑ risk IUGR<br>↑ risk preterm birth |
| Habitual abortion | ↑ emotional or psychologic distress<br>↑ possibility diagnostic workup | ↑ risk abortion |
| Cesarean birth | ↑ possibility repeat cesarean birth | ↑ risk preterm birth<br>↑ risk respiratory distress |
| Rh or blood group sensitization | ↑ financial expenditure for testing | Hydrops fetalis<br>Icterus gravis<br>Neonatal anemia<br>Kernicterus<br>Hypoglycemia |
| Large baby | ↑ risk cesarean birth<br>↑ risk gestational diabetes | Birth injury<br>Hypoglycemia |
| *Current Pregnancy* | | |
| Rubella (first trimester) | | Congenital heart disease<br>Cataracts<br>Nerve deafness<br>Bone lesions<br>Prolonged virus shedding |
| Rubella (second trimester) | | Hepatitis<br>Thrombocytopenia |
| Cytomegalovirus | | IUGR<br>Encephalopathy |
| Herpesvirus type 2 | Severe discomfort<br>Concern about possibility of cesarean birth, fetal infection | Neonatal herpesvirus type 2<br>2% hepatitis with jaundice<br>Neurologic abnormalities |
| Syphilis | ↑ incidence abortion | ↑ fetal demise<br>Congenital syphilis |
| Abruptio placenta and placenta previa | ↑ risk hemorrhage<br>Bed rest<br>Extended hospitalization | Fetal or neonatal anemia<br>Intrauterine hemorrhage<br>↑ fetal demise |
| Preeclampsia or eclampsia (pregnancy-induced hypertension) | See hypertension | ↓ placental perfusion<br>→ low birth weight |
| Multiple gestation | ↑ risk postpartum hemorrhage<br>↑ risk preterm labor | ↑ risk preterm birth<br>↑ risk fetal demise |
| Elevated hematocrit<br>>41% (white)<br>>38% (black) | Increased viscosity of blood | Fetal death rate 5 times normal rate |
| Spontaneous premature rupture of membranes | ↑ uterine infection | ↑ risk preterm birth<br>↑ fetal demise |

## Initial Prenatal Assessment

The prenatal assessment focuses on the woman holistically by considering physical, cultural, and psychosocial factors that influence her health. At the initial visit the woman may be concerned primarily with the diagnosis of pregnancy. However, during this visit she and her primary support person are also evaluating the health team she has chosen. The establishment of the nurse-client relationship will help the woman evaluate the health team and also provide the nurse with a basis for developing an atmosphere that is conducive to interviewing, support, and education. Because many women are excited and anxious at the first antepartal visit, the initial psychosocial-cultural assessment is general.

As part of the initial psychosocial-cultural assessment, the nurse discusses with the woman any religious or spiritual, cultural, or socioeconomic factors that influence the woman's expectations of the childbearing experience. It is especially helpful if the nurse is familiar with common practices of the members of various religious and cultural groups who reside in the community. Gathering these data in a tactful, caring way can help make the childbearing woman's experience a positive one.

After obtaining the history, the nurse prepares the woman for the physical examination. The physical examination begins with assessment of vital signs; then the woman's body is examined. The pelvic examination is performed last.

Before the examination, the woman should provide a clean urine specimen. When her bladder is empty, the woman is more comfortable during the pelvic examination and the examiner can palpate the pelvic organs more easily. After emptying her bladder, the nurse asks the woman to disrobe and gives her a gown and sheet or some other protective covering.

Increasing numbers of nurses, such as CNMs and other nurses in advanced practice, are prepared to perform complete physical examinations. The nurse who has not yet fully developed advanced assessment skills assesses the woman's vital signs, explains the procedures to allay apprehension, positions her for examination, and assists the examiner as necessary. Each nurse is responsible for operating at the expected standard for someone with that individual nurse's skill and knowledge base.

Thoroughness and a systematic procedure are the most important considerations when performing the physical portion of an antepartal examination (see Assessment Guide: Initial Prenatal Assessment, starting on page 179). To promote completeness, the Assessment Guide: Initial Prenatal Assessment is organized in three columns that address the areas to be assessed (and normal findings), the variations or alterations that may be observed, and nursing responses to the data. The nurse should be aware that certain organs and systems are assessed concurrently with others during the physical portion of the examination.

Nursing interventions based on assessment of the normal physical and psychosocial changes of pregnancy, evaluation of the cultural influences associated with pregnancy, and client teaching and counseling needs that have been mutually defined are discussed further in Chapter 9.

### HINTS FOR PRACTICE

In a clinic or office setting, gowns and goggles for the health care provider are usually not necessary because splashing of body fluids is unlikely. Gloves are worn for procedures that involve contact with body fluids such as drawing blood for lab work, handling urine specimens, and conducting pelvic examinations.

### Determination of Due Date

Childbearing families generally want to know the "due date," or the date around which childbirth will occur. Historically the due date has been called the *estimated date of confinement (EDC).* The concept of confinement is, however, rather negative, and there is a trend in the literature to avoid it by referring to the due date as the EDD or estimated date of delivery. Childbirth educators often stress that babies are not "delivered" like a package; they are *born.* In keeping with a view that emphasizes the normalcy of the process, this text refers to the due date as the **estimated date of birth (EDB).**

To calculate the EDB it is helpful to know the date of the LMP. However, some women have episodes of irregular bleeding or fail to keep track of menstrual cycles. Thus other techniques also help to determine how far along a woman is in her pregnancy—that is, at how many weeks' gestation she is. Techniques that can be used include evaluating uterine size, determining when quickening occurs, and auscultating fetal heart rate with a Doppler device or ultrasound and later a fetoscope.

#### Nägele's Rule

The most common method of determining the EDB is **Nägele's rule.** To use this method, one begins with the first day of the last menstrual period, subtracts 3 months, and adds 7 days. For example,

| | | |
|---|---|---|
| First day of LMP | | November 21 |
| Subtract 3 months | − | 3 months |
| | | August 21 |
| Add 7 days | + | 7 days |
| EDB | | August 28 |

Text continues on page 187.

## ASSESSMENT GUIDE: INITIAL PRENATAL ASSESSMENT

| Physical Assessment/ Normal Findings | Alterations and Possible Causes* | Nursing Responses to Data† |
|---|---|---|
| **Vital Signs** | | |
| *Blood pressure (BP):* 90–140/60–90 mm Hg | High BP (essential hypertension; renal disease; pregestational hypertension; apprehension or anxiety associated with pregnancy diagnosis, exam, or other crises; PIH if initial assessment not done until after 20 weeks' gestation) | BP > 140/90 requires immediate consideration; establish woman's BP; refer to physician if necessary. Assess woman's knowledge about high BP; counsel on self-care and medical management. |
| *Pulse:* 60–90 beats/min; rate may increase 10 beats/min during pregnancy | Increased pulse rate (excitement or anxiety, cardiac disorders) | Count for 1 full minute; note irregularities. |
| *Respiration:* 16–24 breaths/min (or pulse rate divided by four); pregnancy may induce a degree of hyperventilation; thoracic breathing predominant | Marked tachypnea or abnormal patterns | Assess for respiratory disease. |
| *Temperature:* 36.2–37.6°C (98–99.6°F) | Elevated temperature (infection) | Assess for infection process or disease state if temperature is elevated; refer to physician or CNM. |
| **Weight** | | |
| Depends on body build | Weight < 45 kg (100 lb) or > 91 kg (200 lb); rapid, sudden weight gain (PIH) | Evaluate need for nutritional counseling; obtain information on eating habits, cooking practices, foods regularly eaten, income limitations, need for food supplements, pica and other abnormal food habits. Note initial weight to establish baseline for weight gain throughout pregnancy. |
| **Skin** | | |
| *Color:* Consistent with racial background; pink nail beds | Pallor (anemia); bronze, yellow (hepatic disease; other causes of jaundice) | The following tests should be performed: complete blood count (CBC), bilirubin level, urinalysis, and blood urea nitrogen (BUN). |
| | Bluish, reddish, mottled; dusky appearance or pallor of palms and nail beds in dark-skinned women (anemia) | If abnormal, refer to physician. |
| *Condition:* Absence of edema (slight edema of lower extremities is normal during pregnancy) | Edema (PIH); rashes, dermatitis (allergic response) | Counsel on relief measures for slight edema. Initiate PIH assessment; refer to physician. |
| *Lesions:* Absence of lesions | Ulceration (varicose veins, decreased circulation) | Further assess circulatory status; refer to physician if lesion is severe. |
| Spider nevi common in pregnancy | Petechiae, multiple bruises, ecchymosis (hemorrhagic disorders; abuse) | Evaluate for bleeding or clotting disorder. Provide opportunities to discuss abuse if suspected. |
| Moles | Change in size or color (carcinoma) | Refer to physician. |
| *Pigmentation:* Pigmentation changes of pregnancy include linea nigra, striae gravidarum, chloasma | | Assure woman that these are normal manifestations of pregnancy and explain the physiologic basis for the changes. |
| Café-au-lait spots | Six or more (Albright's syndrome or neurofibromatosis) | Consult with physician. |

***Possible causes of alterations were placed in parentheses.**

**†This column provides guidelines for further assessment and initial nursing intervention.**

## INITIAL PRENATAL ASSESSMENT *continued*

| Physical Assessment/ Normal Findings | Alterations and Possible Causes* | Nursing Responses to Data† |
|---|---|---|
| **Nose** | | |
| *Character of mucosa:* Redder than oral mucosa; in pregnancy nasal mucosa is edematous in response to increased estrogen, resulting in nasal stuffiness (rhinitis of pregnancy) and nosebleeds | Olfactory loss (first cranial nerve deficit) | Counsel woman about possible relief measures for nasal stuffiness and nosebleeds (epistaxis); refer to physician for olfactory loss. |
| **Mouth** | | |
| May note hypertrophy of gingival tissue because of estrogen | Edema, inflammation (infection); pale in color (anemia) | Assess hematocrit for anemia; counsel regarding dental hygiene habits. Refer to physician or dentist if necessary. Routine dental care appropriate during pregnancy (no x-ray studies, no nitrous anesthesia). |
| **Neck** | | |
| *Nodes:* Small, mobile, nontender nodes | Tender, hard, fixed, or prominent nodes (infection, carcinoma) | Examine for local infection; refer to physician. |
| *Thyroid:* Small, smooth, lateral lobes palpable on either side of trachea; slight hyperplasia by third month of pregnancy | Enlargement or nodule tenderness (hyperthyroidism) | Listen over thyroid for bruits, which may indicate hyperthyroidism. Question woman about dietary habits (iodine intake). Ascertain history of thyroid problems; refer to physician. |
| **Chest and Lungs** | | |
| *Chest:* Symmetric, elliptical, smaller anteroposterior (A-P) than transverse diameter | Increased A-P diameter, funnel chest, pigeon chest (emphysema, asthma, chronic obstructive pulmonary disease [COPD]) | Evaluate for emphysema, asthma, pulmonary disease (COPD). |
| *Ribs:* Slope downward from nipple line | More horizontal (COPD)<br>Angular bumps<br>Rachitic rosary (vitamin C deficiency) | Evaluate for COPD. Evaluate for fractures.<br>Consult physician.<br>Consult nutritionist. |
| *Inspection and palpation:* No retraction or bulging of intercostal spaces (ICS) during inspiration or expiration; symmetrical expansion | ICS retractions with inspiration, bulging with expiration; unequal expansion (respiratory disease) | Do thorough initial assessment. Refer to physician. |
| Tactile fremitus | Tachypnea, hyperpnea, Cheyne-Stokes respirations (respiratory disease) | Refer to physician. |
| *Percussion:* Bilateral symmetry in tone | Flatness of percussion, which may be affected by chest wall thickness | Evaluate for pleural effusions; consolidations, or tumor. |
| Low-pitched resonance of moderate intensity | High diaphragm (atelectasis or paralysis), pleural effusion | Refer to physician. |
| *Auscultation:* Upper lobes—bronchovesicular sounds above sternum and scapulas; equal expiratory and inspiratory phases | Abnormal if heard over any other area of chest | Refer to physician. |
| *Remainder of chest:* vesicular breath sounds heard; inspiratory phase longer (3:1) | Rales, rhonchi, wheezes; pleural friction rub; absence of breath sounds; bronchophony, egophony, whispered pectoriloquy | Refer to physician. |

***Possible causes of alterations are placed in parentheses.**

**†This column provides guidelines for further assessment and initial nursing intervention.**

## INITIAL PRENATAL ASSESSMENT *continued*

| Physical Assessment/ Normal Findings | Alterations and Possible Causes* | Nursing Responses to Data† |
|---|---|---|
| **Breasts** | | |
| Supple; symmetrical in size and contour; darker pigmentation of nipple and areola; may have supernumerary nipples, usually 5–6 cm below normal nipple line | "Pigskin" or orange-peel appearance, nipple retractions, swelling, hardness (carcinoma); redness, heat, tenderness, cracked or fissured nipple (infection) | Encourage monthly self-examination; instruct woman how to examine own breasts. |
| Axillary nodes unpalpable or pellet sized | Tenderness, enlargement, hard node (carcinoma); may be visible bump (infection) | Refer to physician if evidence of inflammation. |
| *Pregnancy changes:*<br>**1.** Size increase noted primarily in first 20 weeks.<br>**2.** Become nodular.<br>**3.** Tingling sensation may be felt during first and third trimester; woman may report feeling of heaviness.<br>**4.** Pigmentation of nipples and areolas darkens.<br>**5.** Superficial veins dilate and become more prominent.<br>**6.** Striae seen in multiparas.<br>**7.** Tubercles of Montgomery enlarge.<br>**8.** Colostrum may be present after 12th week.<br>**9.** Secondary areola appears at 20 weeks, characterized by series of washed-out spots surrounding primary areola.<br>**10.** Breasts less firm, old striae may be present in multiparas. | | Discuss normalcy of changes and their meaning with the woman. Teach and/or institute appropriate relief measures. Encourage use of supportive, well-fitting brassiere. |
| **Heart** | | |
| Normal rate, rhythm, and heart sounds<br>*Pregnancy changes:*<br>**1.** Palpitations may occur due to sympathetic nervous system disturbance.<br>**2.** Short systolic murmurs that increase in held expiration are normal due to increased volume. | Enlargement, thrills, thrusts, gross irregularity or skipped beats, gallop rhythm or extra sounds (cardiac disease) | Complete an initial assessment. Explain normalcy of pregnancy-induced changes. Refer to physician if indicated. |
| **Abdomen** | | |
| Normal appearance, skin texture, and hair distribution; liver nonpalpable; abdomen nontender<br>*Pregnancy changes:*<br>**1.** Purple striae may be present (or silver striae on a multipara) as well as linea nigra.<br>**2.** Diastasis of the rectus muscles late in pregnancy. | Muscle guarding (anxiety, acute tenderness); tenderness, mass (ectopic pregnancy, inflammation, carcinoma) | Assure client of normalcy of diastasis. Provide initial information about appropriate prenatal and postpartum exercises. Evaluate client anxiety level. Refer to physician if indicated. |

***Possible causes of alterations are placed in parentheses.**

**†This column provides guidelines for further assessment and initial nursing intervention.**

# INITIAL PRENATAL ASSESSMENT *continued*

| Physical Assessment/ Normal Findings | Alterations and Possible Causes* | Nursing Responses to Data† |
|---|---|---|
| **Abdomen** *continued* | | |
| 3. Size: Flat or rotund abdomen; progressive enlargement of uterus due to pregnancy.<br>10–12 weeks: Fundus slightly above symphysis pubis.<br>16 weeks: Fundus halfway between symphysis and umbilicus.<br>20–22 weeks: Fundus at umbilicus.<br>28 weeks: Fundus three finger breadths above umbilicus.<br>36 weeks: Fundus just below ensiform cartilage. | Size of uterus inconsistent with length of gestation (intrauterine growth restriction [IUGR], multiple pregnancy, fetal demise, hydatidiform mole) | Reassess menstrual history regarding pregnancy dating. Evaluate increase in size using McDonald's method. Use ultrasound to establish diagnosis. |
| 4. Fetal heartbeats: 120–160 beats/min may be heard with Doppler at 10–12 weeks' gestation; may be heard with fetoscope at 17–20 weeks. | Failure to hear fetal heartbeat with Doppler (fetal demise, hydatidiform mole) | Refer to physician. Administer pregnancy tests. Use ultrasound to establish diagnosis. |
| 5. Fetal movement palpable by a trained examiner after the 18th week. | Failure to feel fetal movements after 20 weeks' gestation (fetal demise, hydatidiform mole) | Refer to physician for evaluation of fetal status. |
| 6. Ballottement: During fourth to fifth month fetus rises and then rebounds to original position when uterus is tapped sharply. | No ballottement (oligohydramnios) | Refer to physician for evaluation of fetal status. |
| **Extremities** | | |
| Skin warm, pulses palpable, full range of motion; may be some edema of hands and ankles in late pregnancy; varicose veins may become more pronounced; palmar erythema may be present | Unpalpable or diminished pulses (arterial insufficiency); marked edema (PIH) | Evaluate for other symptoms of heart disease; initiate follow-up if woman mentions that her rings feel tight. Discuss prevention and self-treatment measures for varicose veins; refer to physician if indicated. |
| **Spine** | | |
| *Normal spinal curves:* Concave cervical, convex thoracic, concave lumbar | Abnormal spinal curves; flatness, kyphosis, lordosis | Refer to physician for assessment of cephalopelvic disproportion (CPD). |
| In pregnancy lumbar spinal curve may be accentuated | Backache | May have implications for administration of spinal anesthetics; see Chapter 9 for relief measures. |
| Shoulders and iliac crests should be even | Uneven shoulders and iliac crests (scoliosis) | Refer very young women to a physician; discuss back-stretching exercises with older women. |
| **Reflexes** | | |
| Normal and symmetrical | Hyperactivity, clonus (PIH) | Evaluate for other symptoms of PIH. |
| **Pelvic Area** | | |
| *External female genitals:* Normally formed with female hair distribution; in multiparas, labia majora loose and pigmented; urinary and vaginal orifices visible and appropriately located | Lesions, hematomas, varicosities, inflammation of Bartholin's glands; clitoral hypertrophy (masculinization) | Explain pelvic examination procedure (Procedure 4–1). Encourage woman to minimize her discomfort by relaxing her hips. Provide privacy. |

***Possible causes of alterations are placed in parentheses.**

**†This column provides guidelines for further assessment and initial nursing intervention.**

## INITIAL PRENATAL ASSESSMENT *continued*

| Physical Assessment/ Normal Findings | Alterations and Possible Causes* | Nursing Responses to Data† |
|---|---|---|
| **Pelvic Area *continued*** | | |
| *Vagina:* Pink or dark pink; vaginal discharge odorless, nonirritating; in multiparas, vaginal folds smooth and flattened; may have episiotomy scar | Abnormal discharge associated with vaginal infections | Obtain vaginal smear. Provide understandable verbal and written instructions about treatment for woman and partner, if indicated. |
| *Cervix:* Pink color; os closed except in multiparas, in whom os admits fingertip | Eversion, reddish erosion, nabothian or retention cysts, cervical polyp; granular area that bleeds (carcinoma of cervix); lesions (herpes, human papillomavirus [HPV]) Presence of string or plastic tip from cervix (intrauterine device [IUD] in uterus) | Provide woman with a hand mirror and identify genital structures for her; encourage her to view her cervix if she wishes. Refer to physician if indicated. Advise woman of potential serious risks of leaving an IUD in place during pregnancy; refer to physician for removal. |
| *Pregnancy changes:*<br>1–4 weeks' gestation: Enlargement in anteroposterior diameter<br>4–6 weeks' gestation: Softening of cervix (Goodell's sign), softening of isthmus of uterus (Hegar's sign); cervix takes on bluish coloring (Chadwick's sign)<br>8–12 weeks' gestation: Vagina and cervix appear bluish violet in color (Chadwick's sign) | Absence of Goodell's sign (inflammatory conditions, carcinoma) | Refer to physician. |
| *Uterus:* Pear shaped, mobile; smooth surface | Fixed (pelvic inflammatory disease [PID]); nodular surface (fibromas) | Refer to physician. |
| *Ovaries:* Small, walnut shaped, nontender (ovaries and fallopian tubes are located in the adnexal areas) | Pain on movement of cervix (PID); enlarged or nodular ovaries (cyst, tumor, tubal pregnancy, corpus luteum of pregnancy) | Evaluate adnexal areas; refer to physician. |
| **Pelvic Measurements** | | |
| *Internal measurements:*<br>**1.** Diagonal conjugate at least 11.5 cm (Figure 8–5) | Measurement below normal | Vaginal birth may not be possible if deviations are present. |
| **2.** Obstetric conjugate estimated by subtracting 1.5–2 cm from diagonal conjugate | Disproportion of pubic arch | |
| **3.** Inclination of sacrum | Abnormal curvature of sacrum | |
| **4.** Motility of coccyx; external intertuberosity diameter > 8 cm | Fixed or malposition of coccyx | |
| **Anus and Rectum** | | |
| No lumps, rashes, excoriation, tenderness; cervix may be felt through rectal wall | Hemorrhoids, rectal prolapse; nodular lesion (carcinoma) | Counsel about appropriate prevention and relief measures; refer to physician for further evaluation. |
| **Laboratory Evaluation** | | |
| *Hemoglobin:* 12–16 g/dL; women residing in areas of high altitude may have higher levels of hemoglobin | < 12 g/dL (anemia) | Note: Wear gloves when drawing blood. Hemoglobin < 12 g/dL requires nutritional counseling; < 11 g/dL requires iron supplementation. |

***Possible causes of alterations are placed in parentheses.**

**†This column provides guidelines for further assessment and initial nursing intervention.**

# INITIAL PRENATAL ASSESSMENT *continued*

| Physical Assessment/ Normal Findings | Alterations and Possible Causes* | Nursing Responses to Data† |
|---|---|---|
| **Laboratory Evaluation *continued*** | | |
| *ABO and Rh typing:* Normal distribution of blood types | Rh negative | If Rh negative, check for presence of anti-Rh antibodies. Check partner's blood type; if partner is Rh positive, discuss with woman the need for antibody titers during pregnancy, management during the intrapartal period, and possible candidacy for RhIgG. |
| *Complete blood count (CBC)* | | |
| *Hematocrit:* 38%–47% physiological anemia (pseudoanemia) may occur | Marked anemia or blood dyscrasias | Perform CBC and Schilling differential cell count. |
| *Red blood cells (RBC):* 4.2–5.4 million/μL | | |
| *White blood cells (WBC):* 5000–12,000/μL | Presence of infection; may be elevated in pregnancy and with labor | Evaluate for other signs of infection. |
| *Differential* | | |
| Neutrophils: 40%–60% | | |
| Bands: up to 5% | | |
| Eosinophils: 1%–3% | | |
| Basophils: up to 1% | | |
| Lymphocytes: 20%–40% | | |
| Monocytes: 4%–8% | | |
| *Syphilis tests:* Serological tests for syphilis (SIS), complement fixation test, veneral disease research laboratory (VDRL) test—nonreactive | Positive reaction STS—tests may have 25%–45% incidence of biological false-positive results; false results may occur in individuals who have acute viral or bacterial infections, hypersensitivity reactions, recent vaccinations, collagen disease, malaria, or tuberculosis | Positive results may be confirmed with the fluorescent treponemal antibody-absorption (FTA-ABS) tests; all tests for syphilis give positive results in the secondary stage of the disease; antibiotic tests may cause negative test results. |
| *Genorrhea culture:* Negative | Positive | Refer for treatment. |
| *Urinalysis (u/a):* Normal color, specific gravity; pH 4.6–8.0 | Abnormal color (porphyria, hemaglobinuria, bilirubinemia); alkaline urine (metabolic alkalemia, *Proteus* infection, old specimen) | Repeat u/a; refer to physician. |
| Negative for protein, red blood cells, white blood cells, casts | Positive findings (contaminated specimen, kidney disease) | Repeat u/a; refer to physician. |
| *Glucose:* Negative (small degree of glycosuria may occur in pregnancy) | Glycosuria (low renal threshold for glucose diabetes mellitus) | Assess blood glucose level; test urine for ketones. |
| *Rubella titer:* Hemagglutination-inhibition (HAI) test – 1:10 indicates woman is immune | HAI titer < 1:10 | Immunization will be given on postpartum or within 6 weeks after childbirth. Instruct woman whose titers are >1:10 to avoid children who have rubella. |
| *Hepatitis B screen* for hepatitis B surface antigen (HBsAg); negative | Positive | If negative, consider referral for hepatitis B vaccine. If positive, refer to physician. Infants born to women who test positive are given hepatitis B immune globulin soon after birth followed by first dose of hepatitis B vaccine. |

***Possible causes of alterations are placed in parentheses.**

**†This column provides guidelines for further assessment and initial nursing intervention.**

# INITIAL PRENATAL ASSESSMENT *continued*

| Physical Assessment/ Normal Findings | Alterations and Possible Causes* | Nursing Responses to Data† |
|---|---|---|
| **Laboratory Evaluation *continued*** | | |
| *HIV screen:* Offered to all women; encouraged for those at risk; negative | Positive | Refer to physician. |
| *Illicit drug screen:* Offered to all women; negative | Positive | Refer to physician. |
| *Sickle-cell screen for clients of African descent:* Negative | Positive; test results would include a description of cells | Refer to physician. |
| *Pap smear:* Negative | Test results that show atypical cells | Refer to physician. Discuss with the woman the meaning of the findings and the importance of follow-up. |

| Cultural Assessment | Variations to Consider* | Nursing Responses to Data† |
|---|---|---|
| Determine the woman's fluency in English. | Woman may be fluent in a language other than English. | Work with a knowledgeable translator to provide information and answer questions. |
| Ask the woman how she prefers to be addressed. | Some women prefer informality; others prefer to use titles. | Address the woman according to her preference. Maintain formality in introducing oneself if that seems preferred. |
| Determine customs and practices regarding prenatal care: | Practices are influenced by individual preference, cultural expectations, or religious beliefs. | Honor a woman's practices and provide for specific preferences unless they are contraindicated because of safety. |
| • Ask the woman if there are certain practices she expects to follow when she is pregnant. | Some women believe that they should perform certain acts related to sleep, activity, or clothing. | Have information printed in the language of different cultural groups that live in the area. |
| • Ask the woman if there are any activities she cannot do while she is pregnant. | Some women have restrictions or taboos they follow related to work, activity, sexual, environmental, or emotional factors. | |
| • Ask the woman whether there are certain foods she is expected to eat or avoid while she is pregnant. Determine whether she has lactose intolerance. | Foods are an important cultural factor. Some women may have certain foods they must eat or avoid; many women have lactose intolerance and have difficulty consuming sufficient calcium. | Respect the woman's food preferences, help her plan an adequate prenatal diet within the framework of her preferences, and refer to a dietitian if necessary. |
| • Ask the woman whether the gender of her caregiver is of concern. | Some women are comfortable only with a female caregiver. | Arrange for a female caregiver if it is the woman's preference. |
| • Ask the woman about the degree of involvement in her pregnancy that she expects or wants from her support person, mother, and other significant people. | A woman may not want her partner involved in the pregnancy. For some the role falls to the woman's mother or a female relative or friend. | Respect the woman's preferences about her partner or husband's involvement; avoid imposing personal values or expectations. |
| • Ask the woman about her sources of support and counseling during pregnancy | Some women seek advice from a family member, *curandera,* tribal healer, and so forth. | Respect and honor the woman's sources of support. |

***Possible causes of alterations are placed in parentheses.**

**†This column provides guidelines for further assessment and initial nursing intervention.**

# INITIAL PRENATAL ASSESSMENT *continued*

| Psychosocial Assessment | Variations to Consider* | Nursing Responses to Data† |
|---|---|---|
| **Psychologic Status** | | |
| Excitement and/or apprehension, ambivalence | Marked anxiety (fear of pregnancy diagnosis, fear of medical facility) | Establish lines of communication. Active listening is useful. Establish trusting relationship. Encourage woman to take active part in her care. |
| | Apathy; display of anger with pregnancy diagnosis | Establish communication and begin counseling. Use active listening techniques. |
| **Educational Needs** | | |
| May have questions about pregnancy or may need time to adjust to reality of pregnancy | | Establish educational, supporting environment that can be expanded throughout pregnancy. |
| **Support Systems** | | |
| Can identify at least two or three individuals with whom woman is emotionally intimate (partner, parent, sibling, friend) | Isolated (no telephone, unlisted number); cannot name a neighbor or friend whom she can call upon in an emergency; does not perceive parents as part of her support system | Institute support system through community groups. Help woman to develop trusting relationship with health care professionals. |
| **Family Functioning** | | |
| Emotionally supportive<br>Communications adequate<br>Mutually satisfying<br>Cohesiveness in times of trouble | Long-term problems or specific problems related to this pregnancy, potential stressors within the family, pessimistic attitudes, unilateral decision making, unrealistic expectations of this pregnancy or child | Help identify the problems and stressors, encourage communication, and discuss role changes and adaptations. |
| **Economic Status** | | |
| Source of income is stable and sufficient to meet basic needs of daily living and medical needs | Limited prenatal care; poor physical health; limited use of health care system; unstable economic status | Discuss available resources for health maintenance and the birth. Institute appropriate referral for meeting expanding family's needs—food stamps and so forth. |
| **Stability of Living Conditions** | | |
| Adequate, stable housing for expanding family's needs | Crowded living conditions; questionable supportive environment for newborn | Refer to appropriate community agency. Work with family on self-help ways to improve situation. |

***Possible causes of alterations are placed in parentheses.**

**†This column provides guidelines for further assessment and initial nursing intervention.**

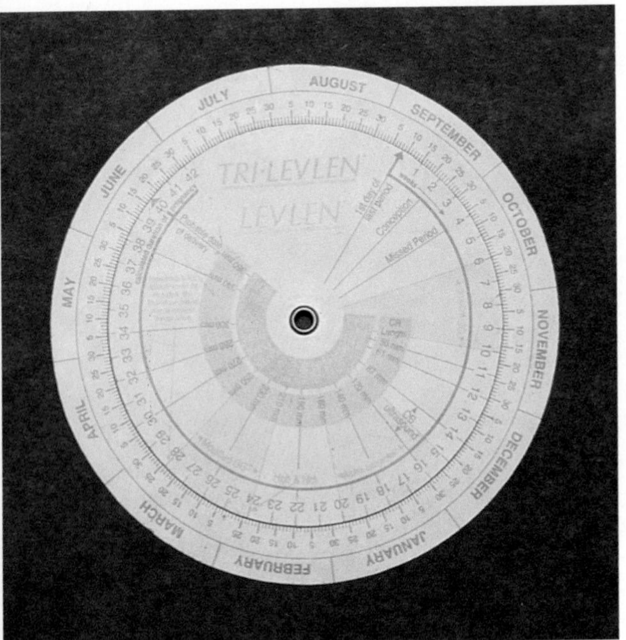

FIGURE 8–2 ♦ The EDB wheel can be used to calculate the due date. To use it, place the last menses began arrow on the date of the woman's LMP. Then read the EDB at the arrow labeled 40. In this case the LMP is September 8 and the EDB is June 17.

It is simpler to change the months to numeric terms:

| | | |
|---|---|---|
| November 21 becomes | | 11-21 |
| Subtract 3 months | − | 3 |
| | | 8-21 |
| Add 7 days | + | 7 |
| EDB | | August 28 |

A gestation calculator or wheel permits the caregiver to calculate the EDB even more quickly (Figure 8–2♦).

If a woman with a history of menses every 28 days remembers her LMP and was not taking oral contraceptives before becoming pregnant, Nägele's rule may be a fairly accurate determiner of the EDB. However, *ovulation usually occurs 14 days before the onset of the next menses, not 14 days after the previous menses.* Consequently, if her cycle is irregular, or 35 to 40 days long, the time of ovulation may be delayed by several days. If she has been using oral contraceptives, ovulation may be delayed several weeks following her last menses. Then, too, a postpartum woman who is breastfeeding may resume ovulating but be amenorrheic for a time, making calculation impossible. Thus Nägele's rule, although helpful, is not foolproof.

## Uterine Assessment

### Physical Examination

When a woman is examined in the first 10 to 12 weeks of her pregnancy and her uterine size is compatible with her menstrual history, uterine size may be the single most important clinical method for dating her pregnancy. In many cases, however, women do not seek maternity care until well into their second trimester, when it becomes much more difficult to evaluate specific uterine size. In obese women it is difficult to determine uterine size early in a pregnancy because the uterus is more difficult to palpate.

### HINTS FOR PRACTICE

When assessing blood pressure, have the pregnant woman sit up with her arm resting on a table so that her arm is at the level of her heart.

Expect a decrease in her blood pressure from baseline during the second trimester because of normal physiologic changes. If this decrease does not occur, evaluate further for signs of pregnancy-induced hypertension.

### Fundal Height

Fundal height may be used as an indicator of uterine size, although this method is less accurate late in pregnancy. A centimeter tape measure is used to measure the distance abdominally from the top of the symphysis pubis to the top of the uterine fundus (McDonald's method) (Figure 8–3♦). Fundal height in centimeters correlates well with weeks of gestation between 22 to 24 weeks and 34 weeks. Thus, at 26 weeks' gestation, fundal height is probably about 26 cm. If the woman is very tall or very short, fundal height will differ. To be most accurate, fundal height should be measured by the same examiner each time. The woman should have voided within ½ hour of the exam and should lie in the same position each time. In the third trimester, variations in fetal weight decrease the accuracy of fundal height measurements.

A lag in progression of measurements of fundal height from month to month and week to week may signal intrauterine growth restriction (IUGR). A sudden increase in fundal height may indicate twins or hydramnios (excessive amount of amniotic fluid).

## Fetal Development

### Quickening

Fetal movements felt by the mother, called *quickening,* may indicate that the fetus is nearing 20 weeks' gestation. However, quickening may be experienced between 16 and 22 weeks' gestation, so this method is not completely accurate.

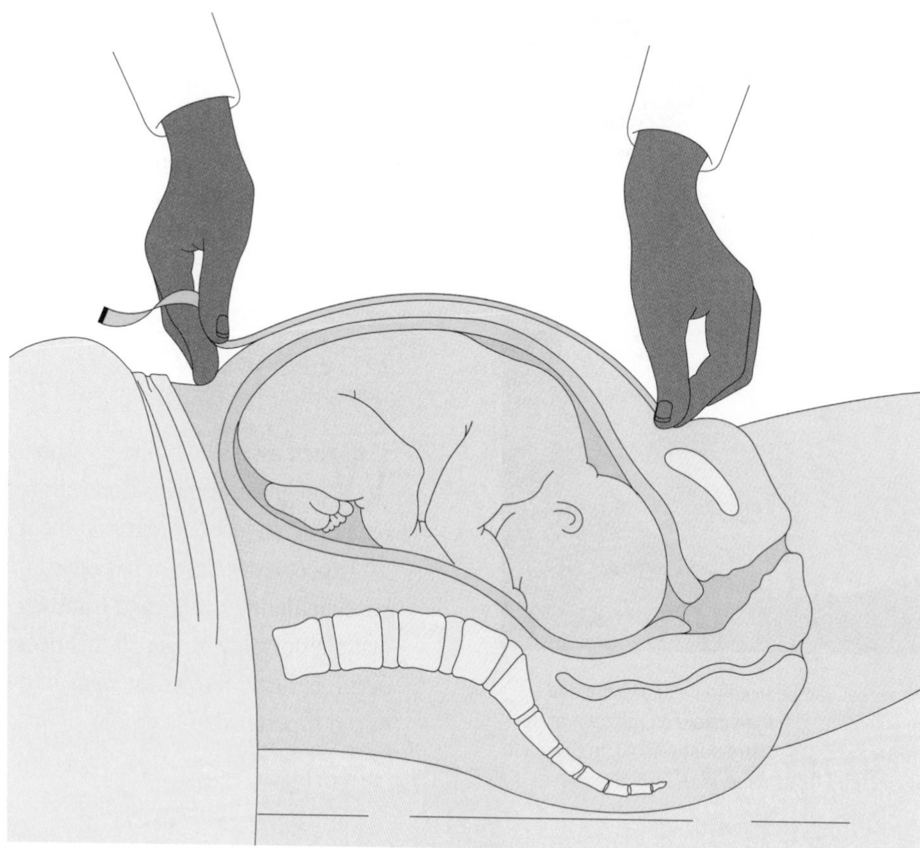

FIGURE 8–3 ♦ A cross-sectional view of fetal position when McDonald's method is used to assess fundal height.

### Fetal Heartbeat

The ultrasonic Doppler device (Figure 8–4♦) is the primary tool for assessing fetal heartbeat. It can detect fetal heartbeat, on average, at 8 to 12 weeks' gestation. If an ultrasonic Doppler is not available, a fetoscope may be used, although in current practice it is seldom necessary. The fetal heartbeat can be detected by fetoscope as early as week 16 and almost always by 19 or 20 weeks' gestation.

### Ultrasound

In the first trimester, ultrasound scanning can detect a gestational sac as early as 5 to 6 weeks after the LMP, fetal heart activity by 6 to 7 weeks, and fetal breathing movement by 10 to 11 weeks of pregnancy. Crown-to-rump measurements can be made to assess fetal age until the fetal head can be visualized clearly. Biparietal diameter (BPD) can then be used. BPD measurements can be made by approximately 12 to 13 weeks and are most accurate between 20 and 30 weeks, when rapid growth in the biparietal diameter occurs. (See Chapter 14 for discussion of fetal ultrasound scanning.)

## Assessment of Pelvic Adequacy (Clinical Pelvimetry)

The pelvis can be assessed vaginally to determine whether its size is adequate for a vaginal birth. This procedure, *clinical pelvimetry,* is performed by physicians or by advanced-

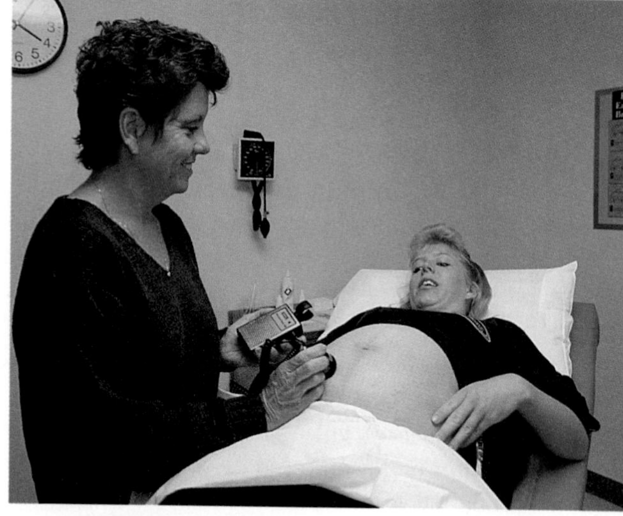

FIGURE 8–4 ♦ Listening to the fetal heartbeat with a Doppler device.

practice nurses such as certified nurse-midwives or nurse-practitioners. Some caregivers assess pelvic adequacy as part of the initial physical examination. Others wait until later in the pregnancy, when hormonal effects are greatest and it is possible to make some determination of fetal size. For a detailed description of clinical pelvimetry, readers are referred to a nurse-midwifery text. This section provides basic information about the assessment of the inlet and outlet (see Figures 8–5 and 8–6♦).

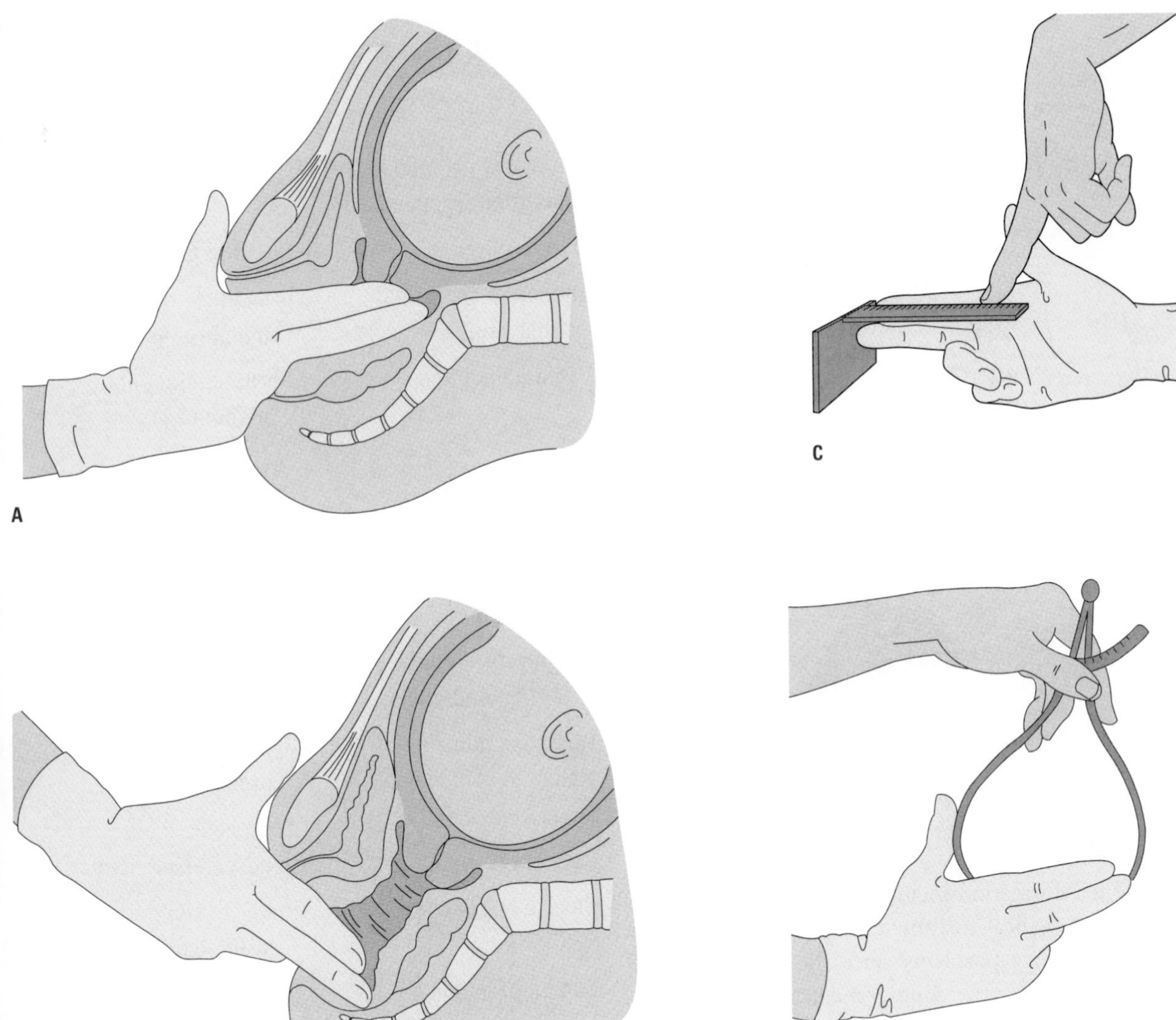


**FIGURE 8–5** ♦ Manual measurement of inlet and outlet. **A,** Estimation of the diagonal conjugate, which extends from the lower border of the symphysis pubis to the sacral promontory. **B,** Estimation of the anteroposterior diameter of the outlet, which extends from the lower border of the symphysis pubis to the tip of the sacrum. **C,** and **D,** Methods that may be used to check the manual estimation of anteroposterior measurements.

1. Pelvic inlet (Figure 8–5♦)
   - **Diagonal conjugate** (the distance from the lower posterior border of the symphysis pubis to the sacral promontory) at least 11.5 cm
   - **Obstetric conjugate** (a measurement approximately 1.5 cm smaller than the diagonal conjugate) 10 cm or more
2. Pelvic outlet (Figures 8–5 and 8–6♦)
   - Anteroposterior diameter, 9.5 to 11.5 cm
   - Transverse diameter (bi-ischial or intertuberous diameter), 8 to 10 cm

The pelvic cavity (midpelvis) cannot be accurately measured by clinical examination. Examiners estimate its adequacy. However, that discussion is also beyond the scope of this text.

## Subsequent Client History

At subsequent prenatal visits the nurse continues to gather data about the course of the pregnancy to date and the woman's responses to it. The nurse also asks about the adjustment of the support person and of other children, if any, in the family. As pregnancy progresses the nurse inquires about the preparations the family has made for the new baby.

The nurse asks specifically whether the woman has experienced any discomfort, especially the kinds of discomfort that are often seen at specific times during a pregnancy. The nurse inquires about physical changes that relate directly to the pregnancy, such as fetal movement. The nurse also asks about the danger signs of pregnancy (see Key Facts to Remember: Danger Signs in Pregnancy, on page 190).

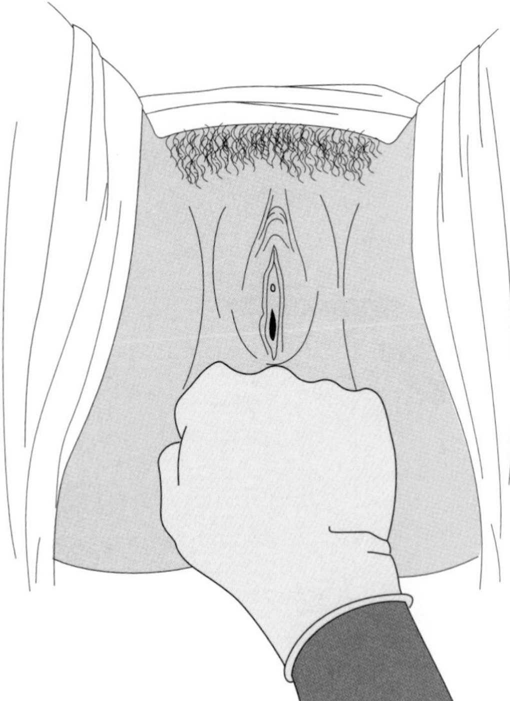

FIGURE 8–6 ♦ Use of a closed fist to measure the outlet. Most examiners know the distance between their first and last proximal knuckles. If they do not, they can use a measuring device.

Other pertinent information includes any exposure to contagious illnesses, medical treatment and therapy prescribed for nonpregnancy problems since the last visit, and any prescription or over-the-counter medications that were not prescribed as part of the woman's prenatal care.

Periodic prenatal examinations offer the nurse an opportunity to assess the childbearing woman's psychological needs and emotional status. If the woman's partner attends the antepartal visits, the nurse can also identify his needs and concerns. The interchange between the nurse and the woman or her partner will be facilitated if it takes place in a friendly, trusting environment. The woman should have sufficient time to ask questions and air concerns. If the nurse provides the time and demonstrates genuine interest, the woman will be more at ease bringing up questions that she may believe are silly or has been afraid to verbalize. The nurse who has an accurate understanding of all the changes of pregnancy is most able to answer questions and provide information. See the foldout color chart, "Maternal-Fetal Development," in the middle of the book for vivid illustrations of some of this information.

The nurse should also be sensitive to religious or spiritual, cultural, and socioeconomic factors that may influence a family's response to pregnancy, as well as to the woman's expectations of the health care system. The nurse can avoid stereotyping clients simply by asking each woman about her expectations for the antepartal period. Although many women's responses may reflect what are thought to be traditional norms, other women will have decidedly different views or expectations that represent a blending of beliefs or cultures.

During the antepartal period, it is essential to begin assessing the readiness of the woman and her partner (if possible) to assume their responsibilities as parents successfully. Table 8–2, on pages 191–192, identifies areas for assessment of parenting ability.

## KEY FACTS TO REMEMBER

### *Danger Signs in Pregnancy*

The woman should report the following danger signs in pregnancy immediately:

| Danger Sign | Possible Cause |
|---|---|
| Sudden gush of fluid from vagina | Premature rupture of membranes |
| Vaginal bleeding | Abruptio placentae, placenta previa<br>Lesions of cervix or vagina<br>"Bloody show" |
| Abdominal pain | Premature labor, abruptio placentae |
| Temperature above 38.3°C (101°F) and chills | Infection |
| Dizziness, blurring of vision, double vision, spots before eyes | Hypertension, preeclampsia |
| Persistent vomiting | Hyperemesis gravidarum |
| Severe headache | Hypertension, preeclampsia |
| Edema of hands, face, legs, and feet | Preeclampsia |
| Muscular irritability, convulsions | Preeclampsia, eclampsia |
| Epigastric pain | Preeclampsia, ischemia in major abdominal vessel |
| Oliguria | Renal impairment, decreased fluid intake |
| Dysuria | Urinary tract infection |
| Absence of fetal movement | Maternal medication, obesity, fetal death |

**TABLE 8–2 Guide to Prenatal Assessment of Parenting**

| *Areas Assessed* | *Sample Questions* |
|---|---|
| I. Perception of complexities of mothering<br>A. Desires baby for itself<br>Positive:<br>1. Feels positive about pregnancy<br>Negative:<br>1. Wants baby to meet own needs such as someone to love her, someone to get her out of unhappy home | 1. Did you plan on getting pregnant?<br>2. How do you feel about being pregnant?<br>3. Why do you want this baby? |
| B. Expresses concern about impact of mothering role on other roles (wife, career, school)<br>Positive:<br>1. Realistic expectations of how baby will affect job, career, school, and personal goals<br>2. Interested in learning about child care<br>Negative:<br>1. Feels pregnancy and baby will make no emotional, physical, or social demands on self<br>2. Has no insight that mothering role will affect other roles or lifestyle | 1. What do you think it will be like to take care of a baby?<br>2. How do you think you life will be different after you have your baby?<br>3. How do you feel this baby will affect your job, career, school, and personal goals?<br>4. How will the baby affect your relationships with your boyfriend or husband?<br>5. Have you done any reading, babysitting, or made any things for a baby? |
| C. Gives up routine habits because "not good for baby" (e.g., quits smoking, adjusts time schedule)<br>Positive:<br>1. Gives up routines not good for baby (quits smoking, adjusts eating habits) | |
| II. Attachment<br>A. Strong feelings regarding sex of baby. Why?<br>Positive:<br>1. Verbalizes positive thoughts about the baby<br>Negative:<br>1. Baby will be like negative aspects of self and partner | 1. Why do you prefer a certain sex? (Is reason inappropriate for a baby?)<br>2. Note comments client makes about baby not being normal and why client feels this way. |
| B. Interested in data regarding fetus (e.g., growth and development, heart tones)<br>Positive:<br>1. As above<br>Negative:<br>1. Shows no interest in fetal growth and development, quickening, and fetal heart tones<br>2. Expresses negative feelings about fetus by rejecting counseling regarding nutrition, rest, hygiene | |
| C. Fantasies about baby<br>Positive:<br>1. Follows cultural norms regarding preparation<br>2. Time of attachment behaviors appropriate to her history of pregnancy loss<br>Negative:<br>1. Bonding conditional depending on sex, age of baby, and/or labor and birth experience<br>2. Woman considers only own needs when making plans for baby<br>3. Exhibits no attachment behaviors after critical period of previous pregnancy<br>4. Failure to follow cultural norms regarding preparation | 1. What did you think or feel when you first felt the baby move?<br>2. Have you started preparing for the baby?<br>3. What do you think your baby will look like; what age do you see your baby?<br>4. How would you like your new baby to look? |

| TABLE 8–2 Guide to Prenatal Assessment of Parenting *continued* | |
|---|---|
| ***Areas Assessed*** | ***Sample Questions*** |
| III. Acceptance of child by significant others | |
| A. Acknowledges acceptance by significant other of the new responsibility inherent in child<br>Positive:<br>1. Acknowledges unconditional acceptance of pregnancy and baby by significant others<br>2. Partner accepts new responsibility inherent with child<br>3. Timely sharing of experience of pregnancy with significant others<br>Negative:<br>1. Significant others not supportively involved with pregnancy<br>2. Conditional acceptance of pregnancy depending on sex, race, age of baby<br>3. Decision making does not take in needs of fetus (eg, spends food money on new car)<br>4. Takes no/little responsibility for needs of pregnancy, woman/fetus | 1. How does your partner feel about this pregnancy?<br>2. How do your parents feel?<br>3. What do your friends think?<br>4. Does your partner have a preference regarding the baby's sex? Why?<br>5. How does your partner feel about being a father?<br>6. What do you think he'll be like as a father?<br>7. What do you think he'll do to help with child care?<br>8. Have you and your partner talked about how the baby might change your lives?<br>9. Who have you told about your pregnancy? |
| B. Concrete demonstration of acceptance of pregnancy/baby by significant others (eg, baby shower, significant other involved in prenatal education)<br>Positive:<br>1. Baby shower<br>2. Significant other attends prenatal class with client | 1. Note if partner attends clinic with client (degree of interest; eg, listens to heart tones). Significant other plans to be with client during labor and birth.<br>2. Is your partner contributing financially? |
| IV. Ensures physical well-being | |
| A. Concerns about having normal pregnancy, labor and birth, and baby<br>Positive:<br>1. Preparing for labor and birth, attends prenatal classes, interested in labor and birth<br>2. Aware of danger signs of pregnancy<br>3. Seeks and uses appropriate health care (eg, time of initial visit, keeps appointments, follows through on recommendations)<br>Negative:<br>1. Denies signs and symptoms that might suggest complications of pregnancy<br>2. Verbalizes extreme fear of labor and birth, refuses to talk about labor and birth<br>3. Fails appointments, fails to follow instructions, refuses to attend prenatal classes | 1. What have your heard about labor and birth?<br>2. Note data about client's reaction to prenatal class. |
| B. Family/client decisions reflect concern for health of mother and baby (eg, use of finances, time)<br>Positive:<br>1. As above | |

*Note:* When "Negative" is not listed in a section, the reader may assume that negative is the absence of positive responses.
*Source:* Modified and used with permission of the Minneapolis Health Department, Minneapolis, MN.

## ASSESSMENT GUIDE: SUBSEQUENT PRENATAL ASSESSMENT

| Physical Assessment/ Normal Findings | Alterations and Possible Causes* | Nursing Responses to Data† |
|---|---|---|
| **Vital Signs** | | |
| *Termperature:* 36.2–37.6°C (98–99.6°F) | Elevated temperature (infection) | Evaluate for signs of infection. Refer to physician. |
| *Pulse:* 60–90/min<br>Rate may increase 10 beats/min during pregnancy | Increased pulse rate (anxiety, cardiac disorders) | Note irregularities. Assess for signs of anxiety and stress. |
| *Respiration:* 16–24/min | Marked tachypnea or abnormal patterns (respiratory disease) | Refer to physician. |
| *Blood pressure:* 90–140/60–90 (falls in second trimester) | >140/90 or increase of 30 mm systolic and 15 mm diastolic (PIH) | Assess for edema, proteinuria, and hyperreflexia. Refer to physician. Schedule appointments more frequently. |
| **Weight Gain** | | |
| *First trimester:* 1.6–2.3 kg (3.5–5 lb)<br>*Second trimester:* 5.5–6.8 kg (12–15 lb)<br>*Third trimester:* 5.5–6.8 kg (12–15 lb) | Inadequate weight gain (poor nutrition, nausea, IUGR)<br>Excessive weight gain (excessive caloric intake, edema, PIH) | Discuss appropriate weight gain.<br>Provide nutritional counseling. Assess for presence of edema or anemia. |
| **Edema** | | |
| Small amount of dependent edema, especially in last weeks of pregnancy | Edema in hands, face, legs, and feet (PIH) | Identify any correlation between edema and activities, blood pressure, or proteinuria. Refer to physician if indicated. |
| **Uterine Size** | | |
| See Assessment Guide: Initial Prenatal Assessment for normal changes during pregnancy | Unusually rapid growth (multiple gestation, hydatidiform mole, hydramnios, miscalculation of EDB) | Evaluate fetal status. Determine height of fundus (page 187). Use diagnostic ultrasound. |
| **Fetal Heartbeat** | | |
| 120–160/min<br>Funic souffle | Absence of fetal heartbeat after 20 weeks' gestation (maternal obesity, fetal demise) | Evaluate fetal status. |
| **Laboratory Evaluation** | | |
| *Hemoglobin:* 12–16 g/dL<br>Pseudoanemia of pregnancy | <12 g/dL (anemia) | Provide nutritional counseling. Hemoglobin is repeated at 7 months' gestation. Women of Mediterranean heritage need a close check on hemoglobin because of possibility of thalassemia. |
| *Triple screen (also called multiple marker screening [MMS])* serum test done at 16-18 weeks' gestation. Evaluates three factors—maternal serum alpha fetoprotein (MSAFP), estriol, and hCG: normal levels | Elevated MSAFP (neural tube defect, underestimated gestational age, multiple gestation, Rh disease). Low level (trisomy 21 [Down syndrome], trisomy 18). Elevated hCG combined with lower than normal estriol and MSAFP (Down syndrome) (ACOG, 2000) | Refer to physician. |

***Possible causes of alterations are placed in parentheses.**

**†This column provides guidelines for further assessment and initial nursing intervention.**

## SUBSEQUENT PRENATAL ASSESSMENT *continued*

| Physical Assessment/ Normal Findings | Alterations and Possible Causes* | Nursing Responses to Data† |
|---|---|---|
| **Laboratory Evaluation *continued*** | | |
| *Indirect Coombs test* done on Rh− women: Negative (done at 28 weeks' gestation) | Rh antibodies present (maternal sensitization has occurred) | If Rh− and unsensitized, RhIgG prophylaxis given (see Chapter 16). If Rh antibodies present, RhIgG *not* given; fetus monitored closely for isoimmune hemolytic disease. |
| *50-g 1-hour glucose screen* (done between 24 and 28 weeks' gestation) | Plasma glucose level > 140 mg/dL (gestational diabetes mellitus [GDM])<br>*Note:* Some facilities use level >130 mg/dL, which identifies 90% of women with GDM (American Diabetes Association, 2000) | Discuss implications of GDM. Refer for a diagnostic 100-g oral glucose tolerance test. |
| *Urinalysis:* See Assessment Guide: Initial Prenatal Assessment for normal findings | See Assessment Guide: Initial Prenatal Assessment for deviations | Repeat urinalysis at 7 months' gestation. Repeat dipstick test at each visit. |
| *Protein:* Negative | Proteinuria, albuminuria (contamination by vaginal discharge, urinary tract infection, PIH) | Obtain dipstick urine sample. Refer to physician if deviations are present. |
| *Glucose:* Negative<br>*Note:* Glycosuria may be present due to physiological alterations in glomerular filtrations rate and renal threshold | Persisent glycosuria (diabetes mellitus) | Refer to physician. |

| Cultural Assessment | Variations to Consider* | Nursing Responses to Data† |
|---|---|---|
| Determine the mother's (and family's) attitudes about the sex of the unborn child. | Some women have no preference about the sex of the child; others do. In many cultures boys are especially valued as firstborn children. | Provide opportunities to discuss preferences and expectations; avoid a judgmental attitude to the response. |
| Ask about the woman's expectations of childbirth. Will she want someone with her for the birth? Whom does she choose? What is the role of her partner? | Some women want their partner present for labor and birth; others prefer a female relative or friend. Some women expect to be separated from their partner once cervical dilatation has occurred (Andrews & Boyle, 1998). | Provide information on birth options but accept the woman's decision about who will attend. |
| Ask about preparations for the baby. Determine what is customary for the woman. | Some women may have a fully prepared nursery; others may not have a separate room for the baby. | Explore reasons for not preparing for the baby. Support the mother's preferences and provide information about possible sources of assistance if the decision is related to a lack of resources. |

| Psychosocial Assessment | Variations to Consider* | Nursing Responses to Data† |
|---|---|---|
| **Expectant Mother** | | |
| *Psychological status*<br>*First trimester:* Incorporates idea of pregnancy; may feel ambivalent, especially if she must give up desired role; usually looks for signs of verification of pregnancy, such as increase in abdominal size or fetal movement | Increased stress and anxiety<br>Inability to establish communication; inability to accept pregnancy; inappropriate response or actions; denial of pregnancy; inability to cope | Encourage woman to make an active part in her care.<br>Establish lines of communication. Establish a trusting relationship. Counsel as necessary. Refer to appropriate professional as needed. |

***Possible causes of alterations are placed in parentheses.**

**†This column provides guidelines for further assessment and initial nursing intervention.**

| Psychosocial Assessment | Variations to Consider* | Nursing Responses to Data† |
|---|---|---|
| **Expectant Mother *continued*** | | |
| *Second trimester:* Baby becomes more real to woman as abdominal size increases and she feels movement; she begins to turn inward, becoming more introspective | | |
| *Third trimester:* Begins to think of baby as separate being; may feel restless and may feel that time of labor will never come; remains self-centered and concentrates on preparing place for baby | Inadequate information | Provide information and counseling. |
| *Educational Needs* | | |
| *Self-care measures and knowledge about the following:* | | |
| Health promotion | | |
| Breast care | | |
| Hygiene | | |
| Rest | | |
| Exercise | | |
| Nutrition | | |
| Relief measures for common discomforts of pregnancy | | |
| Danger signs in pregnancy (Key Facts to Remember, page 190) | | |
| *Sexual activity:* Woman knows how pregnancy affects sexual activity | Lack of information about effects of pregnancy and/or alternative positions during sexual intercourse | Provide counseling. |
| *Preparation for parenting:* Appropriate preparation (Table 8–2) | Lack of preparation (denial, failure to adjust to baby, unwanted child) (Table 8–2) | Counsel. If lack of preparation is due to inadequacy of information, provide information (Chapter 9). |
| *Preparation for Childbirth*<br>*Client aware of the following:*<br>**1.** Prepared childbirth techniques<br>**2.** Normal processes and changes during childbirth | | If couple chooses particular technique, refer to classes (see Chapter 6 for description of childbirth preparation techniques). Encourage prenatal class attendance. Educate woman during visits based on current physical status. Provide reading list for more specific information. |
| **3.** Problems that may occur as a result of drug and alcohol use and of smoking | Continued abuse of drugs and alcohol; denial of possible effect on self and baby | Review danger signs that were presented on initial visit. |
| Woman has met other physician or nurse-midwife who may be attending her birth in the absence of primary caregiver | Introduction of new individual at birth may increase stress and anxiety for woman and partner | Introduce woman to all members of group practice. |

***Possible causes of alterations are placed in parentheses.**

**†This column provides guidelines for further assessment and initial nursing intervention.**

## SUBSEQUENT PRENATAL ASSESSMENT *continued*

| Psychosocial Assessment | Variations to Consider* | Nursing Responses to Data† |
|---|---|---|
| **Expectant Mother** *continued* | | |
| *Impending Labor*<br>*Client knows signs of impending labor:*<br>**1.** Uterine contractions that increase in frequency, duration, and intensity<br>**2.** Bloody show<br>**3.** Expulsion of mucous plug<br>**4.** Rupture of membranes | Lack of information | Provide appropriate teaching, stressing importance of seeking appropriate medical assistance. |
| **Expectant Father** | | |
| *Psychological Status* | | |
| *First trimester:* May express excitement over confirmation of pregnancy and of his virility; concerns move toward providing for financial needs; energetic; may identify with some discomforts of pregnancy and may even exhibit symptoms | Increasing stress and anxiety; inability to establish communication; inability to accept pregnancy diagnosis; withdrawal of support; abandonment of the mother | Encourage expectant father to come to prenatal visits. Establish lines of communication. Establish trusting relationship. |
| *Second trimester:* May feel more confident and be less concerned with financial matters; may have concerns about wife's changing size and shape, her increasing introspection | | Counsel. Let expectant father know that it is normal for him to experience these feelings. |
| *Third trimester:* May have feelings of rivalry with fetus, especially during sexual activity; may make changes in his physical appearance and exhibit more interest in himself; may become more energetic; fantasizes about child but usually imagines older child; fears mutilation and death of woman and child | | Include expectant father in pregnancy activities as he desires. Provide education, information, and support. Increasing numbers of expectant fathers are demonstrating desire to be involved in many or all aspects of prenatal care, education, and preparation. |

*** Possible causes of alterations are placed in parentheses.**

**†This column provides guidelines for further assessment and initial nursing intervention.**

# Subsequent Prenatal Assessment

The Assessment Guide: Subsequent Prenatal Assessment (starting on page 193) provides a systematic approach to the regular physical examinations the pregnant woman should undergo for optimal antepartal care and also provides a model for evaluating both the pregnant woman and the expectant father, if he is involved in the pregnancy.

The recommended frequency of antepartal visits in an uncomplicated pregnancy is as follows:

- Every 4 weeks for the first 28 weeks' gestation
- Every 2 weeks until 36 weeks' gestation
- After week 36, every week until childbirth

During the subsequent antepartal assessments, most women demonstrate ongoing psychologic adjustment to pregnancy. However, some women may exhibit signs of possible psychologic problems such as the following:

- Increasing anxiety
- Inability to establish communication
- Inappropriate responses or actions
- Denial of pregnancy
- Inability to cope with stress
- Intense preoccupation with the sex of the baby
- Failure to acknowledge quickening
- Failure to plan and prepare for the baby (e.g., living arrangements, clothing, and feeding methods)
- Indications of substance abuse

If the woman's behavior indicates possible psychologic problems, the nurse can provide ongoing support and counseling and also refer the woman to appropriate professionals.

# Chapter Review

## CHAPTER HIGHLIGHTS

- A complete history forms the basis of prenatal care and is reevaluated and updated as necessary throughout the pregnancy.
- The initial prenatal assessment is a careful and thorough physical examination and cultural and psychosocial assessment designed to identify variations and potential risk factors.
- Laboratory tests completed at the initial visit, such as a complete blood count, ABO and Rh typing, urinalysis, Pap smear, gonorrhea culture, rubella titer, and various blood screens, provide information about the woman's health during early pregnancy and also help detect potential problems.
- The estimated date of birth (EDB) can be calculated by using Nägele's rule. Using this approach, one begins with the first day of the last menstrual period, subtracts 3 months, and adds 7 days. A gestational calculator or "wheel" may also be used to calculate the EDB.
- Accuracy of the EDB may be evaluated by physical exam to assess uterine size, measurement of fundal height, and ultrasound. Perception of quickening and auscultation of fetal heartbeat are also helpful in confirming the gestation of a pregnancy.
- The diagonal conjugate is the distance from the lower posterior border of the symphysis pubis to the sacral promontory. The obstetric conjugate is estimated by subtracting 1.5 cm from the length of the diagonal conjugate.
- The nurse begins evaluating the woman psychosocially during the initial prenatal assessment. This assessment continues and is modified throughout the pregnancy.
- Religious, cultural, and ethnic beliefs may strongly influence the woman's attitudes and apparent cooperation with care during pregnancy.

## CHAPTER REFERENCES


American College of Obstetricians and Gynecologists (ACOG). (2000). *Planning your pregnancy and birth* (3rd ed.). Washington, DC: ACOG.

American Diabetes Association. (2000). Position statement: Gestational diabetes mellitus. *Diabetes Care, 23*(Suppl. 1), 1–6.

Andrews, M. M., & Boyle, J. S. (1998). *Transcultural concepts in nursing care* (2nd ed.). Glenview, IL: Scott, Foresman/Little, Brown.

Varney, H. (1997). *Varney's midwifery* (3rd ed.). Sudbury, MA: Jones and Bartlett.


## CONTEMPORARY MATERNAL-NEWBORN NURSING ON-LINE

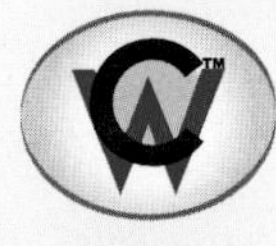

Additional interactive resources including animations and video, for this chapter can be found on the Companion Website at http://www.prenhall.com/ladewig. Click on Chapter 8 and "Begin" to select the activities for this chapter.

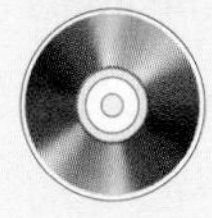

For NCLEX review questions and an audio glossary, access the accompanying CD-ROM in this book.

Chapter 9

# The Expectant Family: Needs and Care

*In my role, I have a very special opportunity to help women and their loved ones prepare for their new baby. I give them information about what to expect and answer their questions so that they can make more informed decisions. Sometimes I have to stop and remind myself to be clear about information that is important for any pregnant woman. Otherwise I might make the mistake of trying to impose my values. It is all too easy to view my way as the only way. When I do that, I fail them and I fail myself.*

—A Registered Nurse Working in a Prenatal Clinic at an Inner-City Hospital

## KEY TERMS



## OBJECTIVES

- Explain the causes of the common discomforts of pregnancy and appropriate measures to alleviate these discomforts.
- Discuss the basic information that the nurse should provide to the expectant family to allow them to carry out appropriate self-care.
- Identify some of the concerns that the expectant couple may have about sexual activity.
- Relate the significance of cultural considerations to the provision of effective prenatal care.
- Describe the medical risks and special concerns of the older expectant woman and her partner.
- Compare similarities and differences in the needs of expectant women in various age groups.

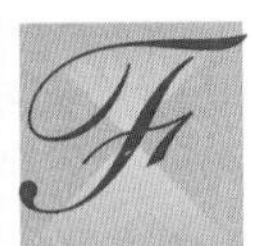

From the moment a woman finds out she is pregnant, she faces a future marked by dramatic changes. Her appearance will alter. Her relationships will change. Even her psychologic state will be affected. In coping with these changes she will need to make adjustments in her daily life. So, too, will her family. Roles and responsibilities of family members may be altered as the woman's ability to perform certain activities changes. The family also must adapt psychologically to the expected arrival of a new member.

The expectant woman and her family will probably have many questions about the pregnancy and its impact on all of them, especially if this is a first pregnancy. The daily activities and health care practices of the woman are important for her well-being and the well-being of the unborn child.

Nurses caring for pregnant women need an up-to-date understanding of pregnancy to be effective in implementing the nursing process as they plan and provide care. With this need in mind, Chapter 7 provided a database for the nurse by presenting material related to the normal physical, social, cultural, and psychologic changes of pregnancy. Chapter 8 then used that database to begin a discussion of nursing care management by focusing on client assessment. This chapter further addresses nursing care management as it relates to the needs of the expectant woman and her loved ones.

# Nursing Care Management

## Nursing Diagnosis during Pregnancy

The nurse may see a pregnant woman only once every 3 to 4 weeks during the first several months of her pregnancy. Therefore a written care plan or critical path that incorporates the database, nursing diagnoses, and client goals is essential to ensure continuity of care.

The nurse can anticipate that, for many women with a low-risk pregnancy, certain nursing diagnoses will be made more frequently than others. The diagnoses will, of course, vary from woman to woman and according to the time in the pregnancy. Examples of common nursing diagnoses include the following:

- ***Constipation*** related to the physiologic effects of pregnancy
- ***Altered sexuality patterns*** related to discomfort during late pregnancy

After formulating an appropriate diagnosis, the nurse and woman establish related goals to guide the nursing plan and interventions.

## Nursing Plan and Implementation during Pregnancy

Once nursing diagnoses have been identified, the next step is to establish priorities of nursing care. Sometimes priorities of care are based on the most immediate needs or concerns expressed by the woman. For example, during the first trimester, when she is experiencing nausea or is concerned about sexual intimacy with her partner, the woman is not likely to want to hear about labor and birth. At other times priorities may develop from findings during a prenatal examination. For example, a woman who is showing signs of preeclampsia (a pregnancy complication discussed in Chapter 13) may feel physically well and find it hard to accept the nurse's emphasis on the need for frequent rest periods. It then becomes the responsibility of medical and nursing professionals to help the woman and her family to understand the significance of a problem and to plan interventions to deal with it.

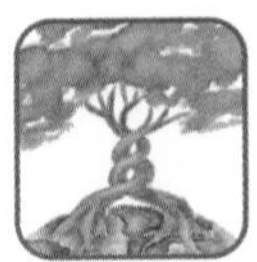

## Community-Based Nursing Care

Prenatal care, especially for women with low-risk pregnancies, is community based, typically in a clinic or a private office. The health care community recognizes the value of providing a primary care nurse in these settings to coordinate holistic care for each childbearing family. The nurse in a clinic or health maintenance organization may be the only source of continuity for the woman, who may see a different physician or certified nurse-midwife at each visit. The nurse can be extremely effective in working with the expectant family by answering their questions; providing complete information about pregnancy, prenatal health care activities, and community resources; and supporting the health care activities of the woman and her family.

Communities often have a wealth of services and educational opportunities available for pregnant women and their families, and the knowledgeable nurse can help expectant mothers to assess and access these services. This approach supports the family's assumption of equal responsibility with health care providers in working toward their common goal of a positive birth experience. See Key Facts to Remember: Key Antepartal Nursing Interventions.

Throughout the prenatal period, the nurse shares information with the family, both verbally and through written materials. This information is designed to help the family to carry out self-care and wellness measures as needed and to report changes that may indicate a health problem. The nurse also provides anticipatory guidance

## KEY FACTS TO REMEMBER

### *Key Antepartal Nursing Interventions*

Antepartal nursing interventions focus on the following:

- Explaining the normal changes of pregnancy to the childbearing family.
- Specifying those signs or symptoms that indicate a problem may be developing.
- Providing appropriate information about self-care measures the pregnant woman may employ to relieve the common discomforts of pregnancy.
- Answering questions about the common concerns that arise during pregnancy.
- Referring the woman for additional or more specialized assistance when necessary.

to help the family plan for changes that will occur after childbirth. The expectant couple is encouraged to identify and discuss issues that could be sources of postpartal stress. Issues to be addressed beforehand may include the sharing of infant and household chores, help in the first few days after childbirth, options for baby-sitting to allow the mother (and couple) some free time, the mother's return to work after the baby's birth, and sibling rivalry. Couples resolve these issues in different ways, but postpartal adjustment tends to be easier for couples who agree on the issues beforehand than for couples who do not confront and resolve these issues.

### Home Care

Home care can be of benefit to any pregnant woman, but it is especially effective in removing barriers for women who have difficulty accessing health care. These barriers may include lack of locally available health care facilities, problems with transportation to the facility, or schedule conflicts with available appointment times because of employment hours or family responsibilities.

In-home nursing assessments vary according to the experience and preparation of the nurse and include current history, vital signs, weight, urine screen, physical activity, dietary intake, reflexes, tests of fetal well-being, and cervical examinations, if indicated. Once the assessments are completed, the nurse can determine the level of follow-up home care or telephone contact needed.

A prenatal home care visit or phone contact can also be useful for women who anticipate a short inpatient stay after childbirth. At the prenatal contact, the nurse explains the postpartum program and answers any questions the woman or her family have. See Chapter 29 for further discussion of home care of the childbearing family.

Currently home care is most often used for women with prenatal complications that can be managed without hospitalization if effective nursing assessment and care are provided in the home (see Chapters 12 and 13).

## Care of the Expectant Father and Siblings

The problems and concerns of the pregnant woman, the relief of her discomforts, and the maintenance of her physical, psychologic, and spiritual health receive much attention. However, her well-being is intertwined with the well-being of those to whom she is closest. Thus the nurse addresses the needs of the woman's family to help maintain the integrity of the family unit. Although the father of the baby is present in most cases, his presence cannot be assumed. If he is not part of the family structure, it is important to assess the woman's support system to determine which significant persons in her life will play a major role during this childbearing experience.

Anticipatory guidance of the expectant father, if he is involved in the pregnancy, is a necessary part of any plan of care. He may need information about the anatomic, physiologic, and emotional changes that occur for both the expectant mother and father during and after pregnancy, the couple's sexuality and sexual response, and the reactions that he is experiencing. He may wish to express his feelings about breast- versus bottle-feeding, the sex of the child, his ability to parent, and other topics.

If it is culturally acceptable to the couple and personally acceptable to him, the nurse refers the couple to expectant parents' classes. These classes provide valuable information about pregnancy and childbirth, using a variety of teaching strategies such as discussion, films, demonstrations with educational models, and written handouts. Some classes even give the father the opportunity to get a "feel" for pregnancy by wearing a pregnancy simulator (Figure 9–1♦). Such classes also offer the couple an opportunity to gain support from other couples.

The nurse assesses the father's intended degree of participation during labor and birth and his knowledge of what to expect. If the couple prefers that his participation be minimal or restricted, the nurse supports the decision. With this type of consideration and collaboration, the father is less apt to develop feelings of alienation, helplessness, and guilt during the pregnancy. As the couple's relationship is strengthened and the father's self-esteem raised, he is better able to provide physical and emotional support to his partner during labor and birth.

In the plan for prenatal care, the nurse also incorporates a discussion about the negative feelings older children may develop. Parents may be distressed to see an older child become aggressive toward the newborn. Parents who

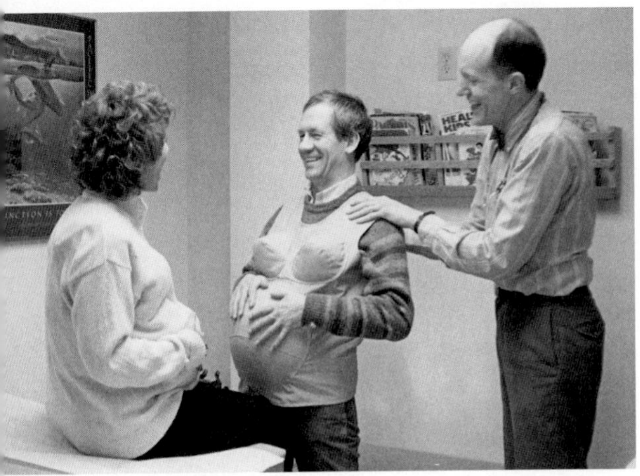

FIGURE 9–1 ♦ The *Empathy Belly* is a pregnancy simulator that allows males and females to experience some of the symptoms of pregnancy. The "belly," which weighs 33 lb, produces symptoms such as shortness of breath, bladder pressure, shift in the center of gravity with resulting waddling gait, increased lordosis and backache, and fatigue. It also can simulate fetal kicking movements. *Source:* Courtesy of Birthways Childbirth Resource Center, Inc.

are unprepared for the older child's feelings of anger, jealousy, and rejection may respond inappropriately in their confusion and surprise. The nurse emphasizes that open communication between parents and children (or acting out feelings with a doll if the child is too young to verbalize) helps children master their feelings. Children may feel less neglected and more secure if they know that their parents are willing to help with their anger and aggressiveness.

# Relief of the Common Discomforts of Pregnancy

The common discomforts of pregnancy result from physiologic and anatomic changes and are fairly specific to each of the three trimesters. Health professionals often refer to these discomforts as minor, but they are not minor to the pregnant woman. They can make her quite uncomfortable and, if they are unexpected, anxious. Table 9–1 on pages 202–203 identifies the common discomforts of pregnancy, their possible causes, and the self-care measures that might relieve the discomfort.

## First Trimester

### Nausea and Vomiting

Nausea and vomiting are early, very common symptoms in pregnancy. These symptoms appear sometime after the first missed menstrual period and usually cease by the fourth missed menstrual period. Some women develop an aversion to specific foods, many experience nausea upon arising in the morning, and others experience nausea throughout the day or in the evening.

The exact cause of nausea and vomiting of pregnancy is unknown, but it is thought to be multifactorial. An elevated human chorionic gonadotropin (hCG) level is believed to be a major factor, but changes in carbohydrate metabolism, fatigue, and emotional factors may also play a role.

In addition to common self-care measures, acupressure applied to a pressure point in the wrist is often helpful (Chez & Murphy, 2000). Some women find 25 mg of pyridoxine (vitamin $B_6$) taken three times a day helpful in reducing symptoms; if $B_6$ is not effective, caregivers often recommend doxylamine (Unisom), an over-the-counter antihistamine (Chez & Niebyl, 2000). A woman should be advised to contact her health care provider if she vomits more than once a day or shows signs of dehydration such as dry mouth and concentrated urine. In such cases, the physician/certified nurse-midwife might order an antiemetic such as promethazine (Phenergan). However, antiemetics should be avoided if possible during this time because of possible harmful effects on embryo development.

### Urinary Frequency

Urinary frequency, a common discomfort of pregnancy, occurs early in pregnancy and again during the third trimester because of pressure of the enlarging uterus on the bladder. Although frequency is considered normal during the first and third trimesters, the woman is advised to report to her health care provider signs of bladder infection such as pain, burning with voiding, or blood in the urine. Fluid intake should never be decreased to prevent frequency. The woman needs to maintain an adequate fluid intake—at least 2000 mL (8 to 10 8-oz glasses) per day. She should also be encouraged to empty her bladder frequently (about every 2 hours while awake).

### Fatigue

Marked fatigue is so common in early pregnancy that it is considered a presumptive sign of pregnancy. It is aggravated if the woman has to arise each night because of urinary frequency. Typically it resolves after the end of the first trimester.

### Breast Tenderness

Sensitivity of the breasts occurs early and continues throughout the pregnancy. Increased levels of estrogen and progesterone contribute to soreness and tingling of the breasts and increased sensitivity of the nipples.

### Increased Vaginal Discharge

Increased whitish vaginal discharge, called **leukorrhea,** is common in pregnancy. It occurs as a result of hyperplasia

**TABLE 9–1 Self-Care Measures for Common Discomforts of Pregnancy**

| *Discomfort* | *Influencing Factors* | *Self-Care Measures* |
|---|---|---|
| **FIRST TRIMESTER** | | |
| Nausea and vomiting | Increased levels of human chorionic gonadotropin<br>Changes in carbohydrate metabolism<br>Emotional factors<br>Fatigue | Avoid odors or causative factors.<br>Eat dry crackers or toast before arising in morning.<br>Have small but frequent meals.<br>Avoid greasy or highly seasoned foods.<br>Take dry meals with fluids between meals.<br>Drink carbonated beverages. |
| Urinary frequency | Pressure of uterus on bladder in both first and third trimesters | Void when urge is felt.<br>Increase fluid intake during the day.<br>Decrease fluid intake *only* in the evening to decrease nocturia. |
| Fatigue | Specific causative factors unknown<br>May be aggravated by nocturia due to urinary frequency | Plan time for a nap or rest period daily.<br>Go to bed earlier.<br>Seek family support and assistance with responsibilities so that more time is available to rest. |
| Breast tenderness | Increased levels of estrogen and progesterone | Wear well-fitting, supportive bra. |
| Increased vaginal discharge | Hyperplasia of vaginal mucosa and increased production of mucus by the endocervical glands due to the increase in estrogen levels. | Promote cleanliness by daily bathing.<br>Avoid douching, nylon underpants, and pantyhose; cotton underpants are more absorbent; powder can be used to maintain dryness if not allowed to cake. |
| Nasal stuffiness and nosebleed (epistaxis) | Elevated estrogen levels | May be unresponsive, but cool-air vaporizer may help; avoid use of nasal sprays and decongestants. |
| Ptyalism (excessive, often bitter salivation) | Specific causative factors unknown | Use astringent mouthwashes, chew gum, or suck hard candy. |
| **SECOND AND THIRD TRIMESTERS** | | |
| Heartburn (pyrosis) | Increased production of progesterone, decreasing gastrointestinal motility and increasing relaxation of cardiac sphincter, displacement of stomach by enlarging uterus, thus regurgitation of acidic gastric contents into the esophagus | Eat small and more frequent meals.<br>Use low-sodium antacids.<br>Avoid overeating, fatty and fried foods, lying down after eating, and sodium bicarbonate. |
| Ankle edema | Prolonged standing or sitting<br>Increased levels of sodium due to hormonal influences<br>Circulatory congestion of lower extremities<br>Increased capillary permeability<br>Varicose veins | Practice frequent dorsiflexion of feet when prolonged sitting or standing is necessary.<br>Elevate legs when sitting or resting.<br>Avoid tight garters or restrictive bands around legs. |
| Varicose veins | Venous congestion in the lower veins that increases with pregnancy<br>Hereditary factors (weakening of walls of veins, faulty valves)<br>Increased age and weight gain | Elevate legs frequently.<br>Wear supportive hose.<br>Avoid crossing legs at the knees, standing for long periods, garters, and hosiery with constrictive bands. |
| Hemorrhoids | Constipation (see following discussion)<br>Increased pressure from gravid uterus on hemorrhoidal veins | Avoid constipation.<br>Apply ice packs, topical ointments, anesthetic agents, warm soaks, or sitz baths; gently reinsert into rectum as necessary. |

**TABLE 9–1 Self-Care Measures for Common Discomforts of Pregnancy *continued***

| *Discomfort* | *Influencing Factors* | *Self-Care Measures* |
|---|---|---|
| **SECOND AND THIRD TRIMESTERS** | | |
| Constipation | Increased levels of progesterone, which cause general bowel sluggishness<br>Pressure of enlarging uterus on intestine<br>Iron supplements<br>Diet, lack of exercise, and decreased fluids | Increase fluid intake, fiber in the diet, and exercise.<br>Develop regular bowel habits.<br>Use stool softeners as recommended by physician. |
| Backache | Increased curvature of the lumbosacral vertebrae as the uterus enlarges<br>Increased levels of hormones, which cause softening of cartilage in body joints<br>Fatigue<br>Poor body mechanics | Use proper body mechanics.<br>Practice the pelvic tilt exercise.<br>Avoid uncomfortable working heights, high-heeled shoes, lifting heavy loads, and fatigue. |
| Leg cramps | Imbalance of calcium/phosphorus ratio<br>Increased pressure of uterus on nerves<br>Fatigue<br>Poor circulation to lower extremities<br>Pointing the toes | Practice dorsiflexion of feet to stretch affected muscle.<br>Evaluate diet.<br>Apply heat to affected muscles.<br>Arise slowly from resting position. |
| Faintness | Postural hypotension<br>Sudden change of position causing venous pooling in dependent veins<br>Standing for long periods in warm area<br>Anemia | Avoid prolonged standing in warm or stuffy environments.<br>Evaluate hematocrit and hemoglobin. |
| Dyspnea | Decreased vital capacity from pressure of enlarging uterus on the diaphragm | Use proper posture when sitting and standing.<br>Sleep propped up with pillows for relief if problem occurs at night. |
| Flatulence | Decrease gastrointestinal motility leading to delayed emptying time<br>Pressure of growing uterus on large intestine<br>Air swallowing | Avoid gas-forming foods.<br>Chew food thoroughly.<br>Get regular daily exercise.<br>Maintain normal bowel habits. |
| Carpal tunnel syndrome | Compression of median nerve in carpal tunnel of wrist<br>Aggravated by repetitive hand movements | Avoid aggravating hand movements.<br>Use splint as prescribed.<br>Elevate affected arm. |

of the vaginal mucosa and increased mucus production by the endocervical glands. The increased acidity of the secretions encourages the growth of *Candida albicans,* so the woman is more susceptible to monilial vaginitis.

### Nasal Stuffiness and Epistaxis

Once pregnancy is well established elevated estrogen levels may produce edema of the nasal mucosa, which results in nasal stuffiness, nasal discharge, and obstruction. Epistaxis (nosebleeds) may also result. Cool-air vaporizers and normal saline nasal sprays may help, but the problem is often unresponsive to treatment. Women experiencing these problems find it difficult to sleep and may resort to using medicated nasal sprays and decongestants. Such interventions may provide initial relief but can actually increase nasal stuffiness over time. Pregnant women should avoid using any medications, if possible.

### Ptyalism

**Ptyalism** is a rare discomfort of pregnancy in which excessive, often bitter saliva is produced. The cause is unknown, and effective treatments are limited.

## Second and Third Trimesters

It is more difficult to classify discomforts as specifically occurring in the second or third trimesters because many problems represent individual variations in women. The discomforts discussed in this section usually do not appear until the third trimester in primigravidas but may occur earlier with each succeeding pregnancy.

## EVIDENCE-BASED PRACTICE

### Fatigue

When you read that fatigue is considered a presumptive sign of pregnancy, you laughed. Maybe, you thought, it should also be considered a presumptive sign of being a nursing student! You decided to learn more about fatigue related to pregnancy because you recognized that fatigue affects attitude, concentration, and decision making.

In your search for literature on the topic, you locate one article that describes previous studies on childbearing fatigue. The authors are nurse researchers who tested two tools to measure fatigue in pregnant women (Pugh, Milligan, Parks, et al., 1999). The definition the researchers used in studying fatigue comes from the North American Nursing Diagnosis Association. It describes childbearing fatigue as "an overwhelming sustained sense of exhaustion and decreased capacity for physical and mental work" (Pugh et al., 1999, p. 74). Such a definition certainly helps to clarify the significance of fatigue to the pregnant woman.

The two fatigue assessment tools are the Fatigue Identification Form and the Fatigue Continuum Form. Both ask 30 questions of the woman, and their content is essentially the same. The difference between the tools is in the design of the questions and the scoring method used by the woman. One is a yes/no (or dichotomous) tool, whereas the other is a scored tool in which the woman rates the degree to which she experiences each symptom.

This article recommends further research on fatigue related to childbearing, particularly using the Fatigue Continuum Form. However, the authors suggest that the Fatigue Identification Form might be helpful in quantifying fatigue during pregnancy and could be used clinically.

This article does not provide a systematic review of the literature in which previous studies are evaluated by specific criteria, nor is it an evidence-based guideline with recommendations made according to the strength of the evidence. However, these limitations do not preclude the use of a fatigue evaluation tool in the clinical setting. With appropriate staff preparation and a method for data gathering and analysis to support understanding of its use in your clinical site, the tool can be an important step in advancing evidence in practice.

Next week you will begin your clinical experience in a prenatal clinic. You plan to determine whether the clinic uses a fatigue assessment tool. It seems like a practical approach to quantify a factor such as fatigue, which can significantly affect a woman's life. You have already learned that research has shown clinicians that the best way to monitor pain is to have clients describe their pain using a 10-point scale. Using a fatigue assessment tool seems equally logical to you.

#### References

Pugh, L. C., Milligan, R., Parks, P. L., Lenz, E. R., & Kitzman, H. (1999). Clinical approaches in the assessment of childbearing fatigue. *Journal of Obstetric, Gynecologic, and Neonatal Nursing, 28*(1), 74–80.

### Heartburn (Pyrosis)

Heartburn is the regurgitation of acidic gastric contents into the esophagus. It creates a burning sensation in the esophagus and sometimes leaves a bad taste in the mouth. Heartburn appears to be primarily a result of the displacement of the stomach by the enlarging uterus. The increased production of progesterone in pregnancy, decreases in gastrointestinal motility, and relaxation of the cardiac (esophageal) sphincter also contribute to heartburn.

Liquid forms of low-sodium antacids are often most effective in providing relief. Women should be advised that antacids containing aluminum may cause constipation, whereas diarrhea is associated with antacids containing magnesium. Sodium bicarbonate (baking soda) and Alka-Seltzer should be avoided because they may lead to electrolyte imbalance.

If maternal heartburn is severe, not relieved by antacids, and accompanied by gastrointestinal reflux, an antisecretory agent ($H_2$-blocker) such as ranitidine (Zantac), cimetidine (Tagamet), or omeprazole (Losec) may be indicated. Research to date has not linked them with an excessive risk of birth defects, preterm birth, or intrauterine growth restriction, and up to 85% of pregnant women use at least one of these medications to control acid reflux ("Good News for Pregnant Women," 1999).

## Ankle Edema

Most women experience ankle edema in the last part of pregnancy because of the increasing difficulty of venous return from the lower extremities. Prolonged standing or sitting and warm weather increase the edema. It is also associated with varicose veins. Ankle edema becomes a concern only when accompanied by hypertension or proteinuria or when the edema is not postural in origin.

## Varicose Veins

Varicose veins are a result of weakening of the walls of veins or faulty functioning of the valves. Poor circulation in the lower extremities predisposes individuals to varicose veins in the legs and thighs, as does prolonged standing or sitting. Pressure of the gravid uterus on the pelvic veins prevents good venous return and may therefore aggravate existing problems or contribute to obvious changes in the veins of the legs (Figure 9–2♦).

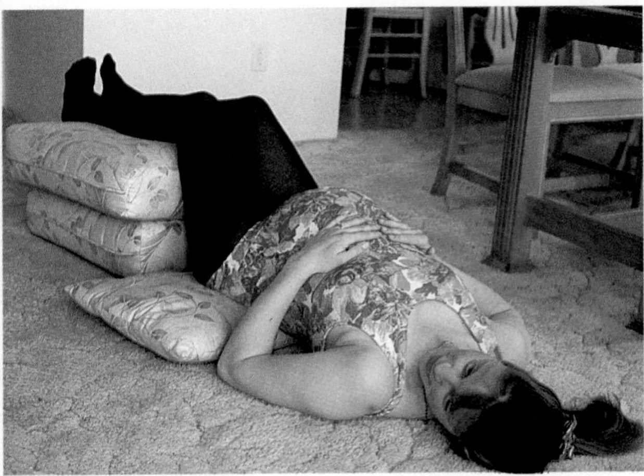

**FIGURE 9–2** ♦ Swelling and discomfort from varicosities can be decreased by lying down with the legs and one hip elevated (to avoid compression of the vena cava).

Surgical correction of varicose veins is not generally recommended during pregnancy (Cunningham, MacDonald, Gant, et al., 1997). The woman can be advised that treatment may be needed after she gives birth because the problem will be aggravated by a succeeding pregnancy.

Although they are less common, varicosities in the vulva and perineum may also develop. They produce aching and a sense of heaviness. Support for vulvar varicosities is sometimes achieved by wearing two sanitary pads inside the underpants. The woman may relieve uterine pressure on the pelvic veins by resting on her side. Blocks may also be placed under the foot of her bed to elevate it slightly.

## Flatulence

Flatulence results from decreased gastrointestinal motility, leading to delayed emptying, and from pressure on the large intestine by the growing uterus. Air swallowing may also contribute to the problem.

## Hemorrhoids

Hemorrhoids are varicosities of the veins in the lower rectum and the anus. During pregnancy, the gravid uterus presses on the veins and interferes with venous circulation. In addition, the straining that accompanies constipation is frequently a contributing cause of hemorrhoids.

Some women may not be bothered by hemorrhoids until the second stage of labor, when the hemorrhoids appear as they push. These hemorrhoids usually become asymptomatic a few days after childbirth. Symptoms of hemorrhoids include itching, swelling, pain, and bleeding. Women who have had hemorrhoids before pregnancy will probably experience difficulties with them during pregnancy.

It is possible to find relief by gently reinserting the hemorrhoid. The woman lies on her side, places some lubricant on her finger, and presses against the hemorrhoids, pushing them inside. She holds them in place for 1 to 2 minutes and then gently withdraws her finger. The anal sphincter should then hold them inside the rectum. The woman will find it especially helpful if she can maintain a side-lying (Sims') position for a time, so this method is best done before bed or prior to a daily rest period.

## Constipation

Conditions that predispose the pregnant woman to constipation include general bowel sluggishness caused by increased progesterone and steroid metabolism; displacement of the intestines, which increases with the growth of the fetus; and the oral iron supplements most pregnant women need. In severe or preexisting cases of constipation, the woman may need stool softeners, mild laxatives, or suppositories as recommended by her caregiver.

## Backache

Many pregnant women experience backache, due primarily to exaggeration of the lumbosacral curve that occurs as the uterus enlarges and becomes heavier. Maintaining good posture and using proper body mechanics throughout pregnancy can help prevent backache. The pregnant woman is advised to avoid bending over at the waist to pick up objects and should bend from the knees instead (Figure 9–3♦). She should place her feet 12 to 18 in apart to maintain body balance. If the woman uses work surfaces that require her to bend, the nurse can advise the woman to adjust the height of the surfaces.

## Leg Cramps

Leg cramps are painful muscle spasms in the gastrocnemius muscles. They occur most frequently after the woman has gone to bed at night but may occur at other times. Extension of the foot can often cause leg cramps. The nurse should warn the pregnant woman not to extend the foot during childbirth preparation exercises or during rest periods. The exact cause of leg cramps is not known, but pressure of the enlarged uterus on pelvic nerves or blood vessels leading to the legs may be a contributing factor (Varney, 1997), especially during the third trimester.

Immediate relief of the muscle spasm is achieved by stretching the muscle. With the woman lying on her back, another person presses the woman's knee down to straighten her leg while pushing her foot toward her leg. The woman may also stand and put her foot flat on the floor. Massage and warm packs can alleviate the discomfort of leg cramps (Figure 9–4♦). In addition, to help prevent leg cramps, the caregiver may recommend a diet that includes daily portions of both calcium and phosphorus (Varney, 1997).

## Faintness

Many pregnant women occasionally feel faint, especially in warm, crowded areas. Faintness is caused by a combination of changes in the blood volume and postural hypotension due to pooling of blood in the dependent veins. Sudden change of position or standing for prolonged periods can also cause this sensation, and fainting can occur.

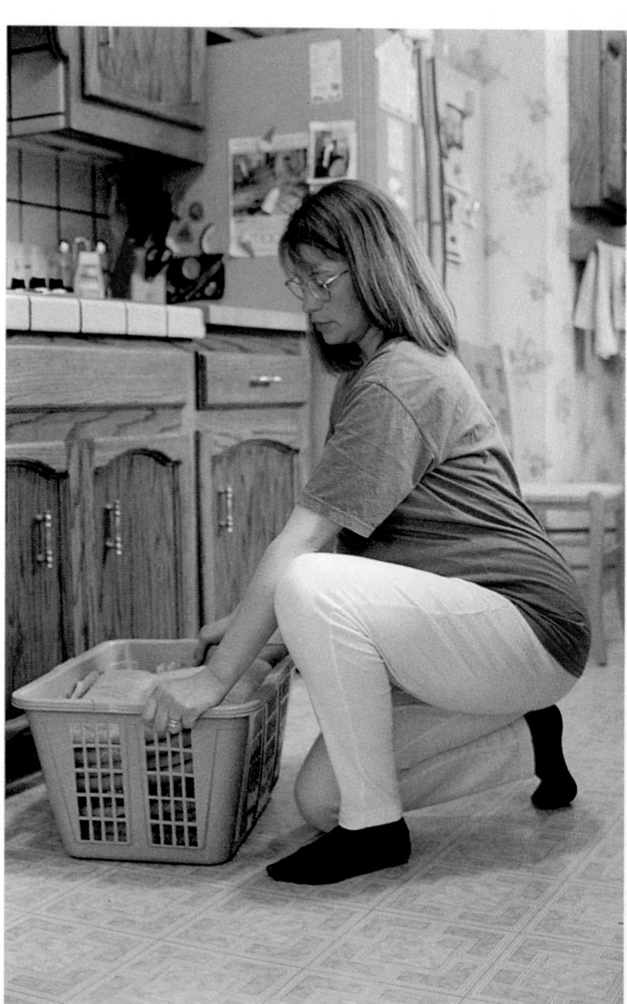

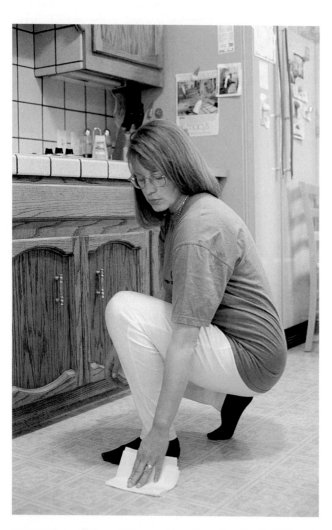

**FIGURE 9–3 ♦** When picking up objects from floor level or lifting objects, the pregnant woman must use proper body mechanics.

If a woman begins to feel faint from prolonged standing or from being in a stuffy room, she should sit down and lower her head between her knees. If this procedure does not help, the woman can be assisted to an area where she can lie down and get fresh air. When arising from a resting position, it is important that she move slowly. Women whose jobs require standing in one place for long periods should march in place regularly to increase venous return from the legs.

### Shortness of Breath (Dyspnea)

Shortness of breath occurs as the uterus rises into the abdomen and causes pressure on the diaphragm. This problem worsens in the last trimester because the enlarged uterus presses directly on the diaphragm, decreasing vital capacity. The primigravida experiences considerable relief from shortness of breath in the last few weeks of pregnancy, when **lightening** occurs, and the fetus and uterus move down in the pelvis. Because the multigravida does not usually experience lightening until labor, she tends to feel short of breath throughout the latter part of her pregnancy.

### Difficulty Sleeping

Many physical factors in late pregnancy may make sleeping difficult. The enlarged uterus may make it difficult to find a comfortable position for sleep, and an active fetus may aggravate the problem. Other discomforts of pregnancy such as urinary frequency, shortness of breath, and leg cramps may also be contributing factors.

### Round Ligament Pain

As the uterus enlarges during pregnancy, the round ligaments stretch and hypertrophy as the uterus rises up in the abdomen. Round ligament pain is attributable to this stretching. The woman may feel concern when she first experiences round ligament pain, because it is often intense and causes a "grabbing" sensation in the lower abdomen and inguinal area. The nurse should warn the pregnant woman of this possible discomfort. Once the caregiver has determined that the cause of the pain is not a medical complication such as appendicitis, the woman may find that applying a heating pad to the abdomen brings relief.

### Carpal Tunnel Syndrome

Carpal tunnel syndrome, characterized by numbness and tingling of the hand near the thumb, occurs in about one-fourth of pregnant women (Cunningham et al., 1997). It is caused by compression of the median nerve in the carpal tunnel of the wrist. The syndrome is aggravated by repetitive hand movements such as typing and may disappear following childbirth. Treatment usually involves splinting and avoiding aggravating movements.

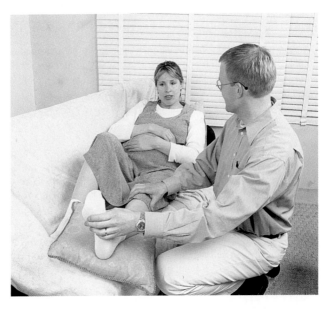

FIGURE 9–4 ♦ The expectant father can help relieve the woman's painful leg cramps by flexing her foot and straightening her leg.

Surgery is indicated in severe cases if more conservative approaches are not effective.

## Promotion of Self-Care during Pregnancy

### Cultural Considerations in Pregnancy

As discussed in Chapter 8, actions during pregnancy are often determined by cultural beliefs. Table 9–2 presents activities encouraged or forbidden by some specific cultures. The table is not meant to be all-inclusive, nor is it meant to imply that all members of a given culture hold these beliefs. Rather, it offers a few examples of cultural activities that may be important to some clients during the prenatal period.

In working with clients of other cultures, the health professional should be open to and respectful of other beliefs. Culturally competent nurses recognize that each childbearing family, shaped by culture and life experience, has expectations of both its members and the health care system during pregnancy and birth.

Language barriers often pose a challenge in providing effective prenatal nursing care. Whenever possible it is important to have an interpreter—family member, friend, or staff person—present at prenatal visits so the nurse can provide basic information about pregnancy and prenatal care. The nurse should also provide opportunities for the woman to ask questions or express concerns. It is essential to have printed material available in the woman's language.

## TABLE 9–2 Cultural Beliefs and Practices during Pregnancy

Here are a few examples of cultural beliefs and practices related to pregnancy. It is important not to make assumptions about a client's beliefs, because cultural norms vary greatly within a culture and from generation to generation. The nurse should observe the client carefully and take the time to ask questions. Clients will benefit greatly from the nurse's increased awareness of their cultural beliefs and practices.

| *Belief or Practice* | *Nursing Consideration* |
|---|---|
| **HOME REMEDIES** | |
| Pregnant women of Native American background may use herbal remedies. An example is the dandelion, which contains a milky juice in its stem believed to increase breast milk flow in mothers who choose to breastfeed (Spector, 2000). Clients of Chinese descent may drink ginseng tea for faintness after childbirth or as a sedative when mixed with bamboo leaves. Some people of African heritage may use self-medication for pregnancy discomforts—for example, laxatives to prevent or treat constipation (Spector, 2000). | Find out what medications and home remedies your client is using and counsel your client regarding overall effects. It is common for individuals to avoid telling health care workers about home remedies; the client may feel her use of home remedies will be judged unfavorably. Phrase your questions in a sensitive, accepting way. |
| **NUTRITION** | |
| Some women of Italian background may believe that it is necessary to satisfy desires for certain foods in order to prevent congenital anomalies. Also, they may believe that they must eat food that they smell, or else the fetus will move "inside," which will result in a miscarriage. Pregnant women of African descent may continue the tradition of eating clay, dirt, or starch, which they believe will benefit the mother and fetus (Spector, 2000). To practice *Tae Kyo,* a set of rules for safe childbirth, pregnant women of Korean descent may practice food taboos by eating particular high-quality foods and avoiding other foods believed to cause an unhealthy fetus (Choi, 1995). | Discuss the client's beliefs and practices in regard to nutrition during pregnancy. Obtain a diet history from the client. Discuss the importance of a well-balanced diet during pregnancy, with consideration of the client's cultural beliefs and practices.<br>In some cases, you might want to suggest remedies that may be more effective—for example, eating high-fiber foods to reduce constipation. If the home remedy is not harmful, there is no reason to ask a client to discontinue this practice. |
| **ALTERNATIVE HEALTH CARE PROVIDERS** | |
| Pregnant women of Mexican background may choose to seek out the care of a *partera* (midwife) for prenatal and intrapartal care. A *partera* speaks their language, shares a similar culture, and can deliver pregnant women at home or in a birthing center instead of a hospital. Some people in Hispanic-American communities may use the *curandero,* the folk healer. The *curandero* frequently uses herbs, massage, and religious artifacts for treatment (Spector, 2000). | Discuss the variety of choices of health care providers available to the pregnant woman. Contrast the benefits and risks of different settings for prenatal care and birth. Provide reassurance that the goal of health care during pregnancy and birth is a healthy outcome for mother and baby, with respect for the specific cultural beliefs and practices of the client. |
| **EXERCISE** | |
| Pregnant women of Italian descent may fear changing their body position in certain ways because they believe doing so may cause the fetus to develop abnormally (Spector, 2000). Some people of Southeast Asian background believe that inactivity during pregnancy will result in a difficult labor (Mattson, 1995). Some people of European, African, and Mexican descent believe that reaching over the head during pregnancy can harm the baby. | Ask your client whether there are any activities she is afraid to do because of the pregnancy. Assure her that reaching over her head will not harm the baby and evaluate other activities related to their effect on the pregnancy. |
| **SPIRITUALITY** | |
| Native Americans of the Navajo tribe may meet with the medicine man 2 months prior to birth, feeling that the prayers will ensure a safe birth and healthy baby. Some people of European background may tend to pay more attention to spirituality in their life to alleviate fears and ensure a safe birth. | Encourage the use of support systems and spiritual aids that provide comfort for the mother. |

## HINTS FOR PRACTICE

At each prenatal visit, focus your teaching on changes or possible discomforts the woman might encounter during the coming month and the next trimester. If the pregnancy is progressing normally, spend a few minutes describing her baby at this stage of development.

## FETAL ACTIVITY MONITORING

Many caregivers encourage pregnant women to monitor their unborn child's well-being by regularly assessing fetal activity beginning at 28 weeks' gestation. Vigorous fetal activity generally provides reassurance of fetal well-being, whereas a marked decrease in activity or cessation of movement may indicate possible fetal compromise that requires immediate evaluation. Fetal activity is affected by fetal sleep, sound, time of day, blood glucose levels, cigarette smoking, and some illicit drugs such as crack and cocaine. At times a healthy fetus may be minimally active or inactive. A variety of methods for tracking fetal activity have been developed. They focus on having the woman keep a **fetal movement record (FMR)** such as the Cardiff Count-to-Ten method. An FMR is a noninvasive technique that enables the pregnant woman to monitor and record movements easily and without expense. See Teaching Guide: What to Tell the Pregnant Woman about Assessing Fetal Activity, on page 211.

## BREAST CARE

Whether the pregnant woman plans to bottle- or breastfeed her infant, support of the breasts is important to promote comfort, retain breast shape, and prevent back strain, particularly if the breasts become large and pendulous. The sensitivity of the breasts in pregnancy is frequently relieved by good support.

A well-fitting, supportive brassiere has the following qualities:

- The straps are wide and do not stretch (elastic straps soon lose their tautness with the weight of the breasts and frequent washing).
- The cup holds all breast tissue comfortably.
- The brassiere has tucks or other devices that allow it to expand, thus accommodating the enlarging chest circumference.
- The brassiere supports the nipple line approximately midway between the elbow and shoulder but is not pulled up in the back by the weight of the breasts.

Cleanliness of the breasts is important, especially as the woman begins producing colostrum. Colostrum that crusts on the nipples can be removed with warm water. The woman planning to breastfeed is advised not to use soap on her nipples because of its drying effect.

**Nipple preparation,** generally begun during the third trimester, helps prevent soreness during the first few days of breastfeeding. Nipple preparation promotes the distribution of the natural lubricants produced by Montgomery's tubercles and helps develop the protective layer of skin over the nipple. Women who are planning to nurse can begin by going braless when possible and by exposing their nipples to sunlight and air. Rubbing the nipples removes protective oils and is best avoided, but rolling the nipple—grasping it between thumb and forefinger and gently rolling it for a short time each day—helps prepare for breastfeeding. A woman with a history of preterm labor is advised not to use this technique because nipple stimulation triggers the release of oxytocin. See Chapter 14 for further discussion of the effects of nipple stimulation on contractions.

Nipple rolling is more difficult for women with flat or inverted nipples, but it can still be a useful preparation for breastfeeding. Breast shields designed to correct inverted nipples can be worn during pregnancy. The shields appear to be the only currently available measure that offers some help to women with inverted nipples (Figure 9–5♦). For further discussion of inverted nipples, see Chapter 24.

Oral stimulation of the nipple by the woman's partner during sex play is also an excellent technique for toughening the nipple in preparation for breastfeeding. Couples who enjoy this stimulation should be encouraged to continue it throughout the pregnancy, except when the woman has a history of preterm labor, as discussed earlier.

## CLOTHING

Clothing in pregnancy is generally an important factor in the woman's feelings about herself and her appearance. Clothes should be loose and nonconstricting Maternity clothes are constructed with fuller lines to allow for the increase in abdominal size during pregnancy. Maternity clothing can be expensive, however, and is worn for a relatively short time. Women may economize by wearing regular clothing, sharing clothes with friends, sewing their own garments, or buying used maternity clothes.

High-heeled shoes tend to aggravate back discomfort by increasing the curvature of the lower back. They are best avoided if the woman experiences backache or has problems with balance. Shoes should fit properly and feel comfortable.

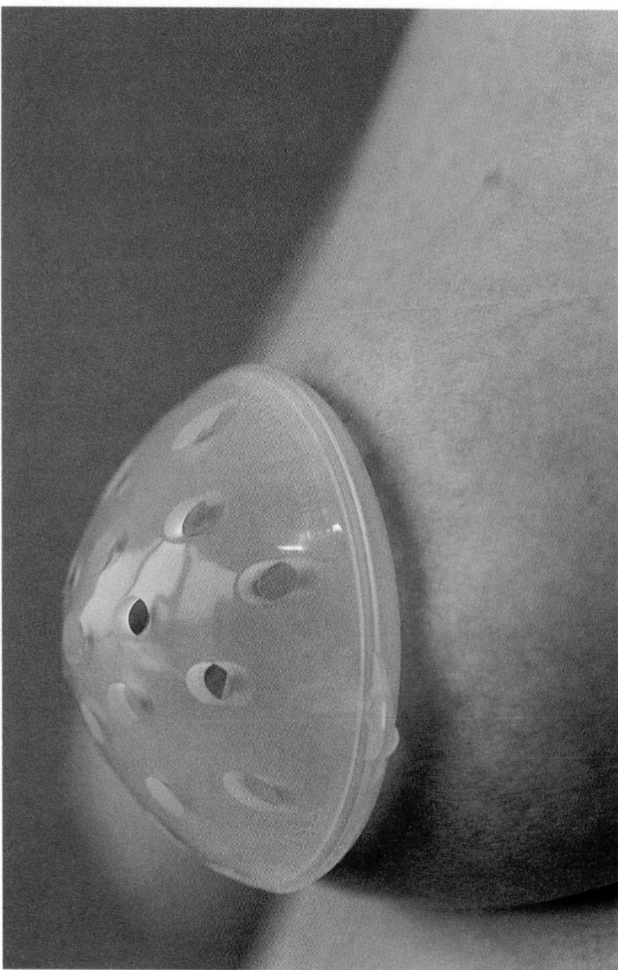

FIGURE 9–5 ♦ This breast shield is designed to increase the protractility of inverted nipples. Worn the last 3 to 4 months of pregnancy, it exerts gentle pulling pressure at the edge of the areola, gradually forcing the nipple through the center of the shield. It may be used after childbirth if still necessary.

## Bathing

Practices related to cleansing the body are often influenced by cultural norms. Perspiration and mucoid vaginal discharge increase during pregnancy. Thus a pregnant woman may choose to cleanse only some portions of her body regularly or may elect to take showers or tub baths. Caution is needed in the tub because balance becomes a problem in late pregnancy. Rubber mats and hand grips are important safety devices. Moreover, vasodilation due to warm water may cause the woman to feel faint when she attempts to get out of the tub. Thus, she may require assistance, especially during the last trimester.

## Employment

Studies of women who are employed outside the home during pregnancy show distinct differences. Women who work in office jobs tend to have slightly lower odds of having a small-for-gestational-age (SGA) baby than unemployed women, for example. This difference may result because they have better access to health care or because these women tend to be healthier as a group. Pregnant women who are employed in jobs that require prolonged standing have a higher incidence of preterm birth (Cunningham et al., 1997).

Overfatigue, excessive physical strain, fetotoxic hazards in the environment, and medical or obstetric complications are the major deterrents to certain types of employment during pregnancy. In the last half of pregnancy, occupations involving balance should be adjusted to protect the mother.

Fetotoxic hazards are always a concern to the expectant couple. The pregnant woman (or the woman contemplating pregnancy) who works in industry should contact her company physician or nurse about possible hazards in her work environment and should do her own reading and research on environmental hazards as well. Similarly, her partner can seek information about hazards in his workplace that might affect his sperm.

## Travel

If medical or pregnancy complications are not present, there are no restrictions on travel. Pregnant women are advised to avoid travel if there is a history of bleeding or pregnancy-induced hypertension or if multiple births are anticipated.

Travel by automobile can be especially fatiguing, aggravating many of the discomforts of pregnancy. The pregnant woman needs frequent opportunities to get out of the car and walk. (A good pattern is to stop every 2 hours and walk around for approximately 10 minutes.) She should wear both lap and shoulder belts; the lap belt should fit snugly and be positioned under the abdomen and across the upper thighs. Seat belts play an important role in preventing maternal mortality with subsequent fetal death (Cunningham et al., 1997). Fetal death in car accidents is also caused by placental separation (abruptio placenta) as a result of uterine distortion. Use of the shoulder belt decreases the risk of traumatic flexion of the woman's body, thus decreasing the risk of placental separation.

As pregnancy progresses, long-distance trips are best taken by plane or train. Availability of medical care at the destination is an important factor for the near-term woman who travels.

## Activity and Rest

Exercise during pregnancy helps maintain maternal fitness and muscle tone, leads to improved self-image, promotes regular bowel function, increases energy, improves sleep, relieves tension, helps control weight gain, and is associated with improved postpartum recovery. Normal participation in exercise can continue throughout an uncomplicated pregnancy and, in fact, is encouraged. The

## TEACHING GUIDE *What to Tell the Pregnant Woman about Assessing Fetal Activity*

### Assessment

The nurse focuses on the woman's prior knowledge and former use of fetal movement assessment methods, the week of gestation, and her communication and ability to understand and process information.

### Nursing Diagnosis

The key nursing diagnosis will probably be

Health-seeking behaviors: information on assessing fetal activity related to an expressed desire to monitor her baby's well-being.

### Nursing Plan and Implementation

The teaching plan provides general information about fetal movement and assessment methods the pregnant woman can use at home.

### Client Goals

At the completion of the teaching session the woman will

- Discuss the types of fetal assessment methods, reasons for assessment, how to accomplish the assessment, and methods of record keeping.
- Demonstrate the use of a fetal movement record.
- Identify resources to call if questions arise.
- Agree to bring the fetal movement record to each prenatal visit.

## *Teaching Plan*

### CONTENT

Explain that fetal movements are first felt around 18 weeks' gestation. From that time the fetal movements get stronger and easier to detect. A slowing or stopping of fetal movement may be an indication that the fetus needs some attention and evaluation.

Explain procedure for Cardiff Count-to-Ten method or for the Daily Fetal Movement Record (DFMR). For both methods, advise the woman to

- Beginning at about 27 weeks' gestation, keep a daily record of fetal movement.
- Try to begin counting at about the same time each day, about 1 hour after a meal if possible.
- Lie quietly in a side-lying position.

Using the Cardiff card, have the woman place an X for each fetal movement until she has recorded 10. Movement varies considerably, but most women feel fetal movement at least 10 times in 3 hours (see Figure 9–6♦).

Using the DFMR have the woman count three times a day for 20 to 30 minutes each session. If there are fewer than three movements in a session, have the woman count for 1 hour or more.

Explain when to contact the care provider:

If there are fewer than 10 movements in 3 hours

If overall the fetus's movements are slowing, and it takes much longer each day to note 10 movements

If there are no movements in the morning

If there are fewer than 3 movements in 8 hours

### TEACHING METHOD

Describe procedures and demonstrate how to assess fetal movement. Sit beside woman and show her how to place her hand on the fundus to feel fetal movement.

Provide a written teaching sheet for the woman's use at home.

Demonstrate how to record fetal movements on Cardiff Count-to-Ten scoring card or on daily fetal movement record.

Watch woman fill out record as examples are provided. Encourage her to complete the record each day and bring it with her to each prenatal visit. Assure her that the record will be discussed at each prenatal visit, and questions may be addressed at that time if desired.

Provide the woman with a name and phone number in case she has further questions.

### EVALUATION

Evaluate learning by having the woman explain the method and by asking the woman to fill the card in using a fictitious situation. At each prenatal visit review the expectant woman's record. Review of the record provides opportunities for questions and clarification.

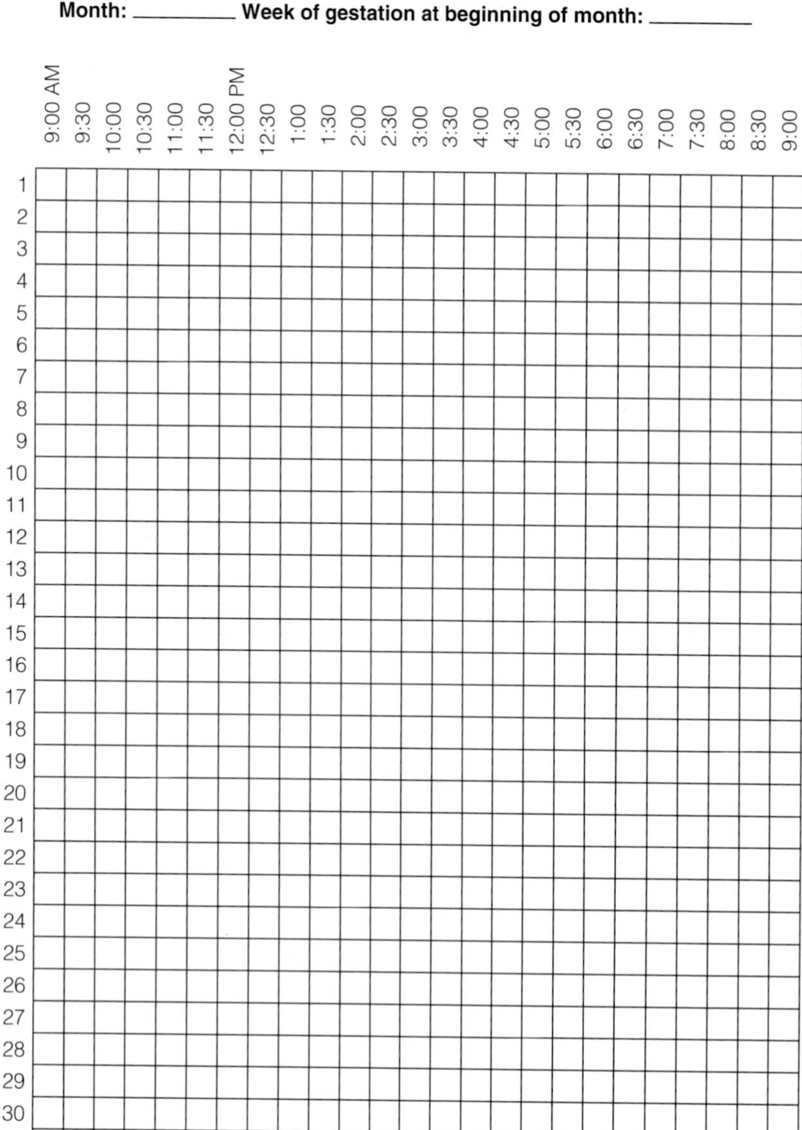

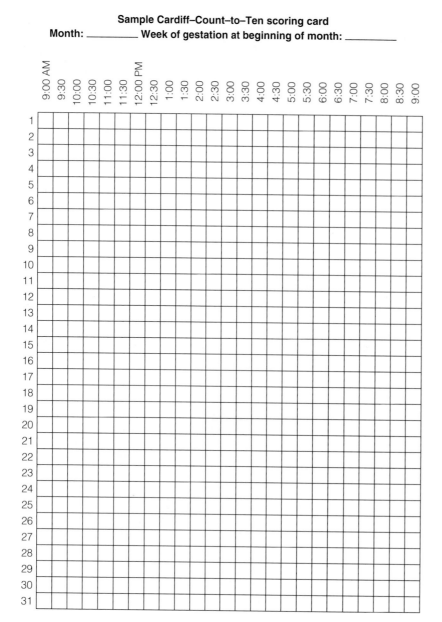

**FIGURE 9–6** ♦ Fetal movement assessment method: the Cardiff Count-to-Ten scoring card (adaptation).

woman can check with her certified nurse-midwife or physician about taking part in strenuous sports, such as skiing and horseback riding. In general, however, the skilled sportswoman is no longer discouraged from participating in these activities if her pregnancy is uncomplicated. However, pregnancy is not the appropriate time to learn a new or strenuous sport.

Certain conditions contraindicate exercise. These conditions include rupture of the membranes, pregnancy-induced hypertension, incompetent cervix or cerclage placement, persistent vaginal bleeding, risk factors for preterm labor, evidence of intrauterine growth restriction, and chronic medical conditions that might be negatively impacted by vigorous exercise (Dickerson & Chez, 1999).

The American College of Obstetricians and Gynecologists (ACOG) has developed the following guidelines about exercise during pregnancy (ACOG, 1994):

- Even mild to moderate exercise is beneficial during pregnancy. Regular exercise, which occurs at least three times a week, is preferred.
- After the first trimester women should avoid exercising in the supine position. In most pregnant women, the supine position is associated with decreased cardiac output. Since uterine blood flow is reduced during exercise as blood is shunted from the visceral organs to the muscles, the remaining cardiac output is further decreased. Similarly, women should also avoid standing motionless for prolonged periods.
- Because decreased oxygen is available for aerobic exercise during pregnancy, women should modify the intensity of their exercise based on their symptoms, should stop when they become

fatigued, and should avoid exercising to the point of exhaustion. Non-weight-bearing exercises such as swimming and cycling are recommended because they decrease the risk of injury and provide fitness with comfort.

- As pregnancy progresses and the center of gravity changes, especially in the third trimester, women should avoid exercises in which the loss of balance could pose a risk to mother or fetus. Similarly, women should avoid any type of exercise that might result in even mild abdominal trauma.
- A normal pregnancy requires an additional 300 kcal per day. Women who exercise regularly during pregnancy should be careful to ensure that they consume an adequate diet.
- To augment heat dissipation, especially during the first trimester, pregnant women who exercise should wear clothing that is comfortable and loose, ensure adequate hydration, and avoid the prolonged overheating associated with vigorous exercise in hot, humid weather because of the possible teratogenic effects of hyperthermia on the fetus (Heffernan, 2000). For the same reason, pregnant women are advised to avoid hot tubs and saunas.
- Women should avoid reaching their maximum physical effort during pregnancy. Thus, as a general rule, their pulse rates should not exceed 140 beats per minute (Shrock, 2000).

The nurse may also suggest that the woman wear a supportive bra and appropriate shoes when exercising. She should be advised to warm up and stretch to help prepare the joints for activity and cool down with a period of mild activity to help restore circulation and avoid pooling of blood. A moderate, rhythmic exercise routine involving large muscle groups such as swimming, cycling, or brisk walking is best. Jogging or running is acceptable for women already conditioned to these activities as long as they avoid exercising at maximum effort and overheating.

Warning signs include pain of any kind, nausea or vomiting, swelling, back pain, decreased or absent fetal movement, difficulty walking, dizziness, blurred vision, palpitations, pubic pain, shortness of breath, tachycardia, uterine contractions, vaginal bleeding, or fluid loss (Heffernan, 2000). The woman should stop exercising if these symptoms occur and modify her exercise program. If the symptoms persist, the woman should contact her caregiver.

Adequate rest in pregnancy is important for both physical and emotional health. Women need more sleep throughout pregnancy, particularly in the first and last trimesters, when they tire easily. Without adequate rest, pregnant women have less resilience. Finding time to rest during the day may be difficult for women who work outside the home or who have small children. The nurse can help the expectant mother examine her daily schedule to develop a realistic plan for short periods of rest and relaxation.

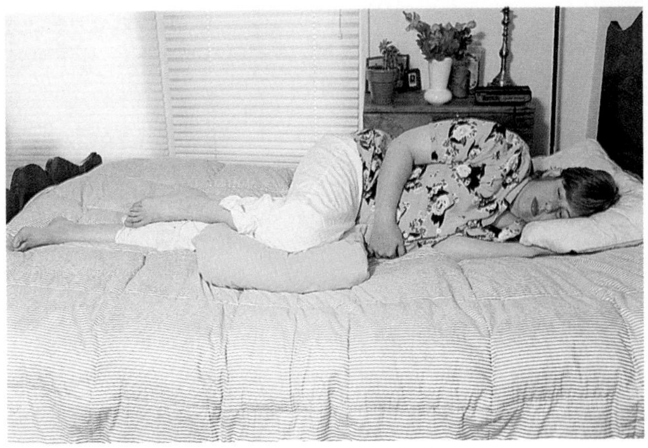

FIGURE 9–7 ♦ Position for relaxation and rest as pregnancy progresses.

Sleeping becomes more difficult during the last trimester because of the enlarged abdomen, increased frequency of urination, and greater activity of the fetus. Finding a comfortable position becomes difficult for the pregnant woman. Figure 9–7♦ shows a position most pregnant women find comfortable. Progressive relaxation techniques similar to those taught in prepared childbirth classes can help prepare the woman for sleep.

## Exercises to Prepare for Childbirth

Certain exercises help strengthen muscle tone in preparation for birth and promote more rapid restoration of muscle tone after birth. Some physical changes of pregnancy can be minimized by faithfully practicing prescribed body-conditioning exercises. Many body-conditioning exercises for pregnancy are taught; a few of the more common ones are discussed here.

The **pelvic tilt,** or pelvic rocking, helps prevent or reduce back strain as it strengthens abdominal muscles. To do the pelvic tilt, the pregnant woman lies on her back and puts her feet flat on the floor. This flexes the knees and helps prevent strain or discomfort. She decreases the curvature in her back by pressing her spine toward the floor. With her back pressed to the floor, the woman tightens her abdominal muscles as she tightens and tucks in her buttocks. The woman can also perform the pelvic tilt on her hands and knees (Figure 9–8♦), while sitting in a chair, or while standing with her back against a wall. The body alignment that results when

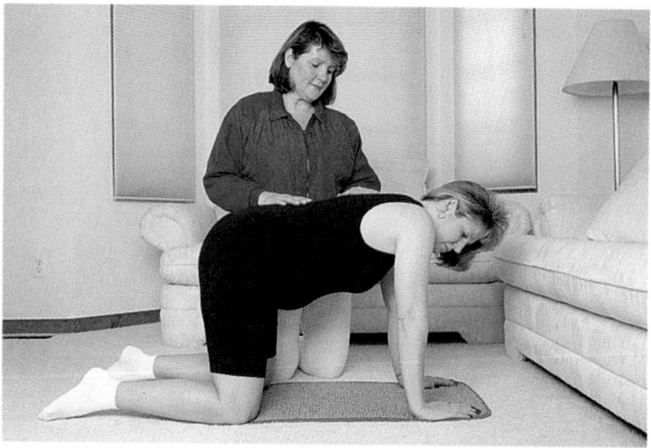

A

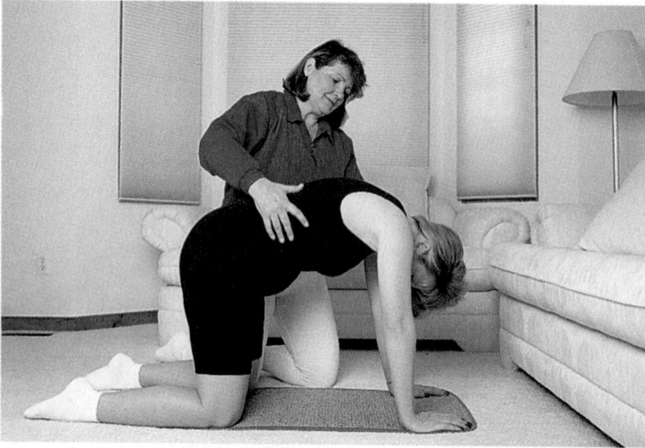

B

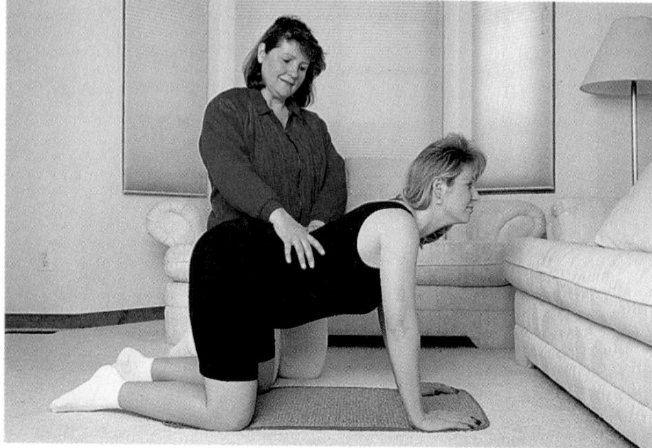

C

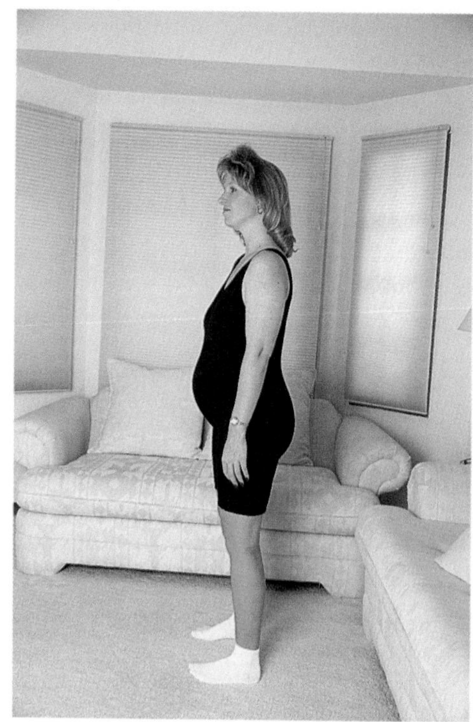

D

FIGURE 9–8 ♦ **A,** Starting position when the pelvic tilt is done on hands and knees. The back is flat and parallel to the floor, the hands are below the head, and the knees are directly below the buttocks. **B,** A prenatal yoga instructor offers pointers for proper positioning for the first part of the tilt: head up, neck long and separated from the shoulders, buttocks up, and pelvis thrust back, allowing the back to drop and release on an inhaled breath. **C,** The instructor helps the woman assume the correct position for the next part of the tilt. It is done on a long exhalation, allowing the pregnant woman to arch her back, drop her head loosely, push away from her hands, and draw in the muscles of her abdomen to strengthen them. Note that in this position the pelvis and buttocks are tucked under, and the buttock muscles are tightened. **D,** Proper posture. The knees are slightly bent but not locked, and the pelvis and buttocks are tucked under, thereby lengthening the spine and helping support the weighty abdomen. With her chin tucked in, this woman's neck, shoulders, hips, knees, and feet are all in a straight line perpendicular to the floor. Her feet are parallel. This is also the starting position for doing the pelvic tilt while standing.

the pelvic tilt is done correctly should be maintained as much as possible throughout the day.

## Abdominal Exercises

A basic exercise to increase abdominal muscle tone is tightening abdominal muscles with each breath. It can be done in any position, but it is best learned while the woman lies supine. With knees flexed and feet flat on the floor, the woman expands her abdomen and slowly takes

## HINTS FOR PRACTICE

Doing the pelvic rock on hands and knees may aggravate back strain. Teach women with a history of minor back problems to do the pelvic rock only in the standing position.

a deep breath. Exhaling slowly, she gradually pulls in her abdominal muscles until they are fully contracted. She relaxes for a few seconds and then repeats the exercise.

Partial sit-ups strengthen abdominal muscle tone and are done according to individual comfort levels. A partial sit-up must be done with the knees flexed and the feet flat on the floor to avoid strain on the lower back. The woman stretches her arms toward her knees as she slowly pulls her head and shoulders off the floor to a comfortable level (if she has poor abdominal muscle tone, she may not be able to pull up very far). She then slowly returns to the starting position, takes a deep breath, and repeats the exercise. To strengthen the oblique abdominal muscles, she repeats the process but stretches the left arm to the side of her right knee, returns to the floor, takes a deep breath, and then reaches with the right arm to the left knee.

These exercises can be done approximately five times in a sequence, and the sequence can be repeated at other times during the day as desired. It is important to do the exercises slowly to prevent muscle strain and overtiring.

### Perineal Exercises

Perineal muscle tightening, also called **Kegel exercises,** strengthens the pubococcygeus muscle and increases its elasticity (Figure 9–9♦). The woman can feel the specific muscle group to be exercised by stopping urination midstream. Doing Kegel exercises while urinating is discouraged, however, because this practice has been associated with urinary stasis and urinary tract infection.

Childbirth educators sometimes use the following technique to teach Kegel exercises. They tell the woman to think of her perineal muscles as an elevator. When she relaxes, the elevator is on the first floor. To do the exercises, she contracts, bringing the elevator to the second, third, and fourth floors. She keeps the elevator on the fourth floor for a few seconds, and then gradually relaxes the area. If the exercise is properly done, the woman does not contract the muscles of the buttocks and thighs.

Kegel exercises can be done at almost any time. Some women use ordinary events—for instance, stopping at a red light—as a cue to remember to do the exercise. Others do Kegel exercises while waiting in a checkout line, talking on the telephone, or watching television.

### Inner Thigh Exercises

The nurse can advise the pregnant woman to assume a cross-legged sitting position whenever possible. This "tailor sit" stretches the muscles of the inner thighs in preparation for labor and birth.

## Sexual Activity

As a result of the physiologic, anatomic, and emotional changes of pregnancy, couples usually have many questions and concerns about sexual activity during pregnancy. Often, these questions are about possible injury to the baby or the woman during intercourse and about changes in the desire each partner feels for the other.

In the past, couples were often warned to avoid sexual intercourse during the last 6 to 8 weeks of pregnancy to prevent complications such as infection or premature rupture of the membranes. However, these fears seem to be unfounded. In a healthy pregnancy, there is no medical reason to limit sexual activity. Intercourse is contraindicated for medical reasons such as multiple pregnancy, threatened abortion, incompetent cervix, partner with sexually transmitted infection, or maternal history of miscarriage following orgasm (Shrock, 2000). Most caregivers also advise against intercourse when the membranes are ruptured and in women with a history of preterm labor.

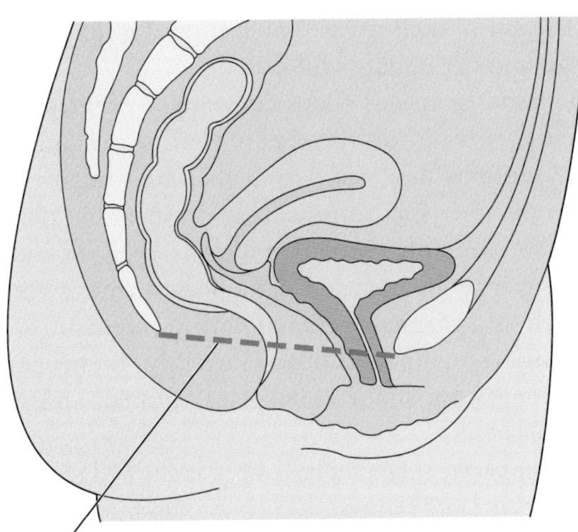


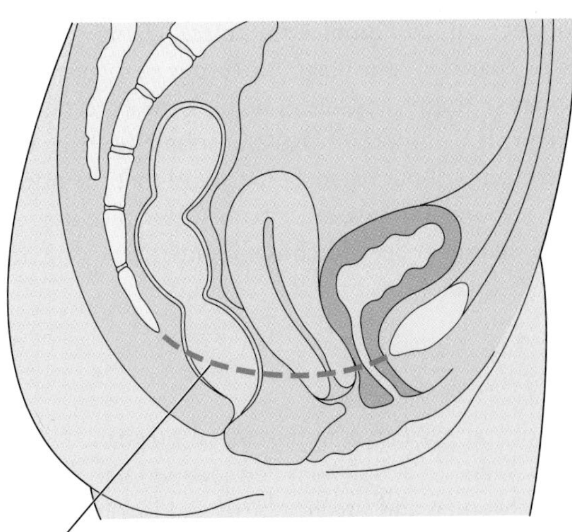


FIGURE 9–9 ♦ Kegel exercises. The woman learns to tighten the pubococcygeus muscle, which improves support to the pelvic organs.

The expectant mother may experience changes in sexual desire and response. Often, these changes are related to the various discomforts that occur throughout pregnancy. For instance, during the first trimester fatigue or nausea and vomiting may decrease desire, and breast tenderness may make the woman less responsive to fondling of her breasts. During the second trimester, many of the discomforts have lessened, and, with the vascular congestion of the pelvis, the woman may experience greater sexual satisfaction than she experienced before pregnancy.

During the third trimester, interest in coitus may again decrease as the woman becomes more uncomfortable and fatigued. In addition, shortness of breath, painful pelvic ligaments, urinary frequency, leg cramps, and decreased mobility may lessen sexual desire and activity. If they are not already doing so, the couple should consider coital positions other than male superior, such as side-by-side, female superior, and vaginal rear entry.

Sexual activity does not have to include intercourse. Many of the nurturing and sexual needs of the pregnant woman can be satisfied by cuddling, kissing, and being held. The warm, sensual feelings that accompany these activities can be an end in themselves. Her partner, however, may choose to masturbate more frequently than before.

The sexual desires of men are also affected by many factors in pregnancy. These factors include the previous relationship with the partner, acceptance of the pregnancy, attitudes toward the partner's change of appearance, and concern about hurting the expectant mother or baby. Some men find it difficult to view their partners as sexually appealing while they are adjusting to the concept of them as mothers. Other men find their partners' pregnancies arousing and experience feelings of increased happiness, intimacy, and closeness.

The expectant couple should be aware of their changing sexual desires, the normality of these changes, and the importance of communicating these changes to each other so that they can make nurturing adaptations. The nurse has an important role in helping the expectant couple adapt. It is important that the couple feel free to express concerns about sexual activity and that the nurse be able to respond and give anticipatory guidance in a comfortable manner. See Teaching Guide: Sexual Activity during Pregnancy, on page 217.

## Dental Care

Proper dental hygiene is important in pregnancy. In fact, research suggests a link between periodontal disease in pregnant women and preterm birth and low-birth-weight infants (Carl, Roux, & Matacale, 2000). In spite of such discomforts as nausea and vomiting, gum hypertrophy and tenderness, possible ptyalism, and heartburn, it is important for pregnant women to maintain regular oral hygiene.

The nurse can encourage the pregnant woman have a dental checkup early in her pregnancy. General dental repair and extractions can be done during pregnancy, preferably under local anesthetic. The second trimester is considered the most appropriate time for dental treatment (Carl et al., 2000). The woman should inform her dentist of her pregnancy so that she is not exposed to teratogenic substances. Dental x-ray examinations and extensive dental work need to be delayed until after the birth when possible.

## Immunizations

All women of childbearing age need to be aware of the risks of receiving certain immunizations if pregnancy is possible. Immunizations with attenuated live viruses, such as rubella vaccine, should not be given in pregnancy because of the teratogenic effect of the live viruses on the developing embryo. Vaccinations using killed viruses may be used, however.

## Complementary and Alternative Therapies (CAM)

As discussed in Chapter 1, many women are electing to use complementary and alternative medicine (CAM) such as homeopathy, herbal medicine, acupressure and acupuncture, biofeedback, therapeutic touch, massage, and chiropractic as part of a holistic approach to their health care regimens. However, they often choose not to report use of alternative approaches to their health care provider (Eisenberg, Davis, Ettner, et al., 1998). It is important that nurses working with pregnant women and childbearing families develop a general understanding of the more commonly used therapies to be able to answer basic questions and to provide resources as needed.

This section focuses on homeopathy and herbal medicine because of their special implications for the pregnant woman and her unborn child.

*Homeopathy* means "like suffering." Homeopathic medicine is based on the theory that a substance can cure symptoms in a sick person that are similar to the symptoms the substance causes in healthy people. Thus, for example, ipecac, which is used to induce vomiting, may be used to treat a person who is vomiting such as a pregnant woman with severe nausea and vomiting (Fontaine, 2000). Currently homeopathic practitioners use about 2000 plant, animal, and mineral substances.

Homeopathic therapies have been identified to address pregnancy-related symptoms such as musculoskeletal disorders, anemia, nausea, ptyalism, pica, threatened miscarriage, and preterm labor. According to homeopathic theory, homeopathic remedies either help an individual or have no effect. However, a healing crisis or aggravation

# TEACHING GUIDE *Sexual Activity during Pregnancy*

## Assessment

Occasionally a woman indicates her beliefs about sexual activity during pregnancy by asking a direct question. Often, however, the nurse must ask some general questions to determine the woman's level of understanding. In many cases teaching about this topic is coupled with ongoing assessment of the woman's understanding of sexual activity during pregnancy.

## Nursing Diagnosis

The key nursing diagnosis will probably be

Health-seeking behaviors: information on sexuality during pregnancy related to the woman's expressed desire for clarification.

## Nursing Plan and Implementation

The teaching plan generally focuses on discussion. The presence of both partners may be beneficial in fostering communication between them and is acceptable unless personal or cultural factors indicate otherwise.

## Client Goals

At the completion of the teaching the woman will be able to

- Relate the changes in sexuality and sexual response that may occur during pregnancy to changes in technique, frequency, and response that may be indicated.
- Explore personal attitudes, beliefs, and expectations about sexual activity during pregnancy.
- Cite maternal factors that would contraindicate sexual intercourse.

## *Teaching Plan*

| CONTENT | TEACHING METHOD |
|---|---|
| Begin by explaining that the pregnant woman may experience changes in desire during the course of pregnancy. During the first trimester, discomforts such as nausea, fatigue, and breast tenderness may make intercourse less desirable for many women. | Universal statements that give permission, such as "Many couples experience changes in sexual desire during pregnancy. What kind of changes have you experienced?" are often effective in starting discussion. Depending on the woman's (or couple's) level of knowledge and sophistication, part or all of this discussion may be necessary. |
| In the second trimester, as symptoms decrease, desire may increase. In the third trimester, discomfort and fatigue may lead to decreased desire in the woman. | |
| Explain that men may notice changes in their level of desire, too. Among other things, this change may be related to feelings about their partner's changing appearance, their belief about the acceptability of sexual activity with a pregnant woman, or concern about hurting the woman or fetus. Some men find the changes of pregnancy erotic; others must adjust to the notion of their partners as mothers. | If the partner is present, approach him in the same nonjudgmental way used above. If not, ask the woman if she has noticed any changes in her partner or if he has expressed any concerns. |
| Explain that the woman may notice that orgasms are much more intense during the last weeks of pregnancy and may be followed by cramping. Because of the pressure of the enlarging uterus on the vena cava, the woman should not lie flat on her back for intercourse after about the fourth month. If the couple prefer that position, a pillow should be placed under her right hip to displace the uterus. Alternate positions such as side-by-side, female superior, or vaginal rear entry may become necessary as her uterus enlarges. | Deal with any specific questions about the physical and psychological changes that the couple may have. |
| Stress that sexual activities that both partners enjoy are generally acceptable. It is not advisable for couples who favor anal sex to go from anal penetration to vaginal penetration because of the risk of introducing *Escherichia coli* into the vagina. | Discussion about various sexual activities requires that you be comfortable with your sexuality and tactful. |
| Suggest that alternative methods of expressing intimacy and affection such as cuddling, holding and stroking each other, and kissing may help maintain the couple's feelings of warmth and closeness. If the man feels desire for further sexual release, his partner may help him masturbate to ejaculation, or he may prefer to masturbate in private. | The couple may be content with these approaches to meeting their sexual needs, or they may require assurance that such approaches are indeed "normal." |

## TEACHING GUIDE *Sexual Activity during Pregnancy continued*

### *Teaching Plan*

Advise the woman who is interested in masturbation as a form of gratification that the orgasmic contractions may be especially intense in later pregnancy.

Stress that sexual intercourse is contraindicated once the membranes are ruptured or if bleeding is present. Women with a history of preterm labor may be advised to avoid intercourse because the oxytocin that is released with orgasm stimulates uterine contractions and may trigger preterm labor. Because oxytocin is also released with nipple stimulation, fondling the breasts may also be contraindicated in those cases.

An explanation of the contraindications accompanied by their rationale provides specific guidelines that most couples find helpful.

A discussion of sexuality and sexual activity should stress the importance of open communication so that the couple feel comfortable expressing their feelings, preferences, and concerns.

Some couples are skilled at expressing their feelings about sexual activity. Others find it difficult and can benefit from specific suggestions. The nurse should provide opportunities for discussion throughout the talk.

Specific handouts on sexual activity are also helpful for couples and may address topics that were not discussed.

### EVALUATION

Evaluate the learning by assessing the woman's (or couple's) response to information throughout the discussion. Ask the woman to express information such as the contraindications to intercourse in her own words. Follow-up sessions and questions from the woman also provide information about teaching effectiveness.

of symptoms can occur if the remedy is given in too high a potency or repeated too frequently (Brennan, 1999).

*Herbal medicine* focuses on the use of therapies derived from plants. Many of these therapies have been used for centuries in different parts of the world and are widely recognized. In fact, countries such as Germany, Canada, England, and France recognize the benefits of scores of herbs and include information about their safety and use as part of formal educational programs for physicians and pharmacists.

In the United States, herbs are categorized as dietary supplements rather than drugs and are often used by pregnant women. Pregnant women interested in using herbs are best advised to follow three basic principles: (1) avoid the use of herbs, even tonic herbs, during the first trimester, whenever possible; (2) avoid standardized or highly concentrated extracts because the risk of side effects tends to be higher than with whole plant extracts; and (3) do not take essential oils internally (Belew, 1999). In addition, pregnant women need to avoid certain categories of herbs such as abortifacient (abortion-inducing) herbs, herbs that induce menstruation, nervous system stimulants, stimulant laxatives, and so forth. Lists identifying common herbs that women are advised to avoid or use with caution during pregnancy and lactation are available.

Nurses caring for pregnant women can develop printed materials describing the use of homeopathic remedies and herbs during pregnancy and identifying those that may present a risk. It is especially important that women choosing these complementary approaches consult someone who is knowledgeable, well trained, and experienced in the specific therapy and that they buy their herbs or homeopathic remedies from reputable manufacturers (Belew, 1999).

## TERATOGENIC SUBSTANCES

Substances that adversely affect the normal growth and development of the fetus are called *teratogens* (see Chapter 3). Many substances are known or suspected teratogens, including, for example, certain medications, psychotropic drugs, and alcohol. The harmful effects of others, such as some pesticides or exposure to x-rays in the first trimester of pregnancy, have also been documented. It is essential to provide pregnant women with information about recognized teratogens and environmental risks.

### MEDICATIONS

The use of medications during pregnancy, including prescriptions, over-the-counter drugs, and herbal remedies, is of great concern. Many pregnant women need medication for therapeutic purposes, such as the treatment of infections, allergies, or other pathologic processes. In these situations, the problem can be very complex. Known teratogenic agents are not prescribed and usually can be replaced by medications considered safe. Even when a woman is highly motivated to avoid taking any medications, she may have taken potentially teratogenic medications before her pregnancy was confirmed, especially if she has an irregular menstrual cycle.

The greatest potential for gross abnormalities in the fetus occurs during the first trimester of pregnancy, when fetal organs are first developing. The classic period of *teratogenesis* in a woman with a 28-day cycle extends from day 31 after the LMP (17 days after fertilization) to day 71 (54 days after fertilization) (Niebyl, 1999). Many factors influence teratogenic effects, including the specific type of teratogen and the dose, the stage of embryo development, and the genetic sensitivity of the mother and fetus (ACOG, 1997c). For example, the commonly prescribed acne medication isotretinoin (Accutane) is associated with a high incidence of spontaneous abortion and congenital malformations if taken early in pregnancy.

To provide information for caregivers and clients, the U.S. Food and Drug Administration (FDA) has developed the following classification system for medications administered during pregnancy:

*Category A:* Controlled studies in women have demonstrated no associated fetal risk. Few drugs fall into this category.

*Category B:* Animal studies show no risk, but there are no controlled studies in women, or animal studies indicate a risk, but controlled human studies fail to demonstrate a risk. The penicillins fall into this category.

*Category C:* Either (1) no adequate animal or human studies are available or (2) animal studies show teratogenic effects, but no controlled studies in women are available. Many drugs fall into this category, which, because of the lack of information, is a problematic one for caregivers. Epinephrine, beta-blockers, and zidovudine (a drug used to decrease perinatal transmission of human immunodeficiency virus) fall into this category.

*Category D:* Evidence of human fetal risk exists, but the benefits of the drug in certain situations are thought to outweigh the risks. Examples of drugs in this category include tetracycline, vincristine, lithium, and hydrochlorothiazide.

*Category X:* The demonstrated fetal risks clearly outweigh any possible benefit. Examples of drugs in this category include isotretinoin (Accutane), the acne medication, which can cause multiple central nervous system (CNS), facial, and cardiovascular anomalies.

If a woman has taken a drug in category D or X, she should be informed of the risks associated with that drug and of her alternatives. Similarly, a woman who has taken a drug in the safer categories can be reassured (Cunningham et al., 1997).

This system, while useful, has been criticized because the use of letters suggests a risk grading that is not necessarily accurate. More importantly, not all drugs in a category have the same risk level. Currently the FDA is working to develop a new labeling system (Whitney, 1999).

Although the first trimester is the critical period for teratogenesis, some medications are known to have a teratogenic effect when taken in the second and third trimesters. For example, tetracycline taken in late pregnancy is commonly associated with staining of teeth in children and has been shown to depress skeletal growth, especially in premature infants. Sulfonamides taken in the last few weeks of pregnancy are known to compete with bilirubin attachment of protein-binding sites, increasing the risk of jaundice in the newborn (Niebyl, 1999).

Pregnant women need to avoid all medication—prescribed, homeopathic, or over-the-counter—if possible. If no alternative exists, it is wisest to select a well-known medication rather than a newer drug whose potential teratogenic effects may not be known. When possible, the oral form of a drug should be used, and it should be prescribed in the lowest possible therapeutic dose for the shortest time possible. Finally, the caregiver needs to consider the multiple components of the medication. Caution is the watchword for nurses caring for pregnant women who have been taking medications. It is essential that pregnant women check with their certified nurse-midwives or physicians about any herbs or medications they were taking when pregnancy occurred and about any nonprescription drugs they are thinking of using. The advantage of using a particular medication must outweigh the risks. Any medication with possible teratogenic effects is best avoided.

### Tobacco

Infants of mothers who smoke cigarettes tend to have a lower birth weight and a higher incidence of preterm birth than infants of mothers who do not smoke (Cunningham et al., 1997). For women with a twin pregnancy, this effect is even more pronounced (Pollack, Lantz, & Frohna, 2000). In addition, mothers who smoke have an increased risk of preterm birth, placenta previa, abruptio placentae, ectopic pregnancy, and premature rupture of the membranes (Castles, Adams, Melvin, et al., 1999). The risk is related to the number of cigarettes smoked. Similarly, smoking has been linked to an increased risk of cleft lip and palate in the newborn (Chung, Kowalski, Kim, et al., 2000). Research also links maternal smoking, both during pregnancy and afterward, with an increased risk of sudden infant death syndrome (SIDS), as well as with an increased risk of acute respiratory illnesses and chronic respiratory symptoms in infants (ACOG, 1997b). The specific mechanism of smoking's effect on the fetus is not known. However, the main ingredients in cigarette smoke that account for adverse effects in the fetus are carbon monoxide and nicotine because they decrease the availability of oxygen to maternal and fetal tissues.

Currently about 12.9% of women smoke during pregnancy. This rate has declined steadily since 1989—a positive trend. Unfortunately, tobacco use by pregnant teens continues to increase (Ventura, Martin, Curtin, et al., 2000). Women who smoke tend to stop smoking or at least reduce their intake once pregnancy is confirmed. However, a majority of women who quit smoking during pregnancy resume following childbirth, although this percentage is lower for women who quit early in pregnancy. This finding suggests that although women are aware of the potential impact of smoking on the fetus, they may be less knowledgeable about the effects of passive smoke on the baby.

Any decrease in smoking during pregnancy most likely improves fetal outcome, and researchers continue to explore approaches designed to help women quit smoking. Pregnancy may be a difficult time for a woman to stop smoking, but the nurse should encourage her to reduce the number of cigarettes she smokes daily. The perceived need to protect her unborn child may increase her motivation.

### Alcohol

Fetuses of women who drink heavily are at increased risk of developing **fetal alcohol syndrome** (Chapter 25). In fact, currently fetal alcohol syndrome, which is characterized by growth retardation, facial anomalies, and central nervous system dysfunction of varying severity, is the major cause of mental retardation in the Western world (Brennan, 1999).

The effects of moderate intake of alcohol during pregnancy are unclear. Research indicates an increased incidence of lowered birth weight and some neurologic effects, such as attention deficit disorder. Evidence suggests that the risk of teratogenic effects increases proportionately with increased average daily intake of alcohol. Although an occasional drink during pregnancy does not carry any known risk, no safe level of drinking during pregnancy has been identified (Niebyl, 1999); thus caregivers recommend that pregnant women abstain from all alcohol during pregnancy. In most cases, once a woman becomes aware of her pregnancy, she decreases her consumption of alcohol. However, the alcohol consumed after conception and before pregnancy is diagnosed remains a cause for concern.

Assessment of alcohol intake is a major part of every woman's medical history, with questions asked in a direct, nonjudgmental manner. All women need to be counseled about the role of alcohol in pregnancy. If heavy consumption is involved, the nurse can refer the pregnant woman immediately to an alcoholic treatment program. Counselors in these programs need to be made aware of a woman's pregnancy before drug therapy is suggested, since certain drugs may be harmful to the developing fetus. For example, the drug disulfiram (Antabuse), often used in conjunction with alcohol treatment, is suspected to be a teratogenic agent.

### Caffeine

Current research reveals no evidence that caffeine has teratogenic effects in humans. However, maternal coffee consumption decreases iron absorption and may increase the risk of anemia (Niebyl, 1999). Until more definitive data are available, nurses can advise women about common sources of caffeine, including coffee, tea, colas, and chocolate, and suggest that they moderate their daily caffeine intake.

### Marijuana

The prevalence of marijuana use in our society raises many concerns about its effect on the fetus, but, to date, no teratogenic effects of marijuana use during pregnancy have been documented (Niebyl, 1999). Research on marijuana use in pregnancy is difficult, however, because it is an illegal drug. Unreliability of reporting, lack of a representative population, inability to determine strength or composition of the marijuana used (including the presence of herbicides), and use of other drugs at the same time are major factors complicating the research being done.

### Cocaine

A woman who uses cocaine during pregnancy is at increased risk for acute myocardial infarction, cardiac arrhythmias, ruptured ascending aorta, seizures, cerebrovascular accidents, hyperthermia, bowel ischemia, and sudden death (Cunningham et al., 1997). Cocaine use during pregnancy has been related to abruptio placentae, preterm birth, fetal distress, low birth weight, neonatal withdrawal, SIDS, and spontaneous pneumothorax (Chan, Pham, & Reece, 1997). Several congenital anomalies in the neonate have also been linked to maternal cocaine use, including, for example, genitourinary anomalies, congenital heart defects, limb reduction defects, and CNS anomalies (Cunningham et al., 1997) (see also Chapter 12).

As the number of women of childbearing age using cocaine increases, health care providers need to become more alert to early signs of cocaine use. It is often difficult for a nurse or physician to face the fact that a client is using cocaine, but ongoing alertness and an open, nonjudgmental approach are important in early detection. Urine screening for cocaine is valuable, but because cocaine is metabolized rapidly, the drug screen is negative within 24 to 48 hours after cocaine use. Thus it is probable that many expectant mothers who use cocaine are not identified.

## Evaluation

Throughout the antepartal period, evaluation is an ongoing and essential part of effective nursing care. As nurses ask questions of the pregnant woman and her family or make observations of physical changes, they are evaluating the results of previous interventions. In evaluating the effectiveness of the interactions, nurses can try creative solutions if they are logical and carefully thought out. Creative solutions are especially important in dealing with families from other cultures. If a practice is important to a woman and not harmful, the culturally competent nurse will not discourage it.

In completing an evaluation, the nurse also recognizes situations that require referral for further evaluation. For example, a woman who has gained 4 lb in a single week does not require counseling about nutrition; she needs further assessment for preeclampsia. The nurse who has a sound knowledge of theory will recognize this need and act immediately.

The ongoing and cyclic nature of the nursing process is especially evident in the prenatal setting. However, throughout the course of pregnancy certain criteria can be used to determine the quality of care provided. In essence, nursing care has been effective if

- The common discomforts of pregnancy are quickly identified and are relieved or lessened effectively.
- The woman is able to discuss the physiologic and psychologic changes of pregnancy.
- The woman implements self-care measures, if they are indicated, during pregnancy.
- The woman avoids substances and situations that pose a risk to her well-being or that of her child.
- The woman seeks regular prenatal care.

## Care of the Expectant Couple over Age 35

Today an increasing number of women are choosing to have their first baby after age 35. In fact, in the United States the rate of first births to women between the ages of 35 and 39 has nearly doubled since 1978, from 19 per 1000 women to 37.4. For women between the ages of 40 and 44, the birth rate increased by over 90% during the same period (Ventura et al., 2000). Many factors have contributed to this trend, including the following:

- The availability of effective birth control methods
- The expanded roles and career options available for women
- The increased number of women obtaining advanced education, pursuing careers, and delaying parenthood until they are established professionally
- The increased incidence of later marriage and second marriage
- The high cost of living, which causes some young couples to delay childbearing until they are more secure financially
- The increased number of women in this older reproductive age group due to the baby boom between 1946 and 1964
- The increased availability of specialized fertilization procedures, which offer opportunities for women who had previously been considered infertile

There are advantages to having a first baby after age 35. Single women or couples who delay childbearing until they are older tend to be well educated and financially secure. Usually their decision to have a baby was deliberately and thoughtfully made (Figure 9–10♦). Compared with younger women, women over age 35 tend to be more emotionally stable and more likely to obtain early prenatal care and demonstrate healthful behaviors during

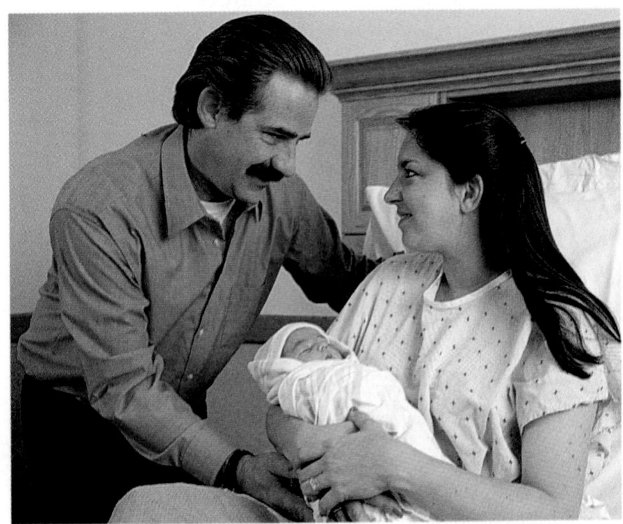

FIGURE 9–10 ♦ For many older couples, the decision to have a child may be very rewarding.

their pregnancy (Catanzarite, Deutchman, Johnson et al., 1995). Because of their greater life experiences, they also are more aware of the realities of having a child and what it means to have a baby at their age (Windridge & Berryman, 1999). Many of the women have experienced fulfillment in their careers and feel secure enough to take on the added responsibility of a child. Some women are ready to make a change in their lives, desiring to stay home with a new baby. Those who plan to continue working typically are able to afford good child care.

## Medical Risks

In the United States, over the past 30 years, the risk of fetal death has declined dramatically for women of all ages because of advances in maternal health and obstetrical practice. However, the risk for fetal death remains highest among teenagers and among women age 40 and older (National Center for Health Statistics, 1999). In addition, women who give birth to a first child after age 40 have a higher risk of preterm birth, preeclampsia, and perinatal mortality (Scholz, Haas, & Petru, 1999), as well as a higher incidence of low-birth-weight infants and infants with congenital malformations (Gilbert, Nesbitt, & Danielson, 1999).

Similarly, in both the United States and Canada, the risk of maternal mortality, though low generally, increases with maternal age. For women age 40 or older, the risk of dying from a pregnancy-related or pregnancy-aggravated cause is 5 times higher than the risk for women ages 20 to 24 years (Hoyert, Danel, & Tully, 2000).

Women over age 35, and, even more, women over age 40, are more likely to have chronic medical conditions that can complicate a pregnancy. Preexisting medical conditions such as hypertension or diabetes probably play a more significant role than age in maternal well-being and the outcome of pregnancy. The frequency of medical complications in pregnant women over age 35 increases in the cardiovascular, neurologic, connective tissue, renal, and pulmonary systems (Cunningham et al., 1997).

The cesarean birth rate is also increased in pregnant women over age 35. This practice may be related to pregnancy complications as well as to increased concern by the woman and physician about the pregnancy outcome (Windridge & Berryman, 1999).

The risk of conceiving a child with Down syndrome increases with age, especially over age 35. Amniocentesis is routinely offered to all women over age 35 to permit the early detection of several chromosomal abnormalities, including Down syndrome. Routine genetic testing has not been offered to couples in whom there is only advanced paternal age because there is not sufficient evidence to determine a specific paternal age at which to start genetic testing. However, advanced paternal age affects autosomal dominant inherited diseases, such as neurofibromatosis, achondroplasia, and Marfan syndrome (ACOG, 1997a).

Research has also focused on the use of multiple marker screening to detect Down syndrome and trisomy 18. A blood test is used to detect levels of specific serum markers—namely, alpha-fetoprotein, human chorionic gonadotropin, and unconjugated estriol. When these tests in combination show certain patterns of increase or decrease, they are considered positive and the woman is advised to consider amniocentesis. Although these tests are not as definite as amniocentesis or chorionic villus sampling in detecting abnormalities, they are safer and less expensive (Rose & Mennuti, 1995).

## Special Concerns of the Expectant Couple over Age 35

No matter what their age, most expectant couples have concerns regarding the well-being of the fetus and their ability to parent. Expectant parents over age 35 often have additional concerns related to their age, especially the closer they are to age 40. Some couples are concerned about whether they will have enough energy to care for a new baby. Of greater concern is their ability to deal with the needs of the child as they age.

The financial concerns of the older couple are usually different from those of the younger couple. The older couple is generally more financially secure than the younger couple. However, when their "baby" is ready for college, the older couple may be close to retirement and might not have the means to provide for their child.

While considering their financial future and future retirement, the older couple may be forced to face their own mortality. Certainly the realization of one's mortality is not uncommon in midlife, but instead of confronting this issue at 40 to 45 years of age or later, the older expectant couple may confront the issue earlier as they consider what will happen as their child grows.

Older couples facing pregnancy following a late or second marriage or after therapy for infertility may find themselves somewhat isolated socially. They may feel different because they are often the only couple in their peer group expecting their first baby. In fact, many of their peers are likely to be parents of adolescents or young adults and may be grandparents as well.

The response of older couples who already have children to learning that the woman is pregnant may vary greatly depending on whether the pregnancy was planned or unexpected. Other factors influencing their response include their children's, family's, and friends' attitudes toward the pregnancy; the impact on their lifestyle; and the financial implications of having another child. Sometimes couples who had previously been married to other mates will choose to have a child together. The concept of blended family applies to situations in which "her" children, "his" children, and "their" children come together as a new family group.

Health care professionals may treat the older expectant couple differently than they would a younger couple. Older women may be offered more medical procedures, such as amniocentesis and ultrasound, than younger women. An older woman may be discouraged from using a birthing room or birthing center even if she is healthy because her age is considered to put her at risk.

The woman who has delayed pregnancy may be concerned about the limited amount of time that she has to bear children. When pregnancy does not occur as quickly as she had hoped, the older woman may become increasingly anxious as time slips away on her "biological clock." When an older woman becomes pregnant but experiences a spontaneous abortion, her grief for the loss of her unborn child is exacerbated by her anxiety about her ability to conceive again in the time remaining to her.

**KEY FACTS TO REMEMBER**

*Pregnancy in Women over Age 35*

- Couples who choose pregnancy at a later age are usually financially secure and have made a thoughtful, planned choice.
- If the woman has no existing health problems, her risk during pregnancy is not appreciably higher than that of the general population.
- The decreased fertility of women over age 35 may make conception more difficult.
- The incidence of Down syndrome increases somewhat in women over age 35 and significantly in those over age 40.
- The couple may choose to have amniocentesis or chorionic villus sampling to gain information about the health of their fetus.

# Nursing Care Management

## Nursing Assessment and Diagnosis

In working with a woman in her late 30s or 40s who is pregnant, the nurse makes the same assessments as are indicated in caring for any woman who is pregnant. The nurse assesses physical status, the woman's understanding of pregnancy and the changes that accompany it, the couple's attitudes about the pregnancy and their expectations of the impact a baby will have on their lives, any health teaching needs, the degree of support the woman has available to her, and the woman's knowledge of infant care.

The nursing diagnoses applicable to pregnant women in general apply to pregnant women over age 35. Examples of other nursing diagnoses that may apply include the following:

- ***Decisional conflict*** related to unexpected pregnancy
- ***Moderate anxiety*** related to uncertainty about fetal well-being

## Nursing Plan and Implementation

Once an older couple has made the decision to have a child, it is the nurse's responsibility to respect and support the couple in this decision. As with any client, the nurse needs to discuss risks, identify concerns, and promote strengths. The woman's age should not be made an issue. It is helpful in promoting a sense of well-being for the nurse to treat the pregnancy as normal unless specific health risks are identified.

As the pregnancy continues, the nurse identifies and discusses concerns the woman may have related to her age or to specific health problems. The older woman who has made a conscious decision to become pregnant often has carefully thought through potential problems and may actually have fewer concerns than a younger woman or one with an unplanned pregnancy.

Childbirth education classes are important in promoting adaptation to the event of childbirth for expectant couples of any age. However, older expectant couples, who are still in the minority, often feel uncomfortable in classes in which most of the participants are much younger. Consequently, classes for expectant parents over age 35 are now available in many communities.

Women who are over age 35 and having their first baby tend to be better educated than other health care consumers. These clients frequently know the kind of care and services they want and may be assertive in their interactions with the health care system. The nurse should neither be intimidated by these individuals nor assume that anticipatory guidance and support are not needed. Instead, the nurse should support the couple's strengths and be sensitive to their individual needs.

In working with older expectant couples or an older single woman, the nurse needs to be sensitive to special needs. A particularly difficult issue these couples face is the possibility of bearing an unhealthy child or a child

## Critical Thinking in Practice

Constance Petrowski, a 24-year-old, GIPO, world-class marathon runner, is 11 weeks pregnant when she sees the nurse-midwife for her first prenatal exam. Because of her low body fat, her menses have always been irregular, and it had not occurred to Constance that she might be pregnant. Constance tells the certified nurse-midwife that she has just begun serious training for a marathon that is to take place when Constance is about 22 weeks pregnant. Constance says she has been told that it is fine to continue any physical activity at which one is proficient and says that she would like to compete in the marathon because she believes she has a chance to come in as one of the top three women runners. What should the nurse tell Constance about competing in the marathon?

Answers can be found in Appendix I.

with a genetic disorder. A triple screening test, also called multiple marker screen (MMS), is useful in assessing for Down syndrome. The test, offered to all pregnant women at about 16 to 18 weeks gestation, is especially important for women over age 35 because of their increased risk of Down syndrome. This blood test evaluates three factors: maternal serum alpha-fetoprotein (MSAFP), estriol, and hCG. If a fetus has Down syndrome, hCG levels tend to be higher than normal while estriol and MSAFP levels tend to be lower than normal. If the levels indicate high risk, further assessments are warranted (ACOG, 2000). Because of the risk of Down syndrome in these families, amniocentesis is often suggested.

For couples who agree to amniocentesis the first few months of pregnancy are a difficult time. Amniocentesis cannot be done until week 14 of pregnancy, and the chromosomal studies take roughly 2 weeks to complete. Their fear that the fetus is at risk may delay the successful completion of the psychologic tasks of early pregnancy.

The nurse can support couples who decide to have amniocentesis by providing information and answering questions about the procedure and by providing comfort and emotional support during the amniocentesis. If the results indicate that the fetus has Down syndrome or another genetic abnormality, the nurse can ensure that the couple has complete information about the condition, its range of possible manifestations, and its developmental implications.

### Evaluation

Anticipated outcomes of nursing care include the following:

- The woman and her partner are knowledgeable about the pregnancy and express confidence in their ability to make appropriate health care choices.
- The expectant couple (and their children) are able to cope with the pregnancy and its implications for the future.
- The woman receives effective health care throughout her pregnancy and during birth and the postpartum period.
- The woman and her partner develop skills in child care and parenting.

# Chapter Review

## CHAPTER HIGHLIGHTS

- Provision of anticipatory guidance about childbirth, the postpartum period, and childrearing is a primary responsibility of the nurse caring for women in an antepartal setting.
- The nurse assesses the expectant father's knowledge level and intended degree of participation and then works with the couple to help ensure a satisfying experience.
- Culturally based practices and proscribed activities may have an impact on the childbearing family.
- The common discomforts of pregnancy occur as a result of physiologic and anatomic changes. The nurse provides the woman with information about self-care activities aimed at reducing or relieving discomfort.
- To make self-care choices and acquire desired healthful habits, a pregnant woman requires accurate information about a range of subjects, from exercise to sexual activity and from bathing to immunization.
- Teratogenic substances are substances that adversely affect the normal growth and development of the fetus.
- A pregnant woman should avoid taking prescribed medications or using over-the-counter preparations during pregnancy.
- Evidence exists that smoking, consuming alcohol, or using "social" drugs such as marijuana or cocaine during pregnancy may be harmful to the fetus.
- Maternal assessment of fetal activity keeps the woman "in touch" with her fetus and provides ongoing assessment of fetal status.
- Childbirth among women over age 35 is becoming increasingly common. It poses fewer health risks than previously believed and seems to offer advantages for the woman or couple who make the choice.
- A major risk for the older expectant couple relates to the increased incidence of Down syndrome in children born to women over age 35 or 40. Amniocentesis can provide information as to whether the fetus has Down syndrome. The couple can then decide whether they wish to continue the pregnancy.

## CHAPTER REFERENCES


American College of Obstetricians and Gynecologists. (1994). *Exercise during pregnancy and the postpartum period* (ACOG Technical Bulletin No. 189). Washington, DC: Author.

American College of Obstetricians and Gynecologists. (1997a). *Advanced paternal age* (ACOG Committee Opinion No. 189). Washington, DC: Author.

American College of Obstetricians and Gynecologists. (2000). *Planning your pregnancy and birth,* (3rd ed.). Washington, DC: ACOG.

American College of Obstetricians and Gynecologists. (1997b). *Smoking and women's health* (ACOG Educational Bulletin No. 240). Washington, DC: Author.

American College of Obstetricians and Gynecologists. (1997c). *Teratology* (ACOG Educational Bulletin No. 236). Washington, DC: Author.

Belew, C. (1999). Herbs and the childbearing woman: Guidelines for midwives. *Journal of Nurse-Midwifery, 44*(3), 231–246.

Brennan, P. (1999). Homeopathic remedies in prenatal care. *Journal of Nurse-Midwifery, 44*(3), 291–299.

Carl, D. L., Roux, G., & Matacale, R. (2000). Exploring dental hygiene and perinatal outcomes. *AWHONN Lifelines, 4*(1), 22–27.

Castles, A., Adams, E. K., Melvin, C. L., Kelsch, C., & Boulton, M. L. (1999). Effects of smoking during pregnancy: Five meta-analyses. *American Journal of Preventive Medicine, 16*(3), 208–215.

Catanzarite, V., Deutchman, M., Johnson, C. A., & Scherger, J. E. (1995, Jan. 15). Pregnancy after 35: What's the real risk? *Patient Care, 29*(1), 41–48, 51.

Chan, L., Pham, H., & Reece, E. A. (1997). Pneumothorax in pregnancy associated with cocaine use. *American Journal of Perinatology, 14*(7), 385–388.

Chez, R. A., & Murphy, P. (2000). Management of nausea and vomiting in pregnancy: Alternative therapies. *Contemporary OB/GYN, 45*(4), 55–64.

Chez, R. A., & Niebyl, J. (2000). Management of nausea and vomiting in pregnancy: Traditional therapies. *Contemporary OB/GYN, 45*(3), 130–136.

Choi, E. C. (1995). A contrast of mothering behaviors in women from Korea and the United States. *Journal of Obstetric, Gynecologic, and Neonatal Nursing, 24*(4), 363–369.

Chung, K. C., Kowalski, C. P., Kim, H. M., & Buchman, S. R. (2000). Maternal cigarette smoking during pregnancy and the risk of having a child with cleft lip/palate. *Plastic and Reconstructive Surgery, 105*(2), 485–491.

Cunningham, F. G., MacDonald, P. C., Gant, N. F., Leveno, K. J., Gilstrap, L. C., III, Hankins, G. D. V., & Clark, S. L. (1997). *Williams obstetrics* (20th ed.). Stamford, CT: Appleton & Lange.

Dickerson, V. M., & Chez, R. A. (1999). Normal pregnancy and prenatal care. In J. R. Scott, P. J. DiSaia, C. B. Hammond, & W. N. Spellacy (Eds.), *Danforth's obstetrics and gynecology* (8th ed.). Philadelphia: Lippincott Williams & Wilkins, pp. 65–90.

Eisenberg, D. M., Davis, R. B., Ettner, S. L., Appel, S., Wilkey, S., Van Rompey, M., & Kessler, R. C. (1998). Trends in alternative medicine use in the United States, 1990–1997. *JAMA, 280,* 1569–1575.

Gilbert, W. M., Nesbitt, T. S., & Danielson, B. (1999). Childbearing beyond age 40: Pregnancy outcome in 24,032 cases. *Obstetrics and Gynecology, 93*(1), 9–14.

Good news for pregnant women with heartburn (1999). *Contemporary OB/GYN, 44*(12), 50.

Heffernan, A. E. (2000). Exercise and pregnancy in primary care. *Nurse Practitioner, 25*(3), 42–60.

Hoyert, D. L., Danel, I., & Tully, P. (2000). Maternal mortality, United States and Canada, 1982–97. *Birth, 27*(1), 4–11.

Mattson, S. (1995). Culturally sensitive perinatal care for Southeast Asians. *Journal of Obstetric, Gynecologic, and Neonatal Nursing, 24*(4), 335–341.

National Center for Health Statistics. (1999, December 15). *Infant mortality rates vary by race and ethnicity.* [News release]. Hyattsville, MD: Author.

Niebyl, J. R. (1999). Teratology and drugs in pregnancy. In J. R. Scott, P. J. DiSaia, C. B. Hammond, & W. N. Spellacy (Eds.), *Danforth's obstetrics and gynecology* (8th ed.). Philadelphia: Lippincott Williams & Wilkins, pp. 197–212.

Pollack, H., Lantz, P. M., & Frohna, J. G. (2000). Maternal smoking and adverse birth outcomes among singletons and twins. *American Journal of Public Health, 90*(3), 395–400.

Rose, N. C., & Mennuti, M. T. (1995). Multiple marker screening for women 35 and older. *Contemporary OB/GYN, 40*(9), 55–68.

Scholz, H. S., Haas, J., & Petru, E. (1999). Do primiparas aged 40 years or older carry an increased obstetric risk? *Preventive Medicine, 29*(4), 263–266.

Shrock, P. (2000). Exercise and physical activity during pregnancy. In J. J. Sciarra (Ed.), *Gynecology and Obstetrics* Vol. 2 Chapter 8. Philadelphia: Lippincott Williams & Wilkins, pp. 1–17.

Spector, R. E. (2000). *Cultural diversity in health and illness* (5th ed.). Upper Saddle River, NJ: Prentice Hall Health.

Varney, H. (1997). *Varney's midwifery* (3rd ed.). Sudbury, MA: Jones and Bartlett.

Ventura, S. J., Martin, J. A., Curtin, S. A., Mathews, T. J., & Parks, M. M. (2000). Births: Final data for 1998. *National Vital Statistic Reports, 48*(3), 1–105.

Whitney, J. L. (1999). Drug labeling and pregnancy update: What has the FDA done lately? *Contemporary OB/GYN, 44*(1), 85–95.

Windridge K. C., & Berryman, J. C. (1999). Women's experiences of giving birth after 35. *Birth, 26*(1), 16–23.


## CONTEMPORARY MATERNAL-NEWBORN NURSING ON-LINE

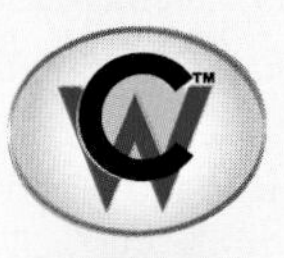

Additional interactive resources, including animations and video, for this chapter can be found on the Companion Website at http://www.prenhall.com/ladewig. Click on Chapter 9 and "Begin" to select the activities for this chapter.

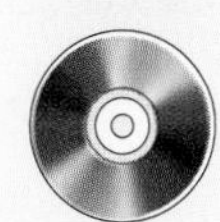

For NCLEX review questions and an audio glossary, access the accompanying CD-ROM in this book.

Chapter 10

# Adolescent Pregnancy

*Sometimes I get discouraged by the terrible reality of children having children. On days when that feeling hits I have to give myself a mental shake and get back into the thick of things. Clinics like ours do make a difference for pregnant teens—we listen, we teach, we care, we accept people where they are, and we never lose sight of the importance of helping the young women who turn to us succeed.*

—A Registered Nurse Working in an Adolescent Pregnancy Clinic

## OBJECTIVES

- Define the scope of the problem of adolescent pregnancy.
- Summarize factors contributing to adolescent pregnancy.
- Discuss the physical, psychologic, and sociologic risks a pregnant adolescent faces.
- Delineate characteristics of the fathers of children of adolescent mothers.
- Discuss the reactions of the adolescent's family and social support groups to her pregnancy.
- Formulate a plan of care to meet the needs of a pregnant adolescent.
- Describe successful community approaches to adolescent pregnancy prevention.

## KEY TERMS

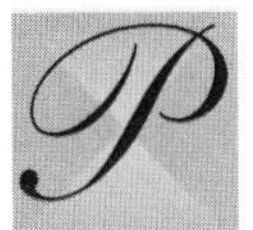

regnancy is a challenging time for a woman as she adjusts to the changes she experiences and prepares to assume a new role as mother of one child or two or more children. Typically this challenge is even greater if the expectant mother is an adolescent. Moreover, depending on her age, her physical development and the developmental tasks of adolescence may be incomplete. Thus both she and her child are at high risk.

In the United States each year almost one million teenage girls become pregnant; 78% of these pregnancies are unintended. Of these pregnancies, nearly two-fifths are terminated by therapeutic abortion, and about 14% end in miscarriage (Alan Guttmacher Institute, 1999). More than half the teens who become pregnant give birth and keep their babies. Very few adolescents give up their babies for adoption (National Campaign to Prevent Teen Pregnancy, 1997).

Although the U.S. birth rate (number of births per 1000 women) for adolescents dropped from 62 per 1000 in 1991 to 51 per 1000 in 1998, the United States continues to have one of the highest levels of adolescent childbearing among industrialized nations—approximately double the rates in Canada and England and over 10 times higher than the level in Japan (Singh & Darroch, 2000). The incidence of sexual activity among teens in many other countries is as high as it is in the United States. Researchers suggest that these countries may have lower adolescent pregnancy rates because of family influences, a greater openness about sexuality, better access to contraceptives, and a more comprehensive approach to sex education.

This chapter explores the issue of adolescent pregnancy and the role of the nurse in meeting the special needs and concerns of pregnant adolescents and their families. It concludes with a discussion of efforts to prevent adolescent pregnancy.

# Overview of the Adolescent Period

## Physical Changes

Puberty—that period during which an individual becomes capable of reproduction—is a maturational process that can last from 1.5 to 6 years. The major physical changes of puberty include a growth spurt, weight change, and the appearance of secondary sexual characteristics. *Menarche,* or the time of the first menstrual period, usually occurs in the last half of this maturational process, with the average age between 12 and 13.

The initial menstrual cycles are usually irregular and often anovulatory, although they are not always so. Thus contraception is important during this time for all adolescents who are sexually active.

## Psychosocial Development

Many writers have described the developmental tasks of adolescence, based on a variety of classic theories. The following are major developmental tasks of this period (Steinberg, 1999):

- Developing a sense of identity
- Gaining autonomy and independence
- Developing truly intimate relationships—that is, relationships characterized by honesty, openness, trust, and self-disclosure
- Developing comfort with one's own sexuality
- Developing a sense of achievement

Resolution of these tasks is a developmental process that occurs over time. This developmental process is reflected in the behaviors of youths during early, middle, and late adolescence. Although average ages for the completion of tasks have been identified, these ages are somewhat arbitrary and are affected by many factors, including culture, religion, and socioeconomic status.

In **early adolescence** (age 14 and under) the teen still sees authority in the parents. However, she begins the process of gaining independence from the family by spending more time with friends. Conformity to peer group standards is important to her. The adolescent in this phase is very egocentric and is a concrete thinker, with only minimal ability to see herself in the future or foresee the consequences of her behavior. She perceives her locus of control as external; that is, her destiny is controlled by others such as parents and school authorities.

**Middle adolescence** (ages 15 to 17 years) is the time for challenging: experimenting with drugs, alcohol, and sex is a common avenue for rebellion. The middle adolescent seeks independence and turns increasingly to her peer group. She is beginning to move from concrete thinking to formal operational thought but is not yet able to anticipate the long-term implications of all her actions. These years are often a time of great turmoil for the family as the adolescent struggles for independence and challenges the family's values and expectations.

In **late adolescence** (ages 18 to 19 years) the teen is more at ease with her individuality and decision-making ability. She can think abstractly and anticipate consequences. The late adolescent is capable of formal operational thought. She is learning to solve problems, to conceptualize, and to make decisions. These abilities help her to see herself as having control, which leads to the ability to understand and accept the consequences of her behavior.

## Factors Contributing to Adolescent Pregnancy

Among American adolescents there is tremendous peer pressure to become sexually active during the teen years. Premarital sexual activity is commonplace, and teenage pregnancy is more socially acceptable today than it was in the past. Sexual innuendo permeates every aspect of the popular media, including music, music videos, television, and movies, but issues of sexual responsibility are commonly ignored. Figure 10–1♦ identifies reasons teens cite for having sex.

Pregnancy risk taking (sexual activity without use of pregnancy prevention measures) is believed to stem from a variety of factors. Many adolescents do not make a conscious decision about being sexually active. In fact, the most common responses by teens when asked why they did not use birth control is that they did not plan or expect to have sex (National Campaign to Prevent Teen Pregnancy, 1997). In addition, pregnancy risk taking has been linked to a lack of knowledge about contraception. Other factors affecting the use of contraception include access or availability, cost of supplies, and concern regarding confidentiality.

Some young teenagers may deliberately plan to get pregnant. The adolescent girl may use pregnancy for various subconscious or conscious reasons: to punish her father and/or mother, to escape from an undesirable home situation, to gain attention, or to feel that she has someone to love and to love her. Pregnancy may also be a young woman's form of acting out.

About three-fourths of adolescents use some form of contraception (often a condom) the first time they have sexual intercourse, and 9 out of 10 sexually active adolescent girls and their partners use contraception, although not always correctly or consistently (Alan Guttmacher Institute, 1999). Statistics have demonstrated an increased use of condoms among the adolescent population, probably because of the tremendous educational efforts related to the human immunodeficiency virus (HIV) (National Campaign to Prevent Teen Pregnancy, 1997).

Compared with other teens, teens with future goals (ie, college or job) tend to use birth control more consistently; if they become pregnant, they are also more likely to have abortions. Adolescents who do not have access to middle-class opportunities tend to maintain their pregnancies, because they see pregnancy as their only option for adult status; 83% of births to unmarried teens occur to those from poor or low-income families (Alan Guttmacher Institute, 1999).

The younger the teen when she first gets pregnant, the more likely she is to have another pregnancy in her teens (East & Felice, 1996). Moreover, the likelihood of repeat pregnancies increases when the teen is living with her sexual partner and has dropped out of school. Daughters of women who had a baby in their early teens are at higher risk for teen pregnancy themselves (Jones & Mondy, 1994).

### Social and Cultural Factors

In the United States, the adolescent birth rate is higher among African-American and Hispanic teens than among white teens. This discrepancy may reflect the fact

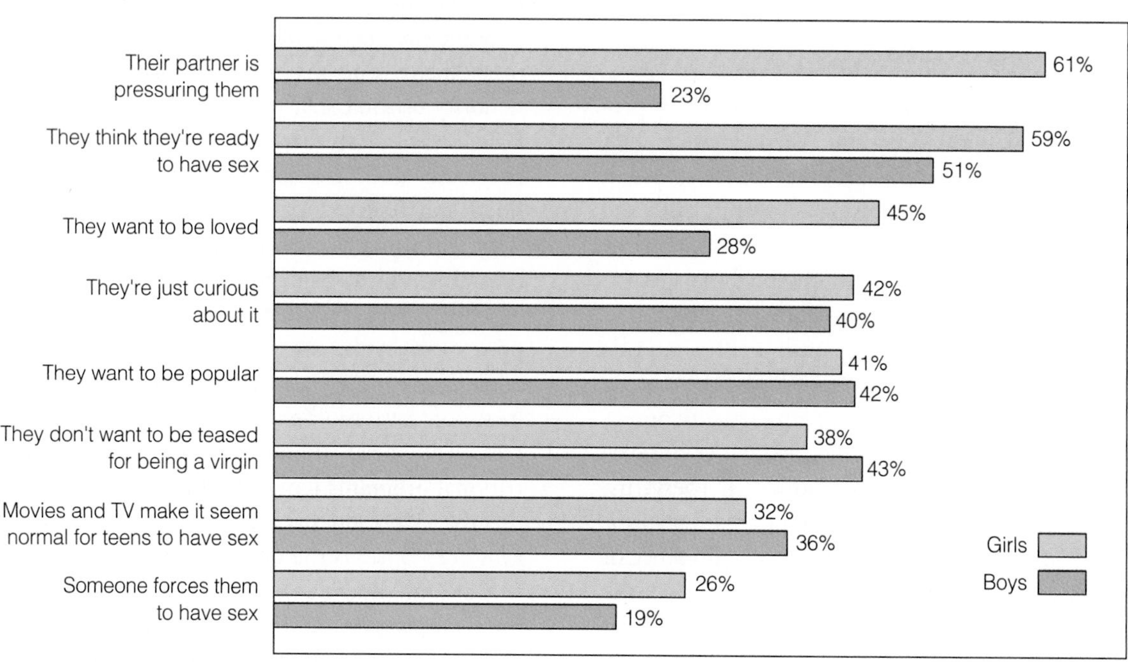


FIGURE 10–1 ♦ Why teens have sex. *Source:* The Kaiser Family Foundation Survey on Teens and Sex: What They Say. *Teens Today Need to Know, and Who They Listen To.* June 1996. Menlo Park, CA: The Harry J. Kaiser Family Foundation.

that a greater percentage of African-American and Hispanic teens are sexually active (Clark, Cohall, & Joffe, 1998). The discrepancy probably also reflects the impact of poverty—a disproportionately higher number of African-American and Hispanic youths live in poverty—and the influence of ethnic or cultural norms.

Internationally, adolescent women are more likely to welcome a pregnancy in a country in which Islam is the predominant religion, where large families are desired, where social change is slow in coming, and where most childbearing occurs within marriage. Early pregnancy is less desired in countries in which the reverse is true. Moreover, throughout the world, the higher a woman's educational level, the more likely she is to delay marriage and childbirth (Alan Guttmacher Institute, 1996).

### Abuse as a Factor

More teens who become pregnant, compared with teens who have not been pregnant, were sexually abused as children. In fact, maltreatment of any kind is a high-risk contributor to early teen pregnancy (Stock, Bell, Boyer, et al., 1997).

Teenage pregnancy can result from an incestuous relationship. In the very young adolescent, incest or sexual abuse should be suspected as a possible cause of pregnancy. Teenage pregnancy could also be caused by other nonvoluntary sexual experiences such as acquaintance rape.

## Risks to the Adolescent Mother

### Physiologic Risks

Adolescents over age 15 who receive early, thorough prenatal care are at no greater risk during pregnancy than women over age 20. Unfortunately, many adolescents fail to seek early prenatal care and fail to cooperate with the recommendations they receive. Thus risks for pregnant adolescents include preterm births, low-birth-weight infants, cephalopelvic disproportion, iron deficiency anemia, and pregnancy-induced hypertension (PIH) and its sequelae. In the adolescent age group, prenatal care is the critical factor that most influences pregnancy outcome.

Teenagers ages 15 to 19 have a high incidence of sexually transmitted infections, including herpesvirus, syphilis, and gonorrhea. The incidence of chlamydial infection is also increased in this age group. The presence of such infections during a pregnancy greatly increases the risk to the fetus (refer to Chapter 13). Other problems seen in adolescents are cigarette smoking and drug use. By the time pregnancy is confirmed in young women, the fetus may already have been harmed by these substances.

### Psychologic Risks

The major psychologic risk to the pregnant adolescent is the interruption of her developmental tasks. Adding to her developmental tasks the tasks of pregnancy creates an overwhelming amount of psychologic work, the completion of which will affect the adolescent's and her newborn's futures.

Table 10–1 suggests typical behaviors of the early, middle, and late adolescent when she becomes aware of her pregnancy. In reviewing these behaviors, the nurse should realize that other factors may influence individual response.

### Sociologic Risks

Being forced into adult roles before completing adolescent developmental tasks causes a series of events that affects the adolescent's entire life. These events may result in a prolonged dependence on parents, lack of stable relationships with the opposite sex, and lack of economic and social stability.

Many teenage mothers drop out of school during their pregnancy. Many never complete their education. Lack of education reduces the quality of jobs available to these individuals. Childbearing at an early age is a strong predictor of the need for public assistance, especially in lower socioeconomic groups and when the pregnant adolescent's family will not support her (National Campaign to Prevent Teen Pregnancy, 1997).

Adolescent mothers frequently fail to establish a stable family, especially if they have a second child while still in their teens. Their family structure tends to be a single-parent, matriarchal family structure, often the same type in which the adolescents themselves were raised.

Some pregnant adolescents choose to marry the father of the baby, who may be a teenager. Unfortunately, the majority of adolescent marriages end in divorce (Roye & Balk, 1996). This fact should not be surprising because pregnancy and marriage interrupt the adolescents' childhood and basic education. Lack of maturity in dealing with an intimate relationship also contributes to marital breakdown in this age group.

The increased incidence of maternal complications, premature birth, and low-birth-weight babies among adolescent mothers also has an impact on society because many of these mothers are on welfare. The need for increased financial support for good prenatal care and nutritional programs remains critical.

Table 10–2 on page 232 identifies the early adolescent's response to the developmental tasks of pregnancy. Middle and older adolescents respond differently, reflecting their progression through the developmental tasks. In addition to her maturational level, the amount of nurturing the pregnant adolescent receives is a critical factor in the way she handles pregnancy and motherhood.

| TABLE 10–1 Initial Reaction to Awareness of Pregnancy | | |
|---|---|---|
| *Age* | *Adolescent Behavior* | *Nursing Implications* |
| Early adolescent (14 and under) | Fears rejection by family and peers. Enters health care system with an adult, most likely mother (parents still seen as locus of control). Value system still closely reflects that of parents, so still turns to parents for decision or approval of decision. Pregnancy probably not result of intimate relationship. Is self-conscious about normal adolescent changes in body. Self-consciousness and low self-esteem likely to increase with rapid breast enlargement and abdominal enlargement of pregnancy. | Be nonjudgmental in approach to care. Focus on needs and concerns of adolescent, but if parent accompanies daughter, include parent in plan of care. Encourage both to express concerns and feelings regarding pregnancy and options: abortion, maintaining pregnancy, and adoption. Be realistic and concrete in discussion implications of each option. During physical exam of adolescent, respect increased sense of modesty. Explain in simple and concrete terms physical changes that are produced by pregnancy versus puberty. Explain each step of physical exam in simple and concrete terms. |
| Middle adolescent (15–17 years) | Fears rejection by peers and parents. Unsure in whom to confide. May seek confirmation of pregnancy on own with increased awareness of options and services, such as over-the-counter pregnancy kits and Planned Parenthood. If in an ongoing, caring relationship with partner (peer), may choose him as confidant. Economic dependence on parents may determine if and when parents are told. Future educational plans and perception of parental support or lack of support are significant factors in decision regarding termination or maintenance of the pregnancy. Possible conflict in parental and own developing value system. | Be nonjudgmental in approach to care. Reassure adolescent that confidentiality will be maintained. Help adolescent identify significant individuals in whom she can confide to help make a decision about the pregnancy. Be aware of state laws regarding requirement of parental notification if abortion intended. Also be aware of state laws regarding requirements for marriage: usually, minimum age for both parties is 18; 16- and 17-year-olds are, in most states, allowed to marry only with consent of parents. Encourage adolescent to be realistic about parental response to pregnancy. |
| Older adolescent (18–19 years) | Most likely to confirm pregnancy on own and at an earlier date due to increased acceptance and awareness of consequences of behavior. Likely to use pregnancy kit for confirmation. Relationship with father of baby, future educational plans, and own value system are among significant determinants of decision about pregnancy. | Be nonjudgmental in approach to care. Reassure adolescent that confidentiality will be maintained. Encourage adolescent to identify significant individuals in whom she can confide. Refer to counseling as appropriate. Encourage adolescent to be realistic about parental response to pregnancy. |

### Risks for Her Child

Children of adolescent parents are at a disadvantage in many ways because teens are not developmentally or economically prepared to be parents. In general, children of teenage mothers are found to be at a developmental disadvantage compared with children whose mothers were older at the time of their birth. Many factors contribute to these differences, especially the adverse social and economic conditions many teenage mothers face. These factors result in high rates of family instability, disadvantaged neighborhoods, and high rates of behavior problems. In addition, these children do not do as well in school and are less likely to complete high school. Children born to adolescent mothers also have higher rates of abuse and neglect, resulting in significantly higher rates of foster care placement (National Campaign to Prevent Teen Pregnancy, 1997).

## Partners of Adolescent Mothers

Almost half of the fathers of infants of adolescent mothers are not teens but are 20 years of age or older (East & Felice, 1996). Of these men, approximately one-fifth are 6 or more years older than the adolescent mother (Taylor, Chavez, Chabra, & Boggess, 1997). The poorer the man's education, the greater the risk that he will father the child of an adolescent, possibly because he is seeking an intellectual and emotional equal. Often the older partners of pregnant adolescents are similar to adolescent fathers socioeconomically. They have experienced early school failure, are unemployed, and are no more likely than adolescent fathers to support the mother (Roye & Balk, 1996).

## TABLE 10–2 The Early Adolescent's Response to the Developmental Tasks of Pregnancy

| *Stage* | *Developmental Tasks of Pregnancy* | *Early Adolescent's Response to Pregnancy* | *Nursing Implications* |
|---|---|---|---|
| First trimester | Pregnancy confirmation. Seeking early prenatal care as a confirmation tool. Begins to evaluate her diet and general health habits. Initial ambivalence common. Usually supportive partner. | May delay confirmation of pregnancy until late part of first trimester or later. Reasons for delay may include lack of awareness that she is pregnant, fear of confiding in anyone, and denial. Rapid enlargement and sensitivity of breasts are embarrassing and frightening to early adolescent—may be perceived as changes of puberty. If confiding in mother, may be experiencing family turmoil in response to pregnancy. | Explain physiologic changes of pregnancy versus those associated with puberty. Explain that ambivalence is normal with any pregnancy, but recognize it as a much greater concern with adolescent pregnancy. Emphasize need for good nutrition as important for her well-being as much as infant's (prevention of PIH and anemia). Use simple explanations and lots of audiovisual aids. Have adolescent listen to fetal heart rate with Doppler. |
| Second trimester | Changes in physical appearance begin, and fetal movement is experienced, causing pregnancy to be experienced as a reality. Begins wearing maternity clothes to accommodate the physical changes. As a result of quickening she perceives her fetus as a real baby and begins preparing for the maternal role and new relationships with her partner and members of her family. | Some teenagers may delay validation of pregnancy until now, with family turmoil occurring at this time. Abdominal enlargement and quickening may be perceived as loss of control over body image. May try to maintain prepregnant weight and wear restrictive clothing to control and conceal changing body. Becomes dependent on her own mother for support. Egocentric; unable to develop a maternal role at this time. | Continue to discuss importance of good nutrition and adequate weight gain as noted above. Discuss ways of utilizing common teenage clothing (large sweatshirts, blouses) to promote comfort but preserve adolescent image to some degree. Discuss plans being made for baby, continued educational plans, and role of teen's parents. |
| Third trimester | At end of second trimester begins to view fetus as separate from self. Buys baby clothes and supplies. Prepares a place for the baby. Realistic about what baby is like. Prepares to give birth to infant. Anxiety increases as labor and birth approach and has concerns about well-being of fetus. | May focus on "wanting it to be over." May have trouble individuating fetus. May have fantasies, dreams, or nightmares about childbirth. Natural fears of labor and birth greater than with older primigravida. Probably has not been in a hospital, and may associate this with negative experiences. | Assess whether adolescent is preparing for baby by buying supplies and preparing a place in the home. Childbirth education is important. Provide hospital tour. Assess for discomforts of pregnancy, such as heartburn and constipation. Adolescent may be uncomfortable mentioning these and other problems. |

Adult paternity also tends to be higher when the teenage mother was born outside the United States. This difference may reflect cultural norms (Taylor et al., 1997).

Adolescent males tend to become sexually active at an earlier age than females, and they have more sexual partners in their teenage years. When the father is an adolescent, he, too, has uncompleted developmental tasks for his age group and is no better prepared psychologically than his female counterpart to deal with the consequences of pregnancy. Consequently, the adolescent who attempts to assume his responsibility as a father faces many of the same psychologic and sociologic risks as the adolescent mother. The mother and father are generally from similar socioeconomic backgrounds and have similar educational levels.

Adolescent fathers tend to achieve less formal education than older fathers, and they enter the workforce earlier. They tend to pursue less prestigious careers and have les job satisfaction. They often marry at a younger age tha older fathers and have more children.

Although they may not be married, many adolescen couples have meaningful relationships. The male partner in such relationships may be very involved in the preg nancy and may be present for the birth. Research suggest that a teen who has a close, satisfying relationship wit her baby's father is more likely than a teen in a stormy re lationship or one who is estranged from the baby's fathe to demonstrate maternal role behaviors during pregnanc and positive maternal attachment after birth (Bloom 1998). Unfortunately, research also indicates that there i decreasing contact with the mother and infant over time even when the father is involved in the birth (Roye & Balk, 1996).

The role of the parents of the adolescent father has not been well studied. Some research indicates that sons are more involved with their babies when they believe that their own mothers expect it. Similarly, the mothers of teen fathers seem to influence the parenting behaviors their sons demonstrate. Adolescent fathers' need for continued parenting and their young age are the main barriers to their ability to perform the parental role (Dallas & Chen, 1999).

Some adolescent fathers face negative reactions from people, including their own families and the families of their young partners. They may experience others' anger, shame, and disappointment. Their relationships with their peers may be altered as well.

The lack of responsibility shown by some unwed fathers has caused a shift in cultural and community attitudes. Fathers are being included on birth certificates far more frequently today than in the past. This inclusion helps ensure the fathers' rights and encourages them to meet their responsibilities to their children. In addition, legal paternity gives children access to military and social security benefits and to medical information about their fathers.

In some situations the pregnant adolescent female may not want to identify or contact the father of the baby, and the male may not readily acknowledge paternity. Those situations include rape, exploitative sexual relations, incest, and casual sexual relations. If health care providers suspect any of the first three causes, further investigation into the situation is important for the well-being of the pregnant adolescent, and referral to other resources should be made as appropriate.

Health care providers should support the adolescent father in his decision to assume responsibility. It is important, however, that the pregnant adolescent have the opportunity to make the decision about whether she wants the father to participate in her health care.

If the adolescents perceive that they have a caring relationship, the adolescent father may want to be supportive and protective but probably does not understand the physical and psychologic changes his female partner is experiencing. The young man will need education regarding pregnancy, childbirth, child care, and parenting.

Although the adolescent father may have been included in the health care of the young woman throughout the pregnancy, it is not unusual for her to want her mother as her primary support person during labor and birth. Younger adolescents are especially likely to choose their mothers for this role. It is important both to support the pregnant adolescent's wishes and to acknowledge and support the adolescent father's wishes as appropriate.

As a part of counseling, the nurse should assess the young man's stressors, his support systems, his plans for involvement in the pregnancy and childbearing, and his future plans. He should be referred to social services for an opportunity for counseling regarding his educational and vocational future. When the father is involved in the pregnancy, the young mother feels less deserted, more confident in her decision making, and better able to discuss her future.

## Reactions of Family and Social Network to Adolescent Pregnancy

The reactions of family members and support groups to adolescent pregnancy are as varied as the motivation and cause of the pregnancy. In families that foster their children's educational and career goals, adolescent pregnancy is often a shock. Anger, shame, and sorrow are common reactions. The majority of pregnant adolescents from these families are likely to use contraception or choose abortion, with the exception of teens whose cultural and religious beliefs prevent them from seeking abortions.

In populations in which adolescent pregnancy is more prevalent and more socially acceptable, family and friends may be more supportive of the adolescent parents. In many cases, the teen's friends and mother are present at the birth. The expectant couple may also have friends who are already teen parents. Some male partners of these adolescent mothers see pregnancy and the birth of a baby as signs of adult status and increased sexual prowess—a source of pride.

The mother of the pregnant adolescent is usually among the first to be told about the pregnancy. She typically becomes involved with decision making, especially with the young adolescent, about issues such as maintaining the pregnancy, abortion, and dealing with the father-to-be and his family.

Once the pregnant adolescent decides how to proceed, it is often the mother who helps the teen access health care and accompanies her to her first prenatal visit. If the pregnancy is maintained, the mother may participate in prenatal care and classes and can be an excellent source of support for her daughter. She should be encouraged to participate if the mother-daughter relationship is positive. If the baby's father is involved in the pregnancy, he and the pregnant adolescent's mother may be able to work together to support the teenage mother. The pregnant adolescent's mother should be updated on childbearing practices to clarify any misconceptions she might have. During labor and birth, the mother may be a key figure for her daughter, offering reassurance and instilling confidence in the teen.

It is commonly believed that the adolescent and her infant will fare better if they live in the same household as the teen's mother, now the grandmother. Increasingly, however, research suggests that the best outcomes for the adolescent and her infant occur when there is regular assistance from the grandmother but they do not live together (Spieker & Bensley, 1994). The wise grandmother gently encourages a balance between helping her daughter to be a parent and allowing her to complete the tasks of adolescence. As her daughter becomes a more confident parent, the grandmother can gradually encourage her independence.

# Nursing Care Management

## Nursing Assessment and Diagnosis

The nurse needs to establish a database to plan interventions for the adolescent mother-to-be and family. Areas of assessment include a history of family and personal physical health, developmental level and impact of pregnancy, and emotional and financial support. The nurse also assesses the family and social support network and the father's degree of involvement in the pregnancy.

As with all pregnant women, it is important to have information on general physical health. This may be the first time the adolescent has ever provided a health history. Consequently, the nurse may find it helpful to ask very specific questions and give examples if the young woman appears confused about a question. The nurse may find that the teen's mother is best able to answer questions about family history because the adolescent is often unaware of this information.

The following areas should be assessed:

- Family and personal health history
- Medical history
- Menstrual history
- Obstetric and gynecologic history
- Substance abuse history

It is important to assess the maturational level of each individual. The adolescent's development level and the impact of pregnancy are reflected in the degree of recognition of the realities and responsibilities involved in teenage pregnancy and parenting. The mother's self-concept (including body image), her relationship with the significant adults in her life, her attitude toward her pregnancy, and her coping methods in the situation are just a few of the significant factors that need to be assessed. The nurse assesses the adolescent's knowledge of, attitude toward, and anticipated ability to care for the coming baby.

The socioeconomic status of the pregnant adolescent often places the baby at risk throughout life, beginning with conception. It is essential to assess family and social support systems, as well as the extent of financial support available.

The nursing diagnoses applicable to pregnant women in general apply to the pregnant adolescents. Other nursing diagnoses are influenced by the adolescent's age, support systems, socioeconomic situation, health, and maturity. Examples of nursing diagnoses specific to the pregnant adolescent include the following:

- Health-seeking behaviors: information about child care related to expressed desire to parent effectively
- Altered nutrition: less than body requirements related to poor eating habits
- Self-esteem disturbance related to unanticipated pregnancy

## Nursing Plan and Implementation

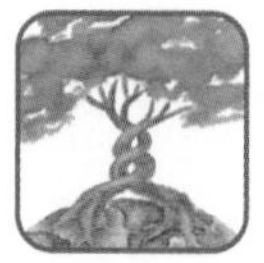

### Community-Based Nursing Care

Early, thorough prenatal care is the strongest and most critical determinant for reducing risk for the adolescent mother and her newborn. The nurse needs to understand the special needs of the adolescent mother to meet this challenge successfully. See Key Facts to Remember: The Pregnant Adolescent.

Many new and innovative community-based programs have evolved to provide care for high-risk clients throughout the childbearing experience and beyond. For example, early research findings suggest that a planned multidimensional approach that includes a combination of preparation for motherhood classes, a series of focused prenatal home visits, and monthly visits for the first year

**KEY FACTS TO REMEMBER**

*The Pregnant Adolescent*

- The rate of adolescent pregnancy in the United States is among the highest of all the developed countries of the world.
- Early, regular, and excellent prenatal care can prevent many of the risks associated with adolescent pregnancy, especially for the young adolescent.
- Prenatal education especially designed for adolescents also plays a significant role in increasing an adolescent's knowledge and in decreasing maternal and perinatal complications.

after childbirth results in a reduced rate of preterm births and fewer days of infant hospitalization (Koniak-Griffin, Mathenge, Anderson, & Verzemnieks, 1999).

Nurses in community-based agencies can help adolescents access the health care system as well as social services and other support services (eg, food banks and the Women, Infants, and Children Program [WIC]). These nurses are also involved extensively in counseling and client teaching.

#### Issue of Confidentiality

Most states in the United States have passed legislation that confirms the right of some minors to assume the rights of adults. These adolescents are referred to as **emancipated minors.** An adolescent may be considered emancipated if he or she is self-supporting and living away from home, married, pregnant, a parent, or in the military service. The pregnant adolescent, even if very young, is generally considered emancipated and has the right and responsibility to consent to health care for herself and, later, for her child. If she is considered emancipated, she is entitled to respect and confidentiality in her dealings with health care providers. Only with her agreement can other adults, including her parents, be included in communication.

#### Development of a Trusting Relationship with the Pregnant Adolescent

The first visit to the clinic or caregiver's office may make the young woman feel anxious and vulnerable. Making this first experience as positive as possible for the young woman will encourage the adolescent to return for follow-up care and to cooperate with her caregivers and will help ensure her recognition of the importance of health care for her and her baby.

Depending on the adolescent's age, this may be her first pelvic examination, an anxiety-provoking experience for any woman. The nurse can provide explanations during the procedure. A gentle and thoughtful examination technique will help the young woman to relax. A mirror is helpful in allowing the client to see her cervix, educating her about her anatomy, and giving her an active role in the exam if she so desires.

Developing a trusting relationship with the pregnant adolescent is essential. Honesty and respect for the individual and a caring attitude promote self-esteem. In developing a trusting relationship with the young woman, the nurse's attitudes about self-care and responsibility affect the adolescent's maturation process.

#### Promotion of Self-Esteem and Problem-Solving Skills

The nurse assists the adolescent in her decision-making and problem-solving skills so that she can proceed with her developmental tasks and begin to assume responsibility for her life and that of her newborn. Many adolescents are not aware of all the legally available options to deal with an unplanned pregnancy. In an open, nonjudgmental way, without imposing personal values, the nurse can educate the teen about her alternatives: maintaining or terminating the pregnancy and parenting the infant or relinquishing the infant for adoption. The nurse can encourage the young woman to share her feelings about each alternative and the projected consequences as they relate to her situation in life. The nurse can also provide information about community resources available to help with each alternative. Once the adolescent has decided on a course of action, health care providers should respect her decision and support her efforts to achieve her goals.

If the adolescent chooses to continue her pregnancy, the nurse summarizes what she can expect over the prenatal period and provides a thorough explanation and rationale for each procedure as it occurs. This overview fosters the adolescent's understanding and gives her some measure of control (Figure 10–2♦).

Early adolescents tend to be egocentric and oriented to the present. They may not regard as important the fact that their health and habits affect the fetus. Thus it is often helpful to emphasize the effects of these practices on the clients themselves. Early adolescents also need help in problem solving and in visualizing the future so they can plan effectively.

Middle adolescents are developing the ability to think abstractly and can recognize that actions may have long-term consequences. They may not yet have acquired assertive communication skills, however, and may be reluctant to ask questions. Thus the nurse should ask teens directly if they have questions. Middle adolescents can absorb more detailed health teaching and apply it.

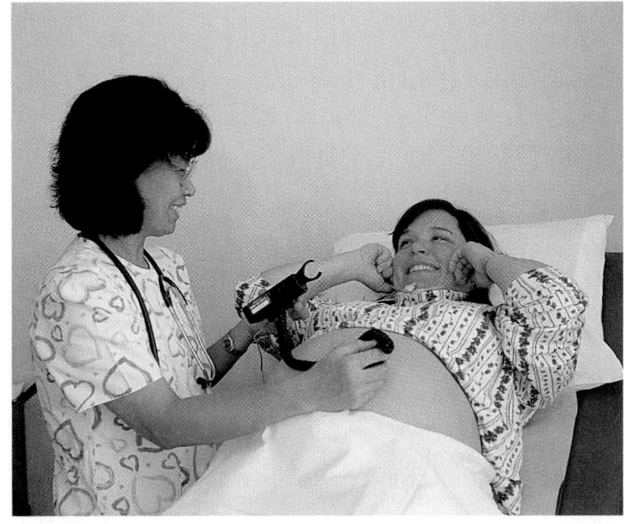

FIGURE 10–2 ♦ The nurse gives this young mother an opportunity to listen to her baby's heartbeat.

Late adolescents can think abstractly, plan for the future, and function in a manner comparable to older pregnant women. They can also handle complex information and apply it.

#### Promotion of Physical Well-Being

Baseline weight and blood pressure measurements are valuable in assessing weight gain and predisposition to pregnancy-induced hypertension. The nurse can encourage the adolescent to take part in her care by measuring and recording her own weight. The nurse may use this time as an opportunity for assisting the young woman in problem solving and encourage her to ask herself the following questions: "Have I gained too much or too little weight?" "What influence does my diet have on my weight?" "How can I change my eating habits?"

Another way to introduce the subject of nutrition is during measurement of baseline and subsequent hemoglobin and hematocrit values. Because the adolescent is at risk for anemia, she will need education regarding the importance of iron in her diet. Indeed, basic education about nutrition is a critical component of care for pregnant teens.

Pregnancy-induced hypertension (PIH) is the most prevalent medical complication of pregnant adolescents. Blood pressure readings of 140/90 mm Hg are not acceptable as the determinant of PIH in adolescents. Women ages 14 to 20 years without evidence of high blood pressure usually have diastolic readings between 50 and 66 mm Hg. Gradual increases from the prepregnant diastolic readings, along with excessive weight gain, must be evaluated as precursors to PIH. Establishment of baseline readings is one reason why early prenatal care is vital to the management of the pregnant adolescent.

Adolescents have an increased incidence of sexually transmitted infections (STIs). The initial prenatal examination should include gonococcal and chlamydial cultures; wet-mount prep for *Candida, Trichomonas,* and *Gardnerella;* and tests for syphilis. Education about STIs is important, as is careful observation of herpetic lesions or other symptoms throughout a young woman's pregnancy. Although today's teens are knowledgeable about HIV/AIDS, they know much less about other STIs, especially with regard to symptoms and risk reduction. If the adolescent's history indicates that she is at increased risk for HIV, she should be given information about it and offered HIV screening.

The nurse should discuss substance abuse with the adolescent. It is important to review the risks associated with the use of tobacco, caffeine, drugs, and alcohol. The young woman should be aware of the ways that these substances affect both her development and that of her fetus.

Ongoing care should include the same assessments that an older pregnant woman receives. The nurse should pay special attention to evaluating fetal growth by determining when quickening occurs and by measuring fundal height, fetal heart rate, and fetal movement. The corresponding dates of auscultating fetal heart tones with the date of last menstrual period and quickening can be helpful in determining correct estimates of time of birth. If there is a question of size-date discrepancy by 2 cm either way when assessing fundal height, an ultrasound is warranted to establish fetal age so that instances of intrauterine growth restriction can be diagnosed and treated early.

#### Promotion of Family Adaptation

The nurse assesses the family situation during the first prenatal visit and discovers the level of involvement the adolescent desires from each of her family members and the father of the child, as well as her perception of their present support. A sensitive approach to the daughter-mother relationship helps motivate their communication. If the mother and daughter agree, the mother should be included in the client's care.

The nurse should also help the mother assess and meet her daughter's needs. Some adolescents become more dependent during pregnancy, and some become more independent. The mother can ease and encourage her daughter's self-growth by understanding how best to respond to and support the adolescent.

The adolescent's relationship with her father is also affected by her pregnancy. The nurse can provide information to the father and encourage his involvement to whatever degree is acceptable to both daughter and father.

Finally, the father of the adolescent's infant should not be forgotten in promoting the family's adaptation to the pregnancy. He should be included in prenatal visits, classes, health teaching, and in the birth itself to the extent that he wishes and that is acceptable to the teenage mother. He should also have the opportunity to express his feelings and concerns and to have his questions answered.

#### Facilitation of Prenatal Education

Some school systems are currently attempting to meet prenatal education needs in a variety of ways. The most effective method appears to be mainstreaming the pregnant adolescent in academic classes with her peers and adding classes appropriate to her needs during pregnancy and initial parenting experiences. Classes about growth and development beginning with the newborn and early infancy periods can help teenage parents to develop realistic expectations of their infants and may help

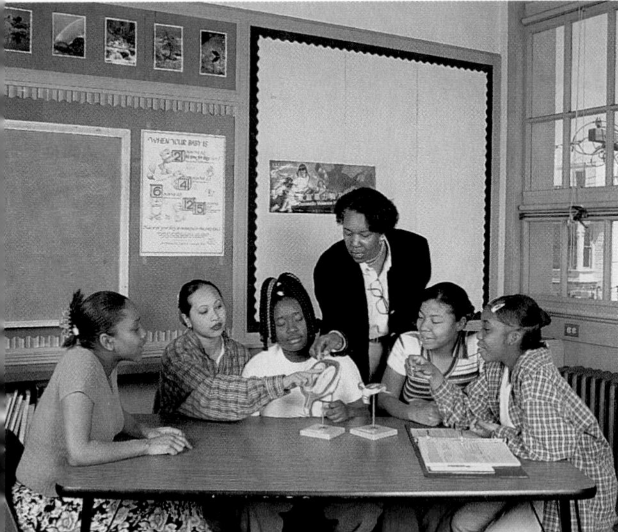

FIGURE 10–3 ♦ Young adolescents may benefit from prenatal classes designed for them.

decrease child abuse. Mainstreaming pregnant adolescents in school is also an ideal way to help them complete their education while learning the skills they need to cope with childbearing and parenting. Vocational guidance in this setting is also beneficial as they plan for their futures.

Most childbirth educators believe that prenatal classes with other teens are preferable, even though these classes can be challenging to teach (Figure 10–3♦). Attendance may be sporadic. The pregnant teen may be accompanied by her mother, her boyfriend, or a girlfriend. Those who bring girlfriends may bring a different one each time, and giggling and side conversations may occur. Such activity reflects the short attention span of the teen and is fairly typical. Thus, to keep the attention of the participants, it is important to use a variety of teaching strategies including age-appropriate audiovisual aids, demonstrations, and games.

Goals for prenatal classes may include the following:

- Providing anticipatory guidance about pregnancy
- Preparing participants for labor and birth
- Helping participants identify the problems and conflicts of teenage pregnancy and parenting
- Promoting increased self-esteem
- Providing information about available community resources
- Helping participants develop adaptive coping skills

Although parenting topics are sometimes included in prenatal classes for adolescents, teens may not retain the information because they tend to be present oriented.

## Critical Thinking in Practice

Cindy Lenz, a 15-year-old G1P0, is 16 weeks pregnant when she arrives for her second prenatal visit. She is drinking diet soda and eating potato chips as she waits for her appointment. Her 18-year-old boyfriend is with her. While reviewing her history the nurse remembers that Cindy had tried to get pregnant for several months. Her boyfriend, a high school dropout, has a part-time job. Cindy is still living at home, although she does not get along with her mother or sister. She plans to stay in school until her baby is born because she has two other friends at school who are also pregnant. As the nurse weighs Cindy, she asks a few questions about her nutritional habits and finds that Cindy eats a lot of junk food and very few vegetables or fruits. How should the nurse discuss Cindy's nutritional needs with her?

Answers can be found in Appendix I.

Parenting skills are crucial, but adolescents generally are not ready to learn about these skills until birth makes the newborn—and thus parenting—a reality.

### Hospital-Based Nursing Care

The adolescent's mother is often present during the teen's labor and birth. The father of the baby may also be involved. Close girlfriends may arrive soon after the teen is admitted. It is important on admission for the nurse to ask the pregnant adolescent who will be her primary support person in labor and who she wants involved in the labor and birth. This information may also be included on her prenatal record.

The adolescent in labor has the same care needs as any pregnant woman. However, she may require more sustained care. The nurse must be readily available and should answer questions simply and honestly, using lay terminology. The nurse can also help the adolescent's support people understand their roles in assisting the teen. If the father of the baby is involved, the nurse can encourage him to work within his own level of comfort to play an active role in all phases of the birth process, perhaps by supporting the teen's relaxation techniques, feeding her ice chips, timing her contractions, and coaching her with her breathing.

The nurse can also recommend hand-holding, back rubs, and supportive touching.

During the postpartum period, most teens do not foresee that they will become sexually active in the near future and are often adamant that they will not become pregnant again for a long time. However, the statistics demonstrate a different reality. Consequently, prior to discharge the nurse's teaching should include information about the resumption of ovulation and the importance of contraception. It is especially helpful to provide this information to both the adolescent mother and her sexual partner. The nurse can encourage the couple to use condoms and spermicide until they choose another method of birth control.

As part of discharge planning, the nurse should ensure that the teen is aware of community resources available to assist her and her family. Postpartum classes, especially with peers, can be particularly beneficial. Such classes address a variety of topics including postpartum adaptation, infant and child development, parenting skills, and the like.

### Evaluation

Expected outcomes of nursing care include the following:

- A trusting relationship is established with the pregnant adolescent.
- The adolescent is able to use her problem-solving abilities to make appropriate choices.
- The adolescent follows the recommendations of the health care team and receives effective health care throughout her pregnancy, the birth, and the postpartum period.
- The adolescent, her partner (if he is involved), and their families are able to cope successfully with the effects of the pregnancy.
- The adolescent is able to discuss pregnancy, prenatal care, and childbirth.
- The adolescent demonstrates developmental and pregnancy progression within established normal parameters.
- The adolescent develops skill in child care and parenting.

## Prevention of Adolescent Pregnancy

A national effort to prevent teen pregnancy was initiated in 1996 with the organization of the National Campaign to Prevent Teen Pregnancy. Its purpose is to reduce teenage pregnancy one-third by 2005 (National Campaign to Prevent Teen Pregnancy, 1997). The National Campaign is a private, nonprofit organization made up of a broad spectrum of religious, political, social, human services, health, and academic organizations. The Association of Women's Health and Neonatal Nurses (AWHONN) is one of the many professional organizations that joined this group and made a commitment to focus on adolescent pregnancy prevention.

Accomplishments in the National Campaign's first year included legislative proposals from bipartisan groups in Congress to allocate money to fund better evaluation of adolescent pregnancy prevention programs and for onetime incentive grants for communities (Cockey, 1997). The National Campaign also has commitments to adolescent pregnancy prevention from such media groups as MTV and ABC Daytime (National Campaign to Prevent Teen Pregnancy, 1997).

One of the first actions of the National Campaign was to commission a task force to do a comprehensive review of the incidence of adolescent pregnancy and its impact in the United States. At the same time, another task force was commissioned to review the research on the effectiveness of pregnancy prevention programs. The purpose of these task forces was to provide accurate information based on fact and research. Not surprisingly, the task forces have found that adolescent pregnancy is a multifaceted problem with no easy answers. The best approach is local and is based on strong, community-wide involvement with a variety of programs directed at the multiple causes of the problem. No one program can be effective by itself in changing the rate of teenage pregnancy (Kirby, 1997).

One of the major problems in local communities continues to be intense conflict among different groups about how to approach adolescent pregnancy prevention. Some groups believe that abstinence is the only answer, whereas others believe that abstinence programs will not work with the many teens who are already sexually active. The latter groups believe that sex education and easy availability of contraception are the answers.

## TABLE 10–3 Community Approaches to Preventing Adolescent Pregnancy

**I. PLANNING**

- Involve all sectors of the community (eg, business groups, religious groups, civic organizations, health and human service providers, schools, media).
- Commit to adequate, long-term funding.
- Include teens in planning effective programs.
- Target high-risk populations within the community.
- Target males as well as females.
- Plan programs that are culturally appropriate and age appropriate as well as locally relevant.

**II. SAMPLE COMPONENTS OF A COMMUNITY PROGRAM**

- Youth development activities, such as tutoring, mentoring, after-school activities, community volunteer work.
- Community-based adolescent health clinics.
- School dropout prevention.
- Opportunities for career counseling and job training.
- Comprehensive sexuality education, which not only includes accurate information about sexually transmitted infections and contraception but also teaches adolescents skills to avoid peer pressure and promote responsible relationships.
- Educational programs for teachers and religious leaders who teach sexuality education.
- Educational programs for parents on communication skills and increasing knowledge.
- Peer training to act as educators and to give support.

**III. EVALUATION**

- Evaluation of the process is essential and should include reports about services that are being delivered plus basic demographics (ie, who attends the program over time).
- Knowledge, attitudes, and intent should also be evaluated; however, these factors have not been found to be significantly related to the adolescents' actual behaviors (Philliber & Namerow, 1995).
- Evaluation of the impact of specific programs may be too expensive for most communities because it involves experimental research that is difficult to implement (ie, large sample size, control groups, random assignment into groups, and long-term follow-up).
- Pregnancy rates and birth rates are not likely to change rapidly (Kirby, 1997; Moore & Sugland, 1996).

Ironically, a comprehensive review of research suggests that neither of the proposed solutions, individually or together, is as effective in reducing the teen pregnancy rate as many believe. The risk factors most closely associated with teen birth rates appear to be poverty, low educational achievement, poor self-esteem, family dysfunction, and high-risk behaviors in general. Thus research suggests that programs to address these societal problems and give teens hope for a different future are more effective than programs narrowly focused on teen sexual activity (Moore & Sugland, 1996; Stevens-Simon, Kelly, Singer, et al., 1996). In teen populations with job accessibility and education, easy, confidential access to sex education and contraception is also important in reducing teen pregnancy rates (Table 10–3).

After visiting communities that have launched programs to prevent adolescent pregnancy, members of the National Campaign concluded that adults must agree to disagree and individual groups must be encouraged to move ahead with their different programs because a variety of approaches are needed.

The cause or motivation for pregnancy varies from one community to another. In inner-city areas, where there are high rates of poverty, low self-esteem, school failure, early behavioral problems, and delinquent behaviors, programs that promote self-esteem, deal with these social ills, and provide hope for these youth are critical. However, the National Campaign's task forces have identified similar characteristics in successful programs, regardless of the type of offering or community. Some of the critical characteristics of effective adolescent pregnancy prevention programs include the following:

- Involvement of adolescents in the planning of programs
- Good role models from the same cultural and racial backgrounds
- Long-term and intensive programs
- Sufficient focus on the adolescent male population

# Chapter Review

## CHAPTER HIGHLIGHTS

- Although the U.S. birth rate (number of births per 1000 women) for adolescents dropped from 62 per 1000 in 1991 to 51 per 1000 in 1998, the United States continues to have one of the highest levels of adolescent childbearing among industrialized nations.
- Many factors contribute to the high teenage pregnancy rate, including earlier age at first experience with sexual intercourse, lack of knowledge about conception, lack of easy access to contraception, lessened stigma associated with adolescent pregnancy in some populations, poverty, early school failure, and early childhood sexual abuse.
- Physical risks of adolescent pregnancy include preterm births, low-birth-weight infants, cephalopelvic disproportion, iron deficiency anemia, and pregnancy-induced hypertension (PIH) and its sequelae.
- In the adolescent age group, prenatal care is the critical factor that most influences pregnancy outcome.
- The major psychologic risk the pregnant adolescent faces is the interruption of her own developmental tasks.
- In general, the children of teenage mothers are found to be at a developmental disadvantage compared with children whose mothers were older at the time of their birth.
- Almost half of the fathers of infants of adolescent mothers are age 20 or older but are often similar to adolescent fathers psychosocially and no more likely to be able to support the mother.
- Factors affecting an adolescent's response to pregnancy include her degree of achievement of the developmental tasks of adolescence (which can be closely associated with age), as well as cultural, religious, and socioeconomic factors.
- Often the adolescent has little understanding of pregnancy, childbirth, or parenting. Consequently, education is a primary responsibility of the nurse.
- Adolescent pregnancy prevention programs should be multifaceted, target males as well as females, and involve community-wide approaches.

## CHAPTER REFERENCES


Alan Guttmacher Institute. (1996). *Issues in brief: Risks and realities of early childbearing.* Washington, DC: Author.

Alan Guttmacher Institute. (1999). *Issues in brief: Teen sex and pregnancy, 1999.* Washington, DC: Author.

Bloom, K. C. (1998). Perceived relationship with the father of the baby and maternal attachment in adolescents. *Journal of Obstetric, Gynecologic, and Neonatal Nursing, 27*(4), 420–430.

Clark, L. R., Cohall, A. T., & Joffe, A. (1998). Beyond the birds and the bees: Talking to teens about sex. *Contemporary OB/GYN, 43*(4), 35–61.

Cockey, C. D. (1997). Preventing teen pregnancy: It's time to stop kidding around. *AWHONN Lifelines, 1*(3), 32–40.

Dallas, C. M., & Chen, S. C. (1999). Perspectives of women whose sons become adolescent fathers. *Maternal-Child Nursing, 24*(5), 247–251.

East, P. L., & Felice, M. E. (1996). *Adolescent pregnancy and parenting: Findings from a racially diverse sample.* Hillsdale, NJ: Erlbaum.

Jones, M. E., & Mondy, L. W. (1994). Lessons for prevention and intervention in adolescent pregnancy: A five-year comparison of outcomes of two programs for school-aged pregnant adolescents. *Journal of Pediatric Health Care, 8*(4), 152–159.

Kirby, D. (1997). *No easy answers: Research findings on programs to reduce teen pregnancy (summary).* Washington, DC: National Campaign to Prevent Teen Pregnancy.

Koniak-Griffin, D., Mathenge, C., Anderson, N. L. R., & Verzemnieks, I. (1999). An early intervention program for adolescent mothers: A nursing demonstration project. *Journal of Obstetric, Gynecologic, and Neonatal Nursing, 28*(1), 51–59.

Moore, K., & Sugland, B. (1996). *Next steps and best bets: Approaches to preventing adolescent childbearing.* Washington, DC: Child Trends.

National Campaign to Prevent Teen Pregnancy. (1997). *Whatever happened to childhood? The problem of teen pregnancy in the United States.* Washington, DC: Author.

Philliber, S., & Namerow, P. (1995). Trying to maximize the odds: Using what we know to prevent teen pregnancy. Paper presented at technical assistance workshop to support the Teen Pregnancy Prevention Program. Division of Reproductive Health, Centers for Disease Control and Prevention, Atlanta, GA, December 13–15, 1995.

Roye, C. F., & Balk, S. J. (1996). The relationship of partner support to outcomes for teenage mothers and their children: A review. *Journal of Adolescent Health, 19*(2), 86–93.

Singh, S., & Darroch, J. E. (2000). Adolescent pregnancy and childbearing: Levels and trends in developed countries. *Family Planning Perspectives, 32*(1), 14–23.

Spieker, S. J., & Bensley, L. (1994). Roles of living arrangements and grandmother social support in adolescent mothering and infant attachment. *Developmental Psychology, 30*(1), 102–111.

Steinberg, L. (1999). *Adolescence* (5th ed.). Boston: McGraw-Hill.

Stevens-Simon, C., Kelly, L., Singer, D., & Cox, A. (1996). Why pregnant adolescents say they did not use contraceptives prior to conception. *Journal of Adolescent Health, 19*(1), 48–53.

Stock, J. L., Bell, M. A., Boyer, D. K., & Connell, F. A. (1997). Adolescent pregnancy and sexual risk-taking among sexually abused girls. *Family Planning Perspectives, 29*(5), 200–203, 227.

Taylor, D., Chavez, G., Chabra, A., & Boggess, J. (1997). Risk factors for adult paternity in births to adolescents. *Obstetrics and Gynecology, 89*(2), 199–205.

## CONTEMPORARY MATERNAL-NEWBORN NURSING ON-LINE

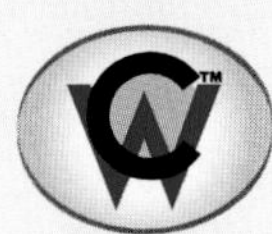

Additional interactive resources, including animations and video, for this chapter can be found on the Companion Website at http://www.prenhall.com/ladewig. Click on Chapter 10 and "Begin" to select the activities for this chapter.

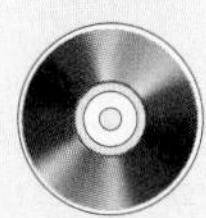

For NCLEX review questions and an audio glossary, access the accompanying CD-ROM in this book.

# Chapter 11

# Maternal Nutrition

*When I was a nursing student I thought nutrition was boring—was I wrong! Now I know how important good nutrition is to every aspect of life, but especially to pregnancy, and I find it endlessly fascinating. When my enthusiasm sparks a response in a pregnant woman I am meeting with, I feel that I am having a long-term impact on the woman's life and hopefully on her family, too.*

—A Nurse Working as a Patient Educator

## OBJECTIVES

- Delineate recommended levels of weight gain during pregnancy.
- Identify the role of specific nutrients in the diet of the pregnant woman.
- Compare nutritional needs during pregnancy, the postpartum period, and lactation with nonpregnant requirements.
- Plan adequate prenatal vegetarian diets based on the nutritional requirements of pregnancy.
- Describe ways in which various physical, psychosocial, and cultural factors can affect nutritional intake and status.
- Compare recommendations for weight gain and nutrient intakes in the pregnant adolescent with those for the mature pregnant adult.
- Discuss basic factors a nurse should consider when offering nutritional counseling to a pregnant adolescent.
- Compare nutritional counseling issues for nursing and nonnursing mothers.
- Formulate a nutritional care plan for pregnant women based on a diagnosis of nutritional problems.

## KEY TERMS

| Term | Page |
|---|---|
| Calorie | 244 |
| Folic acid | 251 |
| Kilocalorie | 244 |
| Lactase deficiency (lactose intolerance) | 253 |
| Lacto-ovovegetarians | 252 |
| Lactovegetarians | 252 |
| Pica | 253 |
| Recommended dietary allowances (RDA) | 243 |
| Vegans | 252 |

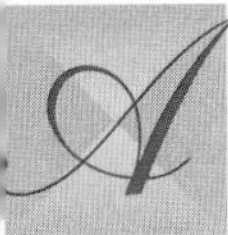

woman's nutritional status before and during pregnancy can significantly influence her health and that of her fetus. In most prenatal clinics and offices, nurses offer nutritional counseling directly or work closely with the nutritionist in providing nutritional assessment and teaching.

This chapter focuses on the nutritional needs of a normal pregnant woman. Special sections consider the nutritional needs of the pregnant adolescent and the woman after giving birth.

Good prenatal nutrition is the result of proper eating for a lifetime, not just during pregnancy. Many factors influence a woman's ability to achieve good prenatal nutrition:

- *General nutritional status prior to pregnancy.* Nutritional deficits present at the time of conception and during the early prenatal period may influence the outcome of the pregnancy.
- *Maternal age.* An expectant adolescent must meet her own growth needs in addition to the nutritional needs of pregnancy.
- *Maternal parity.* The mother's nutritional needs and the outcome of the pregnancy are influenced by the number of pregnancies she has had and the interval between them.

Fetal growth occurs in three overlapping stages: (1) growth by increase in cell number, (2) growth by increases in cell number and cell size, and (3) growth by increase in cell size alone. Nutritional problems that interfere with cell division may have permanent consequences. If the nutritional insult occurs when cells are mainly enlarging, the changes are usually reversible when normal nutrition resumes.

Growth of fetal and maternal tissues requires increased quantities of essential dietary components. These are listed in the **recommended dietary allowances (RDA)** as specific allowances for pregnant and lactating women (Table 11–1). Most of the recommended nutrients can be obtained by eating a well-balanced diet each day. The basic food groups and recommended amounts during pregnancy and lactation are presented in Table 11–2 on page 246.

# Maternal Weight Gain

Maternal weight gain is an important factor in fetal growth and infant birth weight. The optimal weight gain depends on the woman's weight for height (body mass index [BMI]) and her prepregnant nutritional state. An adequate weight gain indicates an adequate caloric intake. It does not, however, ensure that the woman has a sufficient nutrient intake. The pregnant woman must maintain the nutritional quality of her diet as her weight gain progresses.

The Institute of Medicine (1992) recommends weight gains in terms of optimum ranges. Its recommendations are as follows:

- Underweight woman: 28–40 lb (12.5–18 kg)
- Normal-weight woman: 25–35 lb (11.5–16 kg)
- Overweight woman: 15–25 lb (7–11.5 kg)
- Obese woman: ≥15 lb (≥7.0 kg)

The average maternal weight gain is distributed as follows:

| | |
|---|---|
| 11 lb (5.0 kg) | Fetus, placenta, amniotic fluid |
| 2 lb (0.9 kg) | Uterus |
| 4 lb (1.8 kg) | Increased blood volume |
| 3 lb (1.4 kg) | Breast tissue |
| 5–10 lb (2.3–4.5 kg) | Maternal stores |

The ideal pattern of weight gain during pregnancy for a normal-weight woman consists of a gain of 3.5 to 5 lb (1.6 to 2.3 kg) during the first trimester, followed by a gain of about 1 lb (0.5 kg) per week during the second and third trimesters. A normal-weight woman who is expecting twins is advised to gain about 1.5 lb per week during the second and third trimesters of her pregnancy (Brown & Carlson, 2000).

The pattern of weight gain is important. A woman should generally gain 10 to 13 lb (4.5 to 6 kg) by 20 weeks' gestation. If she has not, the nurse should offer further nutritional evaluation and counseling. Sudden, sharp increases (weight gains of 3–5 lb [1.4–2.3 kg] in 1 week) may indicate excessive fluid retention related to pregnancy-induced hypertension (PIH) and should be evaluated. Inadequate gains (less than 2.2 lb [1 kg] per month during the second and third trimesters) or excessive gains (more than 6.6 lb [3 kg] per month) should be assessed and the need for nutritional counseling considered.

Pregnancy is not a time for dieting, and severe weight restrictions during pregnancy can result in maternal ketosis, a threat to fetal well-being. Counseling the pregnant woman to eat according to the Food Guide Pyramid (Figure 11–1♦) on p. 247 places less emphasis on the amount of her weight gain and more on the quality of her intake.

Women who are 10% or more below their recommended weight before conception have an increased risk of giving birth to a low-birth-weight infant and have an increased risk of developing PIH (Institute of Medicine, 1990). Underweight women are generally advised to increase their caloric intake by 500 kilocalories (kcal) above the nonpregnant RDA, as opposed to the 300-kcal increase. They should also consume 20 g additional protein. This is often difficult for underweight women, especially if they have a small appetite, and they will require support and encouragement from family and health care providers.

## TABLE 11–1 Recommended Dietary Allowances (RDAs) for Nonpregnant, Pregnant, and Lactating Females, Revised 1989*

| | | | | | | FAT-SOLUBLE VITAMINS | | | | WATER-SOLUBLE VITAMINS | | |
|---|---|---|---|---|---|---|---|---|---|---|---|---|
| *Age (years) and Sex Group* | *Weight*[†] *kg* | *lb* | *Height*[†] *cm* | *in* | *Protein* | *Vitamin A* | *Vitamin D* | *Vitamin E* | *Vitamin K* | *Vitamin C* | *Thiamine* | *Riboflavi* |
| | | | | | g | μgR[‡] | μg[§] | mg α-TE[‖] | μg | ← mg | mg | mg → |
| Females | | | | | | | | | | | | |
| 11–14 | 46 | 101 | 157 | 62 | 46 | 800 | 10 | 8 | 45 | 50 | 1.1 | 1.3 |
| 15–18 | 55 | 120 | 163 | 64 | 44 | 800 | 10 | 8 | 55 | 60 | 1.1 | 1.3 |
| 19–24 | 58 | 128 | 164 | 65 | 46 | 800 | 10 | 8 | 60 | 60 | 1.1 | 1.3 |
| 25–50 | 63 | 138 | 163 | 64 | 50 | 800 | 5 | 8 | 65 | 60 | 1.1 | 1.3 |
| 51+ | 65 | 143 | 160 | 63 | 50 | 800 | 5 | 8 | 65 | 60 | 1.0 | 1.2 |
| Pregnant | | | | | 60 | 800 | 10 | 10 | 65 | 70 | 1.5 | 1.6 |
| Lactating | | | | | | | | | | | | |
| 1st 6 months | | | | | 65 | 1300 | 10 | 12 | 65 | 95 | 1.6 | 1.8 |
| 2nd 6 months | | | | | 62 | 1200 | 10 | 11 | 65 | 90 | 1.6 | 1.7 |

*The allowances, expressed as average daily intakes over time, are intended to provide for individual variations among most normal persons as they live in the United States under usual environmental stresses. Diets should be based on a variety of common foods in order to provide other nutrients for which human requirements have been less well defined.

[†]Weights and heights of reference adults are actual medians for the U.S. population of the designated age, as reported by NHANES II. The median weights and heights of those under 19 years of age were taken from Hamill, P.V.V. et al. (1979). Physical growth. National Center for Health Statistics Percentiles. *Am J Clin Nutr 32*, 607. The use of these figures does not imply that the height-to-weight ratios are ideal.

[‡]Retinol equivalents. 1 retinol equivalent = 1 μg retinol or 6 μg β-carotene.

[§]As cholecalciferol. 10 μg cholecalciferol = 400 IU of vitamin D.

[‖]α-Tocopherol equivalents. 1 mg d-α tocopherol = 1 α-TE.

[#]1 niacin equivalent (NE) is equal to 1 mg of niacin or 60 mg of dietary tryptophan.

*Source: Recommended dietary allowances,* 10th ed. 1989. Washington, DC: National Academy of Sciences, National Research Council, Food and Nutrition Board.

# Nutritional Requirements

The RDA for almost all nutrients increases during pregnancy, although the amount of increase varies with each nutrient. These increases reflect the additional requirements of both the mother and the developing fetus (Table 11–1).

Folic acid and iron are the only nutritional supplements generally recommended during pregnancy. The increased need for other vitamins and minerals can usually be met with an adequate diet. To avoid possible deficiencies, however, many health care professionals still recommend a daily vitamin supplement.

## Calories

The term **calorie** (cal) designates the amount of heat required to raise the temperature of 1 g of water 1°C. The **kilocalorie** (kcal) is equivalent to 1000 cal and is the unit used to express the energy value of food.

The RDA for energy requirements during pregnancy recommends no increase during the first trimester but an increase of 300 kcal/day during the second and third trimesters. Prepregnant weight, height, maternal age, health status, and activity level all influence caloric needs, and weight should be monitored regularly during the pregnancy. The Teaching Guide: Helping the Pregnant Woman Add 300 kcal to Her Diet, on page 248, offers suggestions for providing basic nutritional information to pregnant women.

## Carbohydrates

Carbohydrates provide the body's primary source of energy as well as the fiber necessary for proper bowel functioning. If the total caloric intake is not adequate, the body uses protein for energy. Protein then becomes unavailable for growth needs. In addition, protein breakdown leads to ketosis. Ketosis can be a problem, especially in diabetic women, because of glycosuria, reduced alkaline reserves, and lipidemia.

| WATER-SOLUBLE VITAMINS | | | | MINERALS | | | | | | |
|---|---|---|---|---|---|---|---|---|---|---|
| *Niacin* | *Vitamin B₆* | *Folate* | *Vitamin B₁₂* | *Calcium* | *Phosphorus* | *Magnesium* | *Iron* | *Zinc* | *Iodine* | *Selenium* |
| mg NE[#] | mg | ←µg | →µg | ←mg | | | | →mg | ←µg | →µg |
| 15 | 1.4 | 150 | 2.0 | 1200 | 1200 | 280 | 15 | 12 | 150 | 45 |
| 15 | 1.5 | 180 | 2.0 | 1200 | 1200 | 300 | 15 | 12 | 150 | 50 |
| 15 | 1.6 | 180 | 2.0 | 1200 | 1200 | 280 | 15 | 12 | 150 | 55 |
| 15 | 1.6 | 180 | 2.0 | 800 | 800 | 280 | 15 | 12 | 150 | 55 |
| 13 | 1.6 | 180 | 2.0 | 800 | 800 | 280 | 10 | 12 | 150 | 55 |
| 17 | 2.2 | 400 | 2.2 | 1200 | 1200 | 320 | 30 | 15 | 175 | 65 |
| 20 | 2.1 | 280 | 2.6 | 1200 | 1200 | 355 | 15 | 19 | 200 | 75 |
| 20 | 2.1 | 260 | 2.6 | 1200 | 1200 | 340 | 15 | 16 | 200 | 75 |

The carbohydrate and caloric needs of the pregnant woman increase, especially during the last two trimesters. Carbohydrate intake promotes weight gain and growth of the fetus, placenta, and other maternal tissues. Dairy products, fruits, vegetables, and whole-grain cereals and breads all contain carbohydrates and other important nutrients.

## PROTEIN

Protein supplies the amino acids (nitrogen) required for hyperplasia and hypertrophy of maternal tissues, such as the uterus and breasts, and to meet fetal needs. The fetus makes its greatest demands during the last half of pregnancy, when fetal growth is greatest. Protein also contributes to the body's overall energy metabolism.

The protein requirement for the pregnant woman is 60 g/day, an increase of 20% over prepregnancy requirements (Reifsnider & Gill, 2000). Animal products such as meat, fish, poultry, and eggs are sources of high-quality protein. Dairy products are also important protein sources. A quart of milk supplies 32 g of protein, more than half the average daily protein requirement. Milk can be incorporated into the diet in a variety of dishes, including soups, puddings, custards, sauces, and yogurt. Beverages such as hot chocolate and milk-and-fruit drinks can also be included, but they are high in calories. Various kinds of hard and soft cheeses and cottage cheese are excellent protein sources, although cream cheese is categorized as a fat source only.

Women who have allergies to milk, are lactose intolerant, or practice vegetarianism may find soy milk acceptable. It can be used in cooked dishes or as a beverage. Tofu, or soybean curd, can replace cottage cheese.

If the woman consumes little or no protein from animal sources, it is necessary to combine foods of plant origin to obtain the amino acids necessary for a complete protein. Examples of combined proteins are beans and rice, peanut butter on whole-grain bread, and whole-grain cereal and milk. Except in unusual medical situations, the pregnant woman should obtain dietary protein

## TABLE 11–2 Daily Food Plan for Pregnancy and Lactation

| *Food Group* | *Nutrients Provided* | *Food Source* | *Recommended Daily Amount during Pregnancy* | *Recommended Daily Amount during Lactation* |
|---|---|---|---|---|
| Dairy products | Protein; riboflavin; vitamins A, D, and others; calcium; phosphorus; zinc, magnesium | Milk—whole, 2%, skim, dry, buttermilk<br>Cheeses—hard, semisoft, cottage<br>Yogurt—plain, low-fat<br>Soybean milk—canned, dry | Four (8-oz) cups (five for teenagers) used plain or with flavoring, in shakes, soups, puddings, custards, cocoa<br>Calcium in 1 cup milk equivalent to 1½ cups cottage cheese, 1½ oz hard or semisoft cheese, 1 cup yogurt, 1½ cups ice cream (high in fat and sugar) | Four (8-oz) cups (five for teenagers); equivalent amount of cheese, yogurt, and so forth |
| Meat and meat alternatives | Protein; iron; thiamine; niacin, and other vitamins; minerals | Beef, pork, veal, lamb, poultry, animal organ meats, fish, eggs; legumes; nuts, seeds, peanut butter, grains in proper vegetarian combination (vitamin $B_{12}$ supplement needed) | Three servings (one serving = 2 oz), combination in amounts necessary for same nutrient equivalent (varies greatly) | Two servings |
| Grain products, whole grain or enriched | B vitamins; iron; whole grain also has zinc, magnesium, and other trace elements; provides fiber | Breads and bread products such as cornbread, muffins, waffles, hotcakes, biscuits, dumplings, cereals, pastas, rice | Six to eleven servings daily: one serving = one slice bread, ¾ cup or 1 oz dry cereal ½ cup rice or pasta | Same as for pregnancy |
| Fruits and fruit juices | Vitamins A and C; minerals; raw fruits for roughage | Citrus fruits and juices, melons, berries, all other fruits and juices | Two to four servings (one serving for vitamin C): one serving = one medium fruit, ½–1 cup fruit, 4 oz orange or grapefruit juice | Same as for pregnancy |
| Vegetables and vegetable juices | Vitamins A and C; minerals; provides roughage | Leafy green vegetables; deep yellow or orange vegetables such as carrots, sweet potatoes, squash, tomatoes; green vegetables such as peas, green beans, broccoli; other vegetables such as beets, cabbage, potatoes, corn, lima beans | Three to five servings (one serving of dark green or deep yellow vegetable for vitamin A): one serving = ½–1 cup vegetable, two tomatoes, one medium potato | Same as for pregnancy |
| Fats | Vitamins A and D; linoleic acid | Butter, cream cheese, fortified table spreads; cream, whipped cream, whipped toppings; avocado, mayonnaise, oil, nuts | As desired in moderation (high in calories): one serving = 1 tbsp butter or enriched margarine | Same as for pregnancy |
| Sugar and sweets | | Sugar, brown sugar, honey, molasses | Occasionally, if desired | Same as for pregnancy |
| Desserts | | Nutritious desserts such as puddings, custards, fruit whips, and crisps; other rich, sweet desserts and pastries | Occasionally, if desired | Same as for pregnancy |
| Beverages | | Coffee, decaffeinated beverages, tea, bouillon, carbonated drinks | As desired, in moderation | Same as for pregnancy |
| Miscellaneous | | Iodized salt, herbs, spices, condiments | As desired | Same as for pregnancy |

*Note:* The pregnant woman should eat regularly, three meals a day, with nutritious snacks of fruit, cheese, milk, or other foods between meals if desired. (More frequent but smaller meals are also recommended.) Four to six (8-oz) glasses of water and a total of 8 to 10 (8-oz) cups total fluid intake should be consumed daily. Water is an essential nutrient.

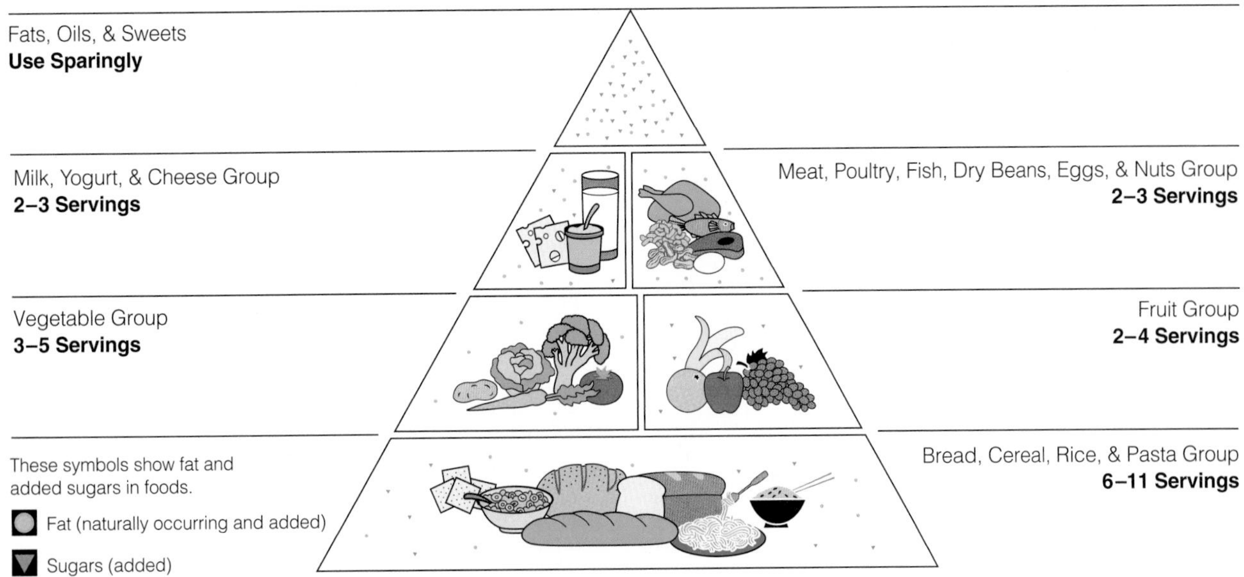


FIGURE 11–1 ♦ The Food Guide Pyramid provides a quick reference for people interested in healthful eating. The largest portion of the pyramid is devoted to grains, rice, bread, and pasta, and the smallest portion of the pyramid is devoted to fats, oils, and sweets, which should be used sparingly. *Source:* U.S. Department of Agriculture; U.S. Department of Health and Human Services

through natural foods and avoid using protein and amino acid supplements.

## Fat

Fats are valuable sources of energy for the body. Fats are more completely absorbed during pregnancy, resulting in a marked increase in serum lipids, lipoproteins, and cholesterol and decreased elimination of fat through the bowel. Fat deposits in the fetus increase from about 2% at midpregnancy to almost 12% at term. The RDA for fat is less than 30% of daily caloric intake, of which less than 10% should be saturated fat.

## Minerals

Increased minerals needed for the growth of new tissue during pregnancy are obtained by improved mineral absorption and an increase in mineral allowances.

### Calcium and Phosphorus

Calcium and phosphorus are involved in the mineralization of fetal bones and teeth, energy and cell production, and acid-base buffering. Calcium is absorbed and used more efficiently during pregnancy. Some calcium and phosphorus are required early in pregnancy, but most fetal bone calcification occurs during the last 2 to 3 months. Teeth begin to form at about 8 weeks' gestation and are formed by birth. The 6-year molars begin to calcify just before birth.

The RDA for calcium for the pregnant or lactating woman, regardless of age, is 1200 mg/day. If calcium intake is low, fetal needs will be met at the mother's expense by demineralization of maternal bone.

A diet that includes 4 cups of milk or an equivalent dairy alternative will provide sufficient calcium. Smaller amounts of calcium are supplied by legumes, nuts, dried fruits, and dark green leafy vegetables (such as kale, cabbage, collards, and turnip greens). It is important to remember that some of the calcium in beet greens, spinach, and chard is bound with oxalic acid, which makes it less available to the body.

The RDA for phosphorus is the same as the RDA for calcium: 1200 mg/day for the pregnant or lactating woman. Because phosphorus is so widely available in foods, the daily requirement is readily supplied through calcium- and protein-rich foods.

### Iodine

Iodine is an essential part of the thyroid hormone thyroxine. Inorganic iodine is excreted in the urine during pregnancy. Enlargement of the thyroid gland may occur if iodine is not replaced by adequate dietary intake or an additional supplement. Moreover, cretinism may occur in the infant if the mother has a severe iodine deficiency. The iodine allowance of 175 g/day can be met by using iodized salt. When sodium is restricted, the physician may prescribe an iodine supplement.

### Sodium

The sodium ion is essential for proper metabolism and the regulation of fluid balance. Sodium intake in the form of salt is never entirely curtailed during pregnancy, even when hypertension or PIH is present. The pregnant woman may season food to taste during cooking but

## TEACHING GUIDE *Helping the Pregnant Woman Add 300 kcal to Her Diet*

### Assessment

The nurse recognizes that the notion of "eating for two" may cause a woman to overestimate the amount of food she should consume during pregnancy. The nurse assesses the pregnant woman's knowledge of basic nutrition, including the use of the Food Guide Pyramid (Figure 11–1♦), and assesses her awareness of the best way to increase the nutrients in her diet.

### Nursing Diagnosis

The key nursing diagnosis will probably be health-seeking behaviors: information on recommended dietary changes in pregnancy related to an expressed desire to maintain good nutrition.

### Nursing Plan and Implementation

The teaching plan focuses on providing information about the Food Guide Pyramid and about the most effective way to use the additional 300 kcal that a woman needs daily during pregnancy.

### Client Goals

At the completion of the teaching the woman will be able to

1. Identify the Food Guide Pyramid categories and the foods included in each.
2. Cite the increase in kilocalories indicated during pregnancy.
3. Discuss the most nutritionally sound way to use the additional calories.
4. Use the information she has gained to plan a nutritionally sound sample menu.

## *Teaching Plan*

| CONTENT | TEACHING METHOD |
| --- | --- |
| Describe the basic food groups, which include the following:<br>Grains: 6 to 11 servings (one serving = 1 slice bread, ½ hamburger roll, 1 oz dry cereal, 1 tortilla, ½ cup pasta, rice, grits)<br>Fruits: Two to four servings; one should be a good source of vitamin C (one serving = 1 medium-sized piece of fruit, ½ cup juice).<br>Vegetables: Three to five servings (one serving = 1 cup raw vegetable, 1 cup green leafy vegetable, ½ cup cooked vegetable)<br>Dairy: Two to three servings (one serving = 1 cup milk or yogurt, 1.5 oz hard cheese, 2 cups cottage cheese, 1 cup pudding made with milk)<br>Meats and alternatives: Two to three servings (one serving = 2 oz cooked lean meat, poultry, or fish; 2 eggs; ½ cup cottage cheese; 1 cup cooked legumes [kidney, lima, garbanzo, or soybeans, split peas]; 6 oz tofu; 2 oz nuts or seeds; 4 tbsp peanut butter) | Ask woman if she has received nutritional information using this approach before. Discuss her understanding of it. Use that information to plan the amount of detail you will use.<br>Use a chart or colorful handout to explain the basic food groups and to give examples of equivalent foods. |
| Point out that not all foods that are nutritionally equivalent have the same number of calories; it is important to consider that when making food choices. | Use a calorie-counting guide to compare the calories in a variety of foods that are equivalent, such as 2 oz beef and 2 oz fish or 1 cup low-fat milk and 1 cup whole milk. |
| Explain the Food Guide Pyramid.<br>The Food Guide Pyramid is designed to represent the food groups needed to make a balanced diet. The grain, fruit, and vegetable groups are at the base of the pyramid and should account for the majority of the food selections. Fewer servings of dairy and meat or meat alternative are required in the diet, and these groups fall in the middle portion of the pyramid. The very top of the pyramid represents fats, oils, and sweets. These items do not have a high nutritional value and should be used sparingly. | Use a similar approach to evaluate the calories in fats, oils, and sweets, but also evaluate their nutrient content, especially levels of nutrients such as vitamin C, iron, and calcium. |
| Emphasize that a woman only has to add 300 kcal/day during pregnancy. This can be achieved by adding two milk servings and one serving of meat or alternative. Because of the varying caloric value a woman needs to consider the advisability of using low-fat milk, lean cuts of meat, or fish broiled or baked instead of fried. | In planning the woman's diet to get optimum nutrition without too many additional calories, it is often helpful to ask her to plan and evaluate a sample menu. |
| Foods can be combined. For example, 1 cup spaghetti with a 2 oz meatball would count as 1 serving meat, ¾ cup spaghetti = 1 grain, and ¼ cup tomato sauce = ½ serving vegetable. | Provide handouts on which the woman can list the foods she has eaten and check off the corresponding nutrient categories. Have her bring her completed handouts to a subsequent visit. |

## EVALUATION

Evaluate the learning by providing time for discussion, questions, and practice using the calorie-counting guide.

Teaching has been effective if all the identified goals are achieved and if the woman seems comfortable planning her diet to provide for the best nutrition possible.

should avoid using extra salt at the table. She can avoid excessive intake by eliminating salty foods such as potato chips, ham, sausages, and sodium-based seasonings.

### Zinc

Zinc is involved in protein metabolism and the synthesis of DNA and RNA. It is essential for normal fetal growth and development as well as milk production during lactation. The RDA during pregnancy is 15 mg/day. Sources include meats, shellfish, poultry, whole grains, and legumes. Zinc deficiency during pregnancy may be associated with maternal and fetal morbidity (Prasad, 1996).

### Magnesium

Magnesium is essential for cellular metabolism and structural growth. The RDA for pregnancy is 320 mg/day. Good sources include milk, whole grains, dark green vegetables, nuts, and legumes.

### Iron

Iron requirements increase during pregnancy because of the growth of the fetus and placenta and the expansion of maternal blood volume. Anemia in pregnancy is mainly caused by low iron stores, although it may also be caused by inadequate intake of other nutrients, such as vitamins $B_6$ and $B_{12}$, folic acid, ascorbic acid, copper, and zinc. Iron deficiency anemia is generally defined as a decrease in the oxygen-carrying capacity of the blood. Anemia leads to a significant reduction in hemoglobin in the volume of packed red cells per deciliter of blood (hematocrit) or in the number of erythrocytes. Iron deficiency anemia may be associated with preterm birth and higher maternal morbidity (Wenstrom & Malee, 1999).

Fetal demands for iron further contribute to symptoms of anemia in the pregnant woman. The fetal liver stores iron, especially during the third trimester. The infant needs this stored iron during the first 4 months of life to compensate for the normally inadequate levels of iron in breast milk and non-iron-fortified formulas.

To prevent anemia, the woman must balance iron requirements and intake. Adequate iron intake is a problem for nonpregnant women and a greater one for pregnant women. By carefully selecting foods high in iron, the woman can increase her daily iron intake considerably. Lean meats, dark green leafy vegetables, eggs, and whole-grain and enriched breads and cereals are the usual food sources of iron. Other iron sources include dried fruits, legumes, shellfish, and molasses.

Iron absorption is generally higher for animal products than for vegetable products. However, the woman can enhance absorption of iron from nonmeat sources by combining them with meat or a food rich in vitamin C. The RDA for iron during pregnancy is 30 mg/day, but this intake is almost impossible to achieve through diet alone. Thus the pregnant woman should take a supplement of simple iron salt, such as ferrous gluconate, ferrous fumarate, or ferrous sulfate. The Centers for Disease Control and Prevention (CDC) recommend a daily supplement of 30 mg elemental iron beginning at the first prenatal visit (CDC, 1998). Unfortunately iron supplements often cause gastrointestinal discomfort, especially if taken on an empty stomach. However, taking the iron supplement after a meal may help reduce this discomfort. Iron supplements may also cause constipation, so an adequate fluid intake is especially important in pregnancy.

## Vitamins

Vitamins are organic substances necessary for life and growth. They are found in small amounts in specific foods and generally cannot be synthesized by the body in adequate amounts.

Vitamins are grouped according to solubility. Vitamins that dissolve in fat are A, D, E, and K; those soluble in water include vitamin C and the B complex. An adequate intake of all vitamins is essential during pregnancy; however, several are required in larger amounts to fulfill specific needs.

## Fat-Soluble Vitamins

The fat-soluble vitamins, A, D, E, and K, are stored in the liver and thus are available if the dietary intake becomes inadequate. The major complication related to these vitamins is not deficiency but toxicity due to overdose. Unlike water-soluble vitamins, excess amounts of vitamins A, D, E, and K are not excreted in the urine. Symptoms of vitamin toxicity include nausea, gastrointestinal upset, dryness and cracking of the skin, and loss of hair.

*Vitamin A* is involved in the growth of epithelial cells, which line the entire gastrointestinal tract and compose the skin. Vitamin A plays a role in the metabolism of carbohydrates and fats. In the absence of vitamin A, the body cannot synthesize glycogen, and the body's ability to handle cholesterol is also affected. The protective layer of tissue surrounding nerve fibers does not form properly if vitamin A is lacking.

Probably the best-known function of vitamin A is its effect on vision in dim light. A person's ability to see in the dark depends on the eye's supply of retinol, a form of vitamin A. In this manner, vitamin A prevents night blindness. Vitamin A is associated with the formation and development of healthy eyes in the fetus.

If maternal stores of vitamin A are adequate, the overall effects of pregnancy on the woman's vitamin A requirements are not remarkable. The blood serum level of vitamin A decreases slightly in early pregnancy, rises in late pregnancy, and falls before the onset of labor. The RDA for vitamin A does not increase during pregnancy.

Although routine supplementation with vitamin A is not recommended, supplementation with 5000 international units (IU) is indicated for women whose dietary intake may be inadequate, specifically strict vegetarians and recent emigrants from countries where deficiency of vitamin A is endemic (American College of Obstetricians and Gynecologists [ACOG], 1998).

Excessive intake of preformed vitamin A is toxic to both children and adults. There are indications that excessive intake of vitamin A in the fetus can cause birth defects.

Rich plant sources of vitamin A include deep green, deep orange, and yellow vegetables; animal sources include egg yolk, cream, butter, and fortified margarine and milk. Liver has long been identified as a source of vitamin A. However, because of today's animal feeding practices, animal liver now contains exceptionally high doses of vitamin A; in fact, a single serving may contain twice the recommended daily allowance. Thus, to avoid toxicity, researchers now recommend that women who are pregnant or trying to conceive avoid eating liver and liver products, including liver sausage and pâté (Doyle, 1998).

*Vitamin D* is best known for its role in the absorption and use of calcium and phosphorus in skeletal development. To supply the needs of the developing fetus, the pregnant woman should have a vitamin D intake of 10 mg/day.

Main food sources of vitamin D include fortified milk, margarine, butter, liver, and egg yolks. Drinking a quart of milk daily provides the vitamin D needed during pregnancy.

Excessive intake of vitamin D is not usually a result of eating but of taking high-potency vitamin preparations. Overdoses during pregnancy can cause hypercalcemia, or high blood calcium levels, due to withdrawal of calcium from the skeletal tissue. Symptoms of toxicity are excessive thirst, loss of appetite, vomiting, weight loss, irritability, and high blood calcium levels.

The major function of *vitamin E,* or tocopherol, is antioxidation. Vitamin E takes on oxygen, thus preventing another substance from undergoing chemical change. For example, vitamin E helps spare vitamin A by preventing its oxidation in the intestinal tract and in the tissues. It decreases the oxidation of polyunsaturated fats, thus helping to retain the flexibility and health of the cell membrane. In protecting the cell membrane, vitamin E affects the health of all cells in the body.

Vitamin E is also involved in certain enzymatic and metabolic reactions. It is an essential nutrient for the synthesis of nucleic acids required in the formation of red blood cells in the bone marrow. Vitamin E is beneficial in treating certain types of muscular pain and intermittent claudication, in surface healing of wounds and burns, and in protecting lung tissue from the damaging effects of smog. These functions may help explain the abundant claims and cures attributed to vitamin E, many of which have not been scientifically proved.

The recommended intake of vitamin E increases from 8 IU for nonpregnant females to 10 IU for pregnant women. The vitamin E requirement varies with the polyunsaturated fat content of the diet. Vitamin E is widely distributed in foodstuffs, especially vegetable fats and oils, whole grains, greens, and eggs.

Some pregnant women use vitamin E oil on the abdominal skin to make it supple and possibly prevent permanent stretch marks. It is questionable whether taking high doses internally will accomplish this goal or satisfy any other claims related to vitamin E's role in reproduction or virility. Excessive intake of vitamin E has been associated with abnormal coagulation in the newborn.

*Vitamin K,* or menadione (as used synthetically in medicine), is an essential factor for the synthesis of prothrombin; its function is thus related to normal blood clotting. Synthesis occurs in the intestinal tract by the *Escherichia coli* bacteria normally inhabiting the large intestine. However, the body's need for vitamin K is not totally met by synthesis. Green leafy vegetables and liver are excellent sources. The RDA for vitamin K does not increase during pregnancy.

Intake of vitamin K is usually adequate in a well-balanced prenatal diet. Secondary problems may arise if an illness is present that results in malabsorption of fats or if antibiotics are used for an extended period, which would inhibit vitamin K synthesis by destroying intestinal *E. coli.*

### Water-Soluble Vitamins

Water-soluble vitamins are excreted in the urine. Since only small amounts are stored, there is little protection from dietary inadequacies. Thus adequate amounts must be ingested daily. During pregnancy, the concentration of water-soluble vitamins in the maternal serum falls, whereas high concentrations are found in the fetus.

The RDA for *vitamin C (ascorbic acid)* increases in pregnancy from 60 to 70 mg. The major function of vitamin C is to aid in the formation and development of connective tissue and the vascular system. Ascorbic acid is essential to the formation of collagen, which binds cells together. If the collagen begins to disintegrate because of a lack of ascorbic acid, cell functioning is disturbed and cell structure breaks down, resulting in muscular weakness, capillary hemorrhage, and eventual death. These are symptoms of scurvy, the disease caused by vitamin C deficiency. Infants fed mainly cow's milk become deficient in vitamin C, and they are the main population that develops these symptoms. Surprisingly, newborns of women who have taken megadoses of vitamin C may experience a rebound form of scurvy.

Maternal plasma levels of vitamin C progressively decline during pregnancy, with values at term being about half those at midpregnancy. It appears that ascorbic acid concentrates in the placenta; levels in the fetus are 50% or more above maternal levels.

A nutritious diet should meet the pregnant woman's needs for vitamin C without additional supplementation. Common food sources of vitamin C include citrus fruit, tomatoes, cantaloupe, strawberries, potatoes, broccoli, and other leafy greens. Ascorbic acid is readily destroyed by water and oxidation. Therefore, foods containing vitamin C must be stored and cooked properly.

The B vitamins include thiamine ($B_1$), riboflavin ($B_2$), niacin, folic acid, pantothenic acid, vitamin $B_6$, and vitamin $B_{12}$. These vitamins serve as vital coenzyme factors in many reactions such as cell respiration, glucose oxidation, and energy metabolism. The quantities needed, therefore, invariably increase as caloric intake increases to meet the metabolic and growth needs of the pregnant woman.

The *thiamine* requirement increases from the prepregnant level of 1.1 mg/day to 1.5 mg/day. Sources include pork, liver, milk, potatoes, and enriched breads and cereals.

*Riboflavin* deficiency is manifested by cheilosis (fissures and cracks of the lips and corners of the mouth) and other skin lesions. During pregnancy women may excrete less riboflavin and still require more because of increased energy and protein needs. An additional 0.3 mg/day is recommended. Sources include milk, liver, eggs, enriched breads, and cereals.

*Niacin* intake should increase 2 mg/day during pregnancy and 5 mg/day during lactation. Sources of niacin include meat, fish, poultry, liver, whole grains, enriched breads, cereals, and peanuts.

**Folic acid,** or folate, is required for normal growth, reproduction, and lactation and prevents the macrocytic, megaloblastic anemia of pregnancy. Megaloblastic anemia due to folate deficiency is rarely found in the United States, but it does occur.

Even more significantly, an inadequate intake of folic acid has been associated with neural tube defects (NTDs) (spina bifida, meningomyelocele) in the fetus or newborn. Because the average daily intake of folic acid from dietary sources is only about half the recommended daily requirement (0.4 mg), in 1999 the CDC, the March of Dimes Birth Defects Foundation, and the National Council on Folic Acid began a national campaign to educate women about the importance of consuming folic acid daily. Specifically, the U.S. Public Health Service recommends that all women of childbearing age (15 to 45 years) consume 0.4 mg of folic acid daily because half of all U.S. pregnancies are unplanned and NTDs occur very early in pregnancy (3 to 4 weeks after conception), before most women realize they are pregnant (Mersereau, 2000). The CDC estimates that 50% to 70% of NTDs could be prevented if this recommendation was followed, especially before conception and during early pregnancy (first trimester) (CDC, 2000).

Large-dose supplementation (4.0 mg/day) is recommended *only* for women who have had a previous NTD-affected pregnancy and are planning another pregnancy (ACOG, 1996).

The best food sources of folates are fresh green leafy vegetables, liver, peanuts, and whole-grain breads and cereals. Folic acid can be made inactive by oxidation, ultraviolet light, and heating. It can easily be lost during improper storage and cooking. To prevent unnecessary loss, foods should be stored covered to protect them from light, cooked with only a small amount of water, and not overcooked.

No allowance has been set for *pantothenic acid* in pregnancy, but 5 mg/day is considered a safe, adequate intake. Sources include meats, egg yolk, legumes, and whole-grain cereals and breads.

*Vitamin $B_6$ (pyridoxine)* is associated with amino acid metabolism; thus a higher-than-average protein intake requires increased pyridoxine intake. The RDA for vitamin $B_6$ during pregnancy is 2.2 mg, an increase of 0.6 mg over the allowance for nonpregnant women. Generally, the slightly increased need can be supplied by dietary sources, which include wheat germ, yeast, fish, liver, pork, potatoes, and lentils.

*Vitamin $B_{12}$*, or *cobalamin*, is the cobalt-containing vitamin found only in animal sources. Women of reproductive age rarely have a $B_{12}$ deficiency. Vegans (see later discussion on vegetarian diets) can develop a deficiency, however, so it is essential that their dietary intake be supplemented with this vitamin. Occasionally vitamin $B_{12}$ levels decrease during pregnancy but increase again after childbirth. The RDA during pregnancy is 2.2 mg/day. A deficiency may be due to a congenital inability to absorb vitamin $B_{12}$, resulting in pernicious anemia. Infertility is a complication of this type of anemia.

### FLUID

Water is essential for life, and it is found in all body tissues. It is necessary for many biochemical reactions. It also serves as a lubricant, as a medium of transport for carrying substances in and out of the body, and as an aid in temperature control. A pregnant woman should consume at least 8 to 10 (8-oz) glasses of fluid each day, of which 4 to 6 glasses should be water.

Because of their sodium content, diet sodas should be consumed in moderation. Caffeinated beverages have a diuretic effect, which is counterproductive to increasing fluid intake.

## Vegetarianism

Vegetarianism is the dietary choice of many people for religious, health, or ethical reasons. There are several types of vegetarians. **Lacto-ovovegetarians** include milk, dairy products, and eggs in their diet. **Lactovegetarians** include dairy products but no eggs in their diets. **Vegans** are "pure" vegetarians who will not eat any food from animal sources.

The expectant woman who is vegetarian must eat the proper combination of foods to obtain adequate nutrients. If her diet allows, a woman can obtain ample and complete proteins from dairy products and eggs. An adequate, pure vegan diet contains protein from unrefined grains (brown rice, whole wheat), legumes (beans, split peas, lentils), nuts in large quantities, and a variety of cooked and fresh vegetables and fruits. Seeds may provide adequate protein in the vegetarian diet if the quantity is large enough. If the vegetarian woman's diet contains sufficient calories, it will also contain sufficient protein if she follows the recommendations for complementing proteins. Figure 11–2♦ depicts the vegetarian food pyramid.

Because vegans use no animal products, a daily supplement of 4 mg of vitamin $B_{12}$ is necessary. If the woman uses soy milk, only partial supplementation may be needed. If she uses no soy milk, she needs daily supplements of 1200 mg of calcium and 10 mg of vitamin D.

Because the best sources of iron and zinc are animal products, vegan diets may also be low in these minerals. In addition, a high fiber intake may reduce mineral (calcium, iron, and zinc) bioavailability. The nurse should emphasize the use of foods containing these nutrients. A vegetarian food group guide appears in Table 11–3.

## Factors Influencing Nutrition

Besides having knowledge of nutritional needs and food sources, the nurse must be aware of other factors that af-

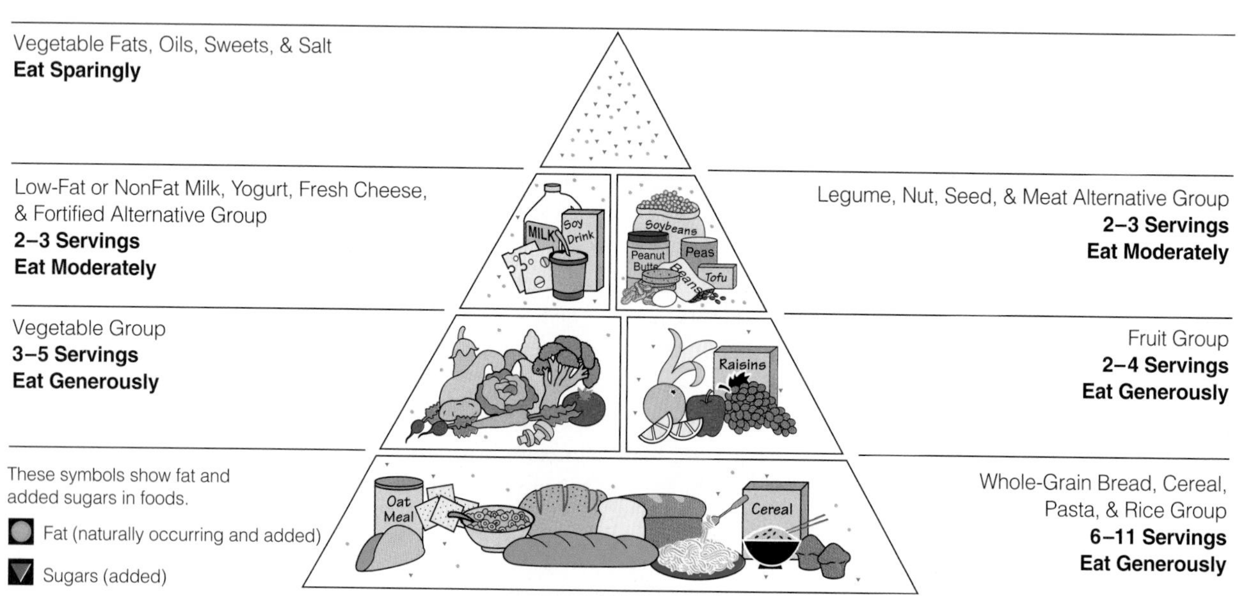


**FIGURE 11–2 ♦** The vegetarian food pyramid. *Source:* Adapted from the Health Connection, 55 West Oak Ridge Drive, Hagertown, MD 21740-7390.

**TABLE 11–3 Vegetarian Food Groups**

| *Food Group* | *Mixed Diet* | *Lacto-ovovegetarian* | *Lactovegetarian* | *Vegan* |
|---|---|---|---|---|
| Grain | Bread, cereal, rice, pasta | Bread, cereal, rice, pasta | Bread, cereal, rice, pasta | Bread, cereal, rice, pasta |
| Fruit | Fruit, fruit juices | Fruit, fruit juices | Fruit, fruit juices | Fruit, fruit juices |
| Vegetable | Vegetables, vegetable juices | Vegetables, vegetable juices | Vegetables, vegetable juices | Vegetables, vegetable juices |
| Dairy and dairy alternatives | Milk, yogurt, cheese | Milk, yogurt, cheese | Milk, yogurt, cheese | Fortified soy milk, rice milk |
| Meat and meat alternatives | Meat, fish, poultry, eggs, legumes, tofu, nuts, nut butters | Eggs, legumes, tofu, nuts, nut butters | Legumes, tofu, nuts, nut butters | Legumes, tofu, nuts, nut butters |

fect a client's nutrition. What are the age, lifestyle, and culture of the pregnant woman? What food beliefs and habits does she have? What a person eats is determined by availability, economics, and symbolism. These factors and others influence the expectant mother's acceptance of the nurse's intervention.

## Lactase Deficiency (Lactose Intolerance)

Some individuals have difficulty digesting milk and milk products. This condition, known as **lactase deficiency (lactose intolerance),** results from an inadequate amount of the enzyme lactase, which breaks down the milk sugar lactose into smaller digestible substances.

Lactase deficiency is found in many people of African, Mexican, Native American, Ashkenazic Jewish, and Asian descent. People who are not affected are mainly of northern European heritage. Symptoms include abdominal distention, discomfort, nausea, vomiting, loose stools, and cramps.

In counseling pregnant women who might be intolerant of milk and milk products, the nurse should be aware that even one glass of milk can produce symptoms. Milk in cooked form, such as custards, is sometimes tolerated, as are cultured or fermented dairy products such as buttermilk, some cheeses, and yogurt. In some instances, the enzyme lactase may be taken to alleviate this problem. It is available as a chewable tablet to be taken before ingesting milk products or as a liquid to add to milk itself. Lactase-treated milk is also available commercially in some grocery stores.

## Eating Disorders

In any given client population, it is probable that about 3% will have an eating disorder (Herrin, 1999). Two serious eating disorders, *anorexia nervosa* and *bulimia nervosa,* develop most commonly in adolescent girls but often continue into adulthood. Both conditions are psychologic disorders that can have a major impact on physiologic well-being.

Anorexia nervosa is an eating disorder characterized by an extreme fear of weight gain and fat. People with this problem have distorted body images and perceive themselves as fat even when they are extremely underweight. Their dietary intake is very restrictive in both variety and quantity. They may also engage in excessive exercise to prevent weight gain.

Bulimia is characterized by bingeing (secretly consuming large amounts of food in a short time) and purging. Self-induced vomiting is the most common method of purging; laxatives and/or diuretics may also be used. Individuals with bulimia nervosa often maintain normal or near-normal weight for their height, so it is difficult to know whether bingeing and purging occur.

Individuals with anorexia nervosa do not often become pregnant because of the physiologic changes that affect their reproductive systems. Women with bulimia can become pregnant. Their self-induced vomiting may produce many of the same complications as hyperemesis gravidarum. In both anorexia nervosa and bulimia, a multidisciplinary approach to treatment, involving medical, nursing, psychiatric, and dietetic practitioners, is indicated. Pregnant women with eating disorders need to be closely monitored and supported throughout their pregnancies.

## Pica

**Pica** is the persistent eating of substances such as dirt, clay, starch, freezer frost, burned matches, or ashes that are not ordinarily considered edible or nutritionally valuable. Most women who practice pica in pregnancy eat such substances only during that time.

Iron-deficiency anemia is the most common concern in pica. The ingestion of laundry starch or certain types of clay may contribute to iron deficiency because they interfere with iron absorption. The ingestion of large quantities of clay could fill the intestine and cause fecal impaction, and the ingestion of starch may be associated with excessive weight gain.

Nurses should be aware of pica and its implications for the woman and fetus. Assessment for pica is an important part of a nutritional history. However, a woman may be embarrassed about her cravings or reluctant to discuss them for fear of criticism. Using a nonjudgmental approach, the nurse can provide the woman with information that is useful in helping her to decrease or eliminate this practice.

## Common Discomforts of Pregnancy

Gastrointestinal functioning can be altered at various times throughout pregnancy, resulting in discomforts such as nausea, vomiting, heartburn, and constipation. Although these changes can be uncomfortable for the woman, they are seldom a major problem. These discomforts and dietary modifications that may provide relief are discussed in Chapter 9.

## Cultural, Ethnic, and Religious Influences

Cultural, ethnic, and occasionally religious backgrounds determine one's experiences with food and influence food preferences and habits (Figure 11–3♦). People of different nationalities are accustomed to eating different foods because of the kinds of foodstuffs available in their countries of origin. The way food is prepared varies, depending on the customs and traditions of the ethnic and cultural group. In addition, the laws of certain religions sanction particular foods, prohibit others, and direct the preparation and serving of meals.

In each culture, certain foods have symbolic significance. Generally these symbolic foods are related to major life experiences such as birth, death, or developmental milestones. Although generalizations have been made about the food practices of ethnic and religious groups, there are many variations. The extent to which individuals continue to consume traditional ethnic foods and follow food-related ethnic customs is affected by the extent of exposure to other cultures; the availability, quality, and cost of traditional foods; and the recency of immigration.

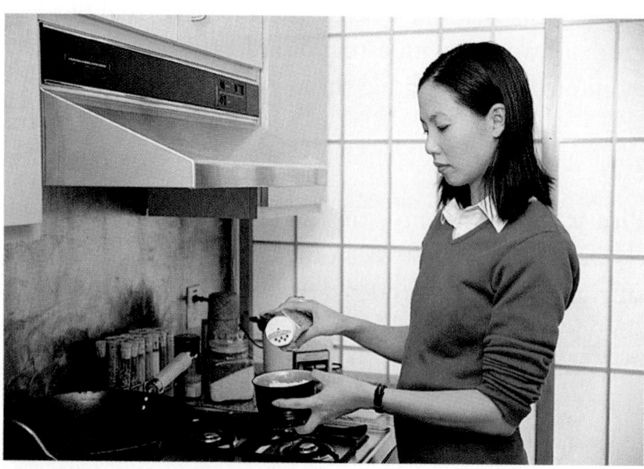

FIGURE 11–3 ♦ Food preferences and habits are affected by cultural factors.

It is common for health care providers to give dietary advice from their own cultural context. When working with pregnant women from any ethnic background, it is important for the nurse to understand the impact of the woman's cultural beliefs on her eating habits and to identify any beliefs she may have about food and pregnancy. Talking with the client can help the nurse determine the level of influence that traditional food customs exert. Dietary advice can then be given in a manner that is meaningful to the woman and her family.

## Psychosocial Factors

The nurse should be aware of the various psychosocial factors that influence a woman's food choices. The sharing of food has long been a symbol of friendliness, warmth, and social acceptance in many cultures. Some foods and food practices are associated with status. Some foods are prepared "just for company"; others are served only on special occasions or holidays.

Socioeconomic level may be a determinant of nutritional status. Poverty-level families cannot afford the same foods that higher-income families can. Thus pregnant women with low incomes are frequently at risk for poor nutrition.

Knowledge about the basic components of a balanced diet is essential. Often educational level is related to economic status, but even people on very limited incomes can prepare well-balanced meals if their knowledge of nutrition is adequate.

The expectant woman's attitudes and feelings about her pregnancy influence her nutritional status. For example, foods may be used as a substitute for the expression of emotions, such as anger or frustration, or as a way of expressing feelings of joy. The woman who is depressed or does not wish to be pregnant may manifest these feelings in loss of appetite or overindulgence in certain foods.

# Nutritional Care of the Pregnant Adolescent

Nutritional care of the pregnant adolescent is of particular concern to health care professionals. Many adolescents are nutritionally at risk because of a variety of complex and interrelated emotional, social, and economic factors. Important nutrition-related factors to assess in pregnant adolescents include low prepregnant weight, low weight gain during pregnancy, young age at menarche, smoking, excessive prepregnant weight, anemia, unhealthy lifestyle (drugs or alcohol use), chronic disease, and history of an eating disorder.

Estimates of the nutritional needs of adolescents are generally determined by using the RDA for nonpregnant teenagers (ages 11 to 14 or 15 to 18) and adding nutrient amounts recommended for all women (see Table 11–1). If mature (more than 4 years since menarche), the pregnant adolescent's nutritional needs approach those reported for pregnant adults. However, adolescents who become pregnant less than 4 years after menarche are at high biologic risk due to their physiologic and anatomic immaturity. They are more likely than older adolescents to still be growing, which can impact the fetus's development. Thus young adolescents (age 14 and under) need to gain more weight than older adolescents (18 years and older) to produce babies of equal size.

In determining the optimal weight gain for the pregnant adolescent, the nurse adds the recommended weight gain for an adult pregnancy to that expected during the postmenarcheal year in which the pregnancy occurs. If the teenager is underweight, additional weight gain is recommended to bring her to a normal weight for her height.

## Specific Nutrient Concerns

Caloric needs of pregnant adolescents vary widely. Major factors in determining caloric needs include whether growth has been completed and the physical activity level of the individual. Figures as high as 50 kcal/kg have been suggested for young, growing teens who are very active physically. A satisfactory weight gain usually confirms an adequate caloric intake.

An inadequate iron intake is a major concern with the adolescent diet. Iron needs are high for the pregnant teen due to the requirement for iron by the enlarging maternal muscle mass and blood volume. Iron supplements—providing between 30 and 60 mg of elemental iron—are definitely indicated.

Calcium is another nutrient that demands special attention from pregnant adolescents. Inadequate intake of calcium is frequently a problem in this age group. To provide for these needs, an intake of 1200 mg/day of calcium is recommended to promote bone mineralization in the adolescent and support fetal skeletal growth. This is 400 mg/day more than the recommended amount for pregnant adults. An extra serving of dairy products is usually suggested for teenagers. Calcium supplementation is indicated for teens with an aversion to milk, unless other dairy products or significant calcium sources are consumed in sufficient quantities.

Because folic acid plays a role in cell reproduction, it is also an important nutrient for pregnant teens. As previously indicated, a supplement is usually recommended for all pregnant females, whether adult or teenager.

Other nutrients and vitamins must be considered when evaluating the overall nutritional quality of the teenager's diet. Nutrients that have frequently been found to be deficient in this age group include zinc and vitamins A, D, and $B_6$. Inclusion of a wide variety of foods—especially fresh and lightly processed foods—is helpful in obtaining adequate amounts of trace minerals, fiber, and other vitamins.

## Dietary Patterns

Healthy adolescents often have irregular eating patterns. Many skip breakfast, and most tend to be frequent snackers. Teens rarely follow the traditional three-meals-a-day pattern. Their day-to-day intake often varies drastically, and they eat food combinations that may seem bizarre to adults. Despite these practices, adolescents usually achieve a better nutritional balance than most adults would expect.

Adolescent food choices are influenced by a variety of factors including hunger, food cravings, time and convenience, appeal of food, food availability, parental influence (including family religion and culture), food benefits, mood, body image, habit, media, cost, vegetarian beliefs, and situation-specific factors. Barriers adolescents cite to increased consumption of vegetables, fruits, and dairy products and decreased consumption of high-fat foods include taste preferences for other foods, a lack of a sense of urgency about personal health, and the cost of more healthful foods. In addition, the places adolescents typically eat when away from home—school and fast-food restaurants—do not offer these foods or they fail to make them appealing (Neumark-Sztainer, Story, Perry, et al., 1999).

In assessing the diet of the pregnant adolescent, the nurse should consider the eating pattern over time, not simply a single day's intake. Once the pattern is identified, counseling can be directed toward correcting deficiencies.

## Counseling Issues

Counseling about nutrition and healthy eating practices is an important element of care for pregnant teenagers that nurses can effectively provide in a community setting. This counseling may be individualized, involve other teens, or provide a combination of both approaches. If an adolescent's family member does most of the meal preparation, it may be useful to include that person in the discussion if the adolescent agrees. Clinics and schools often offer classes and focused activities designed to address this topic.

The pregnant teenager will soon become a parent, and her understanding of nutrition will influence not only her well-being but also that of her child. However, teens tend to live in the present, and counseling that stresses long-term changes may be less effective than more concrete approaches. In many cases group classes are effective, especially those with other teens. In a group atmosphere, adolescents often work together to plan adequate meals including foods that are special favorites.

# Postpartum Nutrition

Nutritional needs change following childbirth. Nutrient requirements vary depending on whether the mother decides to breastfeed. An assessment of postpartal nutritional status is necessary before nutritional guidance is given.

## Postpartal Nutritional Status

Determination of postpartal nutritional status is based primarily on the new mother's weight, hemoglobin and hematocrit levels, clinical signs, and dietary history. As mentioned previously, an ideal weight gain during pregnancy is 25 to 35 lb (11.5 to 16 kg). After birth there is a weight loss of approximately 10 to 12 lb. Additional weight loss is most rapid during the next few weeks as the body adjusts to the completion of pregnancy. The mother's weight will then begin to stabilize. Weight stabilization may take 6 months or longer.

The increased weight gain now recommended during pregnancy may have important implications for women postpartally unless they receive adequate counseling. Women who gain between 25 and 35 lb while pregnant have a net gain of about 3.5 lb (1.6 kg) 6 months after childbirth. Furthermore, multiparous women tend to lose less weight postpartally than primiparas; women who return to work outside the home tend to lose more weight than those who do not. The mother's weight should be considered in terms of ideal weight, prepregnancy weight, and weight gain during pregnancy. Women who desire information about weight reduction can be referred to a dietitian.

Hemoglobin and erythrocyte levels should return to normal within 2 to 6 weeks after childbirth. Hematocrit levels gradually rise due to hemoconcentration as extracellular fluid is excreted. Iron supplements are generally continued for 2 to 3 months following childbirth to replenish stores depleted by pregnancy.

The nurse assesses clinical symptoms the new mother may be experiencing. Constipation, in particular, is a common problem following birth. The nurse can encourage the woman to maintain a high fluid intake to keep the stool soft. Dietary sources of fiber, such as whole grains, fruits, and vegetables, are also helpful in preventing constipation.

The nurse obtains specific information on dietary intake and eating habits directly from the woman. Visiting the mother during mealtimes provides an opportunity for unobtrusive nutritional assessment. Which foods has the woman selected? Is her diet nutritionally sound? A comment focusing on a positive aspect of her meal selection may initiate a discussion of nutrition.

The nurse needs to inform the dietitian of any woman whose cultural or religious beliefs require specific foods so appropriate meals can be prepared for her. The nurse may also refer women with unusual eating habits or numerous questions about good nutrition to the dietitian. In addition, the nurse provides literature on nutrition so that the woman will have a source of appropriate information at home.

## Nutritional Care of Nonnursing Mothers

After birth, the nonnursing mother's dietary requirements return to prepregnancy levels (see Table 11–1). If the mother has a good understanding of nutritional principles, it is sufficient to advise her to reduce her daily caloric intake by about 300 kcal and to return to prepregnancy levels for other nutrients.

If the mother has a limited understanding of nutrition, now is the time to teach her the basic principles and the importance of a well-balanced diet. Her eating habits and dietary practices will eventually be reflected in the diet of her child.

If the mother has gained excessive weight during pregnancy (or perhaps was overweight before pregnancy) and wishes to lose weight, a referral to the dietitian is appropriate. The dietitian can design weight-reduction diets to meet nutritional needs and food preferences. Weight loss goals of 1 to 2 lb/week are usually suggested.

In addition to meeting her own nutritional needs, the new mother is usually interested in learning how to provide for her infant's nutritional needs. A discussion of infant feeding that includes topics such as selecting infant formulas, formula preparation, and vitamin and mineral supplementation is appropriate and generally well received.

## Nutritional Care of Nursing Mothers

Nutrient needs are increased during breastfeeding. Table 11–1 lists the RDA during breastfeeding for specific nutrients. Table 11–2 provides a sample daily food guide for lactating women. It is especially important for the nursing mother to consume sufficient calories, because inadequate caloric intake can reduce milk volume. However, milk quality generally remains unaffected. The nursing mother should increase her calories by about 200 kcal over her pregnancy requirement, or 500 kcal over her prepregnancy requirement. In the woman who breastfeeds exclusively, caloric requirements usually peak at 6 months postpartum because after that time infants generally begin to eat supplemental foods (Reifsnider & Gill, 2000).

Because protein is an important ingredient in breast milk, an adequate intake while breastfeeding is essential. An intake of 65 g/day during the first 6 months of breastfeeding and 62 g/day during the second 6 months is recommended. As in pregnancy, it is important to consume adequate nonprotein calories to prevent the use of protein as an energy source.

Calcium is an important ingredient in milk production, and requirements during lactation remain the same as during pregnancy—an increase of 1200 mg/day. If the intake of calcium from food sources is not adequate, calcium supplements are recommended.

Because iron is not a principal mineral component of milk, the needs of lactating women are not substantially different from those of nonpregnant women. As previously mentioned, however, supplementation for 2 to 3 months after childbirth is advisable to replenish maternal stores depleted by pregnancy.

Liquids are especially important during lactation, since inadequate fluid intake may decrease milk volume. Fluid recommendations while breastfeeding are 8 to 10 (8-oz) glasses daily, including water, juice, milk, and soups.

In addition to counseling nursing mothers on how to meet their increased nutrient needs during breastfeeding, it is important to discuss a few issues related to infant feeding. For example, many mothers are concerned about how specific foods they eat will affect their babies during breastfeeding. Generally the nursing mother need not avoid any foods except those to which she might be allergic. Occasionally, however, some nursing mothers find that their babies are affected by certain foods. Onions, turnips, cabbage, chocolate, spices, and seasonings are commonly listed as offenders. The best advice to give the nursing mother is to avoid those foods she suspects cause distress in her infant. For the most part, however, she should be able to eat any nourishing food she wants without fear that her baby will be affected. For further discussion of successful infant feeding, see Chapter 24.

# Nursing Care Management

## Nursing Assessment and Diagnosis

The nurse needs to assess nutritional status in order to plan an optimal diet with each woman. From the woman's chart and by interviewing her, the nurse gathers information about (1) the woman's height and weight, as well as her weight gain during pregnancy; (2) pertinent laboratory values, especially hemoglobin and hematocrit; (3) clinical signs that have possible nutritional implications, such as constipation, anorexia, or heartburn; and (4) dietary history to evaluate the woman's views on nutrition as well as her specific nutrient intake.

While gathering data, the nurse has an opportunity to discuss important aspects of nutrition within the context of the family's needs and lifestyle. The nurse also seeks information about psychologic, cultural, and socioeconomic factors that may influence food intake.

The nurse can use a nutritional questionnaire to gather and record important facts. This information provides a database the nurse can use to develop an intervention plan to fit the woman's individual needs. The sample questionnaire shown in Figure 11–4♦ has been filled in to demonstrate this process.

Once the nurse obtains the data, he or she begins to analyze the information, formulate appropriate nursing diagnoses, and, with the woman, develop goals and desired outcomes. For a woman during the first trimester, for example, the diagnosis may be "altered nutrition: less than body requirements related to nausea and vomiting." In other cases, the diagnosis may be related to excessive weight gain. In such situations the diagnosis might be "altered nutrition: more than body requirements related to excessive caloric intake." Although these diagnoses are broad, the nurse needs to be specific in addressing issues such as inadequate intake of nutrients including iron, calcium, or folic acid; problems with nutrition because of a limited food budget; problems related to physiologic alterations including anorexia, heartburn, or nausea; and behavioral problems related to excessive dieting, binge eating, and so on. At other times the diagnosis "health-seeking behaviors" may seem most appropriate, especially if the woman asks for information about nutrition.

## Nursing Plan and Implementation

After determining the nursing diagnosis, the nurse can plan an approach to address any nutritional deficiencies or improve the overall quality of the diet. To be truly effective, this plan must be made in cooperation with the woman. The following example demonstrates ways in which the nurse can plan with the woman based on the nursing diagnosis.

Diagnosis: Altered nutrition: less than body requirements related to low intake of calcium

Client goal: The woman will increase her daily intake of calcium to the minimum RDA levels

## NUTRITIONAL QUESTIONNAIRE

Name Susan Longmont Date 1-4-98

Age 20

Ethnic group Caucasian

Religion Protestant

Gravida 1 Para 0 EDB 8-10-98

Age of youngest child? NA

Birth weights of previous children? NA

Usual nonpregnant weight 115 Present weight 125

Weight gain during last pregnancy? NA

Vitamin supplements? none

Current medications? aspirin for headache

Do you smoke? yes How much per day? 1-1½ packs

Eating patterns:

1. How many meals per day? 2 when 12:30 pm 6:30 pm
2. How many snacks per day? 3 when 10:30 am 4:00 pm 10:00 pm
3. What other foods are important to your usual diet? chocolate and candy bars
4. Amount per day 4 bars/week
5. Do you have any different food preferences now? no
6. Do you eat nonfoods such as:

| | | Amount |
|---|---|---|
| laundry starch | no | NA |
| ice | yes | 10 cubes/day |
| other (name) | no | NA |

7. What foods do you dislike or do not eat? spinach and dried beans
8. For added information complete a typical daily intake (24 hour recall is suggested).

Do you have special problems in food preparation such as:

1. Physical disability yes ___ no ✔ Explain ___
2. Cooking appliances yes ___ no ✔ Explain ___
3. Refrigeration of food yes ___ no ✔ Explain ___

Who does the meal planning? I do. shopping? We both do.

cooking? I do most of the time but my husband likes to help.

Are there transportation problems? We have only one car but we go in the evening.

Financial situation: My husband is working and going to school. I am not working. Food Stamps yes WIC no

Do you have any previous nutritional problems? No. I have never paid much attention to food before, but now I have lots of questions.

Are there any problems with this pregnancy? Nausea Yes, in the morning.

Constipation No Other NA

Assessment by the nurse following the completion of the questionnaire.

Basic estimated nutrient and caloric value of typical daily intake.

Please circle one of the following:

| | | | |
|---|---|---|---|
| Protein intake was | low | (adequate) | high |
| Caloric intake was | low | adequate | (high) |
| Calcium intake was | (low) | adequate | high |
| Iron intake was | (low) | adequate | high |
| Vitamin C intake was | low | (adequate) | high |

FIGURE 11–4 ♦ Sample nutritional questionnaire used in nursing management of a pregnant woman.

## KEY FACTS TO REMEMBER

### *Prenatal Nutrition*

- The pregnant woman should eat regularly, three meals a day, and snack on fruits, cheese, milk, or other nutritious foods between meals if desired.
- More frequent but smaller meals are also recommended.
- The woman should diet *only* under the guidance of her primary health care provider.
- Water is an essential nutrient. The woman should drink 4–6 (8-oz) glasses of water and a total of 8–10 glasses of fluid daily.
- If the diet is adequate, iron is the only supplement necessary during pregnancy.
- A multivitamin supplement is indicated for women with a poor diet and for those at high nutritional risk.
- To avoid possible deficiencies, many caregivers also recommend a daily vitamin supplement.
- Taking megadoses of vitamins during pregnancy is unnecessary and potentially dangerous.

Implementation:

1. Plan with the woman how to add more milk or dairy products to the diet (specify amounts).
2. Encourage the use of other calcium sources such as leafy greens and legumes.
3. Plan for the addition of powdered milk in cooking and baking.
4. If none of the preceding options are realistic or acceptable, consider the use of calcium supplements.

Most families can benefit from guidance about food purchasing and preparation. Women should be advised to plan food purchases thoughtfully by preparing general menus and a list before shopping. It is also helpful to advise clients to monitor sales, compare brands, and be cautious when purchasing "convenience" foods, which tend to be expensive. Other techniques for keeping food costs down without jeopardizing quality include buying food in season, using bulk foods when appropriate, using whole-grain or enriched products, buying lower-grade eggs (grading has no relation to the egg's nutritional value but indicates color of the shell, delicacy of flavor, and so forth), and avoiding foods from specialty shops and foods in elaborate packaging.

## Critical Thinking in Practice

Jane is 14 weeks pregnant. The rate and total amount of her weight gain during the first trimester have been consistent with recommendations. She has gained an average of 0.5 kg (1 lb) per week during both of the past 2 weeks. Her appetite is good, and she consumes three meals per day and snacks between meals on occasion.

Jane has altered her diet because she is concerned about excessive weight gain. She told the nurse that she has decreased her intake from the bread and dairy groups in order to limit her calorie intake. Because she has omitted most dairy products, she has increased her consumption of salads and broccoli to provide calcium sources.

A diet history revealed the following:

| | |
|---|---|
| Grain | 3–4 servings, mainly cereal and rice |
| Fruit | 2–4 servings, fresh fruit |
| Vegetables | 3–5 servings, salads, peas, corn, broccoli |
| Meat | 4–5 servings, beef, pork, chicken |
| Dairy | occasionally cheese, ice cream, pudding |
| Fats, oils, sweets | occasionally salad dressings, margarine, desserts |
| Beverages | 8–10 servings, soda, juices, water |

After assessing her diet history, what is your evaluation of Jane's diet? How could you counsel her?

Answers can be found in Appendix I.

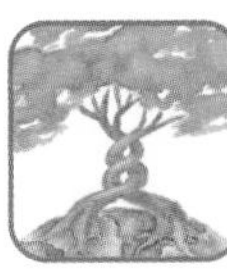

## Community-Based Nursing Care

Food is a significant portion of a family's budget, and meeting nutritional needs may be a challenge for families on limited incomes. Community-based services offered through clinics, local agencies, schools, and volunteer organizations are effective in addressing these needs. Increasingly nurses play an important role in managing such community-based services, especially services focusing on client education. In addition, most communities offer special assistance to qualifying families to meet their nutritional needs. The Food Stamp Program provides stamps or coupons for participating households whose net monthly income is below a specified level. These stamps can be used to purchase food for the household each month.

The Special Supplemental Food Program for Women, Infants, and Children (WIC) is designed to assist pregnant or breastfeeding women with low incomes and their children under 5 years of age. The program provides food assistance, nutrition education, and referrals to health care providers. The food distributed, including dried beans and peas, peanut butter, eggs, cheese, milk, fortified adult and infant cereals, juice, and iron-fortified formula, is designed to provide good sources of iron, protein, and certain vitamins for individuals with an inadequate diet. Research indicates that participation in the WIC program during pregnancy and infancy is associated with a reduced risk of infant death (Moss & Carver, 1998).

### Evaluation

Once a plan has been developed and implemented, the nurse and client may wish to identify ways of evaluating its effectiveness. Evaluation may involve keeping a food journal, writing out weekly menus, returning for weekly weigh-ins, and the like. If anemia is a special problem, periodic hematocrit assessments are also indicated. Key Facts to Remember: Prenatal Nutrition summarizes key points that the pregnant woman should thoroughly understand.

Women with serious nutritional deficiencies are referred to a dietitian. The nurse can then work closely with the dietitian and the client to improve the pregnant woman's health by modification of her diet.

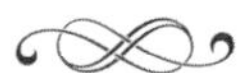

# Chapter Review

## CHAPTER HIGHLIGHTS

- Maternal weight gains averaging 25 to 35 lb (11.5 to 16 kg) for a normal-weight woman are associated with the best reproductive outcomes.
- If the diet is adequate, folic acid and iron are the only supplements generally recommended during pregnancy.
- Because of the risk of NTDs, a national campaign is under way to encourage all women of childbearing age to take a 0.4-mg supplement of folic acid daily.
- Women should not undertake caloric restriction to reduce weight during pregnancy.
- It is most healthful for pregnant women to eat regularly and choose a wide variety of foods, especially fresh and lightly processed foods.
- Taking megadoses of vitamins during pregnancy is unnecessary and potentially dangerous.
- In vegetarian diets, special emphasis is placed on obtaining ample protein, calories, calcium, iron, vitamin D, vitamin $B_{12}$, and zinc through food sources or supplementation if necessary.
- Evaluation of physical, psychosocial, and cultural factors that affect food intake is essential before the nurse can determine nutritional status and plan nutritional counseling.
- Adolescents who become pregnant less than 4 years after menarche have higher nutritional needs than older pregnant adolescents and are considered to be at high biologic risk.
- Weight gains during adolescent pregnancy need to accommodate recommended gains for a normal pregnancy plus necessary gains due to maternal growth.
- After giving birth, the nonnursing mother's dietary requirements return to prepregnancy levels.
- Nursing mothers need an adequate calorie and fluid intake to maintain ample milk volume.

# CHAPTER REFERENCES

American College of Obstetricians and Gynecologists. (1996). *Nutrition and women* (ACOG Educational Bulletin 229). Washington, DC: Author.

American College of Obstetricians and Gynecologists. (1998). *Vitamin A supplementation during pregnancy* (ACOG Committee Opinion 196). Washington, DC: Author.

Brown, J. E., & Carlson, M. (2000). Nutrition and multifetal pregnancy. *Journal of the American Dietetic Association, 100*(3), 343–348.

Centers for Disease Control and Prevention (CDC). (1998, April 3). Recommendations to prevent and control iron deficiency in the United States. *Morbidity and Mortality Weekly Reports,* 47 (No RR-3), 1–36.

Centers for Disease Control and Prevention (CDC). (2000). *Folic acid now.* Birth Defects and Pediatric Genetics Branch, National Center for Environmental Health. Atlanta, GA: Author.

Doyle, W. (1998). Nutrition and pregnancy. *Nursing Times, 94*(Suppl. 16), 22–28.

Herrin, M. (1999). Balancing the scales: Nutritional counseling for women with eating disorders. *AWHONN Lifelines, 3*(4), 26–34.

Institute of Medicine, Subcommittee for a Clinical Application Guide. (1992). *Nutrition during pregnancy and lactation: An implementation guide.* Washington, DC: National Academy Press.

Institute of Medicine, Subcommittee on Dietary Intake and Nutrient Supplements during Pregnancy, Committee on Nutrition Status during Pregnancy and Lactation, Food and Nutrition Board. (1990). *Nutrition during pregnancy: Weight gain and nutrient supplements.* Washington, DC: National Academy Press.

Mersereau, P. W. (2000). Preventing neural tube birth defects: A national campaign. *Small Talk, 12*(2), 1–5.

Moss, N., & Carver, K. (1998). The effect of WIC and Medicaid on infant mortality in the United States. *American Journal of Public Health, 88*(9), 1354–1361.

National Research Council, Food and Nutrition Board. (1989). *Recommended dietary allowances* (10th ed.). Washington, DC: National Academy Press.

Neumark-Sztainer, D., Story, M., Perry, C., & Casey, M. A. (1999). Factors influencing food choices of adolescents: Findings from focus-group discussions with adolescents. *Journal of the American Dietetic Association, 99*(8), 929–938.

Prasad, A. S. (1996). Zinc deficiency in women, infants, and children. *Journal of the American College of Nutrition, 15*(2), 113–120.

Reifsnider, E., & Gill, S. L. (2000). Nutrition for the childbearing years. *Journal of Obstetric, Gynecologic, and Neonatal Nursing, 29*(1), 43–55.

Wenstrom, K. D., & Malee, D. W. (1999). Medical and surgical complications of pregnancy. In J. R. Scott, P. J. DiSaia, C. B. Hammond, & W. N. Spellacy (Eds.), *Danforth's obstetrics and gynecology,* (8th ed.). Philadelphia: Lippincott Williams & Wilkins, 327–362.

# CONTEMPORARY MATERNAL-NEWBORN NURSING ON-LINE

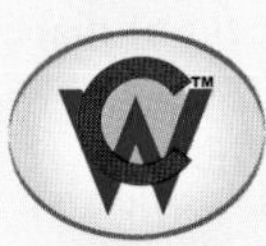

Additional interactive resources, including animations and video, for this chapter can be found on the Companion Website at http://www.prenhall.com/ladewig. Click on Chapter 11 and "Begin" to select the activities for this chapter.

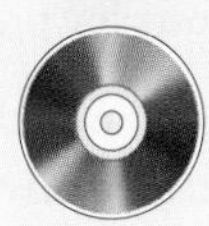

For NCLEX review questions and an audio glossary, access the accompanying CD-ROM in this book.

Chapter 12

# Pregnancy at Risk: Pregestational Problems

*When you work on a high-risk maternity unit, it is sometimes easy to get caught up in technology and procedures, but this area is about* families—*their fears, their pain, their health, their future. We can never lose sight of that reality and remain effective nurses. Never.*

—A Maternity Nurse Working with High-Risk Pregnant Women

## KEY TERMS

| | |
|---|---|
| Acquired immunodeficiency syndrome (AIDS) | 277 |
| Gestational diabetes mellitus | 267 |
| Human immunodeficiency virus (HIV) | 277 |
| Macrosomia | 269 |

## OBJECTIVES

- Summarize the effects of alcohol and illicit drugs on the childbearing woman and her fetus/newborn.
- Relate the pathology and clinical treatment of diabetes mellitus in pregnancy to the implications for nursing care.
- Discriminate among the types of anemia associated with pregnancy regarding signs, treatment, and implications for pregnancy.
- Discuss acquired immunodeficiency syndrome (AIDS), including care of the pregnant woman who has tested positive for the human immunodeficiency virus (HIV), fetal/neonatal implications, and ramifications for the childbearing family.
- Describe the effects of various heart disorders on pregnancy, including their implications for nursing care.
- Delineate the effects of selected pregestational medical conditions on pregnancy.

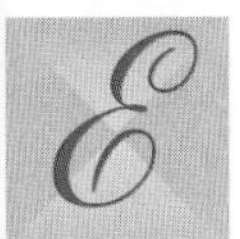

ven though it is a normal process, for some women pregnancy may become a life-threatening event because of potential or existing complications. These complications can be the result of factors such as age, parity, blood type, socioeconomic status, psychologic health, or preexisting chronic illnesses. Effective prenatal care is directed toward identifying factors that increase a pregnant woman's risk and developing supportive therapies that will promote optimal health for the mother and her fetus.

This chapter focuses on women with pregestational medical disorders and the possible effects of these disorders on the pregnancy.

## HINTS FOR PRACTICE

Keep in mind that at least 1 of 10 women in the United States, regardless of socioeconomic status or ethnic background, is currently abusing a substance. If you consider that possibility with every woman, you will ask the important questions about drug use and be alert for signs of substance abuse.

# Care of the Woman with Substance Abuse Problems

Substance abuse occurs when an individual experiences difficulties with work, family, social relations, and health as a result of alcohol or drug use. Research suggests that more than 5% of all pregnant women use illegal drugs during pregnancy, with even higher rates in certain subgroups (Howell, Heiser, & Harrington, 1999). Almost 19% of pregnant women consume alcohol, and more than 20% use tobacco (Andres, 1999).

Drugs that are commonly misused include alcohol, cocaine, marijuana, amphetamines, barbiturates, hallucinogens, heroin, and other narcotics. Table 12–1 on p. 264 identifies common addictive drugs and their effects on the fetus or newborn.

Drug use during pregnancy, particularly in the first trimester, may adversely affect the health of the woman and the growth and development of the fetus. Unfortunately prenatal drug use may be the most frequently missed diagnosis in all of maternity care. Physicians and nurses may fail to ask women about drug and alcohol use because of their own lack of knowledge, discomfort, or biases. Often substance-abusing women wait until late in pregnancy to seek health care. Moreover, the substance-abusing woman who seeks early prenatal care may not voluntarily reveal her addiction, so caregivers should be alert for a history or physical signs that suggest substance abuse.

Providing effective prenatal care to chemically dependent women presents many challenges for clinicians. However, pregnancy represents a period in most women's lives when they recognize the need for and are receptive to caring interventions.

## Substances Commonly Abused during Pregnancy

### Alcohol

Alcohol is a central nervous system (CNS) depressant and a potent teratogen. In fact, the use of alcohol during pregnancy has been described as the leading preventable cause of mental retardation (Andres, 1999). The incidence of alcohol abuse is highest among women ages 20 to 40 years; alcoholism is also seen in teenagers. Chronic abuse of alcohol can undermine maternal health by causing malnutrition (especially folic acid and thiamine deficiencies), bone marrow suppression, increased incidence of infections, and liver disease.

Alcohol is toxic to the fetus, although its exact effects on the fetus are complex and only partly understood. The ethanol of alcohol may interfere with protein synthesis and placental transfer of glucose and amino acids; it may also contribute to vasoconstriction and a resulting hypoxemia in the fetus (Andres, 1999).

The effects of alcohol on the fetus may result in a group of signs known as *fetal alcohol syndrome (FAS)*. The syndrome has characteristic physical and mental abnormalities that vary in severity and combination. (See discussion in Chapter 25.) There is no definitive answer to how much alcohol a woman can safely consume during pregnancy. The expectant woman should avoid alcohol completely during the early weeks of pregnancy, when organogenesis is occurring. During the remainder of pregnancy, an occasional drink carries no currently known risk; however, no alcohol at all is safest (Niebyl, 1999).

As a result of alcohol dependence, a woman may have withdrawal seizures in the intrapartal period as early as 12 to 48 hours after she stops drinking. Delirium tremens may occur in the postpartal period, and the newborn

**TABLE 12–1 Possible Effects of Selected Drugs of Abuse or Addiction on Fetus and Neonate**

| *Maternal Drug* | *Effect on Fetus and Neonate* |
|---|---|
| Depressants | |
| Alcohol | Mental retardation, microcephaly, midfacial hypoplasia, cardiac anomalies, intrauterine growth restriction |
| Narcotics | (IUGR), potential teratogenic effects, fetal alcohol syndrome (FAS), fetal alcohol effects (FAE) |
| Heroin | Withdrawal symptoms, convulsions, death, IUGR, respiratory alkalosis, hyperbilirubinemia |
| Methadone | Fetal distress, meconium aspiration; with abrupt termination of the drug, severe withdrawal symptoms, neonatal death |
| Barbiturates | Neonatal depression, increased anomalies; teratogenic effect (?); withdrawal symptoms, convulsions, hyperactivity, hyperreflexia, vasomotor instability |
| Phenobarbital | Bleeding (with excessive doses) |
| "T's and Blues" (combination of the following) | |
| Talwin (narcotic) | Safe for use in pregnancy; depresses respiration if taken close to time of birth |
| Amytal (barbiturate) | See barbiturates |
| Tranquilizers | |
| Phenothiazine derivatives | Withdrawal, extrapyramidal dysfunction, delayed respiratory onset, hyperbilirubinemia, hypotonia or hyperactivity, decreased platelet count |
| Diazepam (Valium) | Hypotonia, hypothermia, low Apgar score, respiratory depression, poor sucking reflex, possible cleft lip |
| Antianxiety drugs | |
| Lithium | Congenital anomalies, especially Ebstein anomaly; lethargy and cyanosis in the newborn |
| Stimulants | |
| Amphetamines | |
| Amphetamine sulfate (Benzedrine) | Generalized arthritis, learning disabilities, poor motor coordination, transposition of the great vessels, cleft palate |
| Dextroamphetamine sulfate (dexedrine sulfate) | Congenital heart defects, hyperbilirubinemia |
| Cocaine | Cerebral infarctions, microcephaly, learning disabilities, poor state organization, decreased interactive behavior, central nervous system (CNS) anomalies, cardiac anomalies, genitourinary anomalies, sudden infant death syndrome (SIDS) |
| Caffeine (more than 600 mg/day) | Spontaneous abortion, IUGR, increased incidence of cleft palate, other anomalies suspected |
| Nicotine (half to one pack cigarettes/day) | Increased rate of spontaneous abortion, increased incidence of placental abruption, small for gestational age (SGA), small head circumference, decreased length, SIDS |
| Psychotropics | |
| PCP ("angel dust") | Flaccid appearance, poor head control, impaired neurologic development |
| LSD | Chromosomal breakage? |
| Marijuana | IUGR, potential impaired immunologic mechanisms |

may suffer a withdrawal syndrome. The nursing staff in the maternal-newborn unit must be aware of the manifestations of alcohol abuse so they can prepare for the client's special needs. The care regimen includes sedation to decrease irritability and tremors, seizure precautions, intravenous fluid therapy for hydration, and preparation for an addicted newborn. Although high doses of sedatives and analgesics may be necessary for the woman, caution is advised because these medications can cause fetal depression.

Breastfeeding generally is not contraindicated, although alcohol is excreted in breast milk. Excessive alcohol consumption may intoxicate the infant and inhibit the maternal letdown reflex. Discharge planning for the alcohol-addicted mother and newborn needs to be correlated with the social service department of the hospital.

### Cocaine and Crack

Approximately 1 in 10 pregnant women is believed to use cocaine, with even higher rates reported in urban areas

(Kenner & D'Apolito, 1997). Cocaine acts at the nerve terminals to prevent the reuptake of dopamine and norepinephrine, which in turn results in vasoconstriction, tachycardia, and hypertension. Placental vasoconstriction decreases blood flow to the fetus. The onset of cocaine effects occurs rapidly, but the euphoria lasts only about 30 minutes. Euphoria and excitement are usually followed by irritability, depression, pessimism, fatigue, and a strong desire for more cocaine. This pattern often leads the user to take repeated doses to sustain the effect. Cocaine metabolites may be present in the urine of a pregnant woman for as long as 4 to 7 days after use.

Cocaine can be taken by intravenous injection or by snorting the powdered form. *Crack,* a form of freebase cocaine that is made up of baking soda, water, and cocaine mixed into a paste and microwaved to form a rock, can be smoked. Smoking crack leads to a quicker, more intense high because the drug is absorbed through the large surface area of the lungs.

The cocaine user is difficult to identify prenatally. Because cocaine is an illegal substance, many women are reluctant to volunteer information about their drug use. The nurse who is familiar with the woman may recognize subtle signs of cocaine use, including mood swings and appetite changes, and withdrawal symptoms such as depression, irritability, nausea, lack of motivation, and psychomotor changes.

Major adverse maternal effects of cocaine use include seizures and hallucinations, pulmonary edema, cerebral hemorrhage, respiratory failure, and heart problems. Women who use cocaine have an increased incidence of spontaneous abortion, abruptio placentae, preterm birth, and stillbirth.

Exposure of the fetus to cocaine in utero increases the risk of intrauterine growth restriction (IUGR), small head circumference, shorter body length, malformations of the genitourinary tract, and lower Apgar scores. Newborns exposed to cocaine in utero may have neurobehavioral disturbances, marked irritability, an exaggerated startle reflex, labile emotions, and an increased risk of sudden infant death syndrome (SIDS). (See Chapter 25 for further discussion.)

Cocaine crosses into breast milk and may cause symptoms in the breastfeeding infant, including extreme irritability, vomiting, diarrhea, dilated pupils, and apnea. Thus women who continue to use cocaine after childbirth should avoid nursing.

### Marijuana

Estimates of marijuana use during pregnancy vary widely and range from 3% (based on self-report) to 35% (based on urine screen) (Andres, 1999). To date, there is no strong evidence that marijuana has teratogenic effects on the fetus (Niebyl, 1999). However, the impact of heavy marijuana use on pregnancy is difficult to evaluate because of the variety of social factors that may influence the results.

### Heroin

Heroin is an illicit CNS depressant narcotic that alters perception and produces euphoria. It is an addictive drug that is generally administered intravenously, although a snortable form of heroin called Karachi is available. Pregnancy in women who use heroin is considered high risk because of the increased incidence in these women of poor nutrition, iron-deficiency anemia, and preeclampsia. Women addicted to heroin also have a higher incidence of sexually transmitted infection because many rely on prostitution to support their drug habit.

The fetus of a heroin-addicted woman is at increased risk for IUGR, meconium aspiration, and hypoxia. The newborn frequently shows signs of heroin addiction such as restlessness; shrill, high-pitched cry; irritability; fist sucking; vomiting; and seizures. Signs of withdrawal usually appear within 72 hours and may last for several days. (See discussion in Chapter 25.)

### Methadone

Methadone is the most commonly used therapy for women who are dependent on opioids such as heroin. Methadone blocks withdrawal symptoms and reduces or eliminates the craving for narcotics. Dosage should be individualized at the lowest possible therapeutic level. Methadone crosses the placenta and has been associated with preeclampsia, placental problems, and abnormal fetal presentation (Kearney, 1997).

Prenatal exposure to methadone may result in reduced head circumference and lower birth weight. The newborn may experience withdrawal symptoms that are often more severe and longer lasting than those associated with heroin, possibly because of the longer half-life of methadone (Wang, 1999).

## Clinical Therapy

Antepartal care of the pregnant woman with substance abuse problems involves medical, socioeconomic, and legal considerations. A team approach allows for the comprehensive management necessary to provide safe labor and childbirth for the woman and her child.

The management of drug addiction may include hospitalization as necessary to initiate detoxification. "Cold turkey" withdrawal is not advisable during pregnancy because of potential risk to the fetus. Maintenance and support therapy are given during weekly prenatal visits. Urine screening is also done regularly throughout pregnancy if the woman has a known or suspected substance abuse problem. This testing helps to identify the type and amount of drug being abused.

# Nursing Care Management

## Nursing Assessment and Diagnosis

Because of the prevalence of substance abuse in society today, nurses and other care providers should screen all pregnant women for substance abuse during the health history. Several simple screening tools are available. In addition, the nurse needs to be alert for clues in the history or appearance of the woman that suggest substance abuse. If abuse is suspected, the nurse needs to ask direct questions, beginning with less threatening questions about use of tobacco, caffeine, and over-the-counter medications. The nurse can then progress to questions about alcohol consumption and finally to questions focusing on past and current use of illicit drugs. The nurse who is matter-of-fact and nonjudgmental in her or his approach is more likely to elicit honest responses.

Nursing assessment of the woman with a known substance abuse problem focuses on the woman's general health status, with specific attention to nutritional status, susceptibility to infections, and evaluation of all body systems. The nurse also assesses the woman's understanding of the impact of substance abuse on herself and on her pregnancy.

Nursing diagnoses that may apply to a woman at risk because of substance abuse include the following:

- ***Altered nutrition: less than body requirements*** related to inadequate food intake secondary to substance abuse
- ***Risk for infection*** related to use of inadequately cleaned syringes and needles secondary to intravenous (IV) drug use
- ***Knowledge deficit*** related to a lack of information about the impact of substance abuse on the fetus

## Nursing Plan and Implementation

Prevention of substance abuse during pregnancy is the ideal nursing goal and is best accomplished through education. Unfortunately, many women who abuse substances do not receive regular health care and may not seek care until they are far along in pregnancy.

The nurse's role in providing prenatal care for the woman who abuses substances focuses on ongoing assessment and client teaching. The nurse can provide information about the relationship between substance abuse and existing health problems and the implications for the woman's unborn child. By establishing a relationship of trust and support, the nurse may ensure the woman's cooperation. The knowledgeable nurse can discuss possible strategies to help the woman quit (addiction treatment programs, 12-step programs, individual counseling) and suggest a referral for more in-depth assessment by a specialist.

Preparation for labor and birth should be part of prenatal planning. Relief of fear, tension, or discomfort may be achieved through nonnarcotic psychologic support and careful explanation of the labor process. If pain medication is necessary, it should not be withheld; the notion that it will contribute to further addiction is mistaken. Preferred methods of pain relief include the use of psychoprophylaxis and regional blocks such as epidurals or local anesthetics such as pudendal block and local infiltration. Immediate intensive care should be available for the newborn, who is often depressed, small for gestational age (SGA), and premature. (For care of the addicted newborn, see Chapter 25.)

## Evaluation

Expected outcomes of nursing care include the following:

- The woman is able to describe the impact of her substance abuse on herself and her unborn child.
- The woman gives birth to a healthy infant.
- The woman agrees to accept a referral to social services (or another appropriate community agency) for follow-up care after discharge.

# Care of the Woman with Diabetes Mellitus

Diabetes mellitus (DM), an endocrine disorder of carbohydrate metabolism resulting from inadequate production or use of insulin, occurs in about 1% to 14% of all pregnancies, depending on the population served (American Diabetes Association [ADA], 2000a). Insulin, produced by the β-cells of the islets of Langerhans in the pancreas, lowers blood glucose levels by enabling glucose to move from the blood into muscle and adipose tissue cells.

## Carbohydrate Metabolism in Normal Pregnancy

In early pregnancy the rise in serum levels of estrogen, progesterone, and other hormones stimulates increased insulin production by the maternal pancreas and increased tissue response to insulin. Thus an anabolic (building-up) state exists during the first half of pregnancy, with storage of glycogen in the liver and other tissues.

In the second half of pregnancy, placental secretion of human placental lactogen (hPL) and prolactin (from the decidua), as well as elevated cortisol and glycogen levels, cause increased resistance to insulin and decreased glucose tolerance. This decreased effectiveness of insulin results in a catabolic (destructive) state during fasting periods, such as during the night or after meal absorption. Because increasing amounts of circulating maternal glucose and amino acids are diverted to the fetus, maternal fat is metabolized much more readily during fasting periods than in a nonpregnant woman. As a result of this lipolysis (maternal metabolism of fat), ketones may be present in the urine.

The delicate system of checks and balances that exists between glucose production and glucose use is stressed by the growing fetus, who derives energy from glucose taken solely from maternal stores. This stress is known as the *diabetogenic effect* of pregnancy. Thus any preexisting disruption in carbohydrate metabolism is augmented by pregnancy, and any diabetic potential may precipitate gestational diabetes mellitus.

## Pathophysiology of Diabetes Mellitus

In diabetes mellitus, the pancreas does not produce enough insulin to allow necessary carbohydrate metabolism. Without adequate insulin, glucose does not enter the cells and they become energy depleted. Blood glucose levels remain high (hyperglycemia), and the cells break down their stores of fats and protein for energy. Protein breakdown results in a negative nitrogen balance; fat metabolism causes ketosis.

These pathologic developments cause the four cardinal signs and symptoms of diabetes mellitus: polyuria, polydipsia, polyphagia, and weight loss. *Polyuria* (frequent urination) results because water is not reabsorbed by the renal tubules due to the osmotic activity of glucose. *Polydipsia* (excessive thirst) is caused by dehydration from polyuria. *Polyphagia* (excessive hunger) is caused by tissue loss and a state of starvation, which results from the inability of the cells to use the blood glucose. *Weight loss* (seen with marked hyperglycemia) is due to the use of fat and muscle tissue for energy.

## Classification

States of altered carbohydrate metabolism have been classified in several ways. Table 12–2 shows the classification of diabetes mellitus proposed in 1999, which is based on its cause. This classification contains four main categories: type 1 diabetes, type 2 diabetes, other specific types, and gestational diabetes mellitus (GDM). The former classification, developed by the National Diabetes Data Group in 1979, was based to a degree on the type of pharmacologic treatment used. Thus it included type I (insulin-dependent diabetes mellitus [IDDM]) and type II (non-insulin dependent diabetes mellitus [NIDDM]) as well as the broad categories impaired glucose tolerance and gestational diabetes mellitus. During this time of transition, as health care moves to adopt the newer, etiology-based system, the older terms, IDDM and NIDDM, are still being used in some facilities.

**TABLE 12–2 Etiologic Classification of Diabetes Mellitus**

I. Type 1 diabetes* (β-cell destruction, usually leading to absolute insulin deficiency)
   A. Immune mediated
   B. Idiopathic
II. Type 2 diabetes* (may range from predominantly insulin resistance with relative insulin deficiency to a predominantly secretory defect with insulin resistance)
III. Other specific types†
IV. Gestational diabetes mellitus

*Patients with any form of diabetes may require insulin treatment at some stage of their disease. Such use of insulin does not classify the patient.

†The more detailed classification, which can be found in medical-surgical texts and the original source, provides eight subcategories of type.

*Source:* Adapted from the 1999 Report of the Expert Committee on the Diagnosis and Classification of Diabetes Mellitus. *Diabetes Care,* Suppl. 5.

Table 12–3 shows White's classification of diabetes in pregnancy. This classification is useful for describing the extent of the disease.

**Gestational diabetes mellitus** (GDM) is defined as any degree of glucose intolerance that has its onset or is first diagnosed during pregnancy. Except for showing an impaired tolerance to glucose, the woman may remain asymptomatic or may have a mild form of the disease. Diagnosis of GDM is very important, however, because even mild diabetes causes increased risk for perinatal morbidity and mortality. Furthermore, with time, many women with GDM progress to overt type 1 or type 2 diabetes mellitus.

## Influence of Pregnancy on Diabetes

Pregnancy can affect diabetes significantly because the physiologic changes of pregnancy can drastically alter insulin requirements. Pregnancy may also alter the progress of vascular disease secondary to DM. Pregnancy can affect diabetes in the following ways:

- DM may be difficult to control because insulin requirements are changeable.

| TABLE 12–3 | White's Classification of Diabetes in Pregnancy |
|---|---|
| *Class* | *Criterion* |
| A | Chemical diabetes |
| B | Maturity onset (age over 20 years), duration under 10 years, no vascular lesions |
| $C_1$ | Age 10 to 19 years at onset |
| $C_2$ | 10 to 19 years' duration |
| $D_1$ | Under 10 years at onset |
| $D_2$ | Over 20 years' duration |
| $D_3$ | Benign retinopathy |
| $D_4$ | Calcified vessels of legs |
| $D_5$ | Hypertension |
| E | No longer sought |
| F | Nephropathy |
| G | Many failures |
| H | Cardiopathy |
| R | Proliferating retinopathy |
| T | Renal transplant (added by Tagatz and colleagues of the University of Minnesota) |

*Source:* White, P. (1978). Classification of obstetric diabetes. *American Journal of Obstetrics and Gynecology, 130,* 228. Used with permission.

  - During the first trimester, the need for insulin frequently decreases. Levels of hPL, an insulin antagonist, are low, fetal needs are minimal, and the woman may consume less food because of nausea and vomiting.
  - Nausea and vomiting may cause dietary fluctuations and increase the risk of hypoglycemia, formerly called insulin shock.
  - Insulin requirements begin to rise in the second trimester as glucose use and glucose storage by the woman and fetus increase. Insulin requirements may double or quadruple by the end of pregnancy as a result of placental maturation and hPL production.
  - Increased energy needs during labor may require increased insulin to balance intravenous glucose.
  - Usually an abrupt decrease in insulin requirement occurs after the passage of the placenta and the resulting loss of hPL in maternal circulation.
- A decreased renal threshold for glucose leads to a higher incidence of glycosuria.
- The risk of ketoacidosis, which may occur at lower serum glucose levels in the pregnant woman with DM than in the nonpregnant diabetic, increases.
- The vascular disease that accompanies DM may progress during pregnancy.
  - Hypertension may occur, contributing to vascular changes.
  - Nephropathy may result from renal impairment, and retinopathy may develop.

## Influence of Diabetes on Pregnancy Outcome

The pregnancy of a woman who has diabetes carries a higher risk of complications, especially perinatal mortality and congenital anomalies. This risk has been reduced by the recognition of the importance of tight metabolic control (glucose between 70 and 120 mg/dL). New techniques for monitoring blood glucose level, delivering insulin, and monitoring the fetus have also reduced perinatal mortality.

### Maternal Risks

The prognosis for the pregnant woman with gestational, type 1, or type 2 diabetes without significant vascular damage is positive. However, diabetic pregnancy still carries a higher risk of complications than normal pregnancy.

*Hydramnios,* or an increase in the volume of amniotic fluid, occurs in 10% to 20% of pregnant diabetic women. It is thought to be a result of excessive fetal urination because of fetal hyperglycemia (Spellacy, 1999). Premature rupture of membranes and onset of labor may occasionally be a problem with hydramnios.

*Preeclampsia and eclampsia (pregnancy-induced hypertension) (PIH)* occur more often in diabetic pregnancies than in normal pregnancies, especially when vascular changes already exist (Moore, 1999).

Hyperglycemia can lead to *ketoacidosis* as a result of the increase in ketone bodies (which are acidic) released in the blood from the metabolism of fatty acids. Decreased gastric motility and the contrainsulin effects of hPL also predispose the woman to ketoacidosis. Ketoacidosis usually develops slowly but, if untreated, can lead to coma and death for mother and fetus.

The pregnant woman with diabetes is also at increased risk for monilial vaginitis and urinary tract infections because of increased glycosuria, which contributes to a favorable environment for bacterial growth.

### Fetal-Neonatal Risks

Many of the problems of the neonate result directly from high maternal plasma glucose levels. In the presence of untreated maternal ketoacidosis, the risk of fetal death increases to 50% (Spellacy, 1999).

For the general population, the risk of giving birth to a child with a major congenital anomaly is 1% to 2%. For diabetic mothers this risk increases threefold (Spellacy, 1999). Research suggests that this increased incidence of congenital anomalies is related to high glucose levels in early pregnancy (Moore, 1999). Most anomalies involve the heart, central nervous system, and skeletal system. One anomaly, sacral agenesis, appears almost exclusively in infants of diabetic mothers. In sacral agenesis, the sacrum and lumbar spine fail to develop and the lower extremities develop incompletely. To reduce the incidence of congenital anomalies, preconception counseling and strict diabetes control before conception are indicated.

Characteristically, infants of diabetic mothers on insulin therapy (or White's classes A, B, and C; see Table 12–3) are large for gestational age (LGA) as a result of the high maternal levels of blood glucose, from which the fetus derives its glucose. These elevated levels continually stimulate the fetal islets of Langerhans to produce insulin. This hyperinsulin state causes the fetus to use the available glucose, which leads to excessive growth (known as **macrosomia**) and fat deposits. If born vaginally, the macrosomic infant is at increased risk for shoulder dystocia and traumatic birth injuries and may be at increased risk for impaired glucose tolerance in later childhood (Moore, 1999).

After birth the umbilical cord is severed and the generous maternal blood glucose supply eliminated. However, continued islet cell hyperactivity leads to excessive insulin levels and depleted blood glucose (hypoglycemia) in 2 to 4 hours. Macrosomia can be significantly reduced by tight maternal blood glucose control.

Infants of mothers with advanced diabetes (vascular involvement) may demonstrate IUGR. IUGR occurs because vascular changes in the diabetic woman decrease the efficiency of placental perfusion and the fetus is not as well sustained in utero.

*Respiratory distress syndrome* appears to result from inhibition, by high levels of fetal insulin, of some fetal enzymes necessary for surfactant production. *Polycythemia* (excessive number of red blood cells) in the newborn is due primarily to the diminished ability of glycosylated hemoglobin in the mother's blood to release oxygen. *Hyperbilirubinemia* is a direct result of the inability of immature liver enzymes to metabolize the increased bilirubin resulting from the polycythemia.

## Clinical Therapy

Until recently, *all* pregnant women were given a 1-hour oral glucose tolerance test (GTT) between 24 and 28 weeks' gestation to screen for gestational diabetes mellitus. The American Diabetes Association no longer recommends universal screening. Rather, the ADA now recommends that women who are at average risk be screened at 24 to 28 weeks using the 1-hour GTT. Women at average risk include the following (ADA, 2000a):

- Age 25 or older
- Obese women of any age
- Family history of DM in a first-degree relative
- Member of an ethnic group with a high prevalence of diabetes (Hispanic, African-American, Native American, Asian-American)
- History of abnormal glucose tolerance
- History of poor obstetric outcome

To do the 1-hour GTT, the woman ingests a 50-g oral glucose solution at any time during the day. One hour later a blood sample is obtained. If the plasma glucose level exceeds 130 mg/dL, a 3-hour oral GTT is necessary (ADA, 2000a).

During pregnancy, gestational diabetes mellitus is diagnosed by using a 3-hour, 100-g oral glucose tolerance test. To do this test, the woman eats a high-carbohydrate (greater than 200 g carbohydrate daily) diet for 3 days before her scheduled test. She then ingests a 100-g oral glucose solution in the morning after an overnight fast of between 8 and 14 hours. Plasma glucose levels are determined fasting and at 1, 2, and 3 hours. Gestational diabetes is diagnosed if two or more of the following values are equaled or exceeded:

| | |
|---|---|
| Fasting | 95 mg/dL |
| 1 hour | 180 mg/dL |
| 2 hour | 155 mg/dL |
| 3 hour | 140 mg/dL |

Pregnant women considered at high risk for DM should have a blood glucose screening as soon as possible. A fasting plasma glucose level >126 mg/dL or a casual (any time of the day) plasma glucose level >200 mg/dL is diagnostic of GDM if confirmed on a subsequent day. If not confirmed, the 3-hour GTT is indicated. Women at high risk for GDM but with negative initial findings should be retested at 24 to 28 weeks (ADA, 2000a).

The World Health Organization (WHO), on the other hand, recommends a 75-g, 2-hour oral GTT for diagnosing GDM. In the WHO system, a 2-hour value >162 mg/dL is considered diagnostic (Curet, 2000).

### Laboratory Assessment of Long-Term Glucose Control

Measurement of glycosylated hemoglobin levels provides information about the long-term (previous 4 to 8 weeks) control of hyperglycemia. It measures the percentage of glycohemoglobin in the blood. Glycohemoglobin, or $HbA_{1c}$, is the hemoglobin to which a glucose molecule is attached. Because glycosylation is a rather slow and essentially irreversible process, the test is not reliable for screening for gestational diabetes or for close daily control. Women with abnormal $HbA_{1c}$ values of 9.2% to 11.1% have a 23% risk of having an infant with a malformation (Moore, 1999).

### Antepartal Management of Diabetes Mellitus

The major goals of clinical care for all pregnant women with diabetes are (1) to maintain a physiologic equilibrium of insulin availability and glucose utilization during pregnancy and (2) to ensure an optimally healthy mother and newborn. To achieve these goals, good prenatal care using a team approach must be a top priority. The woman with gestational diabetes may find the diagnosis shocking and upsetting. She needs clear explanations and teaching to enlist her cooperation in ensuring a good outcome. The nurse educator plays a major role in this counseling. The woman with pregestational diabetes needs to understand what changes she can expect during pregnancy; she should receive such teaching in preconception counseling.

### Dietary Regulation

The pregnant woman with diabetes needs to increase her caloric intake by about 300 kcal/day. During the first trimester she generally requires about 30 kcal/kg of ideal body weight (IBW). During the second and third trimesters she needs about 35 kcal/kg IBW (Spellacy, 1999). Approximately 40% to 50% of the calories should come from complex carbohydrates, 15% to 20% from protein, and 30% from fats (Curet, 2000). The food is divided among three meals and three snacks. The bedtime snack is the most important and should include both protein and complex carbohydrates to prevent nighttime hypoglycemia. A nutritionist should work out meal plans with the woman based on the woman's lifestyle, culture, and food preferences. The woman needs to be familiar with the use of food exchanges so she can plan her own meals.

### Glucose Monitoring

Glucose monitoring is essential to determine the need for insulin and assess glucose control. Many physicians have the woman come in for weekly assessment of her fasting glucose levels and one or two postprandial levels. In addition, frequent self-monitoring of glucose levels is paramount in maintaining good glucose control. Self-monitoring is discussed on page 274.

### Insulin Administration

Many women with gestational diabetes require insulin to maintain normal glucose levels. Individuals with pregestational diabetes typically are already on insulin. In either case, human insulin should be used because it is the least likely to cause an allergic reaction. Insulin is given either in multiple injections or by continuous subcutaneous infusion. Multiple injections are more common and generally produce excellent results. Most women receive a combination of intermediate and regular insulin. Recently, some clinicians have moved away from the use of regular human insulin, replacing it with a fast-acting human analog called lispro. Lispro is associated with better glucose control (Jovanovic, 2000). Often a four-dose approach is used, with regular insulin or lispro taken before each meal and NPH or Lente insulin added at bedtime (Curet, 2000). Other clinicians vary the NPH and regular insulin patterns slightly but still prefer a four-dose approach.

Oral hypoglycemics are never used during pregnancy because women using them often break away from their control and become severely hyperglycemic, which places the fetus at high risk; their use has been associated with prolonged fetal hypoglycemia; and they may be teratogenic (Spellacy, 1999).

### Evaluation of Fetal Status

Information about the well-being, size, and maturation of the fetus is important for planning the course of pregnancy and the timing of birth. Because pregnancies complicated by diabetes are at increased risk of neural tube defects such as spina bifida in the fetus, *maternal serum alpha-fetoprotein (AFP) screening* is done at 16 to 20 weeks' gestation (see Chapter 14).

Ultrasound is done at 18 weeks to establish gestational age and detect anomalies. It is then repeated at 28 weeks to monitor fetal growth for IUGR or macrosomia. Some agencies do *fetal biophysical profiles (BPP)* (ultrasound evaluation of fetal well-being in which fetal breathing movements, fetal activity, reactivity, muscle tone, and amniotic fluid volume are assessed) as part of an ongoing evaluation of fetal status.

Daily maternal evaluation of fetal activity is begun at about 28 weeks. Twice weekly nonstress testing (NST) using a fetal monitor is begun at 32 weeks for women with preexisting DM and for women with GDM who require insulin. Other clinicians delay beginning NST until closer to term in women with GDM (Landon, 2000). If the NST is nonreactive, a fetal biophysical profile or contraction stress test is performed. (For an explanation of these tests, see Chapter 14.)

## Intrapartal Management of Diabetes Mellitus

During the intrapartal period, medical therapy focuses on the following:

- *Timing of birth.* Most pregnant women with diabetes, regardless of the type, are allowed to go to term, with elective induction of labor and vaginal birth planned at 38 to 40 weeks' gestation. Cesarean birth may be indicated if evidence of fetal distress exists. Birth before term may be indicated for diabetic women with vascular changes and worsening hypertension or if evidence of IUGR exists (Landon, 2000). To determine fetal lung maturity, amniotic fluid (obtained by amniocentesis) is evaluated for lecithin/sphingomyelin (L/S) ratio and the presence of phosphatidylglycerol (PG) (see Chapter 14). Preterm induced birth, often by cesarean, must be considered if prenatal testing indicates that the fetal condition is deteriorating.

- *Labor management.* Frequently maternal insulin requirements decrease dramatically during labor. Consequently maternal glucose levels are measured hourly to determine insulin need. The primary goal in controlling maternal glucose levels intrapartally is to prevent neonatal hypoglycemia (Curet, 2000). Often two intravenous lines are used, one with a 5% dextrose solution and one with a saline solution. The saline solution is then available for piggybacking insulin or if a bolus is needed. Because insulin clings to plastic IV bags and tubing, the tubing should be flushed with insulin before the prescribed amount is added. During the second stage of labor and the immediate postpartal period, the woman may not need additional insulin. The intravenous insulin is discontinued with the completion of the third stage of labor.

### Postpartal Management of Diabetes Mellitus

Generally maternal insulin requirements fall significantly during the postpartal period for all diabetic women, regardless of the type of diabetes, because, with placental separation, hormone levels fall and the antiinsulin effect ceases. For the first 24 hours postpartum women with preexisting diabetes typically require very little insulin. They are usually managed with a sliding scale. Afterward, a more regular insulin dosage pattern can be reestablished. Women with mild diabetes not requiring insulin often have sufficient glucose control and do not require any therapy while they are hospitalized. Antihyperglycemics are contraindicated during breastfeeding. Consequently a nursing woman with diabetes that is not controlled by diet alone may need insulin for a time (Kjos, 2000).

Women with GDM who did not require insulin during pregnancy generally do not need it during the postpartum period. Clinicians routinely discontinue insulin for women with GDM following childbirth and then monitor blood glucose levels. If elevated glucose levels develop, oral antihyperglycemic agents may be tried if the woman is not breastfeeding (Curet, 2000). The woman should be reassessed 6 weeks postpartum to determine whether her glucose levels are normal. If the levels are normal, she should be reassessed at a minimum of 3-year internals (ADA, 2000a).

The establishment of parent-child relationships is a high priority during the postpartum period for all women with DM and their families. If the newborn requires a special-care nursery, the parents need ongoing information, support, and encouragement to visit and be involved in the newborn's care.

Breastfeeding is encouraged as beneficial to both mother and baby. Evidence suggests that breastfed infants have a lower risk of developing diabetes than infants who are bottle-fed (Moore, 1999). Calorie needs increase during lactation to 500 to 800 kcal above prepregnant requirements, and insulin must be adjusted accordingly. Home blood glucose monitoring should continue for the insulin-dependent diabetic.

The woman and her partner, if he is involved, should also receive information on family planning. Barrier methods of contraception (diaphragm, cervical cap, condom) used with a spermicide are safe, effective, and economical and are the method of choice for insulin-dependent diabetic women. The use of oral contraceptives (OCs) by diabetic women is somewhat controversial. Many physicians who prescribe low-dose OCs to women with diabetes restrict them to women who have no vascular disease and do not smoke. The progesterone-only pill has a higher failure rate but is otherwise safer. Many couples who have completed their families choose elective sterilization.

## Nursing Care Management

The Critical Pathway for a woman with diabetes mellitus, on page 272, summarizes nursing management during the antepartum, intrapartum, and postpartum periods.

### Nursing Assessment and Diagnosis

Whether diabetes has been diagnosed before pregnancy occurs or the diagnosis is made during pregnancy (GDM), careful assessment of the disease process and the woman's understanding of diabetes is important. Thorough physical examination—including assessment for vascular complications of the disease, any signs of infectious conditions, and urine and blood testing for glucose—is essential on the first prenatal visit. Follow-up visits are usually scheduled twice a month during the first two trimesters and once a week during the last trimester.

Assessment also yields vital information about the woman's ability to cope with the combined stress of pregnancy and diabetes and to follow a recommended regimen of care. It is necessary to determine the woman's knowledge about diabetes and self-care before formulating a teaching plan.

# CRITICAL PATHWAY: *For A Woman With Diabetes Mellitus*

| Category | Antepartal Management | Intrapartal Management* | Postpartal Management* |
|---|---|---|---|
| **Referral** | • Perinatologist<br>• Endocrinologist<br>• Neonatologist<br>• Social worker<br>• Psych clinical nurse practitioner<br>• Diabetes nurse educator<br>• Dietary/nutritionist<br>• Physical therapy, occupational therapy | • Obtain prenatal record | • Home nursing referral if indicated<br>• Diabetes nurse educator<br>**Expected Outcomes**<br>Appropriate resources identified and utilized |
| **Assessment** | • Electronic fetal monitoring as indicated<br>• Nonstress test as indicated<br>• Ultrasound as indicated<br>• Amniocentesis for lung maturity at 34–36 weeks<br>• Alpha-fetoprotein (done usually at 16 weeks) | • Assess for (s/sx) of hypoglycemia (sweating, periodic tingling, disorientation, shakiness, pallor, clammy skin, irritability, hunger, headache, and blurred vision) during labor<br>• Continuous electronic fetal monitoring<br>• Assess glucose levels with glucometer as ordered or if s/sx of hypoglycemia occur | • Assess glucose levels with glucometer—generally insulin requirements fall significantly in the postpartum phase<br>• Continue normal postpartum assessment q8h<br>• Feeding technique with newborn: should be progressing<br>• Vital signs assessment: q8h; all WNL report temperature >38°C (100.4°F)<br>• Continue assessment of comfort level<br>**Expected Outcomes**<br>Assessment findings indicate control of blood sugar levels with related complications minimized; fetal growth and development unimpaired |
| **Teaching/ psychosocial** | • Room orientation<br>• Notify RN of s/sx of hyper/hypoglycemia, uterine contractions, decreased fetal movement, vaginal leaking and/or bleeding, dysuria<br>• Assess family status and/or additional psychosocial needs<br>• Evaluation of client learning needs<br>• Importance of following diet<br>• Tour of ICN<br>• Prebirth teaching for vaginal and/or cesarean (CS)<br>• Evaluation of teaching effectiveness | • Evaluation of teaching effectiveness<br>• Continuing evaluation of ongoing learning needs | • Complete normal postpartum teaching<br>**Expected Outcomes**<br>Client verbalizes/demonstrates understanding of diabetic and health care education |
| **Nursing care management and reports** | • CBC<br>• UA/dipstick for protein and ketones<br>• Biochemistry profile<br>• Glycosylated hemoglobin level ($Hb_{A1C}$) daily<br>• 24-hour urine for protein and creatinine clearance<br>• Fingerstick blood sugar (BS), every am, before meals, and 2 hours after meals<br>• Vital signs q4h<br>• Fundal height weekly<br>• Daily weight | • Glucose levels monitored as directed | • Continue sitz bath prn<br>• May shower if ambulating without difficulty<br>• DC heparin lock if present<br>**Expected Outcomes**<br>Labs/reports reflect stable, controlled blood sugar<br>Maternal and fetal well-being maintained.<br>Active involvement of client in plan of care for diabetic management |
| **Activity** | • Bed rest with bathroom privileges<br>• Diversional activity | • Bed rest as tolerated | • Up ad lib<br>**Expected Outcomes**<br>Level of activity has not exacerbated condition |
| **Comfort** | • Assess for discomfort<br>• Provide comfort measures as needed | • Assess for discomfort<br>• Provide comfort measures as needed | • Continue with pain management techniques<br>**Expected Outcomes**<br>Optimal comfort maintained |

| Category | Antepartal Management | Intrapartal Management* | Postpartal Management* |
|---|---|---|---|
| **Nutrition** | • American Dietetic Association (ADA) per order<br>• Encourage fluids | • Ice chips<br>Hard candy, PRN | • Encourage breastfeeding<br>• Increase calorie needs 500–800 kcal<br>• Continue diet and fluids<br>**Expected Outcomes**<br>Nutritional needs met, with emphasis on diabetic control |
| **Elimination** | • Review measures to prevent UTI | **Expected Outcomes**<br>Monitor and record intake and output | **Expected Outcomes**<br>Intake and output within normal limits |
| **Medications** | • IV ____ @ ____ mLh/r/heparin lock<br>• Insulin as ordered →________<br>• Prenatal vitamins and iron | • Two IV lines are usually used, one with 5% dextrose solution and one with a saline solution (saline line is used for insulin if needed)<br>• The IV insulin is usually discontinued with completion of 3rd stage of labor | • May take own prenatal vitamins<br>• Rh immune globulin (RhoGAM) and rubella vaccine administered if indicated<br>**Expected Outcomes**<br>BS levels within acceptable medical parameters |
| **Discharge planning/ home care** | • Explain purpose of scheduled tests and procedures<br>• Include family in diabetic teaching<br>• Assess family support | • Assess family support | • Review discharge instruction sheet and check list<br>• Describe postpartum warning signs and when to call CNM/physician<br>• Provide prescriptions<br>• Gift pack given to woman<br>• Arrangements made for baby pictures if desired<br>• Postpartum visit scheduled<br>• Newborn check scheduled<br>**Expected Outcomes**<br>Discharge teaching completed with emphasis on follow-up health care needs and adequate support network |
| **Family involvement** | • Identify available support persons<br>• Assess family perceptions of situation | • Involve support persons in care | • Evidence of parental bonding behaviors apparent<br>• Involve support persons in care: teaching<br>• Plans being made for providing support to mother following discharge<br>**Expected Outcomes**<br>Family utilizes resources |
| **Date** | | | |

*Interventions for a woman with a normal labor and birth and during the early postpartum period may be found in those appropriate critical pathways.

*Note:* BS, blood sugar; heparin lock, intravenous catheter that allows intermittent access; CBC=complete blood count, ICN, intensive care nursery; IV, intravenous; PRN, as needed or as desired; q8h - every 8 hours; Q4h every 4 hours; RN registered nurse; s/sx, signs/symptoms; UA, urinalysis UTI, urinary tract infection; WNL, within normal limits.

Nursing diagnoses that may apply to the pregnant woman with diabetes include the following:

- ***Risk for altered nutrition:*** more than body requirements related to imbalance between intake and available insulin
- ***Risk for injury*** related to possible complications secondary to hypoglycemia or hyperglycemia
- ***Altered family processes*** related to the need for hospitalization secondary to diabetes mellitus

## Nursing Plan and Implementation

For the woman with preexisting diabetes, a nurse and a physician may provide prepregnancy counseling using a team approach. Ideally they see the couple before

## Critical Thinking in Practice

Patti Chang is a 35-year-old, gravida 3, para 2, well-educated, active Chinese-American woman with no history of glucose intolerance. Her two children were born healthy at 36 weeks' gestation. She receives the usual 50-g glucose tolerance test at 26 weeks' gestation, and her plasma level is 160 mg/dL. She seems irritated and frustrated when her obstetrician tells her that it would be best to perform a 3-hour fasting glucose tolerance test. After the physician leaves the room, Patti asks the nurse the following questions: Will the glucose hurt my baby? What will the treatment be? How will the nurse answer the questions? Why does Patti seem so upset?

Answers can be found in Appendix I.

pregnancy so that the DM can be evaluated. The outlook for pregnancy is good if the diabetes is of recent onset without vascular complications, provided that glucose levels can be controlled.

For women with GDM, nursing care focuses heavily on client education about the condition, its implications, and its management.

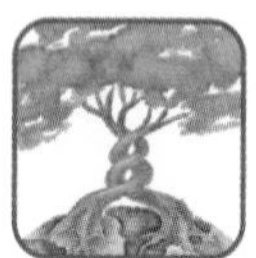

## Community-Based Nursing Care

In many cases, women with gestational diabetes mellitus are stabilized in the hospital and necessary teaching for self-care is begun. Women with preexisting diabetes may also require hospitalization for stabilization of their diabetes. In either case, the majority of ongoing teaching and supervision of pregnant women with diabetes is then carried out by nurses in clinics, community agencies, and the women's homes.

### Effective Insulin Use

The nurse ensures that the woman and her partner understand the purpose of insulin, the types of insulin to be used, and the correct procedure for administering it. The woman's partner is also instructed about insulin administration in case it becomes necessary for the partner to give it. For some highly motivated women whose glucose levels are not well controlled with multiple injections, the continuous infusion pump may improve glucose control.

The nurse teaches the woman how and when to monitor her blood glucose level, the desired range of blood

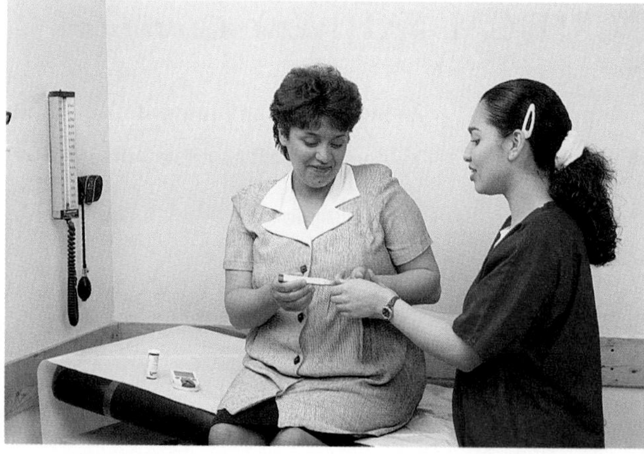

**FIGURE 12–1** ♦ The nurse teaches the pregnant woman with gestational diabetes mellitus how to do home glucose monitoring.

glucose levels, and the importance of good control (Figure 12–1). Most women use a glucose meter to monitor blood sugar level because the meter is more accurate, but some women use a visual method of monitoring. With either method, the nurse teaches the woman to follow the manufacturer's directions exactly; to wash her hands thoroughly before puncturing her finger; to touch the blood droplet, not her finger, to the test pad on the strip; and to store the test strips as directed and discard them after the expiration date.

The nurse can provide the following tips regarding finger puncture: (1) various spring-loaded devices are available that make puncturing easier; (2) letting the arm hang down for 30 seconds increases blood flow to the fingers; and (3) the sides of fingers should be punctured instead of the ends because the ends contain more pain-sensitive nerves.

Diabetic clients need to keep a record of each blood sugar reading as a guide for management. Specific record sheets are available for this purpose.

### Planned Exercise Program

Regardless of the type of diabetes, unless otherwise medically contraindicated, exercise is encouraged for the woman's overall well-being. If she is used to a regular exercise program, the nurse encourages her to continue. In addition, the nurse advises the woman to exercise after meals when blood sugar levels are high, to wear diabetic identification, to carry a simple sugar such as hard candy (because of the possibility of exercise-induced hypoglycemia), to monitor her blood glucose levels regularly, and to avoid injecting insulin into an extremity that will soon be used during exercise.

If the woman has not been following a regular exercise plan, the nurse can encourage her to begin gradually. Due to alterations in metabolism with exercise, the woman's blood glucose should be well controlled before she begins an exercise program.

### *Teaching for Self-Care*

Using the information gained during the nursing assessment of the pregnant woman with diabetes, the nurse provides appropriate teaching to the woman and her family so that the woman can meet her own health care needs as much as possible.

- *Glucose monitoring.* Home monitoring of blood glucose levels is the most accurate and convenient method to determine insulin dose and assess control. Women are taught self-monitoring techniques that they perform four to six times a day according to a specified schedule. They then regulate their insulin dosage based on blood glucose values and anticipated activity level. Women are encouraged to maintain blood glucose levels in normal ranges as follows: before meals, 70 to 100 mg/dL; 2 hours after a meal, <120 mg/dL (ADA, 2000b).
- *Symptoms of hypoglycemia and ketoacidosis.* The pregnant diabetic woman must recognize symptoms of changing glucose levels and take appropriate action by immediately checking her capillary blood glucose level. If it is less than 60 mg/dL, she is advised to take 20 g of carbohydrate, wait 20 minutes, and then retest her glucose level. The necessary carbohydrate can be obtained by drinking 14.5 oz whole milk, 12 oz orange or apple juice, or 13.3 oz cola (Mandeville, 1992). Many people overtreat their symptoms by continuing to eat, but doing so can cause rebound hyperglycemia. The woman should carry a snack at all times and should have other fast sources of glucose (simple carbohydrates) at hand to treat an insulin reaction when milk is not available. Family members are also taught how to inject glucagon in case food does not work or is not feasible (eg, in the presence of severe morning sickness).
- *Smoking.* Smoking has harmful effects on both the maternal vascular system and the developing fetus and is contraindicated for both pregnancy and diabetes.
- *Travel.* Insulin can be kept at room temperature while traveling. Insulin supplies should be kept with the traveler and not packed in the baggage. Special meals can be arranged by notifying most airlines a few days before departure. The woman should wear a diabetic identification bracelet or necklace and should check with her physician for any instructions or advice before traveling.
- *Support groups.* Many communities have diabetes support groups or education classes that are helpful to women with newly diagnosed diabetes.
- *Cesarean birth.* Chances for a cesarean birth increase if the pregnant woman is diabetic. The possibility should be anticipated; caregivers may suggest enrollment in cesarean birth preparation classes. Many hospitals offer classes, and information is available through state or national organizations. The couple may prefer simply to discuss cesarean birth with the nurse and their obstetrician and read some books on the topic.

### *Hospital-Based Nursing Care*

Hospitalization may become necessary during the pregnancy to evaluate blood glucose levels and adjust insulin dosages. In such cases, the nurse monitors the woman's status and continues to provide teaching so that the woman is knowledgeable about her condition and its management.

During the intrapartal period, the nurse continues to monitor the woman's status, maintains her intravenous fluids, is alert for signs of hypoglycemia, and provides the care indicated for any woman in labor. If a cesarean birth becomes necessary, the nurse provides appropriate care, as described in Chapter 20.

## Evaluation

Expected outcomes of nursing care include the following:

- The woman is able to discuss her condition and its possible impact on her pregnancy, labor and birth, and postpartal period.
- The woman participates in developing a health care regimen to meet her needs and follows it throughout her pregnancy.
- The woman avoids developing hypoglycemia or hyperglycemia.
- The woman gives birth to a healthy newborn.
- The woman is able to care for her newborn.

# Care of the Woman with Anemia

Anemia indicates inadequate levels of hemoglobin (Hb) in the blood. During pregnancy, anemia is defined as hemoglobin less than 10 g/dL (Wenstrom & Malee, 1999). The common anemias of pregnancy are due either to insufficient hemoglobin production related to nutritional deficiency in iron or folic acid during pregnancy or to hemoglobin destruction in an inherited disorder such as sickle cell anemia. Table 12–4 describes these common anemias.

TABLE 12–4 Anemia and Pregnancy

| *Condition* | *Brief Description* | *Maternal Implications* | *Fetal/Neonatal Implications* |
|---|---|---|---|
| Iron deficiency anemia | Condition caused by inadequate iron intake resulting in hemoglobin levels below 11g/dL. To prevent this, most women are advised to take supplemental iron during pregnancy. | Pregnant woman with this anemia tires easily, is more susceptible to infection, has increased chance of PIH and postpartal hemorrhage, and cannot tolerate even minimal blood loss during birth. | Risk of low birth weight, prematurity, stillbirth, and neonatal death increases in women with severe iron deficiency anemia (maternal Hb less than 6 g/dL). Fetus may be hypoxic during labor due to impaired uteroplacental oxygenation. |
| Sickle cell anemia | Recessive autosomal disease present in about 1 in 600 African-Americans in the US (the sickle cell trait is carried by 8%) (Scioscia, 1999). The disease is characterized by sickling of the RBCs in the presence of decreased oxygenation. Condition may be marked by crisis with profound anemia, jaundice, high temperature, infarction, and acute pain. Crisis is treated by partial exchange transfusion, rehydration with intravenous fluids, antibiotics, and analgesics. The fetus is monitored throughout. | Pregnancy may aggravate anemia and bring on more crises. Risk of developing preeclampsia increases. Risk of urinary tract infection, pneumonia, congestive heart failure, and pulmonary infarction also increases. The goal of treatment is to reduce the anemia and maintain good health. Oxygen supplementation should be used continuously during labor. Additional blood should be available if transfusion is necessary following birth. | Abortion, fetal death, and prematurity may occur. IUGR is also a characteristic finding in newborns of women with sickle-cell anemia. |
| Folic acid deficiency anemia | Folic acid deficiency is the most common cause of megaloblastic anemia. In the absence of folic acid, immature RBCs fail to divide, become enlarged (megaloblastic), and are fewer in number. Increased folic acid metabolism during pregnancy and lactation can result in deficiency. Because the condition is difficult to diagnose, the best approach is prevention. All women who could become pregnant should take a multivitamin containing 400 μg (0.4 mg) daily (generally found in prenatal vitamins) before conception and through at least the first trimester of pregnancy (Mersereau, 2000). Some authorities recommend increasing the amount of synthetic folate to 0.6 mg daily once pregnancy is confirmed (Institute of Medicine, 1998). The condition is treated with 1.0 mg folate daily (see Chapter 11). | Folate deficiency is the second most common cause of anemia in pregnancy. Severe deficiency increases the risk that the mother may need a blood transfusion following birth due to anemia. She also has an increased risk of hemorrhage due to thrombocytopenia and is more susceptible to infection. Folic acid is readily available in foods such as fresh leafy green vegetables, red meat, fish, poultry, and legumes, but it is easily destroyed by overcooking or cooking with large quantities of water. | Maternal folic acid deficiency has been associated with an increased risk of neural tube defects (NTDs) such as spina bifida, meningomyelocele, and anencephaly in the newborn. Adequate folic acid intake can reduce the incidence of NTDs by 50% to 70% (CDC, 1999c). Folic acid may also help prevent other birth defects, including cleft lip and cleft palate (March of Dimes [MOD], 1999).<br><br>Women who have already had one baby with a NTD are generally advised to take a larger dose of folic acid daily—typically 4.0 mg (MOD, 1999). |

## Care of the Woman with HIV Infection

**Human immunodeficiency virus (HIV)** infection is one of today's major health concerns. It leads to a progressive disease that ultimately results in the development of **acquired immunodeficiency syndrome (AIDS).** As of June 2000, 753,907 cases of AIDS has been reported in the United States (Centers for Disease Control and Prevention [CDC], 2000). From 1996 to the present, the incidence of AIDS has been decreasing, although the rate of decrease has slowed; concurrently the number of people living with AIDS has increased. These changes have been attributed to the effect of new treatment options (CDC, 2000). Homosexual and bisexual men still make up the largest group of infected individuals. Women account for 17% of cases. Although less than one-fourth of U.S. women are African-American and Latino, these groups accounted for 77% of all female AIDS cases in 2000. Moreover, HIV remains the third leading cause of death for all women ages 25 to 44, but it is the leading cause of death for African-American women of the same age group (Hoffman-Terry, 1999). Cases of perinatal AIDS have also decreased significantly in the past several years primarily because of the use of zidovudine (ZDV) therapy in pregnant women with HIV (Lindegren, Byers, Thomas, et al., 1999).

### Pathophysiology of HIV and AIDS

HIV, which causes AIDS, typically enters the body through blood, blood products, or other body fluids such as semen, vaginal fluid, and breast milk. HIV affects specific T cells, thereby decreasing the body's immune responses. This makes the affected person susceptible to opportunistic infections such as *Pneumocystis carinii,* which causes a severe pneumonia, candidiasis, cytomegalovirus, tuberculosis, and toxoplasmosis.

Once infected with the virus, the individual develops antibodies that can be detected with the enzyme-linked immunosorbent assay (ELISA) and confirmed with the Western blot test. Antibodies usually develop within 6 to 12 weeks after exposure, although in some people this latent period is longer. An asymptomatic period of approximately 5 to 11 years follows seroconversion (Minkoff, 1999). The majority of pregnant women fall into this category.

The diagnosis of AIDS is made when an individual is HIV positive and is identified as having one of several specific opportunistic infections.

### Maternal Risks

AIDS-defining diseases that are more common in women than in men include wasting syndrome, esophageal candidiasis, and herpes simplex virus disease. Non-AIDS-defining gynecologic disorders, such as candidiasis or cervical pathology, are prevalent among women in all stages of HIV.

Many women who are HIV positive choose to avoid pregnancy because of the risk of infecting the fetus and the likelihood of dying before the child is raised. Women who become pregnant should be advised that pregnancy is not believed to accelerate the progression of HIV/AIDS, that the use of ZDV during pregnancy significantly reduces the risk of transmitting the HIV to the fetus, and that most medications used to treat HIV can be taken during the pregnancy (Minkoff, 1999).

### Fetal-Neonatal Risks

AIDS may develop in infants whose mothers are seropositive, usually due to perinatal transmission. Perinatal transmission occurs transplacentally, at birth when the infant is exposed to maternal blood and vaginal secretions, and via breast milk. The risk to infants born to mothers who are HIV positive is estimated to be about 25%. When the pregnant woman receives ZDV therapy, that risk decreases to 5% to 8%. When ZDV therapy is combined with a scheduled cesarean birth, the risk is further reduced to about 2% (American College of Obstetricians and Gynecologists [ACOG], 1999).

Often infants have a positive antibody titer for up to 15 months due to the passive transfer of maternal antibodies. For further discussion of the infant who is HIV positive, see Chapter 25.

### Clinical Therapy

The goal for antenatal care is identification of the pregnant woman at risk for HIV infection. All women who are pregnant or planning a pregnancy should be offered voluntary HIV antibody testing using ELISA. If the results are positive, the Western blot test is used to confirm the diagnosis. Women who test positive should be counseled about the implications of the diagnosis for themselves and their fetus to ensure an informed reproductive choice. The care of the woman who chooses to continue her pregnancy focuses on stabilizing the disease, preventing opportunistic infections and the transmission of the virus from mother to fetus, and providing psychosocial and educational support. ZDV therapy should be recommended to all infected pregnant women to reduce the rate of perinatal transmission. This therapy involves administration of ZDV during pregnancy and labor and to the newborn for the first 6 weeks of life (Mofenson, 1999).

The woman infected with HIV should be evaluated and treated for other sexually transmitted infections and for conditions occurring more commonly in women with

HIV, such as tuberculosis, cytomegalovirus, toxoplasmosis, and cervical dysplasia. If there is no history of hepatitis B, she should receive the hepatitis vaccine, as well as the pneumococcal vaccine and an annual flu shot. In addition to routine prenatal laboratory tests, a platelet count and a complete blood count with differential should be obtained at the first prenatal visit and repeated each trimester to identify anemia, thrombocytopenia, and leukopenia, which are associated with both HIV infection and antiviral therapy.

At each prenatal visit, asymptomatic, HIV-infected women are monitored for early signs of complications, such as weight loss in the second or third trimesters or fever. The mouth is inspected for signs of infections such as thrush (candidiasis) or hairy leukoplakia; the lungs are auscultated for signs of pneumonia; and the lymph nodes, the liver, and the spleen are palpated for signs of enlargement. Each trimester the woman should have a visual examination and a fundoscopic examination of the retina to detect such complications as toxoplasmosis.

In addition to routine prenatal testing, the woman who is HIV positive should be assessed regularly for serologic changes indicating that HIV/AIDS is progressing. This assessment includes the absolute CD4 lymphocyte count, which provides the number of helper T4 cells. When the CD4 count reaches a level of 200/mm$^3$ or lower, opportunistic infections are more likely to develop.

A pregnancy complicated by HIV infection, even if asymptomatic, is considered high risk, and the fetus is monitored closely. Weekly nonstress testing is begun at 32 weeks' gestation, and serial ultrasounds are done to detect IUGR. Biophysical profiles are also indicated (see Chapter 14). Invasive procedures such as amniocentesis are avoided when possible to prevent the contamination of a noninfected infant.

Because cesarean birth further reduces the risk of transmission of HIV vertically from mother to baby, ACOG recommends that birth by scheduled cesarean be offered to all HIV-infected women. To decrease the risk of rupture of the membranes before the onset of labor, the cesarean is best done at 38 completed weeks of gestation. Intravenous ZDV prophylaxis should be given before surgery (ACOG, 1999). Intrapartal care is similar to that for all pregnant women having a cesarean, although strict adherence to universal precautions is crucial to avoid nosocomial infection.

Women who are HIV positive are at increased risk for complications such as intrapartal or postpartal hemorrhage, postpartal infection, poor wound healing, and infections of the genitourinary tract. Thus they need careful monitoring and appropriate therapy as indicated. Research suggests that breastfeeding increases the risk of HIV transmission to the newborn. Consequently, the HIV-positive woman should be cautioned against breastfeeding her infant.

Because of the profound implications of HIV infection for the woman, her family, the child, and her health care providers, screening is recommended for women who are at increased risk, including the following: IV drug users; prostitutes; women whose current or previous sexual partners have been bisexual, have abused IV drugs, have hemophilia, or have tested positive for HIV; and women from countries where heterosexual transmission is common. In addition, clinical facilities that are located in areas with a large population of people who test positive for HIV may require routine HIV screening of all prenatal clients.

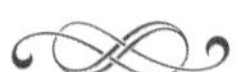

## Nursing Care Management

### Nursing Assessment and Diagnosis

A woman who tests positive for HIV may be asymptomatic or may present with any of the following signs or symptoms: fatigue, anemia, malaise, progressive weight loss, lymphadenopathy, diarrhea, fever, neurologic dysfunction, cell-mediated immunodeficiency, or evidence of Kaposi's sarcoma (purplish, reddish brown lesions either externally or internally).

If a woman tests positive for HIV or is involved in a relationship that places her at high risk, the nurse should assess the woman's knowledge level about the disease, its implications for her and her fetus, and self-care measures the woman can take.

Examples of nursing diagnoses that might apply for a pregnant woman who tests positive for HIV include the following:

- ***Knowledge deficit*** related to lack of information about HIV/AIDS and its long-term implications for the woman and her unborn child
- ***Risk for infection*** related to altered immunity secondary to HIV infection
- ***Ineffective family coping*** related to the implications of a positive HIV test in one of the family members

### Nursing Plan and Implementation

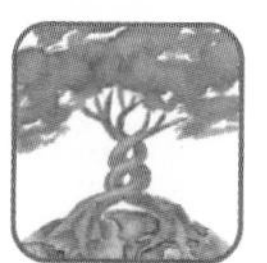

#### Community-Based Nursing Care

Nurses need to help women understand that HIV/AIDS is a fatal disease. HIV infection can be avoided if women practice safe sex, including insisting that their partners wear a latex condom for each act of intercourse, and avoid sharing IV drug needles.

Women at high risk for HIV/AIDS should be offered premarital and prepregnancy screening for HIV antibodies (ACOG, 1997). In many instances, the nurse will be responsible for counseling the woman about the test and its implications for her, her partner, and her child if she becomes pregnant.

In monitoring the asymptomatic pregnant woman who is HIV positive, the nurse needs to be alert for nonspecific symptoms such as fever, weight loss, fatigue, persistent candidiasis, diarrhea, cough, skin lesions, and behavior changes. These may be signs of developing symptomatic HIV infection. Laboratory findings such as decreased hemoglobin, hematocrit, and CD4 lymphocytes; elevated erythrocyte sedimentation rate (ESR); and abnormal complete blood count, differential, and platelets may indicate complications such as infection or progression of the disease.

Education about optimal nutrition and maintenance of wellness is important, and the information should be reviewed frequently with the woman. The woman should also receive information about her ZDV prophylaxis and the importance of following the established regimen for herself during pregnancy and for her newborn after birth.

### Hospital-Based Nursing Care

The Critical Pathway for a woman with HIV/AIDS beginning on page 280 summarizes essential nursing management during the antepartum, intrapartum, and postpartum periods.

In 1987 the CDC stated that the increasing prevalence of HIV/AIDS and the risk of exposure faced by health care workers is significant enough that precautions *should be taken with all clients* (not only those with known HIV infection), especially in dealing with blood and body fluids. These precautions are called *universal precautions.*

Nurses who deal with childbearing families are exposed frequently to blood and body fluids and need to pay careful attention to the CDC guidelines, which are addressed in introductory nursing courses as a preparation for clinical practice. See Key Facts to Remember: The Pregnant Woman with HIV Infection.

Protocols have been established for postexposure treatment of a caregiver who experiences a needlestick or exposure to body fluids of a person with HIV or a person whose HIV status is unknown. The effectiveness of the therapy, usually a combined drug approach, depends on starting therapy rapidly (Catanzarite, Piacquadio, Stanco, et al, 1999). Thus such exposure should be reported immediately.

### Teaching for Self-Care

The psychologic implications of HIV/AIDS for the childbearing family are staggering. The woman is faced with the knowledge that she and her newborn, if infected, have a decreased life expectancy. If her infant is not infected, she must face the probability that others will raise her

## KEY FACTS TO REMEMBER

### *The Pregnant Woman with HIV Infection*

- Following initial infection, antibodies usually become detectable within about 6–12 weeks, but it may take 6 months or longer. *Despite this, the woman is infected, and infectious.*
- HIV infection is spread primarily through sexual contact, exposure to contaminated blood, and (perinatally) from infected mother to child.
- Many women who are HIV positive are asymptomatic and may be unaware they have the infection. *Universal precautions are indicated in caring for all pregnant women.*
- A pregnant woman found to be HIV positive should receive prenatal counseling about the possible implications of HIV for the fetus so that she can make an informed choice about continuing her pregnancy. Her choice should be supported.
- During pregnancy, caregivers should be alert to nonspecific symptoms such as weight loss and fatigue, which may indicate progression of HIV disease.
- The incidence of vertical transmission of HIV infection from mother to baby has decreased significantly because of the administration of ZDV to the mother prenatally and during labor and to the newborn for a specified period following birth.
- The American College of Obstetricians and Gynecologists (1999) recommends scheduled cesarean birth at 38 completed weeks of gestation to reduce the risk of vertical transmission even more.
- Invasive procedures during the intrapartal period increase the risk of exposure to HIV for the fetus (who may be uninfected) and should be undertaken only after carefully weighing the advantages and risks.
- **The cardinal rule in caring for pregnant women is: if it's wet and it's not yours, use protection when handling it!**

# CRITICAL PATHWAY: *For A Woman With HIV/AIDS*

| Category | Antepartal Management | Intrapartal Management* | Postpartal Management* |
|---|---|---|---|
| **Referral** | • Perinatologist<br>• Internist<br>• Social worker<br>• Psych clinical nurse practitioner<br>• Dietary/nutritionist<br>• Infectious disease consult | • Obtain prenatal record | • Home nursing referral if indicated<br>**Expected Outcomes**<br>Appropriate resources identified and utilized |
| **Assessment** | • Obtain course of present pregnancy<br>• Assess estimated gestational age<br>• Assess any sensitivity to medications<br>• Obtain history of any infections<br>• Obtain complete physical examination to include:<br>  • Fetal size, fetal status (FHR), and fetal maturity<br>  • Signs of fatigue, weakness, recurrent diarrhea, pallor, night sweats<br>  • Lymphadenopathy<br>  • Present weight and amount of weight gain or weight loss<br>  • Presence of nonproductive cough, fever, sore throat, chills, shortness of breath (*Pneumocystis carinii* pneumonia)<br>  • Dark purplish marks or lesions, especially on the lower extremities (Kaposi's sarcoma)<br>  • Oral, gingival lesions<br>• Obtain diagnostic studies:<br>  • Ultrasound<br>  • Fetal maturity studies (L/S ratio, PG creatinine)<br>  • Hemoglobin and hematocrit<br>  • WBC<br>  • HIV-I<br>  • CD4+ T lymphocyte count<br>  • ESR<br>  • Differential<br>  • Platelet count | • Assess for signs of infection | • Monitor daily Hct<br>• Continue normal postpartum assessment q8h<br>• Feeding technique with newborn: should be progressing<br>• TPR assessment: q8h; all WNL; report temperature >38°C (100.4°F)<br>• Continue assessment of comfort level<br>**Expected Outcomes**<br>Potential/actual health problems and complications identified and minimized |
| **Teaching/ psychosocial** | • Room orientation<br>• Explain signs and symptoms of worsening disease and importance of notifying RN<br>• Explain s/sx of labor<br>• Increase pt awareness of fetal monitoring<br>• Evaluation of client teaching | • Tour of ICN<br>• Discuss with woman:<br>  a. Mode of childbirth<br>  b. Postpartum expectation | • Implement normal postpartum teaching and psychosocial support<br>**Expected Outcomes**<br>Client verbalizes/demonstrates understanding and incorporation of teaching |
| **Nursing care management and reports** | • Assess emotional response so that support and teaching can be planned accordingly<br>• Weigh woman<br>• Obtain food history<br>• Establish rapport<br>• Provide opportunities to talk without interruption<br>• Monitor for signs of infection<br>• Maintain appropriate isolation precautions | • Ongoing monitoring of blood pressure<br>• Electronic fetal monitoring in place<br>• Try to have same nurses caring for woman during her hospitalization<br>• Maintain appropriate BSI precautions<br>• Monitor for signs of infection<br>Provide supportive care | • Continue sitz baths prn<br>• May shower if ambulating without difficulty<br>• DC buffalo cap (heparin lock) if present<br>• Maintain appropriate isolation precautions<br>• Monitor for signs of infection<br>**Expected Outcomes**<br>Maternal and fetal well-being maximized<br>Active involvement of client in plan of care to include physical, emotional, and spiritual needs |
| **Activity** | • Decreased stimulation in room<br>• Limit visitors | Encourage position change and activity as tolerated | • Up ad lib<br>**Expected Outcome**<br>Level of activity has not exacerbated condition |

| Category | Antepartal Management | Intrapartal Management* | Postpartal Management* |
|---|---|---|---|
| **Comfort** | • Assess for discomfort<br>• Provide comfort measures as needed | • Assess for discomfort<br>• Provide comfort measures as needed | • Continue with pain management techniques<br>**Expected Outcome**<br>Optimal comfort maintained |
| **Nutrition** | • Plan high-protein, high-calorie diet | • Ice chips; popsicles | • Continue diet and fluids<br>**Expected Outcome**<br>Nutritional needs met with emphasis on appetite enhancement and reduction of deficiencies |
| **Elimination** | | | **Expected Outcome**<br>Intake and output WNL |
| **Medications** | | • Continuous IV infusion | • May take own prenatal vitamins<br>• Rh immune globulin (RhoGAM) administered if indicated<br>• Rubella vaccine administered if indicated<br>**Expected Outcomes**<br>Perfusion and hydration supported<br>Ongoing treatments maintained |
| **Discharge planning/ home care Family** | • Assess home care needs<br>• If the client is asymptomatic, the primary nursing activity is client teaching regarding<br>  • Disease process<br>  • Screening and health care for sex partners as appropriate<br>  • Impact of disease on pregnancy<br>  • Methods of HIV transmission<br>  • Precautions to take in preventing the spread of infection<br>  • Options in regard to pregnancy<br>  • Available community resources<br>  • Signs and symptoms to report to health care provider including common discomforts of pregnancy such as nausea and fatigue and complications such as premature rupture of membranes, vaginal bleeding, and preterm labor<br>  • Importance of regular prenatal visits<br>• Provide teaching regarding nutritional needs<br>• Refer to community resources<br>• Discuss disease process, impact on pregnancy, and pregnancy options<br>• Provide support and counseling | | • Review discharge instruction sheet and checklist<br>• Describe postpartum warning signs and when to call CNM/physician<br>• Provide prescriptions and gift pack<br>• Arrangements made for baby pictures<br>• Postpartum visit scheduled<br>• Newborn check scheduled<br>• Discuss the implications of breastfeeding (current information suggests that the virus may be spread in breast milk)<br>• Provide information on transmission of HIV and measures to prevent infection. Discuss household safety issues (eg, it is acceptable to use same dishes, safe to sleep in same bed, safe to use same bathroom, can hold and hug children, should avoid sharing razors and toothbrushes and should wear gloves and use 10% bleach solution to clean spills of body fluids or disinfect bathroom). Inform the woman that sexual abstinence is safest; otherwise latex condoms should be used.<br>**Expected Outcomes**<br>Discharge teaching completed with emphasis on follow-up continuing health care needs, adequate support network |
| **Involvement** | • Assess woman's major concerns regarding losing fetus, relationship with other children, relationship with partner<br>• Assess support systems | • Encourage family member to stay with the woman as long as possible throughout labor and childbirth | • Family members urged to visit<br>• Continue to involve support persons in teaching<br>• Shows parental bonding behaviors<br>• Plans made for providing support to mother following discharge. Support persons verbalize understanding of need for woman to rest, eat nutritionally, recover.<br>**Expected Outcomes**<br>Family demonstrates resource utilization, integration of newborn into family, helpful coping skills |
| **Date** | | | |

*Interventions for a woman with a normal labor and birth and during the early postpartum period may be found in those appropriate critical pathways.

BSI, body substance isolation; ESR erythrocyte sedimentation rate; FHR, fetal heart rate; hct hematocrit ICN, intensive care nursery; IV, intravenous; L/S ratio, Lecithin/sphingomyelin ratio; PG, phosphotidyl glycerol; Q8h every 8 hours; s/sx, signs/symptoms; WBC, white blood count; WNL, within normal limits.

child. The couple must deal with the impact of the illness on the partner, who may or may not be infected, and on other children. The woman and her family may have feelings of fear, helplessness, anger, and isolation.

The nonjudgmental, supportive nurse plays an essential role in preserving confidentiality and the client's right to privacy. The nurse can help ensure that the woman receives complete, accurate information about her condition and ways she might cope. The nurse also teaches transmission prevention using the specific language and parlance of the woman and her partner. In addition the nurse ensures that the woman is referred to a comprehensive program that includes social services, psychologic support, and appropriate health care (Sinclair, 1999/2000).

### Evaluation

Expected outcomes of nursing care include the following:

- The woman discusses the implications of her HIV infection (or diagnosis of AIDS), its implications for her unborn child and for herself, the method of transmission, and the treatment options.
- The woman uses information about social services (or other agency referral) for follow-up assistance and counseling.
- The woman begins to verbalize her feelings about her condition and its implications for her and her family.

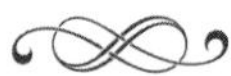

## Care of the Woman with Heart Disease

Pregnancy results in increased cardiac output, heart rate, and blood volume. The normal heart is able to adapt to these changes without undue difficulty. The woman with heart disease, however, has decreased cardiac reserve, making it more difficult for her heart to accommodate the higher workload of pregnancy.

Approximately 4% of pregnant women of childbearing age have preexisting heart disease (Wenstrom & Malee, 1999). The pathology found in a pregnant woman with heart disease varies with the type of disorder. The more common conditions are discussed briefly here.

Congenital heart defects now account for most cases of heart disease in women of reproductive age (Wenstrom & Malee, 1999). Congenital heart defects most commonly seen in pregnant women include atrial septal defect, ventricular septal defect, patent ductus arteriosus, coarctation of the aorta, and tetralogy of Fallot.

For women with congenital heart disease, the implications of pregnancy depend on the specific defect. If the heart defect has been surgically repaired and no evidence of organic heart disease remains, pregnancy may be undertaken with confidence. Because many cardiac lesions are susceptible to subacute bacterial endocarditis, even in cases where the lesion was surgically repaired, antibiotic prophylaxis is often recommended at the time of birth. Women with congenital heart disease who experience cyanosis should be counseled to avoid pregnancy because the risk to mother and fetus is high.

Rheumatic fever, which may develop in untreated group A β-hemolytic streptococcal infections, is an inflammatory connective tissue disease that can involve the heart, joints, central nervous system, skin, and subcutaneous tissue. Once it occurs, rheumatic fever can recur; it is serious primarily because of the permanent damage it can do to the heart—*rheumatic heart disease.* Fortunately, rheumatic heart disease has declined rapidly in the past four decades, primarily because of prompt identification of pharyngeal infections caused by streptococcus and the availability of antibiotics for treatment.

Rheumatic heart disease results when recurrent inflammation from bouts of rheumatic fever causes scar-tissue formation on the valves. The scarring results in stenosis (failure of the valve to open completely), regurgitation due to failure of the valve to close completely, or a combination of both, thereby increasing the workload of the heart. Although mitral valve stenosis is the most commonly seen lesion, the aortic and tricuspid valves may also be affected.

The increased blood volume of pregnancy, coupled with the pregnant woman's need for increased cardiac output, stresses the heart of a woman with mitral stenosis and increases her risk of developing congestive heart failure. Even the woman who has no symptoms at the onset of her pregnancy is at risk.

*Mitral valve prolapse (MVP)* is usually an asymptomatic condition that is commonly found in women of childbearing age. The condition is more common in women than in men and seems to run in families. In MVP, the mitral valve leaflets tend to prolapse into the left atrium during ventricular systole because the chordae tendineae that support them are long, stretched, and thin. This produces a characteristic systolic click on auscultation. In more pronounced cases of MVP, mitral valve regurgitation occurs, producing a systolic murmur.

Women with MVP usually tolerate pregnancy well. Most women require assurance that they can continue with normal activities. A few women experience symptoms—primarily palpitations, chest pain, and dyspnea—which are often due to arrhythmias. They are usually treated with propranolol hydrochloride (Inderal). Limiting caffeine intake also helps decrease palpitations. Prophylactic antibiotics at the time of birth to prevent bacterial endocarditis are not usually necessary for women whose only sign of MVP is a systolic click. Antibiotics are recommended, however, for women with a systolic murmur (Shabetai, 1999).

*Peripartum cardiomyopathy* is a dysfunction of the left ventricle that occurs in the last month of pregnancy or the first 5 months postpartum in a woman with no previous history of heart disease. The cause is unknown, but the mortality rate is as high as 25% to 50% (Sheffield & Cunningham, 1999). The symptoms are similar to those of congestive heart failure: dyspnea, orthopnea, fatigue, cough, chest pain, palpitations, and edema. The woman may have an enlarged heart, tachycardia, rales, and a third heart sound. Treatment includes digoxin, diuretics, vasodilators as necessary, anticoagulants, and strict bed rest (Wenstrom & Malee, 1999). The condition may resolve with bed rest as the heart gradually returns to normal size. Subsequent pregnancy is strongly discouraged because the disease tends to recur during pregnancy.

## Clinical Therapy

The primary goal of clinical therapy is early diagnosis and ongoing management of the woman with cardiac disease. Echocardiogram, chest x-ray, auscultation of heart sounds, and sometimes cardiac catheterization are essential for establishing the type and severity of the heart disease. The severity of the disease can also be determined by the individual's ability to perform ordinary physical activity. The following classification of functional capacity has been standardized by the Criteria Committee of the New York Heart Association (1979):

- Class I. Asymptomatic. No limitation of physical activity.
- Class II. Slight limitation of physical activity. Asymptomatic at rest; symptoms occur with heavy physical activity.
- Class III. Moderate to marked limitation of physical activity. Symptomatic during less-than-ordinary physical activity.
- Class IV. Inability to carry on any physical activity without discomfort. Even at rest the person experiences symptoms of cardiac insufficiency or anginal pain.

Women in classes I and II usually experience a normal pregnancy and have few complications, whereas those in classes III and IV are at risk for more severe complications. Because anemia increases the work of the heart, it should be diagnosed early and treated if present. Infections, even if minor, also increase cardiac workload and should be treated.

### Drug Therapy

The pregnant woman with heart disease may need drug therapy in addition to the iron and vitamin supplements ordinarily prescribed to maintain health during pregnancy. Antibiotics, usually penicillin if not contraindicated by allergy, are used during pregnancy to prevent recurrent bouts of rheumatic fever and subsequent heart valve damage. Antibiotics are also recommended during labor and the early postpartum period to prevent bacterial endocarditis in women with either acquired or congenital disease. If the woman develops coagulation problems, the anticoagulant heparin may be used. Heparin offers the greatest safety to the fetus because it does not cross the placenta. The thiazide diuretics and furosemide (Lasix) may be used to treat congestive heart failure if it develops. Digitalis glycosides and common antiarrhythmic drugs may be used to treat cardiac failure and arrhythmias. These agents cross the placenta but have no reported teratogenic effect.

### Labor and Birth

Spontaneous natural labor with adequate pain relief is usually recommended for women in classes I and II. Special attention should be given to the prompt recognition and treatment of any signs of heart failure. Those in classes III and IV may have labor induced and may need to be hospitalized before the onset of labor for cardiac stabilization. They also require invasive cardiac monitoring during labor.

Use of low forceps provides the safest method of birth, with lumbar epidural anesthesia to reduce the stress of pushing. Cesarean birth is used only if fetal or maternal indications exist, not on the basis of heart disease alone.

# Nursing Care Management

## Nursing Assessment and Diagnosis

The nurse assesses the stress of pregnancy on the functional capacity of the heart during every antepartal visit. The nurse notes the category of functional capacity assigned to the woman; takes the woman's pulse, respirations, and blood pressure; and compares the findings with the normal values expected during pregnancy. The nurse then determines the woman's activity level, including rest, and any changes in the pulse and respirations that have occurred since previous visits. Because it is also an early sign of decompensation, the nurse asks the woman about any increased fatigue with activity at every prenatal visit. The nurse also identifies and evaluates other factors that would increase strain on the heart. These factors might include anemia, infection, anxiety, lack of a support system, and household and career demands.

The following signs and symptoms, if they are progressive, are indicative of congestive heart failure:

- Cough (frequent, with or without blood-stained sputum [hemoptysis])
- Dyspnea (progressive, on exertion)
- Edema (progressive, generalized, including extremities, face, eyelids)
- Heart murmurs (heard on auscultation)
- Palpitations
- Rales (auscultated in lung bases)
- Weight gain (related to fluid retention)

Progressiveness of the cycle is the critical factor because some of these same behaviors are seen to a minor degree in a pregnancy without cardiac problems.

Nursing diagnoses that might apply to the pregnant woman with heart disease include the following:

- ***Decreased cardiac output:*** easy fatigability
- ***Impaired gas exchange*** related to pulmonary edema secondary to cardiac decompensation
- ***Fear*** related to the effects of the maternal cardiac condition on fetal well-being

## Nursing Plan and Implementation

Nursing care is directed toward maintaining a balance between cardiac reserve and cardiac workload.

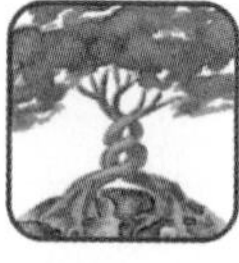

## Community-Based Nursing Care

#### Antepartal Nursing Care

Nursing actions are designed to meet the physiologic and psychosocial needs of the pregnant woman with heart disease. The priority of nursing action varies based on the severity of the disease process and the individual needs of the woman determined by the nursing assessment.

The woman and her family should thoroughly understand her condition and its management and should recognize signs of potential complications; this level of understanding will decrease their anxiety. When the nurse provides thorough explanations, uses printed material, and provides frequent opportunities to ask questions and discuss concerns, the woman is better able to meet her own health care needs and seek assistance appropriately.

As part of health teaching, the nurse explains the purposes of the dietary and activity changes that are required. A diet is instituted that is high in iron, protein, and essential nutrients but low in sodium, with adequate calories to ensure normal weight gain. Such a diet best meets the nutrition needs of the client with cardiac disease. To help preserve her cardiac reserves, the woman may need to restrict her activities. In addition, 8 to 10 hours of sleep with frequent daily rest periods, are essential. Because upper respiratory infections may tax the heart and lead to decompensation, the woman must avoid contact with sources of infection.

During the first half of pregnancy, the woman is seen approximately every 2 weeks to assess cardiac status. During the second half of pregnancy, the woman is seen weekly. These assessments are especially important between weeks 28 and 30, when the blood volume reaches its maximum. If symptoms of cardiac decompensation occur, prompt medical intervention is indicated to correct the cardiac problem.

### *Hospital-Based Nursing Care*

#### Intrapartum Period

Labor and birth exert tremendous stress on the woman and her fetus. This stress could be fatal to the fetus of a woman with cardiac disease, because the fetus may be receiving a decreased oxygen and blood supply. Thus the intrapartal care of a woman with cardiac disease is aimed at reducing physical exertion and the accompanying fatigue.

The nurse evaluates maternal vital signs frequently to determine the woman's response to labor. A pulse rate greater than 100 beats per minute or respirations greater than 25 per minute may indicate the onset of cardiac decompensation and require further evaluation. The nurse also auscultates the woman's lungs frequently for evidence of rales and carefully observes for other signs that she is developing decompensation.

To ensure cardiac emptying and adequate oxygenation, the nurse encourages the laboring woman to assume either a semi-Fowler's or side-lying position, with her head and shoulders elevated. Oxygen by mask, diuretics to reduce fluid retention, sedatives and analgesics, prophylactic antibiotics, and digitalis may also be used as indicated by the woman's status.

The nurse remains with the woman to support her. It is essential that the nurse keep the woman and her family informed of labor progress and management plans, collaborating with them to fulfill their wishes for the birth experience as much as possible. The nurse needs to maintain an atmosphere of calm to lessen the anxiety of the woman and her family.

Continuous electronic fetal monitoring is used to provide ongoing assessment of the fetal response to labor. To prevent overexertion and the accompanying fatigue, the nurse encourages the woman to sleep and relax between

Text continues on page 287.

## TABLE 12–5 Less Common Medical Conditions and Pregnancy

| *Condition* | *Brief Description* | *Maternal Implications* | *Fetal/Neonatal Implications* |
|---|---|---|---|
| Rheumatoid arthritis | Chronic inflammatory disease believed to be caused by a genetically influenced antigen-antibody reaction. Symptoms include fatigue, low-grade fever, pain and swelling of joints, morning stiffness, pain on movement. Treated with salicylates, physical therapy, and rest. Corticosteroids used cautiously if not responsive to above. | Usually there is remission of rheumatoid arthritis symptoms during pregnancy, often with a relapse postpartum. Anemia may be present due to blood loss from salicylate therapy. Mother needs extra rest, particularly to relieve weight-bearing joints, but needs to continue range-of-motion exercises. If in remission, may stop medication during pregnancy. | Possibility of prolonged gestation and longer labor with heavy salicylate use. Possible teratogenic effects of salicylates. |
| Epilepsy | Chronic disorder characterized by seizures; may be idiopathic or secondary to other conditions, such as head injury, metabolic and nutritional disorders such as phenylketonuria (PKU) or vitamin $B_6$ deficiency, encephalitis, neoplasms, or circulatory interferences. Treated with anticonvulsants. | Vast majority of pregnancies in women with seizure disorders are uneventful and have an excellent outcome. Women with more frequent seizures before pregnancy may have exacerbations during pregnancy, but this may be related to lack of cooperation with drug regimen or sleep deprivation. During pregnancy the woman should continue to be treated with the medication that best controls her seizures. Folic acid therapy should be started prior to conception if possible. Folic acid and vitamin D are indicated throughout pregnancy (Samuels, 1996b). | There is an increased incidence of stillbirth in women with epilepsy. Also, anticonvulsant medications are associated with an increased incidence of congenital anomalies, especially cleft lip and heart defects, although the incidence has decreased in recent years. This may be due to the fact that the current ability to determine blood levels of medications has led to more accurate dosages and the resultant use of a single medication; consequently multiple medications are used less often (Samuels, 1996b). |
| Hepatitis B | Hepatitis B, caused by the hepatitis B virus (HBV), is a major, growing health problem. Groups at risk include those from areas with a high incidence (primarily developing countries), illegal intravenous (IV) drug users, prostitutes, homosexuals, those with multiple sex partners, or occupational exposure to blood, although many infected people have no identifiable source of infection. HBV transmission is blood borne, primarily sexually and perinatally transmitted. Because of the dramatic increase and the difficulty of vaccinating high-risk individuals before they become infected, the CDC now recommend (1) testing all pregnant women for the presence of hepatitis B surface antigen (HBsAg), (2) routine vaccination of all newborns, (3) vaccination of older children at high risk for hepatitis B, (4) vaccination of children ages 11–12 years who have not previously received the vaccine, and (5) vaccination of adolescents and adults at high risk for infection (CDC, 1998). | Hepatitis B does not usually affect the course of pregnancy. However, chronic HBV carriers have a great potential for infecting others when exposure to blood and body fluids occurs. In addition, chronic carriers may develop long-term sequelae, such as chronic liver disease and liver cancer. Approximately 4000 to 5000 deaths are caused annually by liver disease associated with chronic HBV infection. It is now recommended that all pregnant women be tested for the presence of HBsAg. A woman who tests negative may be given the hepatitis vaccine. | Perinatal transmission most often occurs at or near the time of childbirth. Infants infected perinatally have a 90% risk of becoming chronically infected if not treated (CDC, 1998). Recommendations now include routine vaccination of all neonates born to HBsAg-negative women and immunoprophylaxis to all newborns of HBsAg-positive women. |
| Hyperthyroidism (thyrotoxicosis) | Enlarged, overactive thyroid gland; increased T4: thyroid-binding globulin (TBG) ratio and increased basal metabolic rate (BMR) Symptoms include muscle wasting, tachycardia, excessive sweating, and exophthalmos. Treatment by antithyroid drug propylthiouracil (PTU) while monitoring free T4 levels. Surgery used only if drug intolerance exists. | Mild hyperthyroidism is not dangerous. Increased incidence of PIH and postpartum hemorrhage if not well controlled. Serious risk related to thyroid storm characterized by high fever, tachycardia, sweating, and congestive heart failure. Now occurs rarely. When diagnosed during pregnancy, may be transient or permanent. | Neonatal thyrotoxicosis is rare. Even low doses of antithyroid drug in mother may produce a mild fetal/neonatal hypothyroidism; higher dose may produce a goiter or mental deficiencies. Fetal loss not increased in euthyroid women. If untreated, rates of abortion, intrauterine death, and stillbirth increase. Breastfeeding contraindicated for women on antithyroid medication because it is excreted in the milk (may be tried by woman on low dose if neonatal T4 levels are monitored). |

## TABLE 12–5 Less Common Medical Conditions and Pregnancy *continued*

| *Condition* | *Brief Description* | *Maternal Implications* | *Fetal/Neonatal Implications* |
|---|---|---|---|
| Hypothyroidism | Characterized by inadequate thyroid secretions (decreased T4:TBG ratio), elevated thyroid-stimulating hormone, lowered BMR, and enlarged thyroid gland (goiter). Symptoms include lack of energy, excessive weight gain, cold intolerance, dry skin, and constipation. Treated by thyroxine replacement therapy. | Long-term replacement therapy usually continues at same dosage during pregnancy as before. Weekly nonstress test (NST) after 35 weeks' gestation. | If mother untreated, fetal loss 50%; high risk of congenital goiter or true cretinism. Therefore newborns are screened for T4 level. Children of mothers with even mild deficiency may show evidence of negative impact on neuropsychologic development (Haddow, Palomaki, Allan, et al., 1999). |
| Maternal phenylketonuria (PKU) (hyperphenylalaninemia) | Inherited recessive single gene anomaly causing a deficiency of the liver enzyme needed to convert the amino acid phenylalanine to tyrosine, resulting in high serum levels of phenylalanine. Brain damage and mental retardation occur if not treated early. | Low phenylalanine diet is mandatory before conception and during pregnancy. The woman should be counseled that her children will either inherit the disease or be carriers, depending on the zygosity of the father for the disease. Treatment at a PKU center is recommended. | Risk to fetus if maternal treatment is not begun preconception. In untreated women increased incidence of fetal mental retardation, microcephaly, congenital heart defects, and growth retardation. Fetal phenylalanine levels are approximately 50% higher than maternal levels. |
| Multiple sclerosis | Neurologic disorder characterized by destruction of the myelin sheath of nerve fibers. The condition occurs primarily in young adults, more commonly in females, and is marked by periods of remission; progresses to marked physical disability in 10 to 20 years. | Associated with remission during pregnancy but with slightly increased relapse rate postpartum (Confavreux, Hours, et al., 1998). Rest is important; help with child care should be planned. Uterine contraction strength is not diminished, but because sensation is frequently lessened, labor may be almost painless. | Increased evidence of a genetic predisposition. Therefore reproductive counseling is recommended. |
| Systemic lupus erythematosus (SLE) | Chronic autoimmune collagen disease, characterized by exacerbations and remissions; symptoms range from characteristic rash to inflammation and pain in joints, fever, nephritis, depression, cranial nerve disorders, and peripheral neuropathies. | Women are generally advised that SLE should be in remission for at least 5–7 months before conceiving. Pregnancy does not appear to alter the long-term prognosis of women with SLE, but maternal morbidity and mortality increase. They also face an increased risk of permanent renal or central nervous system (CNS) deterioration after pregnancy (Classen, Paulson, & Zacharias, 1998). Most maternal deaths occur in the postpartal period and are caused by pulmonary hemorrhage or lupus pneumonitis (Samuels, 1996a). | Increased incidence of spontaneous abortion, stillbirth, prematurity, and IUGR. Infants born to women with SLE may have characteristic skin rash, which usually disappears after 6 months. Infants are at increased risk for complete congenital heart block, a condition that can be diagnosed prenatally. Women with SLE and certain antibodies are at risk. A fetal echocardiogram is done between 18 and 24 weeks of gestation and treatment is started if necessary (Reichlin, 1998). |
| Tuberculosis (TB) | Infection caused by *Mycobacterium tuberculosis;* inflammatory process causes destruction of lung tissue, increased sputum, and coughing. Associated primarily with poverty, crowded living spaces, and malnutrition and may be found among refugees form countries where TB is prevalent. Pregnant women with active TB are treated with triple therapy: isoniazid, rifampin, and ethambutol; breastfeeding women receive the three drugs plus pyrazinamide in a four-agent therapy (Newton, 2000). | The incidence of tuberculosis has begun to increase significantly since the late 1980s, and it is increasingly associated with HIV infection (Newton, 2000). If TB is inactive due to prior treatment, relapse rate is no greater than for nonpregnant women. When isoniazid is used during pregnancy, the woman should take supplemental pyridoxine (vitamin $B_6$). Extra rest and limited contact with others is required until disease becomes inactive. | If maternal TB is inactive, mother may breastfeed and care for her infant. If TB is active and mother is *not* receiving treatment at the time of birth, both mother and infant are treated. Some physicians advocate separating mother and infant for first week of therapy. Others feel the benefits do not outweigh the hardship of separation (Newton, 2000). Isoniazid crosses the placenta, but most studies show no teratogenic effects. Rifampin crosses the placenta; possibility of harmful effects are still being studied. |

contractions and provides her with emotional support and encouragement. Epidural anesthesia is often used to decrease exertion. During pushing, the nurse encourages the woman to use shorter, more moderate open-glottis pushing, with complete relaxation between pushes. Forceps or vacuum extraction may be used if pushing is too difficult. Vital signs are monitored closely during the second stage.

**Postpartum Period**

The postpartum period is a significant time for the woman with cardiac disease. As extravascular fluid returns to the bloodstream for excretion, cardiac output and blood volume increase. This physiologic adaptation places great strain on the heart and may lead to decompensation, especially in the first 48 hours after birth.

So that the health team can detect any possible problems, the woman remains in the hospital for approximately a week to rest and recover. Her vital signs are monitored frequently, and she is assessed for signs of decompensation. She stays in the semi-Fowler's or side-lying position, with her head and shoulders elevated, and begins a gradual, progressive activity program. Appropriate diet and stool softeners facilitate bowel movement without undue strain.

The postpartum nurse gives the woman opportunities to discuss her birth experience and helps her deal with any feelings or concerns that distress her. The nurse also encourages maternal-infant attachment by providing frequent opportunities for the mother to interact with her child.

No evidence exists that breastfeeding compromises cardiac output. Thus the only concern about breastfeeding for women with cardiovascular disease is related to medications the mother may be taking (Friedman & Polifka, 1996). These should be evaluated for the likelihood of passing into the milk or affecting lactation. The nurse can assist the breastfeeding mother to a comfortable side-lying position, with her head moderately elevated, or to a semi-Fowler's position. To conserve the mother's energy, the nurse should position the newborn at the breast and be available to burp the baby and reposition him or her at the other breast.

In addition to providing the normal postpartum discharge teaching, the nurse should ensure that the woman and her family understand the signs of possible problems from her heart disease or other postpartal complications. The nurse also plans an activity schedule with the woman and her family. Visiting nurse referrals may be necessary, depending on the woman's health status.

### Evaluation

Expected outcomes of nursing care include the following:

- The woman is able to discuss her condition and its possible impact on pregnancy, labor and birth, and the postpartal period.
- The woman participates in developing an appropriate health care regimen and follows it throughout her pregnancy.
- The woman gives birth to a healthy infant.
- The woman avoids congestive heart failure, thromboembolism, and infection.
- The woman is able to identify signs and symptoms of possible postpartum complications.
- The woman is able to care effectively for her newborn infant.

## Other Medical Conditions and Pregnancy

A woman with a preexisting medical condition needs to be aware of the possible impact of pregnancy on her condition, as well as the impact of her condition on the successful outcome of her pregnancy. Table 12–5 discusses some of the less common medical conditions in relation to pregnancy. The Evidence-Based Practice Box on Hepatitis B provides further information about one of these conditions.

## EVIDENCE-BASED PRACTICE

### Hepatitis B

You and your colleagues see a variety of problems working nights in the small emergency room (ER) of your rural hospital. Your hospital does not offer maternity services, but last week a woman without prenatal care gave birth in your ER and you cared for her. You believed all the outcomes were good. Then your local health department queried regarding her unknown hepatitis B status and the physician's failure to

## EVIDENCE-BASED PRACTICE

### Hepatitis B *continued*

prescribe immune globulin for the baby. This query resulted in an investigation of your hospital's ER protocols for childbirth. The review clearly showed a lack of awareness of the hepatitis B problem and the recommendations of the Centers for Disease Control and Prevention (CDC) to prevent perinatal transmission of the hepatitis B virus.

Hepatitis B is a major public health problem. There are an estimated 20,000 births to hepatitis B–positive women each year. These infants are at high risk for the disease and its complications (CDC, 1999b). A woman without prenatal care should be a flag to the nurse because screening for hepatitis B is routinely performed as part of prenatal care. Since the woman's status for hepatitis infection was unknown, her baby was potentially at risk. There is a 90% chance that babies exposed perinatally will contract the disease. Therefore, babies of mothers with unknown status should receive Recombivax HB or Engerix-B within 12 hours of birth (Stevenson, 1999). Additionally, you should have drawn the mother's blood so her hepatitis B surface antigen (HBsAg) status could be determined.

The public health department is attempting to locate this mother and baby to complete the testing. If the mother tests positive for the antigen, the baby needs to receive passive immunity in the form of hepatitis B immune globulin (HBIG) by 1 week of age, a second dose of the vaccine at 1 to 2 months, and a third dose at 6 months.

Finally, the health department provided the CDC bulletin that describes the importance of using the preservative-free form of the vaccine in newborns. The preservative thimerosal may have negative effects. Both Recombivax HB and Engerix-B are now producing forms of the vaccine without thimerosal (CDC, 1992a).

#### References


Centers for Disease Control. (1999b, May 2). Program to prevent perinatal hepatitis B virus transmission. *Mortality and Morbidity Weekly Report, 46* (17), 378–380.

Stevenson, A. (1999). Immunizations for women and infants. *Journal of Obstetric, Gynecologic, and Neonatal Nursing, 28* (5), 534–544.

Centers for Disease Control. (1992a, September 10). Availability of hepatitis B vaccine that does not contain thimerosal as a preservative. *Mortality and Morbidity Weekly Report, 48* (35), 780–782.


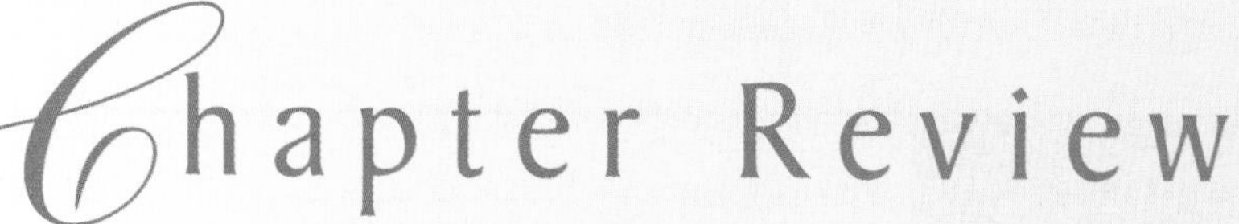

# Chapter Review

## CHAPTER HIGHLIGHTS

- Almost any health problem that a person can have when not pregnant can coexist with pregnancy. Some problems, such as anemias, may be exacerbated by pregnancy. Others, such as collagen disease, may go into temporary remission with pregnancy. Regardless of the health problem, careful health care is needed throughout pregnancy to improve the outcome for mother and fetus.

- The diagnosis of high-risk pregnancy can shock an expectant couple. Providing emotional support, teaching about the condition and prognosis, and educating for self-care are important nursing measures that help clients cope.
- Substance abuse (either drugs or alcohol) not only is detrimental to the mother's health but also may have profound, lasting effects on the fetus. Nurses need to be alert to signs of substance abuse and nonjudgmental in their care of women with substance abuse problems.
- The key point in the care of the pregnant diabetic is scrupulous maternal plasma glucose control. This is best achieved by home blood glucose monitoring, multiple daily insulin injections, and a careful diet.
- To reduce the incidence of congenital anomalies and other problems in the newborn, the woman should maintain a normal blood glucose level before conception and throughout the pregnancy. Diabetics more than most other clients need to be educated about their condition and involved with their own care.
- HIV infection, which is transmitted via blood and body fluids, may also be transmitted vertically from the mother to the fetus. Currently there is no definitive treatment for HIV/AIDS.
- Vertical transmission of HIV infection has been reduced dramatically with the administration of ZDV to the mother prenatally and during labor and to the newborn. The incidence can be reduced even further by the use of scheduled cesarean birth before the onset of labor or rupture of the membranes.
- Nurses should employ blood and body fluid precautions (universal precautions) in caring for all women to avoid potential spread of infection.
- Cardiac disease during pregnancy requires careful assessment, limitation of activity, and knowing and reporting signs of impending cardiac decompensation by both client and nurse.

# CHAPTER REFERENCES


American College of Obstetricians and Gynecologists. (1997). *Human immunodeficiency virus infections in pregnancy* (ACOG Technical Bulletin 232). Washington, DC: Author.

American College of Obstetricians and Gynecologists. (1999). *Scheduled cesarean delivery and the prevention of vertical transmission of HIV infection* (ACOG Committee Opinion 219). Washington, DC: Author.

American Diabetes Association. (2000a). Position statement: Gestational diabetes mellitus. *Diabetes Care, 23* (Suppl. 1), S77–S79.

American Diabetes Association. (2000b). Position statement: Preconception care of women with diabetes. *Diabetes Care, 23* (Suppl. 1), S65–S68.

Andres, R. L. (1999). Social and illicit drug use in pregnancy. In R. K. Creasy & R. Resnik (Eds.), *Maternal-fetal medicine* (4th ed.). Philadelphia: Saunders, 145–164.

Catanzarite, V. A., Piacquadio, K. M., Stanco, L. M., Kollisch, N., Chinn, R., & Gardner, S. (1999). Preventing transmission of AIDS and hepatitis to obstetric-care workers. *Contemporary OB/GYN, 44*(8), 39–55.

Centers for Disease Control and Prevention. (1998). 1998 guidelines for the treatment of sexually transmitted disease. *Morbidity and Mortality Weekly Report, 47* (RR-1).

Centers for Disease Control and Prevention. (2000). *HIV/AIDS Surveillance Report, 12*(1), 1–18.

Centers for Disease Control and Prevention. (1999c). *National Folic Acid Program of the National Center for Environmental Health* (NCEH Publication No. 99-0082). Atlanta, GA: Author.

Classen, S. R., Paulson, P. R., & Zacharias, S. R. (1998). Systemic lupus erythematosis: Perinatal and neonatal implications. *Journal of Obstetric, Gynecologic, and Neonatal Nursing, 27*(5), 493–500.

Confavreux, C., Hutchinson, M., Hours, M. M., Cortinovis-Tourniaire, P., & Moreau, T. (1998). Rate of pregnancy-related relapse in multiple sclerosis. *New England Journal of Medicine, 339*(5), 339–340.

Criteria Committee of the New York Heart Association. (1979). *Nomenclature and criteria for diagnosis of diseases of the heart and great vessels* (8th ed.). New York: New York Heart Association.

Curet, L. B. (2000). Obstetric management of diabetes mellitus in pregnancy. In J. J. Sciarra, (Ed.), *Maternal and fetal medicine* Chapter 14 (Vol. 3, pp. 1–10).

Friedman, J. M., & Polifka, J. E. (1996). *The effects of drugs on the fetus and nursing infant.* Baltimore: Johns Hopkins University Press.

Haddow, J. E., Palomaki, G. E., Allan, W. C., Williams, J. R., Knight, G. J., Gagnon, J., O'Heir, C. E., Mitchell, M. L., Hermos, R. J., Waisbren, S. E., Faix, J. D., & Klein, R. Z. (1999). Maternal thyroid deficiency during pregnancy and subsequent neuropsychological development of the child. *New England Journal of Medicine, 341*(8), 549–555, 601–602.

Hoffman-Terry, M. L. (October, 1999). Defining the epidemic in American women. 1999 National

Conference on Women and HIV/AIDS: Navigating into the New Millennium through Collaboration. Los Angeles.

Howell, E. M., Heiser, N., & Harrington, M. (1999). A review of recent findings on substance abuse treatment for pregnant women. *Journal of Substance Abuse Treatment, 16*(3), 195–219.

Institute of Medicine, Standing Committee on the Scientific Evaluation of Dietary Reference Intakes, Food and Nutrition Board. (1998, April 7). *Dietary reference intakes: Folate, other B vitamins, and choline.* Washington, DC: National Academy Press.

Jovanovic, L. (2000). Role of diet and insulin treatment of diabetes in pregnancy. *Clinical Obstetrics and Gynecology, 43*(1), 46–55.

Kearney, M. H. (1997). Drug treatment for women: Traditional models and new directions. *Journal of Obstetric, Gynecologic, and Neonatal Nursing, 26*(4), 459–468.

Kenner, C., & D'Apolito, K. (1997). Outcomes for children exposed to drugs in utero. *Journal of Obstetric, Gynecologic, and Neonatal Nursing, 26*(5), 595–603.

Kjos, S. L. (2000). Postpartum care of the woman with diabetes. *Clinical Obstetrics and Gynecology, 43*(1), 75–82.

Landon, M. B. (2000). Obstetric management of pregnancies complicated by diabetes mellitus. *Clinical Obstetrics and Gynecology, 43*(1), 65–74.

Lindegren, M. L., Byers, R. H., Thomas, P., Davis, S. F., Caldwell, B., Rogers, M., Gwinn, M., Ward, J. W., & Fleming, P. L. (1999). Trends in perinatal transmission of HIV/AIDS in the United States. *JAMA, 282*(6), 531–540.

Mandeville, L. K. (1992). Diabetes mellitus in pregnancy. In L. K. Mandeville & N. H. Troiano (Eds.), *High-risk intrapartum nursing.* Philadelphia: Lippincott. 165–186.

March of Dimes. 1999. *Folic acid.* Wilkes-Barre, PA: Author.

Mersereau, P. W. (2000). Preventing neural tube defects: A national campaign. *Small Talk, 12*(2), 1–5.

Minkoff, H. L. (1999). Human immunodeficiency virus and other perinatal infections. In J. R. Scott et al. (Eds.), *Danforth's obstetrics and gynecology* (8th ed.). Philadelphia: Lippincott Williams & Wilkins, 393–406.

Mofenson, L. M. (1999). Can perinatal HIV infection be eliminated in the United States? *JAMA, 282*(6), 577–579.

Moore, T. R. (1999). Diabetes in pregnancy. In R. K. Creasy & R. Resnik (Eds.), *Maternal-fetal medicine* (4th ed.). Philadelphia: Saunders, 964–995.

Newton, E. R. (2000). Tuberculosis and pregnancy. In J. J. Sciarra (Ed.), *Maternal and fetal medicine* (Vol. 3, chapter 49, 1–15).

Niebyl, J. R. (1999). Teratology and drugs in pregnancy. In J. R. Scott et al. (Eds.), *Danforth's obstetrics and gynecology* (8th ed.). Philadelphia: Lippincott Williams & Wilkins, 197–212.

Reichlin, M. (1998). Systemic lupus erythematosis and pregnancy. *Journal of Reproductive Medicine, 43*(4), 355–360.

Samuels P. (1996a). Collagen vascular diseases. In S. G. Gabbe, J. R. Niebyl, & J. L. Simpson (Eds.), *Obstetrics: Normal and problem pregnancies* (3rd ed.). New York: Churchill-Livingstone, 1101–1118.

Samuels, P. (1996b). Neurologic disorders. In S. G. Gabbe, J. R. Niebyl, & J. L. Simpson (Eds.), *Obstetrics: Normal and problem pregnancies* (3rd ed.). New York: Churchill-Livingstone, 1135–1154.

Scioscia, A. L. (1999). Prenatal genetic diagnosis. In R. K. Creasy & R. Resnik (Eds.), *Maternal-fetal medicine* (4th ed.). Philadelphia: Saunders, 918–926.

Shabetai, R. (1999). Cardiac diseases. In R. K. Creasy & R. Resnik (Eds.), *Maternal-fetal medicine* (4th ed.). Philadelphia: Saunders,. 927–941.

Sheffield, J. S., & Cunningham, F. G. (1999). Diagnosing and managing cardiomyopathy. *Contemporary OB/GYN, 44,* 74–78.

Sinclair, B. P. (1999/2000). HIV and women: Understand your responsibilities; reduce your risk. *AWHONN Lifelines, 3*(6), 35–38.

Spellacy, W. N. (1999). Diabetes mellitus and pregnancy. In J. R. Scott et al. (Eds.), *Danforth's obstetrics and gynecology* (8th ed.). Philadelphia: Lippincott Williams & Wilkins, 301–308.

Wang, E. C. (1999). Methadone treatment during pregnancy. *Journal of Obstetric, Gynecologic, and Neonatal Nursing, 28*(6), 615–622.

Wenstrom, K. D., & Malee, M. P. (1999). Medical and surgical complications of pregnancy. In J. R. Scott et al. (Eds.), *Danforth's obstetrics and gynecology* (8th ed.). Philadelphia: Lippincott Williams & Wilkins, 327–362.

## CONTEMPORARY MATERNAL-NEWBORN NURSING ON-LINE

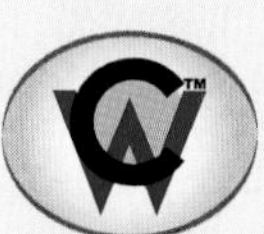

Additional interactive resources, including animations and video, for this chapter can be found on the Companion Website at http://www.prenhall.com/ladewig. Click on Chapter 12 and "Begin" to select the activities for this chapter.

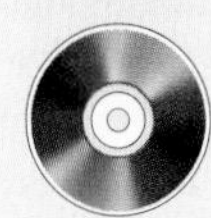

For NCLEX review questions and an audio glossary, access the accompanying CD-ROM in this book.

Chapter 13

# Pregnancy at Risk: Gestational Onset

*Working with women who are dealing with high-risk pregnancies has given me a much deeper appreciation of the stress a family faces when their unborn child is threatened or when the mother is ill. Some families seem so strong and resilient—they use me as a resource, and I am delighted to assist them in that way. Other families seem to crumble and have such needs. I do my best to help them gain the tools they need to cope. When I succeed, I am elated. When they can't seem to cope, no matter what any of us do, I feel such a sense of sadness for the family and their future.*

—A Perinatal Nurse Practitioner (PNNP)

## OBJECTIVES

- Contrast the etiology, medical therapy, and nursing interventions for the various bleeding problems associated with pregnancy.
- Identify the medical therapy and nursing interventions indicated in caring for a woman with an incompetent cervix.
- Discuss the medical therapy and nursing care of a woman with hyperemesis gravidarum.
- Delineate the nursing care needs of a woman experiencing premature rupture of the membranes or preterm labor.
- Describe the development and course of hypertensive disorders associated with pregnancy.
- Explain the cause and prevention of hemolytic disease of the newborn secondary to Rh incompatibility.
- Compare Rh incompatibility to ABO incompatibility with regard to occurrence, treatment, and implications for the fetus or newborn.
- Summarize the effects of surgical procedures on pregnancy and explain ways in which pregnancy may complicate diagnosis.
- Discuss the impact of trauma due to an accident on the pregnant woman or her fetus.
- Explain the needs and care of the pregnant woman who experiences abuse.
- Describe the effects of infections on the pregnant woman and her unborn child.

## KEY TERMS

| Term | Page |
|---|---|
| Abortion | 292 |
| Eclampsia | 310 |
| Ectopic pregnancy | 294 |
| Erythroblastosis fetalis | 319 |
| Gestational trophoblastic disease (GTD) | 296 |
| HELLP syndrome | 309 |
| Hydatidiform mole | 296 |
| Hydrops fetalis | 319 |
| Hyperemesis gravidarum | 298 |
| Incompetent cervix | 298 |
| Miscarriage | 292 |
| Preeclampsia | 308 |
| Pregnancy-induced hypertension (PIH) | 308 |
| Premature rupture of membranes (PROM) | 299 |
| Preterm labor | 302 |
| Rh immune globulin (RhoGAM) | 319 |
| Tocolysis | 303 |

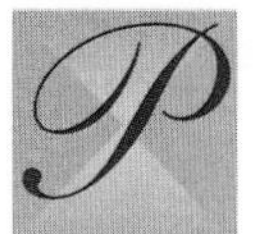regnancy is usually an uncomplicated experience. In some cases, however, problems arise that place the pregnant woman and her unborn child at risk. Regular prenatal care serves to detect these potential complications quickly so that effective care can be provided. This chapter focuses on problems that primarily occur during pregnancy, those with a *gestational onset.*

## Care of the Woman with a Bleeding Disorder

During the first and second trimesters of pregnancy, the major cause of bleeding is **abortion.** This is the expulsion of the fetus prior to viability, which is considered to be 20 weeks' gestation or weight of less than 500 g (Cunningham, MacDonald, Gant, et al., 1997). Abortions are either spontaneous (occurring naturally) or induced (occurring as a result of artificial or mechanical interruption). Because the term *abortion* may have a negative connotation for some, spontaneous abortion is often called **miscarriage.**

Other complications that can cause bleeding in the first half of pregnancy are ectopic pregnancy and gestational trophoblastic disease, discussed shortly. In the second half of pregnancy, particularly in the third trimester, the two major causes of bleeding are placenta previa and abruptio placentae. (They are discussed in detail in Chapter 19.) However, regardless of the cause of bleeding, the nurse has certain general responsibilities in providing nursing care.

### General Principles of Nursing Intervention

Spotting is relatively common during pregnancy and usually occurs following sexual intercourse or exercise because of trauma to the highly vascular cervix. However, the woman is advised to report for evaluation of any spotting or bleeding that occurs during pregnancy.

It is often the nurse's responsibility to make the initial assessment of bleeding. In general, the following nursing measures should be implemented for pregnant women being treated for bleeding disorders:

- Monitor blood pressure and pulse frequently.
- Observe the woman for behaviors indicative of shock, such as pallor, clammy skin, perspiration, dyspnea, or restlessness.
- Count and weigh pads to assess amount of bleeding over a given time period; save any tissue or clots expelled.
- If pregnancy is of 12 weeks' gestation or beyond, assess fetal heart tones with a Doppler.
- Prepare for intravenous therapy. There may be standing orders to begin intravenous (IV) therapy on bleeding clients.
- Prepare equipment for examination.
- Have oxygen available.
- Collect and organize all data, including antepartal history, onset of bleeding episode, and laboratory studies (hemoglobin, hematocrit, hormonal assays) for analysis.
- Obtain an order to type and cross match for blood if evidence of significant blood loss exists.
- Assess coping mechanisms of woman in crisis. Give emotional support to enhance her coping abilities by continuous, sustained presence; by clear explanation of procedures; and by communicating her status to her family. Prepare the woman for possible fetal loss. Assess her expressions of anger, denial, silence, guilt, depression, or self-blame.

### Spontaneous Abortion (Miscarriage)

Many pregnancies end in the first trimester because of spontaneous abortion. Often the woman assumes she is having a heavy menstrual period when she is really having an early abortion. Thus statistics are inaccurate. The incidence is about 10% to 20% for clinically recognized pregnancies but may be as high as 60% for overall pregnancy loss (Carter, 1999).

A majority of early spontaneous abortions are related to chromosomal abnormalities. Other causes include teratogenic drugs, faulty implantation due to abnormalities of the female reproductive tract, a weakened cervix, placental abnormalities, chronic maternal diseases, endocrine imbalances, and maternal infections. Research does not support the belief that accidents and psychic trauma are primary causes of spontaneous abortion.

Spontaneous abortion can be extremely distressing to the couple desiring a child. Chances for carrying the next pregnancy to term after one spontaneous abortion are as good as they are for the general population. Thereafter, however, chances of successful pregnancy decrease with each succeeding spontaneous abortion.

#### Classification

Spontaneous abortions, or miscarriages, are subdivided into the following categories:

- *Threatened abortion.* The embryo or fetus is jeopardized by unexplained bleeding, cramping, and backache. The cervix is closed. Bleeding may persist for days. It may be followed by partial or complete expulsion of the embryo or fetus, placenta, and membranes (sometimes called the "products of conception") (Figure 13–1♦).

- *Imminent abortion.* Bleeding and cramping increase. The internal cervical os dilates. Membranes may rupture. The term *inevitable abortion* also applies.
- *Complete abortion.* All the products of conception are expelled.
- *Incomplete abortion.* Some of the products of conception are retained, most often the placenta. The internal cervical os is dilated slightly.
- *Missed abortion.* The fetus dies in utero but is not expelled. Uterine growth ceases, breast changes regress, and the woman may report a brownish vaginal discharge. The cervix is closed. If the fetus is retained beyond 6 weeks, the breakdown of fetal tissues results in the release of thromboplastin, and disseminated intravascular coagulation (DIC) may develop.
- *Habitual abortion.* Abortion occurs consecutively in three or more pregnancies.
- *Septic abortion.* Presence of infection. May occur with prolonged, unrecognized rupture of the membranes, pregnancy with an intrauterine device (IUD) in utero, or attempts by unqualified individuals to terminate a pregnancy.

### Clinical Therapy

One of the more reliable indicators of potential spontaneous abortion is the presence of pelvic cramping and backache. These symptoms are usually absent in bleeding caused by polyps, ruptured cervical blood vessels, or cervical erosion. Ultrasound scanning may be used to detect the presence of a gestational sac or cardiac activity if the cause of bleeding is unclear. Results of human chorionic gonadotropin (hCG) levels are not particularly helpful because hCG levels fall slowly after fetal death and therefore cannot confirm a live embryo or fetus. Hemoglobin and hematocrit are obtained to assess blood loss. Blood is typed and crossmatched for possible replacement needs.

The therapy prescribed for the pregnant woman with bleeding is bed rest, abstinence from coitus, and perhaps sedation. If bleeding persists and abortion is imminent or incomplete, the woman may be hospitalized, IV therapy or blood transfusions may be started to replace fluid, and dilatation and curettage (D&C) or suction evacuation is performed to remove the remainder of the products of conception. If the woman is Rh negative and not sensitized, Rh immune globulin (RhoGAM) is given within 72 hours (see discussion on Rh sensitization later in this chapter).

In missed abortions, the products of conception eventually are expelled spontaneously. Diagnosis is based on

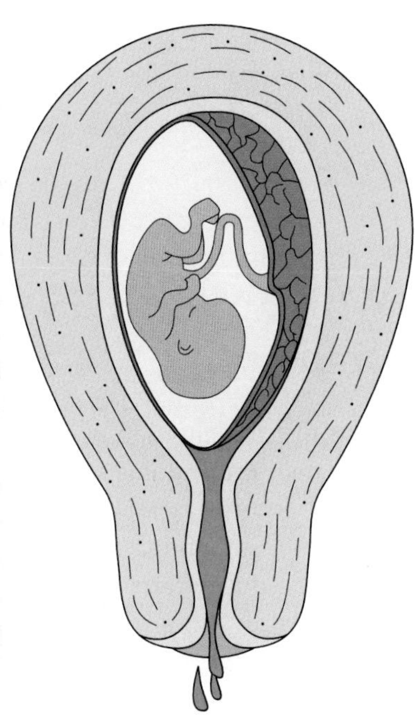


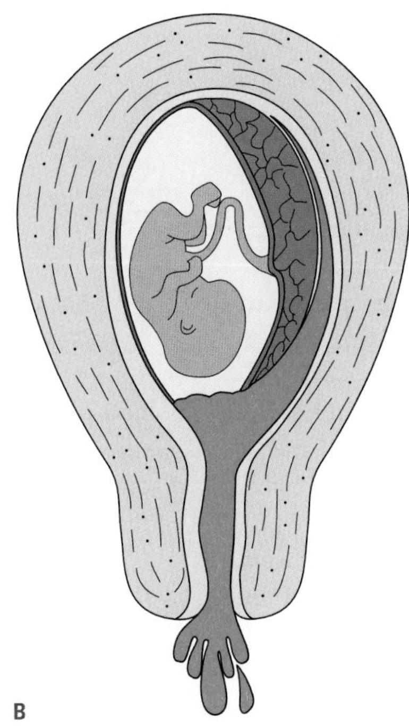


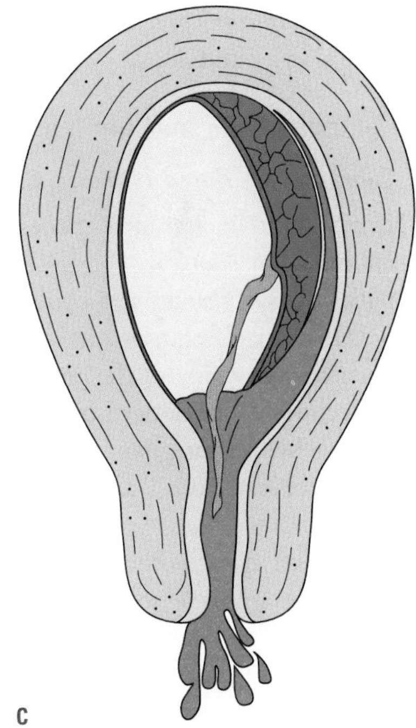


FIGURE 13–1 ♦ Types of spontaneous abortion. **A**, Threatened. The cervix is not dilated, and the placenta is still attached to the uterine wall, but some bleeding occurs. **B**, Imminent. The placenta has separated from the uterine wall, the cervix has dilated, and the amount of bleeding has increased. **C**, Incomplete. The embryo or fetus has passed out of the uterus, but the placenta remains.

history, pelvic examination, and a negative pregnancy test and may be confirmed by ultrasound if necessary. If this does not occur within 4 to 6 weeks after embryo or fetal death, hospitalization is necessary. Dilatation and curettage or suction evacuation is done if the pregnancy is in the first trimester. In the second trimester, labor is induced using intravaginal prostaglandin $E_2$ or misoprostol (Cytotec) applied to the external cervical os. Alternately, dilatation and evacuation (D&E) may be used (Scott, 1999).

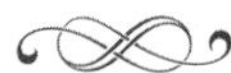

# Nursing Care Management

## Nursing Assessment and Diagnosis

The nurse assesses the woman's vital signs, amount and appearance of any bleeding, level of comfort, and general physical health. If the pregnancy is 10 to 12 weeks or more, fetal heart rates should be assessed by Doppler. The nurse also assesses the responses of the woman and her family to this crisis and evaluates their coping mechanisms and ability to comfort each other.

Examples of nursing diagnoses that may apply include the following:

- ***Pain*** related to abdominal cramping secondary to threatened abortion
- ***Anticipatory grieving*** related to expected loss of unborn child

## Nursing Plan and Implementation

### *Community-Based Nursing Care*

If a woman in her first trimester of pregnancy begins cramping or spotting, she is often evaluated on an outpatient basis. The nurse provides analgesics for pain relief if the woman's cramps are severe and explains what is occurring throughout the process.

Feelings of shock or disbelief are normal. Couples who approached the pregnancy with feelings of joy and a sense of expectancy now also feel grief, sadness, and possibly anger.

Because many women, even with planned pregnancies, feel some ambivalence initially, guilt is also a common emotion. These feelings may be even stronger for women who were negative about their pregnancies. The women may harbor negative feelings about themselves or even believe that the abortion may be a punishment for some wrongdoing.

The nurse can offer invaluable psychologic support to the woman and her family by encouraging them to talk about their feelings, allowing them the privacy to grieve, and listening sympathetically to their concerns about this pregnancy and future ones. The nurse may help decrease feelings of guilt or blame by informing the woman and her family about the causes of spontaneous abortion. The nurse can also refer them to other health care professionals for additional help as necessary. The grieving period following a spontaneous abortion usually lasts 6 to 24 months. Many couples can be helped during this period by an organization or support group established for parents who have lost a fetus or newborn.

### *Hospital-Based Nursing Care*

A woman with an incomplete or missed abortion may need a D&C or other procedure, which is typically done on an outpatient basis. Barring any complications, the woman can return home a few hours after the procedure. The nurse monitors the woman's condition closely and provides instruction for self-care. The nurse also administers Rh immune globulin if it is indicated.

## Evaluation

Expected outcomes of nursing care include the following:

- The woman is able to explain spontaneous abortion, the treatment measures employed in her care, and long-term implications for future pregnancies.
- The woman suffers no complications.
- The woman and her partner begin verbalizing their grief and acknowledge that the grieving process lasts several months.

# Care of the Woman with an Ectopic Pregnancy

**Ectopic pregnancy (EP)** is the implantation of the fertilized ovum in a site other than the endometrial lining of the uterus. It has many causative factors including tubal damage caused by pelvic inflammatory disease (PID), previous tubal surgery, congenital anomalies of the tube, endometriosis, previous ectopic pregnancy, presence of an IUD, and in utero exposure to diethylstilbestrol (DES). Other contributing factors include cigarette smoking, menstrual reflux, and the use of progesterone-only methods of contraception, which decrease the normal movement of the cilia in the tubes (Carter, 1999).

The incidence of EP has increased dramatically in the past several years. Currently there are about 20 ectopic

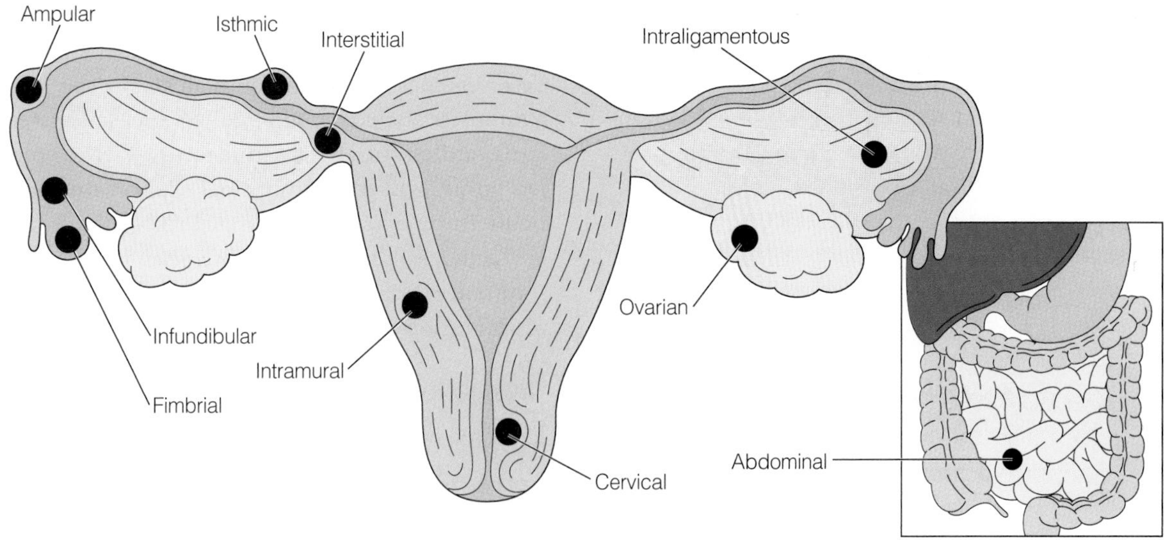


**FIGURE 13–2** ♦ Various implantation sites in ectopic pregnancy. The most common site is within the fallopian tube, hence the name "tubal pregnancy."

pregnancies for every 1000 pregnancies in the United States (American College of Obstetricians and Gynecologists [ACOG], 1998a). EP occurs when the fertilized ovum is prevented or slowed in its passage through the tube and thus implants before it reaches the uterus. The most common location for implantation is the ampulla of the fallopian tube. Figure 13–2♦ identifies other implantation sites.

Initially the normal symptoms of pregnancy may be present, specifically amenorrhea, breast tenderness, and nausea. The hormone hCG is present in the blood and urine. As the pregnancy progresses, the chorionic villi grow into the wall of the tube or site of implantation and a blood supply is established. When the embryo outgrows this space, the tube ruptures and there is bleeding into the abdominal cavity. This bleeding irritates the peritoneum, causing the characteristic symptoms of sharp, one-sided pain, syncope, and referred shoulder pain. The woman may also experience lower abdominal pain. Vaginal bleeding occurs when the embryo dies and the decidua begins to slough.

Physical examination usually reveals adnexal tenderness. (The adnexae are the areas of the lower abdomen located over each ovary and fallopian tube.) An adnexal mass is palpable about half the time. Bleeding tends to be slow and chronic, and the abdomen gradually becomes rigid and very tender. With extensive bleeding into the abdominal cavity, pelvic examination causes extreme pain, and a mass of blood may be palpated in the cul-de-sac of Douglas.

Laboratory tests may reveal low hemoglobin and hematocrit levels and rising leukocyte levels. The hCG titers are lower than in intrauterine pregnancy.

## Clinical Therapy

Diagnosis of ectopic pregnancy begins with an assessment of menstrual history, including the last menstrual period (LMP), followed by a careful pelvic exam to identify any abnormal pelvic masses and tenderness. Serum β-hCG levels are drawn and reassessed in 48 hours if necessary. A woman with EP tends to have abnormally low hCG levels. Moreover, in normal pregnancy, hCG levels double every 48 to 72 hours. Nondoubling hCG levels occur in ectopic pregnancy and in nonviable uterine pregnancies. If the β-hCG levels are above 1500 IU/L, transvaginal ultrasound is used to check for a uterine pregnancy or an adnexal mass. Confirming a uterine pregnancy nearly eliminates the diagnosis of EP (Tulandi, 1999).

Treatment may be medical or surgical. Medical treatment using methotrexate is indicated for the woman who desires future pregnancy if her ectopic pregnancy is unruptured and of 3.5 cm size or less and if her condition is stable. In addition, there must be no fetal cardiac motion and the woman must have no evidence of a blood disorder or kidney or liver disease. The methotrexate is administered intramuscularly. As an outpatient, the woman is monitored for increasing abdominal pain. Serum β-hCG titers are also monitored regularly. Typically the hCG levels increase for 1 to 4 days and then decrease. If they do not, the woman may need a second dose of methotrexate or surgery (ACOG, 1998a).

If surgery is indicated and the woman desires future pregnancies, treatment involves salpingostomy via a laparoscope. With this method, a linear incision is made and the products of conception are gently removed. The surgical incision is left open and allowed to close by secondary intention (Tulandi, 1999). If the tube is ruptured or if future childbearing is not an issue, laparoscopic salpingectomy (removal of the tube) is performed, leaving the ovary in place unless it is damaged.

With both medical and surgical therapies for EP, the Rh-negative nonsensitized woman is given Rh immune globulin to prevent sensitization.

# Nursing Care Management

## Nursing Assessment and Diagnosis

When the woman with a suspected ectopic pregnancy is admitted to the hospital, the nurse assesses the appearance and amount of vaginal bleeding and monitors vital signs for evidence of developing shock.

The nurse assesses the woman's emotional state and coping abilities and determines the couple's informational needs. The woman may experience marked abdominal discomfort, so the nurse also determines the woman's level of pain. If surgery is necessary, the nurse performs the ongoing assessments appropriate postoperatively.

Nursing diagnoses that may apply for a woman with an ectopic pregnancy include the following:

- ***Pain*** related to abdominal bleeding secondary to tubal rupture
- ***Health-seeking behaviors:*** request for information about treatment of ectopic pregnancy and its long-term implications related to stated unfamiliarity with the condition

## Nursing Plan and Implementation

### *Community-Based Nursing Care*

Women with EP are often seen initially in a clinic or office setting. Nurses need to be alert to the possibility of ectopic pregnancy if a woman presents with complaints of abdominal pain and lack of menses for 1 to 2 months. If a woman is to receive medical treatment using methotrexate, she is followed as an outpatient. The nurse advises the woman that some abdominal pain is common following the injection, but generally it is mild and lasts only 24 to 48 hours. More severe pain might indicate treatment failure and should be evaluated. The woman should also report heavy vaginal bleeding, dizziness, or tachycardia (ACOG, 1998a). The nurse stresses the need to return for follow-up hCG testing.

### *Hospital-Based Nursing Care*

Once a diagnosis of ectopic pregnancy is made and surgery is scheduled, the nurse starts an IV as ordered and begins preoperative teaching. The nurse should immediately report signs of developing shock. If the woman is experiencing severe abdominal pain, the nurse can administer analgesics and evaluate their effectiveness.

Regardless of the treatment used, the woman and her family will need emotional support during this difficult time. Their feelings and responses to this crisis are generally similar to those that occur in cases of spontaneous abortion. As a result, similar nursing actions are required.

## Evaluation

Expected outcomes of nursing care include the following:

- The woman is able to explain ectopic pregnancy, treatment alternatives, and implications for future childbearing.
- The woman and her caregivers detect possible complications early and manage them successfully.
- The woman and her partner are able to begin verbalizing their loss.

# Care of the Woman with Gestational Trophoblastic Disease

**Gestational trophoblastic disease (GTD)** includes hydatidiform mole, invasive mole (chorioadenoma destruens), and choriocarcinoma.

**Hydatidiform mole** (molar pregnancy) is a disease in which (1) abnormal development of the placenta occurs, resulting in a fluid-filled, grapelike cluster; and (2) the trophoblastic tissue proliferates. The disease results in the loss of the pregnancy and the possibility, though remote, of developing choriocarcinoma, a form of cancer, from the trophoblastic tissue.

Molar pregnancies are classified into two types, complete and partial, both of which meet the previously mentioned criteria. In the United States, complete moles are more common than partial moles and occur in about 1 in every 1500 to 2000 pregnancies. The incidence is far higher in women of Asian descent (Hammond, 1999). A complete mole develops from an ovum containing no maternal genetic material, an "empty egg," which is fertilized by a normal sperm. The embryo dies very early, no circulation is established, the hydropic vesicles are avascular, and no embryonic tissue or membranes are found. Choriocarcinoma seems to be associated exclusively with the complete mole.

The partial mole usually has a triploid karyotype (69 chromosomes), generally because of failure of either the ovum or sperm to undergo the first meiotic division. There may be a fetal sac or even a fetus with a heartbeat. The fetus has multiple anomalies because of the triploidy and little chance for survival. The villi are often vascularized and may be hydropic in only portions of the placenta. Often partial moles are recognized only after spontaneous abortion, and they may go unnoticed even then.

Invasive mole (chorioadenoma destruens) is similar to a complete mole, but it involves the uterine myometrium. Treatment is the same as for complete mole.

## Clinical Therapy

Initially the clinical picture is similar to that of pregnancy. However, classic signs soon appear. Vaginal bleeding occurs almost universally. It is often brownish (like prune juice) due to liquefaction of the uterine clot, but it may be bright red. Uterine enlargement greater than expected for gestational age is a classic sign, present in about 50% of cases. In the remainder of cases, the uterus is appropriate or small for the gestational age. Hydropic vesicles may be passed; if so, they are diagnostic. With a partial mole the vesicles are often smaller and may not be noticed. In addition, because serum hCG levels are higher with molar pregnancy than with normal pregnancy, the woman may experience hyperemesis gravidarum. Anemia occurs frequently due to blood loss and poor nutrition secondary to hyperemesis. Symptoms of pregnancy-induced hypertension (PIH) prior to 24 weeks' gestation strongly suggest a molar pregnancy. No fetal heart tones are heard, and no fetal movement is palpated. The advent of transvaginal ultrasound has led to earlier diagnosis of molar pregnancy, often in the first trimester.

Therapy begins with suction evacuation of the mole and curettage of the uterus to remove all fragments of the placenta. Early evacuation decreases the possibility of other complications. If the woman is older and has completed her childbearing, or if there is excessive bleeding, hysterectomy may be the treatment of choice to reduce the risk of choriocarcinoma.

Because of the risk of persistent GTD and choriocarcinoma, the woman treated for hydatidiform mole should receive extensive follow-up therapy, typically for up to a year. Follow-up care includes baseline chest x-ray exam to detect metastasis, physical exam including pelvic exam, and regular measurements of serum hCG levels. The woman avoids pregnancy during that time because the elevated hCG levels associated with pregnancy would cause confusion about whether choriocarcinoma had developed (Hammond, 1999).

Continued high or rising hCG titers are abnormal. If they occur, dilatation and curettage is performed, and the tissue is examined. If malignant cells are found, treatment at a center specializing in GTD is advised. Chemotherapy for choriocarcinoma is started using methotrexate alone or in combination with other chemotherapy agents. Persistent GTD is almost 100% curable if diagnosed early and treated appropriately.

If, after a year of monitoring, the hCG serum titers are within normal limits, a couple may be assured that subsequent normal pregnancy can be anticipated, with a low probability of recurring hydatidiform mole.

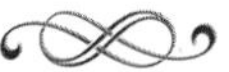

# Nursing Care Management

## Nursing Assessment and Diagnosis

It is important for nurses involved in antepartal care to be aware of symptoms of hydatidiform mole and observe for them at each antepartal visit. The classic symptoms used to diagnose molar pregnancy are found more frequently with the complete than with the partial mole. Before evacuation, the partial mole may be difficult to distinguish from a missed abortion. If a molar pregnancy is diagnosed, the nurse should assess the woman's (or the couple's) understanding of the condition and its implications.

Nursing diagnoses that may apply to a woman with a hydatidiform mole include the following:

- ***Fear*** related to the possible development of choriocarcinoma
- ***Anticipatory grieving*** related to the loss of the pregnancy secondary to GTD

## Nursing Plan and Implementation

### *Community-Based Nursing Care*

When a molar pregnancy is suspected, the woman needs emotional support. The nurse can relieve some of the woman's anxiety by answering questions about the condition and explaining what ultrasound and other diagnostic procedures will entail. If a molar pregnancy is diagnosed, the nurse supports the parents as they deal with their grief about the lost pregnancy. Health care counselors, a member of the clergy, or a professional counselor may be able to help them deal with this loss.

### *Hospital-Based Nursing Care*

When the woman is hospitalized for evacuation of the mole, the nurse must monitor vital signs and vaginal bleeding for evidence of hemorrhage. In addition, the nurse determines whether abdominal pain is present and evaluates the woman's emotional state and coping ability. Typed and crossmatched blood must be available for surgery because of previous blood loss and the potential for hemorrhage. Oxytocin is administered to keep the uterus contracted and prevent hemorrhage. If the woman is Rh negative and not sensitized, she is given Rh immune globulin to prevent antibody formation.

The woman needs to understand the importance of the follow-up visits. She is advised to delay becoming pregnant again until after the follow-up program is completed.

### Evaluation

Expected outcomes of nursing care include the following:

- The woman has a smooth recovery following successful evacuation of the mole.
- The woman is able to explain GTD and its treatment, follow-up, and long-term implications for pregnancy.
- The woman and her partner are able to begin verbalizing their grief at the loss of their anticipated child.
- The woman can discuss the importance of follow-up care and indicates her willingness to cooperate with the regimen.

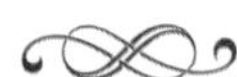

## Care of the Woman with an Incompetent Cervix

**Incompetent cervix** refers to the premature dilatation of the cervix, usually in the fourth or fifth month of pregnancy. It is associated with repeated second-trimester abortions. Possible causes include cervical trauma, infection, congenital cervical or uterine anomalies, or increased uterine volume (as with a multiple gestation).

Diagnosis is established by eliciting a positive history of repeated, relatively painless and bloodless second-trimester abortions. Serial pelvic exams early in the second trimester reveal progressive effacement and dilatation of the cervix and bulging of the membranes through the cervical os. If incompetent cervix is suspected, serial ultrasound provides information on dilatation of the internal cervical os before a dilated external os is detected.

Incompetent cervix is managed surgically with a Shirodkar-Barter operation (cerclage)—or a modification of it by McDonald—which reinforces the weakened cervix by encircling it at the level of the internal os with suture material. A purse-string suture is placed in the cervix in the first trimester or early in the second trimester. Once the suture is in place, a cesarean birth may be planned (to prevent repeating the procedure in subsequent pregnancies) or the suture may be released at term and vaginal birth permitted. The woman must understand the importance of contacting her physician immediately if her membranes rupture or labor begins. The physician can remove the suture to prevent possible complications.

## Care of the Woman with Hyperemesis Gravidarum

**Hyperemesis gravidarum,** a relatively rare condition, is excessive vomiting during pregnancy. It may be mild at first, but true hyperemesis may progress to a point at which the woman not only vomits everything she swallows but also retches between meals.

Although the exact cause of hyperemesis is unclear, increased levels of hCG may play a role. Other variables under investigation include a possible dysfunction of the pituitary-adrenal axis, a transient increase in thyroid function, and psychologic factors (Wenstrom & Malee, 1999).

In severe cases, the pathology of hyperemesis begins with dehydration, which leads to fluid-electrolyte imbalance and alkalosis from loss of hydrochloric acid. Hypovolemia, hypotension, tachycardia, increased hematocrit and blood urea nitrogen (BUN), and decreased urine output can also occur. If untreated, metabolic acidosis may develop. Severe potassium loss may disrupt cardiac functioning. Starvation causes muscle wasting and severe protein and vitamin deficiencies. Fetal or embryonic death may result, and the woman may suffer irreversible metabolic changes or death.

### Clinical Therapy

The goals of treatment include control of vomiting, correction of dehydration, restoration of electrolyte balance, and maintenance of adequate nutrition; 1% to 5% of women with hyperemesis require hospitalization (Simon & Schwartz, 1999). Initially the woman is given nothing by mouth (NPO), and intravenous fluids are administered. Potassium chloride is typically added to the IV infusion to prevent hypokalemia. Agents commonly used to control the nausea and vomiting of hyperemesis gravidarum include the phenothiazines (prochlorperazine, chlorpromazine, promethazine) and antihistamines such as meclizine and dimenhydrinate. Typically the woman remains NPO for 48 hours. If her condition does not improve, total parenteral nutrition may be needed. She then begins controlled oral feedings.

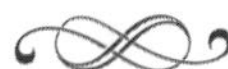

## Nursing Care Management

### Nursing Assessment and Diagnosis

When a woman is hospitalized for control of vomiting, the nurse regularly assesses the amount and character of any emesis, intake and output, fetal heart rate, evidence of jaundice or bleeding, and the woman's emotional state.

Nursing diagnoses that may apply to a woman with hyperemesis gravidarum include the following:

- ***Altered nutrition: less than body requirements*** related to persistent vomiting secondary to hyperemesis
- ***Fear*** related to the effects of hyperemesis on fetal well-being

### Nursing Plan and Implementation

#### *Community-Based Nursing Care*

Parenteral therapy provided at home in collaboration with a physician and a registered dietitian is sometimes used to enable the woman to remain in her home. It also gives the nurse an opportunity to observe family interactions and evaluate the home environment. This assessment is often useful in determining the pregnant woman's level of support, any significant stressors in her life, and her understanding of nutrition and self-care measures.

#### *Hospital-Based Nursing Care*

Nursing care is supportive and directed at maintaining a relaxed, quiet environment away from food odors or offensive smells. Once oral feedings resume, food needs to be attractively served. Oral hygiene is important because the mouth is dry and may be irritated from vomitus. Weight is monitored regularly. Because emotional factors have been found to play a major role in this condition, psychotherapy may be recommended. With proper treatment, prognosis is favorable.

### Evaluation

Expected outcomes of nursing care include the following:

- The woman is able to explain hyperemesis gravidarum, its therapy, and its possible effects on her pregnancy.
- The woman's condition is corrected and complications are avoided.

# Care of the Woman with Premature Rupture of Membranes

**Premature rupture of membranes (PROM)** is spontaneous rupture of the membranes and leakage of amniotic fluid prior to the onset of labor. Preterm PROM (PPROM) is the rupture of membranes that occurs before 37 weeks' gestation and is found in about 2% of pregnancies (Parsons & Spellacy, 1999a). PROM is associated with infection, previous history of PROM, hydramnios, multiple pregnancy, urinary tract infection (UTI), amniocentesis, placenta previa, abruptio placentae, trauma, incompetent cervix, bleeding during pregnancy, and maternal genital tract anomalies.

Maternal risk is related to infection, specifically chorioamnionitis (intraamniotic infection resulting from bacterial invasion before birth) and endometritis (postpartal infection of the endometrium). In addition, abruptio placentae occurs more frequently in women with PROM.

Fetal-newborn implications include risk of respiratory distress syndrome (with PPROM), fetal sepsis due to ascending pathogens, malpresentation, prolapse of the umbilical cord, and increased perinatal morbidity and mortality.

## Clinical Therapy

A sterile speculum examination is done to detect the presence of amniotic fluid in the vagina. If fluid is not obviously pooling, the diagnosis can be confirmed with nitrazine paper (which turns deep blue) and a microscopic examination (ferning test). Digital examination increases the risk of infection and is not recommended unless prompt birth is expected (ACOG, 1998c).

Fetal well-being is assessed through a fetal heart rate tracing or biophysical profile. In addition, the gestational age of the fetus is calculated in order to decide on a management plan. The gestational age of the fetus and the presence or absence of infection determine the direction of treatment for PROM. If maternal signs and symptoms of infection are evident, antibiotic therapy (usually by intravenous infusion) is initiated immediately, and the fetus is born vaginally or by cesarean regardless of the gestational age. Prophylactic antibiotics are often administered for the first 48 hours while awaiting culture results. Upon admission to the nursery, the newborn is assessed for sepsis and placed on antibiotics. (Chapter 26 provides further information about the newborn with sepsis.)

Management of PROM in the absence of infection and gestation of less than 37 weeks is usually conservative. The woman is hospitalized on bed rest. On admission, complete blood cell count (CBC), C-reactive protein, and urinalysis are obtained. Continuous electronic fetal monitoring may be ordered at the beginning of treatment but usually is discontinued after a few hours, unless the fetus is estimated to be very low birth weight (VLBW). Regular nonstress tests (NSTs) or biophysical profiles are used to monitor fetal well-being. (These tests are discussed in Chapter 14.) Maternal blood pressure (BP), pulse, and temperature and fetal heart rate (FHR) are assessed every 4 hours. Regular laboratory evaluations are done to detect maternal infection. Vaginal exams are avoided to decrease the chance of infection. As the gestation approaches 34 weeks, fetal lung maturity studies are indicated (American Academy of Pediatrics [AAP] & ACOG, 1997).

Although controversial, after initial treatment and observation, if leaking of fluid ceases, some women (typically those with sufficient amniotic fluid, no infection, and cervical dilatation less than 4 cm) may be followed at home. The woman is advised to continue bed rest (with bathroom privileges), monitor her temperature and pulse four times a day, keep a fetal movement chart, and have regular NSTs (Parsons & Spellacy, 1999a).

Corticosteroid administration to promote fetal lung maturity and prevent respiratory distress syndrome remains controversial because of possible adverse effects on the fetus and mother. Currently corticosteroid use is recommended for women with PROM prior to 30 to 32 weeks' gestation, if there is no intraamniotic infection. ACOG (1998c) recommends that, following the initial course of treatment, repeat doses be given only if needed in cases in which the woman is being retreated for threatened preterm birth (see Drug Guide: Betamethasone).

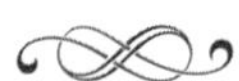

# Nursing Care Management

## Nursing Assessment and Diagnosis

Determining the duration of the rupture of the membranes is a significant component of the intrapartal assessment. The nurse asks the woman when her membranes ruptured and when labor began, because the risk of infection may be directly related to the time involved. Gestational age is determined to prepare for the possibility of a preterm birth. The nurse observes the mother for signs and symptoms of infection, especially by reviewing her white blood cell count (WBC), temperature, pulse rate, and the character of her amniotic fluid. If the mother has a fever, hydration status should be checked. When a preterm or cesarean birth is anticipated, the nurse evaluates the childbirth preparation and coping abilities of the woman and her partner.

Nursing diagnoses that may apply to a woman with PROM include the following:

- ***Risk for infection*** related to premature rupture of membranes
- ***Impaired gas exchange*** in the fetus related to compression of the umbilical cord secondary to prolapse of the cord
- ***Risk for ineffective individual coping*** related to unknown outcome of the pregnancy

## Nursing Plan and Implementation

Nursing actions should focus on the woman, her partner, and the fetus. The nurse monitors for and reports signs of infection to the certified nurse-midwife or physician. Uterine activity and fetal response to the labor are evaluated, but vaginal exams are not done unless absolutely necessary. The woman is encouraged to rest on her left side to promote optimal uteroplacental perfusion. Comfort measures may help promote rest and relaxation. The nurse must also ensure that hydration is maintained, particularly if the woman's temperature is elevated.

Education is another important aspect of nursing care. The woman and her partner, if he is involved, need to understand the implications of PROM and all treatment methods. It is important to address side effects and alternative treatments. The couple needs to know that although the membranes are ruptured, amniotic fluid continues to be produced.

Providing psychologic support for the couple is critical. The nurse may reduce anxiety by listening empathetically, relaying accurate information, and providing explanations of procedures. Preparing the couple for a cesarean birth, a preterm newborn, and the possibility of fetal or newborn demise may be necessary.

## Evaluation

Expected outcomes of nursing care include the following:

- The woman's risk of infection and cord prolapse decrease.
- The couple is able to discuss the implications of PROM and all treatments and alternative treatments.
- The pregnancy is maintained without trauma to the mother or fetus.

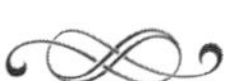

# DRUG GUIDE

## BETAMETHASONE (CELESTONE SOLUPAN)

### *Pregnancy Risk Category: C*

### *Overview of Maternal-Fetal Action*

Studies have provided ample evidence that glucocorticoids such as betamethasone are capable of inducing pulmonary maturation and decreasing the incidence of respiratory distress syndrome in preterm infants. The mechanism by which corticosteroids accelerate fetal lung maturity is unclear, but it is related to the stimulation of enzyme activity by the drug. The enzyme is required for biosynthesis of surfactant by the type II pneumocytes. Surfactant is essential to the proper functioning of the lung in that it decreases the surface tension of the alveoli. Glucocorticoids also increase the rate of glycogen depletion, which leads to thinning of the interalveolar septa and increases the size of the alveoli. The thinning of the epithelium brings the capillaries into closer proximity with the air spaces and improves oxygen exchange.

### *Route, Dosage, Frequency*

Prenatal maternal intramuscular injections of 12 mg of betamethasone are given once a day for 2 days. Dexamethasone may also be given in doses of 6 mg every 6 hours for four doses (Guinn & Lee, 2000). To obtain maximum results, birth should be delayed for at least 24 hours after completing the first round of treatment. The effect of corticosteroids may be transient. Currently, it is suggested by some that the treatment regimen be repeated every week up to 34 weeks' gestation for the undelivered fetus with an immature lung profile, but this approach is controversial (Guinn & Lee, 2000).

### *Contraindications*

Inability to delay birth

Adequate L/S ratio

Presence of a condition that necessitates immediate birth (eg, maternal bleeding)

Presence of maternal infection, diabetes mellitus, hypertension

Gestational age greater than 34 completed weeks

### *Maternal Side Effects*

Increased risk for infection has not been supported in large studies. There may, however, be some increase in the incidence of infection in women with premature rupture of the membranes. Maternal hyperglycemia may occur during corticosteroid administration. Insulin-dependent diabetics may require insulin infusions for several days to prevent ketoacidosis. Corticosteroids may increase the risk of pulmonary edema, especially when used concurrently with tocolytics (Iams, 1996a; National Institutes of Health, 1994).

### *Effects on Fetus or Neonate*

Lowered cortisol levels at birth, but rebound occurs by 2 hours of age

Hypoglycemia

Increased risk of neonatal sepsis

Animal studies have shown serious fetal side effects such as reduced head circumference, reduced weight of the fetal adrenal and thymus glands, and decreased placental weight. Human studies have not shown these effects, however.

### *Nursing Considerations*

Assess for presence of contraindications.

Provide education regarding possible side effects.

Administer betamethasone deep into gluteal muscle, avoiding injection into deltoid (high incidence of local atrophy). (Dexamethasone may be administered IM or IV.)

Periodically evaluate BP, pulse, weight, and edema.

Assess lab data for electrolytes and blood glucose level.

Although concomitant use of betamethasone and tocolytic agents has been implicated in increased risk of pulmonary edema, the betamethasone has little mineral corticoid activity; therefore, it probably does not add significantly to the salt and water retention effects of β-adrenergic agonists. Other causes of noncardiogenic pulmonary edema should also be investigated if pulmonary edema develops during administration of betamethasone to a woman in preterm labor.

## Care of the Woman at Risk Due to Preterm Labor

Labor that occurs between 20 and 37 completed weeks of pregnancy is called **preterm labor.** Prematurity continues to be the number one perinatal and neonatal problem in the United States, with 11% of all live births occurring prematurely (Creasy & Iams, 1999). Often preterm labor is related to multiple risk factors; only rarely is there a single cause. Risk factors can be classified as follows (Aerts & Iams, 1999):

- *Nonrecurrent risk factors:* placenta previa, abruptio placentae, hydramnios, second-trimester bleeding, fetal anomaly or death
- *Recurrent or treatable factors in the mother:* genital tract infection, incompetent cervix, uterine malformations, uterine fibroids, low socioeconomic status, limited prenatal care, poor nutritional status, low prepregnancy weight, tobacco or drug use, occupation or work requirement, sexual activity, anemia (see Evidence-Based Practice: Preterm Birth and Infection).
- *Recurrent but not treatable:* history of preterm birth, race, DES exposure

Maternal implications of preterm labor include psychologic stress related to the baby's condition and physiologic stress related to medical treatment for preterm labor.

Fetal-neonatal implications include increased morbidity and mortality, especially due to respiratory distress syndrome (RDS), increased risk of trauma during birth, and maturational deficiencies (fat storage, heat regulation, immaturity of organ systems).

### Clinical Therapy

Women who are at risk for preterm labor are taught to recognize the symptoms associated with preterm labor and, if any symptoms are present, to notify their certified nurse-midwife or physician immediately. Prompt diagnosis is necessary to stop preterm labor before it progresses to the point at which intervention will be ineffective.

## EVIDENCE-BASED PRACTICE

### Preterm Birth and Infection

The health maintenance organization where you work in the women's health clinic is reviewing its management protocols for prevention of preterm birth. Currently, the clinic has a program that includes written material, a video, and educational sessions on preventing preterm birth. Women who have one of the indicators on the clinic profile also receive case management.

Now the medical director and nurse administrator are looking at the evidence related to vaginal infections, particularly bacterial vaginosis, and preterm birth. Exactly how bacterial vaginosis triggers preterm labor is not yet understood; however, seven studies have reported an increased risk for preterm birth in women with bacterial vaginosis, and five studies have shown that treatment of this infection lowers the preterm birth rate (Paige, Augustyn, Adih, et al., 1998). Since 50% of women with this infection are asymptomatic, your organization is considering a screening and treatment pathway. You have an opportunity to review the screening model reported by Hauth, Goldenber, Andrews, et al. (1995) and the medication treatment options. You learn that treatment with metronidazole at 500 mg twice a day for 7 days demonstrates the same degree of effectiveness as one 2-g dose. Because first-trimester treatment with metronidazole is contraindicated, the group will also look at Clindamycin cream, which can be applied intravaginally once a day (Paige et al., 1998). You decide to survey your clinic clients about the way they prefer to take their medications. Your survey of client preferences will yield important data to consider in the decision regarding treatment routes, since client acceptance of treatment increases the potential for improved outcomes.

#### References

Paige, D., Augustyn, M., Adih, W., et al. (1998). Bacterial vaginosis and preterm birth: A comprehensive review of the literature. *Journal of Nurse-Midwifery, 43*(2), 83–89.

Hauth, J., Goldenber, R., Andrews, W., et al. (1995). Reduced incidence of preterm delivery with metronidazole and erythromycin in women with bacterial vaginosis. *New England Journal of Medicine, 333*, 1732–1736.

Three tests are useful both in screening high-risk women and in helping confirm a diagnosis of preterm labor:

- *Fetal fibronectin (fFN).* Fetal fibronectin is a protein normally found in the fetal membranes and decidua. It is found in the cervicovaginal fluid in early pregnancy but is not usually present in significant quantities between 18 and 36 weeks' gestation. A positive fFN test (fFN found in the cervicovaginal fluid) during this time puts the woman at increased risk for preterm birth. Conversely, a negative test is over 99% accurate for predicting no preterm birth within 7 days. The procedure for collecting a sample is similar to that of the Pap smear; results can be available within 1 hour (Chez, 1999).
- *Salivary estriol.* Research indicates that maternal estriol levels rise about 3 weeks before birth, either preterm or term. Estriol can be measured in the maternal blood or saliva, although saliva is preferred because it is a stable method and no venipuncture is necessary. Salivary estriol levels are most reliable in predicting preterm birth after 30 weeks' gestation. The saliva sample should be collected during the day (estriol levels are elevated at night) but not within 30 minutes of eating (Chez, 1999).
- *Transvaginal ultrasound (sonography) (TVS).* The length of the cervix can be measured fairly reliably after 16 weeks' gestation using an ultrasound probe inserted into the vagina. A cervix that is shorter than expected may be useful in assisting a physician to identify the need for a cerclage to prevent preterm birth because of incompetent cervix. In general, cervical length less than 25 mm prior to term is abnormal (Aerts & Iams, 1999).

Diagnosis of preterm labor is confirmed if the pregnancy is between 20 and 37 weeks, there are documented uterine contractions (four in 20 minutes or six to eight in 1 hour), documented cervical change of 1 cm or more, cervical dilatation of more than 2 cm, or a positive fFN level (Creasy & Iams, 1999).

Labor is not interrupted if one or more of the following conditions are present: severe preeclampsia or eclampsia, chorioamnionitis, hemorrhage, maternal cardiac disease, poorly controlled diabetes mellitus or thyrotoxicosis, severe abruptio placentae, fetal anomalies incompatible with life, fetal death, acute fetal distress, or fetal maturity.

The goal of clinical therapy is to prevent preterm labor from advancing to the point that it no longer responds to medical treatment. The initial management of preterm labor is directed toward maintaining good uterine blood flow, detecting uterine contractions, and quieting the fetus. The mother is asked to lie on her side to increase profusion, and an IV infusion is started to promote maternal hydration.

**Tocolysis** is the use of medications in an attempt to stop labor. Drugs currently used as *tocolytics* include the β-adrenergic agonists (also called β-mimetics), magnesium sulfate ($MgSO_4$), prostaglandin synthetase inhibitors, and calcium channel blockers. The β-mimetics (ritodrine [Yutopar] and terbutaline sulfate [Brethine]) and $MgSO_4$ are the most widely used tocolytics. Ritodrine is approved by the U.S. Food and Drug Administration (FDA) for tocolysis; however, it is much less frequently used than terbutaline, which is not approved by the FDA for this use.

Although tocolytic drugs suppress uterine contractions and allow pregnancy to continue, they may cause maternal side effects; the most serious is maternal pulmonary edema. Reducing the dose and duration of therapy sometimes reduces the side effects.

Because it is effective and has fewer side effects than the β-mimetics, magnesium sulfate administered intravenously is often the initial drug of choice for therapy. Therapy with $MgSO_4$ is indicated in women with cardiopulmonary disease, diabetes, or infection. In all other cases, the selection of $MgSO_4$ or β-mimetics depends on the experience of the health care providers. The use of oral tocolytics for ongoing therapy on an ambulatory basis is of questionable benefit (Parsons & Spellacy, 1999b).

For $MgSO_4$, the recommended loading dose is 4 to 6 g IV using an infusion pump over 20 minutes, followed by a maintenance dose of 1 to 4 g/hr titrated to response and side effects (Creasy & Iams, 1999). The therapy is continued for 12 to 24 hours at the lowest rate that maintains cessation of contractions.

Side effects with the loading dose may include flushing, a feeling of warmth, headache, nystagmus, nausea, and dizziness. Other side effects include lethargy, sluggishness, and pulmonary edema (see Drug Guide: Magnesium Sulfate). Fetal side effects may include hypotonia and lethargy that persists for 1 or 2 days following birth.

One calcium channel blocker, nifedipine, is becoming increasingly popular as a tocolytic because it is easily administered orally or sublingually and has few serious maternal side effects. It decreases smooth muscle contractions by blocking the slow calcium channels at the cell surface. The most common side effects are related to arterial vasodilation and include hypotension, tachycardia, facial flushing, and headache. Nifedipine may be coadministered with the β-mimetics. However, it should not be used with magnesium because both drugs block calcium and simultaneous administration

# DRUG GUIDE

## MAGNESIUM SULFATE ($MgSO_4$)

### *Pregnancy Risk Category: B*

### *Overview of Obstetric Action*

$MgSO_4$ acts as a central nervous system (CNS) depressant by decreasing the quantity of acetylcholine released by motor nerve impulses and thereby blocking neuromuscular transmission. This action reduces the possibility of convulsion, which is why $MgSO_4$ is used in the treatment of preeclampsia. Because magnesium sulfate secondarily relaxes smooth muscle, it may decrease the blood pressure, although it is not considered an antihypertensive. $MgSO_4$ may also decrease the frequency and intensity of uterine contractions; as a result it is also used as a tocolytic in the treatment of preterm labor.

### *Route, Dosage, Frequency*

$MgSO_4$ is generally given intravenously to control dosage more accurately and prevent overdosage. An occasional physician still prescribes intramuscular administration. However, it is painful and irritating to the tissues and does not permit the close control that intravenous (IV) administration does. The intravenous route allows for immediate onset of action. It must be given by infusion pump for accurate dosage.

### *For Treatment of Preterm Labor*

Loading dose: 4–6 g $MgSO_4$ in 250 mL solution administered over a 20-minute period.

Maintenance dose: 1–4 g/hr via infusion pump (Creasy & Iams, 1999).

### *For Treatment of Preeclampsia*

Loading dose: 2–4 g $MgSO_4$ is administered over a 5-minute period.

Maintenance dose: 1 g/hr via infusion pump (Roberts, 1999).

*Note:* $MgSO_4$ is excreted via the kidneys. Because women i preterm labor typically have normal renal function, they ger erally require higher levels of magnesium to achieve a the apeutic range than women who have preeclampsia and ma have compromised renal function. Maintenance dose ma need to be adjusted based on serum magnesium levels.

### *Maternal Contraindications*

Diagnosed maternal myasthenia gravis is the only absolut contraindication to the administration of $MgSO_4$. A histor of myocardial damage or heart block is a relative cor traindication to use of the drug because of the effects o nerve transmission and muscle contractility. Extreme car is necessary in administration to women with impaire renal function because the drug is eliminated by the kid neys, and toxic magnesium levels may develop quickly.

### *Maternal Side Effects*

Most maternal side effects are dose related. Lethargy an weakness related to neuromuscular blockade are com

has been implicated in serious maternal side effects related to low calcium levels.

Prostaglandin synthesis inhibitors (PSIs) such as indomethacin (Indocin) are being used for tocolysis in selected instances. However, potential fetal side effects, such as constriction of the ductus arteriosus, have been reported, especially in pregnancies at 32 weeks' gestation and beyond. Consequently, indomethacin use is limited to pregnancies <32 weeks' gestation; the duration of therapy should be <72 hours, if possible (Vermillion & Scardo, 2000).

A course of antenatal corticosteroids (ACS) (typically betamethasone administered intramuscularly (IM) every 24 hours for two doses or dexamethasone IM every ( hours for four doses) appears to have a beneficial effec on fetal lung maturation. However, controversy exists about the value of multiple courses of ACS because o potential complications in the newborn (Guinn & Lee 2000). ACS is recommended for use before 34 weeks' gestation for all women who are eligible for tocolysis, regardless of fetal gender or race (National Institutes of Health, 1994). (See Drug Guide: Betamethasone, on page 301.)

mon. Sweating, a feeling of warmth, flushing, and nasal congestion may be related to peripheral vasodilation. Other common side effects include nausea and vomiting, constipation, visual blurring, headache, and slurred speech. Signs of developing toxicity include depression or absence of reflexes, oliguria, confusion, respiratory depression, circulatory collapse, and respiratory paralysis. Rapid administration of large doses may cause cardiac arrest.

### Effects on Fetus or Neonate

The drug readily crosses the placenta. Some authorities suggest that transient decrease in fetal heart rate (FHR) variability may occur; others report that no change occurred. In general $MgSO_4$ therapy does not pose a risk to the fetus. Occasionally, the newborn may demonstrate neurologic depression or respiratory depression, loss of reflexes, and muscle weakness. Ill effects in the newborn may actually be related to fetal growth retardation, prematurity, or perinatal asphyxia.

### Nursing Considerations

1. Monitor the blood pressure closely during administration.
2. Monitor maternal serum magnesium levels as ordered (usually every 6–8 hours). Therapeutic levels are in the range of 4.8–9.6 mg/dL. Reflexes often disappear at serum magnesium levels of 8–12 mg/dL; respiratory depression occurs at levels of 15–17 mg/dL; cardiac arrest occurs at levels above 30 mg/dL (Sibai, 1996; Silver, 1996).
3. Monitor respirations closely. If the rate is less than 12/minute, magnesium toxicity may be developing, and further assessments are indicated. Many protocols require stopping the medication if the respiratory rate falls below 12/minute.
4. Assess knee jerk (patellar tendon reflex) for evidence of diminished or absent reflexes. Loss of reflexes is often the first sign of developing toxicity. Also note marked lethargy or decreased level of consciousness and hypotension.
5. Determine urinary output. Output less than 30 mL/hr may result in the accumulation of toxic levels of magnesium.
6. If the respirations or urinary output fall below specified levels or if the reflexes are diminished or absent, no further magnesium should be administered until these factors return to normal.
7. The antagonist of magnesium sulfate is calcium. Consequently, an ampule of calcium gluconate should be available at the bedside. The usual dose is 1 g given IV over a period of about 3 minutes.
8. Monitor fetal heart tones continuously with IV administration.
9. Continue $MgSO_4$ infusion for approximately 24 hours after birth as prophylaxis against postpartum seizures if given for pregnancy-induced hypertension (PIH).
10. If the mother has received $MgSO_4$ close to birth, the newborn should be closely observed for signs of magnesium toxicity for 24–48 hours.

*Note:* Protocols for magnesium sulfate administration may vary somewhat according to agency policy. Consequently, individuals are referred to their own agency protocols for specific guidelines.

# Nursing Care Management

## Nursing Assessment and Diagnosis

During the antepartal period, the nurse identifies the woman at risk for preterm labor by noting the presence of predisposing factors. During the intrapartal period, the nurse assesses the progress of labor and the physiologic impact of labor on the mother and fetus.

Nursing diagnoses that may apply to the woman with preterm labor include the following:

- ***Fear*** related to risk of early labor and birth
- ***Ineffective individual coping*** related to need for constant attention to pregnancy

## Nursing Plan and Implementation

### *Community-Based Nursing Care*

Once the woman at risk for preterm labor has been identified, she needs to be taught about the importance of recognizing the onset of labor (see Teaching Guide: Preterm Labor). This teaching is often provided by clinic nurses or home care nurses.

Home uterine activity monitoring transmitted by telemetry to review stations combined with daily telephone

## TEACHING GUIDE *Preterm Labor*

### Assessment

During the antepartal period, the woman is usually screened for factors that place her at risk for preterm labor. The nurse then assesses the woman's understanding of the danger of preterm labor, the signs of preterm labor, and the actions she can take to prevent it. If she is on a home monitoring program, the woman's understanding of the purpose and rationale for the program is also assessed.

### Nursing Diagnosis

The key nursing diagnosis will probably be health-seeking behaviors: information about preterm labor related to an expressed desire to prevent preterm labor if possible and identify it promptly, if it develops.

### Nursing Plan and Implementation

Teaching focuses on the risks of preterm labor, the functions of and procedures for home monitoring, and self-care activities to decrease the risk of preterm labor.

### Client Goals

At the completion of the teaching the woman will be able to

1. Discuss the risks of preterm labor.
2. Describe the purpose of home monitoring.
3. Demonstrate the correct procedures for doing home monitoring.
4. Explain self-care measures that help decrease the risk of preterm labor.

### *Teaching Plan*

| CONTENT | TEACHING METHOD |
|---|---|
| Describe the dangers of preterm labor, especially the risk of prematurity in the infant, and all the potential problems. | Discuss the risks specifically. Many people understand in a general way that prematurity can be dangerous, but they fail to understand how the baby is affected. |
| Stress the value of home monitoring in evaluating uterine activity on a regular basis. Emphasize that many of the early symptoms of labor, such as backache and increased bloody show, may be subtle initially. Home monitoring can often detect increased uterine activity in the early stages before cervical changes progress to the point where it is impossible to stop labor. Studies have demonstrated that home uterine-monitoring programs offer little or no significant difference in preterm delivery compared with clients followed by daily contact with the nurse and no home uterine monitoring (Iams, 1996b). | Use handouts during the discussion. Help the woman clearly understand the value of the program because, to be successful, it requires a real commitment on her part. |
| If the woman is to be part of a home monitoring program, the monitoring nurse will usually do the initial teaching. Be prepared to reinforce the information provided and answer questions that may arise. | Teach the woman how to palpate for uterine contractions. Demonstrate and ask for a return demonstration. |
| Summarize self-care measures, such as maintaining generous fluid intake (2 to 3 quarts daily), voiding every 2 hours, avoiding lifting and overexertion, avoiding nipple stimulation or orgasm, limiting sexual activity, and cooperating with activity restrictions and bed rest requirements. | Use a handout during the discussion. Provide opportunities for discussion. If the woman has concerns about certain recommendations, try to modify the approach to best meet her needs. |

Evaluation

At the end of the teaching session the woman will be able to discuss the risks of preterm labor, demonstrate home monitoring techniques and explain their rationale, and implement self-care activities to decrease the risks of preterm labor.

calls from a nurse to offer support and advice had been a common approach to care following discharge. However, research has yet to document its value, and its use is not recommended (ACOG, 1996). Nevertheless, periodic home visits by a home care nurse are still an important part of care.

During these visits the nurse completes physical assessments similar to those done in the hospital and assesses the woman's emotional state. The nurse can also provide information about support groups and other community resources for women at risk for preterm birth.

Increasing the woman's awareness of the subtle symptoms of preterm labor is one of the most important teaching objectives of the nurse. The signs and symptoms of preterm labor include the following:

- Uterine contractions that occur every 10 minutes or less, with or without pain
- Mild menstrual-like cramps felt low in the abdomen
- Constant or intermittent feelings of pelvic pressure that feel like the baby pressing down
- Rupture of membranes
- Constant or intermittent low, dull backache
- A change in the vaginal discharge (an increase in amount, a change to more clear and watery, or a pinkish tinge)
- Abdominal cramping with or without diarrhea

The woman is also taught to evaluate contraction activity once or twice a day. She does so by lying down tilted to one side with a pillow behind her back for support. The woman places her fingertips on the fundus of the uterus, which is above the umbilicus (navel). She checks for contractions (hardening or tightening in the uterus) for about 1 hour. It is important for the pregnant woman to know that uterine contractions occur occasionally throughout the pregnancy. If they occur every 10 minutes for 1 hour, however, the cervix could begin to dilate, and labor could ensue.

The nurse ensures that the woman knows when to report signs and symptoms. If contractions occur every 10 minutes (or more frequently) for 1 hour, if any of the other signs and symptoms are present for 1 hour, or if clear fluid begins leaking from the vagina, the woman should telephone her physician or certified nurse-midwife, clinic, or hospital birthing unit and make arrangements to be checked for ongoing labor. Caregivers need to be aware that the woman's call must be taken seriously. When a woman is at risk for preterm labor, she may have many episodes of contractions and other signs or symptoms. If she is treated positively, she will feel freer to report problems as they arise.

Preventive self-care measures are also very important. The nurse has a vital role in communicating the self-care measures described in Table 13–1.

| TABLE 13–1 Self-Care Measures to Prevent Preterm Labor |
|---|
| Rest two or three times a day lying on your left side. |
| Drink 2 to 3 quarts of water or fruit juice each day. Avoid caffeine drinks. Filling a quart container and drinking from it will eliminate the need to keep track of numerous glasses of fluid. |
| Empty your bladder at least every 2 hours during waking hours. |
| Avoid lifting heavy objects. If small children are in the home, work out alternatives for picking them up, such as sitting on a chair and having them climb onto your lap. |
| Avoid prenatal breast preparation such as nipple rolling or rubbing nipples with a towel. This is not meant to discourage breastfeeding but to avoid the potential increase in uterine irritability. |
| Pace necessary activities to avoid overexertion. |
| Sexual activity may need to be curtailed or eliminated. |
| Find pleasurable ways to help compensate for limitations of activities and to boost the spirits. |
| Try to focus on 1 day or 1 week at a time rather than on longer periods of time. |
| If on bed rest, get dressed each day and rest on a couch rather than becoming isolated in the bedroom. |

*Source:* Prepared in consultation with Susan Bennett, RN, ACCE, Coordinator of the Prematurity Prevention Program.

### *Hospital-Based Nursing Care*

Supportive nursing care is important to the woman in preterm labor during hospitalization. This care consists of promoting bed rest, monitoring vital signs (especially blood pressure and respirations), measuring intake and output, and continuous monitoring of FHR and uterine contractions. Placing the woman on her left side facilitates maternal-fetal circulation. Vaginal examinations are kept to a minimum. If tocolytic agents are being administered, the mother and fetus are monitored closely for any adverse effects.

Whether preterm labor is arrested or proceeds, the woman and her partner, if he is involved, experience intense psychologic stress. Decreasing the anxiety associated with the risk of a preterm newborn by providing emotional support is a primary aim of the nurse. The nurse also recognizes the stress of prolonged bed rest and of lack of sexual contact and helps the couple find satisfactory ways of dealing with those stresses. With empathetic communication, the nurse can assist the couple to express their feelings, which commonly include guilt and anxiety, thereby helping the couple identify and implement coping mechanisms. The nurse also keeps the couple informed about the labor progress, the treatment regimen, and the status of the fetus. In the event of imminent vaginal or cesarean birth, the couple should be offered brief but ongoing explanations to prepare them for the actual birth process and the events following the birth.

## Evaluation

Expected outcomes of nursing care include the following:

- The woman is able to discuss the cause, identification, and treatment of preterm labor.
- The woman states that she feels comfortable in her ability to cope with her situation and has resources to call on.

- The woman can describe appropriate self-care measures and can identify characteristics that need to be reported to her caregiver.
- The woman successfully gives birth to a healthy infant.

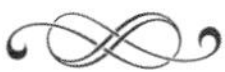

## Care of the Woman with a Hypertensive Disorder

A number of hypertensive disorders can occur during pregnancy. Various attempts have been made to classify these disorders. The following classification is recommended by ACOG (Branch & Porter, 1999):

- Preeclampsia and eclampsia
- Chronic hypertension (of any etiology preceding pregnancy)
- Chronic hypertension with superimposed preeclampsia or eclampsia
- Transient hypertension

Some authorities use the term **pregnancy-induced hypertension (PIH)** to group preeclampsia-eclampsia and transient hypertension. In reality, distinguishing between the two entities is often possible only after the fact, so transient hypertension is typically treated as preeclampsia (Branch & Porter, 1999). Throughout this text, the terms *preeclampsia* or *eclampsia* and *PIH* are used interchangeably.

### Preeclampsia and Eclampsia

**Preeclampsia** is the most common hypertensive disorder in pregnancy. It is characterized by the development of hypertension, proteinuria, and edema. Because only hypertension may be present early in the disease process, that finding is therefore the basis for diagnosis.

The definition of preeclampsia is an increase in systolic blood pressure of 30 mm Hg and/or an increase in diastolic blood pressure of 15 mm Hg over baseline. These blood pressure changes must be noted on at least two occasions 6 hours or more apart for the diagnosis to be made. In the absence of baseline values, a blood pressure of 140/90 mm Hg has been accepted as hypertension (Roberts, 1999).

Preeclampsia, typically categorized as mild or severe, is a progressive disorder. In its most severe form, **eclampsia,** generalized seizures or coma develop. If a woman has a seizure, she is considered eclamptic. Most often preeclampsia is seen in the last 10 weeks of gestation, during labor, or in the first 48 hours after childbirth. Although birth of the fetus is the only known cure for preeclampsia, it can be controlled with early diagnosis and careful management. Preeclampsia occurs in about 7% of all pregnancies in the United States. However, the incidence is significantly higher among primigravidas (Roberts, 1999). Preeclampsia is seen more often in teenagers and in women over age 35, especially if they are primigravidas. Women with a history of preeclampsia are at increased risk, as are women with a large placental mass associated with multiple gestation, GTD, Rh incompatibility, and diabetes mellitus.

#### Pathophysiology of Preeclampsia

The cause of preeclampsia-eclampsia remains unknown, despite decades of research. The condition was previously called "toxemia" because of a theory that a toxin produced in a pregnant woman's body caused the disease. This term is no longer used because the theory has not been substantiated.

Preeclampsia affects all the major systems of the body. The following pathophysiologic changes are associated with the disease:

- In normal pregnancy, the lowered peripheral vascular resistance and the increased maternal resistance to the pressor effects of angiotensin II result in lowered blood pressure. In preeclampsia, blood pressure begins to rise after 20 weeks' gestation, probably due to a gradual loss of resistance to angiotensin II. This response has been linked to the ratio between the prostaglandins prostacyclin and thromboxane. Prostacyclin is a potent vasodilator. It is decreased in preeclampsia, often several weeks before symptoms develop. This changes the ratio between the two prostaglandins, allowing the potent vasoconstriction and platelet-aggregating effects of thromboxane to dominate. This effect is intensified in the later weeks of preeclamptic pregnancy when levels of thrombaxane increase (Mills, DerSimonian, Raymond, et al., 1999).
- In addition, nitric oxide, a potent vasodilator, plays a role in the pregnant woman's resistance to vasopressors. Decreased nitric oxide production in women with PIH may contribute to the development of hypertension (Branch & Porter, 1999).
- The loss of normal vasodilation of uterine arterioles and the concurrent maternal vasospasm result in decreased placental perfusion. The effect on the fetus may be growth restriction, decrease in fetal movement, and chronic hypoxia or fetal distress.

- In preeclampsia, normal renal perfusion is decreased. With a reduction of the glomerular filtration rate (GFR), serum levels of creatinine, BUN, and uric acid begin to rise from normal pregnant levels, while urine output decreases. Sodium is retained in increased amounts, which results in increased extracellular volume, increased sensitivity to angiotensin II, and edema. Stretching of the capillary walls of the glomerular endothelial cells allows the large protein molecules, primarily albumin, to escape in the urine, decreasing serum albumin levels. The decreased serum albumin concentration causes decreased plasma colloid osmotic pressure. This lowered pressure results in a further movement of fluid to the extracellular spaces, which also contributes to the development of edema.
- The decreased intravascular volume causes increased viscosity of the blood and a corresponding rise in hematocrit.

**HELLP syndrome** (***h**emolysis, **e**levated **l**iver enzymes, and **l**ow **p**latelet count*) is sometimes associated with severe preeclampsia. Women who experience this multiple-organ-failure syndrome have high morbidity and mortality rates, as do their offspring.

The hemolysis that occurs is termed *microangiopathic hemolytic anemia.* It is thought that red blood cells are distorted or fragmented during passage through small, damaged blood vessels. Elevated liver enzymes occur from blood flow that is obstructed due to fibrin deposits. Hyperbilirubinemia and jaundice may also be seen. Liver distention causes epigastric pain. Thrombocytopenia (low platelet count) is a frequent finding in preeclampsia. Vascular damage is associated with vasospasm, and platelets aggregate at sites of damage, resulting in low platelet count (less than 100,000/mm$^3$). Symptoms may include nausea, vomiting, flulike symptoms, or epigastric pain.

Women with HELLP syndrome are best cared for in a tertiary care center. Initially the mother's condition should be assessed and stabilized, especially if her platelet counts are very low. Platelet transfusions are indicated for platelet counts below 20,000/mm$^3$. The fetus is also assessed, using a nonstress test and biophysical profile. Once HELLP syndrome is diagnosed and the woman's condition is stable, expeditious birth of the child is indicated. Research suggests that if HELLP syndrome is diagnosed early, before there is multiple-organ injury, the woman may benefit from treatment with dexamethasone given intravenously (Martin & Magann, 1999).

### Maternal Risks

Central nervous system changes associated with PIH are hyperreflexia, headache, and seizures. Hyperreflexia may be due to increased intracellular sodium and decreased intracellular potassium levels. Cerebral vasospasm causes headaches, and cerebral edema and vasoconstriction are responsible for seizures.

Women with severe preeclampsia or eclampsia are at increased risk for renal failure, abruptio placentae, DIC, ruptured liver, and pulmonary embolism.

### Fetal-Neonatal Risks

Infants of women with hypertension during pregnancy tend to be small for gestational age (SGA). The cause is related specifically to maternal vasospasm and hypovolemia, which result in fetal hypoxia and malnutrition. In addition, the neonate may be premature because of the necessity for early birth. Perinatal mortality associated with preeclampsia is approximately 10%, and that associated with eclampsia is 20%.

At birth, the newborn may be oversedated because of medications administered to the mother. The newborn may also have hypermagnesemia due to treatment of the woman with large doses of magnesium sulfate.

### Clinical Therapy

The goals of medical management are prompt diagnosis of the disease; prevention of cerebral hemorrhage, seizures, hematologic complications, and renal and hepatic diseases; and birth of an uncompromised newborn as close to term as possible. Reduction of elevated blood pressure is essential in accomplishing these goals.

#### Clinical Manifestations and Diagnosis

**Mild Preeclampsia** Women with mild preeclampsia may exhibit few if any symptoms. The blood pressure is elevated to 140/90 mm Hg or higher or increases 30 mm Hg systolic and 15 mm Hg diastolic above baseline. Thus a young woman who normally has a blood pressure of 90/60 would be hypertensive at 120/76. Therefore, a baseline blood pressure obtained early in the pregnancy is essential.

Generalized edema, seen as puffy face or hands, and in dependent areas such as the ankles, may be present. Edema is identified by a weight gain of more than 3.3 lb (1.5 kg) per month in the second trimester or more than 1.1 lb (0.5 kg) per week in the third trimester. Edema is assessed on a 1+ to 4+ scale. Urine testing may show a 1+ to 2+ albumin, although proteinuria is often the last of the three cardinal signs to appear.

**Severe Preeclampsia** Severe preeclampsia may develop suddenly. Edema becomes generalized and readily apparent in hands, face, sacral area, lower extremities, and the abdominal wall. Edema is also characterized by an excessive weight gain of more than 2 lb (0.9 kg) over a couple of days to a week. Blood pressure is 160/110 mm Hg or higher, a dipstick albumin measurement is 3+ to 4+, and the 24-hour urine protein level is ≥5 g/L. Hematocrit, serum creatinine, and uric acid levels are elevated. Other characteristic symptoms are frontal headaches, blurred vision, scotomata (spots before the eyes), nausea, vomiting, irritability, hyperreflexia, cerebral disturbances, oliguria (≤500 mL of urine in 24 hours), pulmonary edema with moist breath sounds and dyspnea, cyanosis, retinal edema (retinas appear wet and glistening), narrowed segments on the retinal arterioles when examined with an ophthalmoscope, and, finally, epigastric pain. Epigastric pain is often the sign of impending convulsion and is thought to be caused by increased vascular engorgement of the liver.

**Eclampsia** Eclampsia, characterized by a grand mal convulsion or coma, may occur before the onset of labor, during labor, or early in the postpartal period. Some women experience only one seizure; others have several. Unless they occur quite frequently, the woman often regains consciousness between seizures.

### Antepartal Management

The clinical therapy for PIH depends on the severity of the disease.

**Home Care of Mild Preeclampsia** In general, women with preeclampsia are admitted to the hospital. However, for some women with mild preeclampsia, home care is now an option. The mother and fetus are evaluated twice weekly, and the mother is encouraged to set aside at least two 2- to 3-hour blocks of time for rest in a side-lying position. It is extremely important to advise the woman to report to the doctor if she develops signs of worsening preeclampsia (Branch & Porter, 1999).

**Hospital Care of Mild Preeclampsia** The woman is placed on bed rest, primarily on her left side, to decrease pressure on the vena cava, thereby increasing venous return, circulatory volume, and placental and renal perfusion. Improved renal blood flow helps decrease angiotensin II levels, promotes diuresis, and lowers blood pressure.

Diet should be well balanced and moderate to high in protein (80 to 100 g/day, or 1.5 g/kg/day) to replace protein lost in the urine. Sodium intake should be moderate, not to exceed 6 g/day. Excessively salty foods should be avoided, but sodium restriction and diuretics are no longer used in treating preeclampsia.

To achieve a safe outcome for the fetus, tests to evaluate fetal status are done more frequently as preeclampsia progresses. The following tests are used:

- Fetal movement record
- NST
- Ultrasonography every 3 or 4 weeks for serial determination of growth
- Biophysical profile
- Serum creatinine determinations
- Amniocentesis to determine fetal lung maturity
- Doppler velocimetry beginning at 30 to 32 weeks to screen for fetal compromise

**Severe Preeclampsia** If the uterine environment is considered detrimental to fetal well-being, birth may be the treatment of choice for both mother and fetus, even if the fetus is immature. Other medical therapies for severe preeclampsia include the following:

- *Bed rest.* Bed rest must be complete. Stimuli that may bring on a seizure should be reduced.
- *Diet.* A high-protein, moderate-sodium diet is given as long as the woman is alert and has no nausea or indication of impending seizure.
- *Anticonvulsants.* Magnesium sulfate ($MgSO_4$) is the treatment of choice for convulsions. Its depressant action on the central nervous system (CNS) reduces the possibility of seizure (see Drug Guide: Magnesium Sulfate).
- *Fluid and electrolyte replacement.* The goal of fluid intake is to achieve a balance between correcting hypovolemia and preventing circulatory overload. Fluid intake may be oral or supplemented with intravenous therapy. Intravenous fluids may be started "to keep lines open" in case they are needed for drug therapy even when oral intake is adequate. Electrolytes are replaced as indicated by daily serum electrolyte levels.
- *Sedative.* A sedative such as diazepam (Valium) or phenobarbital is sometimes given to encourage quiet bed rest.
- *Antihypertensives.* Hydralazine (Apresoline) and labetalol (Normodyne) are the antihypertensive medications most commonly used (Branch & Porter, 1999). In general, antihypertensive therapy is given for diastolic blood pressures of 110 mm Hg or above only in cases where the gestational age of the fetus is critical (25 to 30 weeks). Otherwise, for women beyond 30 weeks, childbirth is induced (Roberts, 1999).

**Eclampsia** An eclamptic seizure requires immediate, effective treatment. A bolus of 4 to 6 g magnesium sulfate is given intravenously over 5 minutes to control convulsions. A sedative such as diazepam or amobarbitol is used only if the seizures are not controlled by magnesium sulfate. Dilantin may be used for seizure prevention. The lungs are auscultated for pulmonary edema. The woman is observed for circulatory and renal failure and signs of cerebral hemorrhage. Furosemide (Lasix) may be given for pulmonary edema; digitalis may be given for circulatory failure. Intake and output are monitored hourly.

The woman is observed for signs of labor. She is also checked every 15 minutes for evidence of vaginal bleeding and abdominal rigidity, which might indicate abruptio placentae. While she is comatose, she is positioned on her side with the side rails up.

Because of the severity of her condition, the woman is often cared for in an intensive care unit. Invasive hemodynamic monitoring of either central venous pressure (CVP) or pulmonary artery wedge pressure may be started using a Swan-Ganz catheter. When the condition of the woman and the fetus are stabilized, induction of labor is considered, because birth is the only known cure for PIH. The woman and her partner should be given a careful explanation about her status and that of her unborn child and the treatment they are receiving. Plans for further treatment and for birth must be discussed with them.

#### Intrapartal Management

Labor may be induced by IV oxytocin when there is evidence of fetal maturity and cervical readiness. In very severe cases, cesarean birth may be necessary even if the fetus is immature.

The woman may receive intravenous oxytocin and magnesium sulfate simultaneously. Infusion pumps should be used, and bags and tubing must be carefully labeled.

Meperidine (Demerol) or fentanyl may be given intravenously for labor. A pudendal block is often used for vaginal birth. An epidural block may be used if it is administered by a skilled anesthesiologist who is knowledgeable about preeclampsia.

Birth in the Sims' or semisitting position should be considered. If the lithotomy position is used, a wedge should be placed under the right buttock to displace the uterus. The wedge should also be used if birth is by cesarean. Oxygen is administered to the woman during labor if the need is indicated by fetal response to the contractions.

A pediatrician or neonatal nurse practitioner must be available to care for the newborn at birth. This caregiver must be informed of all amounts and times of medication the woman has received during labor.

#### Postpartum Management

The woman with PIH usually improves rapidly after giving birth, although seizures can still occur during the first 48 hours postpartum. When the hypertension is severe, the woman may continue to receive hydralazine or magnesium sulfate postpartally.

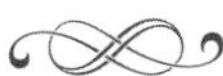

## Nursing Care Management

See the Critical Pathway for a woman with preeclampsia or eclampsia for a detailed summary of nursing care management.

### Nursing Assessment and Diagnosis

Blood pressure is taken and recorded during each antepartal visit. If the blood pressure rises, or if the normal slight decrease in blood pressure expected between 8 and 28 weeks of pregnancy does not occur, the woman should be followed closely. The woman's urine is checked for proteinuria at each visit.

If hospitalization becomes necessary, the nurse then assesses the following:

- *Blood pressure.* Blood pressure should be assessed every 1 to 4 hours, or more frequently if indicated by medication or other changes in the woman's status.
- *Temperature.* Temperature should be taken every 4 hours, or every 2 hours if elevated.

Text continues on page 314.

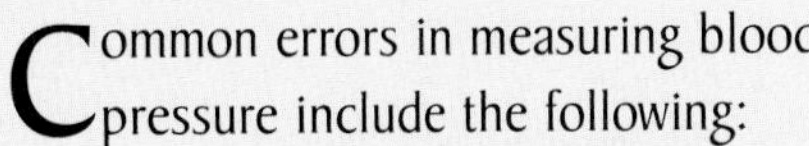

## HINTS FOR PRACTICE

Common errors in measuring blood pressure include the following:

1. Incorrect cuff size—a cuff that is too small results in a falsely elevated blood pressure, whereas one that is too large falsely lowers blood pressure.
2. Elevating the arm above the level of the heart, such as occurs when a woman lies on her left side using her right arm for a blood pressure measurement, will falsely lower the blood pressure 10 to 20 mm Hg.
3. Korotkoff's phase—when blood pressure is checked during pregnancy, the disappearance of sound (phase V) may be unusually low. To standardize measurements, the muffling of sound (phase IV) is the preferred indicator.
4. Anxiety and exercise can elevate blood pressure. Wait 10 minutes after the woman's arrival to check a resting blood pressure.

# CRITICAL PATHWAY *For a Woman with Pregnancy-Induced Hypertension*

| Category | Antepartal Management | Intrapartal Management* | Postpartal Management* |
|---|---|---|---|
| **Referral** | • Perinatologist<br>• Internist<br>• Social worker<br>• Psych clinical nurse practitioner<br>• Dietary/nutritionist | • Obtain prenatal record | • Home nursing referral if indicated<br>**Expected Outcomes**<br>Appropriate resources identified and utilized |
| **Assessment** | • Electronic fetal monitoring (EFM) ____ q 4h ____ q8h ____ Continuous<br>• NST ____ qd<br>• Ultrasound as indicated<br>• Assess for headache, visual disturbances, epigastric pain, edema, DTRs, clonus, and protein in urine | • Assess prenatal BP readings and compare to baseline reading<br>• Assess for headache, visual disturbances, epigastric pain, edema, DTRs, clonus, and protein in urine | • BP q4h for first 48 h then q8h until discharge<br>• Monitor daily hematocrit<br>• Continue normal postpartum assessment q8h<br>• Feeding technique with newborn: should be progressing<br>• TPR assessment: q8h; all WNL: report temperature >38C (100.4F)<br>• Continue assessment of comfort level<br>• Assess for headache, visual disturbances, epigastric pain, edema, DTRs, clonus, and protein in urine<br>**Expected Outcomes**<br>Findings indicate hypertension reduced or stabilized<br>Unstable or escalating hypertension identified in timely manner |
| **Teaching/ psychosocial** | • Room orientation<br>• Explain s/sx of worsening disease and importance of notifying RN<br>• Explain s/sx of labor<br>• Increase pt awareness of fetal monitoring, importance of bed rest and lying on left side<br>• Evaluation of client teaching | • Tour of ICN<br>• Discuss with woman:<br>a. Mode of childbirth<br>b. Progression of disease and possible use of $MgSO_4$ prior to birth<br>c. Postpartum expectation | • Implement normal postpartum teaching and psychosocial support (see Chapter 28)<br>**Expected Outcomes**<br>Verbalizes or otherwise demonstrates understanding of teaching<br>Incorporates teaching of BP management into self-care |
| **Nursing care management and reports** | • CBC daily<br>• Biochemical profile<br>• U/A/dipstick for protein and ketones with each void as well as specific gravity<br>• 24-hour urine for total protein and creatinine clearance<br>• VS q4h or more frequently if indicated<br>• I&O q8h; fluid restriction ____ mL as ordered<br>• DTRs and clonus q4h; report 3+ or 4+ results<br>• Daily weight<br>• Seizure precautions<br>• Headache, visual distress, epigastric pain: report abnormal findings<br>• Assess for edema (ongoing)<br>• Auscultate lungs for moist respirations and report<br>• Assess hourly for vaginal bleeding and/or uterine irritability or contractions<br>• Observe for alertness, mood changes, and signs of impending convulsion or coma<br>• Assess emotional response so that support and teaching can be planned accordingly | • Ongoing monitoring of blood pressure<br>• Ongoing monitoring of edema<br>• Assess urine for proteinuria every shift<br>• Electronic fetal monitoring in place<br>• Assess woman for worsening signs of PIH (placental separation, pulmonary edema, renal failure, and fetal distress)<br>• Try to have same nurses caring for woman during her hospitalization | • Continue sitz bath prn<br>• May shower if ambulating without difficulty<br>• DC buffalo cap (heparin lock) if present<br>• Continue to monitor VS, breath sounds, edema, epigastric pain, DTRs, clonus, and protein in urine until return to normal limits<br>**Expected Outcomes**<br>Hypertension reduced or controlled<br>Maternal-fetal complications quickly identified and minimized<br>Feels safe in environment and remains injury free |

## CRITICAL PATHWAY *Continued*

| Category | Antepartal Management | Intrapartal Management* | Postpartal Management* |
|---|---|---|---|
| **Comfort** | • Assess for discomfort<br>• Provide comfort measures as needed | • Assess for discomfort<br>• Provide comfort measures as needed | • Continue with pain management techniques<br>**Expected Outcomes**<br>Comfort level is maintained |
| **Activity** | • Bedrest with BRP<br>• Decreased stimulation in room<br>• Limit visitors<br>• Encourage left lateral recumbent position | • Positioned on side<br>• Encouraged to push while lying on side<br>• Birth is in a side-lying position if possible | • Up ad lib when VS have stabilized<br>**Expected Outcomes**<br>Level of activity has not exacerbated condition |
| **Nutrition** | • Regular diet | • Ice chips | • Continue diet and fluids<br>**Expected Outcomes**<br>Nutritional needs met |
| **Elimination** | • Report urine output <30 mL/hr or urine or specific gravity >1.040 | • Monitor urine output | • Monitor urine output<br>• I/O recorded for 48h after birth<br>**Expected Outcomes**<br>Intake and output WNL |
| **Medications** | • Heparin lock or IV<br>• If gestational age indicates:<br>  • Celestone Soluspan<br>  • TRH<br>• $MgSO_4$ per infusion pump if indicated<br>• Assess home care needs | • Continuous IV infusion<br>• $MgSO_4$ infusion pump if indicated | • Continue $MgSO_4$ as indicated<br>• May take own prenatal vitamins<br>• Rh immune globulin and rubella vaccine administered if indicated<br>**Expected Outcomes**<br>Hypertensive crisis prevented<br>Pain level controlled<br>Perfusion of tissues supported |
| **Discharge planning/ home care** | | | • Review discharge instruction and checklist<br>• Describe postpartum warning signs and when to call CNM/physician<br>• Provide prescriptions; gift pack given to woman<br>• Arrangements made for baby pictures if desired<br>• Postpartum visit scheduled<br>• Newborn check scheduled<br>**Expected Outcomes**<br>Discharged with plan for follow-up health care and blood pressure monitoring<br>Support network identified |
| **Family involvement** | • Assess woman's major concerns (eg, fear for fetus, relationship with other children, relationship with partner) | • Encourage family members to stay with the woman as long as possible throughout labor and childbirth | • Family members urged to visit<br>• Continue to involve support persons in teaching<br>• Evidence of parental bonding behaviors apparent<br>• Plans being made for providing support to mother following discharge; support persons verbalize understanding of need for woman to rest, eat nutritionally, recover<br>**Expected Outcomes**<br>Family able to participate as desired |
| **Date** | | | |

*Interventions for a woman with a normal labor and birth and during the early postpartum period may be found in those appropriate critical pathways.

Abbreviations used: BP, blood pressure; BRP, bathroom privileges; CBC, complete blood count; CNM/physician, certified nurse-midwife/physician; DTRs, deep tendon reflexes; Hct, hematocrit; Heparin lock, intravenous catheter that allows intermittent access; ICN, intensive care nursery; I&O, intake and output; IV, intravenous; NST, nonstress test; PRN, as needed or as desired; s/sx, signs and symptoms; TPR, temperature, pulse, respiration; VS, vital signs; WNL, within normal limits.

- *Pulse and respirations.* Pulse rate and respirations should be determined along with blood pressure.
- *Fetal heart rate.* The fetal heart rate should be checked with the blood pressure or monitored continuously with the electronic fetal monitor if the situation indicates.
- *Urinary output.* Every voiding should be measured. The woman frequently has an indwelling catheter. In this case, urine output can be assessed hourly. Output should be 700 mL or greater in 24 hours, or at least 30 mL/hr.
- *Urine protein.* Urinary protein is evaluated hourly if an indwelling catheter is in place or with each voiding. Readings of 3+ or 4+ indicate loss of 5 g or more of protein in 24 hours.
- *Urine specific gravity.* Specific gravity of the urine should be checked hourly or with each voiding. Readings over 1.040 correlate with oliguria and proteinuria.
- *Edema.* The face (especially eyelids and cheekbone area), fingers, hands, arms (ulnar surface and wrist), legs (tibial surface), ankles, feet, and sacral area are inspected and palpated for edema. The degree of pitting is determined by pressing over bony areas.
- *Weight.* The woman is weighed daily at the same time, wearing the same robe or gown and slippers. Weighing may be omitted if the woman is to maintain strict bed rest.
- *Pulmonary edema.* The woman is observed for coughing. The lungs are auscultated for moist respirations.
- *Deep tendon reflexes.* The woman is assessed for evidence of hyperreflexia in the brachial, wrist, patellar, or Achilles tendons (Table 13–2). The patellar reflex is the easiest to assess (Procedure 13–1). Clonus should also be assessed by vigorously dorsiflexing the foot while the knee is held in a fixed position. Normally no clonus is present. If it is present, it is measured as beats and recorded as such.
- *Placental separation.* The woman should be assessed hourly for vaginal bleeding and/or uterine rigidity.
- *Headache.* The woman should be questioned about the existence and location of any headache.
- *Visual disturbance.* The woman should be questioned about any visual blurring or changes or scotomata. The results of the daily fundoscopic exam should be recorded on the chart.

**TABLE 13–2 Deep Tendon Reflex Rating Scale**

| *Rating* | *Assessment* |
|---|---|
| 4+ | Hyperactive; very brisk, jerky, or clonic response; abnormal |
| 3+ | Brisker than average; may not be abnormal |
| 2+ | Average response; normal |
| 1+ | Diminished response; low normal |
| 0 | No response; abnormal |

- *Epigastric pain.* The woman should be asked about any epigastric pain. It is important to differentiate it from simple heartburn, which tends to be familiar and less intense.
- *Laboratory blood tests.* Daily tests of hematocrit to measure hemoconcentration; BUN, creatinine, and uric acid levels to assess kidney function; clotting studies for any indication of thrombocytopenia or DIC; liver enzymes; and electrolyte levels for deficiencies are all indicated.
- *Level of consciousness.* The woman is observed for alertness, mood changes, and any signs of impending convulsion or coma.
- *Emotional response and level of understanding.* The woman's emotional response should be carefully assessed so that support and teaching can be planned accordingly.

## HINTS FOR PRACTICE

When caring for a woman with PIH who is receiving IV magnesium sulfate, it is imperative that you follow protocols for monitoring blood levels of magnesium. You are probably already aware of the common signs of increasing magnesium levels, such as diminished reflexes and decreased respiratory rate. However, there are some subtle clues you can also watch for that may suggest either the therapeutic or toxic range. When a woman's magnesium level is in the therapeutic range, she usually has some slurring of speech, awkwardness of movement, and decreased appetite. If the woman begins to have difficulty swallowing and begins to drool, she may be approaching the toxic range.

# Procedure 13–1 Assessing Deep Tendon Reflexes and Clonus

## Nursing Action

**OBJECTIVE: ASSEMBLE AND PREPARE EQUIPMENT.**
Obtain a percussion hammer. If one is not available, the side of the hand is also useful in assessing deep tendon reflexes (DTRs).

## Rationale

*A percussion hammer permits accurate delivery of a brisk tap.*

**OBJECTIVE: PREPARE WOMAN.**
Explain the procedure, indications for it, and information that will be obtained. At a minimum, check the patellar reflex. Most nurses check a second reflex, such as the biceps, triceps, or brachioradialis.

*Explanation decreases anxiety and increases cooperation. DTRs are assessed to gain information about CNS status and to assess the effects of $MgSO_4$ if the woman is receiving it.*

**OBJECTIVE: ELICIT REFLEXES.**
Patellar reflex. The woman is positioned with her legs hanging over the edge of the bed (feet should not be touching the floor) (Figure 13–3♦). She may also lie supine with her knees slightly flexed and supported by the nurse. The nurse briskly strikes the patellar tendon, which is located just below the patella. Normal response is extension or a thrusting forward of the foot.

Biceps reflex. The woman's arm is flexed at the elbow with the nurse's thumb placed on the biceps tendon. The nurse's thumb is struck in a slightly downward motion and response is assessed. Normal response is flexion of the arm.

*Correct positioning and technique are essential to elicit the reflex. The correct position causes the muscle to be slightly stretched. Then when the tendon is stretched with the tap, the muscle should contract.*

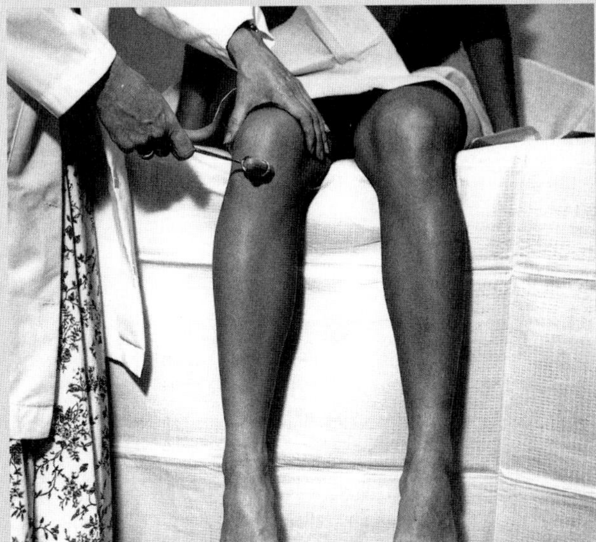

FIGURE 13–3 ♦ Correct sitting position for eliciting patellar reflex.

**OBJECTIVE: GRADE REFLEXES.**
Reflexes are graded on a scale of 0 to 4+. See Table 13–2 on page 314.

*Normally reflexes are 1+ or 2+. With CNS irritation, hyperreflexia may be present; with high magnesium levels, reflexes may be diminished or absent.*

*(Continued)*

## Procedure 13–1 Assessing Deep Tendon Reflexes and Clonus

*continued*

| *Nursing Action* | *Rationale* |
|---|---|
| **Objective: Assess for clonus.**<br>With the knee flexed and the leg supported, vigorously dorsiflex the foot, maintain the dorsiflexion momentarily, and then release (Figure 13–4♦).<br>Normal response: The foot returns to its normal position of plantar flexion. Clonus is present if the foot "jerks" or taps against the examiner's hand. If so, the number of taps or beats of clonus is recorded. | *Clonus indicates more pronounced hyperreflexia and is indicative of CNS irritability.* |

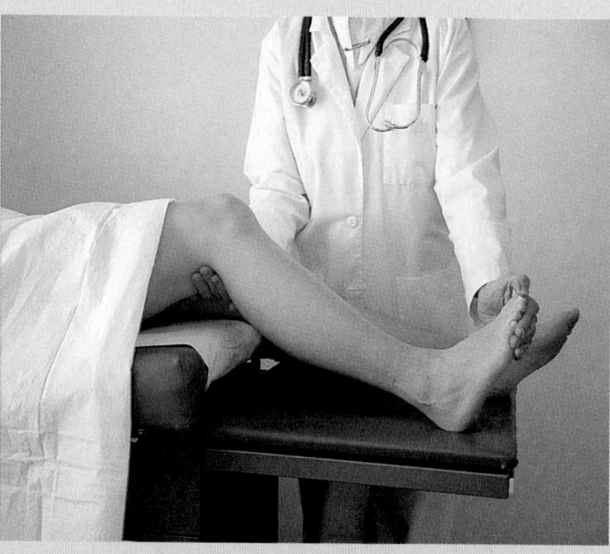

FIGURE 13–4 ♦ To elicit clonus, sharply dorsiflex the foot.

| | |
|---|---|
| **Objective: Report and record findings.**<br>For example: DTRs 2+, no clonus or DTRs 4 +, 2 beats clonus. | *Provides a permanent record.* |

In addition, the nurse continues to assess the effects of any medications administered. Since the administration of prescribed medications is an important aspect of care, the nurse is, of course, familiar with the more commonly used medications and their purpose, implications, and associated untoward or toxic effects.

Examples of nursing diagnoses that might apply to the woman with preeclampsia include the following:

- ***Fluid volume deficit*** related to fluid shift from intravascular to extravascular space secondary to vasospasm
- ***Risk for injury*** related to the possibility of seizure secondary to cerebral vasospasm or edema

### Nursing Plan and Implementation

#### *Community-Based Nursing Care*

A woman with preeclampsia has several major concerns. She may fear losing her fetus, she may worry about her personal relationship with her other children and her personal and sexual relationship with her partner, she may be concerned about finances, and she may also feel bored and a little resentful if she faces prolonged bed rest. If she has small children, she may have trouble providing for their care. The nurse should help the couple identify and discuss these concerns. The nurse can offer information and explanations if certain aspects of therapy cause difficulty. The nurse can also refer the woman and her family o community resources such as support groups or homemaker services as appropriate.

The woman needs to know which symptoms are significant and should be reported at once. Usually the woman with mild preeclampsia is seen once or twice a week, but she may need to come in earlier than her next scheduled appointment if symptoms indicate that her condition is progressing. She must understand her diet plan, which should reflect her culture, finances, and lifestyle.

### *Hospital-Based Nursing Care*

The development of severe preeclampsia is a cause for increased concern for the woman and her family. The most immediate concerns usually are about the prognosis for the woman and her fetus. The nurse can explain medical therapy and its purpose and offer honest, hopeful information. She or he keeps the couple informed of fetal status and discusses other concerns the couple may express. The nurse provides as much information as possible and seeks other sources of information or aid for the family as needed. The nurse can also offer to contact a member of the clergy or hospital chaplain for additional support if the couple so chooses.

The nurse maintains a quiet, low-stimulus environment for the woman. The woman should be placed in a private room in a quiet location where she can be watched closely. Visitors are limited to close family members or main support persons. The woman should maintain the left lateral recumbent position most of the time, with side rails up for her protection. Unlimited phone calls are avoided because the phone ringing unexpectedly may be too jarring. To avoid a sense of isolation, however, some women find it preferable to limit calls to a certain time of day. Bright lights and sudden loud noises may precipitate seizures in the woman with severe preeclampsia.

The occurrence of a convulsion is frightening to any family members who may be present, although the woman will not be able to recall it when she becomes conscious. Therefore, it is essential to offer explanations to the family members and the woman herself later.

A grand mal seizure has both a tonic phase, marked by pronounced muscular contraction and rigidity, and a clonic phase, marked by alternate contraction and relaxation of the muscles, which causes the woman to thrash about wildly. When the tonic phase of the contraction begins, the woman should be turned to her side (if she is not already in that position) to aid circulation to the placenta. Her head should be turned face down to allow saliva to drain from her mouth. Attempting to insert a padded tongue blade is no longer advocated in many facilities; in others, it is used if it can be inserted without force because it may prevent injury to the woman's mouth. The side rails should be padded or a pillow put between the woman and each side rail.

After 15 to 20 seconds the clonic phase starts. When the thrashing subsides, intensive monitoring and therapy begin. An oral airway is inserted, the woman's nasopharynx is suctioned, and oxygen is administered by nasal catheter. Fetal heart tones are monitored continuously. Maternal vital signs are monitored every 5 minutes until they are stable, then every 15 minutes.

#### Nursing Management during Labor and Birth

The laboring woman with preeclampsia must receive all the care and precautions necessary for normal labor, as well as those required for managing preeclampsia. The woman is kept positioned on her left side as much as possible. Both the woman and the fetus are monitored carefully throughout labor. The nurse notes the progress of labor and is alert to signs of worsening PIH or its complications.

During the second stage of labor, the woman is encouraged to push in the side-lying position if possible. If she is unable to do so comfortably or effectively, she can be helped to a semisitting position for pushing and can then resume the lateral position between contractions. Birth is in the side-lying position or in the lithotomy position with a wedge placed under the woman's right hip.

A family member or other support person is encouraged to stay with the woman as much as possible. The woman in labor and the support person should be kept informed of the progress and plan of care. Their wishes concerning the birth experience should be respected whenever possible. Preferably, the woman should be cared for by the same nurses throughout her stay.

#### Nursing Management during the Postpartal Period

Because the woman with preeclampsia is hypovolemic, even normal blood loss can be serious. The amount of vaginal bleeding must be assessed and the woman observed for signs of shock. Blood pressure and pulse are monitored every 4 hours for 48 hours. Hematocrit is checked daily. The woman is assessed for any further signs of preeclampsia. Intake and output are measured. Normal postpartum diuresis helps eliminate edema and is a favorable sign.

Postpartal depression can develop after such a difficult pregnancy. To help prevent it, the nurse provides opportunities for frequent maternal-infant contact and encourages family members to visit. The couple may have many questions, and the nurse should be available for discussion. The couple should be given family-planning information. Oral contraceptives may be used if the woman's blood pressure has returned to normal by the time they are prescribed (usually 4 to 6 weeks after birth).

For a brief summary of PIH, see Key Facts to Remember: Preeclampsia-Eclampsia.

### Evaluation

Expected outcomes of nursing care include the following:

- The woman is able to explain PIH, its implications for her pregnancy, the treatment regimen, and possible complications.
- The woman suffers no eclamptic seizures.
- The woman and her caregivers detect early evidence of increasing severity of the PIH or possible complications so that appropriate treatment measures can be instituted.
- The woman gives birth to a healthy newborn.

**KEY FACTS TO REMEMBER**

*Preeclampsia and Eclampsia*

- Preeclampsia, which occurs after the 20th week of pregnancy, involves elevated BP, edema, and proteinuria. It may be mild or severe.
- A woman with preeclampsia who has a seizure is said to have eclampsia.
- The exact cause of preeclampsia is unknown.
- Vasospasm is responsible for most of the clinical manifestations, including the CNS signs of headache, hyperreflexia, and convulsion. Vasospasm also causes poor placental perfusion, which leads to IUGR.
- The only known cure for preeclampsia is birth of the infant, but symptoms may develop up to 48 hours postpartum.
- Management is supportive and includes anticonvulsant therapy, generally with $MgSO_4$; prevention of renal, hepatic, and hematologic complications; and careful assessment of fetal well-being.
- Nursing care focuses on implementing appropriate interventions based on the data gathered from regular assessment of vital signs, reflexes, degree of edema and proteinuria, response to therapy, fetal status, detection of developing complications, knowledge level, and psychologic state of the woman and her family.

## Chronic Hypertensive Disease

Chronic hypertension exists when the blood pressure is 140/90 mm Hg or higher before pregnancy or before the 20th week of gestation or when hypertension persists indefinitely following childbirth (Branch & Porter, 1999). If the diastolic blood pressure is greater than 80 mm Hg during the second trimester, chronic hypertension should be suspected. The cause of chronic hypertension has not been determined. In most women with chronic hypertension the disease is mild.

The goals of care are to prevent the development of preeclampsia and to ensure normal growth of the fetus. The woman is seen regularly for prenatal care (every 2 weeks until 28 weeks and then weekly until birth).

The woman is taught the importance of daily rest periods in the left lateral recumbent position and also learns to monitor her blood pressure at home. Sodium is limited to about 2 g/day. Antihypertensive medication is continued throughout pregnancy in women with severe chronic hypertension (blood pressure over 160/100 mm Hg). The drug of choice is methyldopa (Aldomet). Serial measurement of hematocrit, serum creatinine, serum uric acid, creatinine clearance, and 24-hour output of urine protein may be necessary (Branch & Porter, 1999).

Nursing care is directed at providing sufficient information so that the woman can meet her health care needs. She is given information about her diet, the importance of regular rest, her medications, the need for blood pressure control, and any procedures used to monitor the well-being of her fetus.

### Chronic Hypertension with Superimposed Preeclampsia

Preeclampsia may develop in a woman previously found to have chronic hypertension. Close monitoring and careful management are indicated if the following signs develop: (1) elevations of systolic blood pressure 30 mm Hg above the baseline or diastolic blood pressure 15 to 20 mm Hg above the baseline, on two occasions at least 6 hours apart; (2) proteinuria; and (3) edema occurring in the upper half of the body. A woman with chronic hypertension who develops superimposed preeclampsia often progresses quickly to eclampsia, sometimes before 30 weeks of pregnancy.

### Late or Transient Hypertension

Late hypertension exists when transient elevation of blood pressure occurs during labor or in the early postpartal period, returning to normal within 10 days after birth.

# Care of the Woman at Risk for Rh Sensitization

The Rh blood group is present on the surface of erythrocytes of a majority of the population. When it is present, a person is designated as Rh positive. Those without the factor are designated as Rh negative. If an Rh-negative individual is exposed to Rh-positive blood, an antigen-antibody response occurs, and the person forms anti-Rh agglutinin and is said to be sensitized. Subsequent exposure to Rh-positive blood can then cause a serious reaction that results in agglutination and hemolysis of red blood cells. Sensitization most commonly occurs when an Rh-negative woman carries an Rh-positive fetus, either to term or to termination by spontaneous or induced abortion. It can also occur if an Rh-negative nonpregnant woman receives an Rh-positive blood transfusion.

The red blood cells (RBCs) from the fetus invade the maternal circulation, thereby stimulating the production of Rh antibodies. Because this transfer of RBCs usually occurs at birth, the first offspring is not affected. In a subsequent pregnancy, however, Rh antibodies cross the placenta and enter the fetal circulation, causing severe hemolysis. The destruction of fetal red blood cells, causing anemia in the fetus, is proportional to the extent of maternal sensitization (Figure 13–5♦).

## Fetal-Neonatal Risks

Although maternal sensitization can now be prevented by appropriate administration of **Rh immune globulin** (**RhoGAM,** or RhIgG), infants still die of Rh hemolytic disease. If treatment is not initiated, the anemia resulting from this disorder can cause marked fetal edema, called **hydrops fetalis.** Congestive heart failure may result; marked jaundice (called *icterus gravis),* which can lead to neurologic damage (*kernicterus*), is also possible. This severe hemolytic syndrome is known as **erythroblastosis fetalis.**

## Screening for Rh Incompatibility and Sensitization

At the first prenatal visit, caregivers (1) take a history of previous sensitization, abortions, blood transfusions, or children who developed jaundice or anemia during the newborn period; (2) determine maternal blood type (ABO) and Rh factor and do a routine Rh antibody screen; and (3) identify other medical complications such as diabetes, infections, or hypertension.

When assessment identifies an Rh-negative woman who may be pregnant with an Rh-positive fetus, an antibody screen (indirect Coombs' test) is done to determine if the woman is sensitized (has developed isoimmunity)

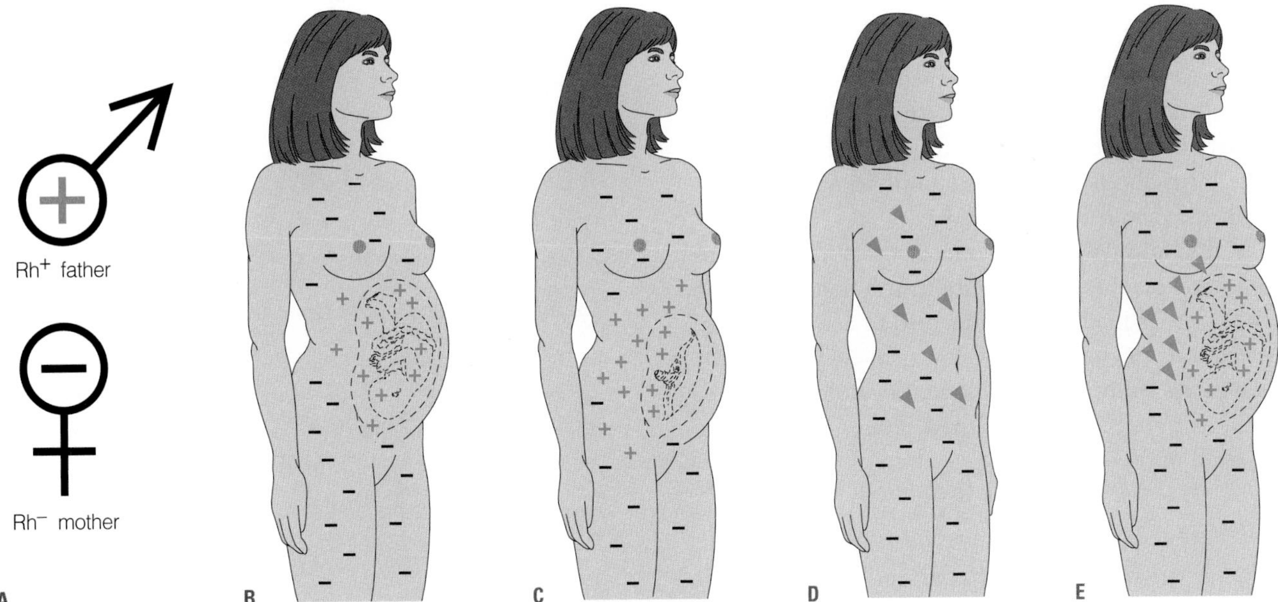


FIGURE 13–5 ♦ Rh isoimmunization sequence. **A,** Rh-positive father and Rh-negative mother. **B,** Pregnancy with Rh-positive fetus. Some Rh-positive blood enters the mother's bloodstream. **C,** As the placenta separates, the mother is further exposed to the Rh-positive blood. **D,** Anti-Rh-positive antibodies (triangles) are formed. **E,** In subsequent pregnancies with an Rh-positive fetus, Rh-positive red blood cells are attacked by the anti-Rh-positive maternal antibodies, causing hemolysis of the red blood cells in the fetus.

to the Rh antigen. The indirect Coombs' test measures the number of antibodies in the maternal blood.

Negative antibody titers and a negative indirect Coombs' test can consistently identify the fetus not at risk. However, the titers cannot reliably point out the fetus in danger, since titer level does not correlate with the severity of the disease. Antibody titers are determined periodically throughout the pregnancy. If the maternal antibody titer is 1:16 or greater, an optical density (ΔOD) analysis of the amniotic fluid is performed. This optical density analysis measures the amount of pigment from the breakdown of red blood cells and can determine the severity of the hemolytic process.

Ultrasound should be done at 14 to 16 weeks to determine gestational age. Then serial ultrasounds and amniotic fluid analysis can be used to follow fetal progress. Ascites and subcutaneous edema are signs of severe fetal involvement. Other indicators of the fetal condition include an increase in fetal heart size and hydramnios.

## Clinical Therapy

The goals of clinical management are the early identification and treatment of maternal conditions that predispose to hemolytic disease, identification and evaluation of the Rh-sensitized woman, coordinated obstetric-pediatric treatment for the seriously affected newborn, and prevention of Rh sensitization if none is present.

### Antepartal Management

Two primary interventions can help the fetus whose blood cells are being destroyed by maternal antibodies: early birth and intrauterine transfusion; both carry risks. Ideally, birth should be delayed until fetal maturity is confirmed at about 36 to 37 weeks.

If ΔOD indicates severe anemia or when fetal hydrops is present, percutaneous umbilical blood sampling (PUBS) (see Chapter 14) is performed to determine fetal hematocrit. If the hematocrit is low (generally 25%), the fetus is given an intrauterine blood transfusion (Scott & Branch, 1999). Severely sensitized fetuses may require birth at 32 to 34 weeks.

### Postpartal Management

The Rh-negative mother who has no antibody titer (indirect Coombs' test negative, nonsensitized) and has given birth to an Rh-positive fetus (direct Coombs' test negative) is given an intramuscular injection of Rh immune globulin (RhoGAM). The Rh immune globulin provides passive antibody protection against Rh antigens. This "tricks" the body, which does not then produce antibodies of its own (active immunity). The woman must receive RhoGAM (HypRho-D) within 72 hours of childbirth so she does not have time to produce antibodies to fetal cells that entered her bloodstream when the placenta separated. Administration of Rh immune globulin in a dose of 300 μg generally provides temporary passive immunity to the mother, which prevents the development of permanent active immunity (antibody formation).

When the woman is Rh negative and not sensitized and the father is Rh positive or unknown, Rh immune globulin is also given after each abortion (whether spontaneous or induced), ectopic pregnancy, or amniocentesis. If abortion or ectopic pregnancy occurs in the first

#### KEY FACTS TO REMEMBER

***Rh Sensitization***

When trying to work through Rh problems, the nurse should remember the following:

- A potential problem exists when an Rh− mother and an Rh+ father conceive a child who is Rh+.
- In this situation, the mother may become sensitized or produce antibodies to her fetus's Rh+ blood.

The following tests are used to detect sensitization:

- Indirect Coombs' test—done on the mother's blood to measure the number of Rh+ antibodies.
- Direct Coombs' test—done on the infant's blood to detect antibody-coated Rh+ RBCs.

Based on the results of these tests, the following may be done:

- If the mother's indirect Coombs' test is negative and the infant's direct Coombs' test is negative, the mother is given Rh immune globulin within 72 hours of birth.
- If the mother's indirect Coombs' test is positive and her Rh+ infant has a positive direct Coombs' test, Rh immune globulin is *not* given; in this case the infant is carefully monitored for hemolytic disease.
- It is recommended that Rh immune globulin be given at 28 weeks antenatally to decrease possible transplacental bleeding concerns.
- Rh immune globulin is also administered after each abortion (spontaneous or therapeutic), ectopic pregnancy, or amniocentesis.

trimester, a smaller (50 μg) dose of Rh immune globulin (MICRhoGAM or Mini-Gamulin Rh) is used. A full dose is used following second-trimester amniocentesis (Scott & Branch, 1999).

Since transplacental hemorrhage is possible during pregnancy, an antibody screen is performed on an Rh-negative woman at 28 weeks. If it is negative, Rh immune globulin is administered prophylactically. Rh immune globulin is not given to the newborn or the father. It is not effective for, and should not be given to, a previously sensitized woman. However, sometimes after birth or an abortion the results of the blood test do not clearly show whether the mother is already sensitized to the Rh antigen. In such cases, the Rh immune globulin should be given; it will cause no harm. For the major considerations in caring for an Rh-negative woman, see Key Facts to Remember: Rh Sensitization. (The treatment of the newborn with isoimmune hemolytic disease is discussed in Chapter 25.)

# Nursing Care Management

## Nursing Assessment and Diagnosis

As part of the initial prenatal history, the nurse asks the mother if she knows her blood type and Rh factor. Many women are aware that they are Rh negative and that this status has implications for pregnancy. If the woman knows she is Rh negative, the nurse can assess the woman's knowledge of what that means. The nurse can also ask the woman if she has ever received Rh immune globulin, if she has had any previous pregnancies and what their outcome was, and if she knows her partner's Rh factor. If the partner is Rh negative, there is no risk to the fetus, who will also be Rh negative.

If the woman does not know what Rh type she is, intervention cannot begin until the initial laboratory data are obtained. Once that is done, the nurse plans care based on the findings.

If the woman becomes sensitized during her pregnancy, nursing assessment focuses on the knowledge and coping skills of the woman and her family. The nurse also provides ongoing assessment during procedures to evaluate fetal well-being, such as ultrasound and amniocentesis.

After birth, the nurse reviews data about the Rh type of the fetus. If the newborn is Rh positive, the mother is Rh negative, and no sensitization has occurred, nursing assessment reveals the need to administer Rh immune globulin.

Nursing diagnoses that might apply to the pregnant woman at risk for Rh sensitization include the following:

- ***Health-seeking behaviors:*** information about Rh immune globulin related to an expressed need to understand the implications of being Rh negative and pregnant
- ***Ineffective individual coping*** related to depression secondary to the development of indications of the need for fetal exchange transfusion

## Nursing Plan and Implementation

During the antepartal period the nurse explains the mechanisms involved in isoimmunization and answers any questions the woman and her partner have. It is imperative that the woman understand the importance of receiving Rh immune globulin after every spontaneous or therapeutic abortion or ectopic pregnancy. The nurse also explains the purpose of the Rh immune globulin administered at 28 weeks' gestation if the woman is not sensitized.

If the woman is sensitized to the Rh factor, it poses a threat to any Rh-positive fetus she carries. The nurse provides emotional support to the family to help the members deal with their grief and any feelings of guilt about the infant's condition. If an intrauterine transfusion becomes necessary, the nurse continues to provide emotional support while also assuming responsibility as part of the health care team.

During labor, the nurse caring for an Rh-negative woman who has not been sensitized ensures that the woman's blood is assessed for any antibodies and also has been cross matched for Rh immune globulin. On the postpartum unit the nurse generally is responsible for administering the Rh immune globulin intramuscularly if the newborn is Rh positive (see Procedure 13–2).

## Evaluation

Expected outcomes of nursing care include the following:

- The woman is able to explain the process of Rh sensitization and its implications for her unborn child and for subsequent pregnancies.
- If the woman has not been sensitized, she is able to discuss the importance of receiving Rh immune globulin when necessary and cooperates with the recommended dosage schedule.
- The woman gives birth to a healthy newborn.
- If complications develop for the fetus or newborn, they are detected quickly and therapy is instituted.

# Procedure 13–2 Administration of Rh Immune Globulin (RhIgG) (RhoGAM, HypRho-D)

| *Nursing Action* | *Rationale* |
| --- | --- |
| **Objective: Confirm that Rh immune globulin is indicated.**<br>Confirm that mother is Rh negative by checking her prenatal or intrapartal record. Then confirm that sensitization has not occurred—maternal indirect Coombs' negative.<br>Confirm that infant is Rh positive. (A sample of the infant's cord blood is generally sent to the lab immediately after birth for typing and cross matching.) If infant is Rh positive, confirm that sensitization has not occurred—direct Coombs' negative. | *Sensitization occurs when an Rh-negative woman is exposed to Rh-positive blood. She develops antibodies to the Rh-positive blood. These antibodies can attack the fetal red blood cells, causing profound anemia. If both the direct and indirect Coombs' tests are negative, sensitization has not occurred, and Rh immune globulin is indicated.* |
| **Objective: Confirm that the woman does not have a history of allergy to immune globulin preparations.**<br>Review entries on medication allergies in client chart and ask woman specifically whether she has had any allergic reactions to medications, globulins, or blood products. | *Rh immune globulin is made from the plasma portion of blood. Allergic reactions are possible.* |
| **Objective: Explain purpose and procedure. Have consent signed.**<br>Many agencies require informed consent before administering Rh immune globulin. | *The woman should clearly understand the purpose of the procedure, its rationale, and the procedure itself, including any risks. Generally, the primary side effects are erythema and tenderness at the injection site and allergic responses.* |
| **Objective: Obtain correct medication.**<br>Rh immune globulin is available from the blood bank or pharmacy according to agency policy. Lot numbers for the drug and the cross match should be the same. | *Because blood products are involved in the preparation, careful verification is essential.* |
| **Objective: Confirm client identity and administer medication in deltoid muscle.**<br>Medication is administered intramuscularly within 72 hours of childbirth. The normal dose of 300 μg provides passive immunity following exposure of up to 15 mL of transfused RBCs or 30 mL of fetal blood. If a larger bleed is suspected (as in cases of severe abruptio placentae), additional doses may be administered at one time using multiple sites or at regular intervals as long as all doses are given within 72 hours of childbirth. | *The medication causes passive immunity to occur and "tricks" the body into believing that it is not necessary to develop antibodies. Immunization is indicated any time there is a potential for maternal exposure to Rh-positive blood. It is given prophylactically at 28 weeks' gestation, within 72 hours after the birth of an Rh-positive Coombs' negative child, and following any spontaneous or therapeutic abortion, ectopic pregnancy, or amniocentesis.* |
| **Objective: Complete education for self-care.**<br>Provide opportunities for the woman to ask questions and express concerns. | *Many women, especially primigravidas, are not aware of the risks for an Rh-positive fetus of a sensitized Rh-negative mother. They must understand the importance of receiving medication for each pregnancy to ensure continued protection.* |
| **Objective: Complete client record.**<br>Chart according to agency procedure. Most agencies chart lot number, route, dose, client education. | *Provides a permanent record.* |

## Care of the Woman at Risk Due to ABO Incompatibility

ABO incompatibility occurs in about 20% to 25% of pregnancies, but it rarely causes significant hemolysis (Scott & Branch, 1999). In most cases ABO incompatibility is limited to type O mothers with a type A or B fetus. Group O infants, because they have no antigenic sites on the red blood cells, are never affected regardless of the mother's blood type. The incompatibility occurs as a result of the interaction of antibodies present in maternal serum and the antigen sites on the fetal red blood cells.

Anti-A and anti-B antibodies are naturally occurring; that is, women are naturally exposed to the A and B antigens through the foods they eat and through exposure to infection by gram-negative bacteria. As a result, some women have high serum anti-A and anti-B titers before they become pregnant. Once they become pregnant, the maternal serum anti-A and anti-B antibodies cross the placenta and produce hemolysis of the fetal red blood cells. With ABO incompatibility, the first infant is frequently involved, and no relationship exists between the appearance of the disease and repeated sensitization from one pregnancy to the next.

Unlike Rh incompatibility, antepartal treatment is never warranted. As part of the initial assessment, however, the nurse should note whether the potential for an ABO incompatibility exists (type O mother and type A or B father). This note alerts caregivers so that, following birth, the newborn can be assessed carefully for the development of hyperbilirubinemia (see Chapter 26).

## Care of the Woman Requiring Surgery during Pregnancy

Elective surgery should be delayed until the postpartal period, but essential surgery can generally be undertaken during pregnancy. Surgery poses some risks, however. The incidence of spontaneous abortion is increased for women who have surgery in the first trimester. There is also an increased incidence of fetal mortality and of low-birth-weight (less than 2500 g) infants. Finally, when surgery is necessary, the incidence of preterm labor and intrauterine growth restriction increases.

Although general preoperative and postoperative care is similar for gravid and nongravid women, special considerations must be kept in mind whenever the surgical client is pregnant. The early second trimester is the best time to operate because there is less risk of spontaneous abortion or early labor, and the uterus is not so large as to impinge on the abdominal field.

To prevent uterine compression of major blood vessels while the woman is supine, the caregiver must place a wedge under the woman's right hip to tilt the uterus during both surgery and recovery. The decreased intestinal motility and delayed gastric emptying that occur in pregnancy increase the risk of vomiting when anesthetics are given and during the postoperative period. Thus inserting a nasogastric tube is recommended before a pregnant woman has major surgery. An indwelling urinary catheter prevents bladder distention, decreases risk of injury to the bladder, and permits convenient monitoring of output.

Pregnancy causes increased secretions of the respiratory tract and engorgement of the nasal mucous membrane, often making breathing through the nose difficult. Consequently, pregnant women often need an endotracheal tube for respiratory support during surgery.

Caregivers must guard against maternal hypoxia. During surgery, uterine circulation decreases, and fetal oxygenation may be reduced quickly. Fetal heart rate must be monitored electronically before, during, and after surgery. Blood loss is also closely monitored throughout the procedure and following it.

Postoperatively, the nurse encourages the woman to turn, breathe deeply, and cough regularly and to use any ventilation therapy, such as incentive spirometry, to avoid developing pneumonia. The pregnant woman is at increased risk for thrombophlebitis, so the nurse applies antiembolism stockings, encourages leg exercises while the woman is confined to bed, and introduces ambulation as soon as possible.

Discharge teaching is especially important. The woman and her family should clearly understand what to expect regarding activity level, discomfort, diet, medications, and any special considerations. In addition, they should know the warning signs they need to report to the physician immediately.

## Care of the Woman Suffering Trauma from an Accident

Trauma complicates approximately 1 in every 12 pregnancies; motor vehicle accidents are the most common cause of trauma, accounting for two-thirds of injuries. Falls and direct assaults account for most of the remaining cases. (Domestic violence, which may be the etiology of trauma, is discussed in the next section.) Most accidents produce minor or non-life-threatening injuries and result in pregnancy loss 1% to 5% of the time. Estimates suggest that abruptio placentae is a complication in 40% to 50% of women who sustain severe trauma (ACOG, 1998b).

Late in pregnancy, when balance and coordination are adversely affected, the woman may fall. Her protruding abdomen is vulnerable to a variety of minor injuries. The fetus is usually well protected by the amniotic fluid, which distributes the force of a blow equally in all directions, and by the muscle layers of the uterus and abdominal wall. In early pregnancy, while the uterus is still in the pelvis, it is shielded from blows by the surrounding pelvic organs, muscles, and bony structures.

Trauma that causes concern includes blunt trauma (from an automobile accident, for example); penetrating abdominal injuries, such as knife and gunshot wounds; and the complications of maternal shock, premature labor, and spontaneous abortion. Maternal mortality most often occurs from head trauma or hemorrhage. Uterine rupture is a rare but life-threatening complication of trauma. It may result from strong deceleration forces in an automobile accident, with or without seat belts. Traumatic separation of the placenta can occur; it causes a high rate of fetal mortality. Premature labor, often following rupture of membranes during an accident, is another serious hazard to the fetus. Premature labor can ensue even if the woman is not injured. To help prevent trauma from automobile accidents, all pregnant women should wear both lap seat belts and shoulder harnesses (ACOG, 1998b).

Treatment of major injuries during pregnancy focuses initially on life-saving measures for the woman. Such measures include establishing an airway, controlling external bleeding, and administering intravenous fluid to alleviate shock. The woman must be kept on her left side to prevent further hypotension. Fetal heart rate is monitored. Exploratory surgery may be necessary following abdominal trauma to determine the extent of injuries. If the fetus is near term and the uterus has been damaged, cesarean birth is indicated. If the fetus is still immature, the uterus can often be repaired, and the pregnancy continues until term.

In cases of trauma in which the mother's life is not directly threatened, fetal monitoring for 4 hours should be sufficient if there are no contractions, vaginal bleeding, uterine tenderness, or leaking amniotic fluid. Abruptio placentae may occur following a blow to the abdomen. Increased uterine irritability in the first few hours after trauma helps identify women who may be at risk for this potentially catastrophic complication.

## Care of the Battered Pregnant Woman

*Female partner abuse,* the intentional injury of a woman by her partner, often begins or increases during pregnancy. The incidence of abuse during pregnancy ranges from 1% to 20%; most studies have found an incidence of 4% to 8% (ACOG, 1999a). Physical abuse may result in loss of pregnancy, preterm labor, low-birth-weight infants, and fetal death. Abused women have significantly higher rates of complications such as anemia, infection, low weight gain, and first- and second-trimester bleeding (McFarlane, Parker, Soeken, et al., 1999).

The first step toward helping the battered woman is to identify her. Asking every woman about abuse at various times during pregnancy is crucial because a woman may not disclose abuse until she knows her caregivers better. ACOG (1999a) recommends screening at the first prenatal visit, at least once each trimester, and then again during the postpartum period.

Chronic psychosomatic symptoms can also be an indicator of abuse. The woman may have nonspecific or vague complaints. It is important to assess old scars around the head, chest, arms, abdomen, and genitalia. Any bruising or evidence of pain is also evaluated. The nurse should be especially alert for signs of bruising or injury to the woman's breasts, abdomen, or genitalia because these areas are common targets of violence during pregnancy. Other indicators include a decrease in eye contact; silence when the partner is in the room; and a history of nervousness, insomnia, drug overdose, or alcohol problems. Frequent visits to the emergency room and a history of accidents without understandable causes are possible indicators of abuse.

The goals of treatment are to identify the woman at risk, increase her decision-making abilities to decrease the potential for further abuse, and provide a safe environment for the pregnant woman and her unborn child. An environment that is private, accepting, and nonjudgmental is necessary so the woman can express her concerns. She needs to be aware of community resources available to her, such as emergency shelters; police, legal, and social services; and counseling. Ultimately, it is the woman's decision to either seek assistance or return to old patterns.

Because abuse often begins during pregnancy, it may be a new, unexpected experience for the woman, one she believes is an isolated incident. She needs to know that battering may continue after childbirth and may extend to the child as well. This is an important time for the nurse to provide information and establish a trusted link for the woman with a health professional. (For further discussion see Chapter 4.)

## Care of the Woman with a TORCH Infection

The TORCH group of infectious diseases are those identified as causing serious harm to the embryo-fetus: ***to***xoplasmosis, ***r***ubella, ***c***ytomegalovirus, and ***h***erpes simplex virus type 2. (Some sources identify the *O* as "other infections.") The importance of understanding what these infections are and identifying risk factors cannot be overemphasized. Exposure of the woman during the first 12 weeks of gestation may cause developmental anomalies in the fetus.

## Toxoplasmosis

Toxoplasmosis is caused by the protozoan *Toxoplasma gondii.* It is innocuous in adults, but, when contracted in pregnancy, it can profoundly affect the fetus. The pregnant woman may contract the organism by eating raw or undercooked meat or by contact with the feces of infected cats, either through the cat litter box or by gardening in areas frequented by cats.

### Fetal-Neonatal Risks

The likelihood of fetal infection increases with each trimester of pregnancy, but the risk of serious impact on the fetus decreases. Thus maternal infection contracted during the first trimester is associated with the lowest incidence of fetal infection but the highest risk of severe fetal disease or death. Maternal infection that occurs before conception is rarely associated with congenital effects (Lopez, Dietz, Wilson, et al., 2000). Most infants born with congenital toxoplasmosis are asymptomatic at birth but develop symptoms later. The infection may vary from mild to severe. In mild cases, retinochoroiditis (inflammation of the retina and choroid of the eye) may be the only recognizable damage, and it and other manifestations may not appear until adolescence or young adulthood. Severe neonatal disorders associated with congenital infection include convulsions, coma, microcephaly, and hydrocephalus. The infant with a severe infection may die soon after birth. Survivors are often blind, deaf, and severely retarded.

### Clinical Therapy

The goal of therapy is to identify the woman at risk for toxoplasmosis and to treat the disease promptly if diagnosed. Diagnosis can be made by serologic testing of antibody titers, specifically *Toxoplasma*-specific antibodies IgG and IgM using the indirect fluorescent antibody (IFA) test. Titers become positive within 1 to 2 weeks after infection and may persist for months or years (Minkoff, 1999).

Prenatal diagnosis of toxoplasmosis is possible using a culture of amniotic fluid or ultrasound-guided cordocentesis to obtain a sample of fetal blood, which is then tested for *Toxoplasma*-specific IgM. If diagnosis can be established by physical findings, history, and serologic testing, the woman may be treated with sulfadiazine, pyrimethamine, and spiramycin. Treatment of the mother can reduce the incidence of fetal infection significantly.

If toxoplasmosis is diagnosed before 20 weeks' gestation, pyrimethamine should be avoided unless a therapeutic abortion is planned because the drug can have teratogenic effects.

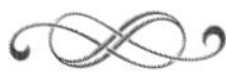

## Nursing Care Management

### Nursing Assessment and Diagnosis

The incubation period for the disease is 10 days. The woman with acute toxoplasmosis may be asymptomatic, or she may develop myalgia, malaise, rash, splenomegaly, and enlarged posterior cervical lymph nodes. Symptoms usually disappear in a few days or weeks.

Nursing diagnoses that might apply to the pregnant woman with toxoplasmosis include the following:

- ***Risk for altered health maintenance*** related to lack of knowledge about ways in which a pregnant woman can contract toxoplasmosis
- ***Anticipatory grieving*** related to potential effects on infant of maternal toxoplasmosis

### Nursing Plan and Implementation

The nurse caring for women during the antepartal period has the primary opportunity to discuss methods of preventing toxoplasmosis. The woman must understand the importance of avoiding poorly cooked or raw meat, especially pork, beef, lamb, and, in the Arctic region, caribou. Fruits and vegetables should be washed. She should avoid contact with the cat litter box and have someone else clean it frequently, since it takes approximately 48 hours for a cat's feces to become infectious. The nurse should also discuss the importance of wearing gloves when gardening and of avoiding garden areas frequented by cats.

### Evaluation

Expected outcomes of nursing care include the following:

- The woman is able to discuss toxoplasmosis, its methods of transmission, the implications for her fetus, and measures she can take to avoid contracting it.
- The woman implements health measures to avoid contracting toxoplasmosis.
- The woman gives birth to a healthy newborn.

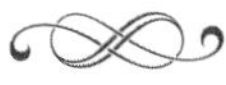

## Rubella

The effects of rubella (German measles) are no more severe for and there are no greater complications in pregnant women than in nonpregnant women of comparable age. However, the effects of this infection on the fetus and newborn are great because rubella causes a chronic infection that begins in the first trimester of pregnancy and may persist for months after birth.

### Fetal-Neonatal Risks

The period of greatest risk for the teratogenic effects of rubella on the fetus is the first trimester. Clinical signs of congenital infection are congenital heart disease, IUGR, and cataracts. Cardiac complications most often seen are patent ductus arteriosus and narrowing of peripheral pulmonary arteries. Cataracts may be unilateral or bilateral and may be present at birth or develop in the newborn period. A petechial rash is seen in some infants, and hepatosplenomegaly and hyperbilirubinemia are frequently seen. Other abnormalities, such as mental retardation or cerebral palsy, may become evident in infancy. Diagnosis in the newborn can be conclusively made in the presence of these conditions and with an elevated rubella IgM antibody titer at birth.

Infants born with congenital rubella syndrome are infectious and should be isolated. These infants may continue to shed the virus for months.

The expanded rubella syndrome relates to effects that may develop for years after the infection. These include an increased incidence of insulin-dependent diabetes mellitus; sudden hearing loss; glaucoma; and a slow, progressive form of encephalitis.

### Clinical Therapy

The best therapy for rubella is prevention. Live attenuated vaccine is available and should be given to all children. Women of childbearing age should be tested for immunity and vaccinated if susceptible once it is established that they are not pregnant.

As part of the prenatal laboratory screen, the woman is evaluated for rubella using hemagglutination inhibition (HAI), a serology test. The presence of a 1:16 titer or greater is evidence of immunity. A titer less than 1:8 indicates susceptibility to rubella.

Because the vaccine is made with attenuated virus, pregnant women are not vaccinated. However, it is considered safe for newly vaccinated children to have contact with pregnant women.

If a woman becomes infected during the first trimester, therapeutic abortion is a legally available alternative.

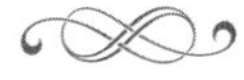

## Nursing Care Management

### Nursing Assessment and Diagnosis

A woman who develops rubella during pregnancy may be asymptomatic or may show signs of a mild infection including a maculopapular rash, lymphadenopathy, muscular achiness, and joint pain. The presence of IgM antirubella antibody is diagnostic of a recent infection. These titers remain elevated for approximately 1 month after infection.

Nursing diagnoses that may apply to the woman who develops rubella early in her pregnancy include the following:

- ***Ineffective family coping*** due to an inability to accept the possibility of fetal anomalies secondary to maternal rubella exposure
- ***Risk for altered health maintenance*** related to lack of knowledge about the importance of rubella immunization before becoming pregnant

### Nursing Plan and Implementation

Nursing support and understanding are vital for the couple contemplating abortion due to a diagnosis of rubella. Such a decision may initiate a crisis for the couple that has planned the pregnancy. The parents need objective data to understand the possible effects on their unborn fetus and the prognosis for the offspring.

### Evaluation

Expected outcomes of nursing care include the following:

- The woman is able to describe the implications of rubella exposure during the first trimester of pregnancy.
- If exposure occurs in a woman who is not immune, she is able to identify her options and make a decision about continuing her pregnancy that is acceptable to her and her partner.
- The nonimmune woman receives the rubella vaccine during the early postpartal period.
- The woman gives birth to a healthy infant.

## Cytomegalovirus

Cytomegalovirus (CMV) belongs to the herpes virus group and causes both congenital and acquired infections referred to as *cytomegalic inclusion disease (CID).* The significance of this virus in pregnancy is related to its ability to be transmitted by asymptomatic women across the placenta to the fetus or by the cervical route during birth.

CMV is the most common cause of congenital infection in the United States (Oshiro, 1999). Nearly half of adults have antibodies for the virus. The virus can be found in virtually all body fluids. It can be passed between humans by any close contact, such as kissing, breastfeeding, and sexual intercourse. Asymptomatic CMV infection is particularly common in children and gravid women. It is a chronic, persistent infection in that the individual may shed the virus continually over many years. The cervix can harbor the virus, and an ascending infection can develop after birth. Although the virus is usually innocuous in adults and children, it may be fatal to the fetus.

Accurate diagnosis in the pregnant woman depends on the presence of CMV in the urine, a rise in IgM levels, and identification of the CMV antibodies within the serum IgM fraction. At present, no treatment exists for maternal CMV or for the congenital disease in the neonate.

Congenital CMV infection afflicts 1% to 2% of all newborns born in the United States. Of these, about 10% have signs of the disease at birth, and 5% to 15% more go on to develop problems (Oshiro, 1999). The mortality rate for newborns with symptomatic disease is 30% (Minkoff, 1999). Subclinical infections in the newborn may produce mental retardation and hearing loss, sometimes not recognized for several months, or learning disabilities not seen until childhood. CMV may be the most common cause of mental retardation.

For the fetus, this infection can result in extensive intrauterine tissue damage that leads to fetal death; in survival with microcephaly, hydrocephaly, cerebral palsy, or mental retardation; or in survival with no damage at all. The infected newborn is often SGA. The principal tissues and organs affected are the blood, brain, and liver. However, virtually all organs are potentially at risk.

## Herpes Simplex Virus

Herpes simplex virus (HSV-I or HSV-2) infection can cause painful lesions in the genital area. Lesions may also develop on the cervix. This condition and its implications for nonpregnant women are discussed in Chapter 4. However, because the presence of herpes lesions in the genital tract may profoundly affect the fetus, herpes infection as it relates to a pregnant woman is discussed here as part of the TORCH complex of infections.

### Fetal-Neonatal Risks

Primary infection poses the greatest risk to both the mother and her infant. Primary infection has been associated with spontaneous abortion, low birth weight, and preterm birth. Transmission to the fetus almost always occurs after the membranes rupture and the virus ascends or during birth through an infected birth canal. Transplacental infection is rare. Approximately 50% of all infants who are born vaginally to a mother who is experiencing a primary genital HSV infection develop some form of herpes infection. Of these infants, about 60% will die in the neonatal period; of the survivors, about half will develop severe problems such as microcephaly, mental retardation, seizures, retinal dysplasia, apnea, and coma (Minkoff, 1999).

The infected infant is often asymptomatic at birth but develops symptoms of fever (or hypothermia), jaundice, seizures, and poor feeding after an incubation period of 2 to 12 days. Approximately half of infected infants develop the characteristic vesicular skin lesions. Vidarabine has been useful in decreasing serious effects from neonatal herpes, but no definitive treatment exists as yet. Some experts treat asymptomatic infants who were exposed to HSV during birth with acyclovir. Positive herpes cultures taken 24 to 48 hours after birth should be obtained before treatment (Centers for Disease Control and Prevention, 1998).

### Clinical Therapy

The vesicular lesions of herpes have a characteristic appearance, and they rupture easily. Definitive diagnosis is made by culturing active lesions.

The ACOG (1999b) recommends antiviral therapy for women with primary HSV infection during pregnancy to decrease viral shedding and promote healing. Women with recurrent infection may also benefit from antiviral therapy. Three medications are available for that purpose: acyclovir, valaclovir, and famciclovir. Acyclovir has been shown to be effective and safe during pregnancy, but it is not as well absorbed as the other two drugs.

If there is no evidence of genital infection, vaginal birth is preferred. However, if the woman has any signs of active genital lesions or prodromal symptoms of infection such as vulvar pain or burning, cesarean birth is indicated. The woman with active HSV infection and ruptured membranes should also give birth by cesarean as soon as the necessary caregivers and equipment can be assembled (ACOG, 1999b).

HSV has not been found in breast milk. Present experience shows that breastfeeding is acceptable if there are no herpes lesions on the mother's breasts and if she washes her hands well to prevent any direct transfer of the virus.

## Critical Thinking in Practice

Your friend Rachel Glassman is 6 months pregnant and mentions to you that she is developing symptoms of a bladder infection. She has had several bladder infections over the past few years and feels she has warded off others by increasing her fluid intake and drinking acidic juices. She tells you she plans to use the same approach this time because she just had her prenatal appointment last week. She assures you that if symptoms persist, she will discuss it with her caregiver at her next prenatal visit. What advice would you give her?

Answers can be found in Appendix I.

# Nursing Care Management

### Nursing Assessment and Diagnosis

During the initial prenatal visit it is important to learn whether the woman or her partner have had previous herpes infections. If so, ongoing assessment is indicated as pregnancy progresses.

Nursing diagnoses that may apply to the pregnant woman with HSV infection include the following:

- ***Sexual dysfunction*** related to unwillingness to engage in sexual intercourse secondary to the presence of active herpes lesions
- ***Ineffective individual coping*** related to depression secondary to the risk to the fetus if herpes lesions are present at birth

### Nursing Plan and Implementation

Nurses need to be particularly concerned with client education about this fast-spreading disease. Women should be informed of the association of HSV infection with spontaneous abortion, newborn mortality and morbidity, and the possibility of cesarean birth. A woman needs to inform all health care providers of her infection. She should also know of the possible association of genital herpes with cervical cancer and the importance of a yearly Pap smear.

The woman who acquired HSV infection as an adolescent may be devastated as a mature young adult who wants to have a family. Clients may be helped by counseling that allows them to express the anger, shame, and depression often experienced by those with herpes. Literature may be helpful and is available from Planned Parenthood and many public health agencies. The American Social Health Association has established the HELP program to provide information and the latest research results on genital herpes. The association has a quarterly journal, *The Helper,* for clients with HSV infection and nurses.

### Evaluation

Expected outcomes of nursing care include the following:

- The woman is able to describe her infection with regard to its method of spread, therapy and comfort measures, implications for her pregnancy, and long-term implications.
- The woman gives birth to a healthy infant.

## Other Infections in Pregnancy

In addition to the TORCH infections, other infections contribute to risk during pregnancy. Spontaneous abortion is frequently the result of a severe maternal infection. Some evidence links infection and prematurity. In addition, if the pregnancy is carried to term in the presence of infection, the risk of maternal and fetal morbidity and mortality increases. Thus it is essential to maternal and fetal health that infection be diagnosed and treated promptly.

Urinary tract, vaginal, and sexually transmitted infections are discussed in detail in Chapter 4. Table 13–3 provides a summary of these infections and their implications for pregnancy.

**TABLE 13–3 Infections that Put Pregnancy at Risk**

| *Condition and Causative Organism* | *Signs and Symptoms* | *Treatment* | *Implications for Pregnancy* |
|---|---|---|---|
| **URINARY TRACT INFECTIONS (UTI)** | | | |
| Asymptomatic bacteriuria (ASB): *Escherichia coli, Klebsiella, Proteus* most common | Bacteria present in urine on culture with no accompanying symptoms. | Oral sulfonamides early in pregnancy, ampicillin and nitrofurantoin (Furadantin) in late pregnancy. | Women with ASB in early pregnancy may go on to develop cystitis or acute pyelonephritis by third trimester if not treated. Oral sulfonamides taken in the last few weeks of pregnancy may lead to neonatal hyperbilirubinemia and kernicterus. |
| Cystitis (lower UTI): Causative organisms same as for ASB | Dysuria, urgency, frequency; low-grade fever and hematuria may occur. Urine culture (clean catch) shows ↑ leukocytes. Presence of $10^5$ (100,000) or more colonies bacteria per ml urine. | Same. | If not treated, infection may ascend and lead to acute pyelonephritis. |
| Acute pyelonephritis: Causative organisms same as for ASB | Sudden onset. Chills, high fever, flank pain. Nausea, vomiting, malaise. May have decreased urine output, severe colicky pain, dehydration. Increased diastolic BP positive fluorescent antibody (FA) test, low creatinine clearance. Marked bacteremia in urine culture, pyuria, WBC casts. | Hospitalization; IV antibiotic therapy. Other antibiotics considered safe during pregnancy include carbenicillin, methenamine, cephalosporins. Catheterization if output is ↓. Supportive therapy for comfort. Follow-up urine cultures are necessary. | Increased risk of premature birth and intrauterine growth restriction (IUGR). These antibiotics interfere with urinary estriol levels and can cause false interpretations of estriol levels during pregnancy. |
| **VAGINAL INFECTIONS** | | | |
| Vulvovaginal candidiasis (yeast infections): *Candida albicans* | Often thick, white, curdy discharge, severe itching, dysuria, dyspareunia. Diagnosis based on presence of hyphae and spores in a wet-mount preparation of vaginal secretions. | Intravaginal insertion of miconazole or clotrimazole suppositories at bedtime for 1 week. Cream may be prescribed for topical application to the vulva if necessary. | If the infection is present at birth and the fetus is born vaginally, the fetus may contract thrush. |
| Bacterial vaginosis: *Gardnerella vaginalis* | Thin, watery, yellow-gray discharge with foul odor often described as "fishy." Wet-mount preparation reveals "clue cells." Application of potassium hydroxide (KOH) to a specimen of vaginal secretions produces a pronounced fishy odor. | Nonpregnant women treated with oral metronidazole (Flagyl). In second and third trimesters, oral metronidazole administered in a lower dose; clindamycin orally and metronidazole vaginal gel are alternatives (CDC, 1998). | Metronidazole has potential teratogenic effects when used in the first trimester. Possible ↑ risk of PROM and preterm birth. Confirmatory studies needed (CDC, 1998). |
| Trichomoniasis: *Trichomonas vaginalis* | Occasionally asymptomatic. May have frothy greenish gray vaginal discharge, pruritus, urinary symptoms. Strawberry patches may be visible on vaginal walls or cervix. Wet-mount preparation of vaginal secretions shows motile flagellated trichomonads. | During early pregnancy symptoms may be controlled with clotrimazole vaginal suppositories. Both partners are treated, but no adequate treatment exists. After first trimester, a single 2-g dose of metronidazole may be used (CDC, 1998). | Metromidazole has potential teratogenic effects. Associated with ↑ risk of PROM and preterm birth (CDC, 1998). |

*(Continued)*

## TABLE 13–3 Infections that Put Pregnancy at Risk *continued*

| Condition and Causative Organism | Signs and Symptoms | Treatment | Implications for Pregnancy |
|---|---|---|---|
| **SEXUALLY TRANSMITTED INFECTIONS** | | | |
| Chlamydial infection: *Chlamydia trachomatis* | Women are often asymptomatic. Symptoms may include thin or purulent discharge, urinary burning and frequency, or lower abdominal pain. Lab test available to detect monoclonal antibodies specific for *Chlamydia.* | Although nonpregnant women are treated with tetracycline, it may permanently discolor fetal teeth. Thus pregnant women are treated with erythromycin ethyl succinate. | Infant of woman with untreated chlamydial infection may develop newborn conjunctivitis, which can be treated with erythromycin eye ointment (but not silver nitrate). Infant may also develop chlamydial pneumonia. May be responsible for premature labor and fetal death. |
| Syphilis: *Treponema pallidum,* a spirochete | Primary stage: chancre, slight fever, malaise. Chancre lasts about 4 weeks, then disappears. Secondary stage: occurs 6 weeks to 6 months after infection. Skin eruptions (condyloma lata); also symptoms of acute arthritis, liver enlargement, iritis, chronic sore throat with hoarseness. Diagnosed by blood tests such as VDRL, RPR, FTA, ABS. Dark-field examination or spirochetes may also be done. | For syphilis less than 1 year in duration: 2.4 million U benzathine penicillin G IM. For syphilis of more than 1 year's duration: 2.4 million U benzathine penicillin G once a week for 3 weeks. Sexual partners should also be screened and treated. | Syphilis can be passed transplacentally to the fetus. If untreated, one of the following can occur: second-trimester abortion, stillborn infant at term, congenitally infected infant, uninfected live infant. |
| Gonorrhea: *Neisseria gonorrhoeae* | Majority of women asymptomatic; disease often diagnosed during routine prenatal cervical culture. If symptoms are present they may include purulent vaginal discharge, dysuria, urinary frequency, inflammation and swelling of the vulva. Cervix may appear eroded. | Nonpregnant women are treated with cefixime orally or ceftriaxone IM plus doxycycline. Pregnant woman are treated with ceftriaxone plus erythromycin (CDC, 1998). If the woman is allergic to ceftriaxone, spectinomycin is used. All sexual partners are also treated. | Infection at time of birth may cause ophthalmia neonatorum in the newborn. |
| Condyloma acuminata: caused by a papovavirus | Soft, grayish pink lesions on the vulva, vagina, cervix, or anus. | Podophyllin not used during pregnancy. Trichloroacetic acid, liquid nitrogen, or cryotherapy $CO_2$ laser therapy done under colposcopy is also successful (CDC, 1998). | Possible teratogenic effect of podophyllin. Large doses have been associated with fetal death. |

# Chapter Review

## CHAPTER HIGHLIGHTS

- Several health problems associated with bleeding arise from the pregnancy itself, such as spontaneous abortion, ectopic pregnancy, and gestational trophoblastic disease. The nurse needs to be alert to early signs of these situations, to guard the woman against heavy bleeding and shock, to facilitate the medical treatment, and to provide educational and emotional support.
- Ectopic pregnancy is the implantation of a fertilized ovum in a site other than the uterus. Treatment may be medical, using IM methotrexate, or surgical.
- Incompetent cervix, the premature dilatation of the cervix, is the most common cause of second-trimester abortion. It is treated surgically with a Shirodkar-Barter operation (cerclage), which involves placing a purse-string suture in the cervix to keep it closed.
- Hyperemesis gravidarum, excessive vomiting during pregnancy, may cause fluid and electrolyte imbalance, dehydration, and signs of starvation in the mother and, if severe enough, death of the fetus. Treatment is aimed at controlling the vomiting, correcting fluid and electrolyte imbalance, correcting dehydration, and improving nutritional status.
- Both premature rupture of the membranes and preterm labor place the fetus at risk. Women with PROM and no signs of infection are managed conservatively with bed rest and careful monitoring of fetal well-being. Women with a history of preterm labor are often placed on home fetal-monitoring programs. If preterm labor develops, tocolytics are often effective in stopping labor, but they have associated side effects.
- Hypertension may exist before pregnancy or, more often, may develop during pregnancy. Preeclampsia can lead to growth retardation for the fetus, and if untreated it may lead to convulsions (eclampsia) and even death for the mother and fetus. A woman's understanding of the disease process helps motivate her to maintain the required rest periods in the left lateral recumbent position. Antihypertensive or anticonvulsive drugs may be part of the therapy.
- Rh incompatibility can exist when an Rh-negative woman and an Rh-positive partner conceive a child who is Rh positive. The use of Rh immune globulin has greatly decreased the incidence of severe sequelae due to Rh because the drug "tricks" the body into thinking antibodies have been produced in response to the Rh antigen.
- The impact of surgery, trauma, or battering on the pregnant woman and her fetus is related to timing in the pregnancy, seriousness of the situation, and other factors influencing the situation.
- Physical violence often begins or continues during pregnancy. The nurse needs to be alert for signs of abuse, including bruising or injury to the breasts, abdomen, or genitalia. The woman should be given information about female partner abuse and about community resources available to assist her.
- TORCH is an acronym standing for toxoplasmosis, rubella, cytomegalovirus, and herpes, all of which pose a grave threat to the fetus.
- Sexually transmitted infections pose less of a threat to the fetus if detected and treated quickly.

# CHAPTER REFERENCES


Aerts, M., & Iams, J. D. (1999). Prevention of spontaneous preterm birth. *Contemporary OB/GYN, 44*(5), 128–136.

American Academy of Pediatrics and American College of Obstetricians and Gynecologists. (1997). Obstetric complications. In *Guidelines for prenatal care* (4th ed, pp. 127–146). Elk Grove Village, IL: Author.

American College of Obstetricians and Gynecologists. (1996). *Home uterine activity monitoring* (ACOG Committee Opinion No. 172). Washington, DC: Author.

American College of Obstetricians and Gynecologists. (1998a). *Medical management of tubal pregnancy* (ACOG Practice Bulletin No. 3). Washington, DC: Author.

American College of Obstetricians and Gynecologists. (1998b). *Obstetric aspects of trauma management* (ACOG Educational Bulletin No. 251). Washington, DC: Author.

American College of Obstetricians and Gynecologists. (1998c). *Premature rupture of membranes* (ACOG Practice Bulletin No. 1). Washington, DC: Author.

American College of Obstetricians and Gynecologists. (1999a). *Domestic violence* (ACOG Educational Bulletin No. 257). Washington, DC: Author.

American College of Obstetricians and Gynecologists. (1999b). *Management of herpes in pregnancy* (ACOG Practice Bulletin No. 8). Washington, DC: Author.

Branch, D. W., & Porter, T. F. (1999). Hypertensive disorders of pregnancy. In J. R. Scott, P. J. DiSaia, C. B. Hammond, & W. N. Spellacy (Eds.), *Danforth's obstetrics and gynecology* (8th ed.). Philadelphia: Lippincott Williams & Wilkins, 309–326.

Carter, S. (1999). Overview of common obstetric bleeding disorders. *Nurse Practitioner, 24*(3), 50–73.

Centers for Disease Control and Prevention. (1998). 1998 sexually transmitted disease treatment guidelines. *Morbidity and Mortality Weekly Report, 47*(RR-1), 1–116.

Chez, R. A. (1999). Prevention of preterm birth: Putting three new tools into practice. *Contemporary OB/GYN, 44*(6), 53–78.

Creasy, R. K., & Iams, J. D. (1999). Preterm labor and delivery. In R. K. Creasy & R. Resnik (Eds.), *Maternal-fetal medicine* (4th ed.). Philadelphia: Saunders, 498–531.

Cunningham, F. G., MacDonald, P. C., Gant, N. F., Leveno, K. J., Gilstrap, L. C., III, Hankins, G. D. V., & Clark, S. L. (1997). *Williams obstetrics* (20th ed.). Stamford, CT: Appleton & Lange.

Guinn, D., & Lee, M. J. (2000). Multiple courses of antenatal corticosteroids: New concerns. *Contemporary OB/GYN, 45*(2), 63–69.

Hammond, C. B.(1999). Gestational trophoblastic neoplasms. In J. R. Scott, P. J. DiSaia, C. B. Hammond, & W. N. Spellacy (Eds.), *Danforth's obstetrics and gynecology* (8th ed.). Philadelphia: Lippincott Williams & Wilkins, 927–938.

Iams, J. (1996a). Preterm birth. In S. G. Gabbe, J. R. Niebyl, & J. L. Simpson (Eds.). *Obstetrics: Normal and problem pregnancies* (3rd ed.). New York: Churchill-Livingstone, 743–820.

Iams, J. (1996b). Tocolysis. In J. T. Queenan & J. C. Hobbins (Eds.), *Protocols for high risk pregnancies.* Cambridge, MA: Blackwell, 539–546.

Lopez, A., Dietz, V. J., Wilson, M., Navin, T. R., & Jones, J. L. (2000, March 31). Preventing congenital toxoplasmosis. *Morbidity and Mortality Weekly Report, 49*(RR02), 57–75.

Martin, J. N., & Magann, E. F. (1999). High-dose dexamethasone: A promising therapeutic option for HELLP. *Contemporary OB/GYN, 44*(11), 55–64.

McFarlane, J., Parker, B., Soeken, K., Silva, C., & Reed, S. (1999). Severity of abuse before and during pregnancy for African American, Hispanic, and Anglo women, *Journal of Nurse-Midwifery, 44*(2), 139–144.

Mills, J. L., DerSimonian, R., Raymond, E., Morrow, J. D., Roberts, L. J., II, Clemens, J. D., Hauth, J. C., Catalano, P., Sibai, B., Curet, L. B., & Levine, R. J. (1999). Prostacyclin and thromboxane changes predating clinical onset of preeclampsia. *JAMA, 282*(4), 356–362.

Minkoff, H. L. (1999). Human immunodeficiency virus and other perinatal infections. In J. R. Scott, P. J. DiSaia, C. B. Hammond, & W. N. Spellacy (Eds.), *Danforth's obstetrics and gynecology* (8th ed.). Philadelphia: Lippincott Williams & Wilkins, 393–406.

National Institutes of Health. (1994, February 28–March 2). *Effect of corticosteroids for fetal maturation on perinatal outcomes.* National Institutes of Health Consensus Development Conference Statement.

Oshiro, B. T. (1999). Cytomegalovirus infection in pregnancy. *Contemporary OB/GYN, 44*(11), 16–24.

Parsons, M. T., & Spellacy, W. N. (1999a). Premature rupture of membranes. In J. R. Scott, P. J. DiSaia, C. B. Hammond, & W. N. Spellacy (Eds.), *Danforth's obstetrics and gynecology* (8th ed.). Philadelphia: Lippincott Williams & Wilkins, 269–278.

Parsons, M. T., & Spellacy, W. N. (1999b). Preterm labor. In J. R. Scott, P. J. DiSaia, C. B. Hammond, & W. N. Spellacy (Eds.), *Danforth's obstetrics and gynecology* (8th ed.). Philadelphia: Lippincott Williams & Wilkins, 257–268.

Roberts, J. M. (1999). Pregnancy-related hypertension. In R. K. Creasy & R. Resnik (Eds.), *Maternal-fetal medicine* (4th ed.). Philadelphia: Saunders, 833–872.

Scott, J. R. (1999). Early pregnancy loss. In J. R. Scott, P. J. DiSaia, C. B. Hammond, & W. N. Spellacy (Eds.), *Danforth's obstetrics and gynecology* (8th ed.). Philadelphia: Lippincott Williams & Wilkins, 143–154.

Scott, J. R., & Branch, D. W. (1999). Immunologic disorders in pregnancy. In J. R. Scott, P. J. DiSaia, C. B. Hammond, & W. N. Spellacy (Eds.), *Danforth's obstetrics and gynecology* (8th ed.). Philadelphia: Lippincott Williams & Wilkins, 363–392.

Sibai, B. M. (1996). Hypertension in pregnancy. In S. G. Gabbe, J. R. Niebyl, & J. L. Simpson (Eds.), *Obstetrics: Normal and problem pregnancies* (3rd ed.). New York: Churchill Livingstone, 935–996.

Silver, H. (1996). Hypertensive disorders. In K. R. Niswander & A. T. Evans (Eds.), *Manual of obstetrics.* Boston: Little, Brown, 283–295.

Simon, E. P., & Schwartz, J. (1999). Medical hypnosis for hyperemesis gravidarum. *Birth, 26*(4), 248–253.

Tulandi, T. (1999). New protocols for ectopic pregnancy. *Contemporary OB/GYN, 44*(10), 42–55.

Vermillion, S. T., & Scardo, J. A. (2000). Using indomethacin as a tocolytic. *Contemporary OB/GYN 45*(7), 102–108.

Wenstrom, K. D., & Malee, M. P. (1999). Medical and surgical complications of pregnancy. In J. R. Scott, P. J. DiSaia, C. B. Hammond, & W. N. Spellacy (Eds.), *Danforth's obstetrics and gynecology* (8th ed.). Philadelphia: Lippincott Williams & Wilkins, 327–362.


## CONTEMPORARY MATERNAL-NEWBORN NURSING ON-LINE

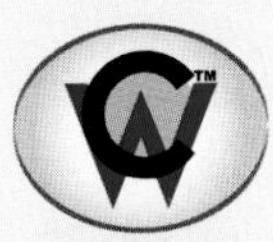

Additional interactive resources, including animations and video, for this chapter can be found on the Companion Website at http://www.prenhall.com/ladewig. Click on Chapter 13 and "Begin" to select the activities for this chapter.

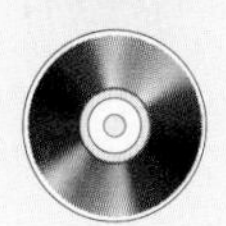

For NCLEX review questions and an audio glossary, access the accompanying CD-ROM in this book.

Chapter 14

# Assessment of Fetal Well-Being

*What makes my job special is the relationships I develop with my patients. Many of the expectant mothers I work with begin coming to our office in early pregnancy and continue on a regular basis until they give birth. I know that some of the diagnostic tests we do can be intimidating, and it's my responsibility to help make those tests understandable. But more than that, I want to really connect with my patients so that when they have questions or fears, I can be the one they are comfortable enough with to express those concerns.*

—Perinatal and Genetics Office Nurse

## KEY TERMS



## OBJECTIVES

- Outline pertinent information to be discussed with the woman regarding her own assessment of fetal activity and methods of recording fetal activity.
- List indications for ultrasonic examination and the information that can be obtained from this procedure.
- Compare and contrast the procedure and information obtained from Doppler velocimetry, nonstress test, contraction stress test, and biophysical profile tests.
- Discuss the use of amniocentesis as a diagnostic tool.
- Describe the tests that can be done on amniotic fluid.

The past few decades have produced a notable increase in the number of techniques used to assess fetal well-being. From the relatively simple maternal assessment of fetal movement to more complex diagnostic tests guided by ultrasound, each technique is used to obtain accurate and helpful data about the growing fetus. For example, specialized diagnostic tests can provide information about the normal growth of the fetus, the presence of congenital anomalies, the location of the placenta, and fetal lung maturity (Table 14–1). At times just one test is done, and in other circumstances a combination of testing is needed.

Some of these diagnostic techniques pose risks to the fetus and possibly to the pregnant woman, and the risk to both should be considered before the decision to perform the test is made. The health care provider must be certain that the advantages outweigh the potential risks and added expense. In addition, the diagnostic accuracy and applicability of these tests may vary. Certainly not all high-risk pregnancies require the same tests. Conditions that indicate a pregnancy at risk include the following:

- Maternal age less than 16 or more than 35 years
- Chronic maternal hypertension, preeclampsia, diabetes mellitus, or heart disease
- Presence of Rh isoimmunization
- A maternal history of unexplained stillbirth
- Suspected intrauterine growth restriction (IUGR)
- Pregnancy prolonged past 42 weeks' gestation
- Multiple gestation

See Chapter 7 for further discussion of prenatal at-risk factors and Chapters 12 and 13 for descriptions of various conditions that may threaten the successful completion of pregnancy.

**TABLE 14–1 Summary of Screening and Diagnostic Tests**

| *Goal* | *Test* | *Timing* |
|---|---|---|
| To validate the pregnancy | Ultrasound: gestational sac volume | 5 and 6 weeks after last menstrual period (LMP) by endovaginal ultrasound |
| To determine how advanced the pregnancy is | Ultrasound: crown–rump length<br>Ultrasound: biparietal diameter, femur length, abdomen circumference | 6 to 10 weeks' gestation<br>13 to 40 weeks' gestation |
| To identify normal growth of the fetus | Ultrasound: biparietal diameter<br>Ultrasound: head/abdomen ratio<br>Ultrasound: estimated fetal weight | Most useful from 20 to 30 weeks' gestation<br>13 to 40 weeks' gestation<br>About 24 to 40 weeks' gestation |
| To detect congenital anomalies and problems | Ultrasound<br>Chorionic villus sampling<br>Amniocentesis<br>Fetoscopy<br>Percutaneous blood sampling<br>Triple test or quadruple test | 18 to 40 weeks' gestation<br>8 to 12 weeks' gestation<br>16 to 18 weeks' gestation<br>18 weeks' gestation<br>Second and third trimesters<br>About 10 weeks' gestation |
| To localize the placenta | Ultrasound | Usually in third trimester or before amniocentesis |
| To assess fetal status | Biophysical profile<br>Maternal assessment of fetal activity<br>Nonstress test<br>Contraction stress test | Approximately 28 weeks to birth<br>About 28 weeks to birth<br>Approximately 28 weeks to birth<br>After 28 weeks |
| To diagnose cardiac problems | Fetal echocardiography | Second and third trimesters |
| To assess fetal lung maturity | Amniocentesis<br>L/S ratio<br>Phosphatidylglycerol<br>Phosphatidylcholine | 33 to 40 weeks<br>33 weeks to birth<br>33 weeks to birth<br>33 weeks to birth |
| To obtain more information about breech presentation | Ultrasound | Just before labor is anticipated or during labor |

**TABLE 14–2 Sample Nursing Approaches to Pretest Teaching**

Assess whether the woman knows the reason the screening or diagnostic test is being recommended.
  Examples:
  "Has your doctor or nurse-midwife told you why this test is necessary?"
  "Sometimes tests are done for many different reasons. Can you tell me why you are having this test?"
  "What is your understanding about what the test will show?"
Provide an opportunity for questions.
  Examples:
  "Do you have any questions about the test?"
  "Is there anything that is not clear to you?"
Explain the test procedure, paying particular attention to any preparation the woman needs prior to the test.
  Example:
  "The test that has been ordered for you is designed to . . ." (Add specific information about the particular test. Give the explanation in simple language.)
Validate the woman's understanding of the preparation.
  Example:
  "Tell me what you will have to do to get ready for this test."
Give permission for the woman to continue to ask questions if needed.
  Example:
  "I'll be with you during the test. If you have any questions at any time, please don't hesitate to ask."

Nursing care for the woman who is undergoing diagnostic testing focuses on outcomes to ensure that she understands the reasons for the test, understands the test results, and has had support during the test (see Table 14–2). In addition, other objectives include completing the tests without complication and ensuring that the safety of the mother and her unborn child has been maintained.

## Maternal Assessment of Fetal Activity

Clinicians now generally agree that vigorous fetal activity provides reassurance of fetal well-being and that marked decrease in activity or cessation of movement may indicate possible fetal compromise (or even death) requiring immediate follow-up (Richardson & Gagnon, 1999). Although there is considerable variation among individuals, the number of daily movements during the third trimester is a maximum of 575 until 32 weeks gestation and then decreases to an average of 280 (12 to 15 gross fetal body movements per hour) (Jasper, 2000). In women with a multiple gestation, daily fetal movements are significantly higher. During the last few weeks of gestation the fetus spends 60% to 70% of its time in an active sleep state (Jasper, 2000).

Fetal activity is affected by many factors, including time of day, sleep states of the fetus, sound, blood glucose levels, cigarette smoking, and drugs. The expectant mother's perception of fetal movements and her commitment to completing a fetal movement record may vary. When a woman understands the purpose of the assessment, how to complete the form, whom to call with questions, and what to report—and has the opportunity for follow-up during each visit—she generally sees completing the fetal activity record as an important activity. The nurse is available to answer questions and clarify areas of concern. (See further discussion and Teaching Guide: What to Tell the Pregnant Woman about Assessing Fetal Activity, in Chapter 9.)

## Ultrasound

Valuable information about the fetus may be obtained from **ultrasound** testing. Intermittent ultrasonic waves (high-frequency sound waves) are transmitted by an alternating current to a transducer, which is applied to the woman's abdomen. The ultrasonic waves deflect off tissues within the woman's abdomen, showing structures of varying densities (Figures 14–1 and 14–2♦).

Diagnostic ultrasound has several advantages. It is noninvasive, painless, and nonradiating to both the woman and the fetus, and it has no known harmful effects to either. Serial studies (several ultrasound tests done over a span of time) may be done for assessment and comparison. Soft tissue masses (such as tumors) can be differentiated, the fetus can be visualized, fetal growth can be followed (especially in the presence of multiple gestation), and a number of potential problems can be averted (Barnhart, Simhan, & Kamelle, 1999). In addition, the ultrasonographer or physician obtains results immediately.

Future research in fetal well-being will be generated and enhanced by the use of the *three-dimensional ultrasound.* It is believed that this new technology will produce more accurate fetal growth and weight assessments (Zelop, 2000).

### Procedures

The two most common methods of ultrasound scanning are transabdominal and endovaginal.

#### Transabdominal Ultrasound

In the transabdominal approach, a transducer is moved across the woman's abdomen. The woman is often scanned with a full bladder; when the bladder is full, the examiner can assess other structures, especially the vagina and cervix, in relation to the bladder. The ability to see the lower portion of

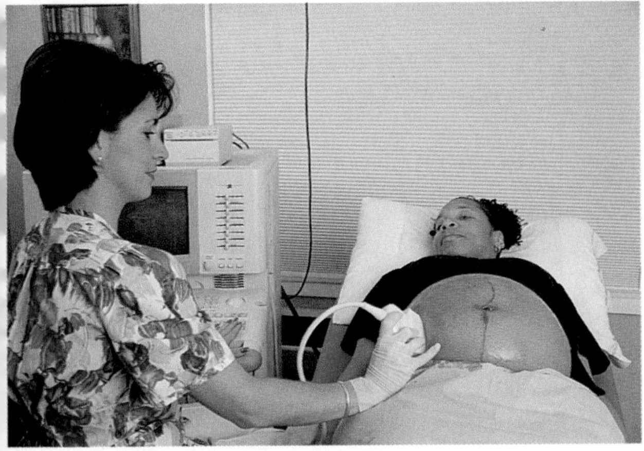

FIGURE 14–1 ♦ Ultrasound scanning permits visualization of the fetus in utero.

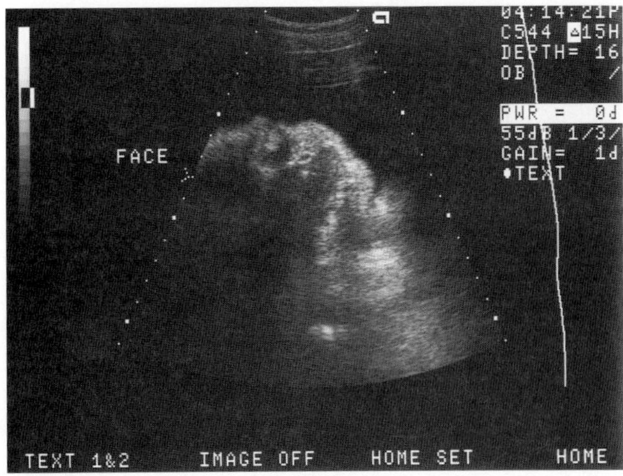


FIGURE 14–2 ♦ Ultrasound of fetal face.

the uterus and cervix is particularly important when vaginal bleeding is noted and placenta previa is the suspected cause. The woman is advised to drink 1 to 1.5 quarts of water approximately 2 hours before the examination, and she is asked to refrain from emptying her bladder. If the bladder is not sufficiently filled, she is asked to drink three to four (8-oz) glasses of water and is rescanned 30 to 45 minutes later. Mineral oil or a transmission gel is generously spread over the woman's abdomen, and the sonographer slowly moves a transducer over the abdomen to obtain a picture of the contents of the uterus. Ultrasound testing takes 20 to 30 minutes. The woman may feel discomfort due to pressure applied over a full bladder. In addition, if the woman lies on her back during the test, shortness of breath can develop. This may be relieved by elevating her upper body during the test.

### Endovaginal Ultrasound

The endovaginal approach uses a probe inserted into the vagina. Once inserted, the endovaginal probe is close to the structures being imaged and so produces a clearer, more defined image. The improved images obtained by endovaginal ultrasound have enabled sonographers to identify structures and fetal characteristics earlier in pregnancy (Owen, Neely, & Northen, 1999). Internal visualization can also be used as a predictor for preterm birth in high-risk cases (Berghella, Daly, Tolosa, et al., 1999). Use of the ultrasound to detect shortened cervical length or funneling (a cone-shaped indentation in the cervical os) is helpful in predicting preterm labor, especially in women who have a history of preterm birth (Andrews, Copper, Hauth, et al., 2000).

After the procedure is fully explained to the woman, she is prepared in the same manner as for a pelvic examination: in the lithotomy position, with appropriate drapes to provide privacy and a female attendant in the room. It is important that her buttocks are at the end of the table so that, once inserted, the probe can be moved in various directions. A small, lightweight vaginal transducer is covered with a specially fitted sterile sheath, a condom, or one finger of a glove. Ultrasound coupling gel is then applied to the covering, making insertion into the vagina easier and providing a medium for enhancing the ultrasound image. The endovaginal procedure can be accomplished with an empty bladder, and most women do not feel discomfort during the exam. The probe is smaller than a speculum, so insertion is usually completed with ease. The woman may feel the movement of the probe during the exam as various structures are imaged. Some women may want to insert the probe themselves to enhance their comfort, whereas others would feel embarrassed even to be asked. The certified nurse-midwife, physician, or ultrasonographer offers the choice based on the rapport she or he has with the woman.

## Clinical Applications

Ultrasound testing can be of benefit in the following ways (Barnhart et al., 1999; Berghella et al., 1999):

- Early identification of pregnancy. (Pregnancy may be detected as early as the fifth or sixth week after the last menstrual period [LMP].)
- Observation of fetal heartbeat and fetal breathing movements (FBMs). FBMs have been observed as early as the 11th week of gestation.
- Identification of more than one embryo or fetus.
- Measurement of the biparietal diameter of the fetal head or the fetal femur length. These measurements help determine the gestational age of the fetus and identify IUGR.

- Clinical estimations of birth weight. This assessment helps to identify macrosomia (infants greater than 4000 g at birth). Macrosomia has been identified as a predictor of birth-related trauma (O'Reilly-Green & Divon, 2000).
- Detection of fetal anomalies such as anencephaly and hydrocephalus.
- Examination of fetal cardiac structures *(echocardiography).*
- Identification of *amniotic fluid index (AFI).* The maternal abdomen is divided into quadrants. The umbilicus is used to divide the upper and lower sections, and the linea nigra divides the right and left sections. The vertical diameter of the largest amniotic fluid pocket in each quadrant is measured. All measurements are totaled to obtain the AFI in centimeters. Women with an AFI of more than 20 cm are considered to have hydramnios, and women with less than 5 cm at term are considered to have oligohydramnios. Both hydramnios and oligohydramnios are associated with increased risk to the fetus (Panting-Kemp, Nguyen, Chang, et al., 1999).
- Location of the placenta. The placenta is located before amniocentesis to avoid puncturing the placenta. Ultrasound is also used to determine the presence of placenta previa.
- Placental grading. As the fetus matures, the placenta calcifies. These changes can be detected by ultrasound and graded according to the degree of calcification (Jasper, 2000).
- Detection of fetal death. Inability to visualize the fetal heart beating and the separation of the bones in the fetal head are signs of fetal death.
- Determination of fetal position and presentation.
- Accompanying procedures such as amniocentesis, periumbilical blood sampling, intrauterine procedures, and other procedures to be discussed shortly.

### Risks of Ultrasound

Ultrasound has been used clinically for over 40 years, and to date no clinical studies verify harmful effects to the mother or the fetus or newborn. The use of ultrasound in pregnancy has spanned nearly three generations. Many pregnant patients themselves received diagnostic ultrasound in utero with no adverse effect (Manning, 1999).

### Nursing Care Management

It is important for the nurse to ascertain whether the woman understands why the ultrasound is being suggested. The nurse provides an opportunity for the woman to ask questions and acts as an advocate if there are questions or concerns that need to be addressed before the ultrasound examination. The nurse explains the preparation needed and ensures that adequate preparation is done. After the test is completed, the nurse can assist with clarifying or interpreting test results for the woman and her partner.

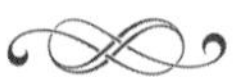

## Doppler Blood Flow Studies (Umbilical Velocimetry)

Umbilical velocimetry, a noninvasive ultrasound test, measures blood flow changes that occur in maternal and fetal circulation in order to assess placental function. An ultrasound beam, like that provided by the pocket Doppler (a handheld ultrasound device), is directed at the umbilical artery (in some cases a maternal vessel such as the arcuate can also be used). The signal is reflected off the red blood cells moving within the vessels and creates a "picture" (waveform) that looks like a series of waves (Figures 14–3 and 14–4♦). The highest-velocity peak of the waves is the systolic measurement, and the lowest point is the diastolic velocity. To interpret the waveforms, the systolic (S) peak is divided by the end-diastolic (D) component. This calculation is called the S/D ratio. The normal S/D ratio is below 2.6 by 26 weeks' gestation and below 3 at term. When uteroplacental perfusion decreases (because of narrowing of the vessels), it causes an increase in placental bed resistance and a decrease in diastolic flow, resulting in an elevated S/D ratio (Trudinger, 1999). Abnormal elevations are considered to be 3.0 and above (Jasper, 2000). Doppler blood flow studies are helpful in assessing and managing pregnancies with suspected uteroplacental insufficiency before asphyxia occurs (Jasper, 2000).

Doppler blood flow studies are relatively easy to obtain. The woman lies supine with a wedge under the left hip (to promote uteroplacental perfusion). Warmed transducer gel is applied to the abdomen, and a pulsed-wave Doppler device is used to ascertain the blood flow. The Doppler flow study takes about 15 to 20 minutes. Doppler flow studies can be initiated at 16 to 18 weeks' gestation and are then scheduled at regular intervals for women at risk.

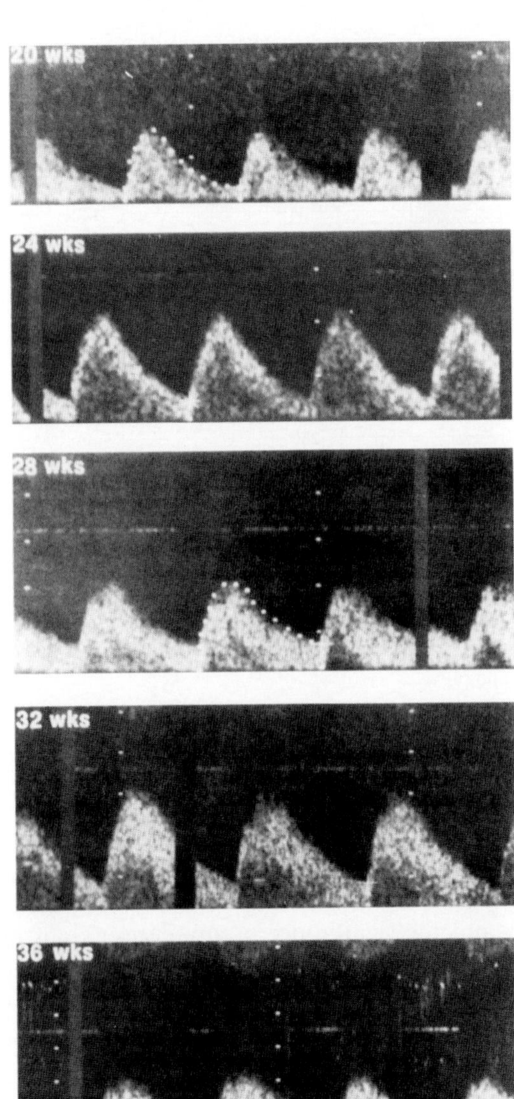


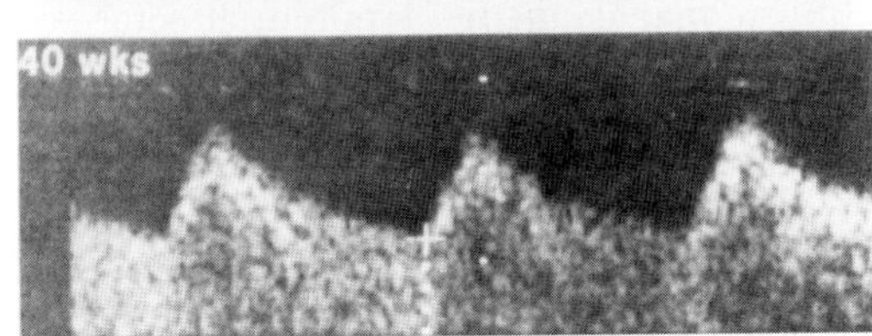


FIGURE 14–3 ♦ Serial studies of the umbilical artery velocity waveforms in a normal pregnancy from one client. *Source:* Cundiff, J. L., Haybrich, K. L., & Hinzman, H. G. (1990). Umbilical artery Doppler flow studies during pregnancy. *Journal of Obstetric, Gynecologic, and Neonatal Nursing,* 19(6), 475, Figure 3.

## Nonstress Test

The **nonstress test (NST),** a widely used method of evaluating fetal status, may be used alone or as part of a more comprehensive diagnostic assessment called a *biophysical profile (BPP).* The nonstress test is based on the knowledge that when the fetus has adequate oxygenation and an intact central nervous system, there are accelerations

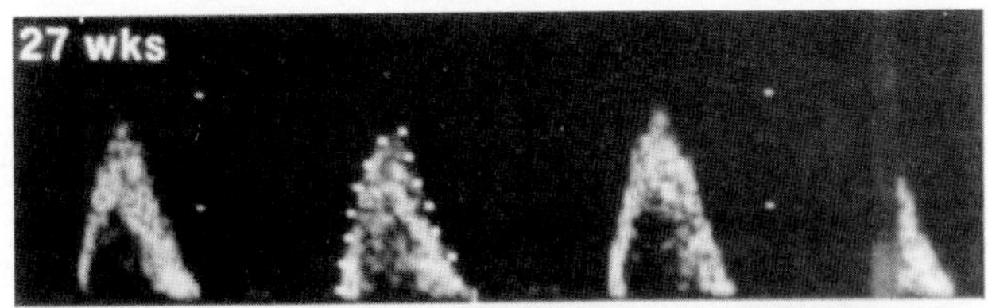


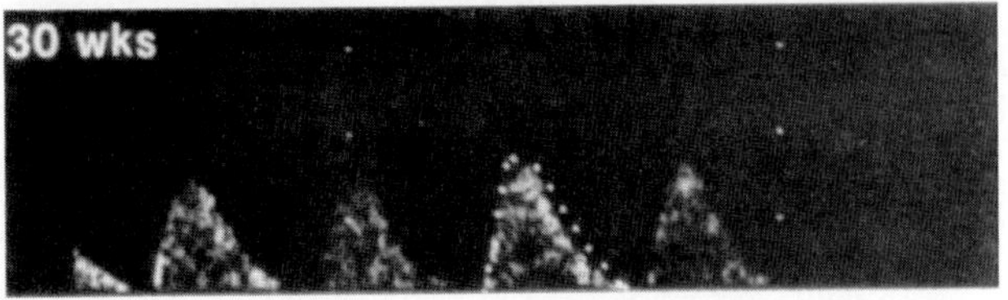


FIGURE 14–4 ♦ Two examples of abnormal umbilical artery velocity waveforms taken from a client with intrauterine growth restriction. *Source:* Cundiff, J. L., Haybrich, K. L., & Hinzman, H. G. (1990). Umbilical artery Doppler flow studies during pregnancy. *Journal of Obstetric, Gynecologic, and Neonatal Nursing,* 19(6), 475, Figure 4.

of the fetal heart rate (FHR) with fetal movement. An NST requires an electronic fetal monitor to observe and record these fetal heart rate accelerations (see discussion of acceleration in Chapter 16). A nonreactive NST is fairly consistent in identifying at-risk fetuses (Murray, 1997). The advantages of the NST are as follows:

- It is quick to perform, permits easy interpretation, and is inexpensive.
- It can be done in an office or clinic setting.
- There are no known side effects.

The disadvantages of the NST include the following:

- It is sometimes difficult to obtain a suitable tracing.
- The woman has to remain relatively still for at least 20 minutes.

### Procedure for NST

The test can be done with the woman in a reclining chair or in bed in a semi-Fowler's or side-lying position. Research has shown that the semi-Fowler's position may shorten the time needed to conduct the NST (Nathan, Haberman, Burgess, et al., 2000). An electronic fetal monitor is used to obtain a tracing of the fetal heart rate (FHR) and fetal movement (FM). The examiner puts two elastic belts on the woman's abdomen. One belt holds a device that detects uterine or fetal movement; the other belt holds a device that detects the FHR. As the NST is done, each fetal movement is documented, so that associated or simultaneous FHR changes can be evaluated. Women with a high-risk factor will probably begin having NSTs at 30 to 32 weeks' gestation and at frequent intervals for the remainder of the pregnancy.

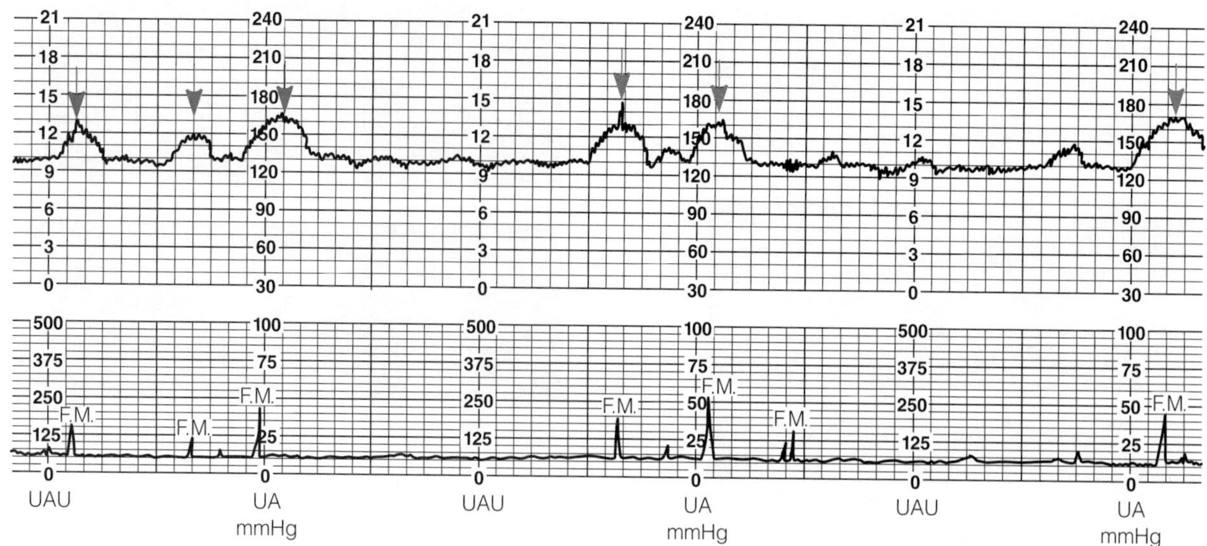


FIGURE 14–5 ♦ Example of a reactive nonstress test (NST). Accelerations of 15 bpm lasting 15 seconds with each fetal movement (FM). Top of strip shows FHR; bottom of strip shows uterine activity tracing. Note that FHR increases (above the baseline) at least 15 beats and remains at that rate for at least 15 seconds before returning to the former baseline.

## Interpretation of NST Results

The results of the NST are interpreted as follows:

- *Reactive test.* A reactive NST shows at least two accelerations of FHR with fetal movements of 15 beats per minute, lasting 15 seconds or more, over 20 minutes (Figure 14–5♦). This is the desired result. (See Key Facts to Remember: Nonstress Test.)
- *Nonreactive test.* In a nonreactive test, the reactive criteria are not met. For example, the accelerations are not as much as 15 beats per minute or do not last 15 seconds (Figure 14–6♦).
- *Unsatisfactory test.* An NST is unsatisfactory if the data cannot be interpreted or there was inadequate fetal activity.

It is important that anyone who performs the NST understand the significance of any decelerations of the FHR during testing. If decelerations are noted, the certified nurse-midwife or physician should be notified for further evaluation of fetal status. (See Chapter 16 for further discussion of FHR decelerations.)

## Clinical Management

The clinical management of potential fetal stress or distress may vary somewhat among clinicians depend-

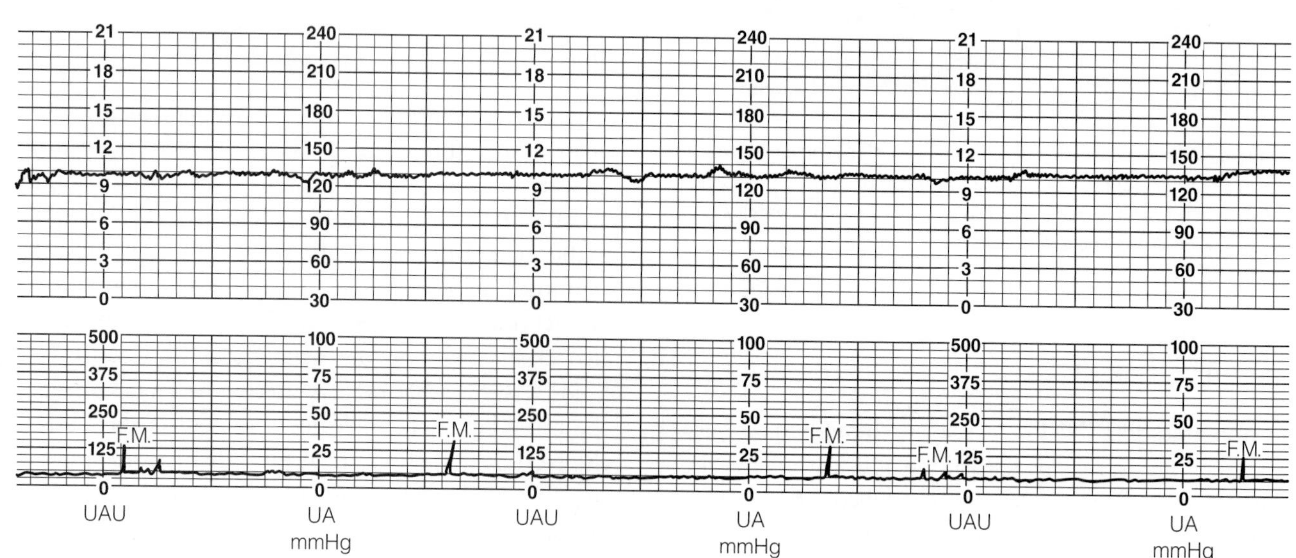


FIGURE 14–6 ♦ Example of a nonreactive NST. There are no accelerations of FHR with FM. Baseline FHR is 130 bpm. The tracing of uterine activity is on the bottom of the strip.

## KEY FACTS TO REMEMBER

### *Nonstress Test*

Diagnostic value: Demonstrates fetus's ability to respond to its environment by acceleration of FHR with movement.

Results:

- Reactive test: Accelerations (at least 2) of 15 bpm above the baseline, lasting 15 sec in a 20-min window, are present, indicating fetal well-being.
- Nonreactive test: Accelerations are not present, indicating that the fetus is at risk or asleep.

ing on the clinical judgment of the care provider. One commonly used protocol is as follows: If the NST is reactive in less than 30 minutes, the test is concluded and rescheduled as indicated by the high-risk condition that is present; if it is nonreactive, the test time is extended for 30 minutes at a time until the results are reactive, and then the test is rescheduled as indicated. If the FHR remains nonreactive, additional testing (such as diagnostic ultrasound and BPP) or immediate birth is considered; if the NST is nonreactive and spontaneous decelerations of the FHR are present, diagnostic ultrasound and BPP are performed and birth is recommended (Figure 14–7♦). Many testing guidelines vary in frequency, recommending a retest either once or twice a week, depending upon the at-risk condition that exists. In some situations, such as preterm premature rupture of membranes, testing may be done daily (Jasper, 2000; Parer, 1999).

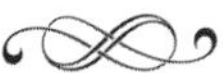

## NURSING CARE MANAGEMENT

The nurse evaluates the woman's understanding of the NST and the possible results. The reasons for the NST and the procedure are reviewed before beginning the test. The nurse administers the NST, interprets the results, and reports the findings to the certified nurse-midwife or physician and the expectant woman.

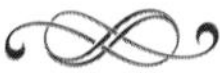

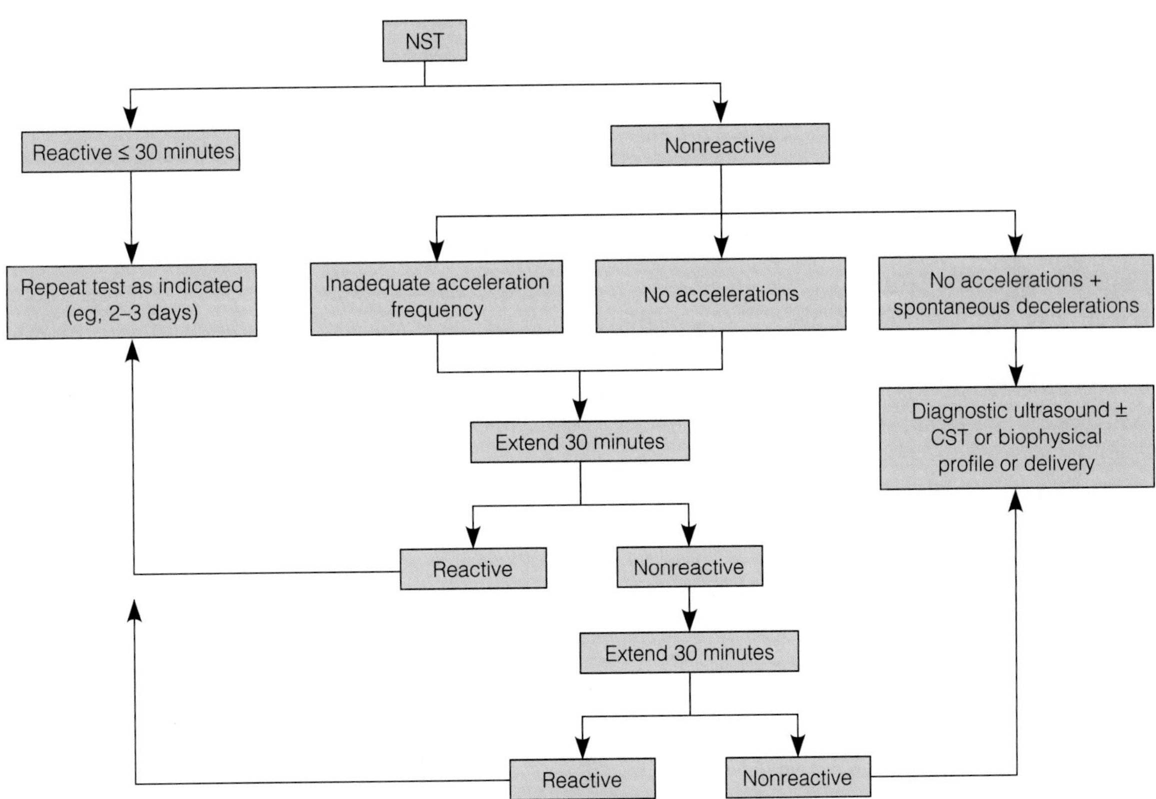


FIGURE 14–7 ♦ NST management scheme. *Source:* Devoe, L. D. (1989). Nonstress and contraction stress testing. In R. Depp, D. A. Eschenbach, & J. J. Sciarri (Eds.), *Gynecology and obstetrics* (Vol. 3, p. 9, Figure 5). Philadelphia: Lippincott.

## Fetal Acoustic Stimulation Test (FAST) and Vibroacoustic Stimulation Test (VST)

Acoustic (sound) and vibroacoustic (vibration and sound) stimulation of the fetus can be used as an adjunct to the NST. A handheld, battery-operated device is applied to the woman's abdomen over the area of the fetal head. This device generates a low-frequency vibration and a buzzing sound that are intended to induce movement and associated accelerations of FHR in fetuses with a nonreactive NST and in fetuses with decreased variability of FHR during labor. (See discussion of variability in Chapter 16.) The sound stimulus persists for 2 to 5 seconds; if no accelerations occur, it is then repeated at 1-minute intervals up to three times (Richardson & Gagnon, 1999; Gegor & Kriebs, 1997). Whether the fetus responds more to the vibration or to the sound is not known. Two FHR accelerations of 15 beats per minute, lasting 15 seconds, in a 10-minute period, indicate a reactive test (Jasper, 2000; Schmidt, 2000). Advantages of the fetal acoustic stimulation test (FAST) and the vibroacoustic stimulation test (VST) are

- Both are noninvasive techniques that are easy to perform.
- Results are rapidly available.
- Time for the NST is shortened.

## Biophysical Profile

The **biophysical profile (BPP)** is a comprehensive assessment of five biophysical variables: fetal breathing movement, fetal movements of body or limbs, fetal tone (extension and flexion of extremities), amniotic fluid volume (visualized as pockets of fluid around the fetus), and reactive FHR with activity (reactive NST). The first four variables are assessed by ultrasound scanning; FHR reactivity is assessed with the NST. By combining these five assessments, the BPP helps to identify the compromised fetus and to confirm the healthy fetus. Specific criteria for normal and abnormal assessments are presented in Table 14–3. A score of 2 is assigned to each normal finding, and 0 to each abnormal one, for a maximum score of 10. The absence of a specific activity is difficult to interpret, since it may be indicative of central nervous system (CNS) depression or simply the resting state of a healthy fetus. Scores of 8 (with normal amniotic fluid) and 10 are considered normal. Such scores have the least chance of being associated with a compromised fetus unless a decrease in the amount of amniotic fluid is noted in which case the infant's birth may be indicated (Jasper 2000). A management protocol regarding BPP is outlined in Table 14–3.

The BPP is indicated when there is risk of placental insufficiency or fetal compromise because of the following

- Intrauterine growth restriction (IUGR)
- Maternal diabetes mellitus
- Maternal heart disease
- Maternal chronic hypertension
- Maternal preeclampsia or eclampsia (pregnancy-induced hypertension [PIH])
- Maternal sickle-cell anemia
- Suspected fetal postmaturity (more than 42 weeks' gestation)
- History of previous stillbirths
- Rh sensitization
- Abnormal estriol excretion
- Hyperthyroidism
- Renal disease
- Nonreactive NST

## Contraction Stress Test

The **contraction stress test (CST)** is a means of evaluating the respiratory function (oxygen and carbon dioxide exchange) of the placenta. It enables the health care team to identify the fetus at risk for intrauterine asphyxia by observing the response of the FHR to the stress of uterine contractions (spontaneous or induced). During contractions, intrauterine pressure increases. Blood flow to the intervillous space of the placenta is reduced momentarily, thereby decreasing oxygen transport to the fetus. A healthy fetus usually tolerates this reduction well and maintains a steady heart rate. If the placental reserve is insufficient, fetal hypoxia, depression of the myocardium, and a decrease in FHR occur.

Although the CST is not currently used as frequently as in the past, it is still utilized in areas where the availability of other technology is reduced (such as during night shifts) or limited (such as at small community hospitals or birthing centers). It may also be used as an adjunct to other forms of fetal assessment. In many areas, however, the CST has given way to the biophysical profile.

The CST is contraindicated if there is third-trimester bleeding from placenta previa or marginal abruptio placentae, previous cesarean with classical incision (vertical incision in the fundus of the uterus), premature rupture of the membranes, incompetent cervix, or multiple gestation.

TABLE 14–3 Biophysical Profile Scoring: Technique and Interpretation

| *Biophysical Variable* | *Normal (Score = 2)* | *Abnormal (Score = 0)* |
|---|---|---|
| Fetal breathing movements | ≥1 episode of ≥30 seconds in 30 minutes | Absent or no episode of ≥30 seconds in 30 minutes |
| Gross body movements | ≥3 discrete body or limb movements in 30 minutes (Episodes of active continuous movement considered as single movement.) | ≤2 episodes of body or limb movements in 30 minutes |
| Fetal tone | ≥1 episode of active extension with return to flexion of fetal limb(s) or trunk (Opening and closing of hand considered normal tone.) | Either slow extension with return to partial flexion or movement of limb in full extension or absent fetal movement |
| Reactive fetal heart rate | ≥2 episodes of acceleration of ≥ 15 bpm and of ≥15 seconds associated with fetal movement in 20 minutes | <2 episodes of acceleration of fetal heart rate or acceleration of <15 bpm in 20 minutes |
| Qualitative amniotic fluid volume | ≥1 pocket of fluid measuring ≥1 cm in two perpendicular planes | Either no pockets or a pocket <1 cm in two perpendicular planes |

*Management Based on Biophysical Profile Score*

| *Attained Score* | *Intervention* |
|---|---|
| 10 of 10 or 8 of 10, with normal amniotic fluid volume | No intervention is needed; normal finding. |
| 8 of 10 with abnormal amniotic fluid volume | If fetal renal function is normal and membranes are intact, delivery is indicated. |
| 6 of 10 with normal amniotic fluid volume | Equivocal. |
| 4 of 10, 2 of 10, or 0 of 10 | Deliver fetus. |

*Source:* Manning, F. (1999). Fetal assessment by evaluation of biophysical variables. In R. K. Creasy & R. Resnik (Eds.) *Maternal-Fetal Medicine* (4th ed. pp. 319–330). Philadelphia: Saunders.

## PROCEDURE

The critical component of the CST is the presence of uterine contractions. They may occur spontaneously (which is unusual prior to the onset of labor), or they may be induced (stimulated) with oxytocin (Pitocin) administered intravenously. Another method of obtaining oxytocin is through the use of breast stimulation (also called nipple self-stimulation); the posterior pituitary produces oxytocin in response to stimulation of the breasts or nipples.

An electronic fetal monitor is used to provide continuous data about the fetal heart rate and uterine contractions. After a 15-minute baseline recording of uterine activity and FHR, the tracing is evaluated for evidence of spontaneous contractions. If three spontaneous contractions of good quality and lasting 40 to 60 seconds occur in a 10-minute window, the results are evaluated, and the test is concluded. If no contractions occur or they are insufficient for interpretation, oxytocin is administered intravenously or breast self-stimulation is done to produce contractions of good quality. (See Chapter 20 for more information on nursing care management of oxytocin induction).

## INTERPRETATION OF CST RESULTS

The CST is classified as follows:

- *Negative.* A negative CST shows three contractions of good quality lasting 40 or more seconds in 10 minutes without evidence of late decelerations. This is the desired result. It implies that the fetus can handle the hypoxic stress of uterine contractions.
- *Positive.* A positive CST shows repetitive persistent late decelerations with more than 50% of the contractions (Figure 14–8♦). This is not a desired result. The hypoxic stress of the uterine contraction causes a slowing of the FHR. The pattern will not improve and will most likely get worse with additional contractions.
- *Equivocal or suspicious.* An equivocal or suspicious test has nonpersistent late decelerations or decelerations associated with hyperstimulation (contraction frequency of <2 minutes or duration of >90 seconds). When this test result occurs, more information is needed.

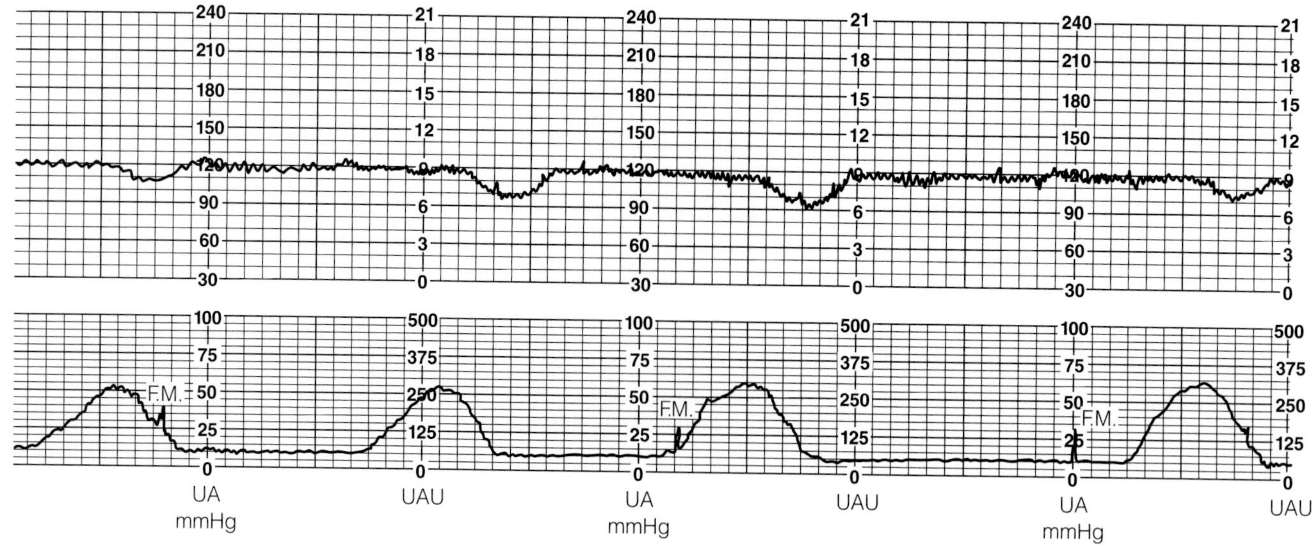


**FIGURE 14–8** ♦ Example of a positive contraction stress test (CST). Repetitive late decelerations occur with each contraction. Note that there are no accelerations of FHR with three fetal movements (FM). The baseline FHR is 120 bpm. Uterine contractions (bottom half of strip) occurred four times in 12 minutes.

## Clinical Application

A negative CST implies that the placenta is functioning normally, fetal oxygenation is adequate, and the fetus will be able to withstand the stress of labor, if it occurs within the ensuing week.

A positive CST with a nonreactive NST presents evidence that the fetus will not likely withstand the stress of labor (Gegor & Kriebs, 1997). Although a negative CST is reliable in predicting fetal status, a positive result needs to be verified. As many as 50% of fetuses with positive CSTs may tolerate labor without any further signs of fetal stress (a false-positive result) (Parer, 1999). (See Key Facts to Remember: Contraction Stress Test).

### KEY FACTS TO REMEMBER

*Contraction Stress Test*

Diagnostic value: Demonstrates reaction of FHR to stress of uterine contraction.

Results:

- Negative test: Stress of uterine contraction does not cause a late deceleration of the FHR.
- Positive test: Stress of uterine contraction is associated with a late deceleration of the FHR.

## Nursing Care Management

The nurse ascertains the woman's understanding of the CST, the reasons for the test, and the possible results before the test begins. Written consent is required in some settings. In this case, the certified nurse-midwife or physician is responsible for fully informing the woman about the test. The nurse administers the CST, interprets the results, and reports the findings to the certified nurse-midwife or physician and the expectant woman. Throughout the procedure, the nurse performs critical assessments and provides continual reassurance to the woman and her support person.

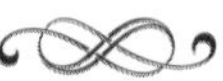

# Amniotic Fluid Analysis

**Amniocentesis** is a procedure used to obtain amniotic fluid for testing. The amniotic fluid is withdrawn by a needle inserted through the abdominal wall into the uterus (Figure 14–9♦). The analysis of amniotic fluid provides valuable information about fetal status. Amniocentesis is a fairly simple procedure, although complications do occur rarely (less than 1% of cases). Procedure 14–1, on page 346, describes the nursing interventions during amniocentesis.

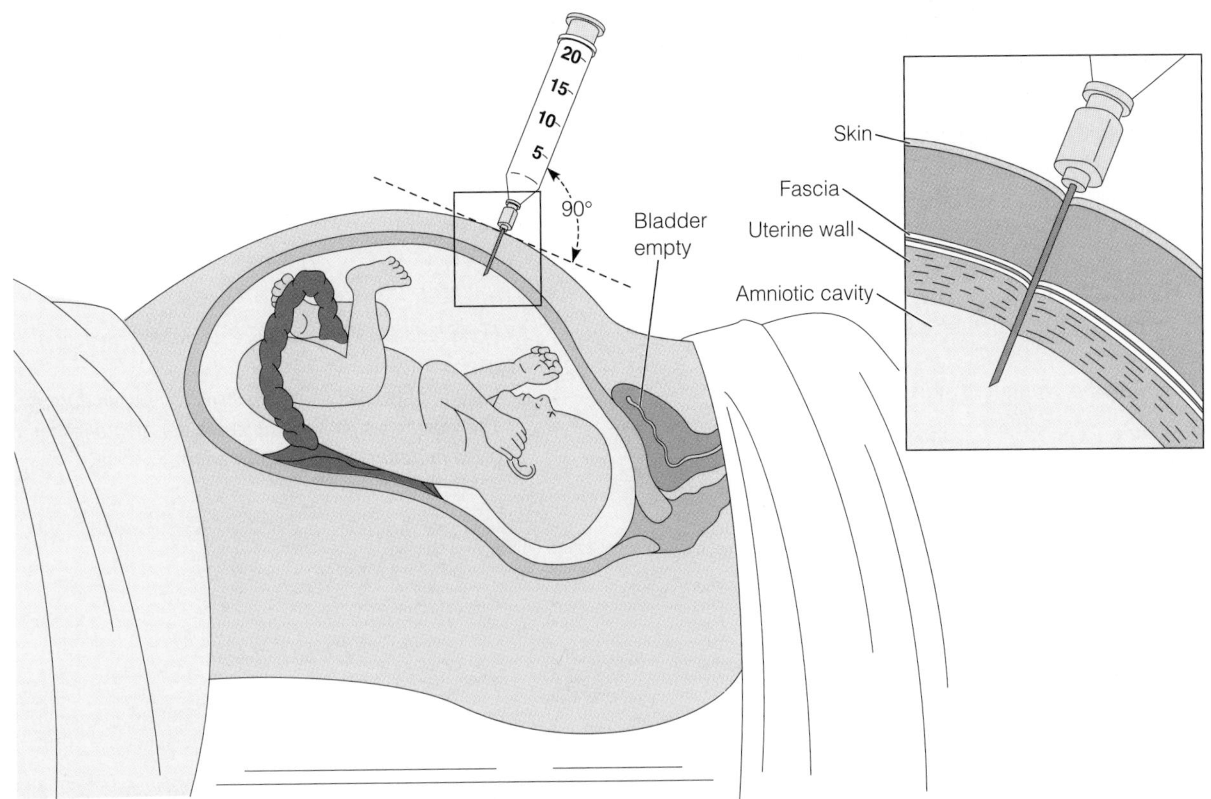


**FIGURE 14–9** ♦ Amniocentesis. The woman is scanned by ultrasound to determine the placental site and to locate a pocket of amniotic fluid. Then the needle is inserted into the uterine cavity to withdraw amniotic fluid.

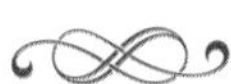

## Nursing Care Management

The nurse assists the physician during the amniocentesis and supports the woman undergoing the procedure. Although the physician has explained the procedure in advance so that the woman can give informed consent, the woman is likely to be apprehensive both about the amniocentesis itself and about the information it may reveal. She may become anxious during the procedure and need additional emotional support. The nurse can provide support by further clarifying the physician's instructions or explanations, by relieving the woman's physical discomfort when possible, and by responding verbally and physically to the woman's need for reassurance.

Following the amniocentesis, the nurse reiterates explanations given by the physician and provides opportunities for questions. The nurse reviews the experience with the woman and presents self-care measures.

## Diagnostic Uses of Amniocentesis

A number of studies can be performed on amniotic fluid following amniocentesis. These tests can provide information about genetic disorders (see Chapter 4), fetal health, and fetal lung maturity. The remainder of this section describes the amniotic fluid studies.

Concentrations of certain substances in amniotic fluid provide information about the health status of the fetus. For example, the **triple test** assesses for appropriate levels of alpha-fetoprotein (AFP), human chorionic gonadotrophin (hCG), and unconjugated estriol (UE3). The triple test is the current standard used to screen for Down syndrome (trisomy 21), trisomy 18, and neural tube defect (NTD). A more sensitive and accurate detector of trisomy 21, the *quadruple screen* (adds measurement of the substance Diameric Inhibin-A), will replace the triple screen as the standard in the near future (McColgin, 1999).

When managing a high-risk pregnancy, the caregiver is faced with the possibility of naturally occurring preterm labor or the need to terminate the pregnancy by induction

# Procedure 14–1 Assisting during Amniocentesis

| *Nursing Action* | *Rationale* |
|---|---|
| **OBJECTIVE: PREPARE THE WOMAN.** | |
| • Explain the procedure and reassure the woman. | *Explanation of the procedure decreases anxiety.* |
| • Ask the woman to sign a consent form. | *It is the physician's responsibility to obtain informed consent. The woman's signature indicates her awareness of risks and gives her consent to the procedure.* |
| **OBJECTIVE: ASSEMBLE THE EQUIPMENT.** Prepare and arrange the following items so they are easily accessible: | |
| • 22-gauge spinal needle with stylet | |
| • 10 and 20-mL syringes | |
| • 1% xylocaine | |
| • Povidone-iodine (Betadine) | |
| • Three 10-mL test tubes with tops (amber colored or covered with tape) | *Amniotic fluid must be shielded from light to prevent breakdown of bilirubin.* |
| **OBJECTIVE: MONITOR THE WOMAN'S VITAL SIGNS.** Obtain baseline data on maternal BP, temperature, pulse, respirations, and FHR; then monitor every 15 minutes. | |
| **OBJECTIVE: LOCATE THE FETUS AND THE PLACENTA.** Assist with real-time ultrasound to assess needle insertion during the procedure. | *Amniocentesis is usually performed laterally in the area of fetal small parts, where pockets of amniotic fluid are often seen. Real-time ultrasound will identify fetal parts and locate pockets of amniotic fluid.* |
| **OBJECTIVE: CLEANSE THE WOMAN'S ABDOMEN.** | *Cleansing the woman's abdomen will decrease the incidence of infection.* |
| **OBJECTIVE: COLLECT THE AMNIOTIC FLUID SPECIMEN.** | |
| • Obtain the test tubes from the physician. | |
| • Label the tubes with the correct identification and send to the lab with the appropriate lab slips. | |
| **OBJECTIVE: MONITOR THE WOMAN AND REASSESS HER VITAL SIGNS.** | *It is important to determine if the fetus was inadvertently punctured.* |
| • Determine the woman's BP, pulse, respirations, and FHR. | |
| • Palpate the woman's fundus to assess for uterine contractions. | |
| • Monitor the woman with an external fetal monitor for 20–30 minutes after the amniocentesis. | |
| • Determine a treatment course to counteract any supine hypotension and to increase venous return and cardiac output. | |

| *Nursing Action* | *Rationale* |
|---|---|
| • Assess the woman's blood type and determine any need for Rh immune globulin. | |
| • Have woman lie on her left side. | |
| **OBJECTIVE: REASSURE THE WOMAN AND PROVIDE SELF-CARE EDUCATION.** | |
| • Instruct the woman to report any of the following side effects to her primary caretaker:<br>a. Unusual fetal hyperactivity or lack of movement<br>b. Vaginal discharge—clear drainage or bleeding<br>c. Uterine contractions or abdominal pain<br>d. Fever or chills | *The woman will know how to recognize side effects or conditions that warrant further treatment.* |
| • Encourage the woman to engage in only light activity for 24 hours. | *A decrease in maternal activity will decrease uterine irritability and increase uteroplacental circulation.* |
| • Encourage the woman to increase her fluid intake. | *Increased hydration will replace the amniotic fluid through the uteroplacental circulation.* |
| **OBJECTIVE: COMPLETE THE CLIENT RECORD.** | *Provides a permanent record.* |
| • Record the type of procedure, the date and time, and the name of the physician who performed the procedure. | |
| • Record the maternal-fetus response, disposition of the specimen, and discharge teaching. | |

of labor or cesarean birth. Indications for early termination of pregnancy include premature rupture of membranes and developing amnionitis (infection of the amnion), severe preeclampsia or eclampsia, bleeding problems (HELLP syndrome, placenta previa, abruptio placenta, and DIC), worsening Rh sensitization, and placental insufficiency. When an infant is born before the lungs are mature, the risk of complications such as respiratory distress syndrome is high.

## EVALUATION OF FETAL MATURITY

Because gestational age, birth weight, and the rate of development of organ systems do not necessarily correspond, amniotic fluid may also be analyzed to determine the maturity of the fetal lungs.

### Lecithin/Sphingomyelin (L/S) Ratio

The alveoli of the lungs are lined with a substance called **surfactant,** which is composed of phospholipids. Surfactant lowers the surface tension of the alveoli when the newborn exhales. When a newborn with mature pulmonary function takes its first breath, a tremendously high pressure is needed to open the lungs. By lowering the alveolar surface tension, surfactant stabilizes the alveoli, and a certain amount of air always remains in the alveoli during expiration. Thus, when the infant exhales, the lungs do not collapse. An infant born before synthesis of surfactant is complete is unable to maintain lung stability. Each breath requires the same effort as the first. This results in underinflation of the lungs and the development of respiratory distress syndrome (RDS).

Fetal lung maturity can be ascertained by determining the **lecithin/sphingomyelin (L/S) ratio**; lecithin and sphingomyelin are two components of surfactant. Early in pregnancy, the sphingomyelin concentration in amniotic fluid is greater than the concentration of lecithin, and so the L/S ratio is low (lecithin levels are low and sphingomyelin levels are high). At about 32 weeks' gestation, sphingomyelin levels begin to fall and the amount of lecithin begins to increase. By 35 weeks' gestation, an L/S ratio of 2:1 (also reported as 2.0) is usually achieved in the normal fetus. A 2:1 L/S ratio indicates that the risk of RDS is very low (Jobe, 1999). Under certain conditions of stress (a physiologic problem in the mother, placenta, and/or fetus), the fetal lungs mature more rapidly.

#### Phosphatidylglycerol

**Phosphatidylglycerol (PG)** is another phospholipid in surfactant. PG is not present in the fetal lung fluid early in gestation. It appears when fetal lung maturity has been attained, at about 35 weeks' gestation. Since the presence of PG is associated with fetal lung maturity, when it is present the risk of RDS is low. PG determination is also useful in blood-contaminated specimens. Since PG is not present in blood or vaginal fluids, its presence is reliable in predicting lung maturity (Jobe, 1999). (See Key Facts to Remember: L/S Ratio and PG.)

> **KEY FACTS TO REMEMBER**
>
> ***L/S Ratio and PG***
>
> Diagnostic value: Provides information to help determine fetal lung maturity.
>
> Results: L/S ratio of 2:1 and presence of PG correlate with 35 weeks' gestation.
>
> An L/S ratio lower than 2:1 and/or an absence of PG may indicate underinflation of lungs and an increased risk for development of respiratory distress syndrome.

## Other Fetal Diagnostic Testing

**Chorionic villus sampling (CVS)** involves obtaining a small sample of chorionic villi from the developing placenta. CVS is performed in some medical centers for first-trimester diagnosis of genetic, metabolic, and deoxyribonucleic acid (DNA) studies. The advantages of this procedure are early diagnosis and short waiting time for results. Whereas amniocentesis is not done until at least 16 weeks' gestation, CVS is performed between weeks 8 and 12 (Scioscia, 1999).

**Percutaneous umbilical blood sampling (PUBS)** is a technique used to obtain a fetal blood sample for a variety of blood disorders, chromosome abnormalities, and certain diseases, as well as fetal karyotyping. This procedure uses ultrasound-guided imaging to locate the fetal umbilical cord. A needle is introduced through the maternal abdomen into the umbilical cord and a blood sample is aspirated.

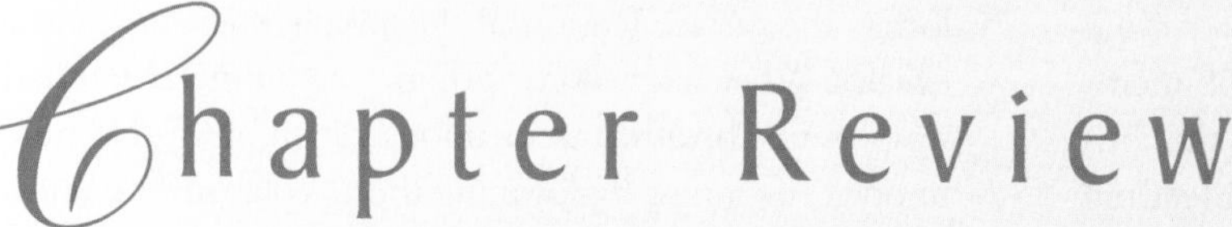

# Chapter Review

## CHAPTER HIGHLIGHTS

- Maternal assessment of fetal activity can be used as a screening tool to provide information about fetal well-being.
- Ultrasound offers a valuable means of assessing intrauterine fetal growth because the growth can be followed over a period of time. It is noninvasive and painless, allows the certified nurse-midwife or physician to study the gestation serially, is nonradiating to both the woman and her fetus, and has no known harmful effects.
- Doppler blood flow studies are used to assess placental function and sufficiency.
- A nonstress test (NST) is based on the knowledge that the FHR normally increases in response to fetal activity and to sound stimulation. The desired result is a reactive test.

- A fetal biophysical profile (BPP) includes five variables (fetal breathing movement, fetal body movement, fetal tone, amniotic fluid volume, and FHR reactivity) to assess the fetus at risk for intrauterine compromise.
- A contraction stress test (CST) provides a method for observing the response of the FHR to the stress of uterine contractions. The desired result is a negative test.
- Amniocentesis can be used to obtain amniotic fluid for a variety of tests, including the L/S ratio and PG.
- The L/S ratio can be used to assess fetal lung maturity. The presence of PG also provides information about fetal lung maturity.
- The triple test (and quadruple screen) measures substances contained in the amniotic fluid that provide information regarding the presence of fetal anomalies, such as neural tube defects and Down syndrome.

## CHAPTER REFERENCES


Andrews, W. W., Copper, R., Hauth, J. C., Goldenberg, R. L., Neely, C., & Dubard, M. (2000). Second-trimester cervical ultrasound associations with increased risk of recurrent early spontaneous delivery. *Obstetrics and Gynecology, 95*(2), 222–226.

Barnhart, K. T., Simhan, H., & Kamelle, S. A. (1999). Diagnostic accuracy of ultrasound above and below the beta-hCG discriminatory zone. *Obstetrics and Gynecology, 94,* 583–586.

Berghella, V., Daly, S. F., Tolosa, J. E., DiVito, M., Chalmers, R., Garg, N., Bhullar, A., & Wapner, R. J., et al. (1999). Prediction of preterm delivery with transvaginal ultrasound of the cervix in patients with high-risk pregnancies: Does cerclage prevent prematurity? *American Journal of Obstetrics and Gynecology, 181,* 809–810.

Gegor, C. L., & Kriebs, J. M. (1997). Fetal assessment. In H. Varney (Ed.), *Midwifery* (3rd ed., pp. 283–316). Sudbury: Jones & Barlett.

Jasper, M. L. (2000). Antepartum fetal assessment. In S. Mattson & J. E. Smith (Eds.), *AWHONN: Maternal newborn nursing* (2nd ed., pp. 127–160). Philadelphia: Saunders.

Jobe, A. H. (1999). Fetal lung development: Tests for maturation, induction of maturation, and treatment. In R. K. Creasy & R. Resnik (Eds.), *Maternal-fetal medicine* (4th ed., pp. 404–422). Philadelphia: Saunders.

Manning, F. (1999). General principles and applications of ultrasound. In R. K. Creasy & R. Resnik (Eds.), *Maternal-fetal medicine.* (4th ed., pp. 169–206). Philadelphia: Saunders.

McColgin, S. W. (1999, November). *Multiple marker screening revisited.* Paper presented at the Memorial Hospitals 3rd Annual Obstetrics Conference, *Update in OB/GYN.* Colorado Springs, CO.

Murray, M. (1997). *Antepartal and intrapartal fetal monitoring.* Albuquerque, NM: Learning Resources International.

Nathan, E. B., Haberman, S., Burgess, T., & Minkoff, H. (2000). The relationship of maternal position to the results of brief nonstress tests: A randomized clinical trial. *American Journal of Obstetrics and Gynecology, 182*(5), 1070–1072.

O'Reilly-Green, C., & Divon, M. (2000). Sonographic and clinical methods of diagnosis of macrosomia. *Clinical Obstetrics and Gynecology, 44,* 309–320.

Owen, J., Neely, C., & Northen, A. (1999). Transperineal versus endovaginal ultrasonography examination of the cervix in the midtrimester: A blended comparison. *American Journal of Obstetrics and Gynecology, 181,* 780.

Panting-Kemp, A., Nguyen, T., Chang, E. Quillen, E., & Castro, L., et al. (1999). Idiopathic polyhydramnios and perinatal outcomes. *American Journal of Obstetrics and Gynecology, 181,* 1079–1082.

Parer, J. T. (1999). Fetal heart rate. In R. K. Creasy & R. Resnik (Eds.), *Maternal-fetal medicine* (4th ed., pp. 270–299). Philadelphia: Saunders.

Richardson, B. S., & Gagnon, R. (1999). Fetal breathing and body movements. In R. K. Creasy & R. Resnik (Eds.) *Maternal-fetal medicine* (4th ed., pp. 231–247). Philadelphia: Saunders.

Schmidt, J. (2000). Intrapartum fetal assessment. In S. Mattson & J. E. Smith (Eds.), *AWHONN: Maternal newborn nursing* (2nd ed., pp. 272–299). Philadelphia: Saunders.

Scioscia, A. L. (1999). Prenatal genetic diagnosis. In R. K. Creasy & R. Resnik (Eds.), *Maternal-fetal medicine* (4th ed., pp. 40–62). Philadelphia: Saunders.

Trudinger, B. (1999). Doppler ultrasound assessment of blood flow. In R. K. Creasy & R. Resnik (Eds.), *Maternal-fetal medicine.* (4th ed., pp. 216–229). Philadelphia: Saunders.

Zelop, C. M. (2000). Prediction of fetal weight with the use of three-dimensional ultrasound. *Clinical Obstetrics and Gynecology, 44,* 321–325.

## CONTEMPORARY MATERNAL-NEWBORN NURSING ON-LINE

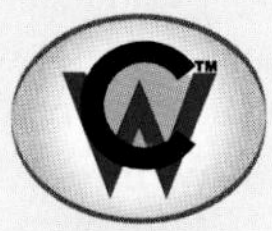

Additional interactive resources, including animations and video, for this chapter can be found on the Companion Website at http://www.prenhall.com/ladewig. Click on Chapter 14 and "Begin" to select the activities for this chapter.

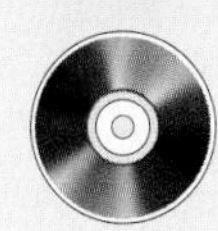

For NCLEX review questions and an audio glossary, access the accompanying CD-ROM in this book.

# Part Four

# Birth and the Family

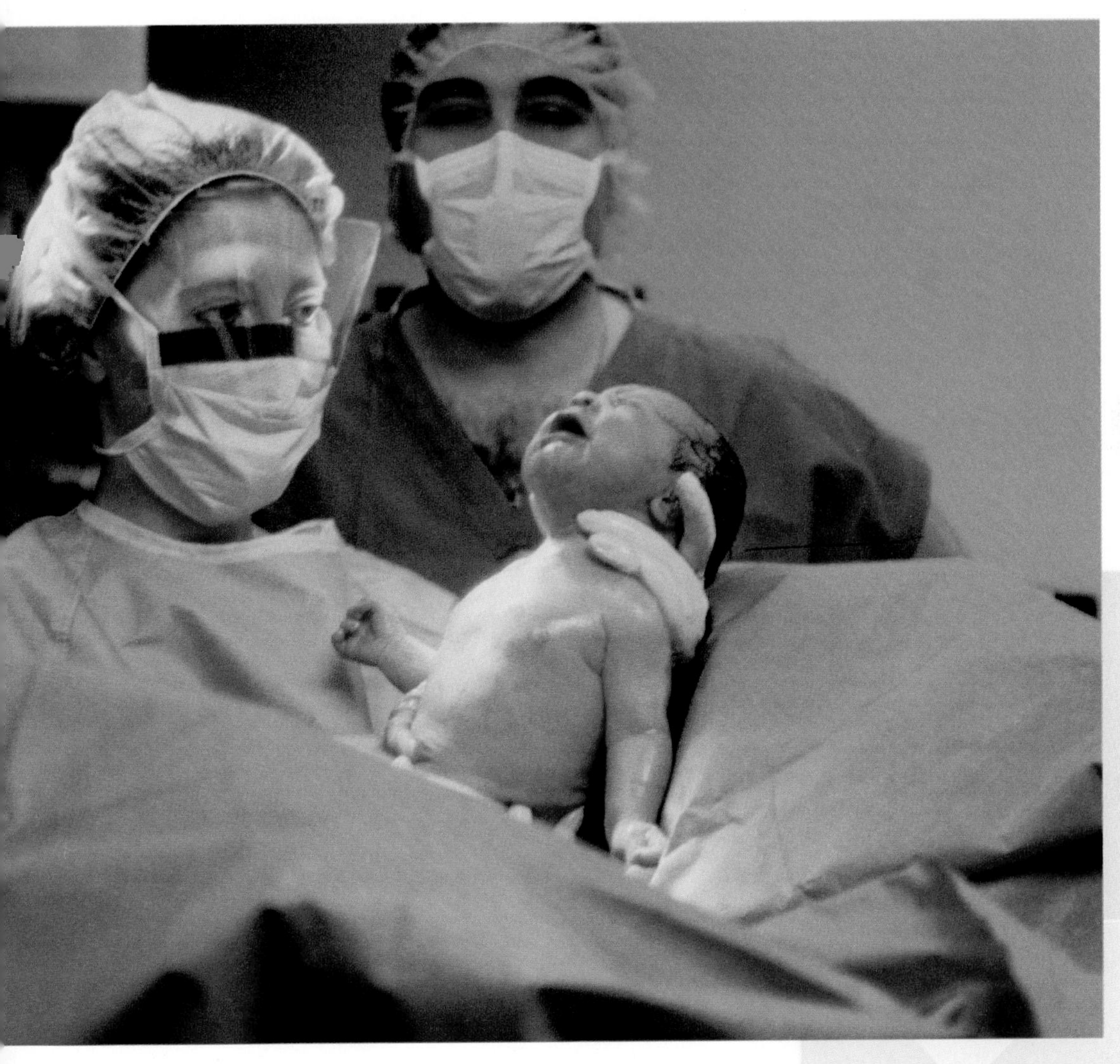

Chapter 15

# Processes and Stages of Labor and Birth

*There is no doubt in my mind that I have the most wonderful job in nursing! What an enormous privilege to be allowed to share in the birth of a new life, in the birth of a new family. The sheer miracle of it never ceases to amaze and humble me. I only hope that I am able to demonstrate that sense of awe and respect even when things don't go as we would expect or like to see them.*

—A Labor and Delivery Nurse

## KEY TERMS



## OBJECTIVES

- Examine the five critical factors that influence labor.
- Describe the physiology of labor.
- Discuss premonitory signs of labor.
- Differentiate between false and true labor.
- Describe the physiologic and psychologic changes occurring in each of the stages of labor.
- Summarize maternal systemic responses to labor.
- Explore fetal responses to labor.

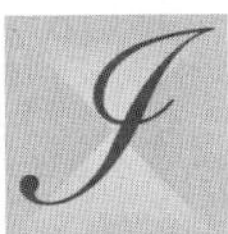

n the final weeks of pregnancy, both mother and baby begin to prepare for birth. The fetus develops and grows in readiness for life outside of the womb. The expectant woman undergoes various physiologic and psychologic changes that gradually prepare her for childbirth and for the role of mother. The onset of labor begins a remarkable change in the relationship between the woman and her baby.

During labor, particularly at the end, a woman instinctively knows she is engaging in one of the most important tasks she will ever do. A precious life is about to emerge. In those hours and moments the birth process may seem to carry all the power in the universe. The mother-to-be and her partner may be stretched beyond all of their normal limits of concentration, purpose, endurance, and pain. The dynamic nature of this experience is what makes the birth of a baby both a physiological and a psychological transition into parenthood (Stern & Bruschweiler-Stern, 1998).

## Critical Factors in Labor

Five factors are important in the process of labor and birth: the passage, the fetus, the relationship between the passage and the fetus, the forces of labor, and the psychosocial considerations. The progress of labor is critically dependent on the complementary relationship of these five factors. Abnormalities that affect any component of these critical forces can alter the outcome of labor and jeopardize both the expectant woman and her baby. These factors are described in this section and are summarized in the accompanying Key Facts to Remember: Critical Forces in Labor. (Complications are discussed in Chapter 19.)

### The Birth Passage

The true pelvis, which forms the bony canal through which the fetus must pass, is divided into three sections: the inlet, the pelvic cavity (midpelvis), and the outlet. (See Chapter 2 for discussion of the pelvis and Chapter 8 for assessment techniques.)

The Caldwell-Moloy classification of pelvises is widely used to differentiate bony pelvis types. The four classic types of pelvis, are *gynecoid, android, anthropoid,* and *platypelloid* (Caldwell & Moloy, 1933) (Figure 15–1♦). The gynecoid, or female, pelvis is most common. All diameters of the gynecoid are adequate for childbirth. Implications of each type of pelvis for childbirth are summarized in Table 15–1.

**KEY FACTS TO REMEMBER**

*Critical Forces in Labor*

1. The birth passage
   - Size of the pelvis (diameters of the pelvic inlet, midpelvis or pelvic cavity, and outlet)
   - Type of pelvis (gynecoid, android, anthropoid, platypelloid, or a combination)
   - Ability of the cervix to dilate and efface and ability of the vaginal canal and the external opening of the vagina (the introitus) to distend
2. The fetus
   - Fetal head (size and presence of molding)
   - Fetal attitude (flexion or extension of the fetal body and extremities)
   - Fetal lie
   - Fetal presentation (the part of the fetal body entering the pelvis first in a single- or multiple-gestation pregnancy)
   - Placenta (implantation site)
3. The relationship between the passage and the fetus
   - Engagement of fetal presenting part
   - Station (location of fetal presenting part within the maternal pelvis)
   - Fetal position (relationship of the presenting part to one of the four quadrants of the maternal pelvis)
4. Primary forces of labor
   - Frequency, duration, and intensity of uterine contractions as the fetus moves through the birth passage
   - Effectiveness of the maternal pushing effort
   - Duration of labor
5. Psychosocial considerations
   - Mental and physical preparation for childbirth
   - Sociocultural values and beliefs
   - Previous childbirth experience
   - Support from significant others
   - Emotional status

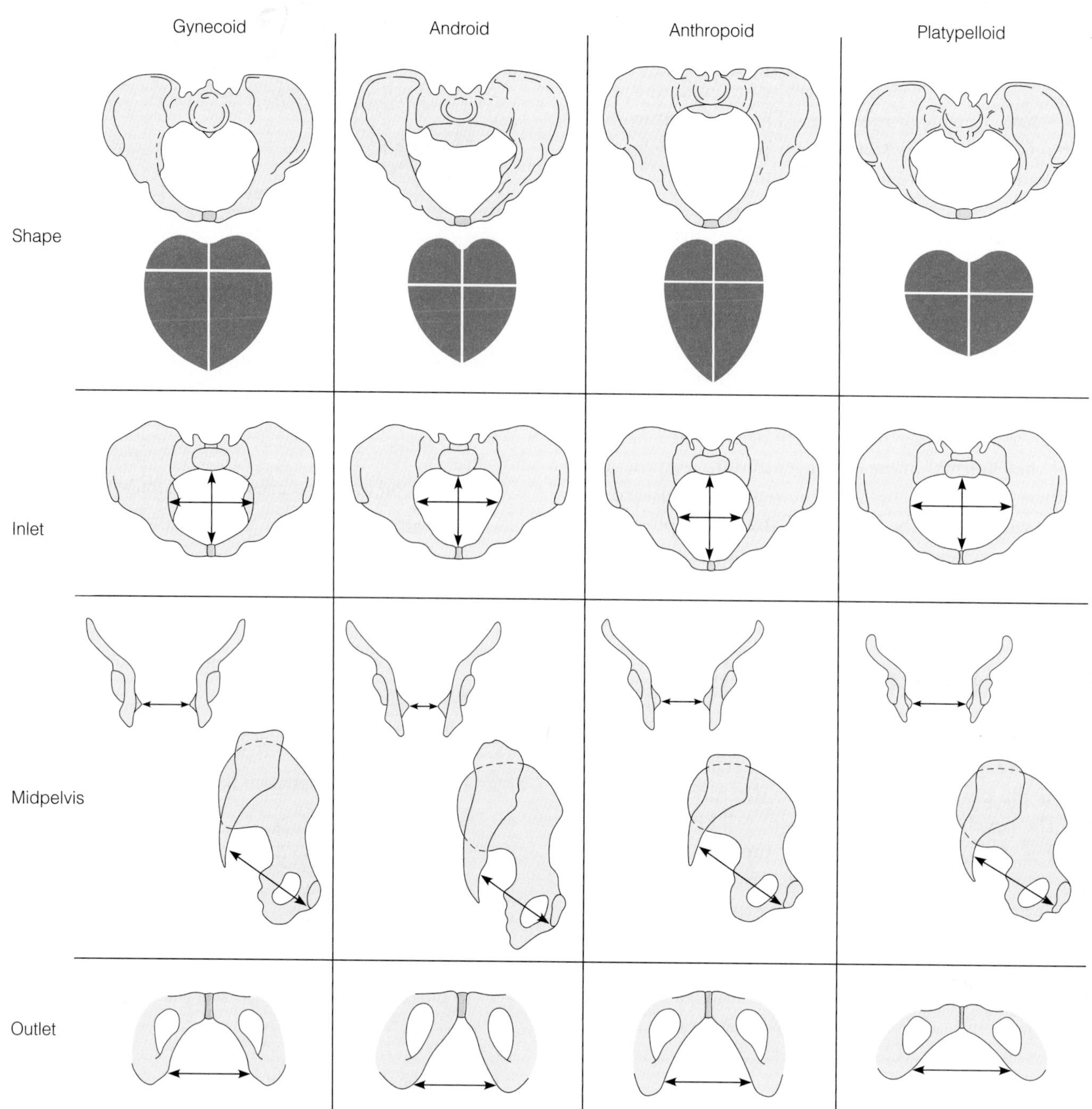


**FIGURE 15–1** ♦ Comparison of Caldwell-Moloy pelvic types.

## The Fetus

### Fetal Head

The fetal head is composed of bony parts that can either hinder childbirth or make it easier. Once the head (the least compressible and largest part of the fetus) has been born, the birth of the rest of the body is rarely delayed. The fetal skull (cranium), has three major parts: the face, the base of the skull, and the vault of the cranium (roof). The bones of the face and cranial base are well fused and essentially fixed. The base of the cranium is composed of the two temporal bones, each with a sphenoid and ethmoid bone. The bones composing the vault are the two frontal bones, the two parietal bones, and the occipital bone (Figure 15–2♦). These bones are not fused, allowing this portion of the head to adjust in shape as the presenting part passes through the narrow portions of the pelvis. The cranial bones overlap under pressure of the powers of labor and the demands of the unyielding pelvis. This overlapping is called **molding.**

The **sutures** of the fetal skull are membranous spaces between the cranial bones. The intersections of the cranial sutures are called **fontanelles.** These sutures allow for molding of the fetal head and help the clinician to

**TABLE 15–1 Implications of Pelvic Type for Labor and Birth**

| *Pelvic Type* | *Pertinent Characteristics* | *Implications for Birth* |
|---|---|---|
| Gynecoid | Inlet rounded with all inlet diameters adequate<br>Midpelvis diameters adequate with parallel side walls<br>Outlet adequate | Favorable for vaginal birth |
| Android | Inlet heart-shaped, with short posterior sagittal diameter<br>Midpelvis diameters reduced<br>Outlet capacity reduced | Not favorable for vaginal birth<br>Descent into pelvis is slow<br>Fetal head enters pelvis in transverse or posterior position, with arrest of labor frequent |
| Anthropoid | Inlet oval in shape, with long anteroposterior diameter<br>Midpelvis diameters adequate<br>Outlet adequate | Favorable for vaginal birth |
| Platypelloid | Inlet oval in shape, with long transverse diameters<br>Midpelvis diameters reduced<br>Outlet capacity inadequate | Not favorable for vaginal birth<br>Fetal head engages in transverse position<br>Difficult descent through midpelvis<br>Frequent delay of progress at outlet of pelvis |

*Note:* Description of pelvic shape is exaggerated for easier comprehension.

identify the position of the fetal head during vaginal examination. The important sutures of the cranial vault are as follows (see Figure 15–2♦):

- *Frontal (mitotic) suture:* located between the two frontal bones; becomes the anterior continuation of the sagittal suture
- *Sagittal suture:* located between the parietal bones; divides the skull into left and right halves; runs anteroposteriorly, connecting the two fontanelles

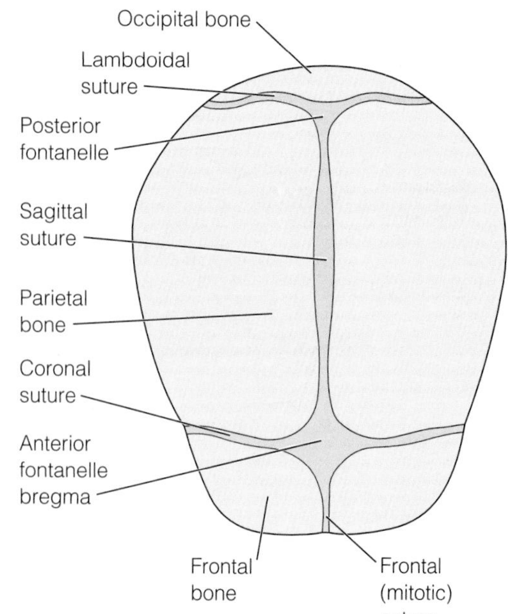


FIGURE 15–2 ♦ Superior view of the fetal skull.

- *Coronal sutures:* located between the frontal and parietal bones; extend transversely left and right from the anterior fontanelle
- *Lambdoidal suture:* located between the two parietal bones and the occipital bone; extends transversely left and right from the posterior fontanelle

The anterior and posterior fontanelles are clinically useful (along with the sutures) in identifying the position of the fetal head in the pelvis and in assessing the status of the newborn after birth. The anterior fontanelle is diamond shaped and measures about 2 by 3 cm. It permits growth of the brain by remaining unossified for as long as 18 months. The posterior fontanelle is much smaller and closes within 8 to 12 weeks after birth. It is shaped like a small triangle and marks the meeting point of the sagittal suture and the lambdoidal suture (Turley, 2000).

Following are several important landmarks of the fetal skull (Figure 15–3♦):

- *Mentum:* fetal chin
- *Sinciput:* anterior area known as the brow
- *Bregma:* large diamond-shaped anterior fontanelle
- *Vertex:* area between the anterior and posterior fontanelles
- *Posterior fontanelle:* intersection between posterior cranial sutures
- *Occiput:* area of the fetal skull occupied by the occipital bone, beneath the posterior fontanelle

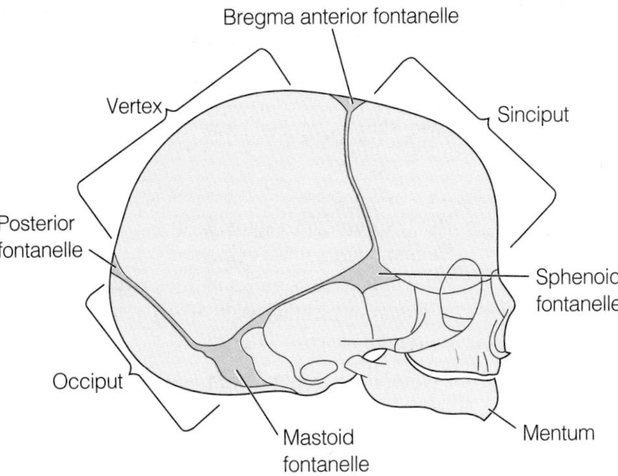


**FIGURE 15–3 ♦** Lateral view of the fetal skull identifying the landmarks that have significance during birth.

The diameters of the fetal skull vary considerably within normal limits. Some diameters shorten and others lengthen as the head is molded during labor. Fetal head diameters are measured between the various landmarks on the skull. For example, the suboccipitobregmatic diameter is the distance from the undersurface of the occiput to the center of the bregma, or anterior fontanelle. Typical fetal skull measurements are given in Figure 15–4♦.

## Fetal Attitude

**Fetal attitude** refers to the relation of the fetal parts to one another. The normal attitude of the fetus is one of moderate flexion of the head, flexion of the arms onto the chest, and flexion of the legs onto the abdomen (Figure 15–5♦).

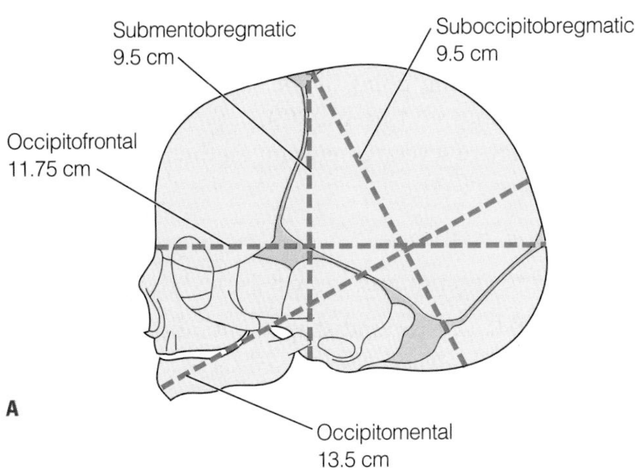


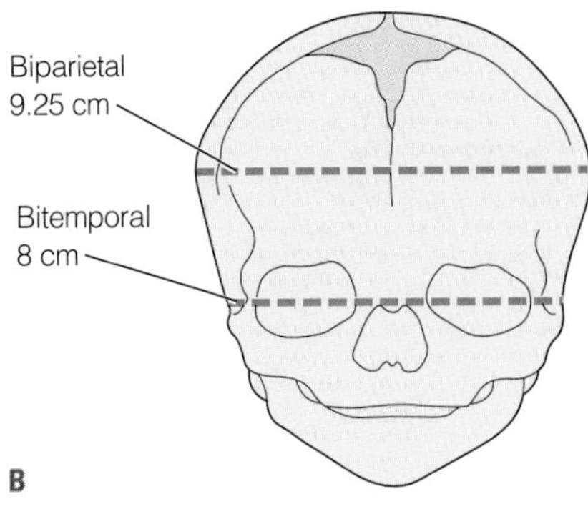


**FIGURE 15–4 ♦ A,** Typical anteroposterior diameters of the fetal skull. When the vertex of the fetus presents and the fetal head is flexed with the chin on the chest, the smallest anteroposterior diameter (suboccipitobregmatic) enters the birth canal. **B,** Transverse diameters of the fetal skull.

## Fetal Lie

**Fetal lie** refers to the relationship of the cephalocaudal (spinal column) axis of the fetus to the cephalocaudal axis of the woman. The fetus may assume either a longitudinal or a transverse lie. A *longitudinal lie* occurs when the cephalocaudal axis of the fetus is parallel to the woman's spine. A *transverse lie* occurs when the cephalocaudal axis of the fetus is at a right angle to the woman's spine.

## Fetal Presentation

**Fetal presentation** is determined by fetal lie and by the body part of the fetus that enters the pelvic passage first. This portion of the fetus is referred to as the **presenting part.** Fetal presentation may be cephalic, breech, or shoulder. The most common presentation is cephalic. When this presentation occurs, labor and birth are likely to proceed normally. Breech and shoulder presentations are associated with difficulties during labor, and labor does not proceed as expected; therefore, they are called **malpresentations** (see Chapter 19 for discussion).

### Cephalic Presentation

The fetal head presents itself to the passage in approximately 97% of term births. The cephalic presentation can be further classified according to the degree of flexion or extension of the fetal head (attitude).

**Vertex Presentation** Vertex is the most common type of presentation. In vertex presentation, the fetal head is completely flexed onto the chest, and the smallest diameter of the fetal head (suboccipitobregmatic) presents to the maternal pelvis (Figure 15–6A♦). The occiput is the presenting part.

**Military Presentation** In military presentation, the fetal head is neither flexed nor extended. The occipitofrontal diameter presents to the maternal pelvis (Figure 15–6B♦); the top of the head is the presenting part.

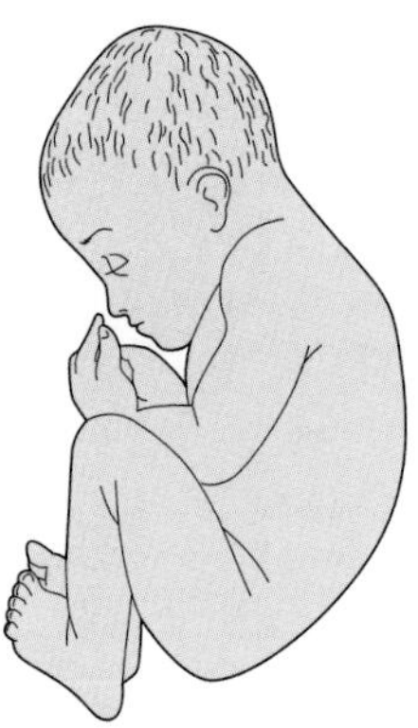

FIGURE 15–5 ♦ Fetal attitude. The attitude (or relationship of body parts) of this fetus is normal. The head is flexed forward, with the chin almost resting on the chest. The arms and legs are flexed.

**Brow Presentation** In brow presentation, the fetal head is partially extended. The occipitomental diameter, the largest anteroposterior diameter, is presented to the maternal pelvis (Figure 15–6C♦); the sinciput is the presenting part (refer to Figure 15–3♦).

**Face Presentation** In face presentation, the fetal head is hyperextended (complete extension). The submentobregmatic diameter presents to the maternal pelvis (Figure 15–6D♦); the face is the presenting part.

### Breech Presentation

Breech presentations occur in 3% of term births. These presentations are classified according to the attitude of the fetus's hips and knees. In all variations of the breech presentation, the sacrum is the landmark to be noted.

**Complete Breech** In complete breech, the fetal knees and hips are both flexed; the thighs are on the abdomen, and the calves are on the posterior aspect of the thighs. The buttocks and feet of the fetus present to the maternal pelvis. (Refer to Chapter 19, Figure 19–7♦.)

**Frank Breech** In frank breech, the fetal hips are flexed, and the knees are extended. The buttocks of the fetus present to the maternal pelvis.

**Footling Breech** In footling breech, the fetal hips and legs are extended, and the feet of the fetus present to the maternal pelvis. In a single footling, one foot presents; in a double footling, both feet present.

### Shoulder Presentation

A shoulder presentation is also called a transverse lie. Most frequently, the shoulder is the presenting part and the acromion process of the scapula is the landmark to be noted. However, the fetal arm, back, abdomen, or side may present in a transverse lie. (See Chapter 19 for further discussion of transverse lie.)

## Functional Relationships of Presenting Part and Passage

### Engagement

**Engagement** of the presenting part occurs when the largest diameter of the presenting part reaches or passes through the pelvic inlet (Figure 15–7♦). Engagement can be determined by vaginal examination. In primigravidas, engagement occurs approximately 2 weeks before term.

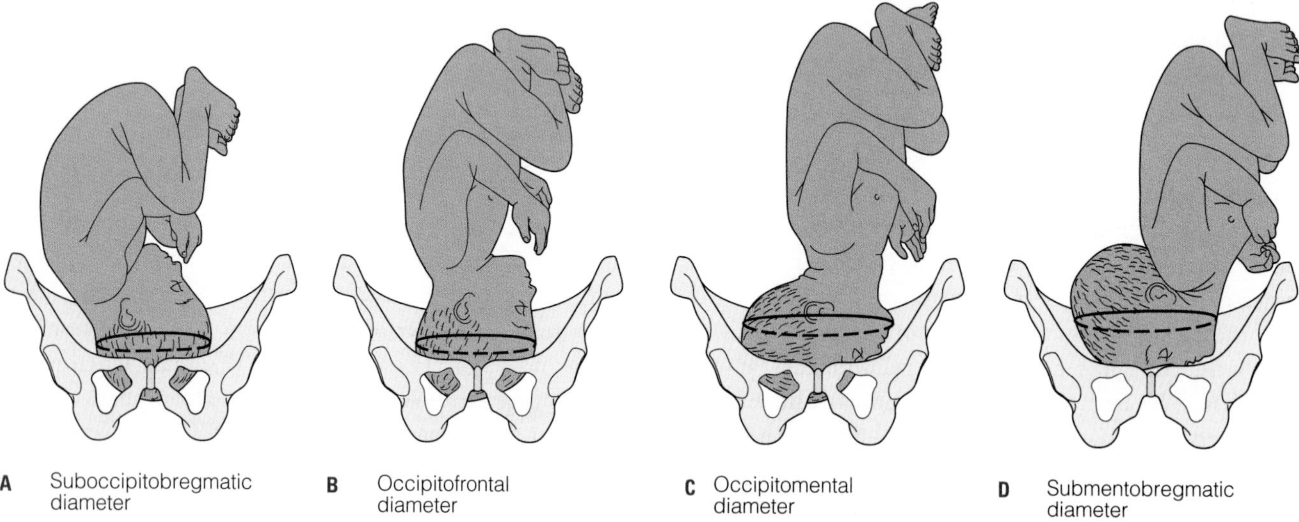


FIGURE 15–6 ♦ Cephalic presentation. **A,** Vertex presentation. Complete flexion of the head allows the suboccipitobregmatic diameter to present to the pelvis. **B,** Military (median vertex) presentation with no flexion or extension. The occipitofrontal diameter presents to the pelvis. **C,** Brow presentation. The fetal head is in partial (halfway) extension. The occipitomental diameter, which is the largest diameter of the fetal head, presents to the pelvis. **D,** Face presentation. The fetal head is in complete extension, and the submentobregmatic diameter presents to the pelvis.

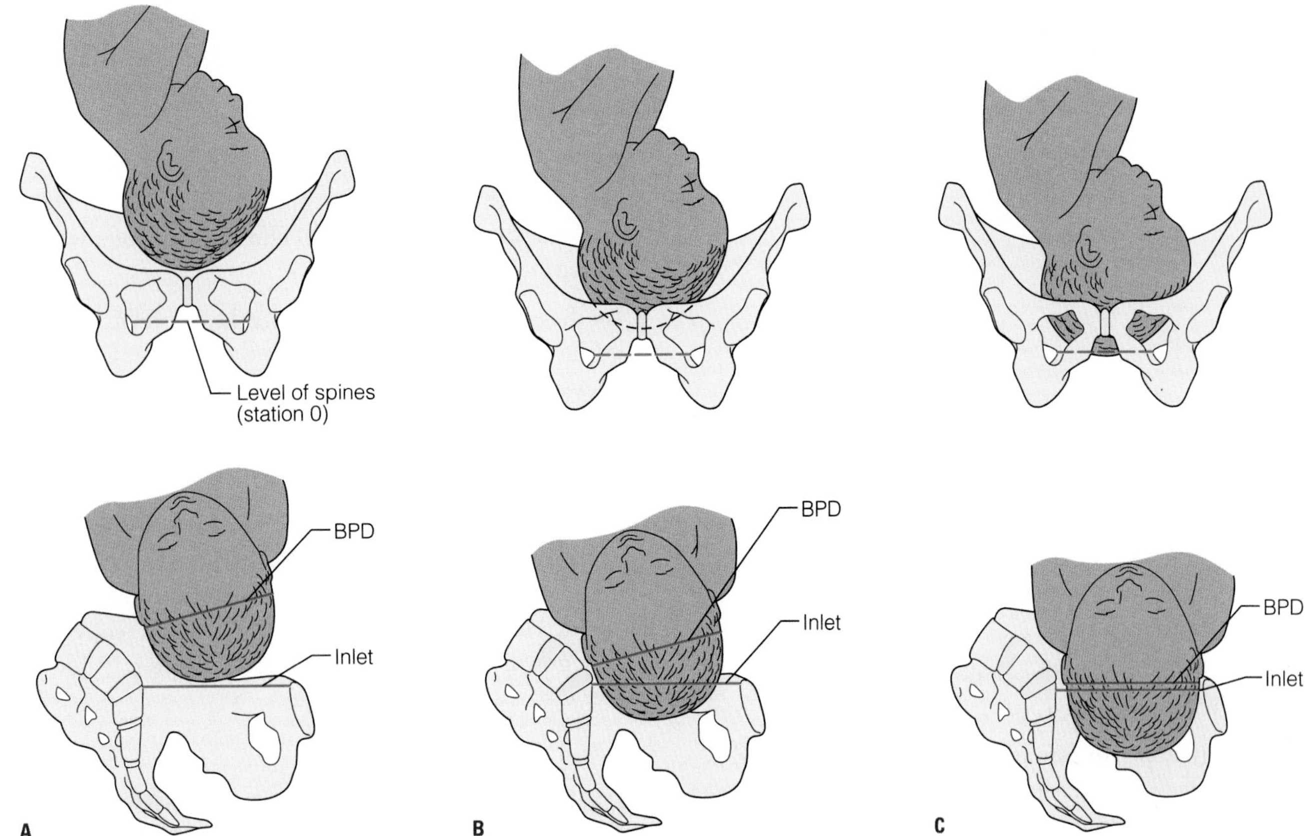


FIGURE 15–7 ♦ Process of engagement in cephalic presentation. **A,** Floating. The fetal head is directed down toward the pelvis but can still easily move away from the inlet. **B,** Dipping. The fetal head dips into the inlet but can be moved away by exerting pressure on the fetus. **C,** Engaged. The biparietal diameter (BPD) of the fetal head is in the inlet of the pelvis. In most instances the presenting part (occiput) is at the level of the ischial spines (zero station).

Multiparas, however, may experience engagement several weeks before the onset of labor or during the process of labor. Engagement confirms the adequacy of the pelvic inlet. Engagement does not, however, indicate whether the midpelvis and outlet are also adequate.

## Station

**Station** refers to the relationship of the presenting part to an imaginary line drawn between the ischial spines of the maternal pelvis. In a normal pelvis, the ischial spines mark the narrowest diameter through which the fetus must pass. These spines are not sharp protrusions that harm the fetus but blunted prominences at the midpelvis. The ischial spines as a landmark have been designated as zero station (Figure 15–8♦). If the presenting part is higher than the ischial spines, a negative number is assigned, noting centimeters above zero station. Positive numbers are used to indicate that the presenting part has passed the ischial spines. Station −5 is at the pelvic inlet, and station +4 is at the outlet. If the presenting part can be seen at the woman's perineum, birth is imminent. During labor, the presenting part should move progressively from the negative stations to the midpelvis at zero station and into the positive stations. Failure of the presenting part to descend in the presence of strong contractions may be due to disproportion between the maternal pelvis and fetal presenting part.

## Fetal Position

**Fetal position** refers to the relationship of a designated landmark on the presenting fetal part to the front, sides, or back of the maternal pelvis. The landmark on the fetal presenting part is related to four imaginary quadrants of the pelvis: left anterior, right anterior, left posterior, and right posterior. These quadrants designate whether the presenting part is directed toward the front, back, left, or right of the passage. The landmark chosen for vertex presentations is the occiput, and the landmark for face presentations is the mentum. In breech presentations, the sacrum is the designated landmark, and the acromion process on the scapula is the landmark in shoulder presentations. If the landmark is directed toward the side of the pelvis, fetal position is designated as *transverse,* rather than anterior or posterior. Three notations are used to describe the fetal position:

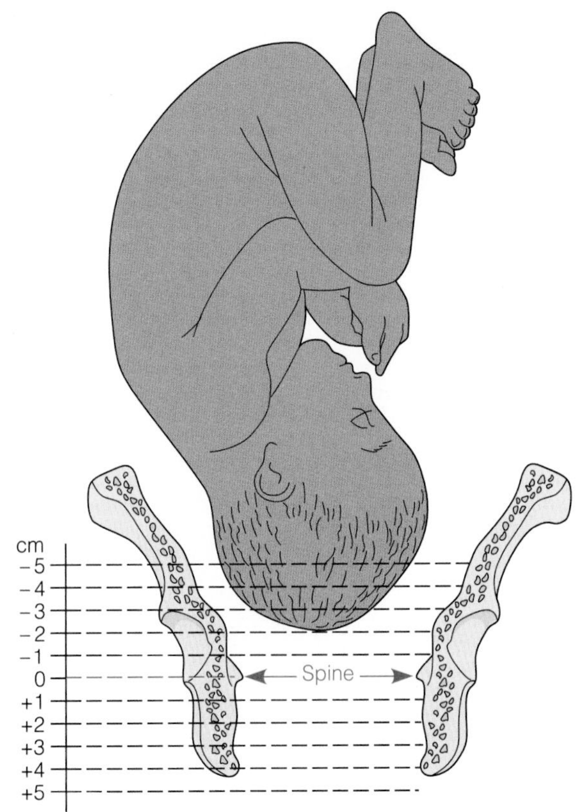


FIGURE 15–8 ♦ Measuring the station of the fetal head while it is descending. In this view the station is −2/−3.

1. Right (R) or left (L) side of the maternal pelvis
2. The landmark of the fetal presenting part: occiput (O), mentum (M), sacrum (S), or acromion process (A)
3. Anterior (A), posterior (P), or transverse (T), depending on whether the landmark is in the front, back, or side of the pelvis

The abbreviations of these notations help the health care team communicate the fetal position. Thus, when the fetal occiput is directed toward the back and to the left of the birth passage, the abbreviation used is LOP (left-occiput-posterior). The term *dorsal* (D) is used when denoting the fetal position in a transverse lie; it refers to the fetal back. Thus RADA indicates that the acromion process of the scapula is directed toward the woman's right and the fetus's back is anterior. The most common occurring positions are illustrated in Figure 15–9♦. The most common fetal position is occiput anterior. When this position occurs, labor and birth are likely to proceed normally. Positions other than occiput anterior are more frequently associated with problems during labor; therefore they are called *malpositions.* (See Chapter 19 for discussion of malpositions and their management.)

Assessment techniques to determine fetal position include inspection and palpation of the maternal abdomen and vaginal examination. They are discussed in Chapter 16.

## The Forces of Labor

Primary and secondary forces work together to achieve birth of the fetus, the fetal membranes, and the placenta. The *primary force* is uterine muscular contractions, which cause the changes of the first stage of labor—complete effacement and dilatation of the cervix. The *secondary force* is the use of abdominal muscles to push during the second stage of labor. The pushing adds to the primary force after full dilatation.

In labor, uterine contractions are rhythmic but intermittent. Between contractions there is a period of relaxation. This allows uterine muscles to rest and provides respite for the laboring woman. It also restores uteroplacental circulation, which is important to fetal oxygenation and adequate circulation in the uterine blood vessels.

Each contraction has three phases: (1) *increment,* the building up of the contraction (the longest phase); (2) *acme,* or the peak of the contraction; and (3) *decrement,* or the letting up of the contraction. When describing uterine contractions during labor, caregivers use the terms *frequency, duration,* and *intensity.* **Frequency** refers to the time between the beginning of one contraction and the beginning of the next contraction. **Duration** is measured from the beginning of a contraction to the completion of that same contraction (Figure 15–10♦ on page 361). **Intensity** refers to the strength of the contraction during acme. In most instances intensity is estimated by palpating the uterine fundus during a contraction, but it may be measured directly with an intrauterine catheter. When estimating intensity by palpation, the nurse determines whether it is mild, moderate, or strong by judging the amount of indentability of the uterine wall during the acme of a contraction. If the uterine wall can be indented easily, the contraction is considered mild. Strong intensity exists when the uterine wall cannot be indented. Moderate intensity falls between these two ranges. When intensity is measured with an intrauterine catheter, the normal resting pressure in the uterus (between contractions) averages 10 to 12 mm Hg. During acme the intensity ranges from 25 to 40 mm Hg in early labor, 50 to 70 mm Hg in active labor, 70 to 90 mm Hg during transition, and 70 to 100 mm Hg while the woman is pushing in the second stage (Varney, 1997). (See Chapter 16 for further discussion of assessment techniques.)

At the beginning of labor, the contractions are usually mild, last about 30 seconds, and occur about every 5 to 7 minutes. As labor progresses, duration of contractions increases to an average of 60 seconds, intensity increases, and frequency is every 2 to 3 minutes. Because the contractions are involuntary, the laboring woman cannot control their duration, frequency, or intensity (Varney, 1997).

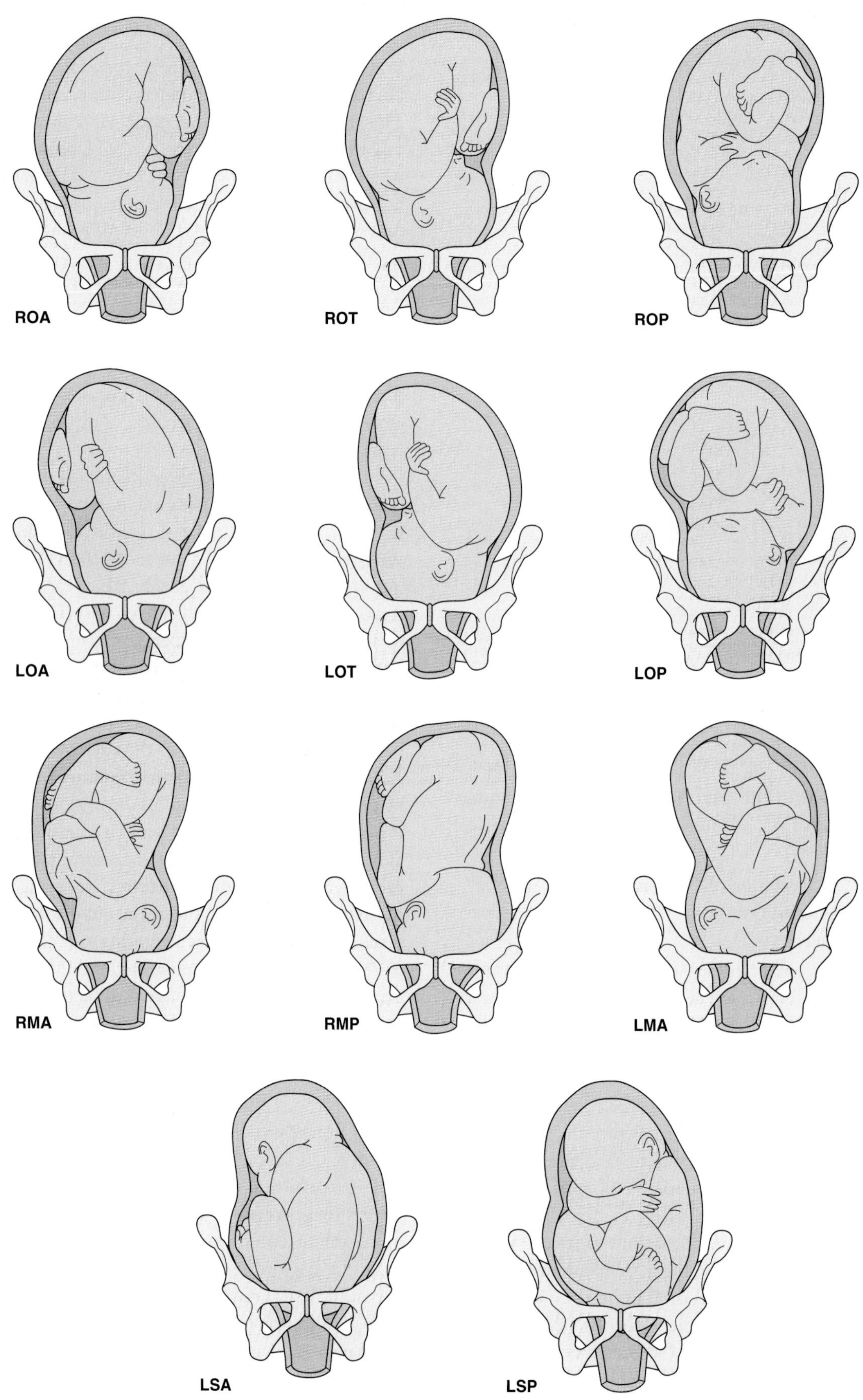


**FIGURE 15–9** ♦ Categories of presentation. *Source:* Courtesy Ross Laboratories, Columbus, OH.

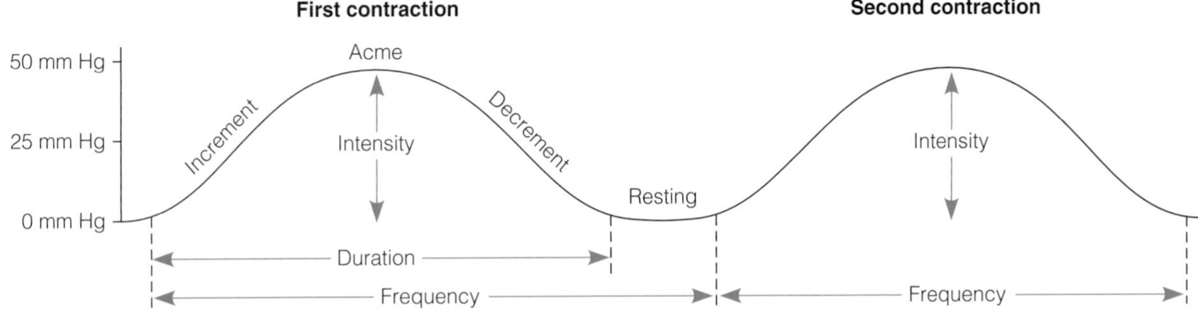


FIGURE 15–10 ♦ Characteristics of uterine contractions.

## Psychosocial Considerations

Similar psychosocial factors affect the mother and the father. Both are making a transition into a new role, and both have expectations of themselves during the labor and birth experience, as caregivers for their child and their new family. Although many prospective mothers and fathers attend childbirth preparation classes, they still tend to be concerned about what labor will be like, whether they will be able to perform the way they expect, whether the discomfort and pain will be more than the mother expects or can cope with, and whether the father can provide helpful support (Mauger, 2000). A common fear expressed in childbirth preparation classes is of "losing it," which often means loss of control or loss of a preconceived image of the "right" way to give birth. It is helpful for the prospective parents to be assured that there is no definitive correct way to approach labor and birth (England & Horowitz, 1998).

Every woman is uncertain about what her labor will be like: A woman approaching her first labor faces a totally new experience, and the woman who has given birth before knows that each labor is unique and different from the past. She wonders if she will live up to her expectations for herself in relation to her friends and relatives, whether she will be physically injured through laceration, episiotomy, or cesarean incision, and whether significant others will be as supportive as she hopes. The woman faces an irrevocable event—the birth of a new family member—and, consequently, disruption of lifestyle, relationships, and self-image. Finally, the woman must deal with concerns about her loss of control of bodily functions, emotional responses to an unfamiliar situation, and reactions to the pain associated with labor.

Various factors influence a woman's reaction to the physical and emotional crisis of labor (Table 15–2). Her accomplishment of the tasks of pregnancy, usual coping mechanisms in response to stressful life events, support system, preparation for childbirth, and cultural influences are all significant factors (Mullaly, 2000).

Expectant women mentally prepare for labor through meaningful action and imaginary rehearsal. The actions frequently consist of "nesting behavior" (housecleaning, decorating the nursery) and a "psyching up" for the labor, which varies depending on the woman's self-confidence, self-esteem, and previous experiences with stress. Specific actions to prepare for labor may focus on becoming better informed and prepared. In addition, just as a woman tries on the maternal role during pregnancy, fantasizing about labor seems to help her understand and become better prepared for it. Fantasies about the excitement of the baby's birth and the sharing of the experience involve the woman in constructive preparation (Mullaly, 2000).

Many women fear the pain of contractions. They not only see the pain as threatening but also associate it with a loss of control over their bodies and emotions. It is important to realize that the discomfort and stresses of labor are an expected part of the process. Assurances that labor is progressing normally can go a long way toward reducing anxiety and thereby reducing pain. A wide variety of coping techniques are available to assist both the laboring

| TABLE 15–2 Factors Associated with a Positive Birth Experience |
|---|
| Motivation for the pregnancy |
| Attendance at childbirth education classes |
| A sense of competence or mastery |
| Self-confidence and self-esteem |
| Positive relationship with mate |
| Maintaining empowerment during labor |
| Support from mate or other person during labor |
| Not being left alone in labor |
| Trust in the medical and nursing staff |
| Having personal control of breathing patterns, comfort measures |
| Choosing a physician or certified nurse-midwife who has a similar philosophy of care |
| Receiving clear information regarding procedures |

woman and her partner, including, for example, relaxation exercises, massage, and patterned breathing. A sometimes underestimated component to feeling empowered and coping in labor is to recognize that maintaining control is not important or even possible (England & Horowitz, 1998).

The laboring woman's support system may also influence the course of labor and birth. Although some women may prefer not to have a support person or family member with them, for many women, the presence of the father and other significant persons (especially the nurse) tends to have a positive effect. A labor partner's presence at the bedside provides a means to enhance communication and to demonstrate feelings of love. Communication needs may include talking and the use of affectionate and understanding words from the partner. Showing love may take the form of holding hands, hugging, or touching (England & Horowitz, 1998).

How the woman views the birth experience in hindsight may have implications for mothering behaviors. A significant relationship exists between the birth experience and mothering behaviors. It appears that any activities by the expectant woman or by health care providers that enhance the birth experience will be beneficial to the mother-baby connection. The father's experience of childbirth and his opportunities for bonding may have important implications for fathering as well (England & Horowitz, 1998).

# The Physiology of Labor

## Possible Causes of Labor Onset

The process of labor usually begins between the 38th and the 42nd week of gestation, when the fetus is mature and ready for birth. Despite medical advances, the exact cause of labor onset is not clearly understood. However, some important aspects have been identified: progesterone relaxes smooth muscle tissue, estrogen stimulates uterine muscle contractions, and connective tissue loosens to permit the softening, thinning and eventual opening of the cervix (R. Smith, 1999). Currently, researchers are focusing on the role of fetal membranes (chorion and amnion), the decidua, and the effect of progesterone withdrawal, of prostaglandin, and of corticotrophin-releasing hormone in relation to labor onset (R. Smith, 1999).

### Progesterone Withdrawal Hypothesis

Progesterone, produced by the placenta, relaxes uterine smooth muscle by interfering with the conduction of impulses from one cell to the next. Therefore during pregnancy, progesterone exerts a quieting effect and the uterus generally is without coordinated contractions. Toward the end of gestation, biochemical changes decrease the availability of progesterone to myometrial cells and may be associated with an antiprogestin that inhibits the relaxant effect but allows other progesterone actions such as lactogenesis (Liggins, 1997). With the decreased availability of progesterone, estrogen is better able to stimulate contractions (Challis, 1999).

### Prostaglandin Hypothesis

Although the exact relationship between prostaglandin and the onset of labor is not yet known, the effect is clinically demonstrated by the successful induction of labor after vaginal application of prostaglandin E. In addition, preterm labor may be stopped by using an inhibitor of prostaglandin synthesis (Challis, 1999; Liggins, 1997).

The amnion and decidua are the focus of research on the source of prostaglandins. Once prostaglandin is produced, stimuli for its synthesis may include rising levels of estrogen, decreased availability of progesterone, and increased levels of oxytocin, platelet-activating factor, and endothelin-1 (Challis, 1999; Liggins, 1997).

### Corticotrophin-Releasing Hormone

Corticotrophin-releasing hormone (CRH) increases throughout pregnancy, with a sharp increase at term, and has a possible role in labor onset. Also, there is an increase in plasma CRH prior to preterm labor, and CRH levels are elevated in multiple gestation. Finally, CRH is known to stimulate the synthesis of prostaglandin F and prostaglandin E by amnion cells (R. Smith, 1999).

## Myometrial Activity

In true labor, with each contraction, the muscles of the upper uterine segment shorten and exert a longitudinal traction on the cervix, causing effacement. **Effacement** is the drawing up of the internal os and the cervical canal into the uterine side walls. The cervix changes progressively from a long, thick structure to a structure that is tissue-paper thin (Figure 15–11♦). In primigravidas, effacement usually precedes dilatation.

The uterus elongates with each contraction, decreasing the horizontal diameter. This elongation causes a straightening of the fetal body, pressing the upper portion against the fundus and thrusting the presenting part down toward the lower uterine segment and the cervix. The pressure exerted by the fetus is called the fetal axis pressure. As the uterus elongates, the longitudinal muscle fibers are pulled upward over the presenting part. This action and the hydrostatic pressure of the fetal membranes cause cervical dilatation. The cervical os and cervical canal widen from less than a centimeter

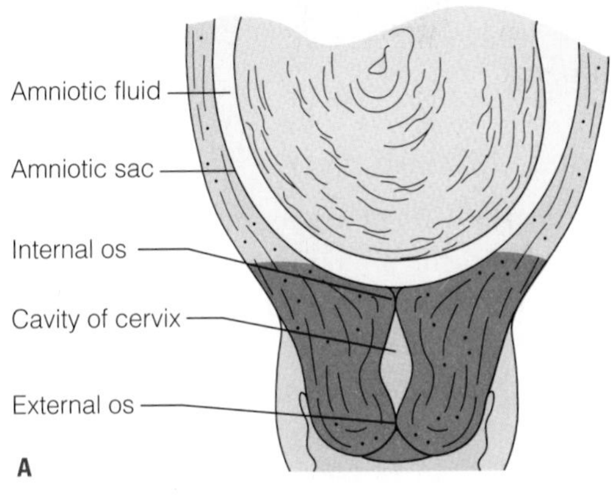


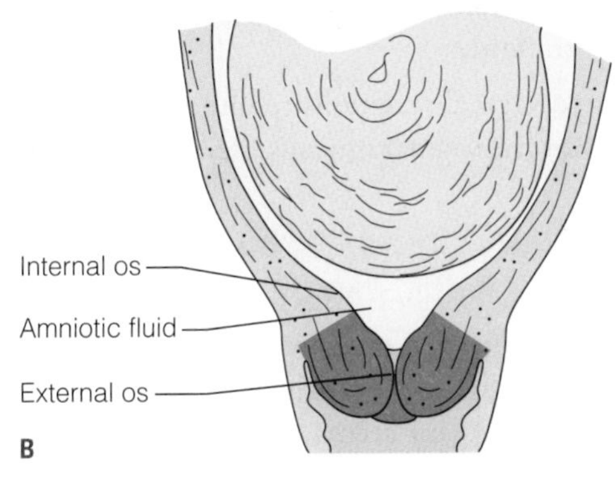


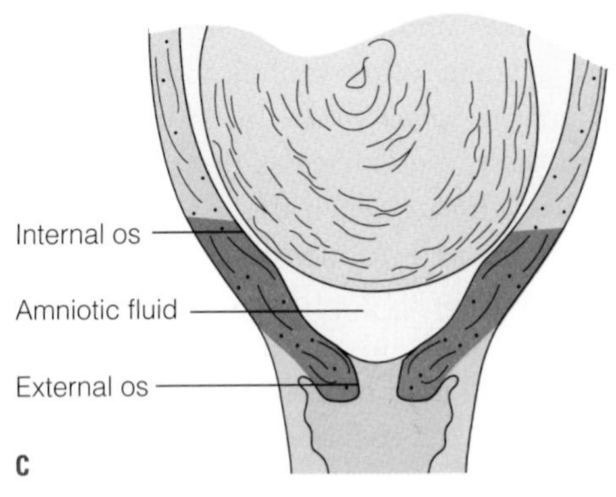


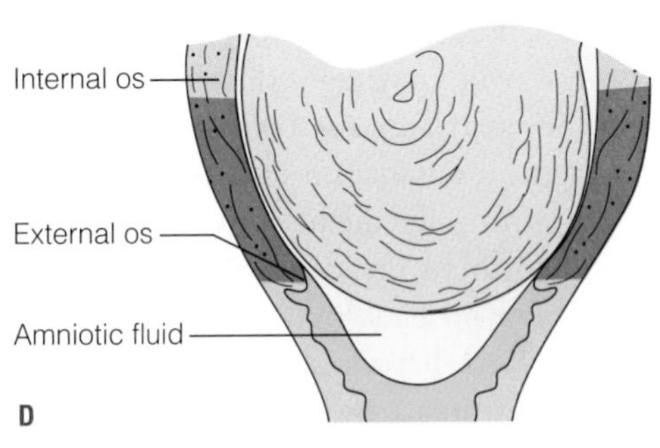


FIGURE 15–11 ♦ Effacement of the cervix in the primigravida. **A,** Beginning of labor. There is no cervical effacement or dilatation. The fetal head is cushioned by amniotic fluid. **B,** Beginning cervical effacement. As the cervix begins to efface, more amniotic fluid collects below the fetal head. **C,** Cervix about one-half effaced and slightly dilated. The increasing amount of amniotic fluid exerts hydrostatic pressure. **D,** Complete effacement and dilatation.

to approximately 10 cm, allowing birth of the fetus. When the cervix is completely dilated and retracted up into the lower uterine segment, it can no longer be palpated. At the same time the round ligament pulls the fundus forward, aligning the fetus with the bony pelvis.

## Intraabdominal Pressure

After the cervix is completely dilated, the maternal abdominal muscles contract as the woman pushes. This pushing action (called bearing down) aids in expulsion of the fetus and placenta. If the cervix is not completely dilated, however, bearing down can cause cervical edema (which retards dilatation), possible tearing and bruising of the cervix, and maternal exhaustion.

## Musculature Changes in the Pelvic Floor

The levator ani muscle and fascia of the pelvic floor draw the rectum and vagina upward and forward with each contraction, along the curve of the pelvic floor. As the fetal head descends to the pelvic floor, the pressure of the presenting part causes the perineal structure, which was once 5 cm in thickness, to thin to less than a centimeter. The anus everts, exposing the interior rectal wall as the fetal head descends forward (Cunningham, MacDonald, Grant, et al., 1997).

## Premonitory Signs of Labor

Most primigravidas and many multiparas experience the following signs and symptoms of impending labor.

### Lightening

**Lightening** describes the effects that occur when the fetus begins to settle into the pelvic inlet (engagement). With fetal descent, the uterus moves downward, and the fundus no longer presses on the diaphragm, which eases breathing. However, with increased downward pressure of the presenting part, the woman may notice the following:

- Leg cramps or pains due to pressure on the nerves that course through the obturator foramen in the pelvis

- Increased pelvic pressure
- Increased venous stasis, leading to edema in the lower extremities
- Increased vaginal secretions resulting from congestion of the vaginal mucous membranes

### Braxton Hicks Contractions

Before the onset of labor, **Braxton Hicks contractions** (the irregular, intermittent contractions that have been occurring throughout the pregnancy) may become uncomfortable. The pain seems to be focused in the abdomen and groin but may feel like the "drawing" sensations experienced by some women with dysmenorrhea. When these contractions are strong enough for the woman to believe she is in labor, she is said to be in *false labor.* False labor is uncomfortable and may be exhausting. Since the contractions can be fairly regular, the woman has no way of knowing if they are the beginning of true labor. She may come to the hospital or birthing center for a vaginal examination to determine if cervical dilatation is occurring. Frequent episodes of false labor, trips back and forth to the certified nurse-midwife or physician's office or hospital, may frustrate or embarrass the woman who feels that she should know when she is really in labor. Reassurance by nursing staff can ease embarrassment.

### Cervical Changes

Considerable change occurs in the cervix during the prenatal and intrapartal period. At the beginning of pregnancy the cervix is rigid and firm, and it must soften so that it can stretch and dilate to allow the fetus passage. This softening of the cervix is called *ripening.*

As term approaches, collagen fibers in the cervix are broken down by the action of enzymes such as collagenase and elastase. As the collagen fibers change, their ability to bind together decreases because of increasing amounts of hyaluronic acid (which loosely binds collagen fibrils) and decreasing amounts of dermatan sulfate (which tightly binds collagen fibrils). The water content of the cervix also increases. All these changes result in a weakening and softening of the cervix.

### Bloody Show

During pregnancy, cervical secretions accumulate in the cervical canal to form a barrier called a mucous plug. With softening and effacement of the cervix, the mucous plug is often expelled, resulting in a small amount of blood loss from the exposed cervical capillaries. The resulting pink-tinged secretions are called **bloody show.** Bloody show is considered a sign that labor will begin within 24 to 48 hours. Vaginal examination that includes manipulation of the cervix may also result in a blood-tinged discharge, which is sometimes confused with bloody show.

### Rupture of Membranes

In approximately 12% of women at term (38 through 41 weeks gestation), the amniotic membranes rupture before the onset of labor. This is called *rupture of membranes (ROM).* After the membranes rupture, 80% of these women experience onset of labor within 24 hours. If membranes rupture and labor does not begin spontaneously within 12 to 24 hours, labor may be induced to decrease the risk of infection. Labor is induced only if the pregnancy is near term (Varney, 1997).

When the membranes rupture, the amniotic fluid may be expelled in large amounts. If engagement has not occurred, there is danger of the umbilical cord washing out with the fluid (*prolapsed cord*). In addition, the open pathway into the uterus increases the risk of infection. Because of these threats, when the membranes rupture, the woman is advised to notify her certified nurse-midwife or physician and proceed to the hospital or birthing center. In some instances, the fluid is expelled in small amounts and may be confused with episodes of urinary incontinence associated with urinary urgency, coughing, or sneezing. The discharge should be checked to determine its source and the appropriate action. (See Chapter 16 for assessment techniques.)

### Sudden Burst of Energy

Some women report a sudden burst of energy approximately 24 to 48 hours before labor. The cause of the energy spurt is unknown. In prenatal teaching the nurse should warn prospective mothers not to overexert themselves during this energy burst to avoid being overtired when labor begins.

### Other Signs

Additional premonitory signs include the following:

- Weight loss of 1 to 3 lb resulting from fluid loss and electrolyte shifts produced by changes in estrogen and progesterone levels
- Diarrhea, indigestion, or nausea and vomiting just before onset of labor

The causes of these signs are unknown.

## Differences between True and False Labor

The contractions of true labor produce progressive dilatation and effacement of the cervix. They occur regularly and increase in frequency, duration, and intensity.

The discomfort of true labor contractions usually starts in the back and radiates around to the abdomen. The pain is not relieved by ambulation (in fact, walking may intensify the pain).

The contractions of false labor do not produce progressive cervical effacement and dilatation. Classically, they are irregular and do not increase in frequency, duration, and intensity. The contractions may be perceived as a hardening or "balling up" without discomfort, or discomfort may occur mainly in the lower abdomen and groin. The discomfort may be relieved by ambulation, changes of position, or a hot shower (Lieberman & Holt, 2000). The woman will find it helpful to know the characteristics of true labor contractions as well as the premonitory signs of ensuing labor. However, many times the only way to differentiate accurately between true and false labor is to assess dilatation. The woman must feel free to come in for accurate assessment of labor and should be counseled not to feel foolish if the labor is false. The nurse must reassure the woman that false labor is common and that it often cannot be distinguished from true labor except by vaginal examination. (See Key Facts to Remember: Comparison of True and False Labor.)

**KEY FACTS TO REMEMBER**

*Comparison of True and False Labor*

| *True Labor* | *False Labor* |
|---|---|
| Contractions are at regular intervals. | Contractions are irregular. |
| Intervals between contractions gradually shorten. | Usually no change. |
| Contractions increase in duration and intensity. | Usually no change. |
| Discomfort begins in back and radiates around to abdomen. | Discomfort is usually in abdomen. |
| Intensity usually increases with walking. | Walking has no effect on or lessens contractions. |
| Cervical dilatation and effacement are progressive. | No change. |

# Stages of Labor and Birth

To assist caregivers, common terms have been developed as benchmarks to subdivide the labor process into *phases* and *stages* of labor. It is important to note, however, that these represent theoretical separations in the process. A laboring woman will not usually experience distinct differences from one to the other.

The first stage begins with the onset of true labor and ends when the cervix is completely dilated at 10 cm. The second stage begins with complete dilatation and ends with the birth of the newborn. The third stage begins with the birth of the newborn and ends with the delivery of the placenta.

Some clinicians identify a fourth stage. During this stage, which lasts 1 to 4 hours after delivery of the placenta, the uterus effectively contracts to control bleeding at the placental site (Cunningham et al., 1997). (The care of the laboring woman is discussed in Chapter 17.)

## First Stage

The first stage of labor is divided into the latent, active, and transition phases. Each phase of labor is characterized by physical and psychologic changes.

### Latent Phase

The latent phase starts with the beginning of regular contractions, which are usually mild. The woman feels able to cope with the discomfort. She may be relieved that labor has finally started and that the end of pregnancy has come. Although she may be anxious, she is able to recognize and express those feelings of anxiety. The woman is often talkative and smiling and is eager to talk about herself and answer questions. Excitement is high, and her partner or other support person is often as elated as she is.

Uterine contractions become established during the latent phase and increase in frequency, duration, and intensity. They may start as mild contractions lasting 15 to 20 seconds with a frequency of 10 to 20 minutes and progress to moderate ones lasting 30 to 40 seconds with a frequency of 5 to 7 minutes. As the cervix begins to dilate, it also effaces, although little or no fetal descent is evident. For a woman in her first labor (nullipara), the latent (or early) phase of the first stage of labor averages 8.6 hours but should not exceed 20 hours. The latent phase in multiparas averages 5.3 hours but should not exceed 14 hours.

At the beginning of labor, the amniotic membranes bulge through the cervix in the shape of a cone. **Spontaneous rupture of membranes (SROM)** generally occurs at the height of an intense contraction with a gush of fluid out of the vagina. In many instances, the membranes are ruptured by the certified nurse-midwife or physician, using an instrument called an amnihook. This procedure is called amniotomy, or **artificial rupture of membranes (AROM).**

### Active Phase

When the woman enters the early *active phase,* her anxiety tends to increase as she senses the intensification of contractions and pain. She begins to fear a loss of control and may use a variety of coping mechanisms. Some women exhibit decreased ability to cope and a sense of helplessness. Women who have support persons and family available may experience greater satisfaction and less anxiety than those without support.

During this phase, the cervix dilates from about 3–4 cm to 8 cm. Fetal descent is progressive. The cervical dilatation averages 1.2 cm/hr in nulliparas and 1.5 cm/hr in multiparas (Varney, 1997).

### Transition Phase

The transition phase is the last part of the first stage of labor. When the woman enters the transition phase, she may demonstrate significant anxiety. She becomes acutely aware of the increasing force and intensity of the contractions. She may become restless, frequently changing position. By the time the woman enters the transition phase, she is inner directed and often tired. She may fear being left alone at the same time the support person may be feeling the need for a break. The nurse should reassure the woman that she will not be left alone. It is crucial that the nurse be available as relief support at this time and keep the woman informed about where her labor support people are, if they leave the room.

During the active and transition phases, contractions become more frequent and longer in duration, and they increase in intensity. By the end of the active phase, contractions have a frequency of 2 to 3 minutes, a duration of 60 seconds, and strong intensity. During transition, contractions have a frequency of about every 2 minutes, a duration of 60 to 90 seconds, and strong intensity (Varney, 1997). Cervical dilatation slows as it progresses from 8 to 10 cm and the rate of fetal descent dramatically increases. The average rate of descent is 1.6 cm/hr and at least 1 cm/hr in nulliparas and 5.4 cm/hr and at least 2.1 cm/hr in multiparas. The transition phase does not usually last longer than 3 hours for nulliparas or longer than 1 hour for multiparas (Varney, 1997).

As dilatation approaches 10 cm, there may be increased rectal pressure and an uncontrollable desire to bear down, increased amount of bloody show, and rupture of membranes (if it has not already occurred). The woman may also fear that she will be "torn open" or "split apart" by the force of the contractions. With the peak of a contraction, she may experience a sensation of pressure so great that it seems to her that her abdomen will burst open with the force. The nurse should inform the woman that what she is feeling is normal. Much of the anxiety experienced may focus on the fear that the powerful forces she feels indicate that something is wrong. The woman may increasingly doubt her ability to cope with labor and may become apprehensive, irritable, and withdrawn. She may be terrified of being left alone, though she does not want anyone to talk to or touch her. However, with the next contraction she may ask for verbal and physical support. Other characteristics of this phase may include the following (Varney, 1997):

- Increasing bloody show
- Hyperventilation, as the woman increases her breathing rate
- Generalized discomfort, including low backache, shaking and cramping in legs, and increased sensitivity to touch
- Increased need for partner's and/or nurse's presence and support
- Restlessness
- Increased apprehension and irritability
- Difficulty understanding directions
- A sense of bewilderment, frustration, and anger at the contractions
- Requests for medication
- Hiccupping, belching, nausea, or vomiting
- Beads of perspiration on the upper lip or brow
- Increasing rectal pressure and feeling the urge to bear down

The woman in this phase is anxious to "get it over with." She may be amnesic and sleep between her now-frequent contractions. Her support persons may start to feel helpless and may turn to the nurse for increased participation as their efforts to alleviate her discomfort seem less effective.

## Second Stage

The second stage of labor begins with complete cervical dilatation and ends with birth of the infant. Traditional thought suggests that the second stage should be completed within 2 hours after the cervix becomes fully dilated for primigravidas; the stage averages 15 minutes for multiparas. Contractions continue with a frequency of about every 2 minutes, a duration of 60 to 90 seconds, and strong intensity (Varney, 1997). Descent of the fetal presenting part continues until it reaches the perineal floor.

TABLE 15–3 Characteristics of Labor

| | First Stage | | | Second Stage |
|---|---|---|---|---|
| | *Latent Phase* | *Active Phase* | *Transition Phase* | |
| Nullipara | 8.6 hr | 4.6 hr | 3.6 hr | Up to 3 hr |
| Multipara | 5.3 hr | 2.4 hr | Variable | 0–30 min |
| Cervical dilatation | 0–3 cm | 4–7 cm | 8–10 cm | |
| Contractions | | | | |
| Frequency | Every 3–30 min | Every 2–3 min | Every 1½–2 min | Every 1½–2 min |
| Duration | 20–40 sec | 40–60 sec | 60–90 sec | 60–90 sec |
| Intensity | Begin as mild and progress to moderate; 25–40 mm Hg by intrauterine pressure catheter (IUPC) | Begin as moderate and progress to strong; 50–70 mm Hg by IUPC | Strong by palpation; 70–90 mm Hg by IUPC | Strong by palpation; 70–100 mm Hg by IUPC |

As the fetal head descends, the woman usually has the urge to push because of pressure of the fetal head on the sacral and obturator nerves. As she pushes, intraabdominal pressure is exerted from contraction of the maternal abdominal muscles. As the fetal head continues its descent, the perineum begins to bulge, flatten, and move anteriorly. The amount of bloody show may increase. The labia begin to part with each contraction. Between contractions the fetal head appears to recede. With succeeding contractions and maternal pushing effort, the fetal head descends farther. **Crowning** occurs when the fetal head is encircled by the external opening of the vagina (introitus), and it means birth is imminent.

A childbirth-prepared woman may feel some relief that the acute pain she felt during the transition phase is over (see Table 15–3). She may also be relieved that the birth is near and she can push. Some women feel a sense of purpose now that they can be actively involved. Others, particularly those without childbirth preparation, may become frightened and fight each contraction. Such behavior may be disconcerting to the woman's support persons. The woman may feel she has lost her ability to cope and become embarrassed, or she may demonstrate extreme irritability toward the staff or her supporters as she attempts to regain control over external forces against which she feels helpless. Most women feel acute, increasingly severe pain and a burning sensation as the perineum distends.

## Spontaneous Birth (Vertex Presentation)

As the fetal head distends the vulva with each contraction, the perineum becomes extremely thin and the anus stretches and protrudes. With time, the head extends under the symphysis pubis and is born. When the anterior shoulder meets the underside of the symphysis pubis, a gentle push by the mother aids in the birth of the shoulders. The body then follows (Figure 15–12♦). (Birth of a fetus in other than a vertex presentation is discussed in Chapter 19.)

## Positional Changes of the Fetus

For the fetus to pass through the birth canal, the fetal head and body must adjust to the passage by certain positional changes. These changes, called **cardinal movements** or mechanisms of labor, are described in the order in which they occur (Figure 15–13♦ on page 369).

### Descent

Descent occurs because of four forces: (1) pressure of the amniotic fluid, (2) direct pressure of the uterine fundus on the breech, (3) contraction of the abdominal muscles, and (4) extension and straightening of the fetal body. The head enters the inlet in the occiput transverse or oblique position because the pelvic inlet is widest from side to side. The sagittal suture is an equal distance from the maternal symphysis pubis and sacral promontory.

### Flexion

Flexion occurs as the fetal head descends and meets resistance from the soft tissues of the pelvis, the muscles of the pelvic floor, and the cervix. As a result of the resistance, the fetal chin flexes downward onto the chest.

### Internal Rotation

The fetal head must rotate to fit the diameter of the pelvic cavity, which is widest in the anteroposterior diameter. As the occiput of the fetal head meets resistance from the levator ani muscles and their fascia, the occiput

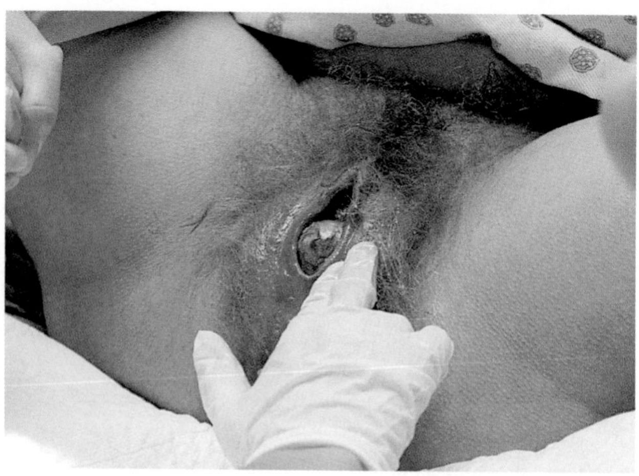
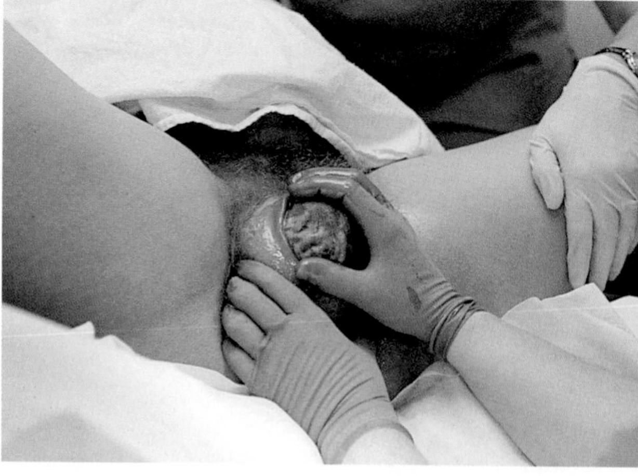
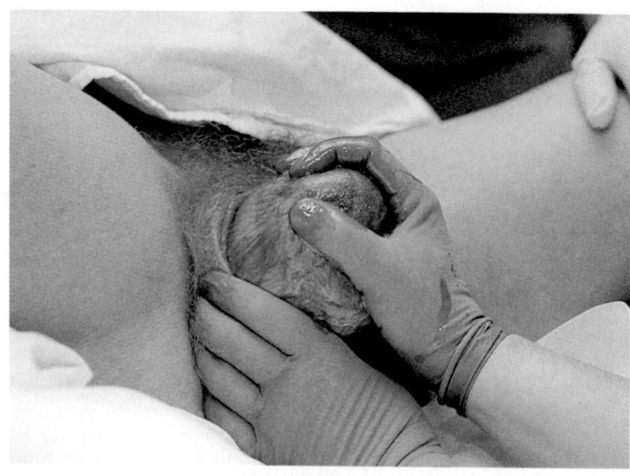
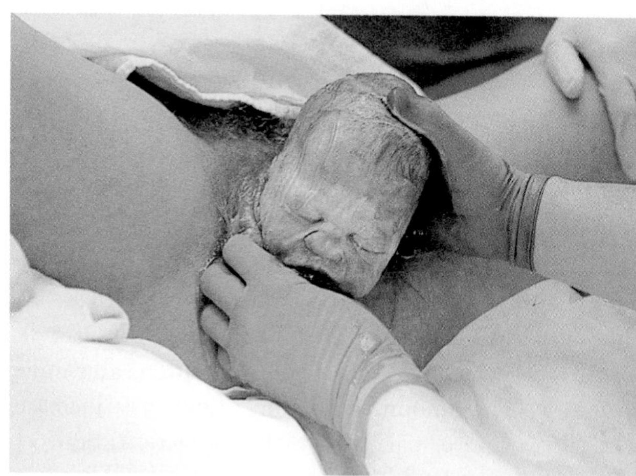
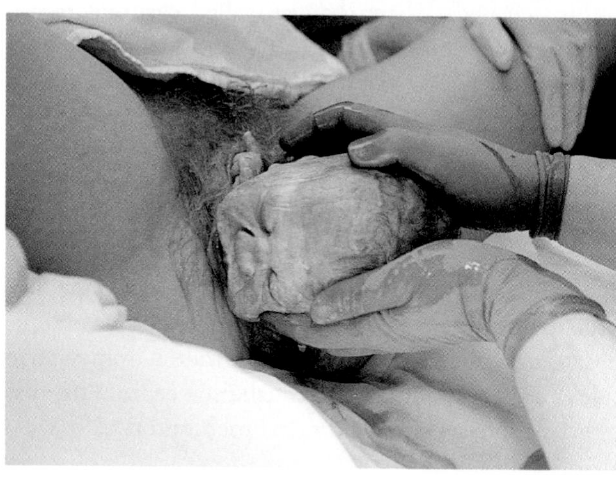
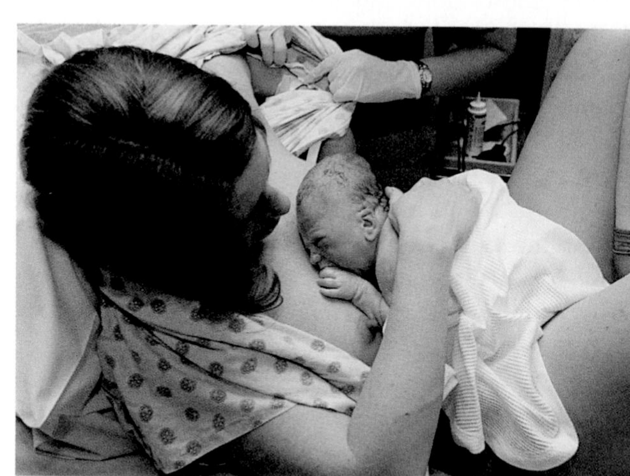

FIGURE 15–12 ♦ The birth sequence.

rotates—usually from left to right—and the sagittal suture aligns in the anteroposterior pelvic diameter.

## Extension

The resistance of the pelvic floor and the mechanical movement of the vulva opening anteriorly and forward assist with extension of the fetal head as it passes under the symphysis pubis. With this positional change, the occiput, then brow and face, emerge from the vagina.

## Restitution

The shoulders of the fetus enter the pelvis inlet obliquely and remain oblique when the head rotates to the anteroposterior diameter through internal rotation. Because of

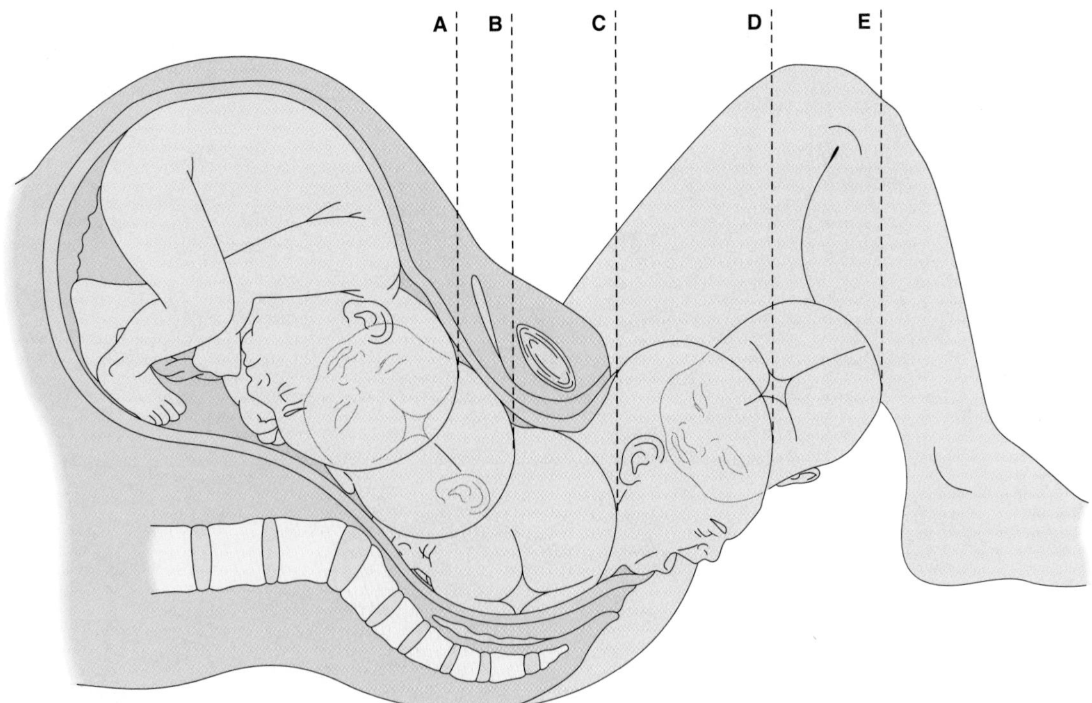


IGURE 15–13 ♦ Mechanisms of labor. **A, B,** Descent. **C,** Internal rotation. **D,** Extension. , External rotation.

nis rotation, the neck becomes twisted. Once the head is orn and is free of pelvic resistance, the neck untwists, urning the head to one side (restitution), and aligns with ne position of the back in the birth canal.

### xternal Rotation

.s the shoulders rotate to the anteroposterior position in ne pelvis, the head turns farther to one side (external roation).

### xpulsion

fter the external rotation, and through the pushing eforts of the laboring woman, the anterior shoulder meets he undersurface of the symphysis pubis and slips under . As lateral flexion of the shoulder and head occurs, the nterior shoulder is born before the posterior shoulder. he body follows quickly.

## THIRD STAGE

### PLACENTAL SEPARATION

fter the infant is born, the uterus contracts firmly, diminishing its capacity and the surface area of placental atachment. The placenta begins to separate because of this ecrease in surface area. As this separation occurs, bleedng results in the formation of a hematoma between the lacental tissue and the remaining decidua. This ematoma accelerates the separation process. The memranes are the last to separate. They are peeled off the terine wall as the placenta descends into the vagina. Signs of placental separation usually appear about 5 minutes after the birth of the newborn. These signs are (1) a globular-shaped uterus, (2) a rise of the fundus in the abdomen, (3) a sudden gush or trickle of blood, and (4) further protrusion of the umbilical cord out of the vagina.

### PLACENTAL DELIVERY

When the signs of placental separation appear, the woman may bear down to aid in placental expulsion. If this fails and the certified nurse-midwife or physician has ascertained that the fundus is firm, gentle traction may be applied to the cord while pressure is exerted on the fundus. The weight of the placenta as it is guided into the placental collection pan aids in the removal of the membranes from the uterine wall. A placenta is considered to be *retained* if 30 minutes have elapsed from completion of the second stage of labor.

If the placenta separates from the inside to the outer margins, it is delivered with the fetal (shiny) side presenting (Figure 15–14♦). This is known as the Schultze mechanism of placental delivery or, more commonly, "shiny Schultze." If the placenta separates from the outer margins inward, it will roll up and present sideways with the maternal surface delivering first. This is known as the Duncan mechanism of placental delivery and is commonly called "dirty Duncan" because the placental surface is rough. (Nursing and medical interventions for the third stage of labor are discussed in Chapter 17.)

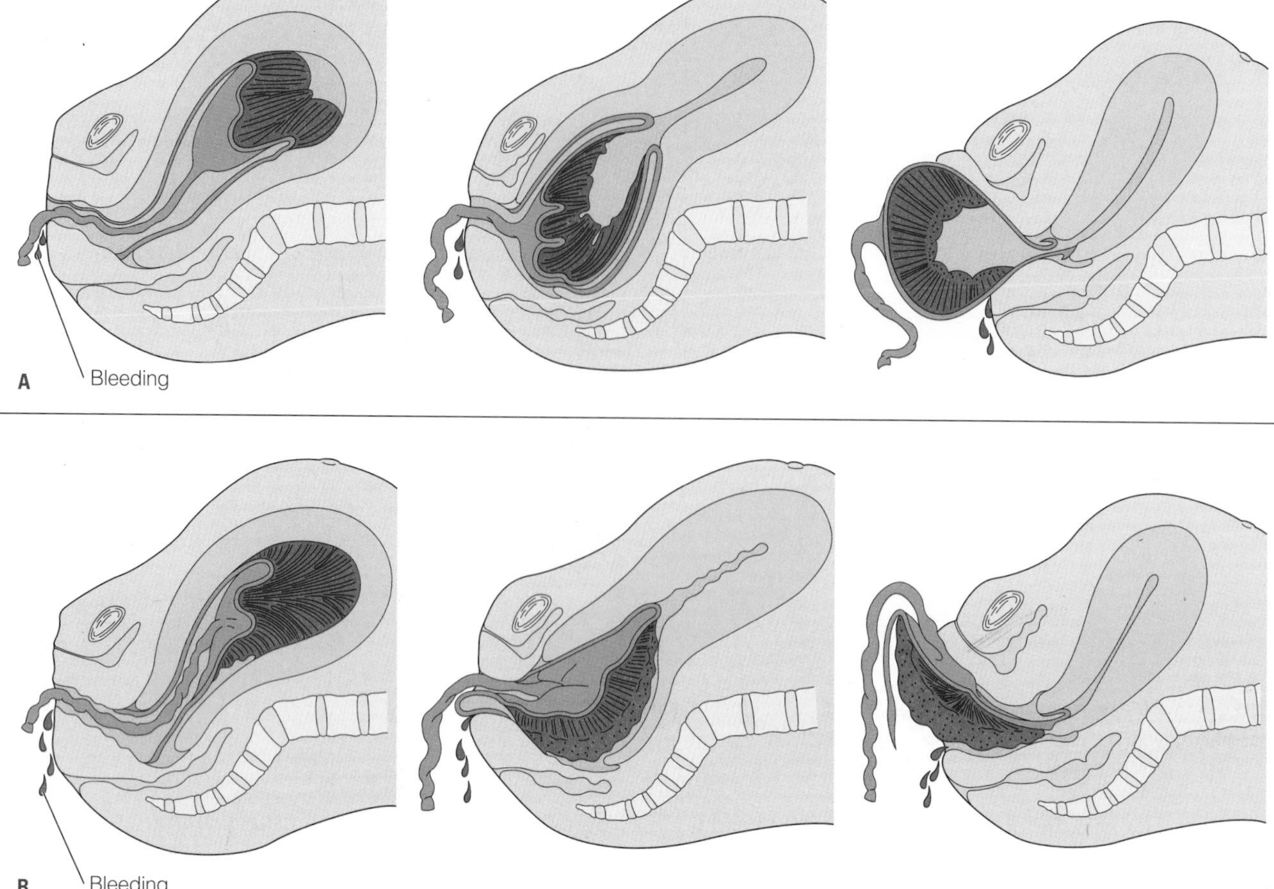


**FIGURE 15–14** ♦ Placental separation and expulsion. **A**, Schultze mechanism. **B**, Duncan mechanism.

## Fourth Stage

The fourth stage of labor is the time, from 1 to 4 hours after birth, during which physiologic readjustment of the mother's body begins. With the birth, hemodynamic changes occur. Blood loss ranges from 250 to 500 mL. With this blood loss and removal of the weight of the pregnant uterus from the surrounding vessels, blood is redistributed into venous beds. This results in a moderate drop in both systolic and diastolic blood pressure, increased pulse pressure, and moderate tachycardia (Cunningham et al., 1997).

The uterus remains contracted in the midline of the abdomen. The fundus is usually midway between the symphysis pubis and umbilicus. Its contracted state constricts the vessels at the site of placental implantation. Immediately after birth of the placenta, the cervix is widely spread and thick.

Nausea and vomiting usually cease. The woman may be thirsty and hungry. She may experience a shaking chill, which is thought to be associated with the ending of the physical exertion of labor. The bladder is often hypotonic due to trauma during the second stage and/or the administration of anesthetics that decrease sensations. Hypotonic bladder can lead to urinary retention. (Nursing care during this stage is discussed in Chapter 17.)

# Maternal Systemic Response to Labor

## Cardiovascular System

The woman's cardiovascular system is stressed both by the uterine contractions and by the pain, anxiety, and apprehension she experiences. During labor there is a significant increase in cardiac output. With each contraction, 300 to 500 mL of blood volume is forced back into the maternal circulation, which results in an increase in cardiac output of as much as 31% (Monga, 1999). Further increases in cardiac output occur as the laboring woman experiences pain with uterine contractions and her anxiety and apprehension increase.

Maternal position also affects cardiac output. In the supine position, cardiac output lowers, heart rate increases, and stroke volume decreases. When the woman turns to a lateral (side-lying) position, cardiac output increases by as much as 25% to 30% (Monga, 1999).

## Blood Pressure

As a result of increased cardiac output, blood pressure (both systolic and diastolic) rises during uterine contractions. In the first stage, systolic pressure increases by 35 mm Hg and diastolic pressure increases by about 25 mm Hg. There may be further increases in the second stage during pushing (Monga, 1999).

## Respiratory System

Oxygen demand and consumption increase at the onset of labor because of the presence of uterine contractions. As anxiety and pain from contractions increase, hyperventilation frequently occurs. With hyperventilation there is a fall in $PaCO_2$, and respiratory alkalosis results (K. Smith, 2000).

By the end of the first stage, most women have developed a mild metabolic acidosis compensated by respiratory alkalosis. As they push in the second stage of labor, the women's $PaCO_2$ levels may rise along with blood lactate levels (due to muscular activity), and mild respiratory acidosis occurs. By the time the baby is born (end of second stage), there is metabolic acidosis uncompensated for by respiratory alkalosis (Blackburn & Loper, 1992).

The changes in acid-base status that occur in labor are quickly reversed in the fourth stage because of changes in women's respiratory rates. Acid-base levels return to pregnancy levels by 24 hours after birth, and nonpregnant values are attained a few weeks after birth (Blackburn & Loper, 1992).

## Renal System

During labor there is an increase in maternal renin, plasma renin activity, and angiotensinogen. This elevation is thought to be important in the control of uteroplacental blood flow during birth and the early postpartal period (Blackburn & Loper, 1992).

Structurally, the base of the bladder is pushed forward and upward when engagement occurs. The pressure from the presenting part may impair blood and lymph drainage from the base of the bladder, leading to edema (Cunningham et al., 1997).

## Gastrointestinal System

During labor, gastric motility and absorption of solid food are reduced. Gastric emptying time is prolonged, and gastric volume (amount of contents that remain in the stomach) remains increased, regardless of the time the last meal was taken (K. Smith, 2000). Some narcotics also delay gastric emptying time and add to the risk of aspiration if general anesthesia is used.

## Immune System and Other Blood Values

The white blood cell count (WBC) increases to 25,000 to $30,000/mm^3$ during labor and the early postpartum period. The change in WBC is mostly due to increased neutrophils resulting from a physiologic response to stress. The increased WBC makes it difficult to identify the presence of an infection.

Maternal blood glucose levels decrease because glucose is used as an energy source during uterine contractions. The decreased blood glucose levels lead to a decrease in insulin requirements (Varney, 1997).

## Pain

According to the *gate-control theory*, pain results from activity in several interacting specialized neural systems. The gate-control theory proposes that a mechanism in the dorsal horn of the spinal column serves as a valve, or gate, that increases or decreases the flow of nerve impulses from the periphery to the central nervous system (CNS). The gate mechanism is influenced by the size of the transmitting fibers and by the nerve impulses that descend from the brain. Psychologic processes such as past experiences, attention, and emotion may influence pain perception and response by activating the gate mechanism. The gates may be opened or closed by CNS activities, such as anxiety or excitement, or selective localized activity.

The gate-control theory has two important implications for childbirth. Pain can be reduced by tactile stimulation and may be modified by activities controlled by the CNS. These activities include back rub, sacral pressure, effleurage, suggestion, distraction, and conditioning.

### Causes of Pain during Labor

The pain associated with the first stage of labor is unique in that it accompanies a normal physiologic process. Even though perception of the pain of childbirth varies among women, there is a physiologic basis for discomfort during labor. Pain during the first stage of labor arises from (a) dilatation of the cervix, which is the primary source of pain; (b) stretching of the lower uterine segment; (c) pressure on adjacent structures; and (d) hypoxia of the uterine muscle cells during contraction (Wesson, 2000). The areas of pain include the lower abdominal wall and the areas over the lower lumbar region and the upper sacrum (Figure 15–15♦).

During the second stage of labor, discomfort is due to (a) hypoxia of the contracting uterine muscle cells, (b) distention of the vagina and perineum, and (c) pressure on adjacent structures. The area of pain increases as shown in Figures 15–16 and 15–17♦.

Pain during the third stage results from uterine contractions and cervical dilatation as the placenta is

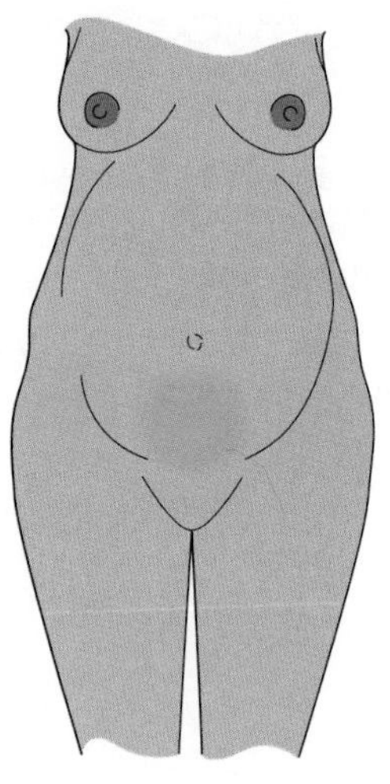

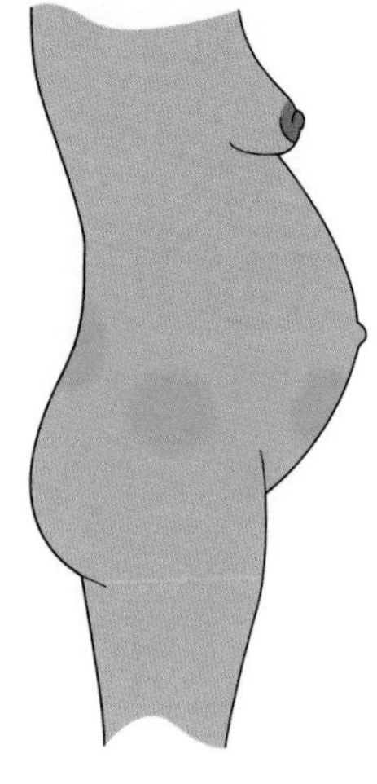

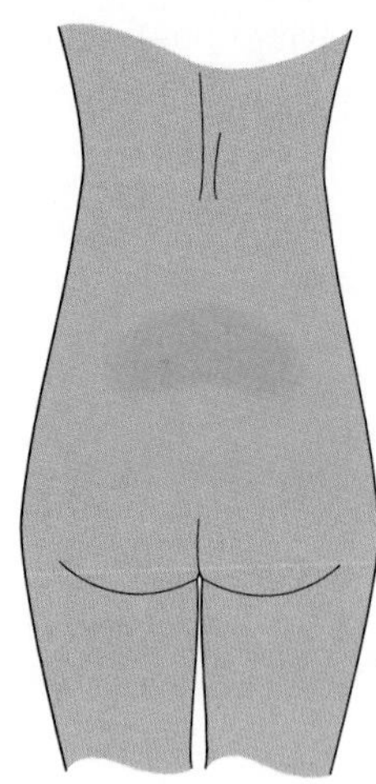

**FIGURE 15–15** ♦ Area of reference of labor pain during the first stage. Pain is the most intense in the darker-colored areas. *Source:* Bonica, J. J. (1972). *Principles and practice of obstetric analgesia and anesthesia* (p. 108). Philadelphia: Davis.

expelled. This stage of labor is short, and after it anesthesia is needed primarily for episiotomy repair.

## Factors Affecting Response to Pain

Many factors affect the individual's perception and response to pain. For example, preparation for childbirth classes may reduce the need for analgesia during labor. In addition, individuals tend to respond to painful stimuli in the way that is acceptable in their culture. In some cultures, it is natural to communicate pain, no matter how mild, whereas members of other cultures stoically accept pain out of fear or because it is expected. Response to pain may also be influenced by fatigue and sleep deprivation. The fatigued woman has less energy and ability t use such strategies as distraction or imagination to dea with pain. As a result, she may lose her ability to cop with labor and choose analgesics or other medications t relieve the discomfort.

The woman's previous experience with pain and anxi ety level also affects her ability to manage current and fu ture pain. Those who have had experience with pain seem more sensitive to painful stimuli than those who have not Unfamiliar surroundings and events can increase anxiety as does separation from family and loved ones. Anticipa

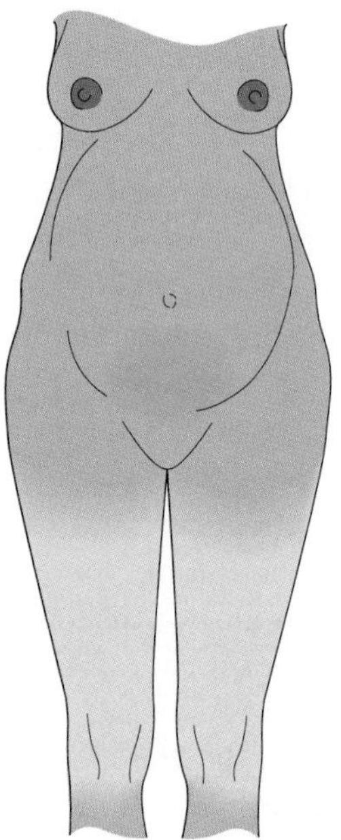

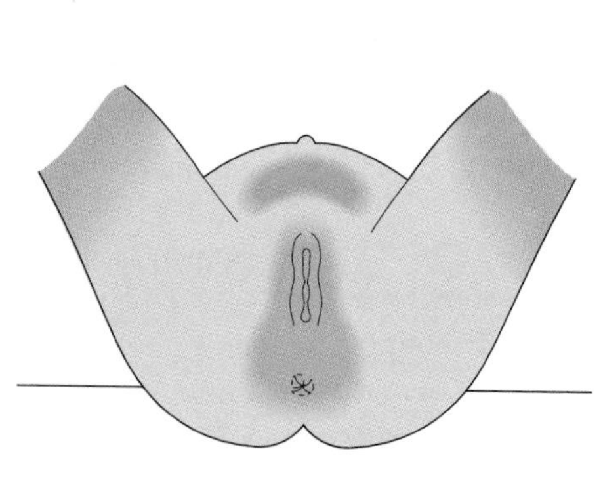

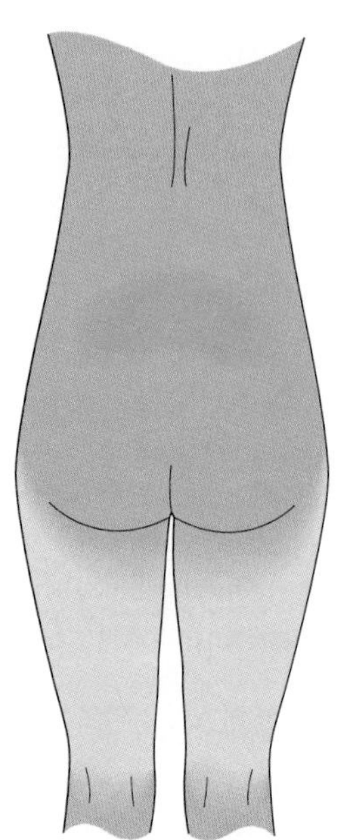

**FIGURE 15–16** ♦ Distribution of labor pain during the later phase of the first stage and early phase of the second stage. The darkest-colored areas indicate the location of the most intense pain, moderate color indicates moderate pain, and lighter color indicates mild pain. The uterine contractions, which at this stage are very strong, produce intense pain. *Source:* Bonica, J. J. (1972). *Principles and practice of obstetric analgesia and anesthesia* (p. 109). Philadelphia: Davis.

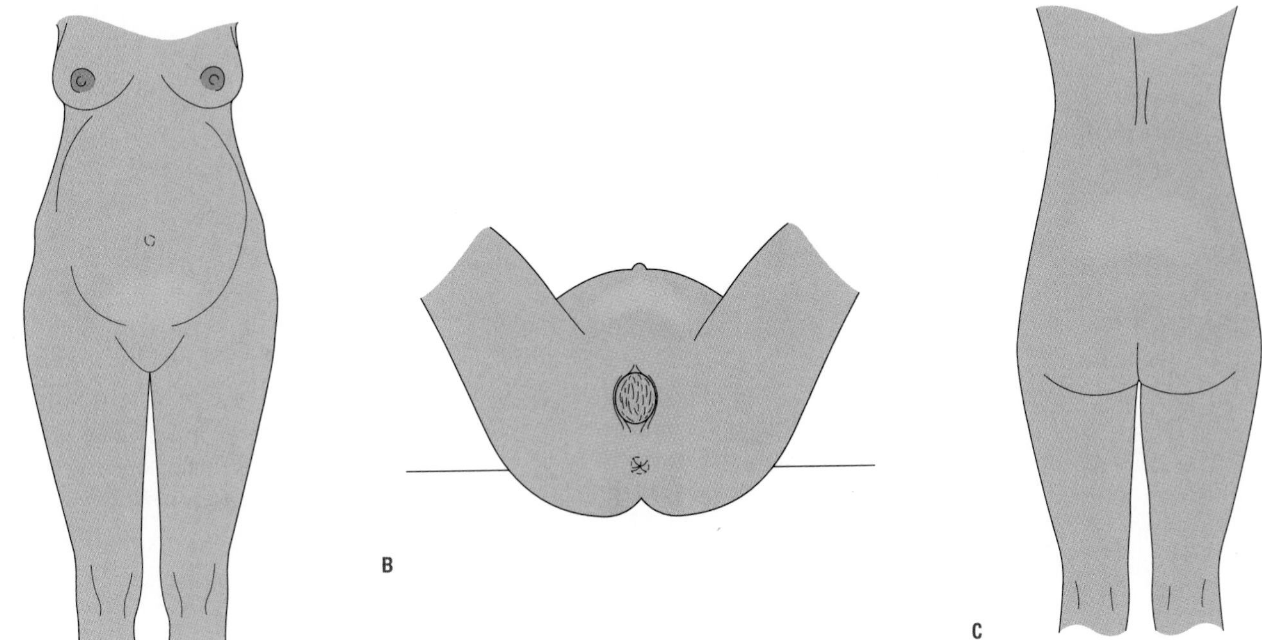


FIGURE 15–17 ♦ Distribution of labor pain during the later phase of the second stage and actual birth. The perineal component is the primary cause of discomfort. Uterine contractions contribute much less to the level of pain. *Source:* Bonica, J. J. (1972). *Principles and practice of obstetric analgesia and anesthesia* (p. 109). Philadelphia: Davis.

tion of discomfort and questions about whether she can cope with the contractions may also increase anxiety.

Both attention and distraction influence the perception of pain. When pain sensation is the focus of attention, the perceived intensity is greater. A sensory stimulus such as a back rub can be a distraction that focuses the woman's attention on the stimulus rather than the pain.

# Fetal Response to Labor

When the fetus is healthy, the mechanical and hemodynamic changes of normal labor have no adverse effects.

## Heart Rate Changes

Early fetal heart rate decelerations can occur with intracranial pressures of 40 to 55 mm Hg, as the head pushes against the cervix. The currently accepted explanation of this early deceleration is hypoxic depression of the central nervous system, which is under vagal control. The absence of these head-compression decelerations in some fetuses during labor is explained by the existence of a threshold that is reached more gradually in the presence of intact membranes and lack of maternal resistance. These early decelerations are harmless in a normal fetus.

## Acid-Base Status

Blood flow is decreased to the fetus at the peak of each contraction, which leads to a slow decrease in pH status. During the second stage of labor, as uterine contractions become longer and stronger and the woman holds her breath to push, the fetal pH decreases more rapidly. The base deficit increases, and fetal oxygen saturation drops approximately 10% (Manning, 1999).

## Hemodynamic Changes

The adequate exchange of nutrients and gases in the fetal capillaries and intervillous spaces depends in part on the fetal blood pressure. Fetal blood pressure is a protective mechanism for the normal fetus during the anoxic periods caused by the contracting uterus during labor. The fetal and placental reserve is usually enough to see the fetus through these anoxic periods unharmed (Meschia, 1999).

## Fetal Sensation

Beginning at about 37 or 38 weeks' gestation (full term), the fetus is able to experience sensations of light, sound, and touch. The full-term fetus is able to hear music and the maternal voice. Even in utero, the fetus is sensitive to light and will move away from a bright light source. Additionally, the term baby is aware of pressure sensations during labor such as the touch of the caregiver during a vaginal exam or pressure on the head as a contraction occurs. Although the fetus may not be able to process this input, it is important to note that as the woman labors the fetus is experiencing the labor as well.

# Chapter Review

## CHAPTER HIGHLIGHTS

- Five factors that continuously interact during the process of labor and birth are the birth passage, the fetus, the relationship between the passage and the fetus, the forces of labor (contractions and pushing efforts), and the emotional components the woman brings to the birth setting (psychosocial status).
- Important parts of the maternal pelvis include the pelvic inlet, pelvic cavity, and pelvic outlet.
- The fetal head contains bones that are not fused. This allows for some overlapping and for a change in the shape of the head called molding to facilitate birth.
- Fetal attitude refers to the relation of the fetal parts to one another. The head is usually moderately flexed at midline, and the extremities are flexed close to the body.
- Fetal lie refers to the relationship of the cephalocaudal axis of the fetus to the maternal spine. The fetal lie is either longitudinal or transverse.
- Fetal presentation is determined by the body part lying closest to the maternal pelvis. Fetal presentation can be cephalic (head down), breech (buttocks or one or both feet), or shoulder.
- Fetal position is the relationship of the landmark on the presenting fetal part to the front, sides, or back of the maternal pelvis.
- Engagement of the presenting part takes place when the largest diameter of the presenting part reaches or passes through the pelvic inlet.
- Station refers to the relationship of the presenting part to an imaginary line drawn between the ischial spines of the maternal pelvis. Negative numbers (−5 through −1) are above the ischial spines, and the fetus is not engaged. Zero (0) station is at the pelvic inlet, and descent below the ishial spines is indicated by positive numbers (+1 through +4).
- Each uterine contraction has an increment, acme, and decrement. Contraction frequency is the time from the beginning of one contraction to the beginning of the next contraction.
- Contraction duration is the time from the beginning to the end of one contraction.
- Contraction intensity is the strength of the contraction during acme. Intensity is termed mild, moderate, or strong.
- Factors that affect the woman's response to labor pain include education, cultural beliefs, fatigue, personal significance of pain, previous experience, anxiety, and availability of coping techniques and support.
- Possible causes of labor include progesterone withdrawal, prostaglandin release, or increased concentrations of CRH.
- Premonitory signs of labor include lightening, Braxton Hicks contractions, cervical softening and effacement, bloody show, sudden burst of energy, weight loss, and sometimes rupture of membranes.
- True labor contractions occur regularly, with an increase in frequency, duration, and intensity over time. The contractions usually start in the back and radiate around the abdomen. The discomfort is not relieved by ambulation or rest. False labor contractions do not produce progressive cervical effacement and dilatation. They are usually irregular and do not increase in intensity. The discomfort may be relieved by changes in activity.
- There are four stages of labor and birth: the first stage is from the beginning of true labor to complete dilatation of the cervix, the second stage is from complete dilatation of the cervix to birth, the third stage is from birth to expulsion of the placenta, and the fourth stage is from expulsion of the placenta to a period of 1 to 4 hours after.

- The fetus accommodates itself to the maternal pelvis in a series of movements called the cardinal movements of labor, which include descent, flexion, internal rotation, extension, external rotation, expulsion, and restitution.
- Placental separation is indicated by lengthening of the umbilical cord, a small spurt of blood, change in uterine shape, and a rise of the fundus in the abdomen.
- The placenta is delivered by the Schultze or Duncan mechanism, which is determined by the way it separates from the uterine wall.
- Maternal systemic responses to labor involve the cardiovascular, respiratory, renal, gastrointestinal, and immune systems.
- The fetus is usually able to tolerate the labor process with no untoward changes.

## CHAPTER REFERENCES


Blackburn, S. T., & Loper, D. L. (1992). *Maternal, fetal, and neonatal physiology.* Philadelphia: Saunders.

Caldwell, W. E., & Moloy, H. C. (1933). Anatomical variations in the female pelvis and their effect on labor with a suggested classification. *American Journal of Obstetrics and Gynecology,* 26, 479.

Challis, J. R. G. (1999). Characteristics of parturition. In R. K. Creasy & R. R. Resnik (Eds.), *Maternal-fetal medicine* (4th ed., pp. 484–497). Philadelphia: Saunders.

Cunningham, F. G., MacDonald, P. C., Grant, N. F., Leveno, K. J., Gilstrap, L. C., Hankins, D. V., & Clark, S. L. (1997). *Williams obstetrics* (20th ed.). Stamford, CT: Appleton & Lange.

England, P., & Horowitz, R. (1998). *Birthing from within.* Albuquerque, NM: Pantera Press.

Lieberman, A. B., & Holt, L. H. (2000). *Nine months and a day.* Boston: Harvard Common Press.

Liggins, G. C. (1997). Biology of parturition. In R. K. Creasy (Ed.), *Management of labor and delivery.* Malden, MA: Blackwell.

Manning, F. (1999). Fetal assessment by evaluation of biophysical variables. In R. K. Creasy & R. R. Resnik (Eds.), *Maternal-fetal medicine* (4th ed., pp. 319–330). Philadelphia: Saunders.

Mauger, B. (2000). *Reclaiming the spirituality of birth: Healing for mothers and babies.* Rochester, VT: Healing Arts Press.

Meschia, G. (1999). Placental respiratory gas exchange and fetal oxygenation. In R. K. Creasy & R. R. Resnik (Eds.), *Maternal-fetal medicine* (4th ed., pp. 260–269). Philadelphia: Saunders.

Monga, M. (1999). Maternal cardiovascular and renal adaptation to pregnancy. In R. K. Creasy & R. R. Resnik (Eds.), *Maternal-fetal medicine* (4th ed., pp. 783–796). Philadelphia: Saunders.

Mullaly, L. M. (2000). Psychology of pregnancy. In S. Mattson & J. E. Smith (Eds.), *AWHONN: Maternal newborn nursing* (2nd ed., pp. 101–114). Philadelphia: Saunders.

Smith, K. (2000). Normal childbirth. In S. Mattson & J. E. Smith (Eds.), *AWHONN: Maternal newborn nursing* (2nd ed., pp. 241–270). Philadelphia: Saunders.

Smith, R. (1999). Corticotrophin-releasing hormone and the fetoplacental clock: An Australian perspective. *American Journal of Obstetrics and Gynecology, 180,* S269–S271.

Stern, D. N., & Bruschweiler-Stern, N. (1998). *The birth of a mother.* New York: Perseus Books.

Turley, G. M. (2000). Essential forces and factors in labor. In S. Mattson & J. E. Smith (Eds.), *AWHONN: Maternal newborn nursing* (2nd ed., pp. 204–240). Philadelphia: Saunders.

Varney, H. (1997). *Nurse-midwifery* (3rd ed.). Boston: Blackwell.

Wesson, N. (2000). *Labor pain: A natural approach to easing delivery.* Rochester, VT: Healing Arts Press.


## CONTEMPORARY MATERNAL-NEWBORN NURSING ON-LINE

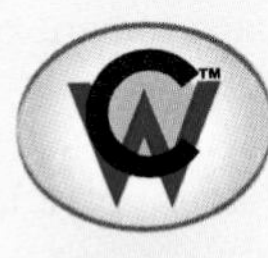

Additional interactive resources, including animations and video, for this chapter can be found on the Companion Website at http://www.prenhall.com/ladewig. Click on Chapter 15 and "Begin" to select the activities for this chapter.

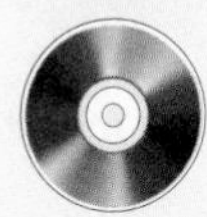

For NCLEX review questions and an audio glossary, access the accompanying CD-ROM in this book.

Chapter 16

# Intrapartal Nursing Assessment

*As charge nurse on a busy birthing unit, sometimes I feel like I'm meeting myself coming and going. At any one time I may be called upon to do a great number of things, seemingly all at once: maintain a safe and adequate staffing, be the extra pair of hands at a high-risk delivery, consult with members of the hospital's support services team, arrange for the smooth transfer of a labor patient to the operating room for a cesarean, help a mom who is having difficulty breastfeeding, or simply cuddle a newborn whose parents (and nurse) need a few minutes of rest. Would I trade this bustle for anything else? Not on your life!*

—Birth Center Charge Nurse

## KEY TERMS

| | |
|---|---|
| Accelerations | 399 |
| Baseline rate | 394 |
| Decelerations | 399 |
| Electronic fetal monitoring (EFM) | 391 |
| Fetal blood sampling (FBS) | 403 |
| Fetal bradycardia | 396 |
| Fetal tachycardia | 396 |
| Intrauterine pressure catheter (IUPC) | 385 |
| Late deceleration | 399 |
| Leopold's maneuvers | 389 |
| Long-term variability (LTV) | 397 |
| Short-term variability (STV) | 397 |
| Variable decelerations | 399 |

## OBJECTIVES

- Discuss high-risk screening and intrapartal assessment of maternal physical and psychosociocultural factors.
- Summarize methods used to evaluate the progress of labor.
- Describe auscultation of fetal heart rate.
- Delineate the procedure for performing Leopold's maneuvers and the information that can be obtained.
- Differentiate between baseline and periodic changes in fetal heart rate monitoring and describe the appearance and significance of each.
- Outline steps to be performed in the systematic evaluation of fetal heart rate tracings.
- Identify nonreassuring fetal heart rate patterns and nursing interventions that should be carried out in the management of fetal stress or distress.
- Delineate the indications for fetal blood sampling and identify related pH values.
- Discuss differing responses to electronic fetal monitoring.

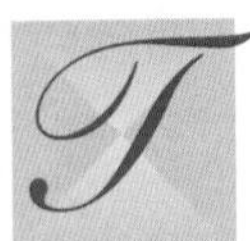he physiologic events that occur during labor call for many adaptations by the mother and fetus. Frequent and accurate assessments are crucial because the changes resulting from these adaptations often occur rapidly and involve two individuals, the expectant mother and her child. The woman's partner or chosen support person is also an integral part of the childbirth experience as new roles are assumed and a new family unit is formed.

In current nursing practice, the traditional assessment techniques of observation, palpation, and auscultation are augmented by the judicious use of technology such as ultrasound and electronic monitoring. These tools may provide more detailed information for assessment, however it is important for the nurse to remember that the technology only provides data; it is the nurse who monitors the mother and her baby.

# Maternal Assessment

## History

The nurse obtains a brief oral history when the woman is admitted to the birthing area. Each agency has its own admission forms, but they usually include the following information:

- Woman's name and age
- Attending physician or certified nurse-midwife (CNM)
- Personal data: blood type; Rh factor; results of serology testing; prepregnant and present weight; allergies to medications, foods, or other substances; prescribed and over-the-counter medications taken during pregnancy; and history of drug and alcohol use and smoking during the pregnancy
- History of previous illness, such as tuberculosis, heart disease, diabetes, convulsive disorders, and thyroid disorders
- Problems in the prenatal period, such as elevated blood pressure, bleeding problems, recurrent urinary tract infections, other infections, or sexually transmitted infections
- Pregnancy data: gravida, para, abortions, and neonatal deaths
- The method chosen for infant feeding
- Type of prenatal education classes (childbirth education classes)
- Woman's preferences regarding labor and birth, such as no episiotomy, no analgesics or anesthetics, or the presence of the father or others at the birth
- Pediatrician or family practice physician
- Additional data: history of special tests such as nonstress test (NST), biophysical profile (BPP), or ultrasound; history of any preterm labor; onset of labor; amniotic fluid membrane status; and brief description of previous labor and birth

Assessment of psychosocial history is a critical component of intrapartal nursing assessment. The nurse begins the assessment when the woman is admitted to the birthing area by obtaining information such as the following:

- Does the woman have a partner? Who are her support people?
- Is she safe in her relationship with the baby's father? Was there any physical or emotional abuse before or during the pregnancy? If so, what interventions were made?

  In questioning the woman about safety and abuse issues, the nurse needs to be aware that abuse affects at least 25% to 30% of pregnant women (McFarland & Gondolf, 1998). It is important to ensure that the woman is alone when the questions are asked so that she can answer freely. If she indicates that there has been a problem, the following information is needed (McFarland & Gondolf, 1998):

  - Have you ever been emotionally or physically abused by your partner or someone important to you?
  - Within the past year, have you been hit, slapped, kicked, or otherwise physically hurt by someone? If yes, by whom? Total number of times?
  - Since you have been pregnant, have you been hit, slapped, kicked, or otherwise physically hurt by someone? If yes, by whom? Total number of times?
  - Within the past year has anyone forced you to have sexual activities? If yes, who? Total number of times?
  - Are you afraid of your partner or anyone you mentioned?
- Has she had difficulty or problems with previous pregnancies, labors, or births that would increase her anxiety now?
- Have emotional problems been present during the past few months? What interventions have occurred (Austin, Gallop, McCay, et al., 1999)?

Given the prevalence of sexual violence against women in our society (the reported incidence is one in three women, regardless of age) the nurse needs to consider that the woman may have experienced sexual violence at some point in her life. In this case she may be anxious about the labor process, or anxiety may arise during labor. Because psychosocial factors may be complex, the impact of the woman's history may not become apparent until later in the labor and birth. The nurse needs to be aware of the following aspects of psychosocial history:

- Has the woman experienced rape or sexual abuse?
- Is there evidence of support between the woman and her partner?
- Is the partner controlling? Does the partner make decisions unilaterally?

It is important for the nurse to obtain the history in a setting that promotes trust and the establishment of a relationship. Some of the questions are straightforward, but others require care and privacy (the nurse and the woman alone together) to ensure that the woman has a safe environment in which to respond.

## HINTS FOR PRACTICE

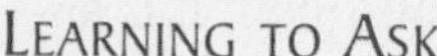

### LEARNING TO ASK

Many nurses have difficulty asking questions about domestic violence, sexual abuse, and drug or alcohol use during pregnancy. However, this information is necessary to provide the best nursing care possible. To create a relationship of trust in which the client feels safe answering uncomfortable questions, the following tips may be helpful:

- Explore your own beliefs and values.
- Use open-ended questions.
- Be receptive of the answers.
- Be accepting of others' life experiences.

## INTRAPARTAL HIGH-RISK SCREENING

Screening for intrapartal high-risk factors is an integral part of assessing the normal laboring woman. (Note that the preceding discussion of abuse is indicative of increased intrapartal risk.) As the history is obtained, the nurse notes the presence of any factors that may be associated with a high-risk condition. For example, the woman who reports a physical symptom such as intermittent bleeding needs further assessment to rule out abruptio placentae or placenta previa before the admission process continues. In addition to identifying the presence of a high-risk condition, the nurse must recognize the implications of the condition for the laboring woman and her fetus. For example, if there is an abnormal fetal presentation, the nurse understands that the labor may be prolonged, prolapse of the umbilical cord is more likely, and the possibility of a cesarean birth is increased.

Although physical conditions are frequently listed as the major factors that increase risk in the intrapartal period, sociocultural variables such as poverty, nutrition, the amount of prenatal care, cultural beliefs regarding pregnancy, and communication patterns may also precipitate a high-risk situation. In addition, recent research indicates that women who suffer from post-traumatic stress disorder (PTSD) may be at increased risk for some pregnancy complications (Seng, Oakley, Samselle, et al., 2001). The nurse can quickly review the prenatal record for number of prenatal visits; weight gain during pregnancy; progression of fundal height; assistance such as Medicaid and the Special Supplemental Food Program for Women, Infants, and Children (WIC); exposure to environmental agents; and history of traumatic life events.

The nurse can begin gathering data about sociocultural factors as the woman enters the birthing area. The nurse observes the communication pattern between the woman and her support person(s) and their responses to admission questions and initial teaching. If the woman and her support person(s) do not speak English and translators are not available among the birthing unit staff, the course of labor and the nurse's ability to interact and provide support and education are affected. The couple must receive information in their primary language to make informed decisions. Communication may also be affected by cultural practices such as beliefs about when to speak, who should ask questions, or whether it is acceptable to let others know about discomfort (Austin et al., 1999).

A partial list of intrapartal risk factors appears in Table 16–1. The factors precede the Intrapartal Assessment Guide because they must be kept in mind during the assessment.

## INTRAPARTAL PHYSICAL AND PSYCHOSOCIOCULTURAL ASSESSMENT

A physical examination is part of the admission procedure and part of the ongoing care of the client. Although the intrapartal physical assessment is not as complete and thorough as the initial prenatal physical examination (Chapter 8), it does involve assessment of some body systems and the actual labor process. The Intrapartal Assessment Guide on pages 380–384 provides a framework the maternity nurse can use when examining the laboring woman.

The physical assessment portion includes assessments performed immediately on admission as well as ongoing assessments. When labor is progressing very quickly, the nurse may not have time for a complete assessment. In that case, the critical physical assessments include maternal vital signs, labor status, fetal status, and laboratory findings.

Text continues on page 385.

## TABLE 16–1 Intrapartal High-Risk Factors

| *Factor* | *Maternal Implications* | *Fetal-Neonatal Implications* |
|---|---|---|
| Abnormal presentation | ↑ Incidence of cesarean birth<br>↑ Incidence of prolonged labor | ↑ Incidence of placenta previa<br>Prematurity<br>↑ Risk of congenital abnormality<br>Neonatal physical trauma<br>↑ Risk of intrauterine growth restriction (IUGR) |
| Multiple gestation | ↑ Uterine distension → ↑ risk of postpartum hemorrhage<br>↑ Risk of cesarean birth<br>↑ Risk of preterm labor | Low birth weight<br>Prematurity<br>↑ Risk of congenital anomalies<br>Feto-fetal transfusion |
| Hydramnios | ↑ Discomfort<br>↑ Dyspnea<br>↑ Risk of preterm labor<br>Edema of lower extremities | ↑ Risk of esophageal or other high-alimentary-tract atresias<br>↑ Risk of CNS anomalies (myelocele) |
| Oligohydramnios | Maternal fear of "dry birth" | ↑ Incidence of congenital anomalies<br>↑ Incidence of renal lesions<br>↑ Risk of IUGR<br>↑ Risk of fetal acidosis<br>↑ Risk of cord compression<br>Postmaturity |
| Meconium staining of amniotic fluid | ↑ Psychologic stress due to fear for baby | ↑ Risk of fetal asphyxia<br>↑ Risk of meconium aspiration<br>↑ Risk of pneumonia due to aspiration of meconium |
| Premature rupture of membranes | ↑ Risk of infection (chorioamnionitis)<br>↑ Risk of preterm labor<br>↑ Anxiety<br>Fear for the baby<br>Prolonged hospitalization<br>↑ Incidence of tocolytic therapy | ↑ Perinatal morbidity<br>Prematurity<br>↓ Birth weight<br>↑ Risk of respiratory distress syndrome<br>Prolonged hospitalization |
| Induction of labor | ↑ Risk of hypercontractility of uterus<br>↑ Risk of uterine rupture<br>↑ Length of labor if cervix not ready<br>↑ Anxiety | Prematurity if gestational age not assessed correctly<br>Hypoxia if hyperstimulation occurs |
| Abruptio placentae/placenta previa | Hemorrhage<br>Uterine atony<br>↑ Incidence of cesarean birth | Fetal hypoxia/acidosis<br>Fetal exsanguination<br>↑ Perinatal mortality |
| Failure to progress in labor | Maternal exhaustion<br>↑ Incidence of augmentation of labor<br>↑ Incidence of cesarean birth | Fetal hypoxia/acidosis<br>Intracranial birth injury |
| Precipitous labor (<3 hours) | Perineal, vaginal, cervical lacerations<br>↑ Risk of PP hemorrhage | Tentorial tears |
| Prolapse of umbilical cord | ↑ Fear for baby<br>Cesarean birth | Acute fetal hypoxia/acidosis |
| Fetal heart aberrations | ↑ Fear for baby<br>↑ Risk of cesarean birth, forceps, vacuum<br>Continuous electronic monitoring and intervention in labor | Tachycardia, chronic asphyxic insult, bradycardia, acute asphyxic insult<br>Chronic hypoxia<br>Congenital heart block |
| Uterine rupture | Hemorrhage<br>Cesarean birth for hysterectomy<br>↑ Risk of death | Fetal anoxia<br>Fetal hemorrhage<br>↑ Neonatal morbidity and mortality |
| Postdates (>42 weeks) | ↑ Anxiety<br>↑ Incidence of induction of labor<br>↑ Incidence of cesarean birth<br>↑ Use of technology to monitor fetus<br>↑ Risk of shoulder dystocia | Postmaturity syndrome<br>↑ Risk of fetal-neonatal mortality and morbidity<br>↑ Risk of antepartum fetal death<br>↑ Incidence or risk of large baby |
| Diabetes | ↑ Risk of hydramnios<br>↑ Risk of hypoglycemia or hyperglycemia<br>↑ Risk of pregnancy-induced hypertension | ↑ Risk of malpresentation<br>↑ Risk of macrosomia<br>↑ Risk of IUGR<br>↑ Risk of respiratory distress syndrome<br>↑ Risk of congenital anomalies |
| Pregnancy-induced hypertension | ↑ Risk of seizures<br>↑ Risk of stroke<br>↑ Risk of HELLP syndrome | ↑ Risk of small-for-gestational-age baby<br>↑ Risk of preterm birth<br>↑ Risk of mortality |
| AIDS/STD | ↑ Risk of additional infections | ↑ Risk of transplacental transmission |

## ASSESSMENT GUIDE: INTRAPARTAL—FIRST STAGE OF LABOR

| Physical Assessment/ Normal Findings | Alterations and Possible Causes* | Nursing Responses to Data† |
|---|---|---|
| **Vital Signs** | | |
| Blood pressure (BP): <130 systolic and <85 diastolic in adult 18 years of age or older or no more than 15–20 mm Hg rise in systolic pressure over baseline BP during early pregnancy | High BP (essential hypertension, preeclampsia, renal disease, apprehension or anxiety)<br>Low BP (supine hypotension) | Evaluate history of preexisting disorders and check for presence of other signs of preeclampsia.<br>Do not assess during contractions; implement measures to decrease anxiety and reassess.<br>Turn woman on her side and recheck BP. Provide quiet environment. |
| Pulse: 60–90 bpm | Increased pulse rate (excitement or anxiety, cardiac disorders, early shock) | Evaluate cause, reassess to see if rate continues; report to physician. |
| Respirations: 14–22/min (or pulse rate divided by 4) | Marked tachypnea (respiratory disease), hyperventilation in transition phase | Assess between contractions; if marked tachypnea continues, assess for signs of respiratory disease. Have $O_2$ available. |
| | Hyperventilation (anxiety) | Encourage slow breaths if woman is hyperventilating. |
| Pulse ox 95% or greater | >90%; hypoxia, hypotension, hemorrhage | Apply $O_2$; notify physician |
| Temperature: 36.2–37.6°C (98–99.6°F) | Elevated temperature (infection, dehydration, prolonged rupture of membranes, epidural regional block) | Assess for other signs of infection or dehydration. |
| **Weight** | | |
| 25–30 lb greater than prepregnant weight | Weight gain >30 lb (fluid retention, obesity, large infant, diabetes mellitus, PIH); weight gain <15 lb (SGA) | Assess for signs of edema.<br>Evaluate pattern from prenatal record. |
| **Lungs** | | |
| Normal breath sounds, clear and equal | Rales, rhonchi, friction rub (infection), pulmonary edema, asthma | Reassess; refer to physician. |
| **Fundus** | | |
| At 40 weeks' gestation located just below xiphoid process | Uterine size not compatible with estimated date of birth (SGA, large for gestational age [LGA], hydramnios, multiple pregnancy) | Reevaluate history regarding pregnancy dating. Refer to physician for additional assessment. |
| **Edema** | | |
| Slight amount of dependent edema | Pitting edema of face, hands, legs, abdomen, sacral area (preeclampsia) | Check deep tendon reflexes for hyperactivity; check for clonus; refer to physician. |
| **Hydration** | | |
| Normal skin turgor, elastic | Poor skin turgor (dehydration) | Assess skin turgor; refer to physician for deviations. Provide fluids per order. |
| **Perineum** | | |
| Tissues smooth, pink color (see Prenatal Initial Physical Assessment Guide, Chapter 25) | Varicose veins of vulva, herpes lesions | Exercise care while doing a perineal prep; note on client record need for follow-up in postpartal period; reassess after birth; refer to physician. |
| Clear mucus; may be blood tinged with earthy or human odor | Profuse, purulent, foul-smelling drainage | Suspected gonorrhea or chorioamnionitis; report to physician; notify neonatal nursing staff and pediatrician. |
| | ***Possible causes of alterations are placed in parentheses.** | **†This column provides guidelines for further assessment and initial nursing intervention.** |

# INTRAPARTAL—FIRST STAGE OF LABOR *continued*

| Physical Assessment/ Normal Findings | Alterations and Possible Causes* | Nursing Responses to Data† |
|---|---|---|
| **Perineum *continued*** | | |
| Presence of small amount of bloody show that gradually increases with further cervical dilatation | Hemorrhage | Assess BP and pulse, pallor, diaphoresis; report any marked changes. (*Note:* Gaping of vagina or anus and bulging of perineum are suggestive signs of second stage of labor.)<br>Follow universal precautions. |
| **Labor Status** | | |
| Uterine contractions: regular pattern | Failure to establish a regular pattern, prolonged latent phase<br>Hypertonicity<br>Hypotonicity | Evaluate whether woman is in true labor; ambulate if in early labor.<br>Evaluate client status and contractile pattern.<br>Obtain a 20-minute EFM strip.<br>Notify physician or CNM. |
| Cervical dilatation: progressive cervical dilatation from size of fingertip to 10 cm (Procedure 16–1) | Rigidity of cervix (frequent cervical infections, scar tissue, failure of presenting part to descend) | Evaluate contractions, fetal engagement, position, and cervical dilatation. Inform client of progress. |
| Cervical effacement: progressive thinning of cervix (Procedure 16–1) | Failure to efface (rigidity of cervix, failure of presenting part to engage); cervical edema (pushing effort by woman before cervix is fully dilated and effaced, trapped cervix) | Evaluate contractions, fetal engagement, and position.<br>Notify physician or CNM if cervix is becoming edematous; work with woman to prevent pushing until cervix is completely dilated.<br>Keep vaginal exams to a minimum. |
| Fetal descent: progressive descent of fetal presenting part from station −5 to +4 (Figure 16–4♦ in Procedure 16–1) | Failure of descent (abnormal fetal position or presentation, macrosomic fetus, inadequate pelvic measurement) | Evaluate fetal position, presentation, and size.<br>Evaluate maternal pelvic measurements. |
| Membranes: may rupture before or during labor | Rupture of membranes more than 12–24 hours before initiation of labor | Assess for ruptured membranes using Nitrazine test tape before doing vaginal exam.<br>Follow BSI precautions.<br>Instruct woman with ruptured membranes to remain on bed rest if presenting part is not engaged and firmly down against the cervix. Keep vaginal exams to a minimum to prevent infection.<br>When membranes rupture in the birth setting, **immediately assess FHR** to detect changes associated with prolapse of umbilical cord (FHR slows). |
| Findings on Nitrazine test tape:<br>Membranes probably intact<br>Yellow pH 5.0<br>Olive pH 5.5<br>Olive green pH 6.0 | False-positive results may be obtained if large amount of bloody show is present, previous vaginal examination has been done using lubricant, or tape is touched by nurse's fingers. | Assess fluid for consistency, amount, odor; assess FHR frequently. Assess fluid at regular intervals for presence of meconium staining.<br>Follow BSI precautions while assessing amniotic fluid. |
| Membranes probably ruptured<br>Blue-green pH 6.5<br>Blue-gray pH 7.0<br>Deep blue pH 7.5 | | Teach woman that amniotic fluid is continually produced (to allay fear of "dry birth").<br>Teach woman that she may feel amniotic fluid trickle or gush with contractions.<br>Change Chux pads often. |
| Amniotic fluid clear, with earthy or human odor, no foul-smelling odor | Greenish amniotic fluid (fetal stress) | Assess FHR; do vaginal exam to evaluate for prolapsed cord; apply fetal monitor for continuous data; report to physician. |
| | Strong or foul odor (amnionitis) | Take woman's temperature and report to physician. |

***Possible causes of alterations are placed in parentheses.**

**†This column provides guidelines for further assessment and initial nursing intervention.**

| Physical Assessment/ Normal Findings | Alterations and Possible Causes* | Nursing Responses to Data† |
|---|---|---|
| **Fetal Status** | | |
| FHR: 120–160 bpm | <120 or >160 bpm (fetal stress); abnormal patterns on fetal monitor: decreased variability, late decelerations, variable decelerations, absence of accelerations with fetal movement | Initiate interventions based on particular FHR pattern. |
| Presentation:<br>Cephalic, 97%<br>Breech, 3% | Face, brow, breech, or shoulder presentation | Report to physician; after presentation is confirmed as face, brow, breech, or shoulder, woman may be prepared for cesarean birth. |
| Position: left-occiput-anterior (LOA) most common | Persistent occipital-posterior (OP) position; transverse arrest | Carefully monitor maternal and fetal status. |
| Activity: fetal movement | Hyperactivity (may precede fetal hypoxia) | Carefully evaluate FHR; apply fetal monitor. |
| | Complete lack of movement (fetal distress or fetal demise) | Carefully evaluate FHR; apply fetal monitor. Report to physician or CNM. |
| **Laboratory Evaluation** | | |
| Hematologic tests<br>Hemoglobin: 12–16 g/dL | <12 g/dL (anemia, hemorrhage) | Evaluate woman for problems due to decreased oxygen-carrying capacity caused by lowered hemoglobin. |
| CBC<br>Hematocrit: 38%–47%<br>RBC: 4.2–5.4 million/mm³<br>WBC: 4500–11,000/mm³, although leukocytosis to 20,000/mm³ is not unusual<br>Platelets: 150,000–400,000/mm³ | Presence of infection or blood dyscrasias, loss of blood (hemorrhage, disseminated intravascular coagulation [DIC]) | Evaluate for other signs of infection or for petechiae, bruising, or unusual bleeding. |
| Serologic testing<br>STS or VDRL test: nonreactive | Positive reaction (Chapter 25, Initial Prenatal Physical Assessment Guide) | For reactive test notify newborn nursery and pediatrician. |
| Rh | Rh-positive fetus in Rh-negative woman | Assess prenatal record for titer levels during pregnancy.<br>Obtain cord blood for direct Coombs' at birth. |
| Urinalysis<br>Glucose: negative | Glycosuria (low renal threshold for glucose, diabetes mellitus) | Assess blood glucose level; test urine for ketones; ketonuria and glycosuria require further assessment of blood sugar levels.‡ |
| Ketones: negative | Ketonuria (starvation ketosis) | |
| Proteins: negative | Proteinuria (urine specimen contaminated with vaginal secretions, fever, kidney disease); proteinuria of 2+ or greater found in uncontaminated urine may be a sign of ensuing preeclampsia | Instruct woman in collection technique; incidence of contamination from vaginal discharge is common. |
| Red blood cells: negative | Blood in urine (calculi, cystitis, glomerulonephritis, neoplasm) | Assess collection technique (may be bloody show). |
| White blood cells: negative | Presence of white blood cells (infection in genitourinary tract) | Assess for signs of urinary tract infection. |
| Casts: none | Presence of casts (nephrotic syndrome) | |

*Possible causes of alterations are placed in parentheses.

†This column provides guidelines for further assessment and initial nursing intervention.

‡Glycosuria should not be discounted. The presence of glycosuria necessitates follow-up.

# INTRAPARTAL—FIRST STAGE OF LABOR *continued*

| Cultural Assessment§ | Variations to Consider | Nursing Responses to Data† |
|---|---|---|
| Cultural influences determine customs and practices regarding intrapartal care | Individual preferences may vary. | |
| Ask the following questions: Who would you like to remain with you during your labor and birth? | She may prefer only her coach to remain or may also want family and/or friends | Provide support for her wishes by encouraging desired people to stay. Provide information to others (with the woman's permission) who are not in the room. |
| What would you like to wear during labor? | She may be more comfortable in her own clothes | Offer supportive materials such as Chux if needed to protect her own clothing. Avoid subtle signals to the woman that she should not have chosen to remain in her own clothes. Have other clothing available if the woman desires. If her clothing becomes contaminated, it will be simple to place it in a plastic bag. The nurse can soak soiled clothing in cool water. The nurse needs to remember to wear disposable gloves and a plastic apron if splashing is anticipated. |
| What activity would you like during labor? | She may want to ambulate most of the time, stand in the shower, sit in the Jacuzzi, sit in a chair or on a stool, remain on the bed, and so forth | Support the woman's wishes; provide encouragement and complete assessments in a manner so her activity and positional wishes are disturbed as little as possible. |
| What position would you like for the birth? | She may feel more comfortable in lithotomy with supports and her upper body elevated, or side-lying or sitting in birthing bed, or standing, or squatting, or on hands and knees | Collect any supplies and equipment needed to support her in her chosen birthing position. Provide information to her partner regarding any changes that may be needed based on the chosen position. |
| Is there anything special you would like? | She may want the room darkened or to have curtains and windows open, music playing, a Leboyer birth, her coach to cut the umbilical cord, to save a portion of the umbilical cord, to save the placenta, to videotape the birth, and so forth | Support requests and communicate requests to any other nursing or medical personnel (so requests can continue to be supported and not questioned). If another nurse or physician does not honor the request, act as advocate for the woman by continuing to support her unless her desire is truly unsafe. |
| Ask the woman if she would like fluids and ask what temperature she prefers | She may prefer clear fluids other than water (tea, clear juice). She may prefer iced, room-temperature, or warmed fluids | Provide fluids as desired. |
| Observe the woman's response when privacy is difficult to maintain and her body is exposed | Some women do not seem to mind being exposed during an exam or procedure; others feel acute discomfort | Maintain privacy and respect the woman's sense of privacy.<br>If the woman is unable to provide specific information, the nurse may draw from general information regarding cultural variation:<br>Southeast Asian woman may not want any family member in the room during exam or procedures. Her partner may not be involved with activities during labor or birth.<br>Saudi women may need to remain covered during the labor and birth and avoid exposure of any body part. The husband may need to be in the room but remain behind a curtain or screen so he does not view his wife at this time. |
| If the woman is to breastfeed, ask if she would like to feed her baby immediately after birth | She may want to feed her baby right away or may want to wait a little while | |

**§These are only a few suggestions. We do not mean to imply that this is a comprehensive cultural assessment; rather, it is a tool to encourage cultural sensitivity.**

**†This column provides guidelines for further assessment and initial nursing intervention.**

| Psychosocial Assessment§ | Variations to Consider | Nursing Responses to Data† |
|---|---|---|
| **Preparation for Childbirth** | | |
| Woman has some information regarding process of normal labor and birth | Some women do not have any information regarding childbirth | Add to present information base. |
| Woman has breathing and/or relaxation techniques to use during labor | Some women do not have any method of relaxation or breathing to use, and some do not desire them | Support breathing and relaxation techniques that client is using; provide information if needed. |
| **Response to Labor** | | |
| Latent phase: relaxed, excited, anxious for labor to be well established | May feel unable to cope with contractions because of fear, anxiety, or lack of information | Provide support and encouragement; establish trusting relationship. |
| Active phase: becomes more intense, begins to tire<br>Transitional phase: feels tired, may feel unable to cope, needs frequent coaching to maintain breathing patterns | May remain quiet and without any sign of discomfort or anxiety; may insist that she is unable to continue with the birthing process | Provide support and coaching if needed. |
| Coping mechanisms: ability to cope with labor through utilization of support system, breathing, relaxation techniques | May feel marked anxiety and apprehension, may not have coping mechanisms that can be brought into this experience, or may be unable to use them at this time | Support coping mechanisms if they are working for the woman; provide information and support if she exhibits anxiety or needs alternative to present coping methods. |
| | Survivors of sexual abuse may demonstrate fear of IVs or needles, may recoil when touched, may insist on a female caregiver, may be very sensitive to body fluids and cleanliness, and may be unable to labor lying down (Burrian, 1995) | Encourage participation of significant other if a supportive relationship seems apparent. Establish rapport and a trusting relationship. Provide information that is true and offer your presence. |
| **Anxiety** | | |
| Some anxiety and apprehension is within normal limits | May show anxiety through rapid breathing, nervous tremors, frowning, grimacing, clenching of teeth, thrashing movements, crying, increased pulse and blood pressure | Provide support, encouragement, and information. Teach relaxation techniques; support controlled breathing efforts. May need to provide a paper bag to breathe into if woman says her lips are tingling. Note FHR. |
| **Sounds during Labor** | | |
| | Some women are very quiet; others moan or make a variety of noises | Provide a supportive environment. Encourage woman to do what is right for her. |
| **Support System** | | |
| Physical intimacy between mother and father (or mother and support person); caretaking activities such as soothing conversation, touching | Some women would prefer no contact; others may show clinging behaviors | Encourage caretaking activities that appear to comfort the woman; encourage support to the woman; if support is limited, the nurse may take a more active role. |
| Support person stays in close proximity | Limited interaction may come from a desire for quiet | Encourage support person to stay close (if this seems appropriate). |
| Relationship between mother and father (or support person): involved interaction | The support person may seem to be detached and maintain little support, attention, or conversation | Support interactions; if interaction is limited, the nurse may provide more information and support. |
| | | Ensure that partner or significant other has short breaks, especially prior to transition. |

**§These are only a few suggestions. We do not mean to imply that this is a comprehensive cultural assessment; rather, it is a tool to encourage cultural sensitivity.**

**†This column provides guidelines for further assessment and initial nursing intervention.**

The cultural assessment portion provides a starting point for this increasingly important aspect of assessment. Individualized nursing care can best be planned and implemented when the values and beliefs of the laboring woman are known and honored (Callister, 2001). Frequently, however, the nurse feels uncertain about what to ask or consider, perhaps because there has been no personal opportunity to become aware of varying cultural values and beliefs.

The final section of the assessment guide addresses psychosocial factors. The laboring woman's psychosocial status is an important part of the total assessment. The woman has previous ideas, knowledge, and fears about childbearing. By assessing her psychosocial status, the nurse can meet the woman's needs for information and support. The nurse can then assist the woman and her partner; in the absence of a partner, the nurse may become the support person.

While performing the intrapartal assessment, it is imperative that the nurse follow Centers for Disease Control and Prevention (CDC) guidelines to prevent exposure to body substances. The nurse can provide information in a factual manner regarding the precautions. A statement such as the following is helpful: "I will be wearing gloves when I change the chux on which you are lying. This is to protect my hands from the discharge you are having and to protect you from any organisms that I may have on my hands." Sharing information with the laboring woman and her support person(s) will promote a supportive, caring environment.

**KEY FACTS TO REMEMBER**

*Contraction and Labor Progress Characteristics*

**Contraction Characteristics**

| | |
|---|---|
| Latent phase: | Every 10–30 min × 20–40 sec; mild, progressing to |
| | Every 5–7 min × 30–40 sec; moderate |
| Active phase: | Every 2–3 min × 40–60 sec; moderate to strong |
| Transition phase: | Every 1½–2 min × 60–90 sec; strong |

**Labor Progress Characteristics**

| | |
|---|---|
| Primipara: | 1.2 cm/hr dilatation |
| | 1 cm/hr descent |
| | <2 hour in second stage |
| Multipara: | 1.5 cm/hr dilatation |
| | 2 cm/hr descent |
| | <1 hour in second stage |

## METHODS OF EVALUATING LABOR PROGRESS

### CONTRACTION ASSESSMENT

Uterine contractions may be assessed by palpation or continuous electronic monitoring.

#### Palpation

The nurse assesses contractions for frequency, duration, and intensity by placing one hand on the uterine fundus. The hand is kept relatively still because excessive movement may stimulate contractions or cause discomfort. The nurse determines the frequency of the contractions by noting the time from the beginning of one contraction to the beginning of the next. If contractions begin at 7:00, 7:04, and 7:08, for example, their frequency is every 4 minutes. To determine contraction duration, the nurse notes the time when tensing of the fundus is first felt (beginning of contraction) and again as relaxation occurs (end of contraction). During the acme of the contraction, intensity can be evaluated by estimating the indentability of the fundus. The nurse should assess at least three successive contractions to provide enough data to determine the contraction pattern. See Key Facts to Remember: Contraction and Labor Progress Characteristics for review of characteristics in different phases of labor.

This is also a good time to assess the laboring woman's perception of pain. How does she describe the pain? What is her affect? Is this contraction more uncomfortable than the last one? Is the nurse's palpation of intensity congruent with the woman's perception? (For instance, the nurse might evaluate a contraction as mild in intensity while the laboring woman evaluates it as very strong.) A nurse's assessment is not complete unless the laboring woman's affect and response to the contractions are also noted and charted.

#### Electronic Monitoring of Contractions

Electronic monitoring of uterine contractions provides continuous data. In many birth settings electronic monitoring is routine for high-risk clients and women who are having oxytocin-induced labor; other facilities monitor all laboring women.

Electronic monitoring may be done externally, with a device that is placed against the maternal abdomen, or internally, with an **intrauterine pressure catheter (IUPC).** When monitoring by external means, the portion of the monitoring equipment called a tocodynamometer, or "toco," is positioned against the fundus of the uterus and held in place with an elastic belt (see Figure 16–1♦). The toco contains a flexible disk that responds to pressure. When the uterus contracts, the fundus tightens and the change in pressure against the toco is amplified and transmitted to the electronic fetal monitor. The monitor displays the uterine contraction as a pattern on graph paper.

External monitoring provides a continuous recording of the frequency and duration of uterine contractions and is noninvasive. However, it does not accurately record the intensity of the uterine contraction, and it is difficult to obtain an accurate fetal heart rate in some women, such as those who are very obese, those who have hydramnios (an abnormally large amount of amniotic fluid), or those whose fetus is very active. In addition, the woman may be bothered by the belt if it requires frequent readjustment when she changes position.

Internal intrauterine monitoring provides the same data and also provides accurate measurement of uterine contraction intensity (the strength of the contraction and the actual pressure within the uterus). After membranes have ruptured, the certified nurse-midwife or physician inserts the IUPC into the uterine cavity and connects it by a cable to the electronic fetal monitor. The pressure within the uterus in the resting state and during each contraction is measured by a small micropressure device located in the tip of the catheter. Internal electronic monitoring is used when it is imperative to have accurate intrauterine pressure readings to evaluate the stress on the uterus.

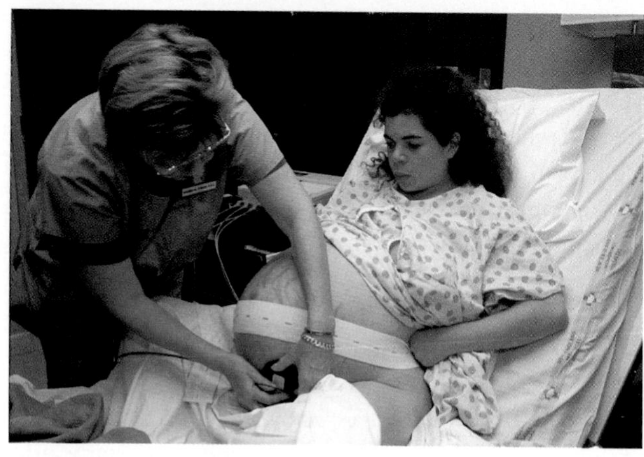

FIGURE 16–1 ♦ Woman in labor with external monitor applied. The tocodynamometer placed on the uterine fundus is recording uterine contractions. The lower belt holds the ultrasonic device that monitors the fetal heart rate. The belts can be adjusted for comfort.

It is important that the nurse also evaluate the woman's labor status by palpating the intensity and resting tone of the uterine fundus during contractions. Technology is a useful tool if used in adjunct to good assessment skills.

### Cervical Assessment

Cervical dilatation and effacement are evaluated directly by vaginal examination (see Procedure 16–1). The vaginal examination can also provide information about membrane status, characteristics of amniotic fluid, fetal position and station.

## *Procedure 16–1* Performing an Intrapartal Vaginal Examination

| *Nursing Action* | *Rationale* |
|---|---|
| **Objective: Assemble the equipment.** | |
| Prepare and arrange the following items so they are easily accessible: | *Organizing the equipment facilitates the examination.* |
| • Clean disposable gloves<br>• Lubricant<br>• Nitrazine test tape<br>• Slide<br>• Sterile cotton-tipped swab (Q-Tip) | *If membranes are ruptured, sterile disposable gloves are used to decrease the chance of introducing bacteria during the examination. When membranes are intact, clean disposable gloves may be used.* |
| **Objective: Prepare the woman.** | |
| • Explain the procedure, the indications for the exam, what the exam may feel like, and that it may cause discomfort. | *By explaining the procedure, the nurse decreases anxiety and increases relaxation.* |

# Procedure 16–1 Performing an Intrapartal Vaginal Examination

continued

| *Nursing Action* | *Rationale* |
| --- | --- |
| • Assess for latex allergies. | *Select nonlatex gloves if woman is allergic.* |
| • Position the woman with her thighs flexed and abducted. Instruct her to put the heels of her feet together. Drape the woman with a sheet, leaving a flap to access the perineum. | *Position provides access to the vulvar area.* *The drape provides privacy.* |
| • Encourage the woman to relax her muscles and legs. | *Relaxation decreases muscle tension and increases comfort.* |
| • Inform the woman prior to touching her. Use gentleness. | *This action communicates regard for the woman and her privacy.* |
| **Objective: Test for amniotic fluid leakage if indicated.** | |
| If fluid leakage has been reported or noted, use Nitrazine test tape and Q-Tip with slide for fern test before performing the exam. | *As long as lubricant has not been used, Nitrazine tape registers a change in pH if amniotic fluid is present.* |
| • Fern test is done by inserting the swab in the pooling of fluid in the posterior vagina and applying the fluid to a slide. | *Digital exam may be deferred if the woman has ruptured membranes and is not actively laboring (AAP & ACOG, 1997).* |
| **Objective: Use aseptic technique during the exam.** | |
| • Pull glove onto dominant hand. | *If sterile exam is needed, both hands will be gloved with sterile gloves.* |
| • Using your gloved hand, position the hand with the wrist straight and the elbow tilted downward. Insert your well-lubricated second and index fingers of the gloved hand into the vagina until they touch the cervix. Use care when positioning your hand. | *This positioning allows the fingertips to point toward the umbilicus and find the cervix.* |
| • If the woman verbalizes discomfort, acknowledge it and apologize. | *This validates the woman's feelings and helps her feel more in control.* |
| **Objective: Determine the status of labor progress.** | |
| • Perform the vaginal examination during and between contractions. | *Cervical dilatation, effacement, and fetal station are affected by the presence of a contraction.* |
| **Objective: Identify the amount of cervical dilatation and effacement (Figure 16–2♦)** | |
| • Palpate for the opening, or a depression, in the cervix. Estimate the diameter of the depression to identify the amount of dilatation. | *Allows determination of effacement and dilatation.* |
| **Objective: Determine the status of the fetal membranes.** | |
| • Observe for expression of amniotic fluid. | *If fluid is expressed, test for amniotic fluid.* |

| *Nursing Action* | *Rationale* |
|---|---|

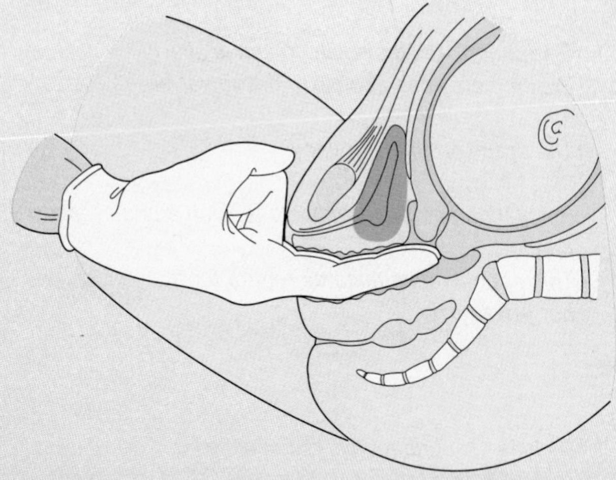

FIGURE 16–2 ♦ To gauge cervical dilatation, the nurse place the index and middle fingers against the cervix and determines the size of the opening. Before labor begins, the cervix is long (approximately 2.5 cm), the sides feel thick, and the cervical canal is closed, so an examining finger cannot be inserted. During labor, the cervix begins to dilate, and the size of the opening progresses from 1 cm to 10 cm in diameter.

| *Nursing Action* | *Rationale* |
|---|---|
| **OBJECTIVE: PALPATE THE PRESENTING PART (FIGURE 16–3♦).** | *Provides information regarding fetal descent and cardinal movements.* |

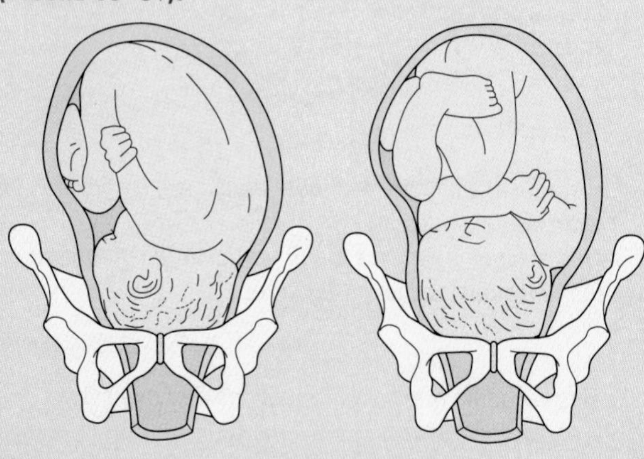

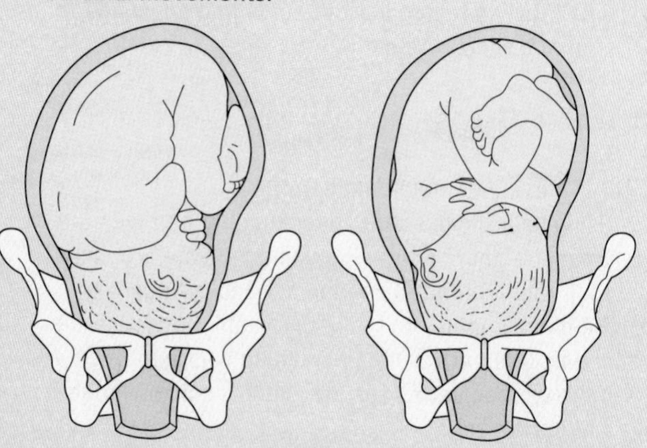

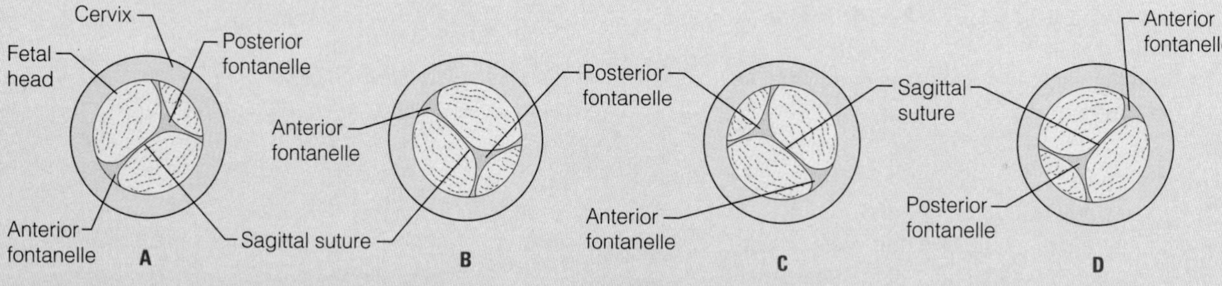


FIGURE 16–3 ♦ Palpating the presenting part (portion of the fetus that enters the pelvis first). **A,** Left occiput anterior (LOA). The occiput (area over the occipital bone on the posterior part of the fetal head) is in the left anterior quadrant of the woman's pelvis. When the fetus is LOA, the posterior fontanelle (located just above the occipital bone and triangular in shape) is in the upper left quadrant of the maternal pelvis. **B,** Left occiput posterior (LOP). The posterior fontanelle is in the lower left quadrant of the maternal pelvis. **C,** Right occiput anterior (ROA). The posterior fontanelle is in the upper right quadrant of the maternal pelvis. **D,** Right occiput posterior (ROP). The posterior fontanelle is in the lower right quadrant of the maternal pelvis. *Note:* The anterior fontanelle is diamond shaped. Because of the roundness of the fetal head, only a portion of the anterior fontanelle can be seen in each of the views, so it appears to be triangular in shape.

| *Nursing Action* | *Rationale* |
|---|---|
| **Objective: Assess the fetal descent (Figure 16–4♦).** | |
| • Assess the station; identify the position of the posterior fontanelle. | *Provides information regarding fetal descent and position.* |

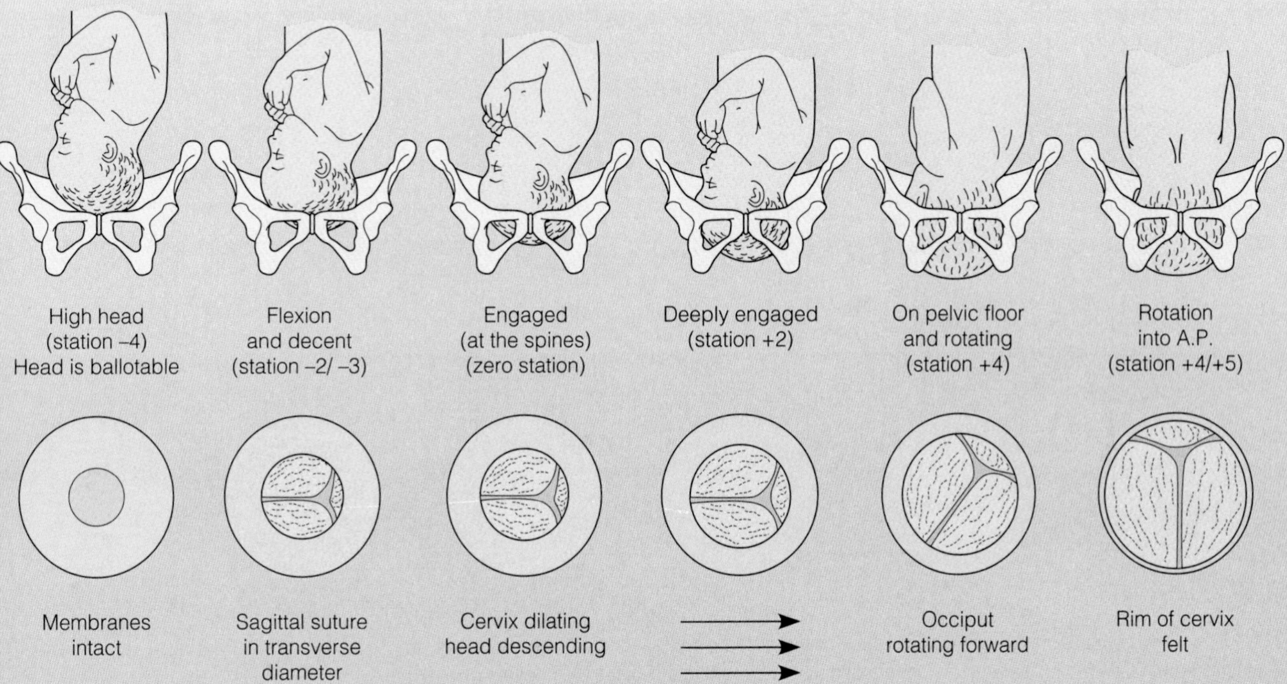


FIGURE 16–4 ♦ Top: The fetal head progressing through the pelvis. Bottom: The changes that the nurse will detect on palpation of the occiput through the cervix while doing a vaginal examination. *Source:* Myles, M. F. (1975). *Textbook for midwives* (p. 246). Edinburgh, Scotland: Churchill-Livingstone.

# Fetal Assessment

## Fetal Position

Fetal position is determined in several ways:

- Inspection of the woman's abdomen
- Palpation of the woman's abdomen
- A vaginal examination to determine the presenting part
- Ultrasound
- Auscultation of fetal heart rate

### Inspection

The nurse should observe the woman's abdomen for size and shape. The lie of the fetus should be assessed by noting whether the uterus projects up and down (longitudinal lie) or left to right (transverse lie).

### Palpation: Leopold's Maneuvers

**Leopold's maneuvers** are a systematic way to evaluate the maternal abdomen. Frequent practice increases the examiner's skill in determining fetal position by palpation. Leopold's maneuvers may be difficult to perform on

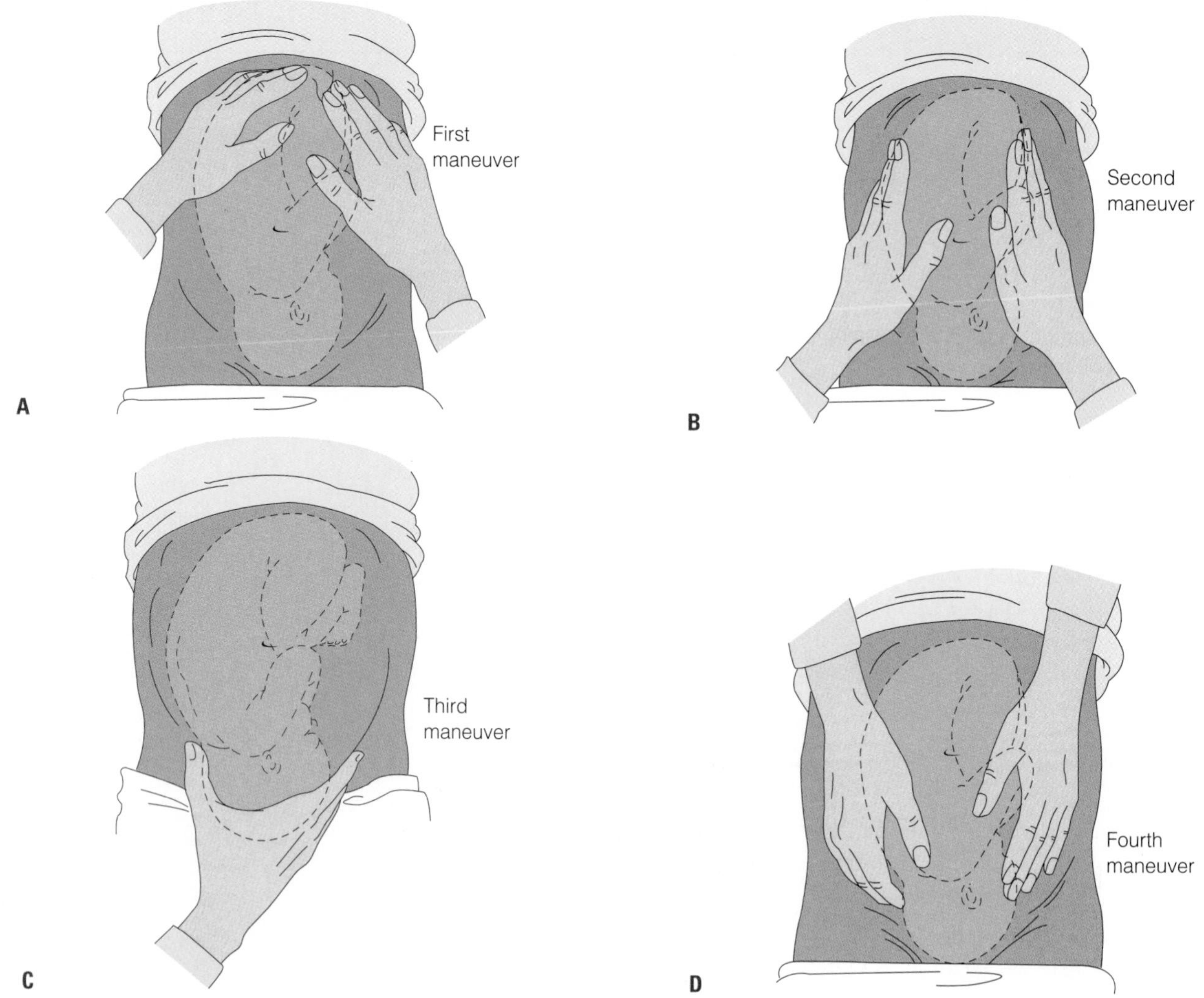


FIGURE 16–5 ♦ Leopold's maneuvers for determining fetal position and presentation. **A,** First maneuver: Facing the woman, palpate the upper abdomen with both hands. Note the shape, consistency, and mobility of the palpated part. The fetal head is firm and round and moves independently of the trunk. The buttock feels softer, and it moves with the trunk. **B,** Second maneuver: Moving the hands on the pelvis, palpate the abdomen with gentle but deep pressure. The fetal back, on one side of the abdomen, feels smooth, and the fetal extremities on the other side feel knobby. **C,** Third maneuver: Place one hand just above the symphysis. Note whether the part palpated feels like the fetal head or the breech and whether it is engaged. **D.** Fourth maneuver: Facing the woman's feet, place both hands on the lower abdomen and move hands gently down the sides of the uterus toward the pubis. Note the cephalic prominence or brow.

an obese woman or on a woman who has excessive amniotic fluid (hydramnios). Before performing Leopold's maneuvers have the woman (1) empty her bladder and (2) lie on her back with her feet on the bed and her knees bent. (See Figure 16–5♦ for technique.)

### Vaginal Examination and Ultrasound

Other assessment techniques to determine fetal position and presentation include vaginal examination and the use of ultrasound to visualize the fetus. During the vaginal examination, the examiner can palpate the presenting part if the cervix is dilated. Information about the position of the fetus and the degree of flexion of its head (in cephalic presentations) can also be obtained (see Procedure 16–1). Visualization by ultrasound is used when the fetal position cannot be determined by abdominal palpation (see Chapter 14).

## Auscultation of Fetal Heart Rate

The fetoscope or handheld Doppler ultrasound is used to auscultate the fetal heart rate (FHR) between, during, and immediately after uterine contractions. Instead of listening haphazardly over the client's abdomen for the FHR, the nurse may choose to perform Leopold's maneuvers first. Leopold's maneuvers not only indicate the probable location of the FHR but also help determine the presence of multiple fetuses, fetal lie, and fetal presentation. The FHR is heard most

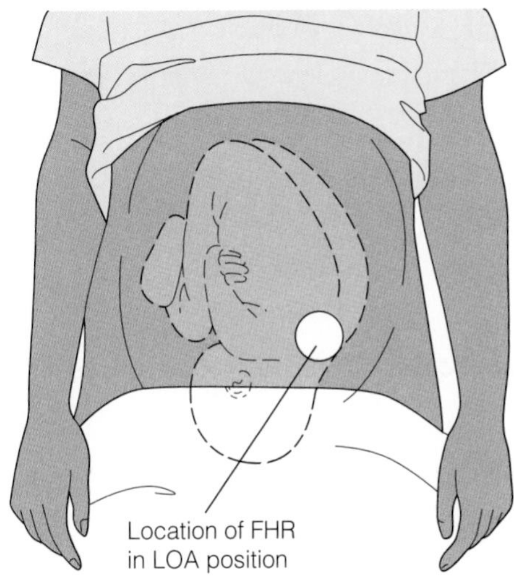


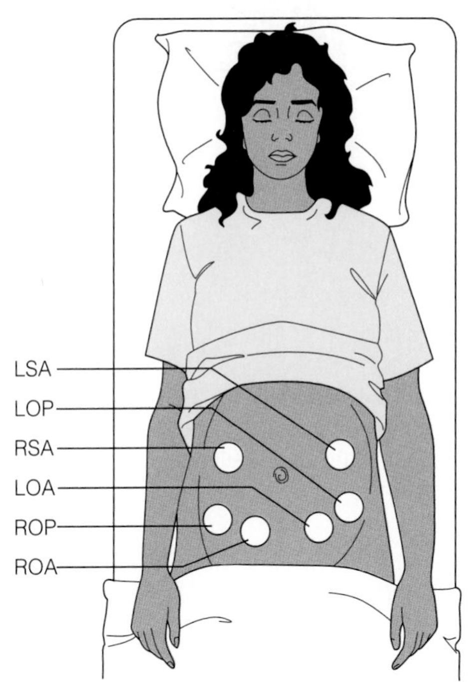


FIGURE 16–6 ♦ Location of FHR in relation to the more commonly seen fetal positions.

clearly at the fetal back (see Figure 16–6♦). Thus, in a cephalic presentation, the FHR is best heard in the lower quadrant of the maternal abdomen. In a breech presentation, it is heard at or above the level of the maternal umbilicus. In a transverse lie, FHR may be heard best just above or just below the umbilicus. As the presenting part descends and rotates through the pelvic structure during labor, the location of the FHR tends to descend and move toward the midline.

After the FHR is located, it is usually counted for 30 seconds and multiplied by 2 to obtain the number of beats per minute. The nurse should occasionally listen for a full minute, through and just after a contraction, to detect any abnormal heart rate, especially if the FHR is over 160 bpm (tachycardia), under 120 bpm (bradycardia), or irregular. If the FHR is irregular or has changed markedly from the last assessment, the nurse should listen for a full minute through and immediately after a contraction. (See Procedure 16–2 and Key Facts to Remember: Frequency of Auscultation for guidelines about how often to auscultate the FHR on page 394.)

It is important to note that intermittent auscultation has been found to be as effective as the electronic method for fetal surveillance. A growing number of health care professionals, doctors and nurses alike, are beginning to question the widespread usage of a technology that has not proven its overall worth (Feinstein, 2000; Parer & King, 2000).

## Electronic Monitoring of Fetal Heart Rate

**Electronic fetal monitoring (EFM)** produces a continuous tracing of the FHR, which allows visual assessment of many characteristics of the FHR. (See Procedure 16–3 on page 395)

### Indications for Electronic Monitoring

If one or more of the following factors are present, the fetal heart rate and contractions are monitored by EFM:

1. Previous history of a stillborn (fetus dies in the uterus) at 38 or more weeks' gestation
2. Presence of a complication of pregnancy (eg, pregnancy-induced hypertension, placenta previa, abruptio placentae, multiple gestation, prolonged or premature rupture of membranes)
3. Induction of labor (labor that is begun as a result of some type of intervention such as an intravenous infusion of pitocin)
4. Preterm labor (gestation less than 37 completed weeks)
5. Decreased fetal movement
6. Fetal stress or distress
7. Meconium staining of amniotic fluid (meconium has been released into the amniotic fluid by the fetus, which may indicate a problem)

### Methods of Electronic Monitoring of FHR

*External monitoring* of the fetus is usually accomplished by ultrasound. A transducer, which emits continuous sound waves, is placed on the maternal abdomen. When placed correctly, the sound waves bounce off the fetal heart and are picked up by the electronic monitor. The actual moment-by-moment FHR is displayed graphically

# *Procedure 16–2* Auscultation of Fetal Heart Rate

| *Nursing Action* | *Rationale* |
|---|---|
| **OBJECTIVE: ASSEMBLE THE EQUIPMENT.**<br>Obtain a fetoscope or a Doppler. | *These devices amplify the fetal heart rate sounds.* |
| **OBJECTIVE: PREPARE THE WOMAN.**<br>• Explain the procedure, the indications for the procedure, and the information that will be obtained.<br>• Uncover the woman's abdomen. | *Explaining the procedure decreases anxiety and increases relaxation.* |
| **OBJECTIVE: USE THE FETOSCOPE OR DOPPLER AS INDICATED AND LISTEN CAREFULLY FOR THE FHR** | |
| **OBJECTIVE: CHECK THE WOMAN'S PULSE, THEN COUNT THE FHR.**<br>• Check the woman's pulse against the fetal sounds you hear. If the rates are the same, you have probably located maternal pulses and you need to readjust the fetoscope or ultrasound device.<br>• If the rates are not similar, count the FHR for 1 full minute. Note that the fetal heart has a double rhythm and just one sound is counted.<br>• If you do not find the FHR, move the fetoscope or ultrasound device laterally.<br>• Explain to the parents what the FHR is and offer to help them listen if they would like to. | |
| **OBJECTIVE: SYSTEMATICALLY EVALUATE THE FHR.**<br>Auscultate between, during, and for 30 seconds following a uterine contraction (UC).<br>*AWHONN (1998) Frequency Recommendations*<br>• Low-risk women: every 1 hour in the latent phase, every 30 minutes in the active phase, and every 15 minutes in the second stage.<br>• High-risk women: every 30 minutes in the latent phase, every 15 minutes in the active phase, and every 5 minutes in the second stage. | *This evaluation provides the opportunity to assess the fetal status and response to the labor process.* |
| **OBJECTIVE: RECORD THE INFORMATION ON THE WOMAN'S CHART.**<br>Document FHR data (rate and rhythm), characteristics of uterine activity, and any actions taken as a result of the FHR. Complete documentation is mandatory.<br><br>Sample recordings follow.<br><br>**SAMPLE DOCUMENTATION**<br>Entry documenting FHR, rhythm, and response to the labor process:<br>1-1-02 FHR 140 by auscultation, regular rhythm, Maternal pulse 78.<br>0730 UC q3min × 60 sec strong. No increase or decrease in FHR noted during or following UC. J Smith RN | |

## *Nursing Action*

**Sample Documentation** ***continued***

Entry documenting FHR, response to UC, nursing intervention, and fetal response:

| | |
|---|---|
| 1-1-02 | FHR 136 by auscultation with slowing to 130 bpm noted during the acme of UC and for |
| 0730 | 10 sec following the UC, STV present, LTV average. Client turned to left side. Maternal pulse 80, FHR 140, regular rhythm with no decrease during or following the next two UC. UC q3min × 60 sec, strong. J Smith RN |

**Using a Fetoscope or a Doppler Ultrasound Device**

*The Fetoscope*

The fetoscope is an older assessment tool; however, some clinicians prefer it because it is "natural" and does not rely on ultrasound.

To use the fetoscope:

- Place the fetoscope earpieces in your ears; use the handpiece to position the bell of the fetoscope on the mother's abdomen.
- Place the diaphragm halfway between the umbilicus and symphysis and in the midline. *You are most likely to hear the FHR in this area.*
- Without touching the fetoscope, listen carefully for the FHR (Figure 16–7A♦).

*The Doppler*

To use the Doppler:

- Place ultrasonic gel on the diaphragm of the Doppler. Gel is used to maintain contact with the maternal abdomen and enhances conduction of ultrasound.
- Place the diaphragm on the woman's abdomen halfway between the umbilicus and symphysis and in the midline. You are most likely to hear the FHR in this area.
- Listen carefully for the FHR (Figure 16–7B♦).

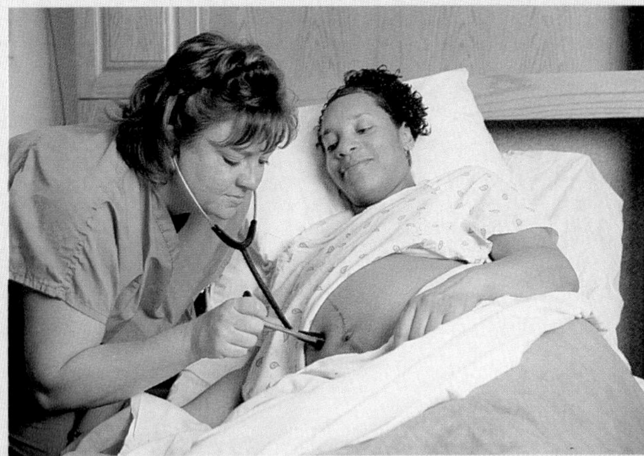

A

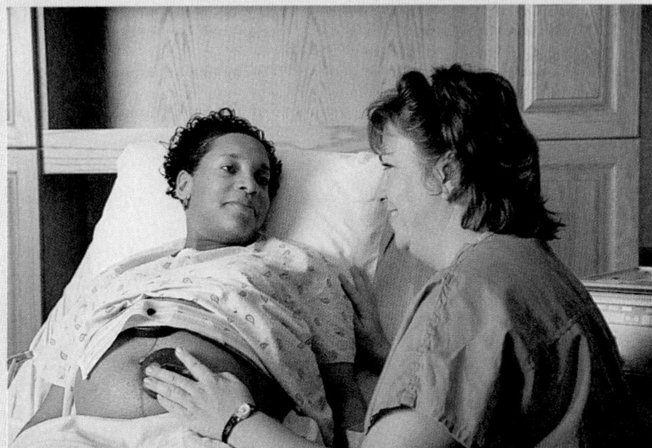

B

C

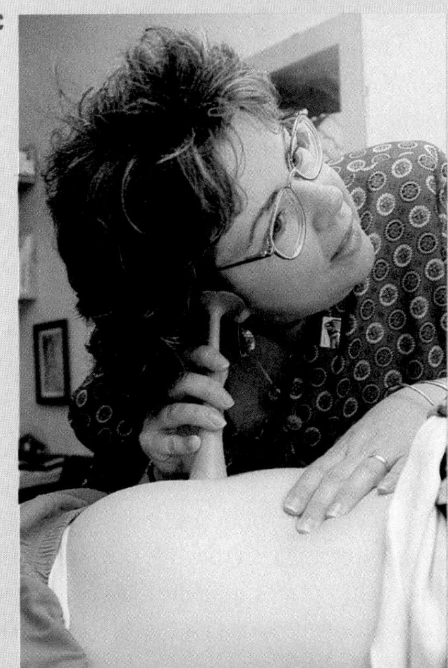

FIGURE 16–7 ♦ **A,** The nurse holds the fetoscope as she places it against the maternal abdomen and then removes her fingers from the fetoscope while counting the fetal heartbeats. **B,** When the fetal heart rate is picked up by the electronic monitor, the sound of the heartbeat can be heard by all persons in the room. **C,** The Penar fetoscope can be easily used in outpatient or community settings.

## KEY FACTS TO REMEMBER

### *Frequency of Auscultation: Assessment and Documentation*

**Low-Risk Patients**

First stage of labor:

q1 hr in latent phase

q30 min in active phase

Second stage of labor:

q15 min

**High-Risk Patients**

First stage of labor:

q30 min in latent phase

q15 min in active phase

Second stage of labor:

q5 min

**Labor Events**

Assess FHR prior to

- Initiation of labor-enhancing procedures (eg, artificial rupture of membranes)
- Periods of ambulation
- Administration of medications
- Administration or initiation of analgesia or anesthesia

**Labor Events *continued***

Assess FHR following

- Rupture of membranes
- Recognition of abnormal uterine activity patterns, such as increased basal tone or tachysystole
- Evaluation of oxytocin (maintenance, increase, or decrease of dosage)
- Administration of medications (at time of peak action)
- Expulsion of enema
- Urinary catheterization
- Vaginal examination
- Periods of ambulation
- Evaluation of analgesia and/or anesthesia (maintenance, increase, or decrease of dosage)

*Source:* AWHONN (1998). *Standards for Professional Nursing Practice in the Care of Women and Newborns* (5th ed.).

on a screen (Figure 16–8♦ see page 397). In some instances, the monitor may track the maternal heart rate instead of the fetal heart rate. However, the nurse can avoid this error by comparing the maternal pulse to the FHR.

Recent advances in technology have led to the development of new ambulatory methods of external monitoring. Using a telemetry system, a small, battery-operated transducer transmits signals to a receiver connected to the monitor. This system, which is held in place with a shoulder strap, allows the woman to ambulate, helping her to feel more comfortable and less confined during labor. In contrast, the system (depicted in Figure 16–8♦ on page 397) requires the woman to remain close to the electrical power source for the monitor.

*Internal monitoring* requires an internal spiral electrode. To place the spiral electrode on the fetal occiput, the amniotic membranes must be ruptured, the cervix must be dilated at least 2 cm, the presenting part must be down against the cervix, and the presenting part must be known (ie, the nurse must be able to detect the actual part of the fetus that is down against the cervix). If all these factors are present, the labor and birth nurse or the physician or CNM inserts a sterile internal spiral electrode into the vagina and places it against the fetal presenting part. The spiral electrode is rotated clockwise until it is attached to the presenting part. Wires that extend from the spiral electrode are attached to a leg plate (which is placed on the woman's thigh) and then attached to the electronic fetal monitor. This method of monitoring the FHR provides more accurate continuous data than external monitoring, because the signal is clearer and movement of the fetus or the woman does not interrupt it (Figure 16–9♦ on page 398).

The FHR tracing at the top of Figure 16–10♦ on page 398 was obtained by internal monitoring with a spiral electrode; the uterine contraction tracing at the bottom of the figure was obtained by external monitoring with a toco. Note that the FHR is variable (the tracing moves up and down instead of in a straight line). In this figure each vertical line represents 1 minute; therefore, contractions are occurring every 2½ to 3 minutes. The FHR is evaluated by assessing an electronic monitor tracing for baseline rate, baseline variability, and periodic changes.

### Baseline Fetal Heart Rate

The **baseline rate** refers to the average FHR observed during a 10-minute period of monitoring. Normal FHR (baseline rate) ranges from 120 to 160 beats per minute. There are two abnormal variations of the baseline rate—those above 160 bpm (tachycardia) and those below 120 bpm (bradycardia). Another change affecting the baseline

# *Procedure 16–3* Electronic Fetal Monitoring

| *Nursing Action* | *Rationale* |
|---|---|
| **Objective: Prepare the woman.**<br>Explain the procedure, the indications for the procedure, and the information that will be obtained. | *Explaining the procedure decreases anxiety and increases relaxation.* |
| **Objective: Place the external fetal monitor.** | |
| • Turn on the monitor. | |
| • Place two elastic belts around the woman's abdomen. | |
| • Place the "toco" over the uterine fundus off the midline on the area palpated to be most firm and secure it with a belt so it fits snugly. | *The uterine fundus is the area of greatest contractility.* |
| • Note the UC tracing. The resting tone tracing (without uterine contraction) should be recording on the 10 or 15 mm Hg pressure line. Adjust the line to reflect that reading. | *If the tracing is on the zero line, there may be a constant grinding noise.* |
| • Apply ultrasonic gel to the diaphragm of the ultrasound transducer. | *Ultrasound gel is used to maintain contact with the maternal abdomen. The ultrasonic beam is directed toward the fetal heart.* |
| • Place the diaphragm on the maternal abdomen in the midline between the umbilicus and the symphysis pubis. | |
| • Listen for the FHR, which will have a whiplike sound. When the FHR is located, attach the elastic belt snugly. Firm contact is necessary to maintain a continuous tracing. | |
| **Objective: Identify the tracing.**<br>Place the following information on the beginning of the fetal monitor paper: date, time, client name, gravida, para, membrane status, physician or CNM name. *Note:* Each birthing area may have specific guidelines regarding additional information to include. | *This ensures accurate identification.* |
| **Objective: Evaluate the EFM tracing.**<br>See the material that follows for evaluation guidelines. | |
| **Objective: Report and record your findings.** | *Reporting provides a permanent record.* |

**Sample Documentation**

Entry documenting reassuring FHR characteristics and response to UCs:

| | |
|---|---|
| 1-1-02 | FHR BL 135–140. STV and LTV present. Two accelerations of 20 bpm × 20 sec with |
| 0700 | fetal movement in 10 min. UC q3min × 50–60 sec of moderate intensity by palpation, resting tone soft. No decelerations noted. B Burch, RNC |

| *Nursing Action* | *Rationale* |
|---|---|
| **Sample Documentation** ***continued***<br>Entry documenting FHR, variability, response of FHR to UC, the intervention used, and subsequent positive fetal response to the intervention.<br>1-1-02 FHR BL 135–140. STV and LTV present. Late decelerations noted with decrease of FHR<br>0730 to 130 bpm for 20 sec. UC q3min × 50–60 sec of moderate intensity by palpation. Client turned to left side. No further deceleration with three subsequent UCs. Two accelerations of 20 bpm × 20 sec noted with fetal movement. Client instructed to remain on left side. B Burch, RNC | |
| **Guidelines for Evaluating the EFM**<br>Evaluating the EFM tracing provides an opportunity to assess the fetal status and response to the labor process. The presence of reassuring characteristics is associated with good fetal outcome. Rapid identification of nonreassuring characteristics allows prompt interventions and the opportunity to determine the fetal response to the interventions. | *For high-risk women, AWHONN (1998) recommends evaluating the EFM tracing every 15 minutes in the first stage and every 5 minutes in the second stage; for low-risk women, every 15–30 minutes in the first stage and every 5–15 minutes in the second stage (as long as the FHR has reassuring characteristics). The time interval for evaluation needs to be shortened if any nonreassuring characteristics occur.* |

is called *variability,* which is a change in FHR over a few seconds to a few minutes.

**Fetal tachycardia** is a sustained rate of 161 bpm or above. Marked tachycardia is 180 bpm or above. Causes of tachycardia include the following (Parer, 1999):

1. Early fetal hypoxia, which leads to stimulation of the sympathetic system as the fetus compensates for reduced blood flow
2. Maternal fever, which accelerates the metabolism of the fetus
3. Maternal dehydration
4. Beta-sympathomimetic drugs such as ritodrine, terbutaline, atropine, and isoxsuprine, which have a cardiac stimulant effect
5. Amnionitis (fetal tachycardia may be the first sign of developing intrauterine infection [Murray, 1997])
6. Maternal hyperthyroidism (thyroid-stimulating hormones may cross the placenta and stimulate fetal heart rate)
7. Fetal anemia (the heart rate is increased as a compensatory mechanism to improve tissue perfusion)

Tachycardia is considered an ominous sign if it is accompanied by late decelerations, severe variable decelerations, or decreased variability. If tachycardia is associated with maternal fever, treatment may consist of antipyretics and/or antibiotics.

**Fetal bradycardia** is a rate less than 110 to 120 beats per minute during a 10-minute period or longer. Causes of fetal bradycardia include the following (Parer, 1999; Schmidt, 2000):

1. Late (profound) fetal hypoxia (depression of myocardial activity)
2. Maternal hypotension, which results in decreased blood flow to the fetus
3. Prolonged umbilical cord compression; fetal baroceptors are activated by cord compression and this produces vagal stimulation, which results in decreased FHR
4. Fetal arrhythmia, which is associated with complete heart block in the fetus

Bradycardia may be a benign or an ominous (preterminal) sign. If there is average long-term variability, the bradycardia is considered benign. When bradycardia is

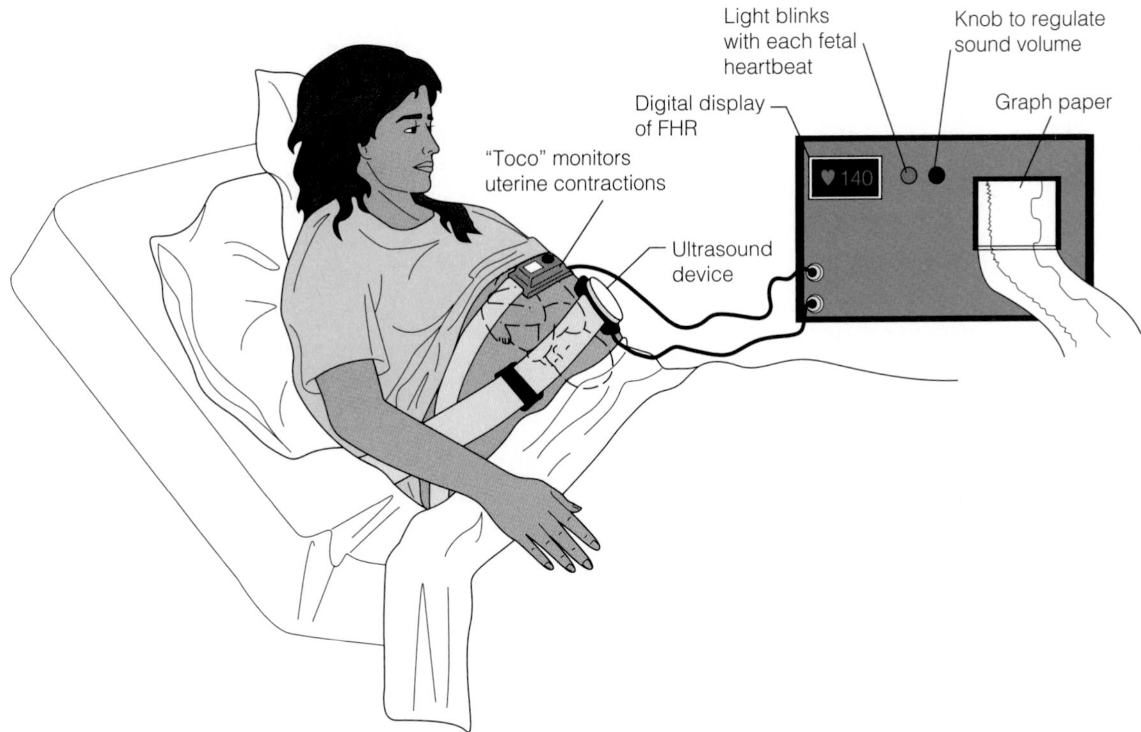


**FIGURE 16–8** ♦ Electronic fetal monitoring by external technique. The tocodynamometer ("toco") is placed over the uterine fundus. The toco provides information that can be used to monitor uterine contractions. The ultrasound device is placed over the area of the fetal back. This device transmits information about the fetal heart rate. Information from both the toco and the ultrasound device is transmitted to the electronic fetal monitor. The fetal heart rate is displayed in a digital display (as a blinking light), on the special monitor paper, and audibly (by adjusting a button on the monitor). The uterine contractions are displayed on the special monitor paper as well.

accompanied by decreased long-term variability and late decelerations, it is considered ominous and a sign of advanced fetal distress (Parer, 1999).

### Variability

*Baseline variability* is a measure of the interplay (the push-pull effect) between the sympathetic and parasympathetic nervous systems. There are two types of fetal heart variability. **Short-term variability (STV)** is the beat-to-beat change in FHR. It represents fluctuations of the baseline. STV can only be measured via internal (scalp electrode) means and is classified as either present or absent. **Long-term variability (LTV)** is the waviness or rhythmic fluctuations (called cycles) of the FHR tracing, which occur three to five times per minute. LTV can be classified as absent, decreased, average, increased, or marked (see Figure 16–11♦). The most important aspect of LTV is that even in the presence of abnormal or questionable FHR patterns, if the variability is normal, the fetus is not suffering from cerebral asphyxia (Murray, 1997).

Causes of decreased variability include the following (Parer, 1999):

1. Hypoxia and acidosis (decreased blood flow to the fetus)
2. Administration of drugs such as meperidine hydrochloride (Demerol), diazepam (Valium), or hydroxyzine (Vistaril), which depress the fetal central nervous system
3. Fetal sleep cycle (during fetal sleep, long-term variability is decreased; fetal sleep cycles usually last for 20 to 30 minutes)
4. Fetus of less than 32 weeks' gestation (fetal neurological control of heart rate is immature)

Causes of increased variability include the following (Parer, 1999):

1. Early mild hypoxia (variability increases as a result of compensatory mechanism)
2. Fetal stimulation (stimulation of autonomic nervous system because of abdominal palpation, maternal vaginal examination, application of spiral electrode on fetal head, or acoustic stimulation)

Decreasing variability that does not appear to be associated with a fetal sleep cycle or the administration of

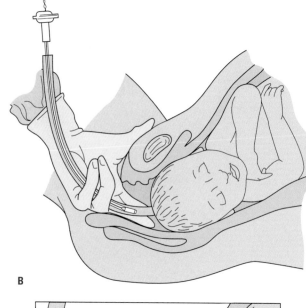

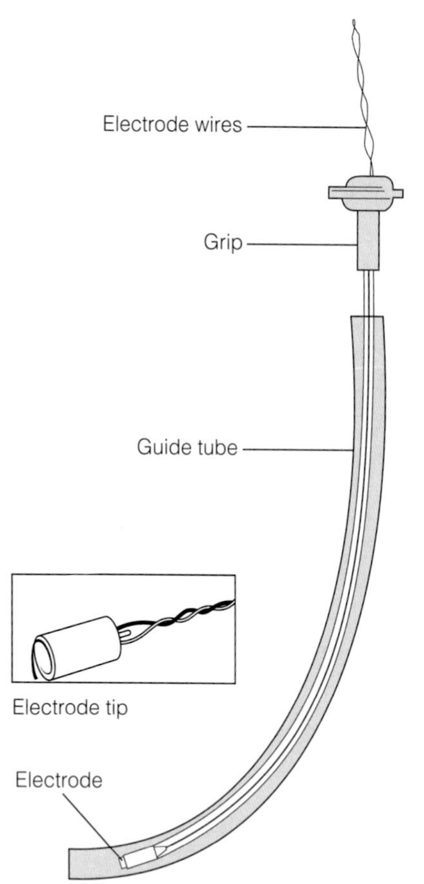


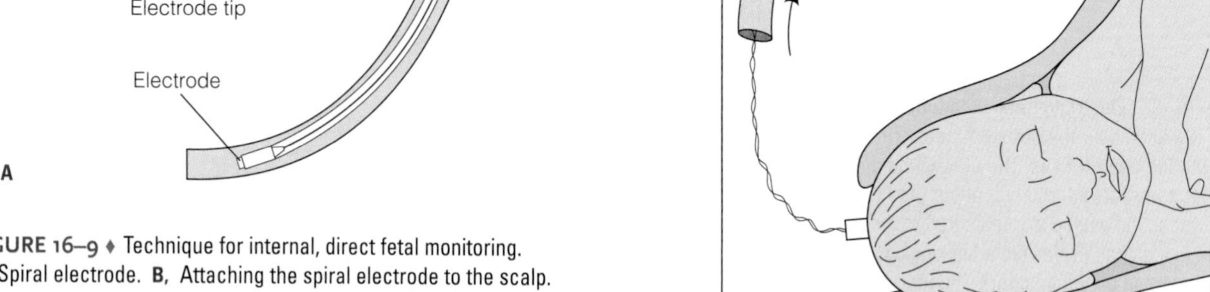


FIGURE 16–9 ♦ Technique for internal, direct fetal monitoring. **A,** Spiral electrode. **B,** Attaching the spiral electrode to the scalp. **C,** Attached spiral electrode with the guide tube removed.

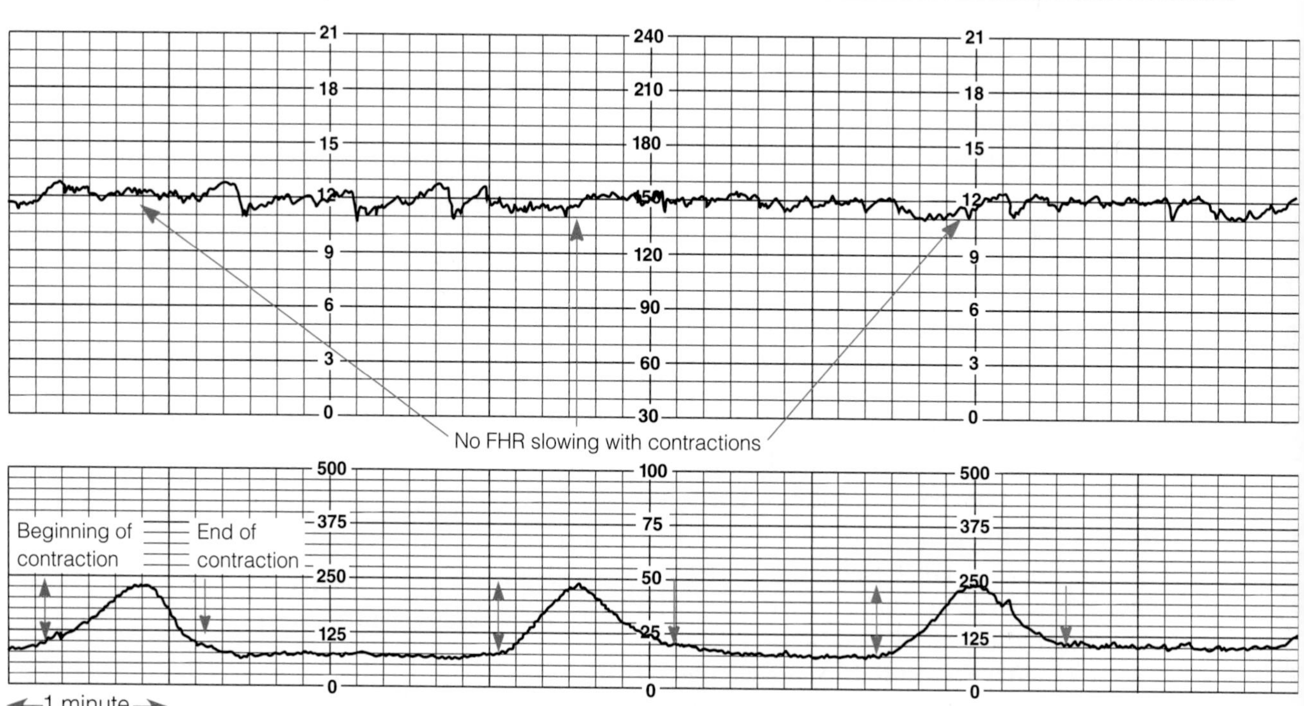


FIGURE 16–10 ♦ Normal fetal heart rate pattern obtained by internal monitoring. Note normal FHR, 140 to 158 beats/min, presence of long- and short-term variability, and absence of deceleration with adequate contractions. Arrows on bottom of tracing indicate beginnings of uterine contractions.

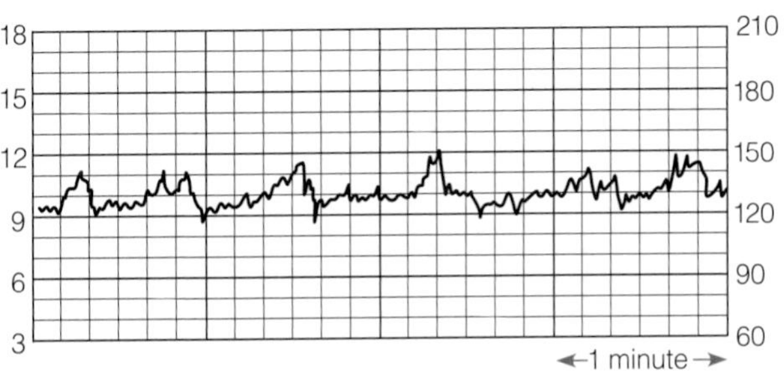


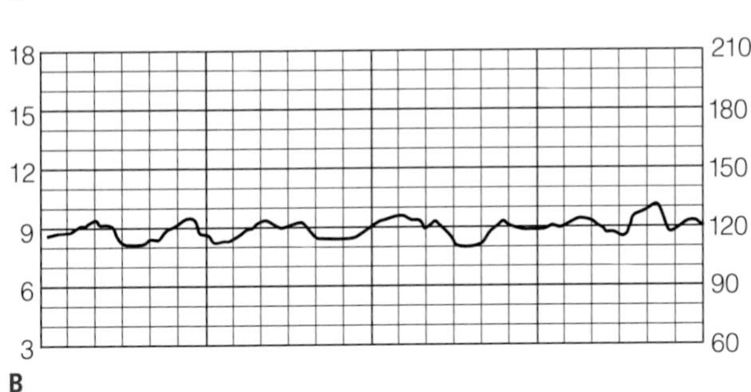


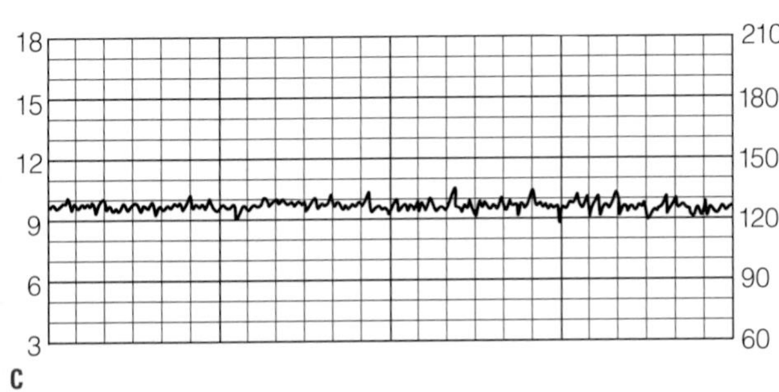


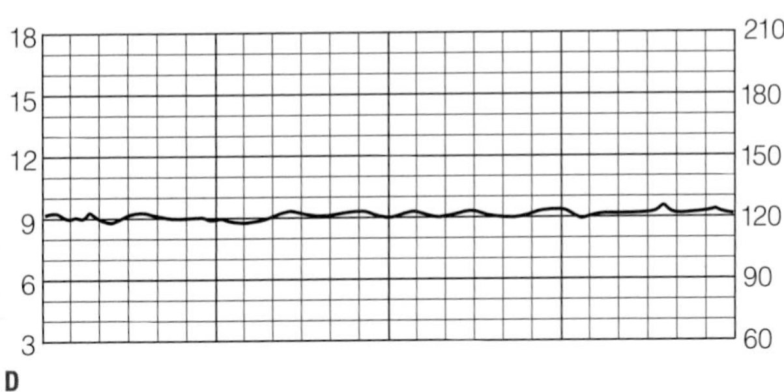


FIGURE 16–11 ♦ Short- and long-term variability. **A,** Increased LTV; STV present. **B,** Average LTV; STV absent. **C,** Absent LTV; STV present. **D,** Absent LTV; STV absent.

drugs is a warning sign of fetal distress. It is especially ominous if decreased variability is accompanied by late decelerations, explained shortly.

External electronic fetal monitoring is not an adequate method to assess short-term variability. If decreased variability is noted on monitoring, application of a spiral electrode should be considered to obtain more accurate information.

## Accelerations

**Accelerations** are transient increases in the FHR normally caused by fetal movement. When the fetus moves, its heart rate increases, just as the heart rates of adults increase during exercise. Often accelerations accompany uterine contractions, usually due to fetal movement in response to the pressure of the contractions. Accelerations of this type are thought to be a sign of fetal well-being and adequate oxygen reserve. The accelerations with fetal movement are the basis for nonstress tests (see Chapter 14).

## Decelerations

**Decelerations** are periodic decreases in FHR from the normal baseline. They are categorized as early, late, and variable according to the time of their occurrence in the contraction cycle and their waveform (Figure 16–12♦). When the fetal head is compressed, cerebral blood flow is decreased, which leads to central vagal stimulation and results in early deceleration. The onset of early deceleration occurs before the onset of the uterine contraction. This type of deceleration is of uniform shape, is usually considered benign, and does not require intervention.

**Late deceleration** is caused by uteroplacental insufficiency resulting from decreased blood flow and oxygen transfer to the fetus through the intervillous spaces during uterine contractions. The onset of the deceleration occurs after the onset of a uterine contraction and is of a uniform shape that tends to reflect associated uterine contractions. The late deceleration pattern is considered a nonreassuring sign but does not necessarily require immediate delivery.

**Variable decelerations** occur if the umbilical cord becomes compressed, thus reducing blood flow between the placenta and fetus. The resulting increase in peripheral resistance in the fetal circulation causes fetal hypertension. The fetal hypertension stimulates the baroreceptors in the aortic arch and carotid sinuses, which slow the FHR. The onset of variable decelerations varies in timing with the onset of the contraction, and the decelerations are variable in shape. This pattern requires further assessment. Nursing interventions for late and variable decelerations in FHR are presented in Table 16–2.

A *sinusoidal pattern* appears similar to a waveform. The characteristics of this pattern include presence of long-term variability, absence of short-term variability, and accelerations with fetal movement. This pattern is associated with Rh isoimmunization, fetal anemia, and a chronic fetal bleed. It may also occur with the administration of medications such as meperidine (Demerol) or butorphanol tartrate (Stadol). When it occurs in association with medication, the pattern is usually temporary (Kang & Boehm, 1999; Murray, 1997) (see Figure 16–13D♦).

## Psychologic Reactions to Electronic Monitoring

Responses to EFM can be varied and complex. Many women have little knowledge of monitoring unless they have attended a prenatal class that dealt with this

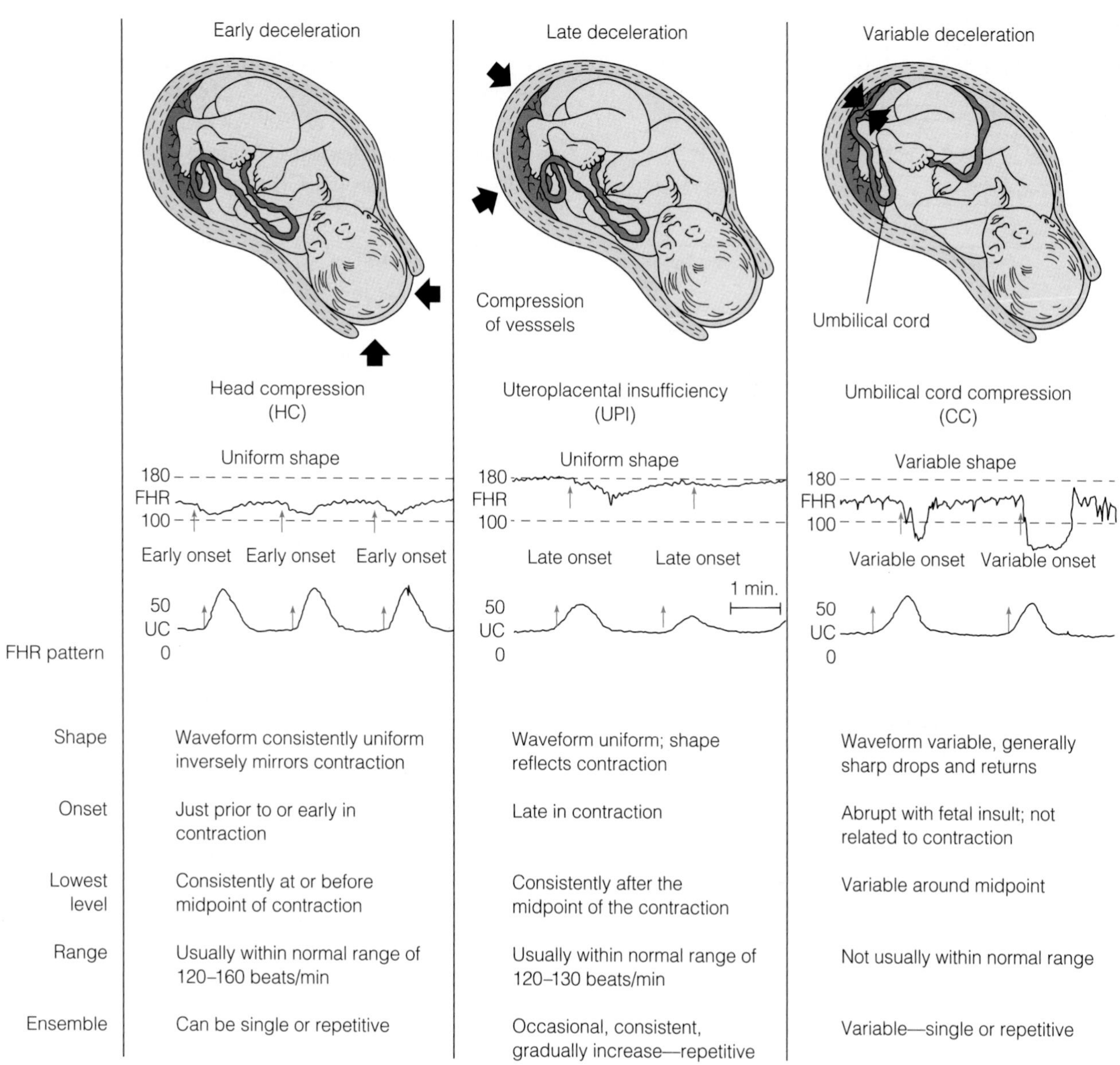

Early deceleration
Late deceleration
Variable deceleration
Compression of vesssels
Umbilical cord
Head compression (HC)
Uteroplacental insufficiency (UPI)
Umbilical cord compression (CC)
Uniform shape
Uniform shape
Variable shape
180
FHR
100
Early onset
Early onset
Early onset
Late onset
Late onset
Variable onset
Variable onset
1 min.
50
UC
0
FHR pattern
Shape
Waveform consistently uniform inversely mirrors contraction
Waveform uniform; shape reflects contraction
Waveform variable, generally sharp drops and returns
Onset
Just prior to or early in contraction
Late in contraction
Abrupt with fetal insult; not related to contraction
Lowest level
Consistently at or before midpoint of contraction
Consistently after the midpoint of the contraction
Variable around midpoint
Range
Usually within normal range of 120–160 beats/min
Usually within normal range of 120–130 beats/min
Not usually within normal range
Ensemble
Can be single or repetitive
Occasional, consistent, gradually increase—repetitive
Variable—single or repetitive


**FIGURE 16–12 ♦ Types and characteristics of early, late, and variable decelerations.** *Source:* Hon, E. (1976). *An introduction to fetal heart rate monitoring* (2nd ed., p. 29). Los Angeles: University of Southern California School of Medicine.

subject. Some women react to electronic monitoring positively, viewing it as a reassurance that "the baby is OK." They may also feel that the monitor helps identify problems that develop in labor. Other women may have ambivalent or even negative feelings about the monitor. They may think that the monitor is interfering with a natural process, and they do not want the intrusion. They may resent the time and attention that the monitor requires, time that could otherwise be spent providing nursing care. Some women may find that the equipment, wires, and sounds increase their anxiety. The discomfort of lying in one position and fear of injury to the baby are other objections.

## Nursing Responsibilities

A key strength of technology is its ability to explain and possibly predict health patterns or problems with precision. However, this advantage has the potential to dehumanize the nurse-client relationship (Bernardo, 1998). Therefore, it is important to recognize that every encounter with the childbearing family offers the nurse an opportunity to provide education and empowerment to the laboring woman and her partner. These encounters include times when technology is utilized. By helping to provide information when needed, answering questions, and encouraging the woman to make decisions, a trusting relationship can be established. Within this bond of

## TABLE 16–2 Guidelines for Management of Variable, Late, and Prolonged Deceleration Patterns

| *Pattern* | *Nursing Interventions* |
|---|---|
| Variable decelerations<br>Isolated or occasional<br>Moderate | Report findings to physician or CNM and document in chart.<br>Provide explanation to woman and partner.<br>Change maternal position to one in which FHR pattern is most improved.<br>Discontinue oxytocin if it is being administered and other interventions are unsuccessful.<br>Perform vaginal examination to assess for prolapsed cord or change in labor progress.<br>Monitor FHR continuously to assess current status and for further changes in FHR pattern. |
| Variable decelerations<br>Severe and uncorrectable | Give oxygen if indicated.<br>Report findings to physician or CNM and document in chart.<br>Provide explanation to woman and partner.<br>Prepare for possible cesarean birth. Follow interventions listed above.<br>Prepare for vaginal birth unless baseline variability is decreasing or FHR is progressively rising—then cesarean, forceps, or vacuum birth is indicated.<br>Assist physician with fetal scalp sampling if ordered.<br>Prepare for cesarean birth if scalp pH shows acidosis or downward trend. |
| Late decelerations | Report findings to physician or CNM and document in chart.<br>Provide explanation to woman and partner.<br>Monitor for further FHR changes.<br>Maintain maternal position on left side.<br>Increase IV fluids to maintain volume and hydration (normal saline or lactated Ringer's).<br>Discontinue oxytocin if it is being administered and late decelerations persist despite other interventions.<br>Administer oxygen by face mask at 7 to 10 L/min.<br>Monitor maternal blood pressure and pulse for signs of hypotension; possibly increase flow rate of IV fluids to treat hypotension.<br>Follow physician's orders for treatment for hypotension if present.<br>Assess labor progress (dilatation and station).<br>Assist physician with fetal blood sampling: If pH stays above 7.25, physician will continue monitoring and resample; if pH shows downward trend (between 7.25 and 7.20) or is below 7.20, prepare for birth by most expeditious means. |
| Late decelerations with tachycardia or decreasing variability | Report findings to physician or CNM and document in chart.<br>Maintain maternal position on left side.<br>Administer oxygen by face mask at 7 to 10 L/min.<br>Discontinue oxytocin if it is being administered.<br>Assess maternal blood pressure and pulse.<br>Increase IV fluids (normal saline or lactated RInger's).<br>Assess labor progress (dilatation and station).<br>Prepare for immediate cesarean birth.<br>Explain plan of treatment to woman and partner.<br>Assist physician with fetal blood sampling (if ordered). |
| Prolonged decelerations | Perform vaginal examination to rule out prolapsed cord or to determine progress in labor status.<br>Change maternal position as needed to try to alleviate decelerations.<br>Discontinue oxytocin if it is being administered.<br>Administer oxygen by face mask at 7 to 10 L/min.<br>Notify physician or CNM of findings and initial interventions and document in chart.<br>Provide explanation to woman and partner.<br>Increase IV fluids (normal saline or lactated Ringer's).<br>Administer tocolytic if hypertonus noted and ordered by physician or CNM.<br>Anticipate normal FHR recovery following deceleration if FHR previously normal.<br>Anticipate intervention if FHR previously abnormal or deceleration lasts >3 minutes. |

trust resides an awareness of the client's whole being and the healing power of each moment. From this framework nothing can be viewed as routine, each moment can be viewed as a teaching opportunity, and each birthing family will rightfully be seen as unique and special.

Technology has been advancing at a rapid rate in the labor and birthing arena, and each new development challenges nurses to understand, include, and balance technology with holistic nursing practice. The use of technology will continue to be an integral part of client care, one that gives rise to many questions about how it changes the nurse's role. However, awareness and the active use of holistic principles that honor the mind, body, and spirit of each individual enhance the nursing care given.

Prior to using the electronic fetal monitor, the nurse needs to fully explain the reason for its use and the information that it can provide. After the monitor is applied, basic information can be recorded on the monitor strip. These data should include the date, client's name, physician or CNM's name, hospital number, age, gravida, para, estimated date of birth (EDB), membrane status, and maternal vital signs. As the monitor strip runs and care is provided, occurrences during labor should be recorded not only in the medical record but also on the monitor strip. This information helps the health care team assess current status and evaluate the tracing.

The following information should be noted on the tracing (American Academy of Pediatrics [AAP] & American College of Obstetricians and Gynecologists, [ACOG], 1997):

1. Vaginal examination (dilatation, effacement, station, position)
2. Amniotomy or spontaneous rupture of membranes, color of amniotic fluid
3. Maternal vital signs
4. Maternal position in bed and changes of position
5. Application of spiral electrode or intrauterine pressure catheter
6. Medications given
7. Oxygen administration
8. Maternal behaviors (emesis, coughing, hiccups)
9. Fetal scalp stimulation or fetal scalp blood sampling
10. Vomiting
11. Pushing
12. Administration of anesthesia blocks

In addition, if the monitor does not automatically add the time on the strip at specific intervals, the time should be included when recording any information on the strip. If more than one nurse is adding information to the monitor strip, it is essential to initial each note. The tracing is considered a legal part of the woman's medical record and is submissible as evidence in court.

It is important for the laboring woman to feel that what is happening to her is the central focus. The nurse can acknowledge this need by always speaking to and looking at the woman when entering the room, before looking at the monitor.

### Evaluation of FHR Tracings

The nurse needs to use a systematic approach in evaluating FHR tracings to avoid interpreting findings on the basis of inadequate or erroneous data. With a systematic approach, the nurse can make a more accurate and rapid assessment; easily communicate data to the woman, physician or CNM, and staff; and have a universal language for documenting in the woman's record.

Evaluation of the electronic monitor tracing begins by looking at the uterine contraction pattern. To evaluate the contraction pattern, the nurse should

1. Determine the uterine resting tone.
2. Assess the contractions: What is the frequency? What is the duration? What is the intensity (if internal monitoring)?

The next step is to evaluate the FHR tracing:

1. Determine the baseline: Is the baseline within the normal range? Is there evidence of tachycardia? Is there evidence of bradycardia?
2. Determine FHR variability: Is short-term variability present or absent? Is long-term variability average? Minimal? Absent? Moderate? Marked?
3. Determine if a sinusoidal pattern is present.
4. Determine if there are periodic changes: Are accelerations present? Do they meet the criteria for a reactive NST? Are decelerations present? Are they uniform in shape? If so, determine if they are early or late decelerations. Are they nonuniform in shape? If so, determine whether they are variable decelerations.

After evaluating the FHR tracing for the factors just listed, the nurse may further classify the tracing as reassuring (normal) or nonreassuring (worrisome). Reassuring patterns contain normal parameters and do not require additional treatment or intervention.

Characteristics of reassuring FHR patterns include the following:

- Baseline rate is 120 to 160 bpm.
- Short-term variability is present.
- Long-term variability ranges from three to five cycles per minute. Periodic patterns consist of accelerations with fetal movement, and early decelerations may be present.

Nonreassuring patterns may indicate that the fetus is becoming stressed and intervention is needed. Characteristics of nonreassuring patterns include the following:

- Severe variable decelerations (FHR drops below 70 bpm for longer than 30 to 45 seconds and is accompanied by rising baseline or decreasing variability or slow return to baseline)
- Late decelerations of any magnitude
- Absence of variability (no short- or long-term variability present)
- Prolonged deceleration (a deceleration that lasts 60 to 90 seconds or more)
- Severe (marked) bradycardia (FHR baseline of 70 bpm or less)

Nonreassuring patterns may require continuous monitoring and more involved treatment and intervention (see Table 16–2).

It is vital to provide information to the laboring woman about the FHR pattern and the interventions, if necessary, that will help her fetus. Most women are aware that something is happening. Sharing information with them provides reassurance that a potential or actual problem is identified and that they are active participants in the interventions. Occasionally a problem arises that requires immediate intervention. In that case, the nurse may say, something like "It is important for you to turn on your left side right now because the baby is having a little difficulty. I'll explain what is happening in just a few moments." This type of response lets the woman know that although an action needs to be accomplished rapidly, information will soon be provided. In the haste to act quickly, nurses and other caregivers must not forget that it is the woman's body and her baby.

## Scalp Stimulation Test

When there is a question regarding fetal status, a scalp stimulation test can be used before the more invasive fetal blood sampling. In this test, the examiner applies pressure to the fetal scalp while doing a vaginal examination. The fetus who is not in any stress or distress responds with an acceleration of the FHR (Cunningham, MacDonald, Gant, et al., 1997).

## Fetal Scalp Blood Sampling

When nonreassuring or confusing FHR patterns are noted, additional information about the acid-base status of the fetus is needed. This information may be obtained by **fetal blood sampling (FBS).** The physician usually draws the blood sample from the fetal scalp but may obtain it from the fetal buttocks if the fetus is in the breech position (Gilstrap, 1999).

Before fetal blood can be sampled, the membranes must be ruptured, the cervix must be dilated at least 2 to 3 cm, and the presenting part must not be above −2 station. Sampling is not done when FHR patterns are ominous. It is contraindicated in acute emergencies and in cases of vaginal bleeding. In these instances, birth by the most expeditious means is indicated.

Normal fetal pH values during labor are above 7.25; 7.20 to 7.25 is considered borderline, warranting further sampling. Values below 7.20 are nonreassuring and necessitate birth without delay (Gilstrap, 1999).

The more information that is available from FHR monitoring, the less need there is for a FBS. Only when FHR patterns are not interpretable, worsening, or suggestive of high risk is this adjunctive procedure indicated. Fetal blood sampling may prevent unnecessary cesarean birth.

# Chapter Review

## CHAPTER HIGHLIGHTS

- Intrapartal assessment includes attention to both the physical and psychosociocultural parameters of the laboring woman, assessment of the fetus, and ongoing assessment for conditions that place the woman and her fetus at increased risk.
- A vaginal examination determines the status of fetal membranes; cervical dilatation and effacement; and fetal presentation, position, and station.
- Uterine contractions may be assessed by palpation or by an electronic monitor.
- Leopold's maneuvers provide a systematic evaluation of fetal presentation and position.
- Fetal presentation and position may also be assessed by vaginal examination or ultrasound.
- The fetal heart rate may be assessed by auscultation (with a fetoscope or Doppler) or by electronic monitoring.
- Electronic fetal monitoring is accomplished by indirect ultrasound or by direct methods that require the placement of a spiral electrode on the fetal presenting part.
- Indications for electronic monitoring include fetal, maternal, and uterine factors; presence of pregnancy complications; regional anesthesia; and elective monitoring.
- Short-term variability of the FHR can only be assessed by direct electronic monitoring.
- Baseline FHR refers to the range of FHR observed between contractions, during a 10-minute period of monitoring.
- The normal range of FHR is 120 to 160 beats per minute.
- Baseline changes of the FHR include tachycardia, bradycardia, and variability.
- Fetal tachycardia is defined as a rate of 161 beats per minute or more for a 10-minute period.
- Fetal bradycardia is defined as a rate of less than 120 beats per minute for a 10-minute period.
- Baseline variability is an important parameter of fetal well-being. It includes both long- and short-term variability.
- Periodic changes are transient decelerations or accelerations of the FHR from the baseline. Accelerations are normally caused by fetal movement; decelerations may be termed early, late, variable, or sinusoidal.
- Early decelerations are due to compression of the fetal head during contractions and are considered reassuring.
- Late decelerations are associated with uteroplacental insufficiency and are considered ominous.
- Variable decelerations are associated with compression of the umbilical cord and require further assessment.
- Sinusoidal patterns are characterized by an undulant sine wave.
- Psychologic reactions to monitoring vary between feelings of relief and feelings of being tied down.
- Birthing room nurses have responsibilities in recognizing and interpreting fetal monitoring patterns, notifying the physician or CNM of problems, and initiating corrective and supportive measures when needed.
- Fetal scalp stimulation can be used when fetal status is in question.
- Fetal acid-base status may be assessed by fetal blood sampling.

## CHAPTER REFERENCES


American Academy of Pediatrics & American College of Obstetricians and Gynecologists. (1997). *Guidelines for perinatal care* (4th ed.).Washington, DC: Author.

Austin, G., Gallop, R., McCay, E., Peternelj-Taylor, C., & Bayer, M. (1999). Culturally competent care for psychiatric clients who have a history of sexual abuse. *Clinical Nursing Research, 8,* 5–25.

AWHONN. (1998). *Standards for Professional Nursing Practice in the Care of Women and Newborns* (5th ed.).

Bernardo, A. (1998). Technology and true presence in nursing. *Holistic Nursing Practice, 12,* 40–49.

Burrian, J. (1995). Helping survivors of sexual abuse through labor. *Maternal-Child Nursing Journal,* 20(5), 252–255.

Callister, L. C. (2001). Culturally competent are of women and newborns: knowledge, attitude, and skills. *Journal of Obstetric, Gynecologic, and Neonatal Nursing, 30*(2), 209–215.

Cunningham, F. G., MacDonald, P. C., Gant, N. F., Leveno, K. J., Gilstrap, L. C., Hankins, D. V., and Clark, S. L. (1997). *Williams obstetrics* (20th ed.). Stamford, CT: Appleton & Lange.

Feinstein, N. (2000). Fetal heart rate auscultation: Current and future practice. *Journal of Obstetric and Gynecological Nurses, 29*(3), 306–314.

Gilstrap, L. (1999). Fetal acid-base balance. In R. K. Creasy & R. Resnik (Eds.), *Maternal-fetal medicine* (4th ed., pp. 331–340). Philadelphia: Saunders.

Kang, A. H., & Boehm, F. H. (1999). The clinical significance of intermittent sinusoidal fetal heart rate. *American Journal of Obstetrics and Gynecology, 180,* 151–152.

McFarland, J., & Gondolf, E. (1998). Preventing abuse during pregnancy: A clinical protocol. *Maternal-Child Nursing Journal, 23,* 22–26.

Murray, M. (1997). *Antepartal and interpartal fetal monitoring* (2nd ed.). Albuquerque, NM: Learning Resources International.

Parer, J. (1999). Fetal heart rate. In R. K. Creasy & R. Resnik (Eds.), *Maternal-fetal medicine* (4th ed., pp. 270–299). Philadelphia: Saunders.

Parer, J., & King, T. (2000). Fetal heart rate monitoring: Is it salvageable? *American Journal of Obstetrics and Gynecology, 182*(4), 982–987.

Schmidt, J. (2000). Intrapartal fetal assessment. In S. Mattson & J. E. Smith (Eds.), *Maternal-newborn nursing* (2nd ed., pp. 271–299). Philadelphia: Saunders.

Seng, J. S., Oakley, D. J., Samselle, C. M., Killion, C., Graham-Bermann, S. & Liberzon, I. (2001). Posttraumatic stress disorder and pregnancy complications. *Obstetrics & Gynecology, 97*(1), 17–22.


## CONTEMPORARY MATERNAL-NEWBORN NURSING ON-LINE

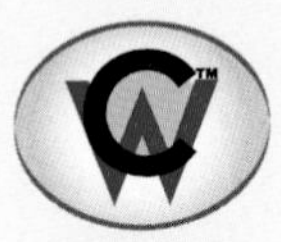

Additional interactive resources, including animations and video, for this chapter can be found on the Companion Website at http://www.prenhall.com/ladewig. Click on Chapter 16 and "Begin" to select the activities for this chapter.

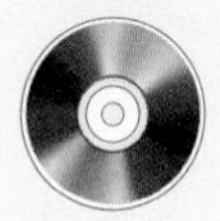

For NCLEX review questions and an audio glossary, access the accompanying CD-ROM in this book.

Chapter 17

# The Family in Childbirth: Needs and Care

*For as long as I can remember I have been fascinated with birth. I began as a hospital volunteer, I have taught childbirth education, and I was a labor nurse before going back to school to become a nurse-midwife. It has been a challenge, and sometimes I wondered if I would make it. But here I am, practicing in the same hospital that I used to volunteer in. I'm still fascinated with birth.*

—A Certified Nurse-Midwife

## KEY TERMS

| | |
|---|---|
| Apgar score | 429 |
| Birthing room | 407 |
| Hyperventilation | 419 |
| Precipitous birth | 435 |

## OBJECTIVES

- Identify the database to be created from information obtained when a woman is admitted to the birthing area.
- Review the nursing care provided at admission.
- Discuss nursing interventions to meet the psychologic and physiologic needs of the woman during each stage of labor.
- Compare and contrast methods of promoting comfort during the first and second stages of labor.
- Summarize the immediate needs of the newborn following birth.
- Delineate management of a precipitous birth.

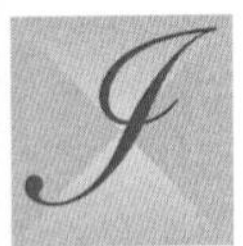t is time for a child to be born. The waiting is over; labor has begun. The dreams and wishes of the past months fade as the mother-to-be or the expectant parents face the reality of the tasks of childbearing and childrearing that are ahead.

The parents are about to undergo one of the most meaningful and stressful events in their lives. The adequacy of their preparation for childbirth, including the coping mechanisms, communication, and support systems that they have established, will be put to the test. In particular, the childbearing woman may feel that her psychologic and physical limits are about to be challenged (Stern & Bruschweiler-Stern, 1998). These events may be even more challenging for the single woman, especially if she lacks a strong support system.

The parents have also been involved in collecting information and making decisions about the setting for childbirth. To reflect the consumer demand for family-centered care, most birthing centers have single-purpose units, which means that the woman stays in the same room for labor, birth, recovery, and possibly the postpartum period. These rooms may be called labor, delivery, recovery, and postpartum (LDRP) rooms or single-room maternity care (SRMC). When speaking to the public, birthing facility spokespersons tend to use the term **birthing room** instead of LDRP or SRMC.

The birthing room atmosphere is more relaxed and families seem to feel more comfortable in it than in a traditional labor room. Not having to be transferred from one area to another for birth helps the laboring woman create her own space to labor in and enhances the family's involvement. Birthing rooms usually have beds that can be adapted for birth by removing a small section near the foot. The decor is designed to produce a homelike atmosphere in which families can feel both safe and at ease.

Maternal-newborn nursing has kept pace with the changing philosophy of childbirth. Nurses who choose positions in a birthing area are presented with opportunities to interact with clients in a wide variety of situations, from a family who wants maximum participation to a single woman who enters alone. In every case, nurses strive to provide high-quality, individualized care.

The previous two chapters provided a database about physiologic and psychologic changes during labor and birth and needed nursing assessments. This chapter presents nursing care during labor and birth and includes an Intrapartal Critical Pathway on page 408.

## Nursing Diagnosis during Labor and Birth

When a plan of care is devised for the intrapartal period, the nurse can develop a general plan that encompasses the total process, from the beginning of labor through the fourth stage, or a plan can be developed for each stage of labor and birth. A general plan presents an overview of the whole process, whereas a plan of care that identifies nursing diagnoses for each stage provides an opportunity to identify more specific nursing care.

In the first stage, examples of appropriate nursing diagnoses may include the following:

- Fear related to discomfort of labor and unknown labor outcome
- Pain related to uterine contractions, cervical dilatation, and fetal descent
- Knowledge deficit related to lack of information about normal labor process and comfort measures

Examples of nursing diagnoses for the second and third stages may include the following:

- Pain related to uterine contractions, birth process, and/or perineal trauma from birth
- Knowledge deficit related to lack of information about pushing methods before birth
- Fear related to outcome of birth process

In the fourth stage, possible nursing diagnoses include the following:

- Pain related to perineal trauma
- Knowledge deficit related to lack of information about the involution process and self-care needs
- Alteration in family process related to incorporation of newborn into the family

## Nursing Care Management during Admission

During her prenatal visits the woman is instructed to come to the birthing unit if any of the following occur:

- Rupture of membranes (ROM)
- Regular, frequent uterine contractions (nulliparas, 5 minutes apart for 1 hour; multiparas, 10 to 15 minutes apart for 1 hour)
- Any vaginal bleeding

# CRITICAL PATHWAY: *For Intrapartal Stages*

| Category | First Stage | Second and Third Stages | Fourth Stage<br>Birth to 1 Hour Past Birth |
|---|---|---|---|
| **Referral** | Review prenatal record<br>Advise CNM/physician of admission | Labor record for first stage | Report to recovery room nurse<br>**Expected Outcomes**<br>Appropriate resources identified and utilized |
| **Assessments** | Admission assessments:<br>Ask about problems since last prenatal visit, labor status (contraction frequency and duration), membrane status (intact or ruptured), coping level, support, woman's desires during labor and birth, ability to verbalize needs, laboratory testing (blood and UA)<br>Intrapartal assessments: cervical assessment—from 1 to 10 cm dilatation; nullipara (1.2 cm/hr), multipara (1.5 cm/hr)<br>Cervical effacement: from 0% to 100%<br>Fetal descent: progressive descent from −4 to +4<br>Membrane assessment: intact or ruptured; when ruptured, Nitrazine positive, fluid clear, no foul odor<br>Comfort level: woman states she is able to cope with contractions<br>Behavioral characteristics: facial expressions, tone of voice and verbal expressions are consistent with comfort and ability to cope<br>Latent phase:<br>• B/P, P, R q1h if in normal range (BP <90–140/60–90 or not >30 mm Hg systolic or 15 mm Hg diastolic over baseline; pulse 60–90; respirations 12–20/min, quiet, easy)<br>• Temp q4h unless >37.6°C (99.6°F) or membranes ruptured, then q2h<br>• Uterine contractions q30min (contractions q5–10 min, 15–40 sec, mild intensity)<br>• FHR q60min (for low-risk women) and q30min (for high-risk women) if reassuring (reassuring FHR has baseline 120–160, STV present, LTV average, accelerations with fetal movement, no late nor variable decelerations); if nonreassuring, position on side, start $O_2$, assess for hypotension, monitor continuously, notify CNM or physician<br>Active phase:<br>• BP, P, R q1h if WNL<br>• Temp as above<br>• Uterine contractions q30min: (contractions q2–3 min, 60 sec, moderate to strong)<br>• FHR q30min (for low-risk women) and q15min (for high-risk women) if reassuring; if nonreassuring institute interventions<br>Transition:<br>• BP, P, R q30min<br>• Uterine contractions q15–30min: (contractions q2min, 60–75 sec, strong)<br>• FHR q30min (for low-risk women) and q15min (for high-risk women) if reassuring; if nonreassuring, see above | Second-stage assessments:<br>• BP, P, R q5–15 min<br>• Uterine contractions palpated continuously<br>• FHR q15min (for low-risk women) and q5min (for high-risk women) if reassuring; if nonreassuring, monitor continuously<br>Fetal descent: descent continues to birth<br>Comfort level: woman states she is able to cope with contractions and pushing<br>Behavioral characteristics: response to pushing, facial expressions, verbalization<br>Third-stage assessments:<br>• BP, P, R q5min<br>• Uterine contractions, palpate occasionally until placenta is delivered, fundus maintains tone, and contraction pattern continues to birth of placenta<br>Newborn assessments:<br>• Assess Apgar score of newborn<br>• Respirations: 30–60, irregular<br>• Apical pulse: 120–160 and somewhat irregular<br>• Temperature: skin temp above 36.5°C (97.8°F)<br>• Umbilical cord: two arteries, one vein (if one artery, assess for anomalies and urine output)<br>• Gestational age: 38–42 weeks | Immediate postbirth assessments of mother q15min, for 1h:<br>• BP: 90–140/60–90; should return to prelabor level<br>• Pulse: slightly lower than in labor; range is 60–90<br>• Respirations: 12–20/min; easy; quiet<br>• Temperature: 36.2–37.6°C (98–99.6°F)<br>• Fundus firm, in midline, at the umbilicus<br>• Lochia rubra; moderate amount; <1 pad/hr; no free flow or passage of clots with massage<br>• Perineum: sutures intact; no bulging or marked swelling; minimal bruising may be present; no c/o severe pain or rectal pain<br>• Bladder nondistended; spontaneous void of >100 mL clear, straw-colored urine; bladder nondistended following voiding<br>• If hemorrhoids present, no tenseness or marked engorgement; <2 cm diameter<br>Comfort level: <3 on scale of 1 to 10<br>Energy level: awake and able to hold newborn<br>Newborn assessments if newborn remains with parents:<br>• Respirations: 30–60; irregular<br>• Apical pulse: 120–160 and somewhat irregular<br>• Temperature: skin temperature above 36.5°C (97.8°F); skin feels warm to touch<br>• Skin color noncyanotic<br>• Mucus: small amount, clear, easily suctioned with bulb syringe without skin color change<br>• Behavioral: newborn opens eyes widely if room is slightly darkened<br>• Movements rhythmic; no hand tremors present<br>**Expected Outcomes**<br>Findings indicate normal progression with absence of complications |

CNM, certified nurse-midwife; BP, blood pressure; FHR, fetal heart rate; STV, short-term variability; LTV, long-term variability; WNL, within normal limits; VS, vital signs; EFM, electronic fetal monitoring; IV, intravenous; I&O, intake & output; IM, intramuscularly; IVP, intravenous push; LDR, labor, delivery and recovery; OOB, out of bed; UA, urinary analysis

| Category | First Stage | Second and Third Stages | Fourth Stage Birth to 1 Hour Past Birth |
|---|---|---|---|
| **Teaching/ psychosocial** | Establish rapport<br>Orient to environment, expected assessments and procedures<br>Answer questions and provide information<br>Orient to EFM if used<br>Teach relaxation, visualization, and breathing pattern if needed<br>Explain comfort measures available<br>Assume advocacy role for woman and family during labor and birth | Orient to expected assessments and procedures<br>Answer questions and provide information<br>Explain comfort measures available<br>Continue advocacy role | Explain immediate assessments and care after this first hour<br>Teach self-massage of fundus and expected findings<br>Instruct to call for assistance if mother desires to get OOB<br>Begin newborn teaching; bulb syringe; positioning; maintaining warmth<br>Assist parents in exploring their newborn<br>Assist with first breastfeeding experience<br>**Expected Outcomes**<br>Client and partner verbalize or demonstrate understanding of teaching |
| **Nursing care management and report** | Straight cath prn if bladder distended<br>If regional block administered monitor BP, FHR, sensation per protocol<br>Provide continuing status reports to CNM or physician<br>Perineal clip per woman's request<br>Small enema per woman's request<br>Perform sterile vaginal examination as indicated | Straight cath prn if bladder distended<br>Continue monitoring VS, FHR, and sensation if regional block has been given | Straight catheter if bladder distended<br>Monitor return of motor ability and sensation if regional block has been given<br>Weigh perineal pads if lochia flow >1 saturated pad in 15 min, presence of boggy uterus and clots: ↓BP, ↑P<br>**Expected Outcomes**<br>• Maternal-fetal well-being maintained and supported<br>• Mother and newborn experience safe labor and birth<br>• Family participates in process as desired |
| **Activity** | Encourage ambulation unless contraindicated<br>Maintain bed rest immediately after administration of IV pain medication or following regional block<br>Woman rests comfortably between contractions | Position comfortably for birth<br>Woman rests comfortably between pushing efforts and while awaiting birth of placenta | Position of comfort<br>**Expected Outcomes**<br>• Activity maintained as desired unless contraindicated<br>• Comfort enhanced by positioning or movement |
| **Comfort** | Institute comfort measures: ambulation, frequent position change, effleurage, focal point, patterned-paced breathing, visualization, therapeutic touch, back rub, moist cloths to face, holding hand, words of encouragement, changing underpad, shower, whirlpool, staying with the woman and family, warmed blanket at back, sacral pressure<br>Offer pain medication or administer if requested<br>Assist with administration of regional block | Institute comfort measures:<br>• Second stage: cool cloth to forehead, encouragement, coaching, help support legs while pushing, position of comfort for pushing and birth<br>• Third stage: cool cloth to forehead, assist parents to see newborn, position mother to hold newborn, provide encouragement | Institute comfort measures:<br>• Perineal discomfort: gently cleanse and apply ice pack; position to decrease pressure on perineum<br>• Uterine discomfort: palpate fundus gently<br>• Hemorrhoids: ice pack<br>• Body tremors: warm blankets<br>• General fatigue: position of comfort, encourage rest<br>• Administer pain medication ____<br>**Expected Outcomes**<br>• Optimal comfort level maintained<br>• Active reduction of pain or discomfort achieved |
| **Nutrition** | Ice chips and clear fluids<br>Evaluate for signs of dehydration<br>Oral intake per order | Ice chips and clear fluids | Regular diet if assessments are WNL<br>Encourage fluids<br>**Expected Outcomes**<br>Nutritional needs met |

of the restrooms, public phones, and nurse-call or emergency call system. These simple steps can go a long way toward helping the couple feel more at ease. The nurse also explains the monitoring equipment or other unfamiliar technology. Every effort needs to be made to demystify the environment for the laboring woman and her support person(s). Some couples prefer to remain together during the admission process, and others prefer to have the partner wait outside. As the nurse helps the woman undress and get into a hospital gown, the nurse can begin to develop rapport and establish a nursing database. The experienced labor and birth nurse can obtain essential information about the woman and her pregnancy within a few minutes after admission, initiate any immediate interventions needed, and establish individualized priorities. A major challenge for nurses is the formulation of realistic objectives for laboring women. Each woman has different coping mechanisms and support systems.

The woman may be facing a number of unfamiliar procedures that are routine for health care providers. It is important to remember that all women have the right to determine what happens to their bodies. The woman's informed consent should be obtained prior to any procedure that involves touching her body.

If indicated, the woman is assisted into bed. A side-lying or semi-Fowler's position rather than a supine position is most comfortable and avoids supine hypotensive syndrome (vena caval syndrome). After obtaining the essential information from the woman and her records, the nurse begins the intrapartal assessment. (Chapter 16 considers intrapartal maternal assessment in depth.) Once the assessment is complete, the nurse can make effective nursing decisions about intrapartal care, such as the following:

- Should ambulation or bed rest be encouraged?
- Is more frequent monitoring needed?
- What does the woman want during her labor and birth?
- Is a support person available?
- What special needs do this woman and her partner have?

The nurse auscultates the fetal heart rate (FHR). (Detailed information on monitoring FHR is presented in Chapter 16.) The nurse determines the woman's blood pressure, pulse, respirations, and oral temperature and assesses contraction frequency, duration, and intensity (possibly while gathering other data). Before the vaginal examination, the nurse informs the woman about the procedure and its purpose; afterward, the nurse conveys the findings. If there are signs of advanced labor (frequent contractions, an urge to bear down, and so on), a vaginal examination must be done quickly. If there are signs of excessive bleeding or if the woman reports episodes of painless bleeding in the last trimester, a vaginal examination should *not* be done.

Results of FHR assessment, uterine contraction evaluation, and the vaginal examination help determine whether the rest of the admission process can proceed at a leisurely pace or whether additional interventions are required. For example, a FHR of 110 beats per minute on auscultation indicates that a fetal monitor should be applied immediately to obtain additional data. The woman's vital signs can be assessed once the monitor is in place.

After the nurse obtains admission data, a clean voided midstream urine specimen is collected. The woman with intact membranes may collect her specimen in the bathroom. If the membranes are ruptured and the presenting part is not engaged, the woman generally remains in bed to avoid prolapse of the umbilical cord. The appropriateness of ambulation when membranes are ruptured varies. The decision is generally based on physical findings, clinician orders, the woman's desires, agency policy, and safety concerns.

The nurse may test the woman's urine for the presence of protein, ketones, and glucose by using a dipstick before sending the sample to the laboratory. This procedure is especially important if edema or elevated blood pressure is noted on admission. Proteinuria of 1+ or more may be a sign of impending preeclampsia. Glycosuria is found frequently in pregnant women because of the increased glomerular filtration rate in the proximal tubules and the inability of these tubules to increase reabsorption of glucose. However, it may also be associated with gestational diabetes and should not be discounted. While the woman is collecting the urine specimen, the nurse can gather the equipment for any preparation procedures ordered by the certified nurse-midwife (CNM) or physician. In the past complete or partial shaving of the pubic area (called a *prep*) was standard. This practice is becoming increasingly rare because the benefit to the woman is questionable (Varney, 1997).

Laboratory tests are done during early admission. Hemoglobin and hematocrit values help determine the oxygen-carrying capacity of the circulatory system and the woman's ability to withstand blood loss at birth. Elevation of the hematocrit indicates hemoconcentration of blood, which occurs with edema or dehydration. A low hemoglobin, in the absence of other evidence of bleeding, suggests anemia. Blood may be typed and cross matched if the woman is in a high-risk category. Additional serological testing may be performed as indicated.

In many hospitals, the admission process also includes signing an informed consent for treatment and providing information regarding advanced directives. In all cases an identification bracelet is attached to the expectant woman's wrist.

Depending on how rapidly labor is progressing, the nurse notifies the CNM or physician before or after completing the admission procedures. The report should include the following information: parity, cervical dilatation and effacement, station, presenting part, status of the membranes, contraction pattern, FHR, vital signs that are not in the normal range, any significant prenatal history, the woman's birth preferences, and her reaction to labor.

A nursing admission note is entered into the computer or the charting system. The admission note should include the reason for admission, the date and time of the woman's arrival and notification of the CNM or physician, the condition of the woman and her baby, and labor and membrane status (American Academy of Pediatrics [AAP] & American College of Obstetricians and Gynecologists [ACOG], 1997).

# Nursing Care Management during the First Stage of Labor

After completing the nursing assessment and diagnosis steps, the nurse creates a plan of care to achieve identified nursing goals. For instance, if the woman and her support person did not have the opportunity to attend preparation for childbirth classes, the nursing goal would be to provide desired information. To accomplish this goal, the nurse would assess the current level of the couple's understanding and then plan to provide brief explanations as labor progresses.

## Integration of Family Expectations

Families come into the birth setting with basic expectations that they will not be harmed and that the labor and birth will be safe for the mother and baby. But what other expectations do they have? What do they want from the nurse who will be with them during this important event in their lives? A study by Hodnett (1996) found that women identify five general categories of nursing support measures that are helpful during labor. The first area is emotional support, which includes physical presence of the nurse, praise, encouragement, reassurance, and companionship. The second area focuses on comfort measures such as the use of touch, providing ice chips and fluids, massage, assistance with care, and a bath or shower. Information and advice constitute the third area and includes offering information regarding procedures, interventions as they occur, and reports of labor progress. The fourth area concerns advocacy. The woman and her partner have goals, hopes, and dreams regarding how the labor and birth will proceed, but they are in an unfamiliar and often intimidating environment. The nurse is able to assist the laboring couple by advocating for them with the certified nurse-midwife or physician or with other caregivers if needed. The last general area centers on support of the partner or husband by providing encouragement, praise for his or her efforts, an opportunity for rest breaks, and role modeling.

## Integration of Cultural Beliefs

Knowledge of values, customs, and practices of different cultures is as important during labor as it is in the prenatal period. Without this knowledge, a nurse is less likely to understand a family's behavior and may attempt to impose personal values and beliefs on them. As cultural sensitivity increases, so does the likelihood of providing high-quality care (Callister, 2001).

The following sections briefly present a few possible cultural responses to labor. It is difficult to present even such a limited discussion in a clear, nonjudgmental way, because once a statement is made it may appear stereotypical, and of course no statement of a specific behavior can accurately reflect the preference of all people in a group. The nurse must always remain aware that an individual example of a birthing practice will never be pertinent to all women in a given group. Within every culture, each person develops his or her own beliefs and value system. General information about any culture or belief system needs to be viewed as background to help caregivers meet each individual's needs and desires.

### Modesty

Modesty is an important consideration for women regardless of culture. However, some women may be more uncomfortable than others with the degree of exposure needed for certain procedures during labor and the birth process. Some women may be particularly uncomfortable when men are present and feel more comfortable with women; others may be uncomfortable with exposure of personal body parts regardless of the gender of the caregivers. The nurse needs to be alert to the woman's responses to examinations and procedures and provide the draping and privacy the woman needs. It is more prudent to assume that embarrassment will occur with exposure and take measures to provide privacy than to assume that it will not matter to the woman if she is exposed during procedures. For example, some Asian women are not accustomed to male physicians and attendants. Modesty is of great concern, and exposure of as little of the woman's body as possible is strongly recommended.

# EVIDENCE-BASED PRACTICE

## Support for Women during Childbirth

The hospital where you work in the labor and delivery unit provides tertiary-level obstetric and neonatal care. After 2 years' experience, you still feel nervous when confronted with more complicated tasks, but you were feeling confident about caring for the woman in normal labor. Then you heard that the hospital's practice-improvement team is reviewing routine care.

The team has provided the nursing staff with research findings on the effectiveness of comfort measures and support for the woman in labor. Fourteen randomized trials that included more than 5000 women have demonstrated that continuous care from a caregiver during labor and birth positively affects patient outcomes. There is less need for pain medication, less operative vaginal delivery, and less likelihood of a cesarean birth. Additionally, the newborn is less likely to have an Apgar score <7 at 5 minutes postbirth (Hodnett, 1999).

You also read two other studies that look at the amount of time a nurse spends providing comfort measures and support to the woman in labor. In both studies, less than 10% of the nurses' time was spent providing comfort measures and support, the activities that have been shown to improve patient outcomes (Gagnon & Waghorn, 1996; McNiven, Hodnett, & Obrien-Pallas, 1992).

How can you address this discrepancy in your busy unit? You already feel overwhelmed with patient care requirements. However, you recognize that if nurses are to demonstrate their contributions to outcome measures, this evidence cannot be ignored.

### References


Gagnon, A. J., & Waghorn, K. (1996). Supportive care by maternity nurses: A work sampling study in an intrapartum unit. *Birth, 23,* 1–6.

Hodnett, E. D. (2000). Caregiver support for women during childbirth. *Cochrane Review, The Cochrane Library,* 1. Oxford: Update Software.

McNiven, P., Hodnett, E., & Obrien-Pallas, S. (1992). Supporting women in labor: A work sampling study of the activities of labor and delivery nurses. *Birth, 19,* 3–9.


### Pain Expression

The manner in which a woman chooses to deal with the discomfort of labor varies widely. Some women seem to turn inward and remain very quiet during the whole process. They speak only to ask others to leave the room or cease conversation. Others may be very vocal, with behaviors such as counting out loud, moaning quietly, crying, or use of loud vocalization. They may also turn from side to side or change positions frequently. In the Asian cultures it is important for individuals to act in a way that will not bring shame on the family. Therefore, the Korean woman may not express pain outwardly for fear of shaming herself or her family, and Filipina women say it is best to lie quietly (Lauderdale, 1999; Wesson, 2000). Hispanic women are encouraged to be patient and not to cry out or the "uterus will rise up" (Lauderdale, 1999). The nurse supports a woman's individual expression, whatever it may be (as long as harm is not done to another), in order to enhance the birthing experience for mother, baby, and family.

### Cultural Beliefs: Some Examples

Some differences among cultures in terms of verbalization, position, food, and drink during labor are apparent. Differing beliefs regarding vocalizations and perception of pain during labor may be exhibited by a Chinese-American woman or a Muslim woman. Silence is valued in Chinese society, so a woman of that heritage is usually quiet and stoic in order to avoid dishonoring herself or her family (Wesson, 2000). South or Central American women may view pain during labor as a symbol of love toward the baby: the more intense the pain, the more intense the love (Scott-Ramos, 1996). Native American women may use meditation, self-control, or indigenous plants throughout their labor (Lipson, Dibble, & Minarik, 1996).

Hmong women from Laos report that squatting during childbirth is common in their culture (Lauderdale, 1999). During labor they may want to be active and move about. The husband is frequently present and actively involved in providing comfort. Traditionally, the woman prefers that the amniotic membranes not be ruptured until just before birth. It is thought that the escape of fluid at this time makes the birth easier. During labor the woman usually prefers only "hot" foods and warm water to drink (Lauderdale, 1999) . As soon as the baby is born, a soft-boiled egg must be given to the mother to restore her energy.

Vietnamese women usually maintain self-control and may even smile throughout labor. They may prefer to walk about during labor and to give birth in a squatting position. The woman may avoid drinking cold water and prefer fluids at room temperature. The newborn is protected from praise to prevent jealousy (Calhoun, 1986).

Latina women have identified expectations of their partners during labor and birth such as wanting their partners to stay with them and to reassure them that everything will be all right. As they labor the women want their partners to show their love and to speak using affectionate words (Khazoyan & Anderson, 1994).

Muslim women may have their husband, a female friend or relative, or a male relative with them during childbirth. Family support may be particularly important but does not preclude the importance of the nurse's presence. The woman may want to retain her head covering (*khimar*), and two long-sleeved gowns can be offered to enhance modesty. It is important for a female nurse, physician, or CNM to perform examinations whenever possible. If a male physician or nurse is involved, the woman may wish for her husband to remain in the room. After the birth Muslim fathers may call praise to Allah (*adhan*) in the newborn's right ear and clean the newborn (Hutchinson & Baqi-Aziz, 1994).

Maternity nurses can provide culturally sensitive care by first becoming acquainted with the beliefs and practices of the various subcultures in their communities. In the birthing situation, the truly effective nurse supports the family's cultural practices as long as it is safe to do so.

## Support of the Adolescent during Birth

As with all women, each adolescent in labor is different. The nurse must assess what each teen brings to the experience by asking the following questions:

- Has the young woman received prenatal care?
- What are her attitudes and feelings about the pregnancy?
- Who will attend the birth and what is the person's relationship to her?
- What preparation has she had for the experience?
- What are her expectations and fears regarding labor and birth?
- How has her culture influenced her?
- What are her usual coping mechanisms?
- Does she plan to keep the newborn?

Any adolescent who has not had prenatal care requires close observation during labor. Fetal well-being is established by fetal monitoring. Adolescent women are at highest risk for pregnancy and labor complications and must be assessed carefully. The nurse should be especially alert for any physiologic complications of labor. The young woman's prenatal record is carefully reviewed for risks, and the adolescent is screened for pregnancy-induced hypertension (PIH), cephalopelvic disproportion (CPD), anemia, drugs ingested during pregnancy, sexually transmitted infections, and size-date discrepancies.

The support role of the nurse depends on the young woman's support system during labor. The adolescent may not be accompanied by someone who will stay with her during childbirth, or she may have her mother, the father of the baby, or a close friend as her labor partner. Regardless of whether the teen has a support person, it is important for the nurse to establish a trusting relationship with her. In this way, the nurse can help the teen understand what is happening to her. Establishing rapport without recrimination for possible inappropriate behavior is essential. The adolescent who is given positive reinforcement for "work well done" will leave the experience with increased self-esteem, despite the emotional problems that may accompany her situation.

If a support person accompanies the adolescent, that person also needs the nurse's encouragement and support. The nurse must explain changes in the young woman's behavior and substantiate her wishes. The nursing staff should reinforce the adolescent's feelings that she is wanted and important.

The adolescent who has taken childbirth education classes is generally better prepared for labor than the adolescent who has not. However, the nurse must keep in mind that the younger the adolescent, the less she may be able to participate actively in the process, even if she has taken prenatal classes.

The very young adolescent (age 14 and under) has fewer coping mechanisms and less experience to draw on than her older counterparts. Because her cognitive development is incomplete, the younger adolescent may have fewer problem-solving capabilities. Her ego integrity may be more threatened by the experience, and she may be more vulnerable to stress and discomfort.

The very young adolescent needs someone to rely on at all times during labor. She may be more childlike and dependent than older teens. The nurse must be sure that instructions and explanations are simple and concrete. During the transition phase, the young teenager may become withdrawn and unable to express her need to be nurtured. Touch, soothing encouragement, and measures to provide comfort help her maintain control and meet her needs for dependence. During the second stage of labor, the young adolescent may feel as if she is losing control and may reach out to those around her. By remaining calm and giving directions, the nurse helps her cope with feelings of helplessness.

The middle adolescent (age 15 to 17 years) often attempts to remain calm and unflinching during labor. If unable to break through the teenager's stoic barrier, the nurse needs to rise above frustration and realize that a caring attitude will still help the young woman. Many older adolescents believe that they "know it all," but they may be no more prepared for childbirth than their younger counterparts. The nurse's reinforcement and nonjudgmental manner will help them save face. If the adolescent has not taken childbirth preparation classes, she may require preparation and explanations. The older teenager's (age 18 to 19) response to the stresses of labor, however, is similar to that of the adult woman (Drake, 1996).

Even if the adolescent is planning to relinquish her newborn, she should be given the option of seeing and holding the infant. She may be reluctant to do this at first, but the grieving process is facilitated if the mother sees the infant. However, seeing or holding the newborn should be the young woman's choice. (See Chapter 28 for further discussion of the relinquishing mother and the adolescent parent.)

## Promotion of Comfort in the First Stage

The first step in planning care is to talk with the woman and her partner (if he is involved) to identify their goals. Usually the couple is concerned with discomfort, so it is helpful to identify factors that may contribute to discomfort. These factors include uncomfortable positions, diaphoresis, continual leaking of amniotic fluid, a full bladder, a dry mouth, anxiety, and fear. Nursing interventions can minimize the effects of these factors. These interventions are described later in this section.

There are many types of responses to pain. As the intensity of the contraction increases with the progress of labor, the woman becomes less aware of the environment and may have difficulty hearing and understanding verbal instructions. The pattern of coping with labor contractions varies from the use of highly structured breathing techniques to turning inward. Low moaning that begins deep in the throat, rocking or swaying, facial grimacing, and using loud vocalizations are all effective means of dealing with the power of labor and birth (England & Horowitz, 1998). Some women feel that making sounds helps them cope and do the work of labor, whereas others make loud sounds only as they lose their perception of control.

The most frequent physiologic manifestations of pain are increased pulse and respiratory rates, dilated pupils, increased blood pressure, and muscle tension. In labor these reactions are transitory because the pain is intermittent. Increased muscle tension is most significant because it may impede the progress of labor. Women in labor frequently tighten skeletal muscles voluntarily during a contraction and remain motionless. This method of dealing with the contractions may actually increase her level of discomfort because of muscular tension, but the woman may believe it is the only acceptable way to cope with the pain.

A woman generally wants touching, massage, effleurage, and other forms of physical contact during the first part of labor, but when she moves into the transition phase, she may rebuff all efforts and pull away. Women may provide verbal and nonverbal signs such as crying, moaning, and beseeching the coach or nurse to hold their hand or rub their back. They may reach out and grasp the support person or indicate their anxiety or fear through eye contact. However, some women are uncomfortable with being touched at all, regardless of the phase of labor. It is important to validate the unique strengths and coping techniques of the individual and to meet each family on their own terms, always keeping in mind that this is *their* experience.

Many nurses like to incorporate touch into their nursing care, and they readily respond to the woman's needs. As the nurse and woman or couple work together to increase comfort during contractions, a ritual of supportive measures begins to develop. The nurse watches for cues and nonverbal behaviors and asks for feedback from the woman. As labor progresses, the nurse and couple will use their prior experience and growing rapport to change comfort measures as needed.

A decrease in the intensity of discomfort is one of the goals of nursing support during labor. Nursing measures used to decrease pain include the following:

- Ensuring general comfort
- Providing information to decrease anxiety
- Using specific supportive relaxation techniques
- Encouraging controlled breathing
- Administering pharmacologic agents as ordered by the physician or CNM

### General Comfort

General comfort measures are of great importance during labor. By relieving minor discomforts, the nurse helps the woman optimize her coping abilities to deal with pain.

The woman is encouraged to ambulate as long as there are no contraindications, such as vaginal bleeding or rupture of membranes (ROM) before the fetus is engaged in the pelvis. Even if the woman prefers not to walk around, upright positions such as sitting in a rocker or leaning against a wall or bed can enhance comfort. If she stays in bed, the nurse can encourage the woman to assume positions that she finds comfortable. A side-lying position is generally the most advantageous for the laboring woman, although frequent position changes seem to achieve more efficient contractions. Care should be taken to support all body parts, with the joints kept slightly flexed. For instance, when the woman is in a side-lying position, pillows may be placed against her chest and under the uppermost arm. A pillow or folded bath blanket is placed between her knees to support the uppermost leg and relieve tension or muscle strain. A pillow placed at the woman's midback also helps provide support. If the woman is more comfortable on her back, the head of the bed should be elevated to relieve the pressure of the uterus on the vena cava. Pillows may be placed under each arm and under the knees to provide support. Since a pregnant woman is at increased risk for thrombophlebitis, excessive pressure behind the knee and calf should be avoided, and the nurse needs to assess pressure points frequently. Back rubs and frequent changes of position contribute to comfort and relaxation (see Figure 17–1♦). Wearing socks or slippers may alleviate cold feet, just as adjusting the room's thermostat can offset excessive warmth. Attention to such details allows the woman to focus on the more important issues of giving birth.

Diaphoresis and the constant leaking of amniotic fluid can dampen the woman's gown and bed linen. Fresh, smooth, dry bed linen promotes comfort. To avoid having to change the bottom sheet following rupture of the membranes, the nurse may replace chux pads at frequent intervals (following body substance isolation [BSI] precautions). The perineal area should be kept as clean and dry as possible to promote comfort and to prevent infection. A full bladder adds to the discomfort during a contraction and may prolong labor by interfering with the descent of the fetus. The bladder should be kept as empty as possible. Even if the woman is voiding, urine may be retained because of the pressure of the fetal presenting part. The nurse can detect a full bladder by palpating directly over the symphysis pubis. Some of the regional procedures for analgesia during labor contribute to the inability to void, and catheterization may be necessary. The woman should be encouraged to empty her bladder every 1 to 2 hours.

Family members also need to be encouraged to maintain their own comfort. Because their attention is directed toward the laboring woman, they may forget their own needs. The nurse may have to encourage them to take breaks, to maintain food and fluid intake, and to rest.

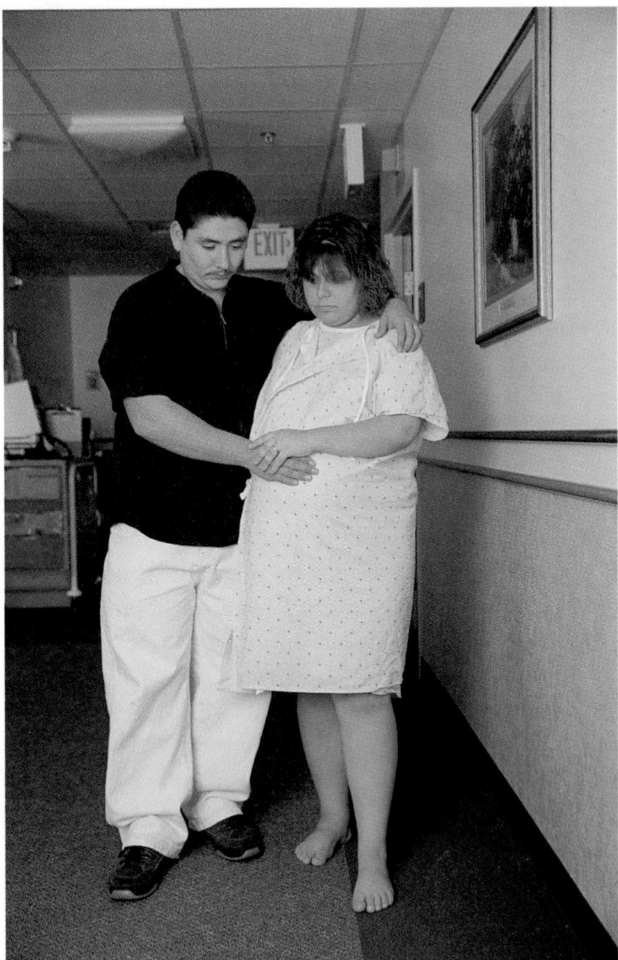


**FIGURE 17–1** ♦ Woman and her partner walking in the hospital during labor.

## Handling Anxiety

The anxiety experienced by women beginning labor is related to a combination of factors inherent to the process. A moderate amount of anxiety about the pain enhances the woman's ability to deal with it. In contrast, an excessive degree of anxiety decreases her ability to cope with the pain. Women in the latent phase of labor who are experiencing increased levels of anxiety about safety and their ability to cope are much more likely to describe their pain as unbearable. They are also more likely to have FHR decelerations in labor, a slow second stage, and/or a cesarean birth, and they are more likely to need pediatric assistance for neonatal resuscitation at birth (Varney, 1997).

Ways to decrease anxiety not related to pain are to give information (which eases fear of the unknown), establish rapport with the couple (which helps them preserve their personal integrity), and express confidence in the couple's ability to work with the labor process. In addition to being a good listener, the nurse must demonstrate genuine concern for the laboring woman. Remaining with the woman as much as possible conveys a caring attitude and dispels fears of abandonment. Praise for breathing, relaxation, and pushing efforts not only encourages repetition of the behavior but also decreases anxiety about the ability to cope with labor (Hodnett, 1996).

### Client Teaching

Providing truthful information about the nature of the discomfort that will occur during labor is important. Stressing the intermittent nature and maximum duration of the contractions can be most helpful. The woman can cope with pain better when she knows that a period of relief will follow. Describing the type of discomfort and specific sensations that will occur as labor progresses helps the woman recognize these sensations as normal and expected when she does experience them.

Descriptions of sensations are best accompanied by information on specific comfort measures. Some women experience the urge to push during transition, when the cervix is not fully dilated and effaced. This sensation can be controlled by panting (it is difficult to pant and bear down at the same time), and the nurse should provide instructions about panting before it is required.

Thorough orientation and explanation of surroundings, procedures, and equipment being used also decrease anxiety, thereby reducing pain. Attachment to an electronic monitor can produce fear because equipment of this type is associated with critically ill people. The nurse can explain beeps, clicks, and other strange noises and give a simplified explanation of the monitor strip. The nurse can emphasize that the use of the fetal monitor provides a way to assess the well-being of the fetus during the course of labor. In addition, the nurse can show the woman and her partner or support person how the monitor can help them identify the beginnings of contractions. At the onset of each contraction, the woman can be encouraged to begin her breathing technique to lessen her perception of pain.

Labor and childbirth may be a critical time for the woman with a history of childhood sexual abuse. Although the literature does not agree about the exact prevalence of sexual abuse, a general consensus is that at least 25% to 35% of all childbearing women have experienced it. To develop a competent plan of care, it is recommended that all women entering the health care arena be evaluated for a history of sexual abuse (Waymire, 1997). However, a woman may or may not be able to address this issue with the nurse, because sharing such personal information with a stranger is difficult. It is therefore especially important for the nurse to be alert for nonverbal cues, such as unexplained anxiety, unrelenting pain, and/or fear during vaginal exams, and to be prepared to offer additional teaching and relaxation support to help offset her anxiety.

### Supportive Relaxation Techniques

Tense muscles increase resistance to the descent of the fetus and contribute to maternal fatigue. This fatigue increases pain perception and decreases the woman's ability to cope with the pain. Comfort measures, massage, techniques for decreasing anxiety, and client teaching can contribute to relaxation. Adequate sleep and rest are also important. The laboring woman needs to be encouraged to use the periods between contractions for rest and relaxation. A prolonged prodromal phase of labor may have prohibited sleeping. An aura of excitement naturally accompanies the onset of labor, making it difficult for the woman to sleep even though the contractions are mild and infrequent.

Distraction is another method of increasing relaxation and coping with discomfort. During early labor, conversation or activities such as light reading or playing cards or other games serve as distractions. One technique that is effective for relieving moderate pain is to have the woman concentrate on a pleasant experience she has had in the past. Other techniques include the use of a specific visual or mental focal point, patterns of breathing and the accompanied sounds, or visualization (England & Horowitz, 1998).

Touch is another type of distraction (Figure 17–2♦). Although some women regard touching as an invasion of privacy or threat to their independence, many want to touch and be touched during a painful experience. Nurses can make themselves available to the woman who desires touch. The nurse can place a hand on the side of the bed within the woman's reach. The person who needs touch will reach out for contact, and the nurse can pick up and follow through with this behavioral cue. Mild to moderate abdominal discomfort during contractions may be relieved or lessened by effleurage. Back pain associated with labor may be relieved by firm pressure on the

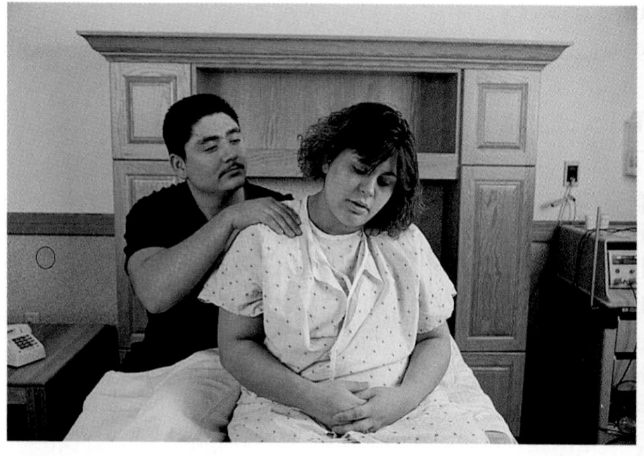

**FIGURE 17–2 ♦** The woman's partner provides support and encouragement during labor.

lower back or sacral area. To apply firm pressure, the nurse places her or his hand or a rolled, warmed towel or blanket in the small of the woman's back. In addition to the measures just described, the nurse can enhance the woman's relaxation by providing encouragement and support for her controlled breathing techniques.

## Breathing Techniques

Breathing techniques may help the laboring woman. Used correctly, they increase the woman's pain threshold, permit relaxation, enhance the woman's ability to cope with the uterine contractions, and allow the uterus to function more efficiently.

Many women learn patterned-paced breathing during prenatal education classes. This type of controlled breathing often has three levels. The woman tends to begin with the first level and then proceed to the next when she feels the need. Regardless of the level of breathing used, a cleansing breath begins and ends each pattern. A cleansing breath involves only the chest. It consists of inhaling through the nose and exhaling through pursed lips (Table 17–1).

### First Pattern

The first pattern may also be called slow, deep breathing or slow-paced breathing. During the breathing movements only the chest moves. The woman inhales slowly through her nose. She moves her chest up and out during the inhalation. She exhales through pursed lips. The breathing rate is six to nine breaths a minute.

### Second Pattern

The second pattern may also be called shallow or modified-paced breathing. The woman begins with a cleansing breath and at the end of the cleansing breath pushes out a short breath. She then inhales and exhales through the mouth at a rate of about four breaths every 5 seconds. This pattern can be altered into a more rapid rate that does not exceed two to two and a half breaths every second.

### Third Pattern

The third pattern is also called pant-blow or patterned-paced breathing. It is similar to modified-paced breathing except the breathing is punctuated every few breaths by a forceful exhalation through pursed lips. A pattern of four breaths may be used to begin. All breaths are kept equal and rhythmic. As the contraction becomes more intense, the woman may adjust the pattern as needed to 3:1, 2:1, and finally 1:1.

If the woman has not learned patterned-paced or another controlled breathing technique, teaching her may be difficult when she is admitted in active labor. In this instance, the nurse can teach abdominal and pant-pant-blow breathing (see Table 17–1). In abdominal breathing, the woman moves the abdominal wall upward as she inhales and downward as she exhales. This method tends to lift the abdominal wall off the contracting uterus and thus may provide some pain relief. The breathing is deep and rhythmic. As transition approaches, the woman may feel the need to breathe more rapidly. To avoid breathing too rapidly, which may occur with deep abdominal breathing, the woman can use the pant-pant-blow breathing pattern.

As the woman uses her breathing technique, the nurse can assess and support the interaction between the woman and her support person or partner. In the absence of a partner, or when the partner desires a less active role in the support of the laboring woman, an additional care provider, often called a *doula,* may be present. The role of the *doula* is to enhance the comfort and decrease the anxiety of the expectant family. A *doula* can be a valuable advocate to the laboring woman, as well as an asset to the labor nurse. For example, the *doula* might support the woman by helping to identify the beginning of each contraction and encouraging her as she breathes through it. A constant presence offering continued encouragement and support with each contraction throughout labor has immeasurable benefits.

**Hyperventilation** is the result of an imbalance of oxygen and carbon dioxide (ie, too much carbon dioxide is exhaled, and too much oxygen remains in the body). Hyperventilation may occur when a woman breathes very rapidly over a prolonged period. The signs and symptoms of hyperventilation are tingling or numbness in the tip of the nose, lips, fingers, or toes; dizziness; spots before the eyes; or spasms of the hands or feet (carpal-pedal spasms). If hyperventilation occurs, the woman should be encouraged to slow her breathing rate and take shallow breaths. With instruction and encouragement, many women are able to change their breathing to correct the problem. Encouraging the woman to relax and counting out loud for her so she can pace her breathing during contractions are also helpful actions. If the signs and symptoms continue or become more severe (they progress from numbness to spasms), the woman can breathe into a paper surgical mask or a paper bag until symptoms abate. Breathing into a mask or bag causes rebreathing of carbon dioxide. The nurse should remain with the woman to reassure her.

In some instances, analgesics or regional anesthetic blocks may be used to enhance comfort and relaxation during labor. (See Chapter 18 for a discussion of analgesia and anesthesia.) Table 17–2 summarizes labor progress, possible responses of the laboring woman, and support measures.

# TABLE 17–1 Nursing Support of Patterned-Paced Breathing

Determine which breathing method the woman (couple) has learned. Provide encouragement as needed in maintaining breathing pattern. Provide support to the labor partner and assist as needed.

## LAMAZE BREATHING PATTERN LEVELS

*First level (slow paced)*

Pattern begins and ends with a cleansing breath (in through the nose and out through pursed lips as if cooling a spoonful of hot food). While inhaling through the nose and exhaling through pursed lips, slow breaths are taken, moving only the chest. The rate should be approximately 6–9/minute or 2 breaths/15 seconds. The partner or nurse may assist by reminding the woman to take a cleansing breath, and then the breaths could be counted out if needed to maintain pacing. The woman inhales as someone counts "one one thousand, two one thousand, three one thousand, four one thousand." Exhalation begins and continues through the same count.

First level for use during uterine contractions (The level begins and ends with a cleansing breath [CB].)

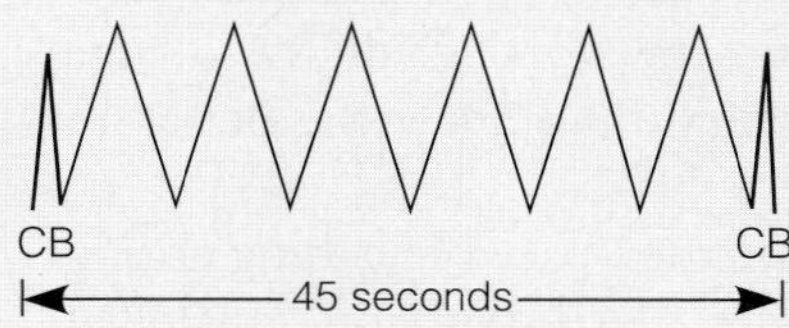


*Second level (modified paced)*

Pattern begins and ends with a cleansing breath. Breaths are then taken in and out silently through the mouth at approximately 4 breaths/5 seconds. The jaw and entire body need to be relaxed. The rate can be accelerated to 2–2 1/2 breaths/second. The rhythm for the breaths can be counted out as "one and two and one and two and . . ." with the woman exhaling on the numbers and inhaling on "and."

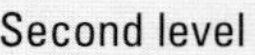

Second level

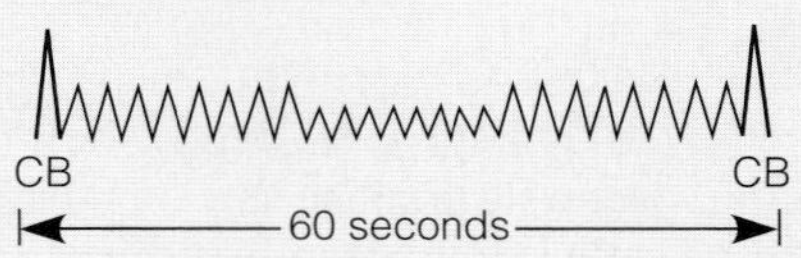


*Third level (pattern paced)*

Pattern begins and ends with a cleansing breath. All breaths are rhythmic, in and out through the mouth. Exhalations are accompanied by a "hee" or "hoo" sound in a varying pattern, 2:1, which begins as 3:1 (hee hee hee hoo) and can change to 2:1 (hee hee hoo) or 1:1 (hee hoo) as the intensity of the contraction changes. The rate should not be more rapid than 2–2 1/2 breaths/second. The rhythm of the breaths would match a "one and two and . . ." count.

Third level (Darkened spike represents "hoo.")

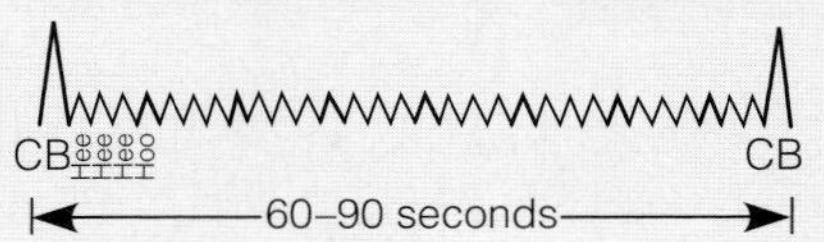


## ABDOMINAL BREATHING PATTERN CUES

The abdomen moves outward during inhalation and downward during exhalation. The rate remains slow, with approximately 6–9 breaths/minute.

Breathing sequence for abdominal breathing

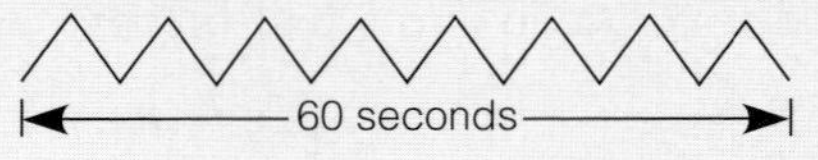


## QUICK METHOD

When the woman has not learned a particular method and is in the active phase of labor, the nurse may teach her a combination of two patterns. Abdominal breathing may be used until labor is more advanced. Then a more rapid pattern consisting of two short blows from the mouth followed by a longer blow can be used. (This pattern is called "pant-pant-blow" even though all exhalations are a blowing motion.)

Pant-pant-blow breathing pattern

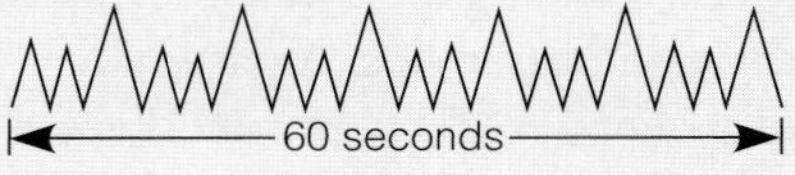

**TABLE 17–2** Normal Progress, Psychologic Characteristics, and Nursing Support during the First and Second Stages of Labor

| Phase | Cervical Dilatation | Uterine Contractions | Woman's Response | Support Measures |
|---|---|---|---|---|
| **STAGE 1** | | | | |
| Latent phase | 1–4 cm | Every 10–20 minutes, 15–20 seconds' duration<br>Mild intensity<br>*progressing to*<br>Every 5–7 minutes, 30–40 seconds' duration<br>Moderate intensity | Usually happy, talkative, and eager to be in labor<br>Exhibits need for independence by taking care of own bodily needs and seeking information | Establish rapport on admission and continue to build during care. Assess information base and learning needs. Be available to consult regarding breathing technique if needed; teach breathing technique if needed and in early labor. Orient family to room, equipment, monitors, and procedures. Encourage woman and partner to participate in care as desired. Provide needed information. Assist woman into position of comfort; encourage frequent change of position; encourage ambulation during early labor. Offer fluids or ice chips. Keep couple informed of progress. Encourage woman to void every 1 to 2 hours. Assess need for an interest in using visualization to enhance relaxation and teach if appropriate. |
| Active phase | 4–7 cm | Every 2–3 minutes, 40–60 seconds' duration<br>Moderate to strong intensity | May experience feelings of helplessness<br>Exhibits increased fatigue and may begin to feel restless and anxious as contractions become stronger<br>Expresses fear of abandonment<br>Becomes more dependent because she is less able to meet her needs | Encourage woman to maintain breathing patterns. Provide quiet environment to reduce external stimuli. Provide reassurance, encouragement, support; keep couple informed of progress. Promote comfort by giving back rubs, sacral pressure, cool cloth on forehead, assistance with position changes, support with pillows, effleurage. Provide ice chips, ointment for dry mouth and lips. Encourage to void every 1 to 2 hours. Offer shower, whirlpool, or warm bath if available. |
| Transition phase | 8–10 cm | Every 2 minutes, 60–75 seconds' duration<br>Strong intensity | Tires and may exhibit increased restlessness and irritability<br>May feel she cannot keep up with labor process and is out of control<br>Physical discomforts<br>Fear of being left alone<br>May fear tearing open or splitting apart with contractions | Encourage woman to rest between contractions. If she sleeps between contractions, wake her at beginning of contraction so she can begin breathing pattern (increases feeling of control). Provide support, encouragement, and praise for efforts. Keep couple informed of progress; encourage continued participation of support persons. Promote comfort as listed earlier but recognize that many women do not want to be touched when in transition. Provide privacy. Provide ice chips, ointment for lips. Encourage to void every 1 to 2 hours. |
| **STAGE 2** | Complete | Every 2 to 5 minutes | May feel out of control, helpless, panicky | Assist woman in pushing efforts. Encourage woman to assume position of comfort. Provide encouragement and praise her efforts. Keep couple informed of progress. Provide ice chips. Maintain privacy as woman desires. |

## Special Assessments and Care throughout the First Stage of Labor

### Latent Phase

As discussed in Chapter 16 the nurse needs to evaluate physical parameters of the woman and her fetus. Maternal temperature is monitored every 4 hours unless the temperature is over 37.5°C (99.6°F); in such cases it is taken every hour. Blood pressure, pulse, and respirations are monitored every hour. If the woman's blood pressure is over 140/90 mm Hg or her pulse is more than 100, the nurse must notify the CNM or physician and reevaluate the blood pressure and pulse more frequently. The nurse palpates uterine contractions for frequency, intensity, and duration and auscultates the FHR every 60 minutes for low-risk women and every 30 minutes for high-risk women as long as it remains between 120 and 160 beats per minute and is reassuring. The FHR should be auscultated throughout one contraction and for about 15 seconds after the contraction to ensure that there are no decelerations. If the FHR baseline is not in the 120 to 160 range or decelerations are heard, continuous electronic monitoring is recommended (Table 17–3).

The nurse should offer fluids in the form of clear liquids or ice chips at frequent intervals, unless complications exist that may necessitate a sudden cesarean birth. Some certified childbirth educators (CBE) advise the woman to bring lollipops to help combat the dryness that occurs with some of the labor breathing patterns. Because gastric emptying time is prolonged during labor, solid foods are usually avoided. However, fasting during labor is a controversial practice. Some providers believe that eating and drinking during labor should be an option. Many nurse-midwifery practices are now encouraging mothers to eat and drink to toleration, based on the current literature (Varney, 1997).

### Active Phase

During the active phase, the contractions have a frequency of 2 to 3 minutes, a duration of 50 to 60 seconds, and a moderate intensity. Contractions need to be palpated every 15 to 30 minutes. As the contractions become more frequent and intense, vaginal exams are done to assess cervical dilatation and effacement and fetal station and position. During the active phase, the cervix dilates from 4 to 7 cm, and vaginal discharge and bloody show increase. Maternal blood pressure, pulse, and respirations should be monitored every hour for low-risk women (unless elevated, as previously noted) and every 30 minutes for high-risk women. The FHR is auscultated and evaluated every 30 minutes for low-risk women and every 15 minutes for high-risk women (AWHONN, 1999).

A woman who has been ambulatory up to this point may now wish to sit in a chair or on a bed (Figure 17–3♦). If the woman wants to lie on the bed, she is encouraged to assume a side-lying position. The nurse can assist her to a position of comfort and may place pillows to support her body. To increase comfort, the nurse can give back rubs or effleurage or place a cool cloth on the woman's forehead or across her neck. Because vaginal discharge increases, the nurse needs to change the chux frequently. Washing the perineum with warm soap and water removes secretions and increases comfort. The nurse needs to wear disposable gloves to avoid exposure to vaginal discharge.

If the amniotic membranes have not ruptured previously, they may do so during this phase. When the membranes rupture, the nurse notes the color, odor, and consistency of the amniotic fluid and the time of rupture and immediately auscultates the FHR. The fluid should be clear, with no odor. Fetal stress leads to intestinal and anal sphincter relaxation, and meconium may be released into the amniotic fluid, which turns the fluid greenish

**TABLE 17–3 Nursing Assessments in the First Stage**

| *Phase* | *Mother* | *Fetus* |
|---|---|---|
| Latent | Blood pressure, respirations each hour if in normal range<br>Temperature every 4 hours unless over 37.5°C (99.6°F) or membranes ruptured, then every hour<br>Uterine contractions every 30 minutes | Fetal heart rate (FHR) every 60 minutes for low-risk women and every 30 minutes for high-risk women if normal characteristics present (average variability, baseline in the 120–160 beats per minute range, without late or variable decelerations) AWHONN, 1998).<br>Note fetal activity.<br>If electronic fetal monitor in place, assess for reactive nonstress test (NST). |
| Active | Blood pressure, pulse, respirations every hour if in normal range<br>Uterine contractions every 30 minutes | FHR every 30 minutes for low-risk women and every 15 minutes for high-risk women if normal characteristics are present (AWHONN, 1998). |
| Transition | Blood pressure, pulse, respirations every 30 minutes | FHR every 30 minutes for low-risk women and every 15 minutes for high-risk women if normal characteristics are present (AWHONN, 1998). |

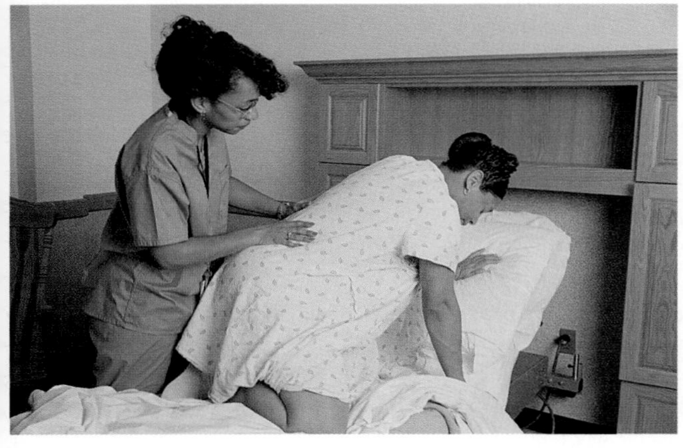

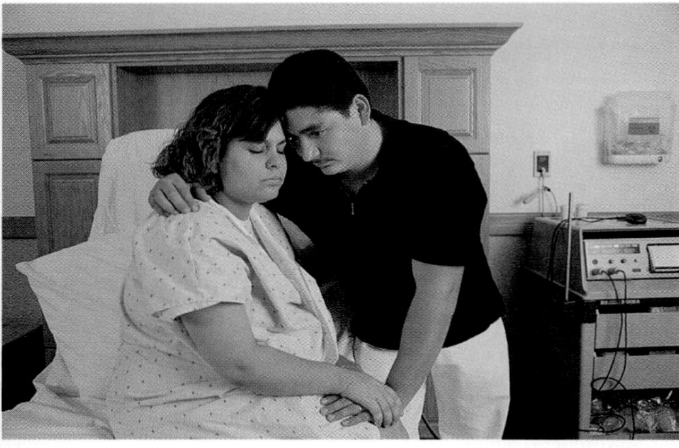

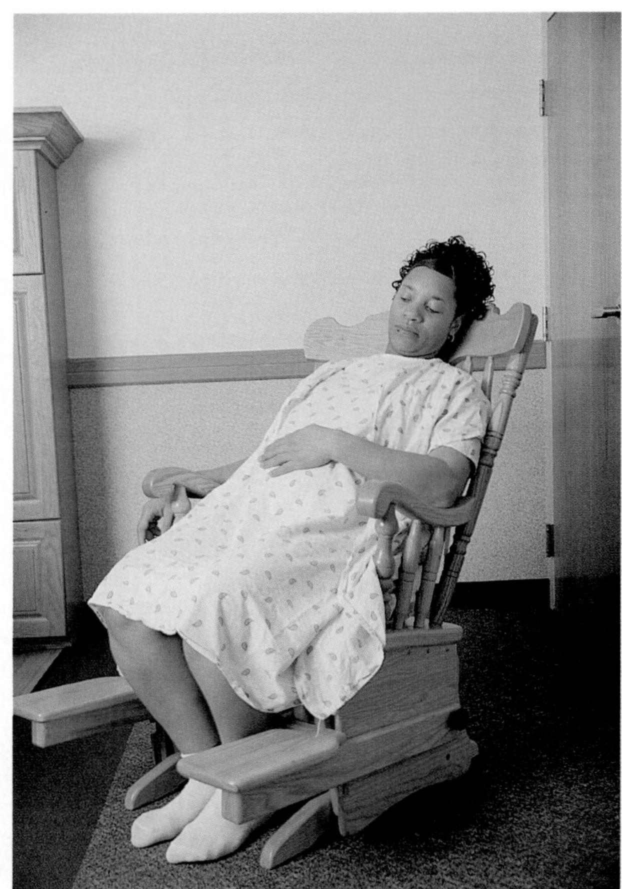

FIGURE 17–3 ♦ The laboring woman is encouraged to choose a position of comfort. The nurse modifies assessments and intervention as necessary.

brown. Whenever the nurse notes meconium-stained fluid, an electronic monitor is applied to assess the FHR continuously. The time of rupture is noted, because current medical practice suggests that birth should occur within 24 hours of ROM.

An additional concern is prolapse of the umbilical cord, which may occur when membranes rupture and the fetus is not engaged. The concern is that the amniotic fluid coming through the cervix will propel the umbilical cord through the cervix (prolapsed cord). The FHR is auscultated because a drop in the rate might indicate an undetected prolapsed cord. Immediate intervention is necessary to remove pressure on a prolapsed umbilical cord (see Chapter 19). (See Table 17–4 for additional deviations from normal.)

### Transition

During transition, the contraction frequency is every 2 to 3 minutes, duration is 60 to 90 seconds, and intensity is strong. Cervical dilatation increases from 8 to 10 cm, effacement is complete (100%), and there is usually a heavy amount of bloody show. Contractions are palpated at least every 15 minutes. Sterile vaginal examinations may be done more frequently because this stage of labor usually is accompanied by rapid change. Maternal blood pressure, pulse, and respirations are taken at least every 30 minutes, and FHR is auscultated every 15 minutes.

Comfort measures become very important in this phase of labor, but continual assessment is required to intervene appropriately. The woman may rapidly change from wanting a back rub and other hands-on care to wanting to be left completely alone. The support person and the nurse need to follow her cues and change interventions as needed. Because the woman is breathing more rapidly, the nurse can increase her comfort by offering small spoons of ice chips to moisten her mouth or by applying petroleum jelly to dry lips. The nurse can encourage the woman to rest between contractions. If analgesics have been administered, a quiet environment enhances the quality of rest between contractions. The nurse can awaken the woman just before another contraction begins so that she can initiate patterned breathing.

Some women have difficulty coping during this time and need help with their breathing. Either the support person or the nurse can breathe along with the woman during each contraction to help her maintain her pattern. It is helpful to encourage the woman and to assure her that she is doing a good job. The woman will begin to feel

**TABLE 17–4 Deviations from Normal Labor Process Requiring Immediate Intervention**

| *Problem* | *Immediate Action* |
|---|---|
| Woman admitted with vaginal bleeding or history of painless vaginal bleeding | Do not perform vaginal examination.<br>Assess fetal heart rate (FHR)<br>Evaluate amount of blood loss.<br>Evaluate labor pattern.<br>Notify physician or certified nurse-midwife (CNM) immediately. |
| Presence of greenish or brownish amniotic fluid | Continuously monitor FHR.<br>Evaluate dilatation of cervix and determine if umbilical cord is prolapsed.<br>Evaluate presentation (vertex or breech).<br>Maintain woman on complete bed rest on left side.<br>Notify physician or CNM immediately. |
| Absence of FHR and fetal movement | Notify physician or CNM.<br>Provide truthful information and emotional support to laboring couple.<br>Remain with the couple. |
| Prolapse of umbilical cord | Relieve pressure on cord manually.<br>Continuously monitor FHR; watch for changes in FHR pattern.<br>Notify physician or CNM.<br>Assist woman into knee-chest position.<br>Administer oxygen. |
| Woman admitted in advanced labor; birth imminent | Prepare for immediate birth.<br>Obtain critical information:<br>Estimated date of birth (EDB)<br>History of bleeding problems<br>History of medical or obstetric problems<br>Past and/or present use or abuse of prescription, over-the-counter (OTC), or illicit drugs<br>Problems with this pregnancy<br>FHR and maternal vital signs<br>Whether membranes are ruptured and how long since rupture<br>Blood type and Rh<br>Direct another person to contact physician or CNM.<br>Do not leave woman alone.<br>Provide support to couple.<br>Put on gloves. |

increased rectal pressure as the fetal presenting part moves down the birth canal. The nurse encourages the woman to refrain from pushing until the cervix is completely dilated. This measure helps prevent cervical edema.

The end of transition and the beginning of the second stage may be indicated by a change in the woman's voice or the sounds she is making. As the fetus moves down and she feels increased pressure and a bearing-down sensation, her voice tends to deepen. A moan during a contraction takes on a more guttural quality. Expert nurses recognize this sound as a sign of changes in the woman.

## Nursing Care Management during the Second Stage of Labor

The second stage is reached when the cervix is completely dilated (10 cm). The uterine contractions continue as in the transition phase. Maternal pulse and blood pressure and FHR are assessed every 5 to 15 minutes.

As the woman pushes during the second stage, she may make a variety of sounds. A low-pitched, grunting sound ("uhhh") usually indicates that the woman is working with the pushing. The nurse who feels comfortable with maternal sounds and stays sensitive to changes in the sounds may be able to detect if the woman is losing her ability to cope. For instance, if the woman feels afraid of the sensations produced by her pushing effort, her sound may change to a high-pitched cry or whimper, and the nurse can then provide extra support (Wesson, 2000). Some nurses and physicians value "staying in control" and may encourage the woman to push harder and not let any breath out. The belief is that making noise decreases the pushing effort, although research disputes this.

During the second stage, the woman may interpret rectal pressure as a need to move her bowels. The instinctive response is to resist and to tighten muscles

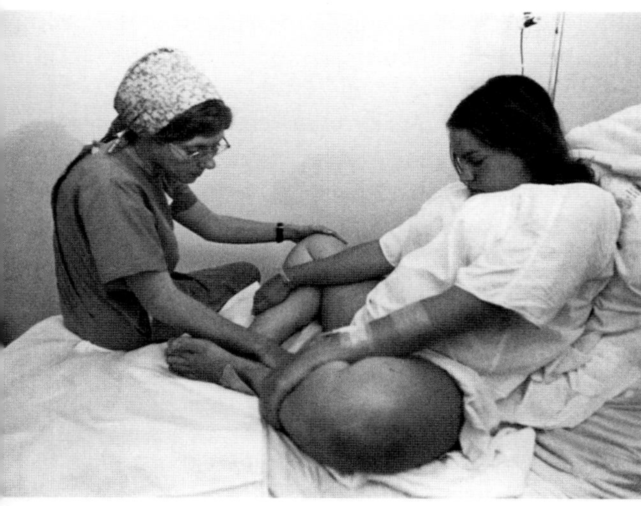

FIGURE 17–4 ♦ The nurse provides support during pushing efforts.

rather than bear down (push). A sensation of splitting apart also occurs in the latter part of the second stage, and the woman may fear the urge to push. The woman who expects these sensations and understands that bearing down contributes to progress at this stage is more likely to do so.

When the urge to bear down becomes uncontrollable and pushing begins, the nurse can help by encouraging her and by assisting with positioning (Figure 17–4♦). The woman may want to be supported with pillows in a semi-reclining position, be side-lying, position herself on her hands and knees, or use a squatting bar. Most women spontaneously push in a very effective manner. However, in many settings sustained, forceful pushing is believed to be necessary. In that case, when the contraction begins, the nurse tells the woman to take a cleansing breath or two, then to take a third large breath and hold it while pushing down with her abdominal muscles (called the *Valsalva maneuver*). A woman may prefer to push when and how she chooses in response to messages from her body. Studies have shown that with this more natural pushing, the second stage of labor is either the same length or shorter than that of women using the Valsalva maneuver (Varney, 1997).

A nullipara is usually prepared for birth when perineal bulging is noted. A multipara usually progresses much more quickly, so she may be prepared for the birth when the cervix is dilated 7 to 8 cm. As the birth approaches, the woman's partner or support person also prepares for the birth. (See Key Facts to Remember: Indications of Imminent Birth.)

The woman's blood pressure and the FHR are monitored between contractions, and the contractions are palpated until the birth. The nurse continues to assist the woman in her pushing efforts, to keep both the woman and the coach informed of procedures and progress, and to support them both throughout the birth.

**KEY FACTS TO REMEMBER**

***Indications of Imminent Birth***

Birth is imminent if the woman shows the following changes:

- Bulging of the perineum
- Uncontrollable urge to bear down
- Increased bloody show

In addition to assisting the woman and her partner, the nurse also assists the physician or certified nurse-midwife in preparing for the birth. The physician or CNM dons a sterile gown and gloves and may place sterile drapes over the woman's abdomen and legs. An episiotomy may be done just before the actual birth if needed. (See the discussion of episiotomy in Chapter 20.)

## Promotion of Comfort in the Second Stage

Most of the comfort measures that have been used during the first stage remain appropriate at this time. Applying cool cloths to the face and forehead may help cool the woman involved in the intense physical exertion of pushing. The woman may feel hot and want to remove some of the covering. Care still needs to be taken to provide privacy even though covers are removed. The woman can be encouraged to rest and relax all muscles during the periods between contractions. The nurse and support person(s) can assist the woman into a pushing position with each contraction to further conserve energy. Sips of fluids or ice chips may be used to provide moisture and relieve dryness of the mouth.

## Assisting during Birth

Shortly before the birth, the birthing room or delivery room is prepared with the equipment and materials that may be needed. Family members do not need to change into other clothing if the birth occurs in a birthing room; they don a disposable scrub suit if the birth is to occur in a delivery room or surgery suite. Good handwashing is required of the nurses and CNM or physician. Nurses who will be in direct contact with the mother at the time of birth need to wear protective clothing such as an apron or gown with a splash apron, disposable gloves, and eye covering. The certified nurse-midwife or physician also needs to wear a plastic apron or a gown with a splash apron, eye covering, and sterile gloves.

If for any reason the laboring woman is to give birth in a location other than the birthing room (such as in the case of a cesarean birth), she is moved on her bed or a cart shortly before birth. It is important that the woman move from one bed to another *between contractions.* During the contraction, the woman feels increased discomfort and may be involved in pushing efforts. Perineal bulging may be occurring, which adds to the discomfort and difficulty in moving. Care should be taken to preserve her privacy during the transfer, and safety must be provided by raising the side rails into a locked position. The labor bed or transfer cart must be carefully braced against the delivery table to ensure the woman's safety during the transfer.

Even though there are differences in the delivery room setting, the family can still be together during the birth. It is important to provide encouragement for family members to participate, because the delivery room environment may be unfamiliar and seem intimidating. The family member may hesitate to continue providing support because of fear of interfering or being in the way.

## Maternal Birthing Positions

The upright posture for birth was considered normal in most societies until modern times. Women variously selected squatting, kneeling, standing, and sitting positions for birth. The recumbent position (lithotomy) became more usual in the Western world because of the convenience it offers in applying new technology. The lithotomy position has thus become the conventional manner in which North American women give birth in hospitals. In searching for alternative positions, consumers and professionals alike are refocusing on the comfort of the laboring woman rather than on the convenience of the CNM or physician (Figures 17–5 and 17–6♦ and Table 17–5).

The woman is usually positioned for birth on a bed with use of leg supports, in a squatting position, or perhaps on her hands and knees. If a birthing bed is used, the back is elevated 30 to 60 degrees to help the woman bear down. Stirrups, if needed and used, are padded to alleviate pressure. If assisting the woman to place her legs in the stirrups, both legs should be lifted simultaneously to avoid strain on abdominal, back, and perineal muscles. The stirrups should be adjusted to fit the woman's legs. The feet are supported in the stirrup holders. The height and angle of the stirrups are adjusted so there is no pressure on the backs of the knees or the calves, which might cause discomfort and postpartal vascular problems.

## Cleansing the Perineum

After the woman has been positioned for the birth, her vulvar and perineal area are cleansed to increase her comfort and to remove the bloody discharge that is present prior to the actual birth. Perineal cleansing methods range from use of warm soapy water to aseptic technique depending on the agency protocol or on physician or CNM orders. Once the cleansing is completed, the woman returns to the desired birthing position.

## Continued Labor Support

Both the woman's partner and the nurse who has been with the woman during the labor continue to provide

A

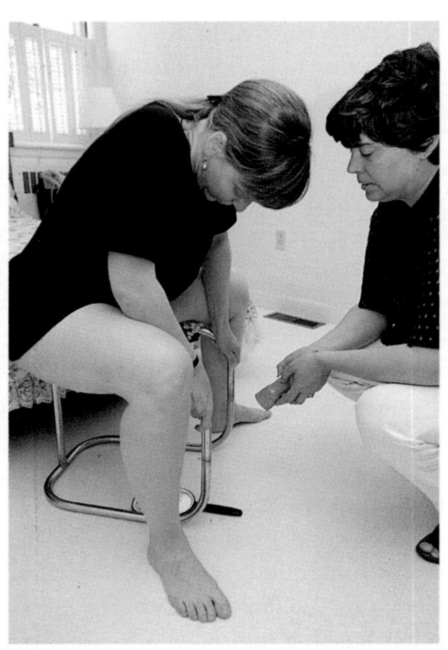

B

FIGURE 17–5 ♦ Birthing positions. **A,** Side-lying position. **B,** Using a birthing stool.

support during contractions. The woman is encouraged to push with each contraction and, as the fetal head emerges, is asked to take shallow breaths or to pant to prevent pushing. While supporting the head, the physician or certified nurse-midwife assesses whether the umbilical cord is around the fetal neck and removes it if it is, then suctions the mouth and nose with a bulb syringe. The mouth is suctioned first to prevent reflex inhalation of mucus when the sensitive nares are touched with the bulb syringe tip. The woman is encouraged to push again as the rest of the newborn's body is born. Figure 17–6♦ depicts an entire birthing experience.

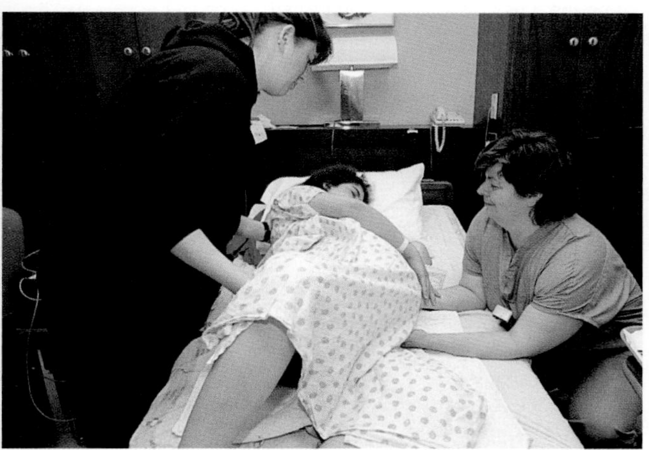

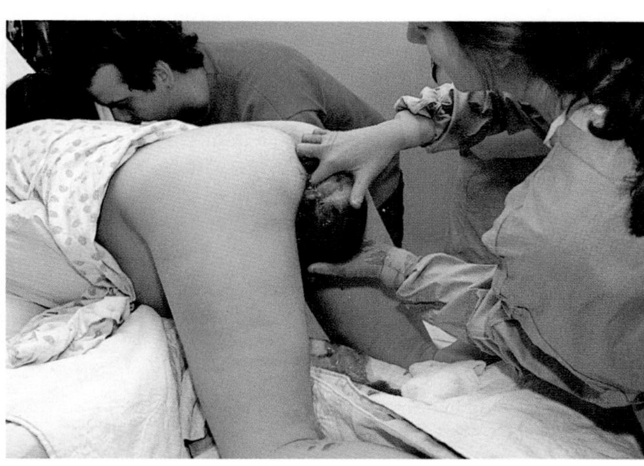

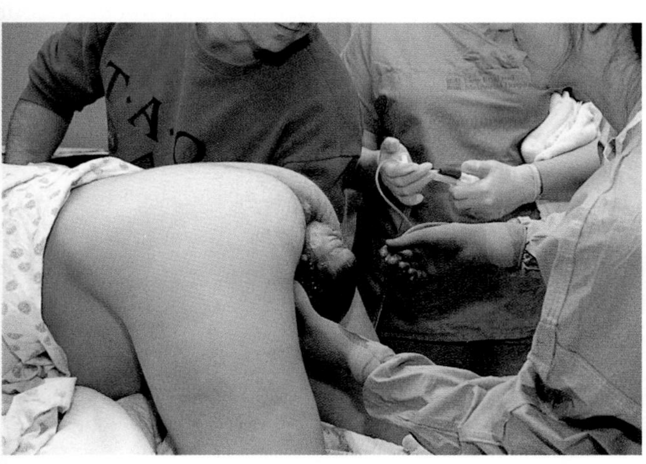

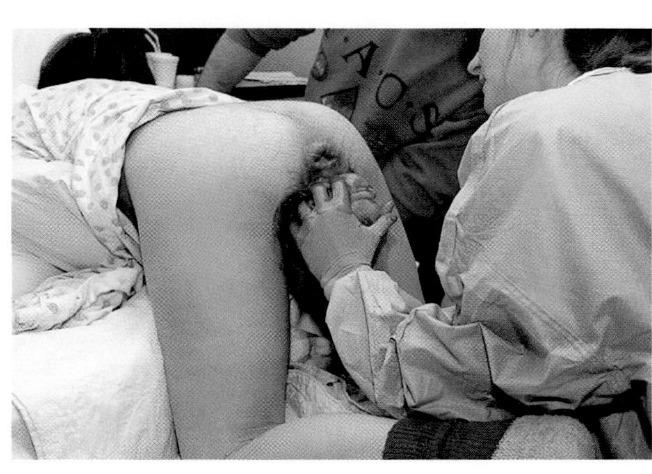

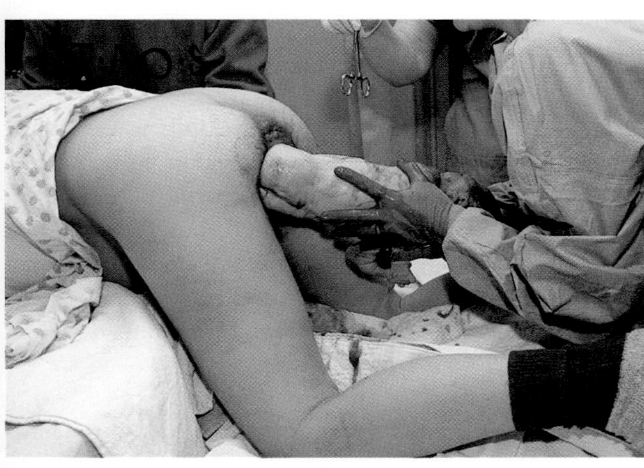

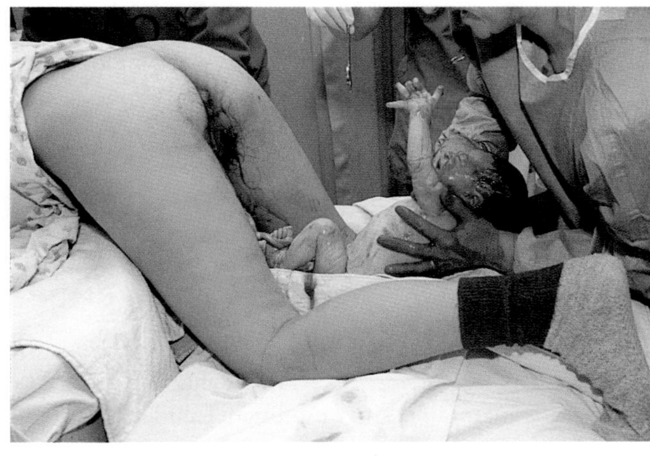

FIGURE 17–6 ♦ A birthing sequence.

| TABLE 17–5 Comparison of Birthing Positions | | | |
|---|---|---|---|
| *Position* | *Advantages* | *Disadvantages* | *Nursing Actions* |
| Sitting on birthing stool | Gravity aids descent and expulsion of infant.<br>Does not compromise venous return from lower extremities.<br>Woman can view birth process. | It is difficult to provide support for the woman's back. | Encourage woman to sit in a position that increases her comfort. |
| Semi-Fowler's | Does not compromise venous return from lower extremities.<br>Woman can view birth process. | If legs are positioned wide apart, relaxation of perineal tissues is decreased. | Assess that upper torso is evenly supported.<br>Increase support of body by changing position of bed or using pillows as props. |
| Left lateral Sims' | Does not compromise venous return from lower extremities.<br>Increases perineal relaxation and decreases need for episiotomy.<br>Appears to prevent rapid descent. | It is difficult for the woman to see the birth. | Adjust position so that the upper leg lies on the bed (scissor fashion) or is supported by the partner or on pillows. |
| Squatting | Size of pelvic outlet is increased.<br>Gravity aids descent and expulsion of newborn.<br>Second stage may be shortened | It may be difficult to maintain balance while squatting. | Help woman maintain balance.<br>Use a birthing bar if available. |
| Sitting in birthing bed | Gravity aids descent and expulsion of the fetus.<br>Does not compromise venous return from lower extremities.<br>Woman can view the birth process.<br>Leg position may be changed at will. | | Ensure that legs and feet have adequate support. |
| Hands and knees | Increases perineal relaxation and decreases need for episiotomy.<br>Increases placental and umbilical blood flow and decreases fetal distress.<br>Improves fetal rotation.<br>Nurse is better able to assess perineum.<br>Nurse has better access to fetal nose and mouth for suctioning at birth.<br>Facilitates birth of infant with shoulder dystocia. | Woman cannot view birth.<br>There is decreased contact with birth attendant.<br>Caregivers cannot use instruments.<br>There may be increased maternal fatigue. | Adjust birthing bed by dropping the foot down.<br>Supply extra pillows for increased support. |

# Nursing Care Management during the Third and Fourth Stages of Labor

## Initial Care of the Newborn

The CNM or physician places the newborn on the mother's abdomen or in the radiant-heated unit. The newborn is maintained in a modified Trendelenburg position. This position aids drainage of mucus from the nasopharynx and trachea by gravity. The newborn is dried immediately. The nurse helps maintain infant warmth by placing warmed blankets over the newborn or by placing the newborn in skin-to-skin contact with the mother. If the newborn is in a radiant-heated unit, he or she is dried, placed on a dry blanket, and left uncovered under the radiant heat. Because radiant heat warms the outer surface of objects, a newborn wrapped in blankets will receive no benefit from radiant heat.

The newborn's nose and mouth are suctioned with a bulb syringe as needed. Most immediate care of the newborn can be accomplished while the newborn is in the parent's arms or in the radiant-heated unit.

| TABLE 17–6 The Apgar Scoring System | | | |
|---|---|---|---|
| | Score | | |
| *Sign* | *0* | *1* | *2* |
| Heart rate | Absent | Slow—below 100 | Above 100 |
| Respiratory effort | Absent | Slow—irregular | Good crying |
| Muscle tone | Flaccid | Some flexion of extremities | Active motion |
| Reflex irritability | None | Grimace | Vigorous cry |
| Color | Pale blue | Body pink, blue extremities | Completely pink |

*Source:* Apgar V: The newborn (Apgar) scoring system, reflections and advice. (1966, August). *Pediatric Clinics of North America,* 13, 645.

## Apgar Scoring System

The Apgar scoring system (Table 17–6) is used to evaluate the physical condition of the newborn at birth. The newborn is rated 1 minute after birth and again at 5 minutes and receives a total score **(Apgar score)** ranging from 0 to 10 based on the following assessments:

1. *Heart rate* is auscultated or palpated at the junction of the umbilical cord and skin. This is the most important assessment. A newborn heart rate of less than 100 beats per minute indicates the need for immediate resuscitation.
2. *Respiratory effort* is the second most important Apgar assessment. Complete absence of respirations is termed *apnea.* A vigorous cry indicates adequate respirations.
3. *Muscle tone* is determined by evaluating the degree of flexion and resistance to straightening of the extremities. A normal newborn's elbows and hips are flexed, with the knees positioned up toward the abdomen.
4. *Reflex irritability* is evaluated by stroking the baby's back along the spine or by flicking the soles of the feet. A cry merits a full score of 2. A grimace is 1 point, and no response is 0.
5. *Skin color* is inspected for cyanosis and pallor. Generally, newborns have blue extremities, with a pink body, which merits a score of 1. This condition is termed *acrocyanosis* and is present in 85% of normal newborns at 1 minute after birth. A completely pink newborn scores a 2, and a totally cyanotic, pale infant scores 0. Newborns with darker skin pigmentation will not be pink in color. Their skin color is assessed for pallor and acrocyanosis, and a score is selected based on the assessment.

A score of 8 to 10 indicates a newborn in good condition who requires only nasopharyngeal suctioning and perhaps some oxygen near the face (called "blow-by" oxygen). If the Apgar score is below 8, resuscitative measures may need to be instituted. (See the discussion in Chapter 25.)

## Care of Umbilical Cord

If the clinician has not placed some type of cord clamp on the newborn's umbilical cord, the nurse must do so. Before applying the cord clamp, the nurse examines the cut end of the cord for the presence of two arteries and one vein. The umbilical vein is the largest vessel, and the arteries are seen as smaller vessels. The number of vessels is recorded on the birth and newborn records. The cord is clamped approximately 1/2 to 1 in from the abdomen to allow room between the abdomen and clamp as the cord dries. Abdominal skin must not be clamped, because this will cause necrosis of the tissue. The most common type of cord clamp is the plastic Hollister cord clamp (Figure 17–7♦). The Hollister clamp is removed in the newborn nursery approximately 24 hours after the cord has dried.

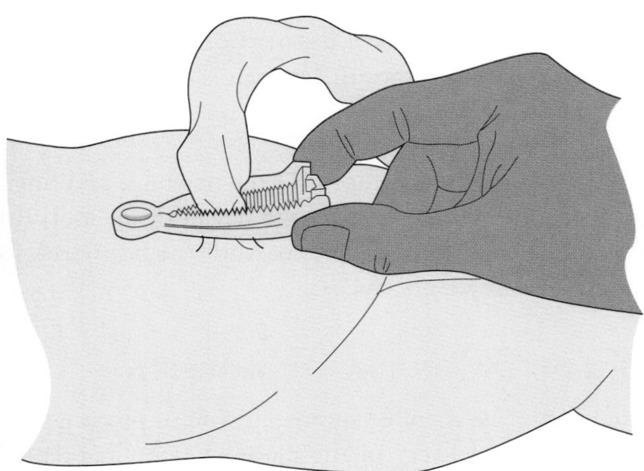


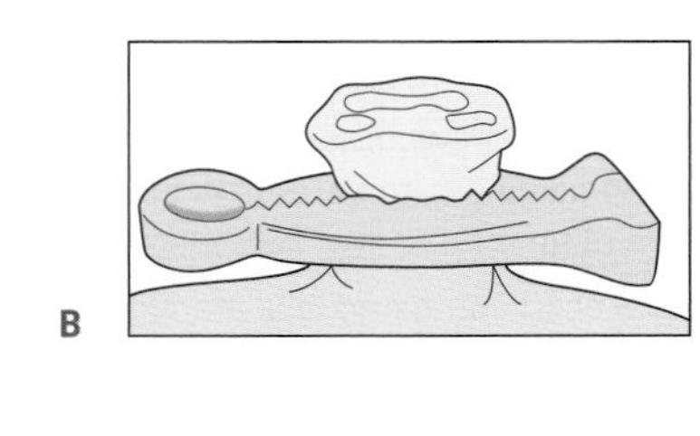


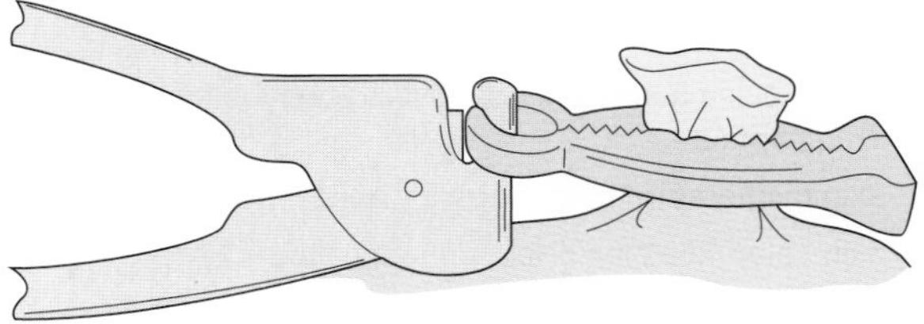


FIGURE 17–7 ♦ Hollister cord clamp. **A**, Clamp is positioned 1/2 to 1 in from the abdomen and then secured. **B**, Cut cord. The one vein and two arteries can be seen. **C**, Plastic device for removing clamp after cord has dried. After the cord is cut, the nurse grasps the Hollister clamp on either side of the cut area and gently separates it.

### Cord Blood Collection for Banking

A growing number of parents are arranging for cord blood banking (see discussion in Chapter 1). Immediately after the newborn's umbilical cord is clamped and cut and the placenta is expelled, the CNM or physician withdraws blood from the remaining umbilical cord and the placenta. The blood is placed in a special container that parents receive from the Cord Blood Registry and bring with them for the birth. The parents should have any special directions that are required for storage and care of the container.

### Physical Assessment of the Newborn

The nurse performs an abbreviated systematic physical assessment in the birthing area to detect any abnormalities (Table 17–7). First, the nurse notes the size of the newborn and the contour and size of the head in relationship to the rest of the body. The newborn's posture and movements indicate tone and neurologic functioning.

The nurse inspects the skin for discoloration, presence of vernix caseosa and lanugo, and evidence of trauma and desquamation (peeling of skin). *Vernix caseosa* is a white, cheesy substance found normally on newborns. It is absorbed within 24 hours after birth. Vernix is abundant on preterm infants and absent on postterm newborns. A large quantity of fine hair (lanugo) is often seen on preterm newborns, especially on their shoulders, foreheads, backs, and cheeks. Desquamation of the skin is seen in postterm newborns.

The nurse observes the nares for flaring and, as the newborn cries, inspects the palate for cleft palate. The nurse looks for mucus in the nose and mouth and removes it with a bulb syringe as needed. The nurse inspects the chest for respiratory rate and the presence of retractions. If retractions are present, the nurse assesses the newborn for grunting or stridor. A normal respiratory rate is 30 to 60 per minute. The nurse auscultates the lungs bilaterally for breath sounds. Absence of breath sounds on one side could mean pneumothorax. Rales may be heard immediately after birth because a small amount of fluid may remain in the lungs; this fluid will be absorbed. Rhonchi indicate aspiration of oral secretions. If there is excessive mucus or respiratory distress, the nurse suctions the newborn with a mucus trap. (See Procedure 17–1 and Figure 17–8♦.) The nurse notes and records elimination of urine or meconium on the newborn record.

**TABLE 17–7 Initial Newborn Evaluation**

| *Assess* | *Normal Findings* |
|---|---|
| Respirations | Rate 36–60, irregular<br>No retractions, no grunting |
| Apical pulse | Rate 120–160 and somewhat irregular |
| Temperature | Skin temp above 36.5°C (97.8°F) |
| Skin color | Body pink with bluish extremities |
| Umbilical cord | Two arteries and one vein |
| Gestational age | Should be 38–42 weeks to remain with parents for extended time |
| Sole creases | Sole creases that involve the heel |

In general, expect scant amount of vernix on upper back, axilla, groin; lanugo only on upper back; ears with incurving of upper 2/3 of pinnae and thin cartilage that springs back from folding; male genitals—testes palpated in upper or lower scrotum; female genitals—labia majora larger; clitoris nearly covered

In the following situations, newborns should generally be stabilized rather than remaining with parents in the birth area for an extended period of time:

- Apgar less than 8 at 1 minute and less than 9 at 5 minutes or baby requires resuscitation measures (other than whiffs of oxygen)
- Respirations below 30 or above 60, with retractions and/or grunting
- Apical pulse below 120 or above 160 with marked irregularities
- Skin temperature below 36.5°C (97.8°F)
- Skin color pale blue or circumoral pallor
- Baby less than 38 or more than 42 weeks' gestation
- Baby very small or very large for gestational age
- Congenital anomalies involving open areas in the skin (meningomyelocele)

### Newborn Identification

The nurse places two bracelets on the newborn—one on the wrist and one on the ankle. The newborn bands must fit snugly to prevent their loss. To ensure correct identification, the nurse gives the mother and partner each a band that matches that of the newborn (while still in the birthing or delivery room). The bands allow access to the infant care areas and must not be removed until the infant is discharged.

Many hospitals also footprint the newborn and fingerprint the mother. To prepare the newborn for footprinting, the nurse wipes the soles of both the newborn's feet to remove any vernix caseosa.

## Delivery of the Placenta

After birth, the certified nurse-midwife or physician prepares for the delivery of the placenta (see Chapter 15). The following signs suggest placental separation:

1. The uterus rises upward in the abdomen.
2. As the placenta moves downward, the umbilical cord lengthens.

# Procedure 17–1 Performing Nasal Pharyngeal Suctioning

| Nursing Action | Rationale |
|---|---|
| **Objective: Clear secretions from the newborn's nose or oropharynx if respirations are depressed or if amniotic fluid was meconium stained.** | |
| • Tighten the lid on the DeLee mucus trap or other suction device collection bottle. | *This avoids spillage of secretions and prevents air from leaking out of the lid.* |
| • Connect one end of the DeLee tubing to low suction. | |
| • Insert the other end of the tubing 3 to 5 in into the newborn's nose or mouth (Figure 17–8♦). | |

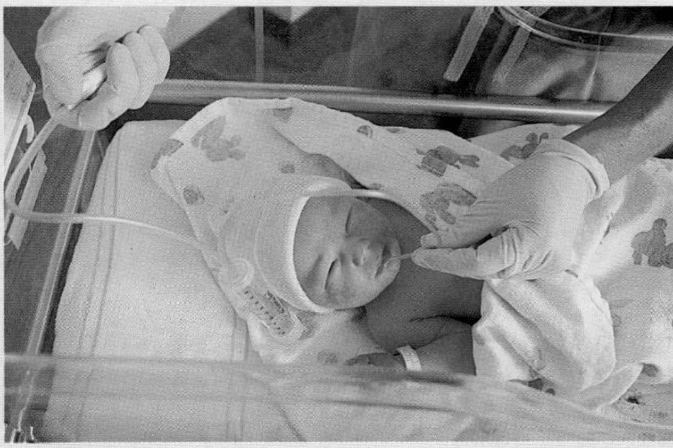

FIGURE 17–8 ♦ DeLee mucus trap.

| Nursing Action | Rationale |
|---|---|
| • Continue suction as you remove the tube. | *This avoids redepositing secretions in the newborn's nasopharynx.* |
| • Continue to reinsert the tube and provide suction for as long as fluid is aspirated. *Note: Excessive suctioning can cause vagal stimulation, which decreases heart rate.* | |
| • If it is necessary to pass the tube into the newborn's stomach to remove meconium secretions that the newborn swallowed before birth, insert the tube into the newborn's mouth and then into the stomach. Provide suction and continue suction as you remove the tube. | |
| **Objective: Record relevant information on the newborn's chart.** | |
| Document completion of the procedure and the amount and type of secretions. | *This provides documentation of intervention and status at birth.* |

3. A sudden trickle or spurt of blood appears.
4. The shape of the uterus changes from a disk to a globe.

While waiting for these signs, the nurse palpates the uterus to check for ballooning caused by uterine relaxation and subsequent bleeding into the uterine cavity. After the placenta has separated, the woman may be asked to bear down to aid delivery of the placenta.

Oxytocics are frequently given at the time of the delivery of the placenta, so the uterus will contract and bleeding will be minimized. Oxytocin (Pitocin), 10 units, may be added to an intravenous (IV) infusion or given intramuscularly or by slow IV push. Some physicians order methylergonovine maleate (Methergine), 0.2 mg, administered intramuscularly, or carboprost tromethamine (Hemabate), 250 ug/mL, administered intramuscularly. In addition to administering the ordered medications, the nurse assesses and records maternal blood pressure before and after administration of oxytocics. For further information, refer to Drug Guide: Oxytocin (in Chapter 20) and Drug Guide: Methylergonovine Maleate (in Chapter 28).

After the delivery of the placenta, the CNM or physician inspects the placental membranes to make sure they are intact and that all cotyledons are present. If there is a defect or a part missing from the placenta, a manual uterine examination is done. The nurse notes on the birth record the time of delivery of the placenta.

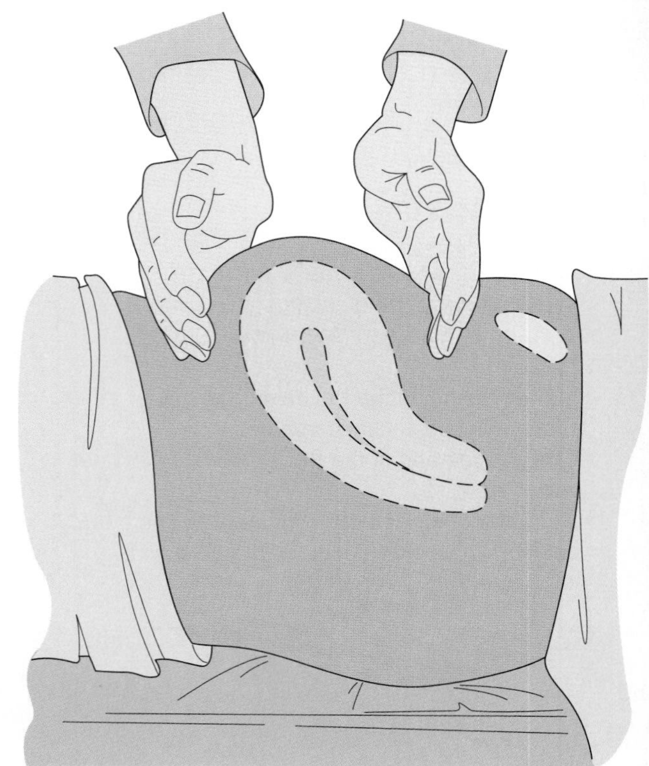

FIGURE 17–9 ♦ Suggested method of palpating the fundus of the uterus during the fourth stage. The left hand is placed just above the symphysis pubis, and gentle downward pressure is exerted. The right hand is cupped around the uterine fundus.

## Special Assessments and Care of the New Mother

The physician or CNM inspects the vagina and cervix for lacerations and makes any necessary repairs. The episiotomy may be repaired now if it has not been done previously (see Chapter 20).

The nurse assesses the fundus for firmness by palpating. The normal position is at the midline and below the umbilicus. A displaced fundus may be caused by a full bladder or blood collected in the uterus. The uterus may be emptied of blood by grasping it with one hand anteriorly and posteriorly and squeezing. The nurse continues to palpate the uterine fundus at frequent intervals for >4 hours to ensure that it remains firmly contracted. It is palpated (Figure 17–9♦) but not massaged unless it is soft (boggy). If it becomes boggy or appears to rise in the abdomen, the fundus is massaged until firm; then the nurse exerts firm pressure on the fundus in an attempt to express retained clots. During all aspects of fundal massage, the nurse uses one hand to provide support for the lower portion of the uterus. The uterus is very tender at this time; all palpation and massage should be done as gently as possible.

The nurse washes the woman's perineum with gauze squares and warmed solution and dries the area well with a towel before placing the maternity pad. If stirrups have been used, the woman's legs are removed from the stirrups at the same time to avoid muscle strain. The woman is encouraged to move her legs gently up and down in a bicycle motion. The woman remains in the same bed or is transferred to a recovery room bed, and the nurse helps her don a clean gown.

During the recovery period (1 to 4 hours) the woman is monitored closely. Frequent checking for deviations from normal in vital signs is required. The maternal blood pressure is monitored at 5- to 15-minute intervals to detect any changes. Blood pressure should return to the prelabor level due to an increased volume of blood returning to the maternal circulation from the uteroplacental shunt. Pulse rate should be slightly lower than it was during labor. Baroreceptors cause a vagal response, which slows the pulse. A rise in blood pressure may be a response to oxytocic drugs or may be caused by PIH. Blood loss may be reflected by a lowered blood pressure and a rising pulse rate (Table 17–8).

The nurse also monitors the woman's temperature. Frequently women have tremors in the immediate postpartum period that may be caused by a difference in internal

| TABLE 17–8 | Maternal Adaptations Following Birth |
|---|---|
| *Characteristic* | *Normal Finding* |
| Blood pressure | Returns to prelabor level |
| Pulse | Slightly lower than in labor |
| Uterine fundus | In the midline at the umbilicus or one to two finger breadths below the umbilicus |
| Lochia | Red (rubra), small to moderate amount (from spotting on pads to 1/4–1/2 of pad covered in 15 minutes) |
| | Does not exceed saturation of one pad in first hour |
| Bladder | Nonpalpable |
| Perineum | Smooth, pink, without bruising or edema |
| Emotional state | Wide variation, including excited, exhilarated, smiling, crying, fatigued, verbal, quiet, pensive, and sleepy |

and external body temperatures (higher temperature inside the body than outside). Another theory is that the woman is reacting to the fetal cells that have entered the maternal circulation at the placental site. A heated bath blanket placed next to the woman tends to alleviate the problem and can be replaced as often as the mother desires.

The nurse inspects the bloody vaginal discharge for amount and charts it as minimal, moderate, or heavy and with or without clots. This discharge, lochia rubra, should be bright red. A soaked perineal pad contains approximately 100 mL of blood. If the perineal pad becomes soaked in a 15-minute period or if blood pools under the buttocks, continuous observation is necessary (see Procedure 17–2). When the fundus is firm, a continuous trickle of blood may signal laceration of the vagina or cervix or an unligated vessel in the episiotomy. (See Key Facts to Remember: Immediate Postbirth Danger Signs.)

If the fundus rises and displaces to the right, the nurse must be concerned about two factors:

1. As the uterus rises, the uterine contractions become less effective and increased bleeding may occur.
2. The most common cause of uterine displacement is bladder distention.

The nurse palpates the bladder to determine whether it is distended. The bladder fills rapidly with the extra fluid volume returned from the uteroplacental circulation (and with any fluid received intravenously during labor and birth). The postpartal woman may not realize that her bladder is full because trauma to the bladder and urethra during childbirth and the use of regional anesthesia decrease bladder tone and the urge to void.

**KEY FACTS TO REMEMBER**

*Immediate Postbirth Danger Signs*

In the immediate postbirth recovery period, the following conditions should be reported to the CNM or physician:

- Hypotension
- Tachycardia
- Uterine atony
- Excessive bleeding
- Hematoma

All measures should be taken to enable the mother to void. The nurse may place a warm towel across the lower abdomen or pour warm water over the perineum to relax the urinary sphincter and facilitate voiding. If the woman is unable to void, catheterization is necessary. The perineum is inspected for edema and hematoma formation. An ice pack often reduces the swelling and alleviates the discomfort of an episiotomy.

The couple may be tired, hungry, and thirsty. Some agencies serve the couple a meal. The tired mother will probably drift off into a welcome sleep. The partner can also be encouraged to rest, since his supporting role is physically and mentally tiring. If the mother is not in a birthing room, she is usually transferred from the birthing unit to the postpartal or mother-baby area after 2 hours or more, depending on agency policy and whether the following criteria are met:

- Stable vital signs
- No bleeding
- Undistended bladder
- Firm fundus
- Sensations fully recovered from any anesthetic agent received during birth

For some women, the childbirth experience has been extremely painful, filled with hours of feeling powerless or out of control. In this circumstance, the woman is at higher risk for developing posttraumatic stress disorder (Reynolds, 1997). (See Chapter 19 for further discussion.)

## Enhancing Attachment

Dramatic evidence indicates that the first few hours and even minutes after birth are an important period for the attachment of mother and infant. If this period of contact can occur during the first hour after birth, the newborn will be in the quiet state and able to interact with

## Procedure 17–2 Evaluating Lochia After Birth

| *Nursing Action* | *Rationale* |
|---|---|
| **OBJECTIVE: PREPARE THE WOMAN.** | |
| Explain the procedure, the reason for performing the procedure, and the information that will be obtained. | *Explaining the procedure decreases anxiety and increases relaxation.* |
| **OBJECTIVE: OBTAIN AND EVALUATE MATERNAL VITAL SIGNS.** | |
| Assess maternal temperature, blood pressure, and pulse. | *This provides information regarding the woman's physiologic status.* |
| **OBJECTIVE: ACCURATELY EVALUATE THE AMOUNT OF LOCHIA AFTER BIRTH.** | |
| • Don disposable gloves.<br>• Lower the perineal pad so that you can visualize the amount of lochia. | *Universal precautions and body substance isolation require use of gloves when exposed to body secretions.* |
| • Palpate the uterine fundus, located in the midline at the umbilicus or one to two finger breadths below the umbilicus, by placing one hand on the fundus and the other hand just over the symphysis pubis and pressing downward. Use your other hand to palpate the fundus. | *Downward pressure exerted just above the symphysis pubis will prevent excessive downward movement of the uterus during assessment.* |
| • Determine the firmness of the fundus.<br>• If the fundus is boggy, massage by rubbing in a circular motion.<br>• Evaluate the color and amount of lochia and observe for clots. | *The uterus must remain firmly contracted to prevent excessive blood loss. Manual pressure stimulates uterine contractions.* |
| *LOCHIA EVALUATION GUIDELINES*<br>Small: Smaller than a 4-in stain on the pad; 10 to 25 mL<br>Moderate: Smaller than a 6-in stain; 25 to 50 mL<br>Large: Larger than a 6-in stain; 50 to 80 mL | |
| If blood loss exceeds the above guidelines, weigh the perineal pads and the Chux to estimate the blood loss more accurately (1 g = 1 mL). | *Weighing the pads and Chux can provide important information. Because some blood loss is normal, care providers may not otherwise detect excessive blood loss.* |

parents by looking at them. Newborns also turn their heads in response to a spoken voice. (See Chapter 21 for further discussion of newborn states.)

The first parent-newborn contact may be brief (a few minutes), to be followed by a more extended contact after uncomfortable procedures (delivery of the placenta and suturing of the episiotomy) are completed. When the newborn is returned to the mother, the nurse can assist her to begin breastfeeding if she so desires. The baby may seek out the mother's breast, and early contact between the two can greatly affect breastfeeding success. Even if the newborn does not actively nurse, he or she can lick, taste, and smell the mother's skin. This activity by the newborn stimulates the maternal release of prolactin, which promotes the onset of lactation.

Darkening the birthing room by turning out most of the lights causes newborns to open their eyes and gaze around. This in turn enhances eye-to-eye contact with the parents. (*Note:* If the physician or CNM needs a light source, the spotlight can be left on.) Treatment of the newborn's eyes may also be delayed. Many parents who establish eye contact with the newborn are content to quietly gaze at their infant. Others may show more active involvement by touching or inspecting the newborn.

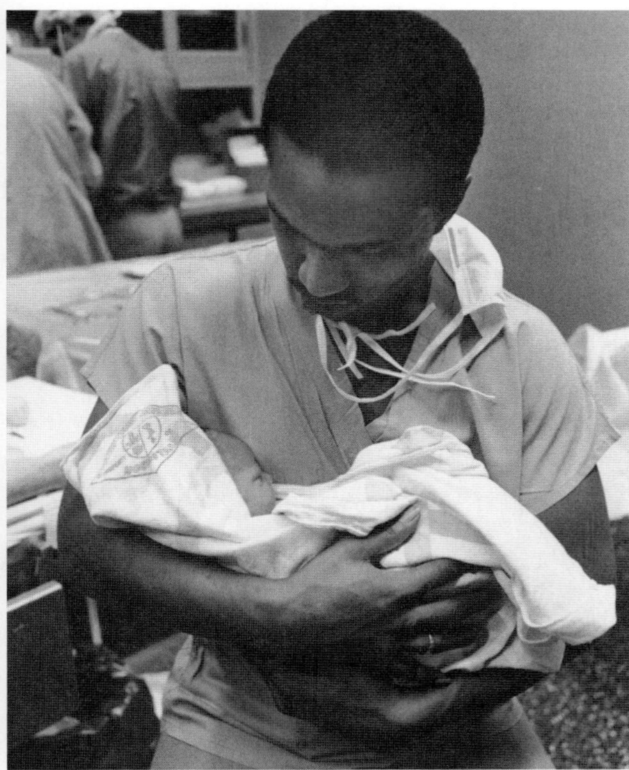

FIGURE 17–10 ♦ A father holds his newborn.

Some mothers talk to their babies in a high-pitched voice, which seems to be soothing to newborns. Some couples verbally express amazement and pride when they see they have produced a beautiful, healthy baby. Their verbalization enhances feelings of accomplishment and ecstasy. Figure 17–10♦ shows a new parent establishing bonds with his newborn son.

Both parents need to be encouraged to do whatever they feel most comfortable doing. Some parents prefer only limited contact with the newborn immediately after birth and instead desire private time together in a quiet environment. In spite of the current zeal for providing immediate attachment opportunities, nursing personnel need to be aware of parents' wishes. The desire to delay interaction with the newborn does not necessarily imply a decreased ability of the parents to bond with their newborn. (See Chapter 26 for further discussion of parent-newborn attachment.)

## Nursing Care Management during Nurse-Attended Birth

Occasionally labor progresses so rapidly that the maternity nurse is faced with the task of assisting in the actual birth of the baby. This is called a **precipitous birth.** The attending maternity nurse has the primary responsibility for providing a physically and psychologically safe experience for the woman and her baby. A woman whose certified nurse-midwife or physician is not present may feel disappointed, frightened, abandoned, angry, and cheated. She may fear what is going to happen and feel that everything is out of her control. In working with the woman, the nurse provides support by keeping her informed about the labor progress and assuring her that the nurse will stay with her. If birth is imminent, the nurse must not leave the mother alone. Auxiliary personnel can be directed to contact the CNM or physician and retrieve the emergency birth pack ("precip pack"). An emergency birth pack should be readily accessible to birthing rooms. A typical pack contains the following items:

1. A small drape that can be placed under the woman's buttocks to provide a sterile field
2. A bulb syringe to clear mucus from the newborn's mouth
3. Two sterile clamps (Kelly or Rochester) to clamp the umbilical cord before applying a cord clamp
4. Sterile scissors to cut the umbilical cord
5. A sterile umbilical cord clamp, either Hesseltine or Hollister
6. A baby blanket to wrap the newborn in after birth
7. A package of sterile gloves

As the materials are being gathered, the nurse must remain calm; the woman is reassured by the composure of the nurse and feels that the nurse is competent. At all times during the birth, the nurse provides suggestions such as when to maintain a controlled breathing pattern and when to push, supports the woman's efforts, and provides reassurance.

The nurse assists in the precipitous birth as follows: The woman is encouraged to assume a comfortable position. If time permits, the nurse scrubs his or her hands with soap and water and puts on sterile gloves. Sterile drapes are placed under the woman's buttocks. The nurse may place an index finger inside the lower portion of the vagina and the thumb on the outer portion of the perineum and gently massage the area to help stretch perineal tissues and prevent perineal lacerations. This procedure is called "ironing the perineum."

When the infant's head crowns, the nurse instructs the woman to pant, which decreases her urge to push. The nurse checks whether the amniotic sac is intact. If it is, the nurse tears the sac so the newborn will not breathe in amniotic fluid with the first breath.

With one hand, the nurse applies gentle pressure against the fetal head to prevent it from popping out rapidly. The nurse does not hold the head back forcibly. Rapid birth of the head may result in tears in the woman's perineal tissues. In the fetus, the rapid change in pressure within the fetal head may cause subdural or dural tears. The nurse supports the perineum with the other hand and allows the head to be born between contractions.

As the woman continues to pant, the nurse inserts one or two fingers along the back of the fetal head to check for the umbilical cord. If there is a nuchal cord (umbilical cord around the neck), the nurse bends her or his fingers like a fish hook, grasps the cord, and pulls it over the baby's head. It is important to check that the cord is not wrapped around the neck more than one time. If the cord is tightly looped and cannot be slipped over the baby's head, two clamps are placed on the cord, the cord is cut between the clamps, and the cord is unwound.

Immediately after birth of the head, the nurse suctions the baby's mouth, throat, and nasal passages. The nurse then places one hand on each side of the head and exerts gentle downward traction until the anterior shoulder passes under the symphysis pubis. Then gentle upward traction aids the birth of the posterior shoulder. The nurse then instructs the woman to push gently so that the rest of the body can be born quickly. The newborn must be supported as she or he emerges.

The newborn is held at the level of the uterus to facilitate blood flow through the umbilical cord. The combination of amniotic fluid and vernix makes the newborn very slippery, so the nurse must be careful to avoid dropping the baby. The nose and mouth of the newborn are suctioned again, using a bulb syringe. The nurse then dries the newborn to prevent heat loss.

As soon as the nurse determines that the newborn's respirations are adequate, the infant can be placed on the mother's abdomen. The newborn's head should be slightly lower than the body to aid drainage of fluid and mucus. The weight of the newborn on the mother's abdomen stimulates uterine contractions, which aid in placental separation. The umbilical cord should not be pulled.

The nurse is alert for signs of placental separation (slight gush of dark blood from the vagina, lengthening of the cord, or a change in uterine shape from discoid to globular). When these signs are present, the mother is instructed to push so that the placenta can be delivered. The nurse inspects the placenta to determine whether it is intact.

The nurse checks the firmness of the uterus. The fundus may be gently massaged to stimulate contractions and decrease bleeding. Putting the newborn to breast also stimulates uterine contractions through release of oxytocin from the pituitary gland.

The umbilical cord may now be cut. The nurse places two sterile Kelly clamps approximately 1 to 3 in from the newborn's abdomen. The cord is cut between the Kelly clamps with sterile scissors. The nurse places a sterile umbilical cord clamp adjacent to the clamp on the newborn's cord, between the clamp and the newborn's abdomen. The clamp must not be placed snugly against the abdomen, because the cord will dry and shrink.

The nurse cleanses the area under the mother's buttocks and inspects her perineum for lacerations. Bleeding from lacerations may be controlled by pressing a clean perineal pad against the perineum and instructing the woman to keep her thighs together.

If the CNM or physician's arrival is delayed or if the newborn is having respiratory distress, the newborn should be transported immediately to the nursery. The newborn must be properly identified before he or she leaves the birth area. The nurse notes and places on a birth record the following information:

1. Position of fetus at birth
2. Presence of cord around neck or shoulder (nuchal cord)
3. Time of birth
4. Apgar scores at 1 and 5 minutes after birth
5. Gender of newborn
6. Time of expulsion of placenta
7. Method of placental expulsion
8. Appearance and intactness of placenta
9. Mother's condition
10. Any medications that were given to mother or newborn (per agency protocol)

## Evaluation

Evaluation provides an opportunity to determine the effectiveness of nursing care. As a result of comprehensive nursing care during the intrapartal period, the following outcomes may be anticipated:

- The mother's physical and psychologic well-being has been maintained and supported.
- The baby's physical and psychologic well-being has been protected and supported.
- The couple have had input into the birth process and have participated as much as they desired.
- The mother and her baby have had a safe birth.

# Chapter Review

## CHAPTER HIGHLIGHTS

- During labor, before procedures are begun, it is important to explain what will be done, the reasons, potential benefits and risks, and possible alternatives. These explanations help the woman determine what happens to her body.
- Behavioral responses to labor vary with the phase of labor, the preparation the woman has had, and her previous experience, cultural beliefs, and developmental level.
- The childbearing family may have a variety of expectations of the nurse during labor and birth. Some families want to make all decisions themselves with limited nursing contact, others want a moderate amount of contact and see the relationship as a cooperative venture, and some families want a lot of involvement and look to the nurse to instill confidence in them that everything will be all right.
- Each woman's cultural beliefs affect her needs for privacy, expression of discomfort, and expectations for the birth and the role she wishes the father to play in the birth event.
- The adolescent mother has special needs in the birth setting. Her developmental needs require specialized nursing care.
- The laboring woman's comfort may be increased by general comfort measures, supportive relaxation techniques, methods of handling anxiety, controlled breathing, and support by a caring person.
- Maternal birthing positions include a wide variety of possibilities, from side-lying to sitting, squatting, and semi-Fowler's.
- Immediate assessments of the newborn include evaluation of the Apgar score and an abbreviated physical assessment. These early assessments help determine the need for resuscitation and whether the newborn's adaptation to extrauterine life is progressing normally. The newborn who is not experiencing problems may remain with the parents for an extended period after birth.
- Immediate care of the newborn also includes maintenance of respirations, promotion of warmth, prevention of infection, and accurate identification.
- The placenta separates from the uterine wall and is expelled with either the maternal or fetal side emerging from the vagina. The maternal side contains the cotyledons, appears rough in texture, and may be associated with retention of placental fragments.
- The fourth stage includes the first 1 to 4 hours following birth. Many physiologic and psychologic changes occur during this period.
- At times a baby is born rapidly without the physician or certified nurse-midwife present. This event is referred to as a precipitous birth. The nurse in the birthing area remains with the woman and attends her during the birth until a CNM or physician can be present.

## CHAPTER REFERENCES


American Academy of Pediatrics & American College of Obstetricians and Gynecologists. (1997). *Guidelines for perinatal care* (4th ed.). Washington, DC: Author.

AWHONN (1998). *Standards for Professional Nursing Practice in the Care of Women and Newborns* (5th ed).

Association of Women's Health, Obstetric, and Neonatal Nurses. (1999). Guidelines for fetal monitoring. In L. K. Mandeville & N. H. Troiano (Eds.), *High-risk & critical care intrapartum nursing.* Philadelphia: Lippincott.

Calhoun, M. A. (1986). The Vietnamese woman: Health/illness attitudes and behaviors. In P. N. Stearn (Ed.), *Women, health, and culture.* Washington, DC: Hemisphere.

Callister, L. C. (2001). Culturally competent care of women and newborns: knowledge, attitude, and skills. *Journal of Obstetric Gynecologic, and Neonatal Nursing, 30*(2) 209–215.

Drake, P. (1996). Addressing developmental needs of pregnant adolescents. *Journal of Obstetric, Gynecologic, and Neonatal Nursing, 25,* 518.

England, P. & Horowitz, R. (1998). *Birthing from within.* Albuquerque, NM: Partera Press.

Hodnett, E. (1996). Nursing support of the laboring woman. *Journal of Obstetric, Gynecologic, and Neonatal Nursing, 25,* 257.

Hutchinson, M. K., & Baqi-Aziz, M. (1994). Nursing care of the childbearing Muslim family. *Journal of Obstetric, Gynecologic, and Neonatal Nursing, 23*(9), 767.

Khazoyan, C. M., & Anderson, N. L. R. (1994). Latinas' expectations for their partners during childbirth. *Maternal-Child Nursing Journal, 19,* 226.

Lauderdale, J. (1999). Childbearing and transcultural nursing care issues. In M. M. Andrews & J. S. Boyle (Eds.), *Transcultural concepts in nursing care* (3rd ed., pp. 81–106). Philadelphia: Lippincott.

Lipson, J. G., Dibble, S. L., & Minarik, P. A. (1996). *Culture and nursing care: A pocket guide.* San Francisco: University of California at San Francisco Nursing Press.

Reynolds, J. L. (1997). Post-traumatic stress disorder after childbirth: The phenomenon of traumatic birth. *Canadian Medical Association Journal, 156,* 831–835.

Scott-Ramos, I. (1996). Culturally sensitive care giving for the Latino woman (Ed.), *Journal of Obstetric, Gynecologic, and Neonatal Nursing, 25,* 67.

Stern, D. N. & Bruschweiler-Stern, N. (1998). *The birth of a mother.* New York: Basic Books.

Varney, H. (1997). *Varney's midwifery* (3rd ed.). Sudbury, MA: Jones & Bartlett.

Waymire, V. (1997). A triggering time: Childbirth may recall sexual abuse memories. *Association of Women's Health, Obstetric, and Neonatal Nursing-Lifelines, 23,* 47–50.

Wesson, N. (2000). *Labor pain: A natural approach to easing delivery.* Rochester, NY: Healing Arts Press.

## CONTEMPORARY MATERNAL-NEWBORN NURSING ON-LINE

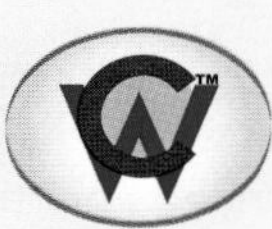

Additional interactive resources, including animations and video, for this chapter can be found on the Companion Website at http://www.prenhall.com/ladewig. Click on Chapter 17 and "Begin" to select the activities for this chapter.

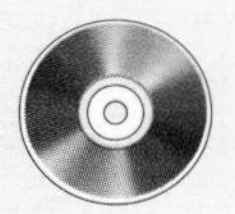

For NCLEX review questions and an audio glossary, access the accompanying CD-ROM in this book.

Chapter 18

# Maternal Analgesia and Anesthesia

*I had the unique opportunity to join the staff of a brand-new women's hospital as it was opening. The team I work with is very tight knit, and we really support each other. Our schedule rotates so that I cover the regular (daytime) surgical cases for 2 days a week and then I have a 24-hour call shift on the birthing unit. I may do 10 to 12 epidurals during that call period, so I really have to be efficient. Still, it's important to me (and the others on my team) to spend as much time as that laboring woman needs, to explain things, and help her feel comfortable with her choice of pain relief.*

–Certified Nurse Anesthetist

## OBJECTIVES

- **Describe the use of systemic drugs to promote pain relief during labor.**
- **Compare the major types of regional analgesia and anesthesia, including area affected, advantages, disadvantages, techniques, and nursing implications.**
- **Discuss the possible complications of regional anesthesia.**
- **Describe the nursing care related to general anesthesia.**
- **Delineate the major complications of general anesthesia.**

## KEY TERMS

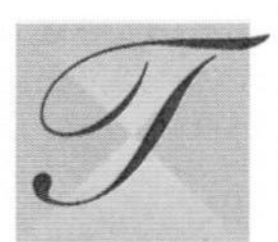

The childbearing woman experiences many demanding sensations and discomforts during labor and birth. The nurse can help her have a positive childbirth experience by providing effective comfort measures. Nursing interventions directed toward pain relief begin with nonpharmacologic measures such as providing information, support, and physical comfort. Measures to promote comfort include back rubs, showers, whirlpools (Jacuzzi), the application of cool cloths to her forehead, and encouragement. Some laboring women need no further interventions. For other women, the progression of labor brings increasing discomfort that interferes with their ability to cope effectively with labor. Pharmacologic agents such as systemic drugs, epidural analgesics, intrathecal narcotics, and regional nerve blocks may be used to decrease discomfort, increase relaxation, and reestablish the woman's sense of balance and control. The methods are not all mutually exclusive, and any of them may be used in combination with other comfort measures.

Although systemic analgesics and regional local anesthetic blocks may affect the fetus, so do the pain and stress experienced by the laboring woman. During labor there is an increase in maternal respirations and oxygen consumption, which decreases the amount of oxygen available to the fetus. In addition, the pain and stress can lead to metabolic acidosis and the release of catecholamine, which causes maternal blood vessels to constrict, lessening oxygen and nutrient supply to the fetus (Russell & Reynolds, 1997).

Many couples who have had childbirth education approach childbirth confident that the techniques they have learned will enable them to cope with the discomforts of labor. There is a good deal of peer pressure on expectant parents to have the "ideal" birth experience. They may plan a natural childbirth, and the need for analgesia may make them feel inadequate and guilty. The nurse has a very special role in helping a woman and her partner to accept alterations in their original plan and to recognize the unique qualities of their birth experience. Reassurance that accepting analgesia for discomfort is not a failure can help maintain the woman's self-esteem. The emphasis should be placed on achieving a healthy, satisfying outcome for the family.

## Systemic Drugs

The goal of pharmacologic analgesia during labor is to provide maximum pain relief at minimum risk for the mother and fetus. To reach this goal, clinicians must consider a number of factors, including the following:

- All systemic drugs used for pain relief during labor cross the placental barrier by simple diffusion, but some drugs cross more readily than others.
- Drug action in the body depends on the rate at which the substance is metabolized by liver enzymes and excreted by the kidneys.
- High drug doses may remain in the fetus for long periods because fetal liver enzymes and kidney excretion are inadequate for metabolizing analgesic agents.

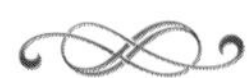

### Nursing Care Management

Analgesic drugs provide pain relief for the laboring woman but also affect the fetus and the labor process. Pain medication given too early may prolong labor and depress the fetus; if given too late it is of minimal use to the woman and may lead to respiratory depression in the newborn. The nurse assesses the mother and fetus and also evaluates the contraction pattern before administering prescribed systemic medications.

#### Maternal Assessment parameters include:

- The woman is willing to receive medication after being advised about it.
- Vital signs are stable.
- Contraindications (such as specific drug allergy, respiratory compromise, or current drug dependence) are not present.

#### Fetal Assessment parameters include:

- The fetal heart rate (FHR) baseline is between 120 and 160 beats per minute, and no late decelerations or nonreassuring FHR patterns are present.
- Short-term variability is present, and long-term variability is average.
- The fetus exhibits normal movement, and accelerations are present with fetal movement.
- The fetus is at term.

#### Assessment of Labor includes:

- Contraction pattern is well established.
- The cervix is dilated at least 4 to 5 cm in nulliparas and 3 to 4 cm in multiparas.
- The fetal presenting part is engaged.
- There is progressive descent of the fetal presenting part.

If normal parameters are absent, the nurse may need to complete further assessments with the physician or certified nurse-midwife (CNM).

Before administering the medication, the nurse once again ascertains whether the woman has a history of any drug reactions or allergies and provides information about the medication. (See Key Facts to Remember: What Women Need to Know about Pain Relief Medications.) After giving the medication, the nurse records the drug name, dose, route, and site, and the woman's blood pressure (BP) and pulse, on the FHR monitor strip and on the woman's records. If the woman is alone, side rails should be raised to provide safety. The nurse assesses the FHR for possible adverse effects of the medication.

When an analgesic medication is administered by intramuscular or subcutaneous route, it takes a few minutes for the effect to be felt. The nurse can continue with other supportive measures to enhance comfort, such as ensuring a quiet environment, providing a back rub or cool cloth, assisting with relaxation and visualization exercises, or providing therapeutic touch until the woman feels the effect of the medication. When the medication begins to take effect, the woman may sleep between contractions. This short period of rest helps her relax and can restore her energy. When an intravenous route is ordered by the certified nurse-midwife/physician, the effect of the drug will be felt within a few minutes, so if any change of position is necessary or if the woman needs to void, the nurse may suggest that these activities be completed before the drug administration. Some women may be so uncomfortable that they do not want anything except the medication. In this case, administering the medication first would be more helpful for the woman.

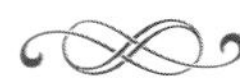

## Narcotic Analgesic: Butorphanol Tartrate (Stadol)

Butorphanol tartrate (Stadol) is a synthetic parenteral analgesic agent that can be given by the intramuscular or intravenous (IV) route. Its onset of action is rapid after IV injection, peak analgesia occurs in 30 to 60 minutes, and the duration is from 3 to 4 hours (Wilson, Shannon, & Strang, 2001). The recommended initial dose is 2 mg administered intramuscularly (IM) every 3 to 4 hours. If it is given IV, the dosage is reduced. Respiratory depression of both the mother and fetus or neonate can occur. The effects of butorphanol can be reversed with naloxone (Narcan). Butorphanol should not be used for women with a known opiate dependency and should be used with caution if drug dependence is suspected because it may precipitate withdrawal (Wilson et al., 2001).

Urinary retention following administration of butorphanol is not common but does occur. Therefore, the nurse should be alert for bladder distension when a woman has received butorphanol for analgesia during labor, has IV fluids infusing, and receives regional anesthesia for the birth. Butorphanol (Stadol) needs to be protected from light and stored at room temperature (Wilson et al., 2001).

### KEY FACTS TO REMEMBER

*What Women Need to Know about Pain Relief Medications*

Before receiving medications, the woman should understand the following:

- Type of medication administered
- Route of administration
- Expected effects of medication
- Implications for fetus or neonate
- Safety measures needed (e.g., remain in bed with side rails up)

## Opiate Antagonist: Naloxone (Narcan)

Since naloxone is an antagonist with little or no agonistic effect, it exhibits little pharmacologic activity in the absence of narcotics. Naloxone can be used to reverse the mild respiratory depression that follows administration of small doses of opiates. The drug is useful for respiratory depression caused by fentanyl, morphine, and meperidine, as well as butorphanol and nalbuphine hydrochloride. *Naloxone is the drug of choice when the depressant is unknown because it will cause no further depression* (Wilson et al., 2001). An initial dose of 0.4 to 2.0 mg may be administered intravenously to the laboring woman. Naloxone may be given to the newborn if needed after birth (Karch, 2001). (See Drug Guide: Naloxone Hydrochloride: Narcan, in Chapter 26.)

When naloxone is given, other resuscitative measures may be indicated, and trained personnel should be readily available. The duration of the drug's effect is shorter than that of the analgesic drug for which it is acting as an antagonist, so the nurse must be alert to the return of respiratory depression and the need for repeated doses. Naloxone should be given with caution in women with known or suspected opiate dependency because it may precipitate severe withdrawal (Way, Fields, & Way, 1998).

## Critical Thinking in Practice

Luisa Silva, a 33-year-old GI PO, is 32 weeks' pregnant. She is trying to decide whether she should accept any analgesia during her labor. She has finished childbirth education classes and wants an unmedicated labor and birth. She says, "I want to do this on my own, but I'm afraid it may be too much. Will it be OK if I need to take something?" What will you tell her?

Answers can be found in Appendix I

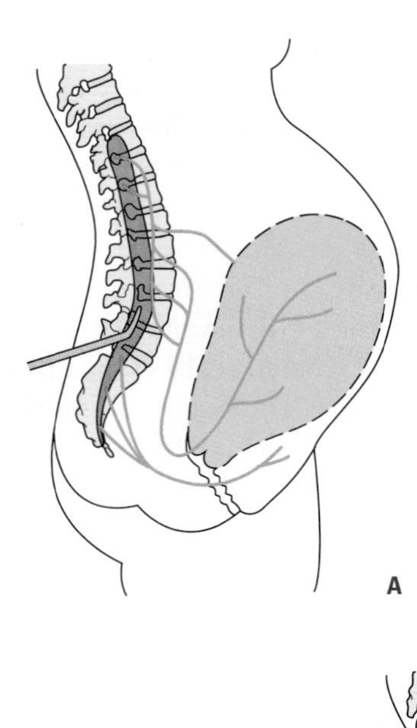


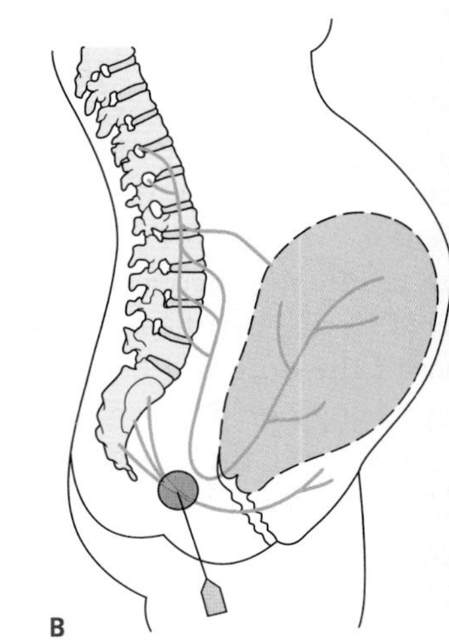


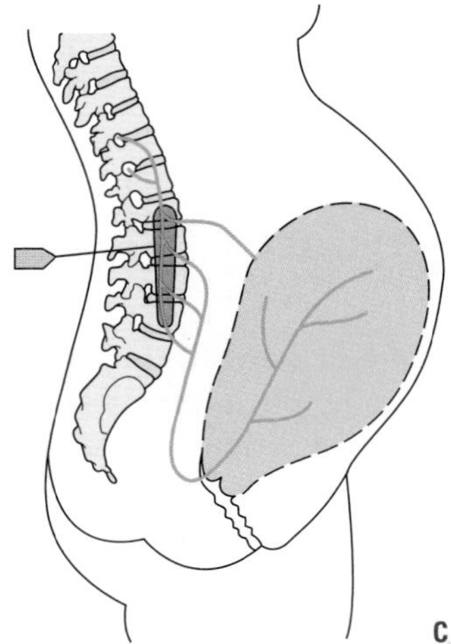


FIGURE 18–1 ♦ Schematic diagram showing pain pathways and sites of interruption. **A,** Lumbar epidural block: the dark area demonstrates peridural (epidural) space and nerves affected, and the gray tube represents a continuous plastic catheter. **B,** Pudendal block: relief of perineal pain. **C,** Lumbar sympathetic (spinal) block: relief of uterine pain only. *Source:* Bonica, J. J. (1972). *Principles and practice of obstetric analgesia and anesthesia* (pp. 492, 512, 521, 614). Philadelphia: Davis.

## Regional Anesthesia and Analgesia

**Regional anesthesia** is the temporary loss of sensation produced by injecting an anesthetic agent (called a local) into direct contact with nervous tissue. Loss of sensation happens because the local agents stabilize the cell membrane, which prevents initiation and transmission of nerve impulses. The regional anesthetic blocks most commonly used in childbirth include the epidural, spinal, and combined epidural-spinal blocks. Epidural blocks may be used for analgesia during labor and vaginal birth and for anesthesia during cesarean birth.

An epidural relieves pain associated with the first stage of labor by blocking the sensory nerves supplying the uterus. Pain associated with the second stage of labor and with birth can be alleviated with epidural, combined epidural-spinal, and pudendal blocks (see Figure 18–1♦).

Until the past few years, the same anesthetic agents used for regional epidurals were also used to produce **regional analgesia** (pain relief) during labor. This practice was problematic because the anesthetic agents used alter the transmission of impulses to the bladder, making voiding difficult. The agents also interfere with blood pressure stability and leg movement. In addition, the descent of the fetus may be slowed because of the woman's decreased ability to push during the second stage of labor (Fishburne, 1999). To address these difficulties, regional analgesia is now obtained by injecting a narcotic such as fentanyl along with only a small amount of local anesthetic agent. This approach relieves the woman's pain while minimizing side effects.

The *intrathecal* injection of narcotics results in another type of regional analgesia. In this case, the narcotic is injected into the subarachnoid space. Fentanyl citrate and preservative-free morphine are the most commonly used drugs. The woman's pain is usually relieved, but she may experience urinary retention, pruritus, nausea, and vomiting (Fishburne, 1999; Karch, 2001).

Nursing care during administration of regional analgesia is directed toward helping the woman void prior to the injection, assisting her with positioning during and after the procedure, monitoring and assessing vital signs and respiratory status, monitoring analgesic effect, and determining fetal well-being. Additional measures may be needed to address pruritus, nausea and vomiting, and urinary retention.

As with other procedures, the woman needs to know how the block is given, the expected effect on her and the fetus, advantages and disadvantages, and possible complications (Pattee, Ballantyne, & Milne, 1997). Many women discuss possible anesthetic blocks with their care provider at some point in the pregnancy. If they have not, it is important to give them an opportunity to ask questions and obtain information before receiving the block while in labor.

## Anesthetic Agents for Regional Blocks

Local anesthetic agents block the conduction of nerve impulses from the periphery to the central nervous system by preventing the propagation of an action potential from the source of pain (Russell & Reynolds, 1997). The types of nerve fibers are differentially sensitive to the various anesthetic agents. In general, the smaller the fiber, the more sensitive it is to local agents. For example, it is possible to block the small C and A delta fibers, which transmit pain and temperature, without blocking the larger A alpha, A beta, and A gamma fibers, which continue to maintain a sense of pressure, muscle tone, position sense, and motor function.

Absorption of local anesthetics depends primarily on the vascularity of the area of injection. The agents themselves contribute to increased blood flow by causing vasodilation. High concentrations of drugs cause greater vasodilation. Good maternal physical condition or a high metabolic rate aids absorption. Malnutrition, dehydration, electrolyte imbalance, and cardiovascular and pulmonary problems increase the potential for toxic effects. The pH of tissues affects the rate of absorption, which has implications for fetal complications such as acidosis. The addition of vasoconstrictors such as epinephrine delays absorption and prolongs the anesthetic effect. Epinephrine decreases uteroplacental blood flow, making it an undesirable additive in many situations. The breakdown of local anesthetics in the body is accomplished by the liver and plasma esterase, and the resulting substance is eliminated by the kidneys. It is important to use the weakest concentration and the smallest amount necessary to produce the desired results.

## Types of Local Anesthetic Agents

Three types of local anesthetic agents are currently available: esters, amides, and opiates. The ester type includes procaine hydrochloride (Novocain), chloroprocaine hydrochloride (Nesacaine), and tetracaine hydrochloride (Pontocaine). Esters are rapidly metabolized; therefore, toxic maternal levels are not as likely to be reached, and placental transfer to the fetus is prevented. Amide types include lidocaine hydrochloride (Xylocaine), mepivacaine hydrochloride (Carbocaine), and bupivacaine hydrochloride (Marcaine). Amide types are more powerful and longer-acting agents. They readily cross the placenta, can be measured in the fetal circulation, and affect the fetus for a prolonged period.

Opioids are used with epidural blocks for labor. Some of the agents used include morphine, fentanyl, butorphanol, and meperidine (Russell & Reynolds, 1997). When only opioids are used epidurally, rather than in combination with another type of agent, the amount of pain relief is not as effective, especially toward the end of labor; therefore, a combination of opioids and a low dose of local are given (Russell & Reynolds, 1997).

## Adverse Maternal Reactions to Anesthetic Agents

Reactions to local anesthetic agents range from mild symptoms to cardiovascular collapse. Mild reactions include palpitations, tinnitus, apprehension, confusion, and a metallic taste in the mouth. Moderate reactions include more severe degrees of mild symptoms plus nausea and vomiting, hypotension, and muscle twitching, which may progress to convulsions. Severe reactions are sudden loss of consciousness, coma, severe hypotension, bradycardia, respiratory depression, and cardiac arrest. Anesthetic agents should not be used unless an intravenous line is in place.

The preferred treatment for a mild toxic reaction is administration of oxygen and IV injection of a short-acting barbiturate to diminish anxiety. Nursing interventions for adverse reactions are included in the Critical Pathway for Epidural Anesthesia.

## Neonatal Neurobehavioral Effects of Anesthesia and Analgesia

Many studies have focused on the neurobehavioral effects on the newborn of pharmacologic agents used during labor and birth. Although analgesic and anesthetic agents

# CRITICAL PATHWAY: *For Epidural Anesthesia*

| Category | First Stage | Second and Third Stages | Fourth Stage<br>Birth to 1 Hour Past Birth |
|---|---|---|---|
| **Referral** | Review prenatal record<br>Advise CNM/physician of admission | Labor record for first stage | Report to recovery room nurse<br>**Expected Outcomes**<br>Appropriate resources identified and utilized |
| **Assessments** | Admission assessments:<br>Ask about problems since last prenatal visit; labor status (contraction frequency and duration cervical dilations, and effacement); membrane status; coping level; support; woman's desires during labor and birth; ability to verbalize needs; laboratory testing (blood and UA)<br>Woman's request for epidural<br>Intrapartal assessment: timing<br>*Latent Phase:*<br>• BP, P, R, q1h if in normal range (BP 90–140/60–90 or no increase >30mm Hg systolic or 15 mm Hg diastolic over baseline; pulse 60–90; respirations 12–20/min, quiet, easy)<br>• Temp q4h unless > 37.6°C (99.6°F) or membranes ruptured; then q2h. Uterine contractions q30min; contractions q5–10 min, 15–40 sec, mild intensity)<br>• FHR q60min (for low-risk women) and q30min for high-risk women if reassuring (FHR baseline 120–160, STV present, LTV average, accelerations with fetal movement, no late or variable decelerations); if nonreassuring, position on side, start $O_2$, assess for hypotension, monitor continuously, notify CNM or physician<br>*Active Phase:*<br>• BP, P, R, q1h if WNL<br>• Temp as in latent phase<br>• Uterine contractions assessed continuously<br>• FHR assessed continuously per EFM<br>• Pulse ox > 95%<br>*Transition:*<br>• BP, P, R, q30min if in normal range<br>• Uterie contractions q15–30 min<br>• FHR q30min (for low-risk women) and q15min (for high-risk women) if reassuring: if nonreassuring, see guidelines for latent phase<br>• Pulse ox > 95%<br>Cervical assessment: from 1 to 10 cm dilation; nullipara (1.2 cm/hr), multipara (1.5 cm/hr)<br>Cervical effacement: from 0% to 100%<br>Fetal descent: progressive descent from −4 to +4<br>Membrane assessment: when ruptured, Nitrazine positive, fluid clear, no foul odor<br>Behavioral characteristics: response to labor process, facial expressions, verbalizations, tone of voice, changes in behavior during contractions, body movement | Second-stage assessments:<br>• BP, P, R q5–15 min<br>• Uterine contractions palpated continuously<br>• FHR q15min (for low-risk women) and q5min (for high-risk women) if reassuring; if nonreassuring, monitor continuously<br>Fetal descent; descent continues to birth<br>Behavioral characteristics: response to pushing, facial expressions, verbalization<br>Third-stage assessments:<br>• BP, P, R q5min<br>• uterine contractions, palpate occasionally until placenta is delivered, fundus maintains tone, and contraction pattern continues to birth of placenta<br>Newborn assessments:<br>• Assess Apgar score of newborn<br>• Respirations: 30–60, irregular<br>• Apical pulse: 120–160 and somewhat irregular<br>• Temperature: skin temperature above 36.5°C (97.8°F)<br>• Umbilical cord: two arteries, one vein (if one artery, assess for anomalies and urine output)<br>• Gestational age: 38 to 42 weeks | Immediate postbirth assessments q15min for one hour<br>• BP: 90–140/60–90; should return to prelabor level<br>• Pulse: slightly lower than in labor; range is 60–90<br>• Respirations: 12–20/min; easy; quiet<br>• Temperature: 36.2–37.6°C (98–99.6°F)<br>• Fundus firm, in midline, at the umbilicus or 1–2 finger breadths below the umbilicus<br>• Lochia rubra; moderate amount; <1pad/hr; no free flow or passage of clots with massage<br>• Perineum; sutures intact; no bulging or marked swelling; minimal bruising may be present; no c/o severe pain or rectal pain<br>• Bladder nondistended; spontaneous void of >100 mL clear, straw-colored urine; bladder nondistended following voiding (catheterize if necessary)<br>• If hemorrhoids present, no tenseness or marked engorgement; <2 cm diameter<br>Comfort level: <3 on scale of 1 to 10<br>Energy level: awake and able to hold newborn<br>Newborn assessments if newborn remains with parents<br>• Respirations: 30–60; irregular<br>• Apical pulse: 120–160 and somewhat irregular<br>• Temperature: skin temp above 36.5°C (97.8°F); skin feels warm to touch<br>• Skin color noncyanotic<br>• Mucus: small amount, clear, easily suctioned with bulb syringe without skin color change<br>• Behavioral: newborn opens eyes widely if room is slightly darkened<br>• Movements rhythmic; no hand tremors present<br>**Expected Outcomes**<br>• Assessment findings indicate labor is progressing WNL, maternal vital signs stable and within establish parameters, and reassuring fetal heart rate<br>• Maternal-fetal well-being unimpaired |

BP, P, R, blood pressure, pulse, respirations; CNM certified nurse-midwife; EFM, electronic fetal monitor; FHR, fetal heart rate; IV, intravenous; IVP, intravenous push; LDR, labor, delivery, recovery; LTV, long-term variability; PRN, as needed or as desired; $O_2$, oxygen; OOB, out of bed; STV, short-term variability; temp, temperature; VS, vital signs; WNL, within normal limits; c/o, complaints of.

# CRITICAL PATHWAY *Continued*

| Category | First Stage | Second and Third Stages | Fourth Stage<br>Birth to 1 Hour Past Birth |
|---|---|---|---|
| **Teaching/psychosocial** | Establish rapport<br>Orient to environment, expected assessments and procedures<br>Answer questions and provide information; give emotional support<br>Orient to EFM<br>Teach relaxation, visualization, and breathing pattern if needed<br>Explain comfort measures available; provide information regarding the reason for the block, possible side effects and nursing care that may be expected<br>Assume advocacy role for woman and family during labor and birth<br>Explain possible delayed effects of anesthetic agents on fetus | Orient to expected assessments and procedures<br>Answer questions and provide information<br>Continue advocacy role<br>Instruct woman to maintain bed rest until full function of lower extremities returns | Explain immediate assessments and care after this first hour<br>Teach self-massage of fundus and expected findings<br>Instruct to call for assistance if mother desires to get OOB<br>Begin newborn teaching; bulb syringe, positioning, maintaining warmth<br>Assist with first breastfeeding experience<br>**Expected Outcomes**<br>Woman verbalizes or demonstrates understanding of teaching |
| **Nursing care management and reports** | Straight cath PRN if bladder is distended<br>If regional block administered monitor BP, FHR, sensation per protocol and obtain consent for procedure<br>Providing continuing status report<br>Perineal clip per woman's request<br>Small enema per woman's request<br>Perform sterile vaginal examination as indicated<br>Position woman correctly for regional block<br>Assess maternal status:<br>• Obtain baseline vital signs before any anesthetic agent is given<br>• Monitor blood pressure q1–2min for 10 min and then q5–15 min following administration of anesthetic agent<br>• Monitor pulse and respiration<br>• Monitor FHR continuously<br>Observe, record, and report complications of anesthesia, including hypotension, fetal stress, respiratory paralysis, changes in uterine contractility, decrease involuntary muscle effort, trauma to extremities, nausea and vomiting, and loss of bladder tone<br>Observe, record, and report symptoms of hypotension, including systolic pressure <100 mm Hg or a 20%–30% fall in systolic pressure, apprehension, restlessness, dizziness, tinnitus, headache<br>Initiate treatment measures:<br>• Place woman in left lateral position or position as directed, with the foot of the bed elevated<br>• Increase IV fluid rate<br>• Administer oxygen by face mask at 7–10 L/min as needed<br>• Administer vasopressors as ordered (usually ephedrine 5–15 mg IV)<br>• Manually displace uterus laterally to left<br>• Keep woman supine (semireclining) for 5–10 min following administration of block to allow drug to diffuse bilaterally; after 5–10 min position woman on side<br>Observe, record, and report fetal bardycardia (FHR <120bpm) and loss of beat-to-beat variability | Straight cath PRN if bladder distended<br>Continue monitoring VS, FHR, and sensation<br>Assess for potential probes of epidural infusion: sedation, nausea, vomiting, pruritus, hypotension, and breakthrough pain | Straight cath if bladder is distended<br>Monitor return of motor ability and sensation if regional block has been given<br>Weigh perineal pads if lochia flow >1 saturated pad in 1 hr; presence of boggy uterus and clots; decreased BP, increased P<br>**Expected Outcomes**<br>Mother and fetus experience safe labor and birth<br>Actual or potential complication identified and minimized<br>Woman and family actively participate in decision making and plan or care |

| Category | First Stage | Second and Third Stages | Fourth Stage Birth to 1 Hour Past Birth |
|---|---|---|---|
| **Activity** | Encourage ambulation unless contraindicated<br>Maintain bed rest immediately after administration of IV pain medication or following regional block<br>Woman rests comfortably between contractions | Position comfortably for birth<br>Woman rests comfortably between pushing efforts and while awaiting birth of placenta | Position of comfort<br>**Expected Outcomes**<br>Activity maintained per protocol; comfort and uterine perfusion enhanced by position or movement |
| **Comfort** | Woman states that she desires regional anesthesia<br>Assist with administration of epidural block | Second stage: assess and inform woman of progress of labor, provide reassurance throughout labor, assist with "sitting dose" reinjection for birth, offer encouragement, help support legs while pushing, ensure position of comfort for pushing and birth.<br>Third stage: cool cloth to forehead, assist parents to see newborn, position mother to hold newborn, provide encouragement | Institute comfort measures<br>Perineal discomfort: gently cleanse and apply ice pack; position to decrease pressure on perineum<br>Uterine discomfort; palpate fundus gently<br>Hemorrhoids: apply ice pack<br>General fatigue: ensure position of comfort, encourage rest<br>Administer pain medication<br>**Expected Outcomes**<br>Optimal comfort maintained |
| **Nutrition** | Ice chips and clear fluids<br>Evaluate for signs of dehydration | Ice chips and clear fluids | Regular diet if assessments are WNL<br>Encourage fluids<br>**Expected Outcomes**<br>Nutrition and hydration needs met |
| **Elimination** | Voids at least q2h; urine clear, straw colored, negative for protein<br>Bladder nondistended; empty before regional block administered<br>May have bowel movement<br>Monitor I & O with IVs | Monitor bladder at frequent intervals | Monitor bladder status with each assessment<br>**Expected Outcomes**<br>Intake and output WNL |
| **Medications** | Hydrate the woman receiving an epidural block with 500–1000 mL fluid prior to procedure (dextrose-free solution is recommended) | Local infiltration of anesthetic agent for birth by CNM or physician<br>Pitocin 10 units IM, IVP per IV tubing, or added to IV fluids | Continue Pitocin infusion<br>Administer pain medication<br>**Expected Outcomes**<br>Perfusion and hydration supported<br>Uterine hemorrhage prevented or successfully treated |
| **Discharge planning/home care** | Evaluate knowledge of labor and birth process<br>Evaluate support system and need for referral after birth | | Provide information if mother is to be moved from LDR room<br>Provide opportunity for parents to ask questions regarding newborn<br>Evaluate knowledge of normal postpartum, newborn care<br>**Expected Outcomes**<br>Individualized discharge teaching completed |
| **Family involvement** | Identify available support person(s)<br>Recognize possible impact of culture on responses<br>Observe interaction between woman and partner<br>Create moment alone with woman to identify possible abuse<br>Assess current parent skills | Provide opportunities for woman and support person(s) to watch newborn assessments<br>Perform newborn assessment on mother's abdomen or chest if possible | Provide opportunity for parents to be with baby<br>Encourage skin-to-skin contact<br>Darken room to encourage eye-to-eye contact<br>Provide quiet time for new family<br>Parenting: demonstrates early culturally expected parenting behaviors<br>**Expected Outcomes**<br>Family demonstrates support of family members<br>Family able to identify supportive resources in the community |
| **Date** | | | |

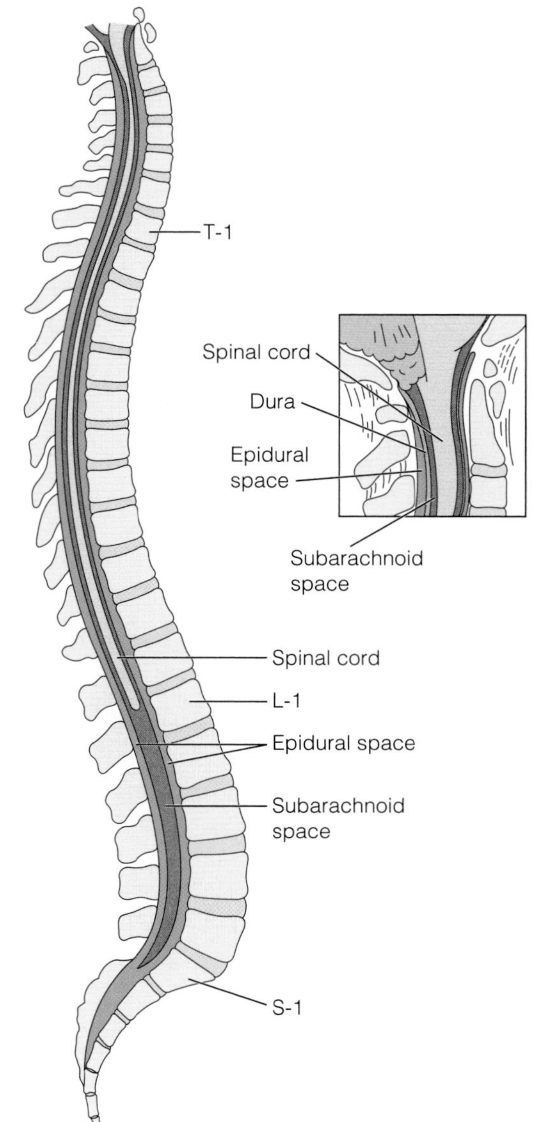


**FIGURE 18–2** ♦ The epidural space is between the dura mater and the ligamentum flavum, extending from the base of the skull to the end of the sacral canal.

may alter the behavioral and adaptive function of the newborn, physiologic factors such as hunger, degree of hydration, and time within the sleep-wake cycle may also exert an influence (Ezekiel, 1997).

## Epidural Block

A lumbar **epidural block** involves injection of an anesthetic agent into the epidural space to provide pain relief throughout labor. The epidural space, a potential space between the dura mater and the ligamentum flavum, is accessed through the lumbar area (Figure 18–2♦). The epidural is most frequently used as a continuous block to provide analgesia and anesthesia from active labor through episiotomy repair (Figure 18–3♦).

Epidurals have become a relatively common method of analgesia and anesthesia during labor and birth in the United States. An epidural can be given as soon as active labor is established (Holt, Diehl, & Wright, 1999). Insurance providers have limited some women's access to epidural anesthesia; however, the American College of Obstetricians and Gynecologists (ACOG) believes that a woman's request is sufficient justification for providing an epidural (ACOG, 1997).

### Advantages

The epidural block relieves discomfort during labor and birth, and the woman is fully awake and a part of the birth process. The continuous epidural allows different blocking for each stage of labor, so that the fetus is able to descend and rotate in the maternal pelvis; many times the woman's urge to bear down is preserved.

### Disadvantages

The most common complication of an epidural block is maternal hypotension, which is generally prevented by intravenous fluid administration, left uterine displacement, and maternal positioning on her side. In some instances, labor progress and fetal descent may be slowed, pushing efforts in the second stage may be less effective, and the use of forceps or a vacuum extractor is more common (Main, Main, & Moore, 2000). Delay in return of bladder sensation may result in the need for catheterization during labor and in the fourth stage.

### Contraindications

The absolute contraindications for epidural block are client refusal, infection at the site of the needle puncture, maternal problems with blood coagulation (coagulopathies), specific drug allergy to the agent being used, and hypovolemic shock (Russell & Reynolds, 1997).

## Nursing Care Management

Assessment of the woman's knowledge level about an epidural block is essential. Before providing information, the nurse determines the woman's current knowledge and evaluates factors related to learning, such as primary language spoken, ability to hear and interpret information, and the presence of anxiety. If the woman is not able to understand because of a language barrier or inability to hear, the nurse must locate and provide an interpreter. Although the nurse is an integral person in providing information, the anesthesiologist is the essential person to provide information to obtain written informed consent.

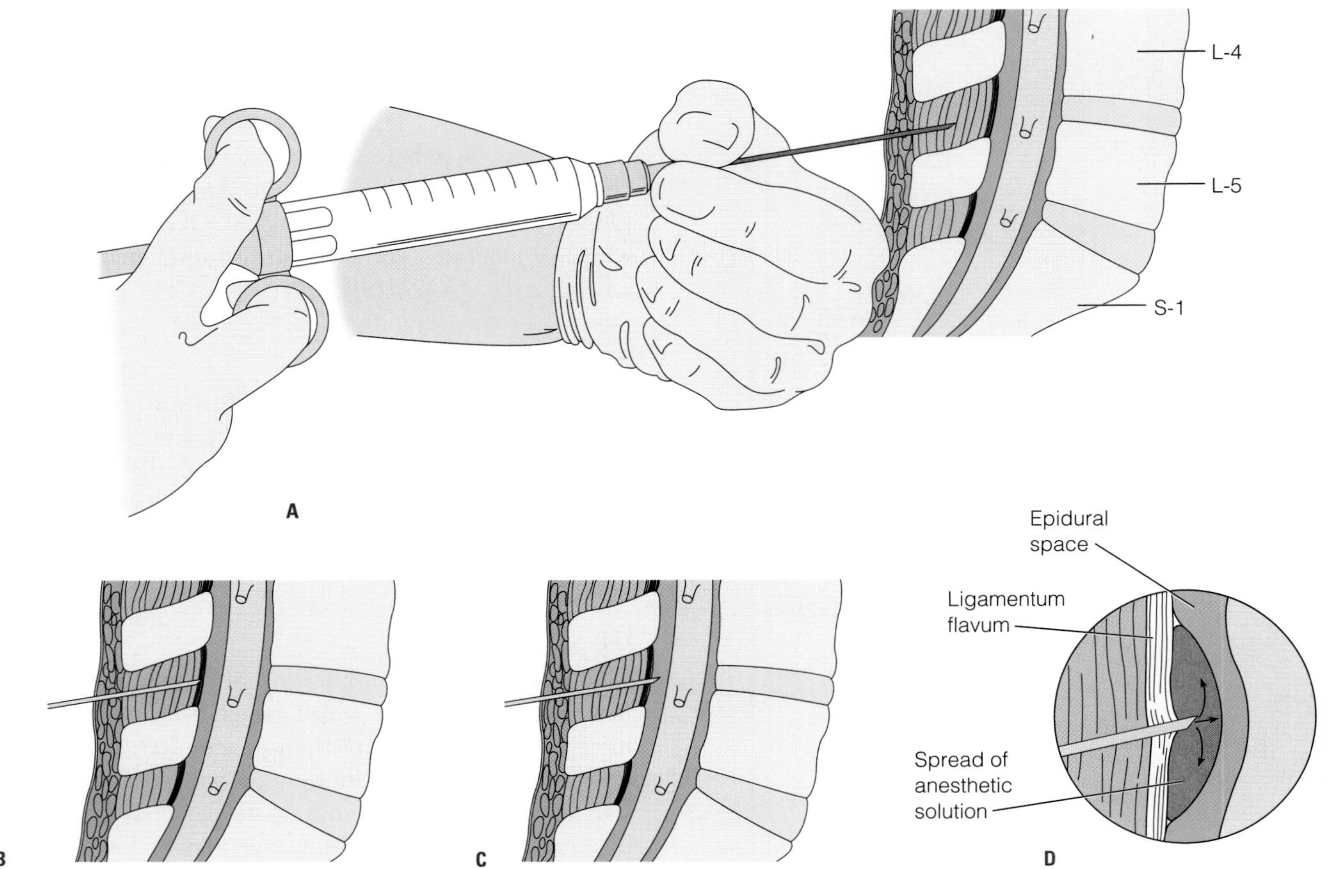


FIGURE 18–3 ♦ Technique for lumbar epidural block. **A,** Proper position of insertion. **B,** Needle in the ligamentum flavum. **C,** Tip of needle in epidural space. **D,** Force of injection pushing dura away from tip of needle. *Source:* Bonica, J. J. (1972). *Principles and practice of obstetric analgesia and anesthesia* (p. 631). Philadelphia: Davis.

In preparation for the epidural, the nurse encourages the woman to empty her bladder, because the block may interfere with her ability to void. The nurse assesses maternal blood pressure, pulse, and respirations and FHR to determine that normal parameters are present and to establish a baseline. Continuous electronic fetal monitoring to assess fetal status and frequent monitoring of maternal blood pressure and pulse for hypotension are essential. An intravenous infusion is usually begun with an 18-gauge plastic indwelling catheter. A large-gauge catheter is used so that IV fluids can be administered quickly if hypotension occurs. A bolus of 500 to 1000 mL of IV fluid is given before beginning the epidural block.

The nurse assists the woman into a side-lying position at the edge of the bed, where the mattress is firmer and provides more support. The woman's head is supported with a small pillow so it remains in alignment with the spine. A pillow may also be placed in front of her chest to provide support for her upper arm. Her back needs to remain straight, with the shoulders square. Her legs are bent and her knees kept together so that the upper hip does not roll forward and cause the spine to twist. The block may also be given with the woman in a sitting position, with her back arched and her feet supported on a stool. After positioning, the nurse continues to provide support and tries to ensure that the woman does not move during the procedure. After the block is administered, maternal vital signs are assessed frequently per protocol until the block wears off. The blood pressure can be monitored by a mechanical blood pressure device or by the nurse directly. The vital signs are recorded on the fetal monitor strip and/or on the client record. The nurse encourages the woman to maintain a side-lying position to maximize uteroplacental blood flow and changes her position (from side to side) frequently to increase circulation, promote comfort, and avoid a one-sided block. The nurse should assess the woman's ability to lift her legs and her level of sensation every 30 minutes to monitor the effects of the nerve block.

The nurse assesses the woman's bladder for distension at frequent intervals because the epidural block lessens the urge to urinate. During the second stage of labor, the woman with an epidural block may need assistance with pushing. The nurse may need to tell the woman when contractions begin and give extra assistance by holding her legs during pushing efforts. The woman's

## HINTS FOR PRACTICE

### Dermatome Sensation Levels

An important assessment following the administration of regional blocks, such as the epidural, is the location and degree of lost sensation. Landmarks (called dermatomes) can be used to measure and document where these sensory levels begin and end. Some useful tips include the following:

- Use dermatome level charts.
- Use a cool alcohol prep pad to check for areas and levels of sensation.
- Assess dermatome levels approximately every 30 minutes.
- Evaluate the level of anesthesia. The anesthesia level is too high if the patient reports numbness in her chest, face, or tongue or any difficulty breathing. Be alert for statements such as "I feel like I can't take a full breath" or "My tongue feels funny."

legs need to be protected from pressure applied to them while sensation is diminished.

The most common side effect of epidural regional block is hypotension. The risk of hypotension can be minimized by a preload fluid bolus of crystalloid solution (Ezekiel, 1997). If hypotension occurs, the nurse increases the IV flow rate (to increase intravascular volume and raise the blood pressure), ensures or verifies left uterine displacement (to increase circulation), and administers oxygen (to improve oxygenation). If blood pressure is not restored in 1 to 2 minutes the nurse administers ephedrine, 5 to 10 mg IV, per physician order (Fishburne, 1999). The nurse also continuously assesses FHR to monitor fetal effects.

The epidural may cause elevation of maternal temperature (pyrexia). Pyrexia may be confused with maternal infection and frequently results in additional testing of the newborn to rule out infection (Bowes, 1999).

Headache (which may occur with spinal blocks) is not a side effect of epidural anesthesia because the dura mater of the spinal canal has not been penetrated and there is no leakage of spinal fluid. Therefore, lying flat for a prescribed number of hours after birth is not necessary. Motor control of the legs is weak but not totally absent after birth. Return of complete sensation and the ability to control the legs are essential before ambulation is attempted. Recovery may take several hours, depending on the anesthetic agent and the dose given.

To assess sensation the nurse can touch various parts of the woman's legs and abdomen bilaterally to determine if the touch can be felt. The nurse can evaluate motor control by asking the woman to raise her knees, to lift her feet (one at a time) off the bed, or to dorsiflex her foot. Even though assessments may indicate that sensation and motor control have returned, the nurse needs to be ready to support the woman's weight as she stands and quickly return her to bed if motor control is inadequate. In addition, blood pressure assessments help the nurse determine the safety of ambulation. The nurse assesses blood pressure while the woman is lying down, then sitting in the bed. As long as blood pressure values remain stable (no evidence of orthostatic hypotension), a standing blood pressure is assessed. It is advisable to have additional assistance when the woman stands for the first time, to maintain safety.

## Continuous Epidural Infusion

Epidural anesthesia may be given with a continuous infusion pump. Some of the benefits include good to excellent analgesia, infrequent nausea, minimal sedation, decreased anxiety, earlier mobilization, retained cough reflex, decreased risk of deep vein thrombosis, decreased myocardial oxygen demand, and ease of administration.

Obviously, ease of administration does not imply lack of need for close observation. Malfunctioning equipment with subsequent overdose is always a possibility. Fortunately, infusion pumps designed specifically for use in epidural anesthesia have safety factors incorporated. Continuous epidural infusions should be administered with the same precautions used for intermittent injections.

Some of the potential problems of epidural infusions include breakthrough pain, sedation, nausea and vomiting, pruritus, and hypotension. Breakthrough pain may occur at any time during the epidural infusion but usually occurs when the infusion rate of the agent is below the recommended therapeutic rate. It may also occur when the infusion pump rate is altered or the integrity of the epidural line is broken. When breakthrough pain occurs, the nurse checks the integrity of the epidural infusion line and notifies the anesthesiologist or nurse anesthetist. There may be standing orders for treatment of breakthrough pain, but it is best to inform the anesthesiologist of any problems that occur.

General sedation and resulting respiratory depression may occur from the systemic effect of the epidural agents as they are absorbed into the circulation. The respiratory rate, along with the quality of respirations, should be assessed no less frequently than every 15 to 30 minutes. The nurse should notify the anesthetist of any significant decreases in respiratory rate or respiratory pattern change. If respiratory rate decreases below 14 respirations per minute, naloxone may be given to counteract the effect of the anesthetic agent; typically respirations then return to a normal rate.

Nausea and vomiting can occur at any time during or after epidural infusion. The nurse should give an antiemetic if one is ordered and notify the anesthesiologist. The nausea and vomiting can make the woman very uncomfortable, and the infusion rate of the epidural may need to be decreased or terminated to alleviate this discomfort.

Pruritus (itching and rash) may occur at any time during the epidural infusion. It usually appears first on the face, neck, or torso and is usually the result of the agent in the epidural infusion. Treatment generally involves administration of diphenhydramine hydrochloride (Benadryl). If no standing order exists, the nurse notifies the anesthetist and identifies the problem. The epidural infusion may need to be decreased or terminated.

Hypotension may occur from hypovolemia or from the effect of the epidural. Treatment involves administering oxygen by mask, administering a bolus of crystalloid fluid, and notifying the anesthetist. Usually standing orders for treatment of hypotension are graded in terms of the degree of hypotension. The epidural infusion may have to be terminated and the woman placed in the Trendelenburg position. See the Critical Pathway for Epidural Anesthesia for further nursing assessment and interventions.

## Epidural Narcotic Analgesia after Birth

To provide analgesia for approximately 24 hours after the birth, the anesthesiologist may inject an opioid, such as morphine sulfate (Duramorph), into the epidural space immediately after the birth. The analgesic effect begins approximately 30 to 60 minutes after the injection. The side effects include pruritus, nausea and vomiting, and urinary retention (*PDR Nurse's Handbook,* 2001).. The onset seems to occur early, and it resolves within 14 to 16 hours after the birth. (See Drug Guide: Postbirth Epidural Morphine.)

## Spinal Block

In a **spinal block,** a local anesthetic agent is injected directly into the spinal fluid in the spinal canal to provide anesthesia for cesarean birth and occasionally for vaginal birth. The technique of administration varies depending on whether the spinal block is being given for a cesarean or vaginal birth (Figure 18–4♦).

### Advantages

The advantages of spinal block are immediate onset of anesthesia, relative ease of administration, a need for smaller drug volume, and maternal compartmentalization of the drug.

### Disadvantages

The primary disadvantage of spinal block is blockade of sympathetic nerve fibers, resulting in a high incidence of hypotension; maternal hypotension may lead to fetal hypoxia. In addition, uterine tone is maintained, which makes intrauterine manipulation difficult.

### Contraindications

Contraindications for spinal block include severe hypovolemia, regardless of the cause; central nervous system disease; infection over the puncture site; allergy to local anesthetic agents; coagulation problems; and client refusal (Cunningham, MacDonald, Gant, et al., 1997).

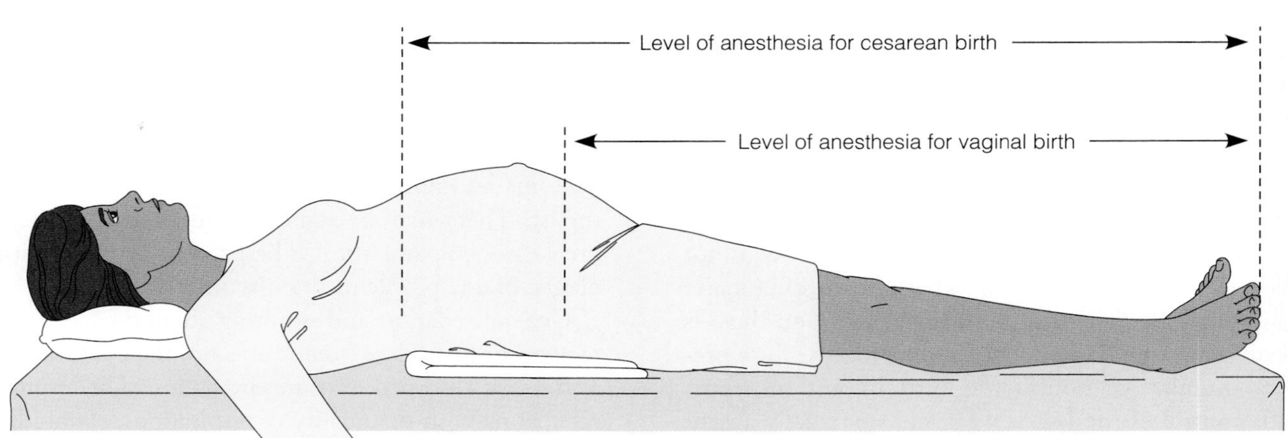


FIGURE 18–4 ♦ Levels of anesthesia for vaginal and cesarean births. *Source:* Reprinted with permission of Ross Laboratories, Columbus, OH. From Clinical Education Aid No. 17.

# DRUG GUIDE

## POSTBIRTH EPIDURAL MORPHINE

### *Overview of Action*

Epidural morphine is used to provide relief of pain associated with cesarean birth, extensive episiotomies (mediolaterals), or third- and fourth-degree lacerations. Epidural morphine pain relief results directly from its effect on the opiate receptors in the spinal cord (it depresses pain impulse transmission). Morphine binds opiate receptors, thereby altering both the perception of and the emotional response to pain. Women experience little or no discomfort or pain during recovery and for up to 24 hours afterward. There is no motor or sympathetic block or associated hypotension. Onset of analgesia is slower, but duration is longer.

### *Dosage, Route*

5–10 mg of morphine is injected through a catheter into the epidural space, providing relief for about 24 hours (Wilson, Shannon, & Strang, 2001).

### *Maternal Contraindications*

Hypersensitivity to opiates

Narcotic addiction

Chronic debilitating respiratory disease

Reduced blood volume

### *Maternal Side Effects*

Late-onset respiratory depression (rare but may occur 8–12 hours after administration)

Nausea and vomiting (occurring between 4 and 7 hours after injection)

Itching (begins within 3 hours and lasts up to 10 hours)

Urinary retention

Somnolence (rarely)

Side effects can be managed with naloxone (Cunningham et al., 1997)

### *Effect on Fetus or Neonate*

No adverse effects since medication is injected after birth of baby

### *Nursing Considerations*

Assess client's sensitivity to narcotics on admission.

Monitor and evaluate analgesic effect. Ask client about comfort level and notify anesthesiologist of inadequate pain relief.

If present, check epidural catheter for obvious knots, breaks, and leakage at insertion site and catheter hub.

Assess for pruritus (scratching and rubbing, especially around the face and neck).

Administer comfort measures for narcotic-induced pruritus, such as lotion, back rubs, cool or warm packs, or diversional activities. If the itching can be tolerated, naloxone should be avoided, especially because it counteracts the pain relief.

If allergic reaction (urticaria, edema, or respiratory difficulties) occurs, administer naloxone or diphenhydramine per physician order.

Provide comfort measures for nausea or vomiting, such as frequent oral hygiene or gradual increase in activity; administration of naloxone, trimethobenzamide, or metoclopramide HCl per physician order.

Assess postural blood pressure and heart rate before ambulation.

Assist client with her first ambulation and then as needed.

Assess respiratory function frequently for the first 24 hours, then every 2–8 hours as needed. Also assess level of consciousness and mucous membrane color. May need to monitor client via apnea monitor for 24 hours and use continuous pulse oximetry.

Monitor urinary output and assess bladder for distension. Assist client to void.

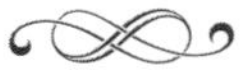

## Nursing Care Management

If an intravenous infusion is not already in place, it is started with a 16- to 18-gauge plastic catheter, and a bolus of 500 to 1000 mL is infused rapidly. The nurse assesses maternal vital signs and the FHR to establish a baseline and then positions the woman in a sitting position (or a side-lying position). The woman sits on the side of the bed or operating room table and places her feet on a stool. The woman places her arms between her knees or up around the nurse's shoulders, bows her head, and arches her back to widen the intervertebral spaces. The nurse supports the woman in this position and palpates the uterus to identify the beginning of uterine contractions (if labor is present). The physician injects the anesthetic agent between contractions. If the anesthetic agent is injected during a contraction, the level of anesthesia obtained is higher and may compromise respirations.

The woman remains in a sitting position for 30 seconds and then returns to a lying position, with a rolled towel or blanket under her right hip to displace the uterus from the vena cava. The nurse monitors maternal blood pressure and pulse frequently per protocol or physician's order. The blood pressure is also reassessed when the woman is moved after birth, because movement may lower blood pressure.

If the spinal block is being used during vaginal birth, the nurse monitors uterine contractions and instructs the woman to bear down during a contraction. The block usually reduces the woman's ability to push, and the birth may be assisted with forceps or vacuum extractor (see Chapter 20).

After birth, the temporary motor paralysis of the woman's legs continues. The nurse needs to exercise caution when moving the woman from the birthing bed (or operating room table) to protect her from injury. The woman remains flat in bed for 6 to 12 hours following the block; she may not regain sensation and control of her bladder for 8 to 12 hours and may need to be catheterized. An indwelling bladder catheter is usually inserted before surgery for women undergoing cesarean birth.

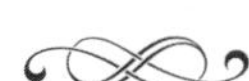

## Combined Spinal-Epidural Block

Spinal anesthesia may be combined with an epidural block. The combined spinal-epidural (CSE) block can be used for labor analgesia and for cesarean birth. The anesthetic and analgesic agents used differ according to the purpose of the CSE block. A CSE is accomplished by inserting an epidural needle into the epidural space. A narrow-gauge atraumatic (24- to 27-gauge pencil point) needle is inserted through the epidural needle, through the dura, and into the cerebral spinal fluid. A small amount of local anesthetic agent, opioid, or both is injected, and the atraumatic needle is withdrawn. An epidural catheter is then threaded through the epidural needle and into the epidural space. The epidural needle is removed, and the epidural catheter is secured.

An advantage of CSE block is that the spinal (intrathecal) anesthetic and/or analgesic agent has a faster onset than medications that are injected into the epidural space. Most drugs are used in low dose, so spinal analgesia may be given in early labor to assist in alleviating labor pain. The epidural is activated when active labor begins (Ezekiel, 1997).

## Pudendal Block

A **pudendal block,** administered by a transvaginal method, intercepts signals to the pudendal nerve. The pudendal block provides perineal anesthesia for the latter part of the first stage of labor, the second stage, birth, and episiotomy repair. The pudendal block relieves the pain of perineal distension but not the discomfort of uterine contractions (Figure 18–5♦).

Advantages of the pudendal block are ease of administration and absence of maternal hypotension. It also may be used to decrease the discomfort of low forceps or vacuum-assisted birth. Because a pudendal block does not alter maternal vital signs or FHR, additional assessments are not necessary. The nurse explains the procedure and answers any questions.

The disadvantages of the pudendal block include possible broad ligament hematoma, perforation of the rectum, and trauma to the sciatic nerve. A moderate dose of anesthetic agent has minimal ill effects on the course of labor, but the urge to push may decrease.

## Local Infiltration Anesthesia

**Local anesthesia** is accomplished by injecting an anesthetic agent into the intracutaneous, subcutaneous, and intramuscular areas of the perineum (Figure 18–6♦). It is generally used at the time of birth, both in preparation for an episiotomy if one is needed and for the episiotomy repair. Women who have followed some type of prepared childbirth method and want minimal analgesia and anesthesia usually do not object to local anesthesia for the episiotomy. The administration procedure is technically uncomplicated and is practically free from complications.

A disadvantage of local infiltration is that large amounts of local anesthetic must be used to infuse the tissues. Although any local anesthetic may by used,

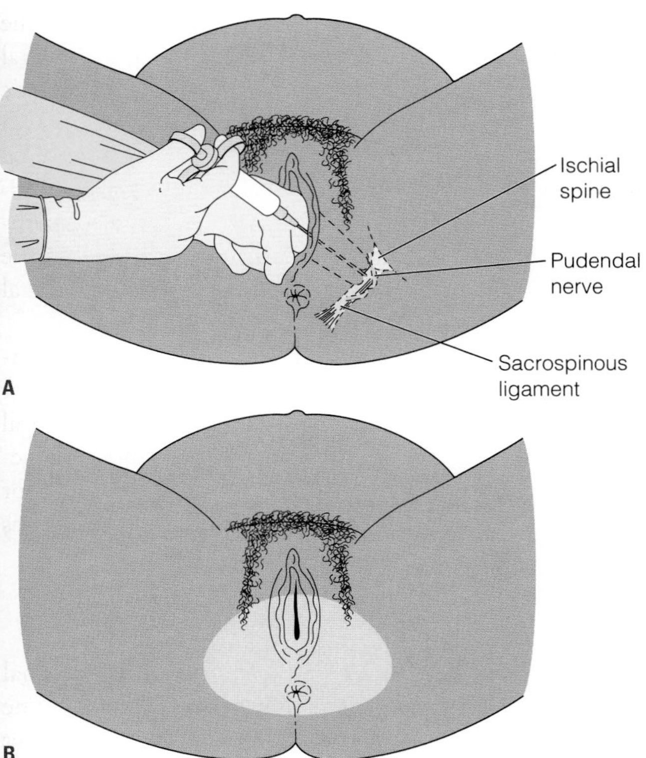


FIGURE 18–5 ♦ **A**, Pudendal block by the transvaginal approach. **B**, Area of perineum affected by pudendal block.

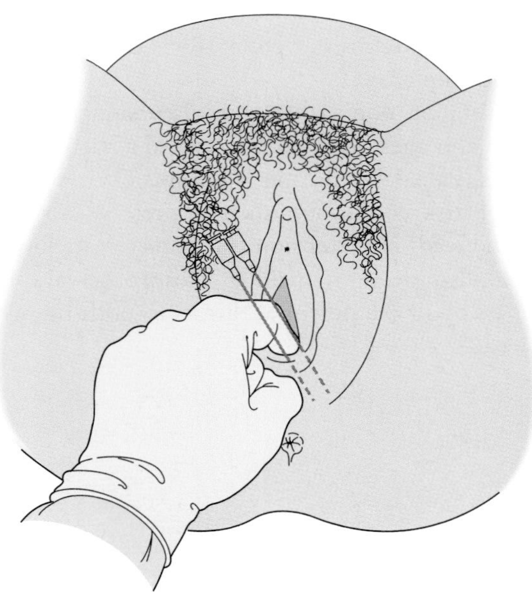

FIGURE 18–6 ♦ Technique of local infiltration for episiotomy and repair. *Source:* Bonica, J. J. (1972). *Principles and practice of obstetric analgesia and anesthesia* (p. 505). Philadelphia: Davis.

chloroprocaine hydrochloride (Nesacaine), lidocaine hydrochloride (Xylocaine), and mepivacaine hydrochloride (Carbocaine) are the agents of choice because of their capacity for diffusion. Because local anesthetic agents have no effect on maternal vital signs or FHR, additional assessments are unnecessary.

# General Anesthesia

Occasionally, **general anesthesia** (induced unconsciousness) may be needed for cesarean birth and for surgical intervention with some complications. The method used to achieve general anesthesia is usually a combination of intravenous injection and inhalation of anesthetic agents.

## Complications of General Anesthesia

A primary danger of general anesthesia is fetal depression. Most general anesthetic agents reach the fetus in about 2 minutes. The depression in the fetus is directly proportional to the depth and duration of the anesthesia. The poor fetal metabolism of general anesthetic agents is similar to that of analgesic agents administered during labor. General anesthesia is not advocated when the fetus is considered to be at high risk, particularly in preterm birth.

The majority of general anesthetic agents cause some degree of uterine relaxation. They may also cause vomiting and aspiration. Since pregnancy results in decreased gastric motility, and the onset of labor halts the process almost entirely, food eaten hours earlier may remain undigested in the stomach. The nurse must find out when the laboring woman last ate and record this information on the client's chart and on her anesthesia record. Even when food and fluids have been withheld, the gastric juice produced during fasting is highly acidic and can cause chemical pneumonitis if aspirated.

## Nursing Care during General Anesthesia

Prophylactic antacid therapy to reduce the acidic content of the stomach before general anesthesia is common practice. A nonparticulate antacid (such as bicitra) is often used. Cimetidine (Tagamet) has also been suggested by some anesthesiologists (Cunningham et al., 1997).

Before induction of anesthesia, the nurse places a wedge under the woman's right hip to displace the uterus and prevent vena caval compression in the supine position. The woman should also be preoxygenated with 3 to 5 minutes of 100% oxygen. Intravenous fluids are started so that access to the intravascular system is immediately available.

During the process of rapid induction of anesthesia, the nurse applies cricoid pressure to occlude the esophagus and prevent possible aspiration; the esophagus is occluded by depressing the cricoid cartilage 2 to 3 cm posteriorly. Cricoid pressure is maintained until the anesthesiologist has placed the endotracheal tube and indicates that the pressure can be released. Figure 18–7♦ shows the appropriate technique.

It should be noted that this discussion of obstetric analgesia and anesthesia applies only to a healthy woman and fetus. Pain relief during labor and birth for women with high-risk conditions, such as preterm labor, pregnancy-induced hypertension or diabetes mellitus, requires skilled decision making, close observation, and awareness of all the potential threats to both the woman and her baby.

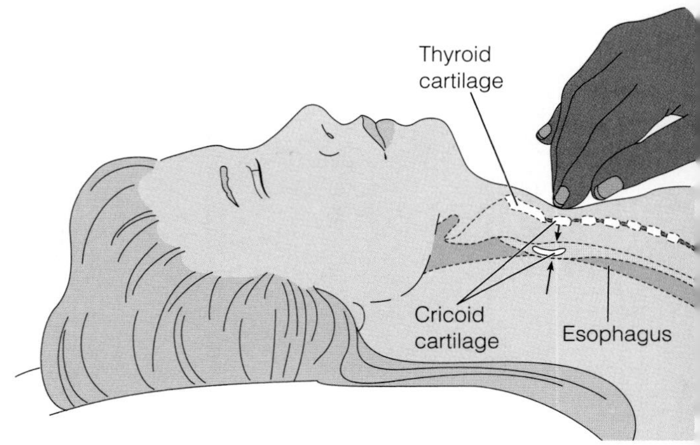


**FIGURE 18–7** ♦ Proper position for fingers in applying cricoid pressure until a cuffed endotracheal tube is placed by the anesthesiologist or certified nurse anesthetist. The cricoid cartilage is depressed 2 to 3 cm posteriorly so that the esophagus is occluded.

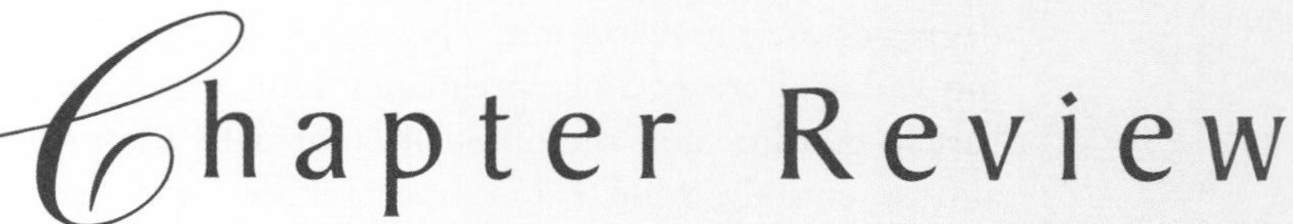

# Chapter Review

## CHAPTER HIGHLIGHTS

- Pain relief during labor may be enhanced by childbirth preparation methods and by the administration of analgesics and/or regional anesthesia blocks.
- The goal of pharmacologic pain relief during labor is to provide maximum analgesia with minimal risk for the mother and fetus.
- The best time for administering analgesia is determined after a complete assessment. An analgesic agent is generally administered to nulliparas when the cervix has dilated 4 to 5 cm and to multiparas when the cervix has dilated 3 to 4 cm.
- Analgesic agents include a variety of drugs, such as butorphanol tartrate (Stadol) and nalbuphine hydrochloride (Nubain).
- Narcotic antagonists (such as naloxone) counteract the respiratory depressant effect of the opiate narcotics by acting at specific receptor sites in the CNS.
- Regional analgesia and anesthesia are achieved by injecting local anesthetic agents into an area that will bring the agent into direct contact with nerve tissue. Methods most commonly used in childbearing include epidural block, spinal block, pudendal block, and local infiltration.
- Three types of local anesthetic agents used in regional blocks are the amides, esters, and opiates.
- Adverse reactions of the woman to local anesthetic agents range from mild symptoms such as palpitations to cardiovascular collapse.
- Complications of general anesthesia include fetal depression, uterine relaxation, vomiting, and aspiration.
- The choice of analgesia and anesthesia for the high-risk woman and fetus requires careful evaluation.

# CHAPTER REFERENCES


American College of Obstetrics and Gynecologists. (1997). *Guidelines for perinatal care* (4th ed.). Washington, DC: Author.

Bowes, W. A. (1999). Clinical aspects of normal and abnormal labor. In R. K. Creasy & R. Resnik (Eds.), *Maternal-fetal medicine* (4th ed., pp. 541–568). Philadelphia: Saunders.

Cunningham, F. G., MacDonald, P. C., Gant, N. F., Leveno, K. J., Gilstrap, L. C., Hankins, D. V., & Clark, S. L. (1997). *Williams obstetrics* (20th ed.). Stamford, CT: Appleton & Lange.

Ezekiel, M. R. (1997). *Handbook of anesthesiology.* Laguna Hills, CA: Current Clinical Strategies Publishing.

Fishburne, J., Jr. (1999). Obstetric analgesia and anesthesia. In J. R. Scott, P. J. DiSaia, C. B. Hammond, & W. N. Spellacy (Eds.), *Danforth's obstetrics and gynecology* (8th ed., pp. 111–129). Philadelphia: Lippincott, Williams & Wilkins.

Holt, R. O., Diehl, S. J., & Wright, J. (1999). Station and cervical dilation at epidural placement in predicting cesarean risk. *Obstetrics and Gynecology, 93,* 281–284.

Karch, A. M. (2001). *Lippincott's nursing drug guide.* Philadelphia: Lippincott Williams & Wilkins.

Main, D. M., Main, E. K., & Moore, D. H. (2000). The relationship between maternal care and uterine dysfunction: A continuous effect throughout reproductive life. *American Journal of Obstetrics and Gynecology, 182* (6), 1312–1317.

*PDR nurse's handbook.* (2001). Montvale, NJ: Demar Publishers.

Pattee, C., Ballantyne, M., & Milne, B. (1997). Epidural analgesia for labour and delivery: Informed consent issues. *Canadian Journal of Anesthesia, 44*(9), 918–923.

Russell, R., & Reynolds, F. (1997). Pain relief and anesthesia during labor. In R. K. Creasy (Ed.), *Management of labor and delivery* (pp. 183–222). Malden, MA: Blackwell.

Way, W., Fields, H. L., & Way, E. L. (1998). Opioid analgesics and antagonists. In B. G. Katzung (Ed.), *Basic and clinical pharmacology* (7th ed., pp. 512–513). Stamford, CT: Appleton & Lange.

Wilson, B. A., Shannon, M. T., & Strang, C. L. (Eds.). (2001). *Nursing drug guide: 2001.* Upper Saddle River, NJ: Prentice-Hall.


# CONTEMPORARY MATERNAL-NEWBORN NURSING ON-LINE

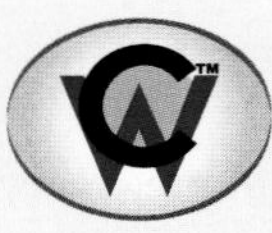

Additional interactive resources, including animations and video, for this chapter can be found on the Companion Website at http://www.prenhall.com/ladewig. Click on Chapter 18 and "Begin" to select the activities for this chapter.

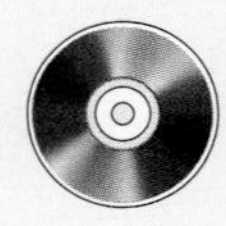

For NCLEX review questions and an audio glossary, access the accompanying CD-ROM in this book.

Chapter 19

# Childbirth at Risk

*I am very conscientious about making sure that I cover "unexpected outcomes" in my childbirth preparation classes. Although everyone hopes and anticipates that labor and birth will proceed normally, unfortunately it sometimes doesn't. At those times, when the family is anxious or afraid, maybe somewhere in the back of their minds is a little seed of reassurance because we have already talked about problems a little.*

—Labor/Delivery Nurse and Childbirth Educator(CBE)

## KEY TERMS

| Term | Page |
|---|---|
| Abruptio placentae | 477 |
| Active management of labor (AMOL) | 460 |
| Amniotic fluid embolism | 484 |
| Cephalopelvic disproportion (CPD) | 489 |
| Dystocia | 457 |
| Hydramnios | 487 |
| Intrauterine fetal death (IUFD) | 475 |
| Intrauterine resuscitation | 472 |
| Macrosomia | 470 |
| Oligohydramnios | 488 |
| Persistent occiput-posterior (POP) position | 464 |
| Placenta previa | 479 |
| Postterm pregnancy | 463 |
| Precipitous labor | 462 |
| Prolapsed umbilical cord | 482 |

## OBJECTIVES

- Describe the psychologic factors that may contribute to complications during labor and birth.
- Explain dysfunctional labor patterns.
- Describe the possible impact of postterm pregnancy on the childbearing family.
- Relate the various types of fetal malposition and malpresentation to the possible associated problems.
- Discuss the identification, management, and care of fetal macrosomia.
- Delineate the nursing care for the woman with more than one fetus.
- Summarize the nursing care indicated for fetal distress.
- Discuss intrauterine fetal death including etiology, diagnosis, management, and the nurse's role in assisting the family.
- Describe abruptio placentae and placenta previa.
- Identify variations that may occur in the umbilical cord and insertion into the placenta.
- Contrast the identification, management, and nursing care of women with amniotic fluid embolus, hydramnios, and oligohydramnios.
- Delineate the effects of pelvic contractures on labor and birth.
- Discuss the complications of third and fourth stages of labor.

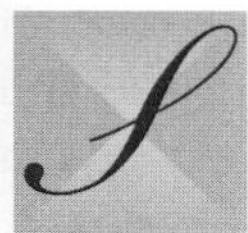

Successful completion of a pregnancy requires the harmonious functioning of five components: emotional factors, contractile forces, fetus, pelvis, and relationship between the fetus and the pelvis. (These components are described in depth in Chapter 15.) Disruptions in any of the five components may affect the others and cause **dystocia** (abnormal or difficult labor). The most common of these disruptions are discussed in this chapter.

# Care of the Woman at Risk due to Anxiety and Fear

Anxiety and fear have an enormous effect on labor, especially when unexpected complications may jeopardize the life or health of the mother and/or fetus. A childbirth experience that was initially approached with expectation and confidence may become fraught with anxiety and uncertainty. In labor, anxiety and fear may exacerbate pain. The resulting increase in catecholamine release in turn increases physical distress and results in myometrial dysfunction and possibly ineffectual labor.

A frequent outcome of increased levels of fear, anxiety, and loss of control in childbirth is the development of posttraumatic stress disorder (PTSD). Women who experience unexpectedly high levels of labor intervention and who feel unsatisfied with their health care are much more likely to exhibit long-term symptoms of PTSD, such as episodes of intense fear, persistent reexperiencing of the traumatic event(s), and recurring feelings of helplessness and horror (Creedy, Shochet, & Horsfall, 2000).

## Clinical Therapy

The goal of clinical therapy is to provide strategies that will help decrease the anxiety of the woman and her partner. Research suggests that if caregivers provide opportunities for the laboring woman to talk about concerns and make choices regarding care, even in situations in which complications exist, the childbirth experience is enhanced (Berg & Dahlberg, 1998). The nurse can use therapeutic communication and sharing of information to allay anxiety for both the woman and her support person. When needed, pharmacologic measures such as sedatives and analgesics may be ordered to help the woman feel calmer.

## Nursing Care Management

### Nursing Assessment and Diagnosis

Unless birth is imminent or severe complications exist, the nurse begins the assessment by reviewing the woman's background. Factors such as age, marital and socioeconomic status, culture, methods of coping, and understanding of the labor process, all contribute to the woman's psychologic response to labor. In addition, if the woman has other children, she may have unresolved concerns or fears related to a previous childbirth experience. As labor progresses, the nurse is alert to the woman's verbal and nonverbal behavioral responses to the pain and anxiety of labor. The woman who is agitated and seems uncooperative or is too quiet and compliant may require further appraisal for posttraumatic stress symptoms (Saito, Ylikorkala, & Halmesmaki, 1999). Verbal cues such as "Is everything okay?" "I'm really nervous," or "What's going on?" usually indicate some degree of anxiety and concern. Other women may be irritable, require frequent explanations, or repeat questions. The nurse further observes for nonverbal cues, including a tense posture, clenched hands, or pain out of proportion to the stage of labor (S. J. Roberts, Reardon, & Rosenfeld, 1999). Recognizing the impact of fatigue on pain and anxiety is another important nursing function.

Nursing diagnoses that may apply to the woman with excessive fear or anxiety include the following:

- Anxiety related to stress of the labor process
- Fear related to unknown outcome of labor
- Pain related to increased anxiety and stress

### Nursing Plan and Implementation

The primary nursing interventions center on providing support to the laboring woman and her partner or family. Families that have had the opportunity to attend prenatal classes may benefit from encouragement as they employ some of the coping techniques they have learned (see Chapter 6). When unexpected events occur (such as fetal stress or distress), the woman may lose confidence in her ability to handle her pain and to maintain a level of control in the situation. The nurse can help the woman regain some balance by providing information and including her in any decision making (see Chapters 17 and 18).

Unprepared couples can be taught a great deal at the time of admission, especially if active labor has not yet begun. The nurse can give clear but succinct information about the labor process, medical procedures, the environment, simple breathing exercises, and relaxation techniques, thereby preventing or relieving some apprehension and fear. Even a woman in active labor who has had no prior preparation can achieve a great deal of relaxation from physical comfort measures, touch, frequent attention, therapeutic interaction, and possibly analgesics.

The nurse's ability to help the woman and her partner cope with the stress of labor is directly related to the rapport they have established. By employing a calm, caring, confident, nonjudgmental approach, the nurse may be able not only to acknowledge the anxiety but also to identify the source of the distress. Once the causative factors are known, the nurse can implement appropriate interventions such as offering information, comfort measures, touch, or therapeutic communication. At times a woman (or couple) experiencing increased anxiety presents so many challenges that the nurse feels reluctant about being in the labor room for prolonged periods. However, the nurse's presence is the single most important factor that women identify as helping them during labor (Dahlberg, Berg, & Lundgren, 1999).

### Evaluation

Anticipated outcomes of nursing care include the following:

- The woman experiences decreased physiologic signs of stress and increased physical and psychologic comfort.
- The fear experienced by the woman and her family decreases.
- The woman is able to verbalize feelings about her labor.

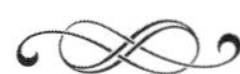

# Care of the Woman with Dystocia Related to Dysfunctional Uterine Contractions

Dystocia, or difficult labor, may be due to a wide variety of problems, the most common of which is dysfunctional (or uncoordinated) uterine contractions. These uncoordinated contractions result in a prolonged labor (Bowes, 1999). Contractions that result in a more normal progression of labor tend to be moderate to strong when palpated and occur regularly (two to four contractions in 10 minutes in early labor and four to five per 10 minutes in later phases). Dysfunctional contractions are typically irregular in strength, timing, or both. These irregular uterine contractions often arrest cervical dilatation.

## Hypertonic Labor Patterns

In hypertonic labor patterns, ineffectual uterine contractions of poor quality occur in the latent phase of labor, and the resting tone of the myometrium increases. Contractions usually become more frequent, but their intensity may decrease (Figure 19–1♦). The contractions are painful but ineffective in dilating and effacing the cervix, and a prolonged latent phase may result.

Maternal risks of hypertonic labor include

- Increased discomfort due to uterine muscle cell anoxia
- Fatigue as the pattern continues and no labor progress results
- Stress on coping abilities
- Dehydration and increased incidence of infection if labor is prolonged

Fetal-neonatal risks include

- Fetal distress because contractions and increased resting tone interfere with the uteroplacental exchange
- Prolonged pressure on the fetal head, which may result in cephalhematoma, caput succedaneum, or excessive molding (Figure 19–2♦)

### Clinical Therapy

Management of hypertonic labor may include bed rest and sedation to promote relaxation and reduce pain. If the hypertonic pattern continues and develops into a prolonged latent phase, oxytocin infusion or amniotomy may be considered (see Chapter 20). These methods are instituted only after cephalopelvic disproportion (CPD) and fetal malpresentation have been ruled out. When an oxytocin infusion is used to stimulate uterine contractions, the physician or certified nurse-midwife (CNM) needs to assess whether vaginal birth is possible (ie, whether the maternal pelvis is large enough for the fetus to pass through). If the maternal pelvic diameters are less than average, or if the fetus is particularly large or is in a malpresentation or malposition, CPD is said to be present. In the presence of true CPD, labor is not stimulated because vaginal birth is not possible.

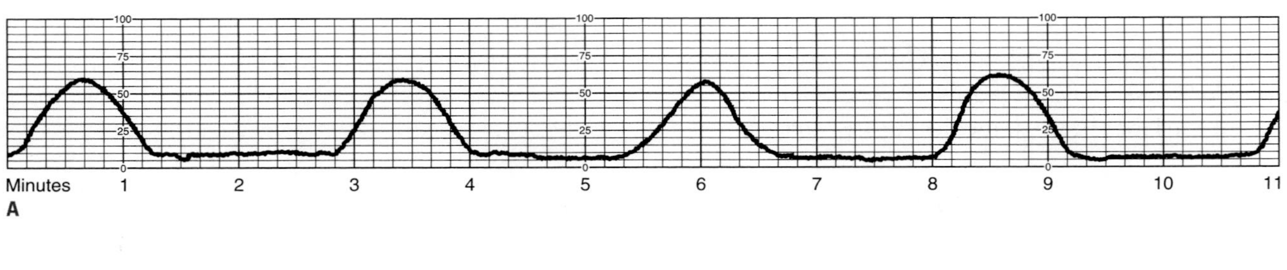


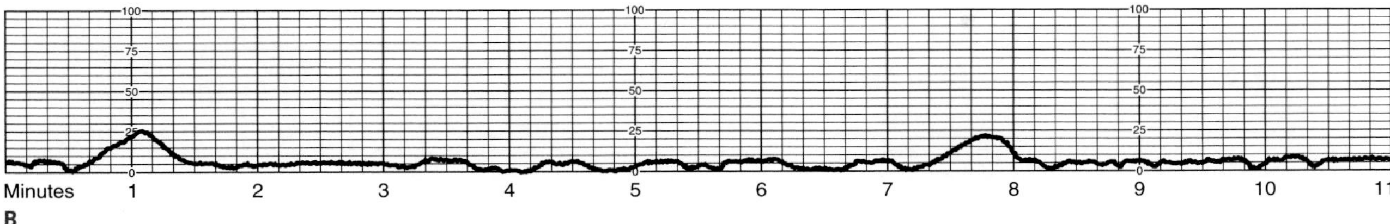


FIGURE 19–1 ♦ Comparison of labor patterns. **A**, Normal uterine contraction pattern. In this example contraction frequency is every 3 minutes; duration is 60 seconds. The baseline resting tone is below 10 mm Hg. **B**, Hypotonic uterine contraction pattern. In this example the contraction frequency is every 7 minutes (with some uterine activity between contractions), duration is 50 seconds, and intensity increases approximately 25 mm Hg during contractions.

# Nursing Care Management

## Nursing Assessment and Diagnosis

As part of the labor assessment, the nurse should evaluate the relationship between the intensity of the pain being experienced and the degree to which the cervix is dilating and effacing. The nurse should also note whether anxiety is negatively affecting labor progress. Evidence of increasing frustration and discouragement on the part of the mother and her partner may indicate that the nurse needs to provide some additional information or assurance.

Nursing diagnoses that may apply to the woman in hypertonic labor include the following:

- Pain related to the woman's inability to relax secondary to hypertonic uterine contractions
- Ineffective individual coping related to ineffectiveness of breathing techniques to relieve discomfort
- Anxiety related to slow labor progress

## Nursing Plan and Implementation

A key nursing responsibility is to provide comfort and support to the laboring woman and her partner. The woman experiencing a hypertonic labor pattern will probably be very uncomfortable because of the increased force of contractions. Her anxiety level and that of her partner may be high. The nurse attempts to reduce the woman's discomfort and promote a more effective labor pattern.

The nurse may suggest supportive measures such as a change of position: left lateral side-lying, high Fowler's, on her knees in the bed with her arms up around the top of the bed while it is in high Fowler's, rocking in a rocking chair, sitting up, and walking. Soothing measures, such as a warm shower, Jacuzzi, quiet environment, use of music the woman finds soothing, back rub, therapeutic touch, and visualization, and comfort measures, such as mouth care, change of linens, effleurage, and relaxation exercises, may also be helpful. If sedation is ordered, the nurse ensures that the environment is conducive to relaxation. The labor partner may also need assistance in helping the woman cope. A calm, understanding approach by the nurse offers the woman and her partner further support. Providing information about the cause of the hypertonic labor pattern and assuring the woman that she is not overreacting to the situation are important nursing actions.

Client education is key for the woman experiencing hypertonic labor. She needs information about the dysfunctional labor pattern and the possible implications for her and her baby. Information will help relieve anxiety and thereby increase relaxation and comfort. The nurse needs to explain treatment options and offer opportunities to ask questions.

## Evaluation

Anticipated outcomes of nursing care include the following:

- The woman has increased comfort and decreased anxiety.

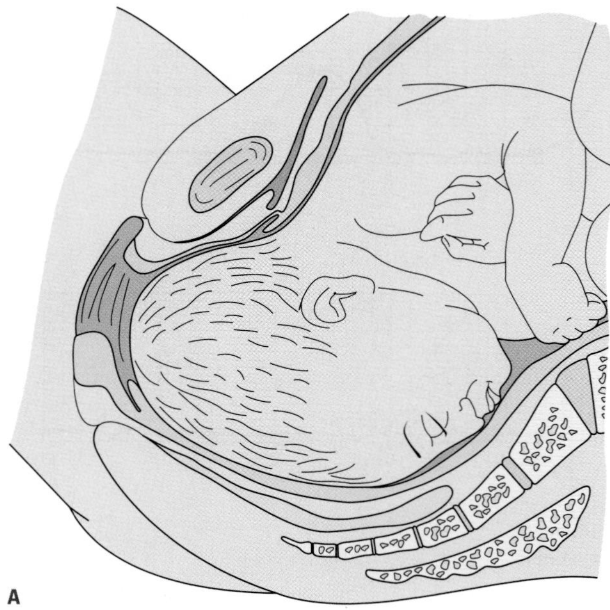


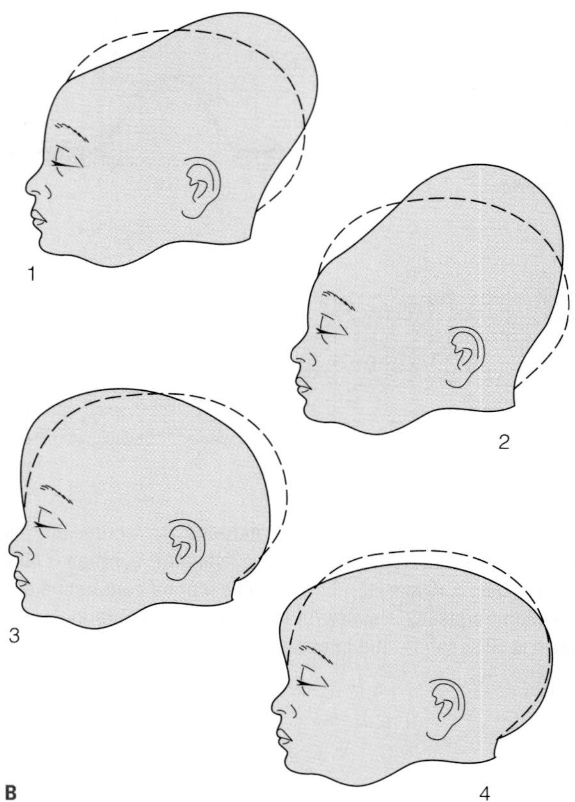


FIGURE 19–2 ♦ Effects of labor on the fetal head. **A**, Caput succedaneum formation. The presenting portion of the scalp area is encircled by the cervix during labor, causing swelling of the soft tissue. **B**, Molding of the fetal head in cephalic presentations: (1) occiput anterior, (2) occiput posterior, (3) brow, (4) face.

- The woman and her partner are able to cope with the labor.
- The woman experiences a more effective labor pattern.

## Hypotonic Labor Patterns

A hypotonic labor pattern usually develops in the active phase of labor, after labor has been well established. Hypotonic labor is characterized by fewer than two to three contractions in a 10-minute period (Figure 19–1B♦, page 459). Hypotonic labor may occur when the uterus is overstretched from a twin gestation, or in the presence of a large fetus, hydramnios, or grand multiparity. Bladder or bowel distention and CPD may also be associated with this pattern. Maternal implications of hypotonic labor patterns include the risk of

- Maternal exhaustion
- Stress on coping abilities
- Postpartal hemorrhage from insufficient uterine contractions following birth
- Intrauterine infection if labor is prolonged

Fetal-neonatal implications include the risk of

- Fetal distress due to prolonged labor pattern
- Fetal sepsis from pathogens that ascend from the birth canal

### Clinical Therapy

Improving the quality of the uterine contractions while ensuring a safe outcome for the woman and her baby are the goals of therapy. Before initiating treatment for hypotonic labor, the physician or CNM validates the adequacy of pelvic measurements and completes tests to establish gestational age if fetal maturity is in question. After CPD, fetal malpresentation, and fetal immaturity have been ruled out, oxytocin (Pitocin) may be given intravenously via an infusion pump to improve the quality of uterine contractions. Intravenous fluid is useful to maintain adequate hydration and prevent maternal exhaustion. Amniotomy may be used to stimulate the labor process.

Some physicians support the use of **active management of labor (AMOL),** a process whereby labor is managed from the beginning with amniotomy, timed cervical exams are performed, and augmentation of labor with intravenous (IV) administration of oxytocin is begun if a specified level of progress is not met. Supporters of AMOL contend that it is a preventative treatment that reduces the chance for protracted labor (Lopez-Zeno, 1997).

An improvement in the quality of uterine contractions is demonstrated by noticeable progress in the labor process. If the labor pattern does not become effective or if other complications develop, further interventions, including cesarean birth, may be necessary.

## EVIDENCE-BASED PRACTICE

### Dystocia

You are a member of a practice-improvement team in your birthing unit. Currently, you are studying the cesarean birth rate, which is 22%. One of your major projects is to gather data on the various diagnoses that prompted the surgery decision. *Dystocia* is one of the chief targets because it is the second most common reason for cesarean in the United States (Spellicy-Gifford, Morton, Fisk, et al., 2000).

You have cared for women who were diagnosed with failure to progress and/or dystocia prior to cesarean birth. Now you will review charts and gather real-time data about the progress of labor. The chart reviews will compare the documented status of the patient with the criteria established by the American College of Obstetricians and Gynecologists (ACOG) for a diagnosis of dystocia.

About 30% of the cesarean births in the United States result from a diagnosis of dystocia, and recent studies have shown that many of the women with dystocia were diagnosed in the latent phase of labor (Spellicy-Gifford et al., 2000). However, a valid dystocia diagnosis cannot be made for a woman in latent labor. The diagnosis of dystocia can be made only when the woman is in active labor, with a cervix dilated 3 to 4 cm, and has no additional cervical dilatation despite adequate labor (Austin & Calderon, 1999).

You realize nurses can directly affect cesarean rates with accurate assessment and use of triage prior to admission into the labor unit. A recent study demonstrated improvements in outcome measures of (1) length of labor, (2) use of analgesia, and (3) augmentation with oxytocin when women were triaged for active labor prior to admission (Austin & Calderon, 1999).

#### References

Austin, D., & Calderon, L. (1999). Triaging patients in the latent phase of labor. *Journal of Nurse Midwifery, 44*(6), 585–591.

Spellicy-Gifford, D., Morton, S., Fisk, M., Keesye, J., et al. (2000). Lack of progress in labor as a reason for cesarean. *Obstetrics and Gynecology, 95*(4), 589–595.

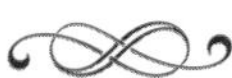

## NURSING CARE MANAGEMENT

### Nursing Assessment and Diagnosis

Assessment of contractions (for frequency and intensity), maternal vital signs, and fetal heart rate (FHR) provides the nurse with data to evaluate maternal-fetal status. The nurse is also alert for signs and symptoms of infection and dehydration. Because of the stress associated with a prolonged labor, observing the woman and her partner's success in implementing coping mechanisms is important, too.

Nursing diagnoses that may apply to the woman in hypotonic labor include the following:

- Pain related to uterine contractions secondary to dysfunctional labor
- Knowledge deficit related to lack of information about dysfunctional labor

### Nursing Plan and Implementation

Nursing measures to promote maternal-fetal physical well-being include frequent monitoring of contractions, maternal vital signs, and FHR. If amniotic membranes are ruptured, the nurse assesses for the presence of meconium (dark green or black stool present in the fetal large intestine). The presence of meconium in the amniotic fluid makes close observation of fetal status more critical because it often indicates that the fetus is experiencing some form of stress. An intake and output record provides a way of determining maternal hydration or dehydration. The woman should be encouraged to void every 2 hours, and her bladder should be checked for distension. Because her labor may be prolonged, the nurse must continue to monitor the woman for signs of infection (elevated temperature, chills, foul-smelling amniotic fluid). Vaginal examinations should be kept to a minimum to decrease the risk of introducing an infection. (The nursing implications of oxytocin infusion are presented in Chapter 20.)

Clients experiencing a hypotonic labor pattern require emotional support. The nurse assists the woman and her partner to cope with the frustration of a lengthy labor process. A warm, caring approach is coupled with techniques to reduce anxiety and discomfort.

The teaching plan must include information regarding the dysfunctional labor process and implications for the mother and baby. Disadvantages of and alternatives to treatment also need to be discussed and understood.

### Evaluation

Anticipated outcomes of nursing care include the following:

- The woman maintains comfort during labor.
- The woman understands the type of labor pattern that is occurring and the treatment plan.

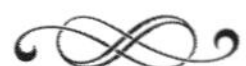

## Precipitous Labor and Birth

**Precipitous labor** is labor that lasts less than 3 hours and results in rapid birth. Contributing factors in precipitous labor are (a) multiparity, (b) large pelvis, (c) previous precipitous labor, and (d) a small fetus in a favorable position. One or more of these factors, plus strong contractions, result in a rapid descent of the infant through the birth canal (Cunningham, MacDonald, Grant, et al., 1997).

Precipitous labor and precipitous birth are not the same. A precipitous birth is an unexpected, sudden, and often unattended birth. (See Chapter 17 for discussion of emergency birth.)

Maternal risks of precipitous labor include

- Loss of coping abilities
- Lacerations of the cervix, vagina, and perineum due to rapid descent and birth of the fetus
- Postpartal hemorrhage due to undetected lacerations or inadequate uterine contractions after birth

Fetal-neonatal implications include

- Fetal distress or hypoxia from decreased uteroplacental circulation due to intense uterine contractions
- Cerebral trauma from rapid descent through the birth canal

### Clinical Therapy

Any woman with a history of precipitous labor requires close monitoring in the last few weeks of pregnancy. If the cervix softens and begins to dilate, the woman may be scheduled for immediate induction of labor.

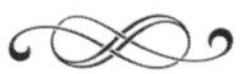

## Nursing Care Management

### Nursing Assessment and Diagnosis

During the intrapartal nursing assessment, the nurse can identify a woman at increased risk of precipitous labor (eg, a previous history of precipitous or short labor places a woman at risk). During labor the presence of one or both of the following factors may indicate potential problems:

- Accelerated cervical dilatation (>2 cm/hr in multigravidas and >1.2 cm/hr in primigravidas) and fetal descent
- Intense uterine contractions with little uterine relaxation between contractions

Nursing diagnoses that may apply to the woman with precipitous labor include the following:

- Risk for injury related to rapid labor and birth
- Pain related to rapid labor process

### Nursing Plan and Implementation

If the woman has a history of precipitous labor, she is closely monitored, and an emergency birth pack is kept at hand. The nurse stays in constant attendance if possible and promotes comfort and rest by assisting the woman to a comfortable position, providing a quiet environment, and administering sedatives as needed. The nurse provides information and support before and after the birth.

To avoid possible precipitous labor and hyperstimulation of the uterus during oxytocin administration, the nurse should be alert to the dangers of oxytocin overdosage (see Drug Guide: Oxytocin, in Chapter 20). If the woman who is receiving oxytocin develops an accelerated labor pattern, the oxytocin is discontinued immediately, and the woman is turned on her left side to improve uterine perfusion. Oxygen may be administered to increase the available oxygen in the maternal circulating blood, which in turn increases the amount available for exchange at the placental site. The fetus is monitored for signs of hypoxia and other indications of fetal distress.

### Evaluation

Anticipated outcomes of nursing care include the following:

- The woman and her baby are closely monitored during labor, and a safe birth occurs.
- The woman maintains optimal comfort.

## Care of the Woman with Postterm Pregnancy

A **postterm pregnancy** is one that extends more than 294 days or 42 weeks past the first day of the last menstrual period. It is important to distinguish between the term *postdates,* which means that the pregnancy has gone beyond the estimated date of birth (EDB), and *postterm* which indicates that the pregnancy has gone at least 1 day beyond 42 complete weeks from the last menstrual period (Martin, 2000). The actual incidence of past-term pregnancies is small, approximately 3% to 7%. The cause of true postterm pregnancy is unknown, but it seems to occur more frequently in primigravidas and women over age 35 (Clausson, Cnattingius, & Axelsson, 1999).

Maternal risks associated with postterm pregnancy include the following (Martin, 2000):

- Probable labor induction
- Increased risk for large-for-gestational-age (LGA) infant
- Increased incidence of forceps-assisted, vacuum-assisted, or cesarean birth
- Increased psychologic stress as the due date passes and concern for the baby increases

Fetal risks include the following (Martin, 2000):

- Decreased perfusion from the placenta
- Oligohydramnios (decreased amount of amniotic fluid), which increases the risk of cord compression
- Meconium aspiration (aspiration of meconium-stained amniotic fluid by the fetus at the time of birth), which is more likely if oligohydramnios and thick meconium are present

Some fetuses continue to grow beyond the 42nd week of pregnancy and can be excessively large at birth (macrosomia). In other cases, the intrauterine environment becomes unfavorable for growth, and at birth the infant has lost muscle mass and subcutaneous fat. The macrosomic fetus is at risk for birth trauma, whereas the small-for-gestational-age (SGA) fetus is at risk for fetal distress during labor because there is frequently associated oligohydramnios (Martin, 2000).

### Clinical Therapy

When the 40th week of gestation is completed and birth has not occurred, most obstetricians begin using the nonstress test (NST) and biophysical profile (BPP) (especially the amniotic fluid volume portion of the BPP) as assessment tools. These tests may be done two to three times a week to help evaluate fetal well-being (Parer, 1999). If at any time the fetal assessment tests indicate a problem, interventions are taken to accomplish the birth.

## Nursing Care Management

### Nursing Assessment and Diagnosis

When the woman is admitted into the birthing area, ongoing assessments of fetal well-being begin as soon as the postterm condition has been verified. The nurse needs to identify reassuring FHR characteristics and evaluate for the presence of nonreassuring patterns, such as nonperiodic variable decelerations (which are associated with cord compression), so that corrective actions can be taken. When the amniotic membranes rupture, the nurse assesses the fluid for meconium. In addition, the nurse assesses the woman's knowledge about the condition, implications for her baby, risks, and possible interventions.

Nursing diagnoses that may apply to the woman with postterm pregnancy include the following:

- Knowledge deficit related to lack of information about postterm pregnancy
- Fear related to the unknown outcome for the baby
- Ineffective individual coping related to anxiety about the status of the baby

### Nursing Plan and Implementation

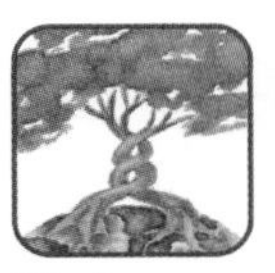

#### Community-Based Nursing Care

If the woman has not been assessing fetal movement every day, the nurse teaches her how to do so. It is vital to stress the importance of identifying inadequate fetal movement and immediately contacting her health care provider. (See Chapter 9 for further discussion of techniques to detect fetal movement.)

Client education about the postterm pregnancy is another important nursing responsibility. The nurse should address the implications and associated risks for the baby, as well as possible treatment plans. The woman and her partner need opportunities to ask questions and clarify information.

### Hospital-Based Nursing Care

Promotion of fetal well-being requires careful assessment of the response of the fetus during labor. If oligohydramnios exists, a continuous FHR tracing is obtained and evaluated frequently. Variable decelerations are often associated with oligohydramnios, because the decreased amount of fluid allows compression of the umbilical cord. If the fetus is macrosomic, careful assessment of labor progress (contraction characteristics, progressive cervical dilatation, fetal descent) is also needed.

Emotional support is a key nursing intervention for women with pregnancies that extend past the due date. Women experiencing postterm pregnancy frequently feel increased stress and anxiety and have difficulty coping. Encouragement, support, and recognition of the woman's anxiety are helpful health personnel strategies.

### Evaluation

Anticipated outcomes of nursing care include the following:

- The woman has knowledge about the postterm pregnancy.
- The woman and her partner feel supported and able to cope with the postterm pregnancy.
- Fetal status is maintained, any abnormalities are quickly identified, and supportive measures are initiated.

# Care of the Woman and Fetus at Risk due to Fetal Malposition

The *occiput-posterior (OP)* position is the most common fetal malposition. When the fetus is OP, the occiput of the fetal head is directed toward the back of the maternal pelvis. During labor, 87% of OP fetuses rotate to an occiput-anterior (OA) position (Rivlin, 2000).

A variation of OP called the **persistent occiput-posterior (POP) position** occurs in 5% of labors. In this case the fetus enters and travels the birth canal, and is born in the OP position. Persistent occiput-posterior is associated with android and anthropoid pelvic shapes. Labor may be prolonged, however most POP fetuses are born without the aid of forceps (Rivlin, 2000).

Maternal risks related to the persistent occiput-posterior position include

- Risk of third- or fourth-degree perineal lacerations during birth
- Risk of extension of a midline episiotomy

Fetal implications do not include an increased mortality risk unless labor is prolonged or additional interventions such as forceps-assisted, vacuum-assisted, or cesarean birth are required.

## Clinical Therapy

Clinical treatment focuses on close monitoring of maternal and fetal status and labor progress to determine whether vaginal or cesarean birth is the safer birth method. A cesarean birth is chosen if maternal or fetal problems make a vaginal birth unwise or if CPD is present. Although the majority of persistent occiput-posterior fetuses are born vaginally, in some cases forceps-assisted birth may be necessary. The forceps can be used to deliver the fetus while it is still in the occiput-posterior position or to rotate the occiput to an anterior position (called Scanzoni's maneuver). A rotation from Left occiput-posterior (LOP) or Right occiput-posterior (ROP) to an anterior position may also be accomplished with a vacuum-assistance device. (See Chapter 20 for further discussion of forceps and vacuum.)

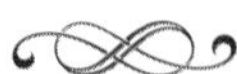

## Nursing Care Management

### Nursing Assessment and Diagnosis

Signs and symptoms of a persistent occiput-posterior position include complaints of intense back pain by the laboring woman, a dysfunctional labor pattern, hypotonic labor (the fetal head does not put adequate pressure on the cervix), arrest of dilatation, or arrest of fetal descent. The back pain is caused by the fetal occiput compressing the sacral nerves. Further assessment may reveal a depression in the maternal abdomen above the symphysis. FHR is typically heard far laterally on the abdomen, and on vaginal examination the certified nurse-midwife/physician finds the wide, diamond-shaped anterior fontanelle in the anterior portion of the pelvis. This fontanelle may be difficult to feel because of molding of the fetal head.

Nursing diagnoses that may apply to women with persistent occiput posterior include the following:

- Pain related to back discomfort secondary to the OP position
- Ineffective individual coping related to unanticipated discomfort and slow progress in labor

### Nursing Plan and Implementation

Changing maternal posture has been used for many years to enhance rotation of OP or occiput-transverse (OT) to OA. A number of position changes may be tried. For instance, the woman may be asked to lie on one side and then asked to move to the other side as the fetus begins to rotate. This side-lying position may promote rotation; it also enables the support person to apply counterpressure on the sacral area to decrease discomfort. A knee-chest position provides a downward slant to the vaginal canal, directing the fetal head downward on descent. A hands-and-knees position is often effective in rotating the fetus. In addition to maintaining a hands-and-knees position on the bed, the woman may try pelvic rocking, and the support person may firmly stroke the abdomen. The stroking begins over the fetal back and swings around to the other side of the abdomen. After the fetus has rotated, the woman lies in a Sims' position on the side opposite the fetal back.

### Evaluation

Anticipated outcomes of nursing care include the following:

- The woman's discomfort is decreased.
- The coping abilities of the woman and her partner are strengthened.

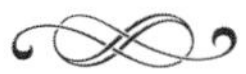

## Care of the Woman and Fetus at Risk due to Fetal Malpresentation

In a normal presentation, the occiput is the presenting part (Figure 19–3A♦). Fetal malpresentations include brow, face, breech, shoulder (transverse lie), and compound presentation.

### Brow Presentation

In a brow presentation, the forehead of the fetus becomes the presenting part. The fetal head is between flexion and extension (military position, Figure 19–3B♦), and the fetal head enters the birth canal with the widest diameter of the head (occipitomental—14 cm) foremost (Figure 19–3C♦).

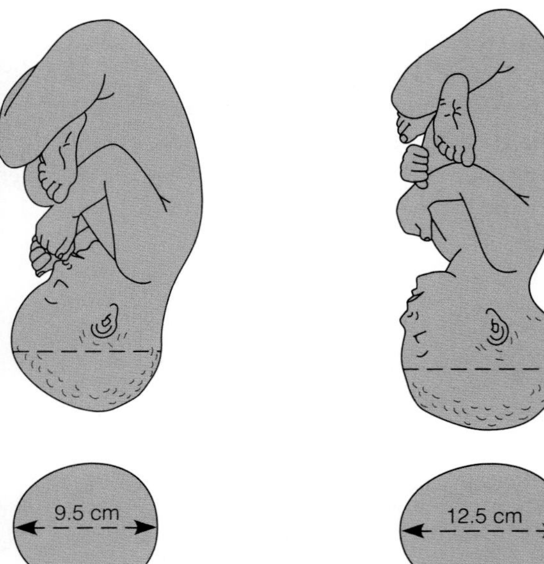


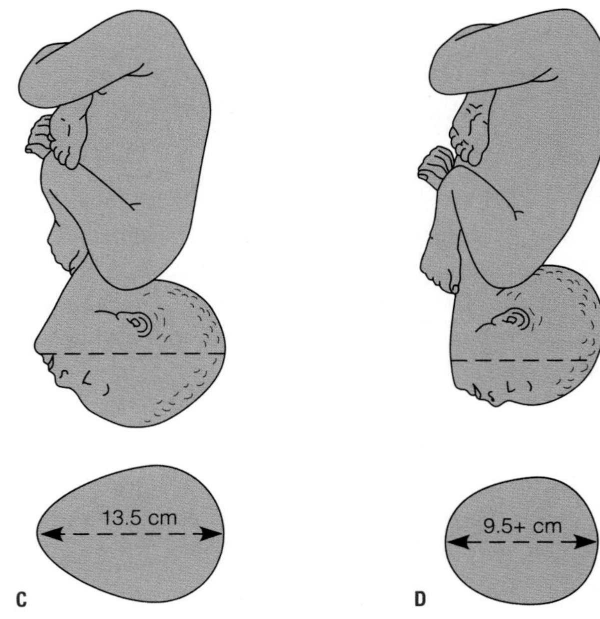


FIGURE 19–3 ♦ Types of cephalic presentations. **A,** The occiput is the presenting part because the head is flexed and the fetal chin is against the chest. The largest anteroposterior (AP) diameter that presents and passes through the pelvis is approximately 9.5 cm. **B,** Military presentation. The head is neither flexed nor extended. The presenting AP diameter is approximately 12.5 cm. **C,** Brow presentation. The largest diameter of the fetal head (approximately 13.5 cm) presents in this situation. **D,** Face presentation. The AP diameter is 9.5 cm.
*Source:* Danforth, D. N., & Scott, J. R. (Eds.). (1990). *Obstetrics and gynecology* (5th ed., p. 170, Figure 8–9♦). New York: Lippincott.

The brow presentation occurs more often in multiparas than in nulliparas and is thought to be due to lax abdominal and pelvic musculature. Many brow presentations spontaneously convert to face or occipital presentations (Bowes, 1999).

Maternal implications of brow presentation include increased risk of

- Longer labor due to ineffective contractions and slow or arrested fetal descent
- Cesarean birth if brow presentation persists

Fetal-neonatal risks include increased mortality because of cerebral and neck compression and damage to the trachea and larynx (Rivlin, 2000). In addition, facial edema and exaggerated molding of the newborn's head may be observed.

#### Clinical Therapy

If a brow presentation fails to convert to occiputal or face presentation, cesarean birth is indicated, in most cases (Rivlin, 2000). If a vaginal birth is attempted, the woman is closely monitored for CPD and will probably need an episiotomy. *Right mediolateral (RML)* or *left mediolateral (LML)* episiotomy is preferable, because the more common *midline (ML)* episiotomy has the risk of extending into the anus and rectum (fourth-degree laceration).

## Nursing Care Management

### Nursing Assessment and Diagnosis

A brow presentation can be detected on vaginal examination (with ultrasound or x-ray confirmation) by palpation of the diamond-shaped anterior fontanelle on one side and orbital ridges and root of the nose on the other side (Rivlin, 2000).

Nursing diagnoses that may apply to a woman with a brow presentation include the following:

- Knowledge deficit related to lack of information about the possible maternal-fetal effects of brow presentation
- Risk for injury to the fetus related to pressure on fetal structures secondary to brow presentation

### Nursing Plan and Implementation

The nurse closely observes the woman for labor problems and the fetus for signs of stress or distress. The fetus should be observed closely during labor for signs of hypoxia, as evidenced by late decelerations and bradycardia.

The nurse also provides emotional support to the family. In this role the nurse explains the fetal position to the woman and her support person or interprets what the CNM or physician has told them. The nurse should stay close at hand to reassure the couple, inform them of any changes, and assist them with labor-coping techniques. In face and brow presentations, the newborn's face may be edematous. The couple may need help in beginning the attachment process because of the newborn's facial appearance. After the infant is inspected for any abnormalities, the pediatrician and nurse can assure the couple that the facial edema is only temporary and will subside in 3 or 4 days and that the molding will be much less visible in a few days (even though completion of the process takes several weeks).

### Evaluation

Anticipated outcomes of nursing care include the following:

- The woman and her partner understand the implications and associated problems of brow presentation.
- The mother and her baby have a safe labor and birth.

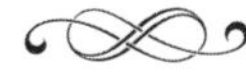

## Face Presentation

In a face presentation, the face of the fetus is the presenting part (Figure 19–4 and Figure 19–3D♦). The fetal head is hyperextended even more than in the brow presentation. Face presentation occurs most frequently in multiparas, in preterm birth, and in the presence of anencephaly. The incidence of face presentation is about 1 in 500 births (Bowes, 1999).

Maternal risks related to face presentation include

- Increased risk of CPD and prolongation of labor
- Increased risk of infection (with prolonged labor)
- Cesarean birth if fetal chin is posterior (mentum posterior)

Fetal-neonatal risks include

- Cephalhematoma of the face
- Edema of the face and throat if the fetal chin is anterior (mentum anterior) and a vaginal birth occurs (may also occur during fetal descent)
- Pronounced molding of the head

#### Clinical Therapy

A vaginal birth may be anticipated if no CPD is present, the chin (mentum) is anterior, the labor pattern is

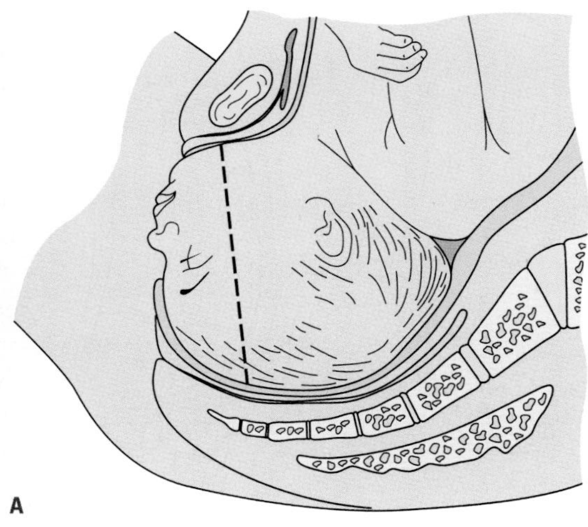


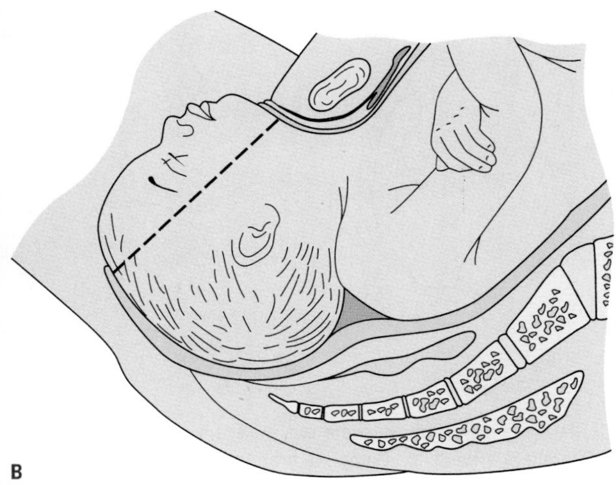


FIGURE 19–4 ♦ Mechanism of birth in face (mentoanterior) position. **A**, The submentobregmatic diameter at the outlet. **B**, The fetal head is born by the movement of flexion.

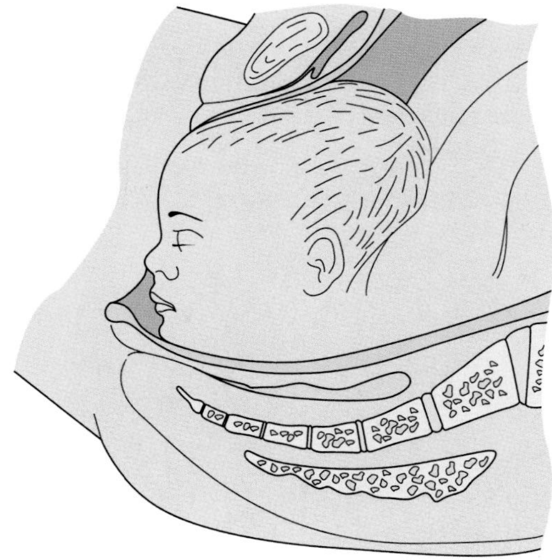

FIGURE 19–5 ♦ Face presentation. Mechanism of birth in mentoposterior position. Fetal head is unable to extend farther. The face becomes impacted.

effective, and no fetal stress or distress is present. If the mentum is posterior a vaginal birth is not possible and a cesarean birth is necessary (Figure 19–5♦).

# Nursing Care Management

## Nursing Assessment and Diagnosis

When performing Leopold's maneuvers, the nurse finds that the back of the fetus is difficult to outline, and a deep furrow can be palpated between the hard occiput and the fetal back (Figure 19–6♦). Fetal heart tones are audible on the side where the fetal feet are palpated. It may be difficult to determine by vaginal examination whether a breech or face is presenting, especially if facial edema is already present. During the vaginal examination, palpation of the saddle of the nose and the gums should be attempted. When assessing engagement, the nurse must remember that the face has to be deep within the pelvis before the biparietal diameters have entered the inlet.

Nursing diagnoses that may apply to the woman with a fetus in face presentation include the following:

- Fear related to unknown outcome of the labor
- Risk for injury to the newborn's face related to edema secondary to the birth process

## Nursing Plan and Implementation

Nursing interventions are the same as those indicated for the brow presentation.

## Evaluation

Anticipated outcomes of nursing care include the following:

- The woman and her partner understand the implications and associated problems of face presentation.
- The mother and her baby have a safe labor and birth.

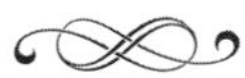

# Breech Presentation

The exact cause of breech presentation (Figure 19–7♦) is unknown. This malpresentation occurs in about 3% to 4% of labors and is frequently associated with preterm birth,

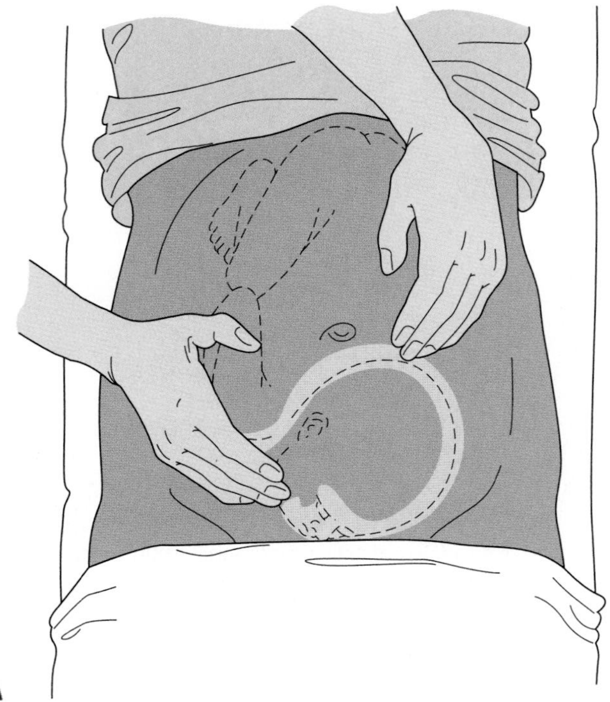


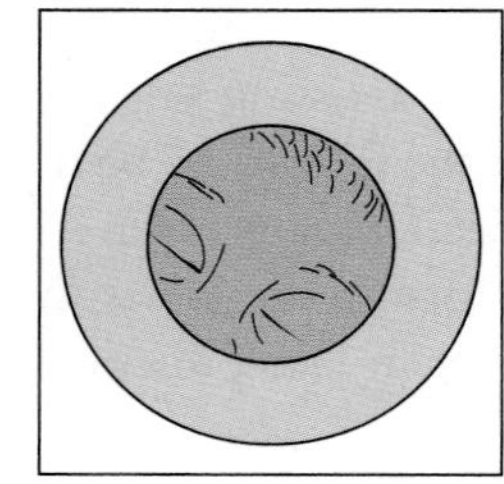


FIGURE 19–6 ♦ Face presentation. **A,** Palpation of the maternal abdomen with the fetus in right mentum posterior (RMP) position. **B,** Vaginal examination may permit palpation of facial features of the fetus.

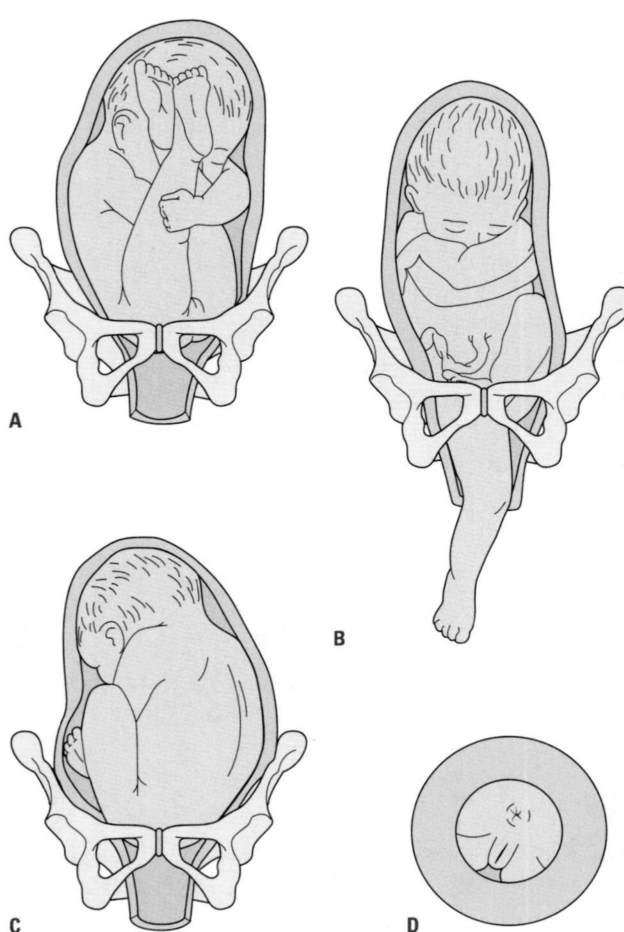


FIGURE 19–7 ♦ Breech presentation. **A,** Frank breech. **B,** Incomplete (footling) breech. **C,** Complete breech in left sacral anterior (LSA) position. **D,** On vaginal examination the nurse may feel the anal sphincter. The tissue of the fetal buttocks feels soft.

placenta previa, hydramnios, multiple gestation, uterine anomalies (such as bicornuate uterus), and fetal anomalies (especially anencephaly and hydrocephaly) (Bofill, 2000).

The maternal implication of breech presentation is a likelihood of cesarean birth. Fetal-neonatal implications include the following (Bowes, 1999):

- Higher perinatal morbidity and mortality rates
- Increased risk of prolapsed cord, especially in incomplete breeches, because space is available between the cervix and presenting part
- Increased risk of cervical cord injuries due to hyperextension of the fetal head during vaginal birth
- Increased risk of birth trauma (especially of the head) during either vaginal or cesarean breech birth

### Clinical Therapy

Current clinical therapy is directed toward converting the breech presentation to a cephalic presentation prior to the beginning of labor. Therefore an external cephalic version (ECV) may be attempted at 36 to 38 weeks' gestation as long as the woman is not in labor (Bowes, 1999; Bowfill, 2000). (See Chapter 20 for discussion of external version.) Opinions differ about the best method of birth for the fetus in a breech presentation. When the fetus is still in breech presentation and labor occurs, the method of birth varies depending on gestational age, estimated fetal weight, type of breech, and physician preference.

## Nursing Care Management

### Nursing Assessment and Diagnosis

Frequently it is the nurse who first recognizes a breech presentation. On palpation the nurse feels the firm fetal head in the uterine fundus and the wider sacrum in the lower part of the abdomen. If the sacrum has not descended, ballottement causes the entire fetal body to move. Furthermore, FHR is usually auscultated above the umbilicus. Passage of meconium into the amniotic fluid due to compression of the fetus's intestinal tract is common (Bofill, 2000).

If membranes are ruptured, the nurse is particularly alert for a prolapsed umbilical cord, especially in footling breeches, because there is space between the cervix and presenting part through which the cord can slip. If the infant is small and the membranes rupture, the danger is even greater. The risk of a prolapsed umbilical cord is one reason why any woman with a history of ruptured membranes should not walk around the birthing area until a full assessment, including vaginal examination, has been performed.

Nursing diagnoses that may apply to a woman with a breech presentation include the following:

- Impaired gas exchange in the fetus related to interruption in umbilical blood flow secondary to compression of the cord
- Knowledge deficit related to lack of information about the implications and associated complications of breech presentation for the mother and fetus

### Nursing Plan and Implementation

During labor, the nurse promotes maternal-fetal physical well-being by frequently assessing fetal and maternal status. Since the fetus is at increased risk for prolapse of the cord, some agency protocols may call for continuous fetal monitoring; however, no current research supports this practice. The nurse provides teaching and information about the breech presentation and the nursing care needed.

Although as many as 90% of infants in breech presentations are born by cesarean birth, a few are born vaginally (Bofill, 2000). The nurse assists with the vaginal birth by including Piper forceps (used to guide the aftercoming fetal head) in the birth table setup. The nurse may assist the physician if forceps are needed for the birth. If the family and certified nurse-midwife (CNM) or physician decide on a cesarean birth, the nurse intervenes as with any cesarean birth.

### Evaluation

Anticipated outcomes of nursing care include the following:

- The woman and her partner understand the implications and associated problems of breech presentation.
- Major complications are recognized early and corrective measures are instituted.
- The mother and baby have a safe labor and birth.

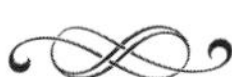

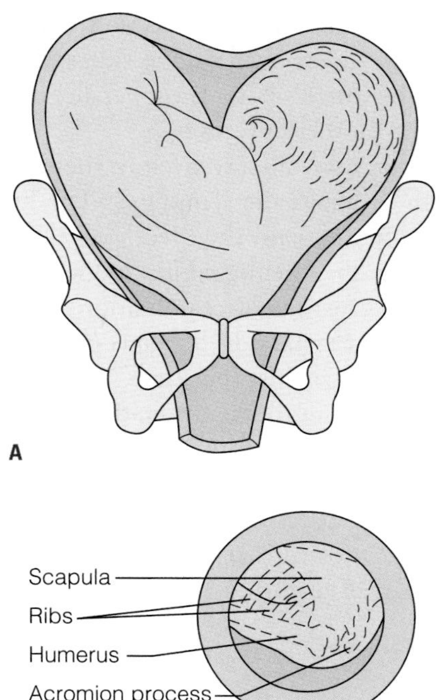


FIGURE 19–8 ♦ Transverse lie. **A**, Shoulder presentation. **B**, On vaginal examination the nurse may feel the acromion process as the fetal presenting part.

## Transverse Lie (Shoulder Presentation) of a Single Fetus

A transverse lie occurs in approximately 1 in 300 term births (Bowes, 1999). Maternal conditions associated with a transverse lie are grand multiparity with relaxed uterine muscles and placenta previa (Figure 19–8♦).

### Clinical Therapy

The management of shoulder presentation depends on the gestational age. If discovered before term, the management is expectant (watchful), because some fetuses may change presentation without any intervention. When a shoulder presentation is still evident at 37 completed weeks of gestation, an external cephalic version attempt (followed, if successful, by induction of labor) is recommended, because the associated risk of prolapsed cord is significant. Intrapartum ECV is often successful, reducing the need for cesarean birth by as much as 50% (Rivlin, 2000).

## Nursing Care Management

The nurse can identify a transverse lie by inspection and palpation of the abdomen, by auscultation of FHR, and by vaginal examination. On inspection the woman's abdomen appears widest from side to side as a result of the long axis of the infant's body lying parallel to the ground and across the mother's uterus.

On palpation no fetal part is felt in the fundal portion of the uterus or above the symphysis. The head may be palpated on one side and the breech on the other. Fetal heart rate is usually auscultated just below the midline of the umbilicus. On vaginal examination, if a presenting part is palpated, it is the ridged thorax or possibly an arm that is compressed against the chest.

The nurse assists in the interpretation of the fetal presentation and provides information and support to the couple. The nurse also assesses maternal and fetal status frequently and prepares the woman for a cesarean birth. (See Chapter 20 for further information about teaching related to cesarean birth.)

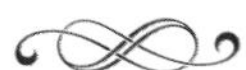

## Compound Presentation

A compound presentation is one in which there are two presenting parts, such as the occiput and fetal hand or the complete breech and fetal hand. Most compound presentations resolve themselves spontaneously, but others require additional manipulation at birth.

# Care of the Woman and Fetus at Risk due to Macrosomia

Fetal **macrosomia** is defined as a newborn weight of more than 4000 g at birth. Some sources suggest that the fetus not be considered macrosomic unless it weighs 4500 g or more and that considerations of ethnic grouping be incorporated as well (Hogg & Kimberlin, 2000). The condition is more common among offspring of large parents and diabetic women and in cases of grand multiparity and postterm gestation (Berkus, Conway, & Langer, 1999).

Maternal implications of macrosomia include increased risk of

- CPD
- Dysfunctional labor
- Soft tissue laceration during vaginal birth
- Postpartal hemorrhage

Fetal-neonatal implications include increased risk of

- Meconium aspiration
- Asphyxia
- Shoulder dystocia, in which, after birth of the head, the anterior shoulder fails to deliver either spontaneously or with gentle traction (Bowes, 1999)
- Upper brachial plexus injury and fractured clavicles

## Clinical Therapy

The occurrence of maternal and fetal problems associated with excessively large infants may be lessened somewhat by identifying macrosomia before the onset of labor. If a large fetus is suspected, the maternal pelvis should be evaluated carefully. Fetal size can be estimated by palpating the crown-to-rump length of the fetus in utero and by ultrasound or x-ray pelvimetry. Clinical studies have demonstrated that palpation and ultrasound are equally effective assessments of fetal weight; both provide accurate estimates in about 65% of cases (O'Reilly-Green & Divon, 2000). Whenever the uterus appears excessively large, hydramnios, an oversized fetus, or multiple pregnancies must be considered as the possible cause.

When fetal weight is estimated to be 4500 g or more, a cesarean birth is usually planned. The best method of birth for an estimated fetal weight of 4000 to 4500 g is debated. The discussion centers primarily on the incidence of shoulder dystocia during vaginal birth and the difficulty in accurately estimating the fetal weight. Unexpected shoulder dystocia during vaginal birth can be a grave problem. As an emergency measure the CNM or physician may ask the nurse to assist the woman into the McRoberts maneuver (sharp flexion of the thighs toward the hips and abdomen) or to apply gentle suprapubic pressure in an attempt to aid in the delivery of the fetal shoulders (Schmidt, 1999).

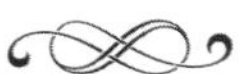

# Nursing Care Management

The nurse assists in identifying women who are at risk for carrying a large fetus or those who exhibit signs of macrosomia. Because these women are prime candidates for dystocia and its complications, the nurse frequently assesses the FHR for indications of fetal stress and evaluates the rates of cervical dilatation and fetal descent.

The fetal monitor is applied for continuous fetal evaluation. Early decelerations (caused by fetal head compression) could mean size disproportion at the bony inlet. Any sign of labor dysfunction or fetal distress is reported to the physician or CNM immediately.

The nurse provides support for the laboring woman and her partner and information about the implications of macrosomia and possible associated problems. During the birth, the nurse continues to provide support and encouragement to the couple.

The nurse inspects macrosomic newborns after birth for cephalhematoma and Erb's palsy and informs the nursery staff of any problems so that the newborn is observed closely for cerebral, neurologic, and motor problems. The presence of a macrosomic fetus means that the uterus has been stretched farther than it would have been with an average-sized fetus. The overstretching may lead to contractile problems during labor or after birth. After birth the overstretched uterus may not contract well (uterine atony) and will feel boggy (soft). In this case, uterine hemorrhage is likely. The fundus of the uterus is massaged to stimulate contraction, and IV oxytocin may be needed. Maternal vital signs are closely monitored for deviation suggestive of shock.

# Care of the Woman with Multiple Gestation

In part due to advances in infertility treatments, the incidence of twins in the United States is approximately 1 in 45 pregnancies, and the overall *multifetal* birth rate has more than doubled since 1991 (Miller, Ransom, Shalhoub, et al., 2000). Spontaneous twin and other multiple-gestation pregnancies can develop either from the fertilization of two (or more) separate ova or from the division of one fertilized ovum. Twins from two separate ova are called *dizygotic* and may be of the same or different sexes. In this type of twinning, there are two amnions (diamniotic) and two chorions (dichorionic). In multiple-gestation pregnancies each fetus usually has its own amniotic sac. The incidence of spontaneous twins varies but is highest in African-Americans, women of greater age and parity, and women who are tall and tend to be heavier. The incidence is low in the Asian population (Benirschke, 1999; Miller et al., 2000).

Twins from one fertilized ovum are called *monozygotic* and are always of the same sex. If the fertilized ovum (zygote) divides within the first 72 hours after fertilization, the siblings will be dichorionic (trichorionic and so on) and diamniotic (triamniotic and so on). The most common monozygotic twins result from division that occurs from the fourth to the eighth day after fertilization; the embryos develop one chorion (monochorionic) and separate amnions (diamniotic or multiamniotic). The relationship of membranes among triplets and other high-order gestations generally follows the same principles as for twins, except that monochorionic and dichorionic amniotic sacs may coexist (Benirschke, 1999; W. E. Roberts, 2000). The terminology is important because the perinatal morbidity and mortality rates differ greatly among different types of multiple-gestation pregnancies (Keith, Papiernik, & Oleszcuzuk, 1998).

During the prenatal period, visualization of two gestational sacs at 5 to 6 weeks, fundal height greater than expected for the length of gestation, and auscultation of heart rates that differ by at least 10 beats per minute, are the most likely clues to multiple-gestation pregnancies. In addition, the alpha-fetoprotein level is usually elevated in twin or multiple-gestation pregnancies and many women experience severe nausea and vomiting (due to elevated levels of the human chorionic gonadotropin [hCG] hormone) (Malone & D'Alton, 1999).

## Maternal Implications

During her pregnancy, the woman may experience physical discomfort such as shortness of breath, dyspnea on exertion, backaches, and pedal edema. Other associated problems include urinary tract infections, pregnancy-induced hypertension (PIH), preterm labor, and placenta previa (Malone & D'Alton, 1999). Complications during labor include abnormal fetal presentations, uterine dysfunction, prolapsed cord, and hemorrhage at birth or shortly after (W. E. Roberts, 2000).

## Fetal-Neonatal Implications

The perinatal mortality rate is approximately 10 times greater for twins than for a single fetus (W. E. Roberts, 2000). The perinatal mortality rate for monoamniotic siblings has been estimated to be as high as 50% to 60% (Benirschke, 1999). Fetal problems include decreased intrauterine growth rate for each fetus, increased incidence of fetal anomalies, increased risk of prematurity and its associated problems, and abnormal presentations (W. E. Roberts, 2000).

## Clinical Therapy

Once the presence of twins has been detected, preventing and treating problems that infringe on the development and birth of normal fetuses is the most significant clinical goal. Prenatal visits are more frequent for women with twins than for those with one fetus. Women with multiple-gestation pregnancies need to understand the nutritional implications of multiple fetuses, the assessment of fetal activity, the signs of preterm labor, and the danger signs of pregnancy.

Serial ultrasounds are used to assess the growth of each fetus and to provide early recognition of intrauterine growth restriction (IUGR). Some physicians believe that bed rest in the lateral position enhances utero-placental-fetal blood flow and decreases the risk of preterm labor. Others question the value of bed rest for the prevention of periodic uterine contractions, which seem to precede preterm labor (W. E. Roberts, 2000). More recent strategies include work leave and lifestyle modifications (Papiernik, Keith, Oleszcuzuk, et al., 1998).

Testing usually begins at 30 to 34 weeks' gestation and may include NST, BPP, and Doppler ultrasound to assess umbilical blood waveforms (Rodis, Arky, Egan, et al., 1999). A reactive NST is associated with good fetal outcome if birth occurs within 1 week of the testing. The NST is done every 3 to 7 days until birth or until results become nonreactive. The BPP is also accurate in assessing fetal status with twin pregnancies. A biophysical profile of 8 or better for each fetus is considered reassuring, and weekly or biweekly BPPs and NSTs continue until birth (Parer, 1999).

Intrapartal management requires careful attention to maternal and fetal status. The mother should have an IV with a large-bore needle in place. Anesthesia and cross-matched blood should be readily available. The twins are monitored by dual electronic fetal monitoring.

The decision about method of birth, which depends on a variety of factors, may not be made until labor occurs. The presence of maternal complications such as placenta previa, abruptio placentae, or severe PIH usually indicates the need for cesarean birth. Fetal factors such as severe IUGR, preterm birth, fetal anomalies, fetal distress, and unfavorable fetal position or presentation also require cesarean birth.

Any combination of presentations and positions can occur with multiple births. Figure 19–9♦ shows some possible presentations of twins. When the presenting fetus is in a nonvertex position cesarean birth is usually indicated (Malone & D'Alton, 1999).

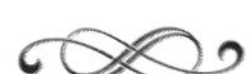

# Nursing Care Management

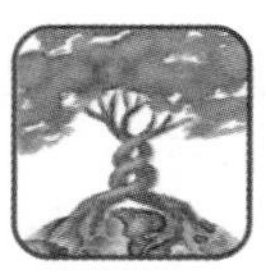

## Community-Based Nursing Care

During pregnancy the woman may need counseling about diet and daily activities. The nurse can help her plan meals to meet her increased needs. A daily intake of 4000 kcal (minimum) and 135 g of protein is recommended for optimal weight gain and fetal growth. A prenatal vitamin and 1 mg of folic acid should also be taken daily. A weight gain of 40 to 50 lb, with a 15- to 20-lb weight gain by 20 weeks, has been recommended for women with multiple-gestation pregnancy (Papiernik et al., 1998).

Counseling about daily activities may include encouraging the woman to plan frequent rest periods during the day. The rest period is most effective if the woman rests in a side-lying position (which increases uteroplacental blood flow) and elevates her lower legs and feet to reduce edema. Back discomfort may be relieved by pelvic rocking, maintaining good posture, and using good body mechanics when lifting objects and moving about.

## Hospital-Based Nursing Care

During labor, the FHRs of the siblings are monitored continuously by electronic fetal monitor (EFM). Electronic monitoring equipment now makes it possible to monitor the fetuses simultaneously, whether by external or internal means. They are monitored throughout labor and vaginal birth or up to the time of abdominal incision if a cesarean is done.

After birth the nurse must prepare to receive two or more newborns instead of one. This means duplicating everything, including resuscitation equipment, radiant warmers, and newborn identification papers and bracelets. Two or more physicians or nurses should be available for newborn resuscitation.

# Care of the Woman and Fetus in the Presence of Fetal Distress

When the oxygen supply is insufficient to meet the physiologic needs of the fetus, fetal distress may result. The condition may be acute, chronic, or a combination of the two. A variety of factors may contribute to fetal distress. The most common are cord compression and uteroplacental insufficiency, possibly caused by preexisting maternal or fetal disease or placental abnormalities. If the resulting hypoxia persists and metabolic acidosis occurs, the situation could cause permanent damage to or be life threatening for the fetus.

The most common early warning signs of fetal distress are meconium-stained amniotic fluid and the presence of ominous FHR patterns such as persistent late decelerations (regardless of the depth of deceleration), persistent severe variable decelerations (especially if the return to baseline is prolonged), and prolonged decelerations (Uckan & Townsend, 1999). When fetal distress is indicated, **intrauterine resuscitation** (corrective measures

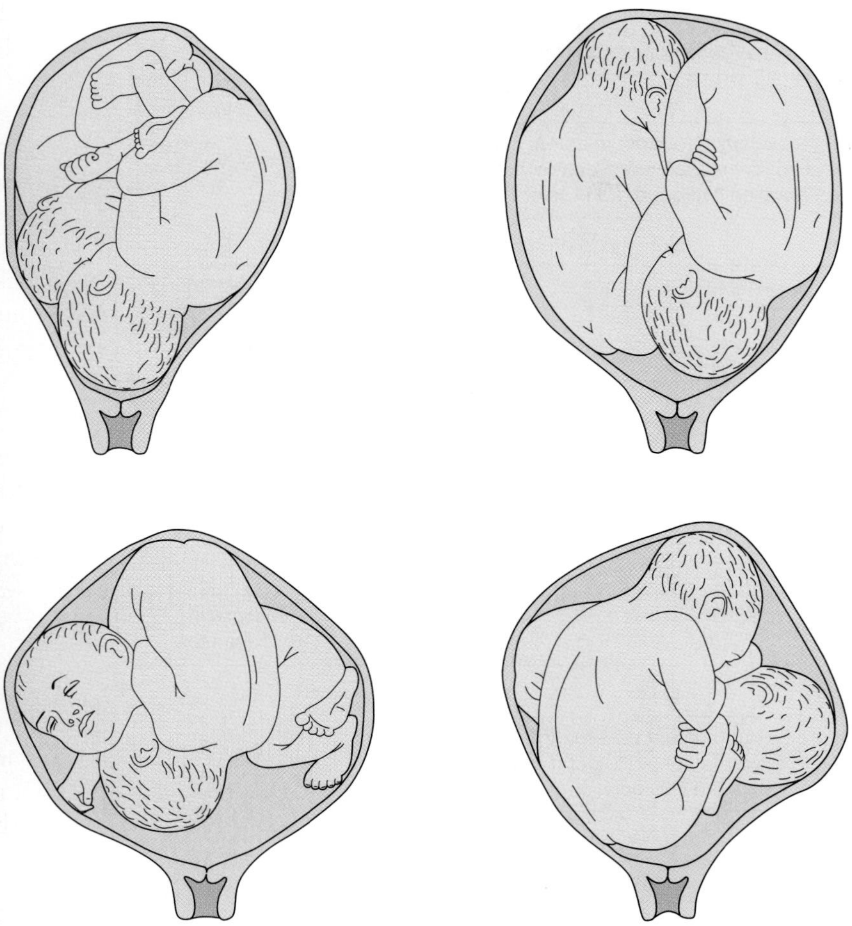

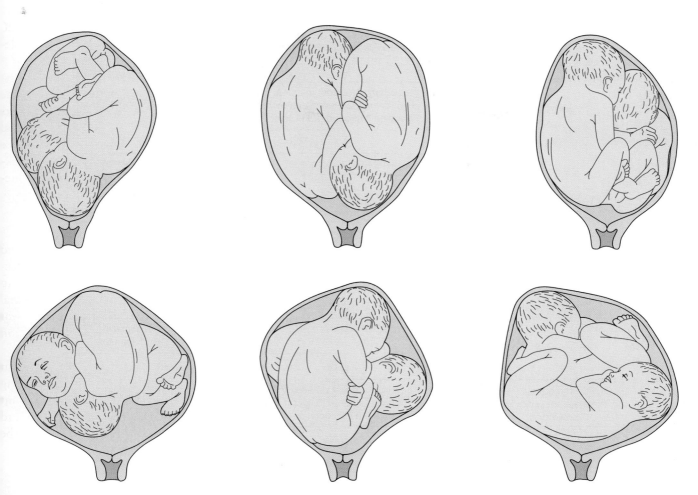

FIGURE 19–9 ♦ Twins may be in any of these presentations while in utero.

used to optimize the oxygen exchange within the maternal-fetal circulation) should be started without delay. Treatment of maternal hypotension involves having the woman turn to a left lateral decubitus position (right lateral decubitus may also be tried), beginning an intravenous infusion or increasing the flow rate if an infusion is already in place, or, if cord prolapse is suspected, having the woman assume a knee-chest position. Uterine activity can be decreased by discontinuing intravenous oxytocin administration or administering a tocolytic agent (such as terbutaline) to decrease contraction frequency and intensity. Oxygen is also administered to the woman via facial mask (Uckan & Townsend, 1999).

Caregivers can obtain additional information about the condition of the fetus by fetal scalp blood sampling, fetal scalp stimulation, or fetal acoustical stimulation (see Chapter 14). The management scheme for fetal distress is illustrated in Figure 19–10♦.

## Maternal Implications

Indications of fetal distress greatly increase the psychologic stress of a laboring woman. Professional staff members

## HINTS FOR PRACTICE

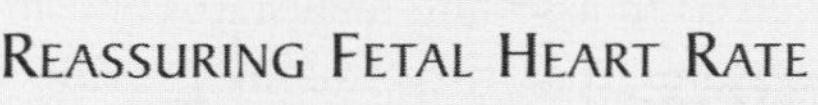

### Reassuring Fetal Heart Rate

To determine whether the fetal heart rate is reassuring, look for the following (Schmidt, 2000):

- Baseline heart rate between 120 and 160 bpm
- Long-term variability is average
- Short-term variability (can only be assessed with an internal EFM device) is present
- Accelerations are spontaneous
- Decelerations are absent or limited to early or occasional variables (see Chapter 14)

Recognition of fetal distress pattern (persistent late decelerations, persistent severe variable decelerations, prolonged deceleratons)*

Intrauterine resuscitation (correct maternal hypotension, reposition woman, decrease uterine contraction frequency and duration if needed, administer $O_2$)

Distress pattern ceases? — Yes → Continue monitoring, watch fetus closely

No ↓

Vaginal birth imminent? — Yes → Vaginal birth (neonatal resuscitation as needed)

No ↓

Bradycardia present? (bl<120 bpm) — Yes → Cesarean birth (neonatal resuscitation as needed)

No ↓

Variability average? (6–10 bpm) — Yes → Reassess in 10–15 minutes → Distress pattern ceases? — Yes → Continue monitoring, watch fetus closely; No → Vaginal birth imminent?

No ↓

FAST and/or SST reassuring? (acceleration with sound or manual stimulation) — No → Cesarean birth (neonatal resuscitation as needed)

No ↓

Fetal scalp blood pH ≥ 7.20 — No → Cesarean birth (neonatal resuscitation as needed)

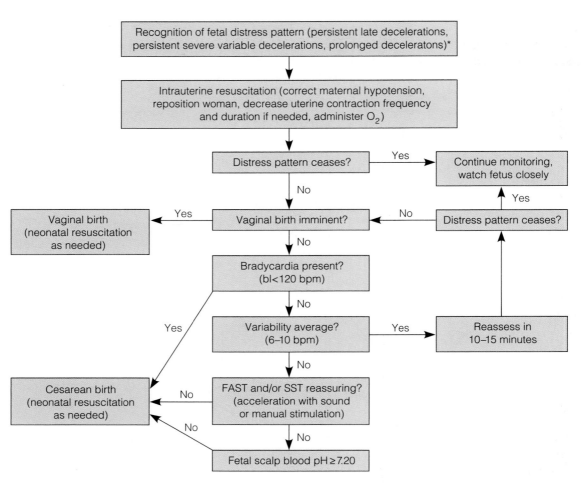

**FIGURE 19–10 ♦** Intrapartum management of fetal distress. Note: bl = baseline; FAST = fetal acoustic stimulation test; SST = scalp stimulation test. *Sources:* Based on information from Strong, T. H. (1990). Fetal distress in the intrapartum period. In E. J. Quilligan & F. P. Zuspan's (Eds.) *Current Therapy in Obstetrics and Gynecology,* (3rd ed.). Philadelphia: Saunders. *Huddleston, J. F. & Freeman, R. K. (1992). Estimation of fetal well-being. In A. A. Fanaroff & R. S. Martin's (Eds.) *Neonatal-Perinatal Medicine: Diseases of the fetus and newborn,* (5th ed.). St. Louis: Mosby-Year Book.

may become so involved in assessing fetal status and initiating corrective measures that they fail to provide the woman and her partner with explanations and emotional support. It is imperative to offer both. In many instances, if birth is not imminent, the woman must undergo cesarean birth. This method of birth may be a source of fear and of frustration, too, if the couple prepared for a shared vaginal birth experience.

## Clinical Therapy

When evidence of possible fetal distress exists, treatment centers on improving the blood flow to the fetus by correcting maternal hypotension, decreasing the intensity and frequency of contractions if present, providing IV fluids to the woman as needed, administering oxygen, and gathering further information about fetal status. Fetal response to intrauterine resuscitation measures dictates subsequent actions.

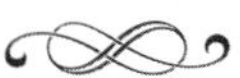

## Nursing Care Management

The nurse reviews the woman's prenatal history and notes the presence of any conditions (such as PIH, diabetes, renal disease, intrauterine growth restriction IUGR) that may be associated with decreased uteroplacental-fetal blood flow. When the membranes rupture, the nurse assesses the FHR immediately and notes the characteristics of the amniotic fluid. As labor progresses, the nurse is especially alert to suspicious changes in the FHR. At all times, the nurse encourages and supports maternal positioning that maximizes utero-placental-fetal blood flow.

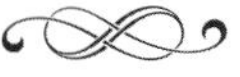

## Care of the Family at Risk due to Intrauterine Fetal Death

**Intrauterine fetal death (IUFD),** often referred to as *fetal demise,* accounts for one-half of perinatal mortality after 20 weeks' gestation. Fetal death results from unknown causes or from a number of physiologic maladaptations including preeclampsia or eclampsia, abruptio placentae, placenta previa, diabetes, infection, congenital anomalies, and isoimmune disease.

Prolonged retention of the dead fetus may lead to the development of *disseminated intravascular coagulation (DIC),* also called consumption coagulopathy, in the mother. After the release of thromboplastin from the degenerating fetal tissues into the maternal bloodstream, the extrinsic clotting system is activated, triggering the formation of multiple tiny blood clots. Fibrinogen and factors V and VII are subsequently depleted, and the woman begins to display symptoms of DIC. Fibrinogen levels begin a linear descent 3 to 4 weeks after the death of the fetus and continue to decrease in the absence of appropriate medical intervention.

### CLINICAL THERAPY

When fetal death has occurred, abdominal x-ray examination may reveal Spalding's sign, an overriding of the fetal cranial bones. In addition, maternal estriol levels fall. Diagnosis of IUFD is confirmed by absence of heart action on ultrasound. Most women have spontaneous labor within 2 weeks of fetal death, and if other complications are not present some physicians wait for labor to begin spontaneously (Anderson, 2000). In the absence of spontaneous labor, induction measures are begun.

## NURSING CARE MANAGEMENT

### Nursing Assessment and Diagnosis

Cessation of fetal movement reported by the mother to the nurse is frequently the first indication of fetal death. It is followed by a gradual decrease in the signs and symptoms of pregnancy. Fetal heart tones are absent, and fetal movement is no longer palpable. Once fetal demise is established, the nurse assesses the family members' ability to adapt to their loss. Open communication between the mother, her partner, and the health team members contributes to a realistic understanding of the medical condition and its associated treatments. The nurse may discuss prior experiences the family has had with stress and what they feel were their perceived coping abilities at that time. Identifying the family's social supports and resources is also important.

Nursing diagnoses that may apply include the following:

- Grief related to death of the fetus
- Ineffective individual and family coping related to depression secondary to loss of a child
- Ineffective family coping related to death of a child

### Nursing Plan and Implementation

The parents of a stillborn infant suffer a devastating experience that precipitates an intense emotional trauma. During the pregnancy, the couple has already begun the attachment process, which now must be terminated through the grieving process. Although enough similarity among individuals exists to identify some common phases in the course of grief, the process is "more fluid than an ordering of discrete phases would seem to imply" (Kay, Roman, & Schulte, 1997, p. 8). Therefore, it is important to recognize and honor the individual, using the three phases of grief that follow, as general guidelines (Kay et al., 1997).

1. Often the first phase is *protest* of the death of the fetus. This is likely to result in immediate shock and numbness, followed by disbelief and denial. In most cases this inability to grasp the reality of the loss is short lived and is followed by distress. When the caregiver first suspects fetal demise, the mother or parents may initially attempt to dismiss the possibility because the loss is too difficult to consider. When the death is confirmed, there may be a brief period during which the family refuses to believe it, followed by development of visible signs of loss such as weeping.
2. The second phase is *disorganization,* which involves developing awareness of the finality of the loss. Feelings of profound sadness and a deep yearning for the lost baby develop. Isolation, loneliness, and meaninglessness manifest into withdrawal from everyone and everything. The most common characteristic of disorganization is preoccupation with painful thoughts and visions of the lost infant.
3. *Reorganization* is the third and final phase. This step in the mourning process is the most individual of all, as the bereaved parents slowly begin to reengage with the world. The time frame varies greatly, but eventually painful memories become less frequent and new activities are begun. However, this phase may be accompanied by transitory feelings of guilt for enjoying life again in spite of the loss.

Some facilities use a checklist to ensure that caregivers address important aspects of working with the parents. The checklist becomes a communication tool as staff members share information particular to the couple. Such a checklist might include the following items:

- When fetal death has been confirmed before admission, inform the staff so they can avoid making inappropriate remarks.
- Allow the woman and her partner to remain together as much as they wish. Provide privacy and a supportive environment.
- Stay with the couple; do not leave them alone and isolated.
- As much as possible, have the same nurse provide care to increase the support for the couple. Develop a care plan to provide for continuity of care.
- Have the most experienced labor and birth nurse auscultate for fetal heart tones to avoid the searching that a more inexperienced nurse might feel compelled to do. Avoid the temptation to listen again "to make sure."
- Listen to the couple; do not offer explanations. They require solace without minimizing the situation.
- Facilitate the participation of the woman and her partner in the labor and birth process. Help them to make decisions about who is present and what rituals will occur during the birth process. Allow the woman to make the decision regarding anesthesia and analgesia during labor and birth.
- Give parents accurate information about plans for labor and birth.
- Provide ongoing opportunities for the couple to ask questions.
- Arrange for the woman to be assigned to a room that is away from new mothers and babies. If early discharge is an option, allow the family to make that decision.
- Encourage the couple to experience the grief that they feel. A couple may have intense feelings that they are unable to share with each other. Encourage them to talk and allow their emotions to show freely. Help them understand that they may each experience different feelings.
- Give the couple an opportunity to see and hold the stillborn infant in a private, quiet location. (Advocates of seeing the stillborn believe that viewing assists in dispelling denial and enables the couple to progress to the next step in the grieving process.) If they choose to see their stillborn infant, prepare the couple for what they will see by saying "the baby is cold," "the baby is blue," "the baby is bruised," or other appropriate statements.
- Some families may elect to bathe or dress their stillborn; support them in their choice.
- Take a photograph of the infant and let the family know it is available if they want it now or some time in the future.
- Offer a card with footprints, crib card, identification band, and possibly a lock of hair to the parents. These items may be kept with the photo if the parents do not want them at this time.
- Prepare the couple to return home. If there are siblings, each will usually progress through age-appropriate grieving. Provide the parents with information about normal mourning reactions, both psychologic and physiologic.
- Furnish the mother with educational materials that discuss the changes she will experience in returning to a nonpregnant state.
- Provide information about community support groups, including group name, contact person (if possible), and phone number. Use materials such as the book *When Hello Means Goodbye* by Schwiebert and Kirk (1985).
- Contact religious support systems if the parents desire.

The nurse experiences many of the same grief reactions as the parents of a stillborn infant. It is important to have support persons and colleagues available for counseling and support.

## HINTS FOR PRACTICE

### Intrauterine Fetal Demise

No matter who you are, or how much nursing experience you have, when an expectant family is in pain because of their loss, you will probably feel that you do not have the right thing to say. "I'm sorry and I don't know what to say" is a start.

## Evaluation

Anticipated outcomes of nursing care include the following:

- Family members express their feelings about the death of their baby.
- Family members participate in the decision of whether to see their baby and other decisions about the baby.
- The family has resources available for continued support.
- Family members know the community resources available and have names and phone numbers to use if they choose.
- The family is moving into and through the grieving process.

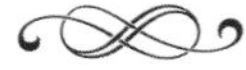

# Care of the Woman and Fetus at Risk due to Placental Problems

The most common types of placental problems are abruptio placentae, placenta previa, and abnormalities in placental formation and structure. Because the placenta is very vascular, problems are usually associated with maternal and possibly fetal hemorrhage. Abruptio placentae is a major emergency in labor and birth and requires rapid, effective interventions. Although placenta previa is primarily an antepartal problem, it is presented here for the sake of comparison. Causes and sources of hemorrhage are highlighted in Key Facts to Remember: Causes and Sources of Hemorrhage.

## ABRUPTIO PLACENTAE

**Abruptio placentae** is the premature separation of a normally implanted placenta from the uterine wall. Premature separation is considered a catastrophic event because of the severity of the resulting hemorrhage. The incidence of abruptio placentae is approximately 1 in 100 births and occurs more frequently in pregnancies complicated by hypertension and cocaine abuse. The risk of recurrence is much higher than for the general population (Scott, 1999).

The cause of abruptio placentae is largely unknown. Theories have been proposed relating its occurrence to decreased blood flow to the placenta through the sinuses during the last trimester. Excessive intrauterine pressure caused by hydramnios or multiple-gestation pregnancy, maternal hypertension, cigarette smoking, alcohol ingestion, increased maternal age and parity, trauma, and sudden changes in intrauterine pressure (as with amniotomy) have been suggested as contributing factors (Scott, 1999).

Abruptio placentae is subdivided into three types (Figure 19–11♦):

- *Marginal.* In this case the placenta separates at its edges, the blood passes between the fetal membranes and the uterine wall, and the blood escapes vaginally (also called marginal sinus rupture).
- *Central.* In this situation, the placenta separates centrally, and the blood is trapped between the placenta and the uterine wall. Entrapment of the blood results in concealed bleeding.
- *Complete.* Massive vaginal bleeding is seen in the presence of total separation.

### KEY FACTS TO REMEMBER

*Causes and Sources of Hemorrhage*

| Causes and Sources | Signs and Symptoms |
|---|---|
| **Antepartal Period** | |
| Abortion | Vaginal bleeding<br>Intermittent uterine contractions<br>Rupture of membranes |
| Placenta previa | Painless vaginal bleeding after seventh month |
| Abruptio placentae | |
| Partial | Vaginal bleeding: no increase in uterine pain |
| Severe | Vaginal bleeding may or may not be present<br>Extreme tenderness of abdominal area<br>Rigid, boardlike abdomen<br>Increase in size of abdomen |
| **Intrapartal Period** | |
| Placenta previa | Bright-red vaginal bleeding |
| Abruptio placentae | Same signs and symptoms listed earlier |
| Uterine atony in stage 3 | Bright-red vaginal bleeding<br>Ineffectual contractility |
| **Postpartal Period** | |
| Uterine atony | Boggy uterus<br>Dark vaginal bleeding<br>Presence of clots |
| Retained placental fragments | Boggy uterus<br>Dark vaginal bleeding<br>Presence of clots |
| Lacerations of cervic or vagina | Firm uterus<br>Bright-red blood |

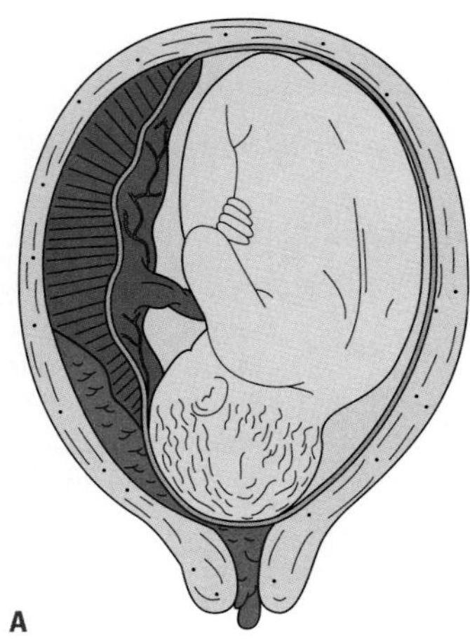


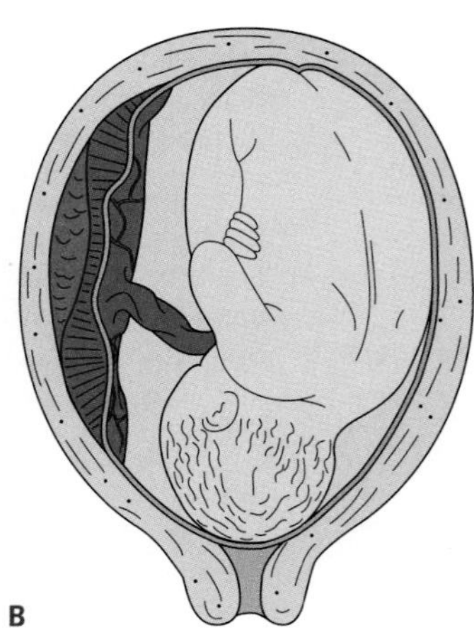


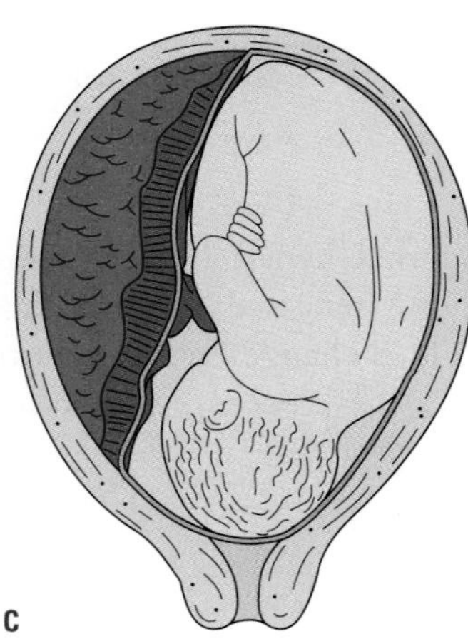


**FIGURE 19–11** ♦ Abruptio placentae. **A,** Marginal abruption with external hemorrhage. **B,** Central abruption with concealed hemorrhage. **C,** Complete separation.

The signs and symptoms of these three types of placental abruption are listed in Key Facts to Remember: Differential Signs and Symptoms of Placenta Previa and Abruptio Placentae. In severe cases of central abruptio placentae, the blood invades the myometrial tissues between the muscle fibers. This occurrence accounts for the uterine irritability that is a significant sign of abruptio placentae. If hemorrhage continues, eventually the uterus turns entirely blue because the muscle fibers are filled with blood. After birth the uterus contracts poorly. This condition is known as *Couvelaire* uterus and frequently necessitates hysterectomy.

As a result of the damage to the uterine wall and the retroplacental clotting with central abruption, large amounts of thromboplastin are released into the maternal blood supply. This thromboplastin in turn triggers the development of DIC and resultant hypofibrinogenemia. Fibrinogen levels, which are ordinarily elevated in pregnancy, may drop in minutes to the point at which blood will no longer coagulate (Perry, 2000a).

### Maternal Implications

Postpartal problems depend in large part on the severity of the intrapartal bleeding, coagulation defects (DIC), hypofibrinogenemia, and time between separation and birth. Moderate to severe hemorrhage results in hemorrhagic shock, which may prove fatal to the mother if it is not rapidly reversed. In the postpartal period, women with this disorder are at risk for hemorrhage and renal failure due to shock, vascular spasm, intravascular clotting, or a combination of these factors (Scott, 1999).

### Fetal-Neonatal Implications

Perinatal mortality associated with abruptio placentae ranges from 25% to 35% (Perry, 2000a). In severe cases, in which most of the placenta has separated, the infant mortality rate is 100%. In less severe separation, fetal outcome depends on the level of maturity. The most serious complications in the newborn arise from preterm labor, anemia, and hypoxia. If fetal hypoxia progresses unchecked, irreversible brain damage or fetal demise may result. Thorough assessment and prompt action on the part of the health team can improve both fetal and maternal outcomes.

## Clinical Therapy

Because of the risk of DIC, evaluating the results of coagulation tests is imperative. In DIC, fibrinogen levels and platelet counts usually decrease; prothrombin times and partial thromboplastin times are normal to prolonged. If the values are not markedly abnormal, serial testing may be helpful in establishing an abnormal trend indicative of coagulopathy. Another test determines levels of fibrin-degradation products; these values rise with DIC.

After establishing the diagnosis, emphasis is placed on maintaining the cardiovascular status of the mother and developing a plan for effecting the birth of the fetus. The birth method selected depends on the condition of the woman and fetus; in many circumstances, cesarean birth may be the safest option.

## KEY FACTS TO REMEMBER

*Differential Signs and Symptoms of Placenta Previa and Abruptio Placentae*

| | Placenta Previa | Abruptio Placentae |
|---|---|---|
| Onset | Quiet and sneaky | Sudden and stormy |
| Bleeding | External | External or concealed |
| Color of blood | Bright red | Dark venous |
| Anemia | = Blood loss | > Apparent blood loss |
| Shock | = Blood loss | > Apparent blood loss |
| Toxemia | Absent | May be present |
| Pain | Only during labor | Severe and steady |
| Uterine tenderness | Absent | Present |
| Uterine tone | Soft and relaxed | Firm to stony hard |
| Uterine contour | Normal | May enlarge and change shape |
| Fetal heart tones | Usually present | Present or absent |
| Engagement | Absent | May be present |
| Presentation | May be abnormal | No relationship |

*Source:* Oxorn, H. (1986). *Human labor and birth* (5th ed., p. 507). Norwalk, CT: Appleton & Lange.

If the separation is mild and the pregnancy is near term, labor may be induced and the fetus born vaginally with as little trauma as possible. If rupture of membranes and oxytocin infusion by pump do not initiate labor, a cesarean birth is required. A long delay would raise the risk of increased hemorrhage, with resulting hypofibrinogenemia. Supportive actions to decrease the risk of DIC include typing and cross matching for blood transfusions (at least four units), evaluating the clotting mechanism, and providing intravenous fluids (Perry, 2000a).

In cases of moderate to severe placental separation, a cesarean birth is done after treatment of hypofibrinogenemia by intravenous infusion of cryoprecipitate or plasma. Vaginal birth is impossible with a Couvelaire uterus, because the uterus would not contract properly in labor. Severe hemorrhage necessitates cesarean birth to allow an immediate hysterectomy to save both the woman and the fetus.

The hypovolemia that accompanies severe abruptio placentae is life threatening and requires the administration of whole blood. If the fetus is alive but in distress, emergency cesarean birth is the method of choice. With a stillborn fetus, vaginal birth is preferable unless maternal shock from hemorrhage is uncontrollable (Perry, 2000a). Central venous pressure (CVP) monitoring may be needed to evaluate intravenous fluid replacement. A normal CVP of 10 cm $H_2O$ is the goal. The CVP is evaluated hourly, and results are communicated to the physician. Elevations of CVP may indicate fluid overload and pulmonary edema. Laboratory testing is ordered to provide ongoing data regarding hemoglobin, hematocrit, and coagulation status. The hematocrit is maintained through the administration of packed red blood cells or whole blood (Perry, 2000a). Measures are taken to stimulate labor to prevent DIC. An amniotomy may be performed, and oxytocin is given to hasten delivery. Progressive dilatation and effacement usually occur (Perry, 2000a).

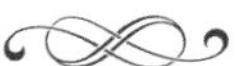

## Nursing Care Management

Electronic monitoring of the uterine contractions and resting tone between contractions provides information about the labor pattern and effectiveness of the oxytocin induction. Since uterine resting tone is frequently increased with abruptio placentae, it must be evaluated frequently for further increase. Abdominal girth measurements may be ordered hourly and are obtained by placing a tape measure around the maternal abdomen at the level of the umbilicus. Another method of evaluating uterine size, which increases as more bleeding occurs at the site of abruption, involves placing a mark at the top of the uterine fundus; the distance from the symphysis pubis to the mark may be measured hourly.

### Placenta Previa

In **placenta previa,** the placenta is implanted in the lower uterine segment rather than the upper portion of the uterus. This implantation may be on a portion of the lower segment or over the internal cervical os. As the lower uterine segment contracts and dilates in the later

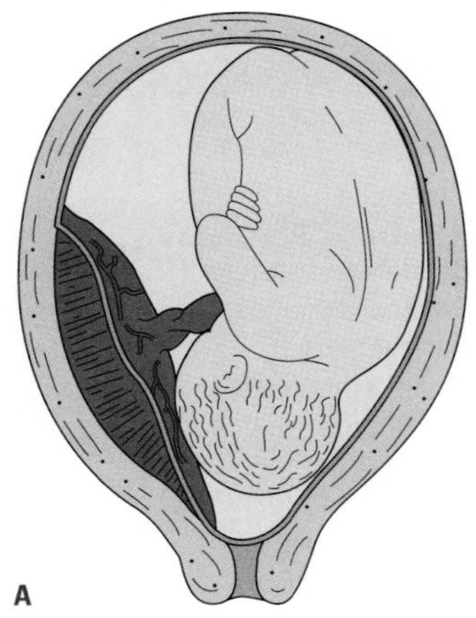

A

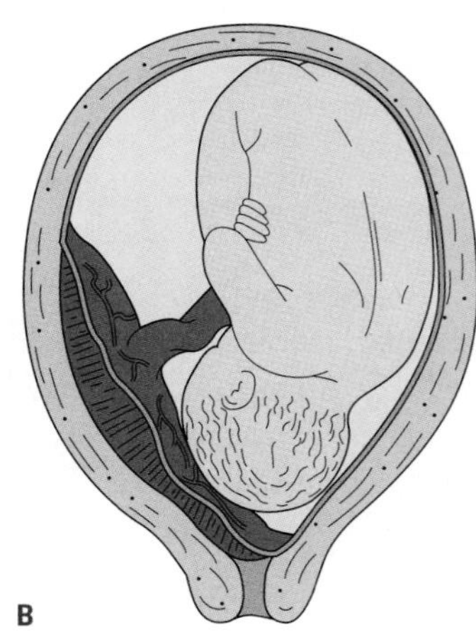

B

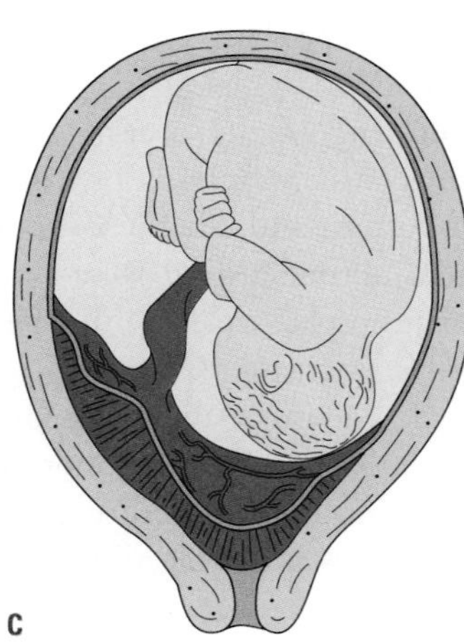

C

**FIGURE 19–12** ♦ Placenta previa. **A,** Low placental implantation. **B,** Partial placenta previa. **C,** Total placenta previa.

weeks of pregnancy, the placental villi are torn from the uterine wall, thus exposing the uterine sinuses at the placental site. Bleeding begins, but because its amount depends on the number of sinuses exposed, initially it may be either scanty or profuse (Figure 19–12♦).

The cause of placenta previa is unknown. Statistically it occurs in about 1 in every 200 births. Women with a previous history of placenta previa have a recurrence rate as high as 10% to 15% (Perry, 2000b). Other factors associated with placenta previa are multiparity, increasing age, placenta accreta, defective development of blood vessels in the decidua, and a large placenta (Perry, 2000b).

### Fetal-Neonatal Implications

The prognosis for the fetus depends on the extent of placenta previa. Changes in the FHR and meconium staining of the amniotic fluid may be apparent. In a profuse bleeding episode, the fetus is compromised and suffers some hypoxia. FHR monitoring is imperative when the woman is admitted, particularly if a vaginal birth is anticipated, because the presenting part of the fetus may obstruct the flow of blood from the placenta or umbilical cord. If fetal distress occurs, cesarean birth is indicated. After birth, blood sampling should be done to determine whether the intrauterine bleeding episodes of the woman have caused anemia in the newborn.

### Clinical Therapy

The goal of medical care is to identify the cause of bleeding and to provide treatment that will ensure birth of a mature newborn. Indirect diagnosis is made by localizing the placenta through tests that require no vaginal examination. The most commonly employed diagnostic test is the ultrasound scan (Figure 19–13♦). If placenta previa is ruled out, a vaginal examination can be performed with a speculum to determine the cause of bleeding (such as cervical lesions).

The differential diagnosis of placental or cervical bleeding takes careful consideration. Partial separation of the placenta may also present with painless bleeding, and

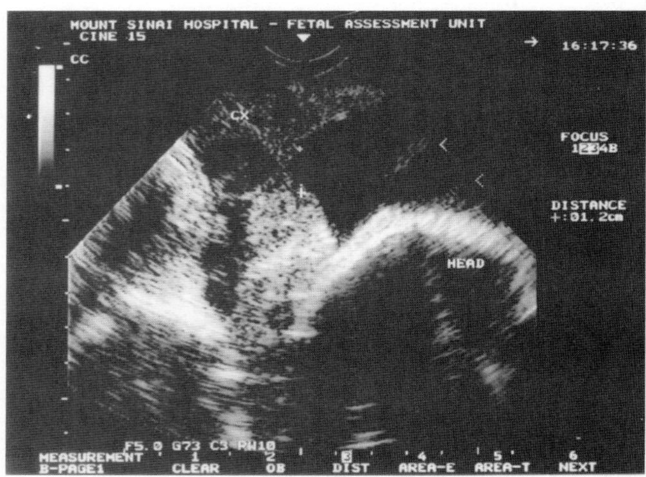


**FIGURE 19–13** ♦ Ultrasound of placenta previa.

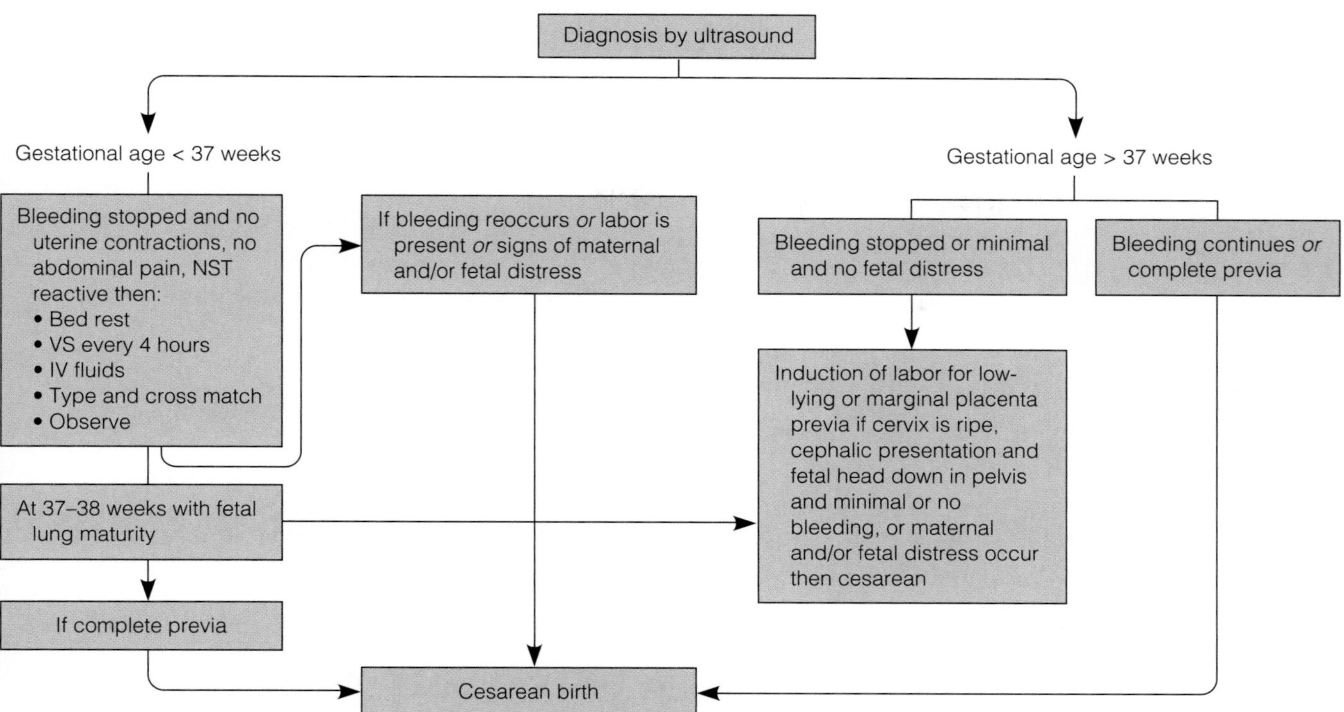


**FIGURE 19–14** ♦ Management of placenta previa. *Source:* Based on information from Barker, R. K., Fields, D. H., & Kaufman, S. A. (1990). *Quick Reference to OB-GYN Procedures,* (3rd ed.) New York: Lippincott/Harper & Row.

true placenta previa may not demonstrate overt bleeding until labor begins, thus confusing the diagnosis.

Care of the woman with painless late-gestational bleeding depends on (1) the week of gestation during which the first bleeding episode occurs and (2) the amount of bleeding (Figure 19–14♦). If the pregnancy is less than 37 weeks' gestation, expectant management is employed to delay birth until about 37 weeks' gestation to allow the fetus to mature. Expectant management involves stringent regulation of the following:

1. Bed rest with bathroom privileges as long as the woman is not bleeding
2. No vaginal exams
3. Monitoring blood loss, pain, and uterine contractility
4. Evaluating FHR with an external fetal monitor
5. Monitoring maternal vital signs
6. Complete laboratory evaluation: hemoglobin, hematocrit, Rh factor, and urinalysis
7. Intravenous fluid (lactated Ringer's solution)
8. Two units of cross-matched blood available for transfusion

If frequent, recurrent, or profuse bleeding persists, or if fetal well-being appears threatened, a cesarean birth may be performed.

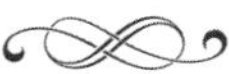

# Nursing Care Management

## Nursing Assessment and Diagnosis

Assessment of the woman with placenta previa must be ongoing to prevent or treat complications that are potentially lethal to the mother and fetus. Painless, bright-red vaginal bleeding is the most accurate diagnostic sign of placenta previa. If this sign develops during the last 3 months of pregnancy, placenta previa should always be considered until ruled out by examination. The first bleeding episode is generally scanty. If no vaginal examinations are performed, it often subsides spontaneously. However, each subsequent hemorrhage is more profuse.

The uterus remains soft, and if labor begins, it relaxes fully between contractions. The FHR usually remains stable unless profuse hemorrhage and maternal shock occur. As a result of the placement of the placenta, the fetal presenting part is often unengaged, and transverse lie is common.

The nurse assesses blood loss, pain, and uterine contractility both subjectively and objectively. Maternal vital signs and the results of blood and urine tests provide the nurse with additional data about the woman's condition. The FHR is evaluated with continuous external fetal monitoring. Another pressing nursing responsibility is to observe and verify the family's ability to cope with the anxiety associated with an unknown outcome.

Nursing diagnoses that may apply include the following:

- Fluid volume deficit related to hypovolemia secondary to excessive blood loss
- Risk for impaired fetal gas exchange related to decreased blood volume and maternal hypotension
- Anxiety related to concern for own personal status and the baby's safety

### Nursing Plan and Implementation

The nurse monitors the woman and her fetus to determine the status of the bleeding and the responses of the mother and baby. Vital signs, intake and output, and other pertinent assessments must be made frequently. The nurse uses the electronic monitor tracing to evaluate fetal status. A whole-blood setup should be ready for intravenous infusion and a patent intravenous line established before caregivers undertake any intrusive procedures. Maternal vital signs should be monitored every 15 minutes in the absence of hemorrhage and every 5 minutes with active hemorrhage. The external tocodynamometer should be connected to the maternal abdomen to monitor uterine activity continuously.

Provision of emotional support for the family is an important nursing care goal. During active bleeding, the assessments and management must be directed toward physical support. However, emotional aspects need to be addressed simultaneously. The nurse can explain the assessments and treatment measures needed. Time can be provided for questions, and the nurse can act as an advocate in obtaining information for the family. Emotional support can also be offered by staying with the family and using touch.

Promotion of neonatal physiologic adaptation is another important nursing responsibility. The newborn's hemoglobin, cell volume, and erythrocyte count should be checked immediately and then monitored closely. The newborn may require oxygen, administration of blood, and admission into a special care nursery. Nursing care of the woman with bleeding is addressed fully in the Critical Pathway for Hemorrhage in Third Trimester and at Birth, on page 485.

### Evaluation

Anticipated outcomes of nursing care include the following:

- The cause of hemorrhage is recognized promptly and corrective measures are taken.
- The woman's vital signs remain in the normal range.
- Any other complications are recognized and treated early.
- The family understands what has happened and the implications and associated problems of placenta previa.
- The woman and her baby have a safe labor and birth.

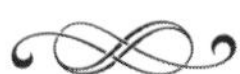

## Other Placental Problems

Other problems of the placenta are presented in Table 19–1.

# Care of the Woman and Fetus with a Prolapsed Umbilical Cord

A **prolapsed umbilical cord** results when the umbilical cord precedes the fetal presenting part. When this occurs, pressure is placed on the umbilical cord as it is trapped between the presenting part and the maternal pelvis. Consequently the vessels carrying blood to and from the fetus are compressed (Figure 19–15♦). Prolapse of the cord may occur with rupture of the membranes if the presenting part is not well engaged in the pelvis.

## Maternal Implications

Although a prolapsed cord does not directly precipitate physical alterations in the woman, her immediate concern for the baby creates enormous stress. The woman may need to deal with some unusual interventions, a cesarean birth, and, in some circumstances, the death of her baby.

## Fetal-Neonatal Implications

Compression of the cord results in decreased blood flow and leads to fetal distress. If labor is under way, the cord is compressed further with each contraction. If the pressure on the cord is not relieved, the fetus will die.

## Clinical Therapy

Preventing the occurrence of prolapse of the cord is the preferred medical approach. A laboring woman with a confirmed rupture of membranes will be kept horizontal, usually in bed, until the fetal head is well engaged and the risk of a prolapse is significantly decreased. If a prolapse

## TABLE 19–1 Placental and Umbilical Cord Variations

| *Placental Variation* | *Maternal Implications* | *Fetal-Neonatal Implications* | |
|---|---|---|---|
| **SUCCENTURIATE PLACENTA**<br>One or more accessory lobes of fetal villi will develop on the placenta. | Postpartal hemorrhage from retained lobe | None, as long as all parts of the placenta remain attached until after birth of the fetus | 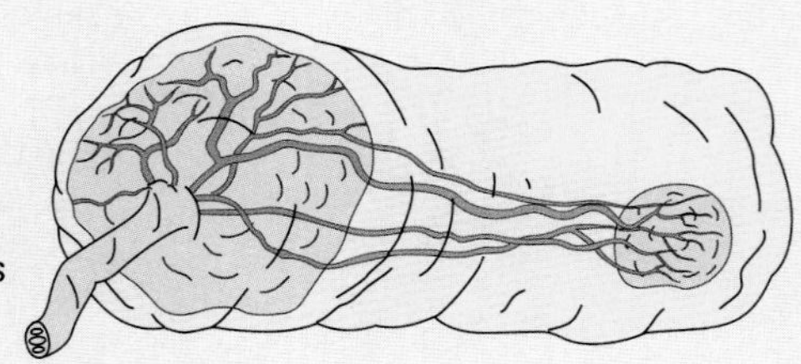 |
| **CIRCUMVALLATE PLACENTA**<br>A double fold of chorion and amnion form a ring around the umbilical cord, on the fetal side of the placenta. | Increased incidence of late abortion, antepartal hemorrhage, and preterm labor | Intrauterine growth restriction, prematurity, fetal death | 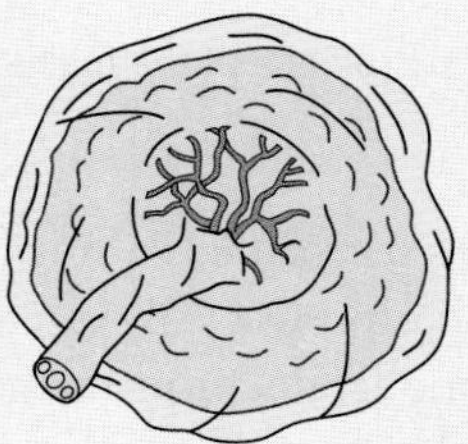 |
| **BATTLEDORE PLACENTA**<br>The umbilical cord is inserted at or near the placental margin. | Increased incidence of preterm labor and bleeding | Prematurity, fetal distress | 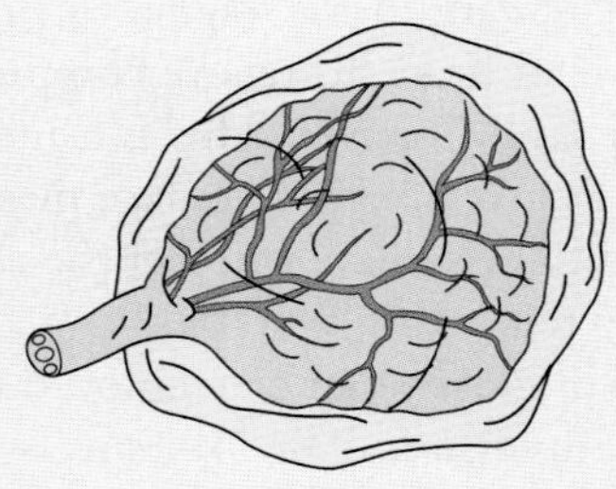 |
| **VELAMENTOUS INSERTION OF THE UMBILICAL CORD**<br>The vessels of the umbilical cord divide some distance from the placenta in the placental membranes. | Hemorrhage if one of the vessels is torn | Fetal distress, hemorrhage | 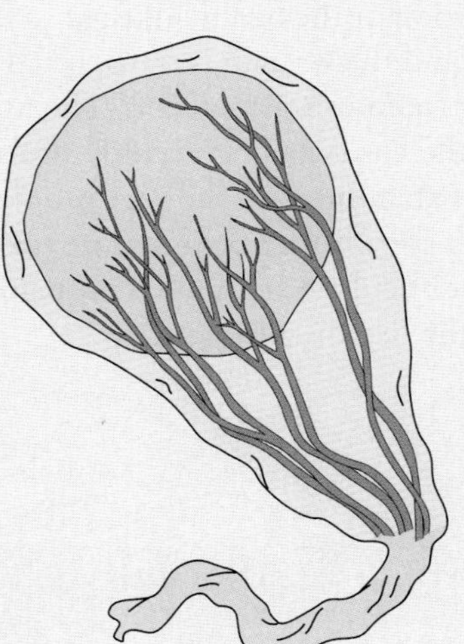 |

occurs, relieving the compression on the cord is critical to fetal outcome. The medical and nursing team must work together to facilitate birth.

Bed rest is indicated for all laboring women with a history of ruptured membranes, until engagement with no cord prolapse has been documented. Furthermore, with spontaneous rupture of membranes or amniotomy, the FHR should be auscultated for at least a full minute and at the beginning and end of contractions for several contractions. If fetal bradycardia is detected on the auscultation, a

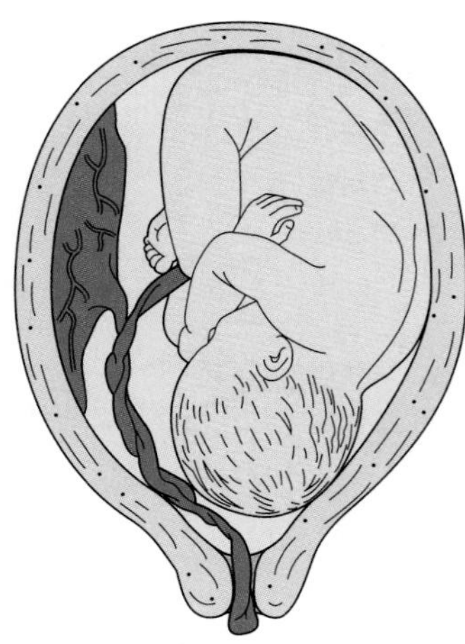

FIGURE 19–15 ♦ Prolapse of the umbilical cord.

vaginal exam is performed to rule out cord prolapse. In the presence of cord prolapse, electronic monitor tracings show severe, moderate, or prolonged variable decelerations with baseline bradycardia. If these patterns are found, the woman is examined vaginally.

If a loop of cord is discovered, the examiner's gloved fingers must remain in the vagina to provide firm pressure on the fetal head (to relieve compression) until the physician or CNM arrives. This is a lifesaving measure. The mother is given oxygen via face mask, and the FHR is monitored to determine whether the cord compression is adequately relieved.

The force of gravity can be employed to relieve umbilical cord compression. The woman assumes the knee-chest position or the bed is adjusted to the Trendelenburg position, and the woman is transported to the delivery or operating room in this position. The nurse must remember that the cord may be occultly prolapsed with an actual loop extending into the vagina or lying alongside the presenting part. It may be pulsating strongly or so weakly that it is difficult to determine on palpation of the cord whether the fetus is alive.

## Nursing Care Management

Because there are few outward signs of cord prolapse, each pregnant woman is advised to call her physician or certified nurse-midwife when the membranes rupture and to go to the office, clinic, or birthing facility. A sterile vaginal examination determines if there is danger of cord prolapse. If the presenting part is well engaged, the risk of cord prolapse is minimal, and the woman may ambulate as desired. If the presenting part is not well engaged, bed rest is recommended to prevent cord prolapse.

Because cord prolapse can be associated with fetal death, some physicians and CNMs insist that bed rest be maintained after rupture of membranes regardless of fetal engagement. This can lead to conflict if the laboring woman and her partner do not hold the same opinions. The nurse can ease this situation by assisting communication between the physician or CNM and the couple.

During labor, any alteration of the FHR or the presence of meconium in the amniotic fluid indicates the need to assess for cord prolapse. Vaginal birth is possible with prolapsed cord if the cervix is completely dilated and pelvic measurements are adequate.

If these conditions are not present, cesarean birth is the method of choice. The woman is taken to the surgical delivery room, and the examiner continues to relieve the pressure on the cord until the infant is born.

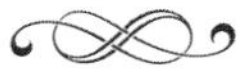

# Care of the Woman and Fetus at Risk due to Amniotic Fluid–Related Complications

## Amniotic Fluid Embolism

In the presence of a small tear in the amnion or chorion high in the uterus, a small amount of amniotic fluid may leak into the chorionic plate and enter the maternal system as an **amniotic fluid embolism.** The fluid can also enter at areas of placental separation or cervical tears. Under pressure from the contracting uterus, the fluid is driven into the maternal circulation and then the maternal lungs. The more debris in the amniotic fluid (such as meconium), the greater the maternal problems. This condition frequently occurs during or after the birth when the woman has had a difficult, rapid labor. Suddenly she experiences respiratory distress, circulatory collapse, acute hemorrhage, and cor pulmonale as the embolism blocks the vessels of the lungs. The woman exhibits a sudden onset of dyspnea, cyanosis, cardiovascular collapse, shock, and coma. Birth must be facilitated immediately to obtain a live fetus.

### Clinical Therapy

Any woman exhibiting chest pain, dyspnea, cyanosis, frothy sputum, tachycardia, hypotension, and massive hemorrhage requires the cooperation of every member of the health team if her life is to be saved. Medical interventions are supportive. Recovery is contingent on return of the mother's cardiovascular and respiratory stability. If necessary, the birth is assisted to enhance the health of the newborn.

# CRITICAL PATHWAY: *For Hemorrhage in Third Trimester and at Birth*

| Category | Immediate Care | Outcomes |
|---|---|---|
| **Referral** | Perinatologist<br>Neonatologist | **Expected Outcomes**<br>Appropriate resources identified and utilized |
| **Assessments** | Obtain history to identify whether any factors are present predisposing the mother to hemorrhage:<br>• Presence of preeclampsia or eclampsia (PIH)<br>• Overdistension of the uterus; multiple pregnancy; hydramnios<br>• Grand multiparity<br>• Advanced age<br>• Uterine contractile problems: hypotonicity; hypertonicity<br>• Painless vaginal bleeding after seventh month<br>• Presence of hypertension<br>• Presence of diabetes<br>• History of previous hemorrhage or bleeding problems, blood coagulation defects, abortion<br>• Retention of placental fragments<br>• Cervical and/or vaginal lacerations<br>Determine religious preference to establish whether client will permit a blood transfusion | **Expected Outcomes**<br>• Potential or actual hemorrhage identified<br>• Related complications minimized |
| **Teaching/psychosocial** | Keep woman informed of present status<br>Provide accurate information<br>Provide opportunities for questions<br>Establish a trusting relationship with client<br>Encourage the woman to participate in decision making if at all possible<br>Instruct client to keep bladder empty<br>Notify nurse if vaginal bleeding or leaking noted, decreased fetal movement, abdominal pain or discomfort, or uterine contractions<br>Report saturation $>$1 pad within 1 hr or less | **Expected Outcomes**<br>Woman verbalizes or demonstrates understanding of teaching |
| **Nursing care management and reports** | Observe, record, and report blood loss<br>Evaluate using the following parameters:<br>• Monitor rate and quality of respirations frequently<br>• Measure pulse rate<br>• Assess pulse quality by direct palpation<br>• Determine pulse deficit by comparing apical-radial rates<br>• Compare present BP with woman's baseline BP; note pulse pressure<br>• Inspect skin for presence of pallor and cyanosis, coldness, and clamminess<br>• Evaluate state of consciousness frequently<br>• Measure central venous pressure (CVP): normal CVP is 5–10 cm $H_2O$<br>• Assess amount of blood loss<br>• Count pads<br>• Weigh pads and Chux (1 g = approximately 1 mL blood)<br>• Record amount in a specific amount of time (eg, 50 mL bright-red blood on pad in 20 minutes)<br>Relieve decreased blood pressure by administering whole blood per physician order<br>While waiting for whole blood to be available, infuse isotonic fluids, plasma, plasma expanders, or serum albumin, per physician order<br>If marginal abruptio placentae is present:<br>• Evaluate blood loss<br>• Assess uterine contractile pattern, tenderness, and height<br>• Start continuous monitoring of uterine contractions by EFM | **Expected Outcomes**<br>Blood loss reduced and controlled or halted<br>Perfusion and oxygenation supported |

BP, blood pressure; CVP, central venous pressure; EFM, electronic fetal monitor; NPO, nothing by mouth; PIH, pregnancy-induced hypertension

| Category | Immediate Care | Outcomes |
|---|---|---|
| **Nursing care management and reports** | • Monitor maternal vital signs<br>• Assess fetal status per continuous EFM<br>• Assess cervical dilatation and effacement to determine labor progress if uterine contractions are present<br>• Rule out placenta previa<br>• Assist with amniotomy and begin oxytocin infusion per physician order if labor does not start immediately or is ineffective<br>• Review and evaluate diagnostic lab tests (hemoglobin, hematocrit, prothrombin time (PT), (APPT), fibrin split products, fibrinogen, platelets)<br>If central abruptio placentae with severe blood loss is present:<br>• Perform same assessments as for marginal abruptio placentae<br>• Monitor CVP<br>• Replace blood loss<br>• Effect immediate birth<br>• Observe for signs and symptoms of DIC<br>Woman is at risk for uterine atony following birth:<br>• Assess contractility of uterus and amount of vaginal bleeding<br>• Assess uterus q15 min × 4, q30 min × 2, q60 min × 2–4; evaluate more frequently if uterus is boggy or not in the midline; administer oxytocin per protocol or physician order | (previous page) |
| **Activity** | Complete bed rest<br>Diversional activity | **Expected Outcomes**<br>No exacerbation of hemorrhage occurs |
| **Comfort** | Assess comfort or woman | **Expected Outcomes**<br>Woman's comfort maintained |
| **Nutrition** | IV fluids infusing<br>NPO | **Expected Outcomes**<br>Optimal hydration and blood volume maintained |
| **Elimination** | Monitor urine output (decrease to less than 30 mL/hr is sign of shock):<br>• Insert Foley catheter<br>• Measure output hourly<br>• Measure specific gravity to determine concentration of urine | **Expected Outcomes**<br>Urinary output maintained |
| **Medications** | IV—lactated Ringer's at 150 mL/hr<br>If premature—betamethasone<br>$O_2$ as indicated | **Expected Outcomes**<br>Circulation and perfusion maintained |
| **Discharge planning/home care** | Determine need for assistance in the home<br>Provide information regarding community resources | **Expected Outcomes**<br>Woman is discharged with plan for follow-up care related to fatigue and blood loss |
| **Family involvement** | Establish a trusting relationship with family | **Expected Outcomes**<br>Family development and newborn attachment unimpaired |
| **Date** | | |

## Nursing Care Management

In the absence of the physician or CNM, the nurse administers oxygen under positive pressure until medical help arrives. An intravenous line is quickly established. If respiratory and cardiac arrest occurs, cardiopulmonary resuscitation (CPR) is initiated immediately.

The nurse readies the equipment necessary for blood transfusion and for the insertion of the CVP line. As the blood volume is replaced, using fresh whole blood to provide clotting factors, the CVP is monitored frequently. In the presence of cor pulmonale, fluid overload could easily occur.

## Hydramnios

**Hydramnios** (also called polyhydramnios) occurs when there is more than 2000 mL of amniotic fluid. The exact cause of hydramnios is unknown; however, in about 20% of cases it is associated with major congenital anomalies (Rosemond, 2000). In addition to the fetal implications, the maternal implications include significantly increased incidence of cesarean birth (Biggio, Wenstrom, Dubarb, et al., 1999).

During the second half of the pregnancy, the fetus begins to swallow and inspire amniotic fluid and to urinate, which contributes to the amount of amniotic fluid present. In cases of hydramnios, no pathology has been found in the amniotic epithelium. However, hydramnios is associated with fetal malformations that affect the fetal swallowing mechanism and neurologic disorders in which the fetal meninges are exposed in the amniotic cavity. This condition is also found in cases of anencephaly, in which the fetus is thought to urinate excessively due to overstimulation of the cerebrospinal centers. When monozygotic twins manifest hydramnios, it is because the twin with the increased blood volume urinates excessively. The weight of the placenta has been found to be increased in some cases of hydramnios, indicating that increased functioning of the placental tissue may be a factor.

There are two types of hydramnios: chronic and acute. In the chronic type, the fluid volume gradually increases and is a problem of the third trimester. Most cases are of this variety. In acute cases, the volume increases rapidly over a period of a few days. The acute type is usually diagnosed between 20 and 24 weeks' gestation.

### Maternal Implications

When the amount of amniotic fluid is 3000 mL or more, the woman experiences shortness of breath and edema in the lower extremities from compression of the vena cava. Milder forms of hydramnios occur more frequently and are associated with minimal symptoms. Hydramnios is associated with maternal disorders such as diabetes and Rh sensitization and with multiple-gestation pregnancies.

If the amniotic fluid is removed rapidly before birth, abruptio placentae can result from too sudden a change in the size of the uterus. Because of overdistension of uterine muscles, uterine dysfunction can occur in the intrapartal period, and the incidence of postpartal hemorrhage increases.

### Fetal-Neonatal Implications

Fetal malformations and preterm birth are common with hydramnios; thus the perinatal mortality rate is fairly high. Prolapsed cord can occur when the membranes rupture, a further complication for the fetus. The incidence of malpresentations also increases.

### Clinical Therapy

Hydramnios is managed with supportive treatment unless the intensity of the woman's distress and symptoms dictates otherwise. If the accumulation of amniotic fluid is severe enough to cause maternal dyspnea and pain, hospitalization and removal of the excessive fluid are required. Fluid can be removed vaginally or by amniocentesis. The dangers of performing the technique vaginally are prolapsed cord and the inability to remove the fluid slowly. If amniocentesis is performed, it should be done with the aid of sonography to prevent inadvertent damage to the fetus and placenta. The fluid should be removed slowly to prevent abruption (Rosemond, 2000).

## Nursing Care Management

Hydramnios should be suspected when the fundal height increases out of proportion to the gestational age. As the amount of fluid increases, the nurse may have difficulty palpating the fetus and auscultating the FHR. In more severe cases, the maternal abdomen appears extremely tense and tight on inspection. On sonography, large spaces can be identified between the fetus and the uterine wall.

When amniocentesis is performed, it is vital to maintain sterile technique to prevent infection. The nurse can offer support to the couple by explaining the procedure to them.

If the fetus has been diagnosed with a congenital defect in utero or is born with the defect, psychologic support is needed to assist the family. Often the nurse collaborates with social services to offer the family this additional help.

## Oligohydramnios

**Oligohydramnios,** in which the amount of amniotic fluid is severely reduced and concentrated, is a rare maternal finding. The exact cause of this condition is unknown. It is found in cases of postmaturity, with IUGR secondary to placental insufficiency, and in fetal conditions associated with major renal malformations, including renal aplasia with dysplastic kidneys and obstructive lesions of the lower urinary tract (Rosemond, 2000). If oligohydramnios occurs in the first part of pregnancy, there is a danger of fetal adhesions (one part of the fetus may adhere to another part).

### Maternal Implications

Labor can be dysfunctional, and progress is slow.

### Fetal-Neonatal Implications

During the gestational period, fetal skin and skeletal abnormalities may occur because fetal movement is impaired as a result of reduced amniotic fluid volume. Because there is less fluid available for the fetus to use during fetal breathing movements, pulmonary hypoplasia may develop. During the labor and birth, the lessened amounts of fluid reduce the cushioning effect for the umbilical cord, and cord compression is more likely to occur. Decreased amniotic fluid also contributes to fetal head compression.

### Clinical Therapy

During the antepartum period oligohydramnios may be suspected when the uterus does not increase in size according to the dates, the fetus is easily palpated and outlined by the examiner, and the fetus is not ballotable. The fetus can be assessed by biophysical profiles, nonstress tests, and serial ultrasound. During labor, the fetus is monitored by continuous EFM to detect cord compression, which is indicated by variable decelerations. Some clinicians advocate the use of an amnioinfusion (a transcervical instillation of 500 mL of warmed sterile saline, followed by a continuous infusion rate of 100 to 200 mL/hr) after membranes have ruptured to decrease the frequency and severity of variable decelerations in the FHR during labor (Rosemond, 2000). The infusion of saline provides more fluid for the umbilical cord to float in and thereby lessens or prevents cord compression.

## Critical Thinking in Practice

A fetal heart rate (FHR) tracing demonstrates the following: baseline heart rate of 140 with variability of 6–10 bpm. When you compare the FHR with the uterine contractions, you note that there is a slowing of the FHR at the time of the contraction and that the FHR tracing looks like the contraction curve, but it is upside down. Based on this tracing, what would you do?

Answers can be found in Appendix 00.

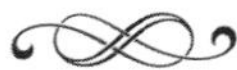

## Nursing Care Management

Continuous electronic fetal monitoring is an important part of the assessment during the labor and birth. The nurse evaluates the EFM tracing for the presence of variable decelerations or other nonreassuring signs (such as increasing or decreasing baseline, decreased variability, presence of late decelerations). If variable decelerations are noted, the woman's position can be changed (to relieve pressure on the umbilical cord), and the CNM or physician needs to be notified. After the birth, the newborn is evaluated for signs of congenital anomalies, pulmonary hypoplasia, and postmaturity.

# Care of the Woman with Cephalopelvic Disproportion (CPD)

The birth passage includes the maternal bony pelvis, beginning at the pelvic inlet and ending at the pelvic outlet, and the maternal soft tissues within these anatomic areas. A contracture (narrowed diameter) in any of the described areas can result in **cephalopelvic disproportion (CPD)** if the fetus is larger than the pelvic diameters. Abnormal fetal presentations and positions occur in CPD as the fetus moves to accommodate its passage through the maternal pelvis.

The gynecoid and anthropoid pelvic types are usually adequate for vertex birth, but the android and platypelloid types are predisposed to CPD. Certain combinations of types also can result in pelvic diameters inadequate for vertex birth. (See Chapter 15 for a description of pelvic types and their implications for childbirth.)

## Types of Contractures

The pelvic inlet is contracted if the shortest anterior-posterior diameter is less than 10 cm or the greatest transverse diameter is less than 12 cm. The anterior-posterior diameter may be approximated by measuring the diagonal conjugate, which in the contracted inlet is less than 11.5 cm. Clinical and x-ray pelvimetry are used to determine the smallest anterior-posterior diameter through which the fetal head must pass.

The treatment goal is to allow the natural forces of labor to push the biparietal diameter of the fetal head beyond the potential interspinous obstruction. Although forceps may be used, they cause difficulty because pulling on the head destroys flexion, and the space is further diminished. A bulging perineum and crowning indicate that the obstruction has been passed.

An interischial tuberous diameter of less than 8 cm constitutes an outlet contracture. Outlet and midpelvic contractures frequently occur simultaneously. Whether vaginal birth can occur depends on the woman's interischial tuberous diameters and the fetal posterosagittal diameter.

## Maternal Implications

Labor is prolonged in the presence of CPD. Membrane rupture can result from the force of the unequally distributed contractions being exerted on the fetal membranes. In obstructed labor, in which the fetus cannot descend, uterine rupture can occur. With delayed descent, necrosis of maternal soft tissues can result from pressure exerted by the fetal head. Eventually, necrosis can cause fistulas from the vagina to other nearby structures. Difficult, forceps-assisted births can also result in damage to maternal soft tissue.

## Fetal-Neonatal Implications

If the membranes rupture and the fetal head has not entered the inlet, there is a danger of cord prolapse. Excessive molding of the fetal head can result. Traumatic, forceps-assisted birth can damage the fetal skull and central nervous system.

## Clinical Therapy

Fetopelvic relationships can be assessed by comparing pelvic measurements obtained by a manual exam before labor and by computed tomography (CT) with estimated weight of the fetus as obtained by ultrasound measurements.

When the pelvic diameters are borderline or questionable, a trial of labor (TOL) may be advised. In this process, the woman continues to labor, and careful, frequent assessments of cervical dilatation and fetal descent are made. As long as there is continued progress, the TOL continues. If progress ceases, the decision for a cesarean birth is made.

# Nursing Care Management

The adequacy of the maternal pelvis for a vaginal birth should be assessed both during and before labor. During the intrapartal assessment, the size of the fetus and its presentation, position, and lie must also be considered. (See Chapter 16 for intrapartal assessment techniques.)

The nurse should suspect CPD when labor is prolonged, cervical dilatation and effacement are slow, and engagement of the presenting part is delayed. The couple may need support in coping with the stresses of this complicated labor. The nurse should keep the couple informed of what is happening and explain the procedures being used. This knowledge reassures the couple that measures are being taken to resolve the problem.

Nursing actions during the TOL are similar to care during any labor except that cervical dilatation and fetal descent are assessed more frequently. Both contractions and the fetus should be monitored continuously. Any signs of fetal distress are reported to the CNM or physician immediately.

The mother may be positioned in a variety of ways to increase the pelvic diameters. Sitting or squatting increases the outlet diameters and may be effective when there is failure of or slow fetal descent. Changing from one side to the other or maintaining a hands-and-knees position may assist the fetus in the occiput-posterior position to change to an occiput-anterior position. The mother may instinctively want to assume one of these positions. If not, the nurse may encourage a change of position.

# Care of the Woman at Risk due to Complications of the Third and Fourth Stages of Labor

## Lacerations

Lacerations of the cervix or vagina may be indicated when bright-red vaginal bleeding persists in the presence of a well-contracted uterus. The incidence of lacerations is higher when the childbearing woman is young or a nullipara, has an epidural, has forceps-assisted birth and an episiotomy, and has not done perineal massage or preparation during pregnancy. Vaginal and perineal lacerations are often categorized in terms of degree, as follows:

- First-degree laceration is limited to the fourchette, perineal skin, and vaginal mucous membrane.
- Second-degree laceration involves the perineal skin, vaginal mucous membrane, underlying fascia, and muscles of the perineal body; it may extend upward on one or both sides of the vagina.
- Third-degree laceration extends through the perineal skin, vaginal mucous membranes, and perineal body and involves the anal sphincter; it may extend up the anterior wall of the rectum.
- Fourth-degree laceration is the same as third-degree but extends through the rectal mucosa to the lumen of the rectum; it may be called a third-degree laceration with a rectal wall extension.

## Placenta Accreta

The chorionic villi attach directly to the myometrium of the uterus in *placenta accreta.* Two other types of placental adherence are *placenta increta,* in which the myometrium is invaded, and *placenta percreta,* in which the myometrium is penetrated. The adherence itself may be total, partial, or focal, depending on the amount of placental involvement. The incidence of placenta accreta is 1 in 2500 (Cunningham et al., 1997). Placenta accreta is the most common type and accounts for 80% of adherent placentas.

The primary complication with placenta accreta is maternal hemorrhage and failure of the placenta to separate following birth of the infant. An abdominal hysterectomy may be necessary, depending on the amount and depth of involvement.

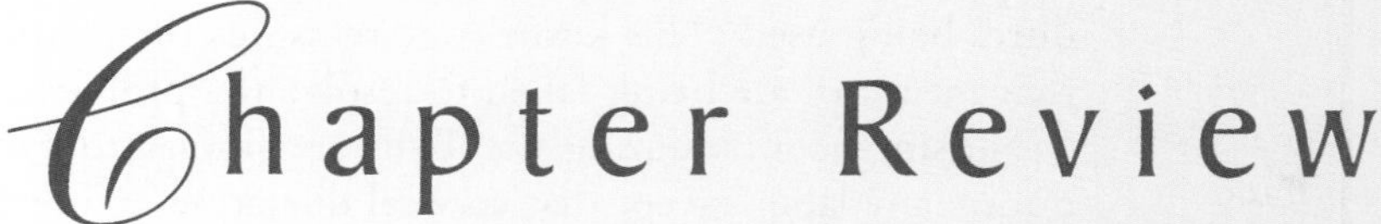


## CHAPTER HIGHLIGHTS

- Anxiety and fear have a profound effect on labor, particularly when complications that might jeopardize the mother or fetus occur.
- A hypertonic labor pattern is characterized by painful contractions that are not effective in effacing and dilating the cervix. It usually leads to a prolonged latent phase.
- Hypotonic labor patterns begin normally and then progress to infrequent, less intense contractions.
- Precipitous labor is extremely rapid labor and birth that lasts less than 3 hours. It is associated with an increased risk to the mother and newborn infant.
- Postterm pregnancy is one that extends more than 294 days, or 42 weeks, past the first day of the last menstrual period.
- The occiput-posterior position of the fetus during labor prolongs the labor process, causes severe back discomfort in the laboring

woman, and predisposes her to vaginal and perineal trauma and lacerations during birth.

- The types of fetal malpresentations include face, brow, breech, and shoulder.
- A fetus or newborn weighing more than 4000 g is termed *macrosomic.* Problems may occur during labor, birth, and the early neonatal period.
- Preventing and treating problems that infringe on the development and birth of normal fetuses are significant medical-nursing activities once the presence of twins or multiple-gestation pregnancies has been detected.
- Fetal distress is indicated by persistent late decelerations, persistent severe variable decelerations, and prolonged decelerations. If fetal distress is recognized and treated appropriately, the fetus may be spared any permanent damage.
- Intrauterine fetal death poses a major nursing challenge to provide support and care for the parents.
- Major bleeding problems in the intrapartal period are abruptio placentae and placenta previa.
- Abruptio placentae is the separation of the placenta from the side of the uterus prior to birth of the infant. Abruptio placentae may be central, marginal, or complete.
- Placenta previa occurs when the placenta implants low in the uterus near or over the cervix. A low-lying or marginal placenta is one that lies near the cervix. In partial placenta previa, part of the placenta lies over the cervix; in complete placenta previa, the cervix is completely covered.
- Prolapsed umbilical cord results when the umbilical cord precedes the fetal presenting part. This places pressure on the umbilical cord and diminishes blood flow to the fetus.
- Amniotic fluid embolism occurs when a bolus of amniotic fluid enters the maternal circulation and then the maternal lungs. The maternal mortality rate is very high with this complication.
- Hydramnios (also called polyhydramnios) occurs when there is more than 2000 mL of amniotic fluid contained within the amniotic membranes. Hydramnios is associated with fetal malformations that affect fetal swallowing and with maternal diabetes mellitus, Rh sensitization, and multiple-gestation pregnancies.
- Oligohydramnios is present when there is a severely reduced volume of amniotic fluid. Oligohydramnios is associated with IUGR, with postmaturity, and with fetal renal or urinary malfunctions. The fetus is more likely to experience variable decelerations because the amniotic fluid is insufficient to keep pressure off the umbilical cord.
- CPD occurs when there is a narrowed diameter in the maternal pelvis. The narrowed diameter is called a contracture and may occur in the pelvic inlet, the midpelvis, or the outlet. If pelvic measurements are borderline, a trial of labor may be attempted. Failure of cervical dilatation or fetal descent necessitates a cesarean birth.
- Third- and fourth-stage complications usually involve hemorrhage. The causes of hemorrhage include lacerations of the birth canal or cervix and placenta accreta.

## CHAPTER REFERENCES


Anderson, G. D. (2000). Fetal demise. In M. E. Rivlin & R. W. Martin (Eds.), *Manual of clinical problems in obstetrics and gynecology* (5th ed., pp. 122–126). Philadelphia: Lippincott.

Benirschke, K. (1999). Multiple gestation: Incidence, etiology, and inheritance. In R. K. Creasy & R. Resnik (Eds.), *Maternal-fetal medicine* (4th ed., pp. 585–597). Philadelphia: Saunders.

Berg, M., & Dahlberg, K. (1998). A phenomenological study of women's experiences of complicated childbirth. *Midwifery, 14,* 23–29.

Berkus, M. D., Conway, D., & Langer, O. (1999). The large fetus. *Clinical Obstetrics and Gynecology, 42*(4), 766–784.

Biggio, J. R., Wenstrom, K. D., Dubarb, M. B., & Cliver, S. P. (1999). Hydramnios: Prediction of adverse perinatal outcomes. *Obstetrics and Gynecology, 94*(5), 762–773.

Bofill, J. A. (2000). Breech presentation. In M. E. Rivlin & R. W. Martin (Eds.), *Manual of clinical problems in obstetrics and gynecology* (5th ed., pp. 143–146). Philadelphia: Lippincott.

Bowes, W. A. (1999). Clinical aspects of normal and abnormal labor. In R. K. Creasy & R. Resnik (Eds.), *Maternal-fetal medicine* (4th ed., pp. 541–568). Philadelphia: Saunders.

Clausson, B., Cnattingius, S., & Axelsson, O. (1999). Outcomes of post-term births: The role of fetal growth restriction and malformations. *Obstetrics and Gynecology, 94*(5), 758–762.

Creedy, D. K., Shochet, I. M., & Horsfall, J. (2000). Childbirth and the development of acute traumatic symptoms: Incidence and contributing factors. *Birth, 27*(2), 104–111.

Cunningham, F. G., MacDonald, P. C., Grant, N. F., Leveno, K. J., Gilstrap, L. C., Hankins, G. D. V., & Clark, S. L. (1997). *Williams obstetrics* (20th ed.). Stamford, CT: Appleton & Lange.

Dahlberg, K., Berg, M., & Lundgren, I. (1999). Commentary: Studying maternal experiences of childbirth. *Birth, 26*(4), 215–217.

Hogg, B. B., & Kimberlin, D. F. (2000). Delivery of the small and large infant. In M. E. Rivlin & R. W. Martin (Eds.), *Manual of clinical problems in obstetrics and gynecology* (5th ed., pp. 179–182). Philadelphia: Lippincott.

Kay, J., Roman, B., & Schulte, H. M. (1997). Pregnancy loss and the grief process. In J. R. Woods & J. L. Esposito (Eds.), *Loss during pregnancy or in the newborn period: Principles of care with clinical cases and analyses* (pp. 5–36). Pittman, NJ: Jannetti Publications.

Keith, L., Papiernik, E., & Oleszcuzuk, J. J. (1998). How should the efficacy of prenatal care be tested in twin gestation? *Clinical Obstetrics and Gynecology, 41,* 85–93.

Lopez-Zeno, J. A. (1997). Active management of labor: The American experience. *Clinical Obstetrics and Gynecology, 40,* 510–515.

Malone, F. D., & D'Alton, M. E. (1999). Multiple gestation: Clinical characteristics and management. In R. K. Creasy & R. Resnik (Eds.), *Maternal-fetal medicine* (4th ed., pp. 598–615). Philadelphia: Saunders.

Martin, J. N. (2000). Postterm pregnancy. In M. E. Rivlin & R. W. Martin (Eds.), *Manual of clinical problems in obstetrics and gynecology* (5th ed., pp. 105–108). Philadelphia: Lippincott.

Miller, V. L., Ransom, S. B., Shalhoub, A., Sokol, R. J. & Evans, M. I. (2000). Multifetal pregnancy reduction: Perinatal and fiscal outcomes. *American Journal of Obstetrics and Gynecology, 182*(6), 1575–1579.

O'Reilly-Green, C., & Divon, M. (2000). Sonographic and clinical methods in diagnosis of macrosomia. *Clinical Obstetrics and Gynecology, 43*(2) 309–325.

Papiernik, E., Keith, L., Oleszcuzuk, J. J., & Cervantes, A. (1998). What interventions are useful in reducing the rate of preterm delivery in twins? *Clinical Obstetrics and Gynecology, 41,* 13–23.

Parer, J. T. (1999). Fetal heart rate. In R. K. Creasy & R. Resnik (Eds.), *Maternal-fetal medicine* (4th ed., pp. 270–299). Philadelphia: Saunders.

Perry, K. G., Jr. (2000a). Abruptio placentae. In M. E. Rivlin & R. W. Martin (Eds.), *Manual of clinical problems in obstetrics and gynecology* (5th ed., pp. 21–23). Philadelphia: Lippincott.

Perry, K. G., Jr. (2000b). Placenta previa. In M. E. Rivlin & R. W. Martin (Eds.), *Manual of clinical problems in obstetrics and gynecology* (5th ed., pp. 18–20). Philadelphia: Lippincott.

Rivlin, M. E. (2000). Nonbreech abnormal presentations, positions, and lies. In M. E. Rivlin & R. W. Martin (Eds.), *Manual of clinical problems in obstetrics and gynecology* (5th ed., pp. 146–149). Philadelphia: Lippincott.

Roberts, S. J., Reardon, K. M., & Rosenfeld, S. (1999). Childbirth sexual abuse: Surveying its impact on primary care. *AWHONN Lifelines, 3,* 39–45.

Roberts, W. E. (2000). Multifetal gestation. In M. E. Rivlin & R. W. Martin (Eds.), *Manual of clinical problems in obstetrics and gynecology* (5th ed., pp. 95–100). Philadelphia: Lippincott.

Rodis, J. F., Arky, L., Egan, J. F. X., Borgida, A. F., Leo, M. V., & Campbell, W. A. (1999). Comprehensive fetal ultrasonography measurements in triplet gestation. *American Journal of Obstetrics and Gynecology, 181*(5), 1128–1132.

Rosemond, R. L. (2000). Hydramnios and oligohydramnios. In M. E. Rivlin & R. W. Martin (Eds.), *Manual of clinical problems in obstetrics and gynecology,* (5th ed., pp. 149–152). Philadelphia: Lippincott.

Saito, T., Ylikorkala, O., & Halmesmaki, E. (1999). Factors associated with fear of delivery in second pregnancies. *Obstetrics and Gynecology, 94*(5), 679–682.

Schmidt, J. (1999). Prolonged labor. In L. K. Mandeville & N. H. Troiano (Eds.), *AWHONN: High risk and critical care intrapartum nursing* (2nd ed., pp. 123–138). Philadelphia: Lippincott.

Schmidt, J. (2000). Intrapartum fetal assessment. In S. Mattson & J. E. Smiths (Eds.), *AWHONN: Maternal newborn nursing* (4th ed., pp. 272–299). Philadelphia: Saunders.

Schwiebert, P., & Kirk, P. (1985). *When hello means goodbye.* Eugene, OR: Health Sciences University.

Scott, J. R. (1999). Placenta previa and abruption. In J. R. Scott, P. J. DiSaia, C. B. Hammond, & W. N. Spellacy (Eds.), *Danforth's obstetrics and gynecology* (8th ed., pp. 407–418). Philadelphia: Lippincott.

Uckan, E. M., & Townsend, N. S. (1999). Fetal adaptation. In L. K. Mandeville & N. H. Troiano (Eds.), *AWHONN: High-risk and critical care intrapartum nursing* (2nd ed., pp. 32–50). Philadelphia: Lippincott.

# CONTEMPORARY MATERNAL-NEWBORN NURSING ON-LINE

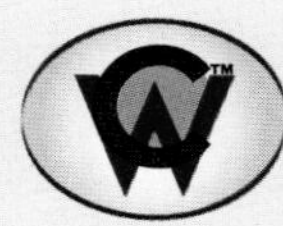

Additional interactive resources, including animations and video, for this chapter can be found on the Companion Website at http://www.prenhall.com/ladewig. Click on Chapter 19 and "Begin" to select the activities for this chapter.

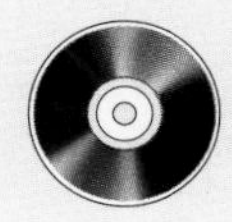

For NCLEX review questions and an audio glossary, access the accompanying CD-ROM in this book.

# Chapter 20

# Birth-Related Procedures

*Labor and birth today are remarkably safe for both the mother and her baby. With all of our advanced technology, we in health care have the ability to make enormous strides toward our outcome goals. But the bigger challenge is to do all of that and still honor the truly life-changing, miraculous nature of the birth experience.*

—Labor and Delivery RNC

## KEY TERMS

| | |
|---|---|
| Amnioinfusion (AI) | 500 |
| Amniotomy | 496 |
| Cervical ripening | 496 |
| Episiotomy | 505 |
| External cephalic version (ECV) | 495 |
| Forceps | 506 |
| Internal version | 495 |
| Labor augmentation | 498 |
| Labor induction | 498 |
| Vacuum-assisted birth | 507 |
| Vaginal birth after cesarean (VBAC) | 512 |

## OBJECTIVES

- **Examine the methods and purpose of external and internal version.**
- **Discuss the use of amniotomy in current maternal-newborn care.**
- **Compare methods for inducing labor, explaining their advantages and disadvantages.**
- **Identify at least two indications for amnioinfusion.**
- **Describe the types of episiotomy performed and the associated nursing interventions.**
- **Summarize the indications for forceps-assisted birth.**
- **Discuss the use of vacuum extraction to assist birth.**
- **Explain the indications for cesarean birth, impact on the family unit, preparation and teaching needs, and associated nursing care.**
- **Discuss vaginal birth following cesarean birth.**

Most births occur without the need for operative obstetric intervention. In some instances, however, procedures are necessary to maintain safety for the woman and the fetus. The most common of these are amniotomy, induction of labor, episiotomy, cesarean birth, and vaginal birth following a previous cesarean birth.

Generally, women are aware of the possible need for an obstetric procedure during their labor and birth. However, some women expect to have a "natural" experience and do not anticipate the need for medical intervention. This conflict between expectation and the need for intervention presents a challenge to maternity nurses. The nurse provides information regarding any procedure to help the woman and her partner understand what is proposed, the anticipated benefits and possible risks, and any alternatives.

# Care of the Woman during Version

*Version,* or turning the fetus, is a procedure used to change the fetal presentation by abdominal or intrauterine manipulation. The most common type of version is **external cephalic version (ECV),** in which the fetus is changed from a breech to a cephalic presentation by external manipulation of the maternal abdomen (Figure 20–1♦). A less common type of version, called **internal** (or *podalic*) **version,** is used only with the second fetus during a vaginal twin birth and only if the twin does not descend readily or shows signs of distress. In an internal version medication is used to relax the uterus and the obstetrician places a hand inside the uterus, grabs the fetus's feet, and draws them down through the cervix.

## External Version

If breech or shoulder presentation (transverse lie) is detected in the later weeks of pregnancy, an external version may be attempted. Before the external version is begun, an ultrasound is used to locate the placenta and to confirm fetal presentation.

The following criteria should be met prior to performing external version:

- The pregnancy is 36 or more weeks' gestation. A version may result in complications that require immediate birth by cesarean (Cruikshank, 1999).
- A nonstress test (NST), obtained immediately prior to performing the version, is reactive. A reactive NST indicates fetal well-being.

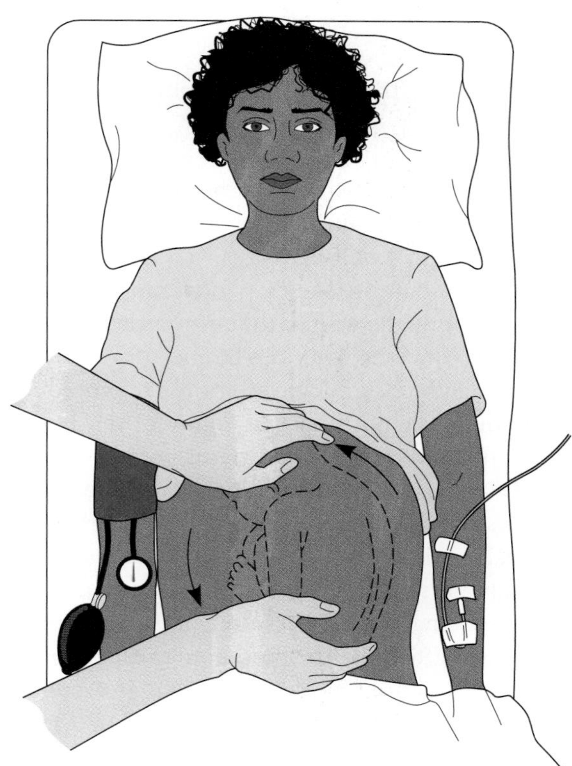

FIGURE 20–1 ♦ External (or cephalic) version of the fetus. A new technique involves pressure on the fetal head and buttocks so that the fetus completes a "backward flip" or "forward roll."

- The fetal breech is not engaged. Once the presenting part is engaged it is difficult, if not impossible, to do a version.

Contraindications include the following (Bowes, 1999):

- Maternal problems, such as uterine anomalies, pregnancy-induced hypertension (PIH), or third-trimester bleeding
- Complications of pregnancy, such as rupture of membranes, oligohydramnios, hydramnios, or placenta previa
- Previous cesarean birth or other significant uterine surgery
- Multiple gestation
- Nonreassuring fetal heart rate (FHR) or other evidence of uteroplacental insufficiency
- Fetal abnormalities, such as intrauterine growth restriction (IUGR) or nuchal cord

Before the external version begins an intravenous line is established to administer medications in case of difficulty. The woman receives terbutaline to relax the uterus. The version is discontinued in the presence of severe maternal pain or significant FHR bradycardia or decelerations.

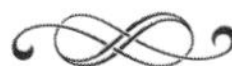

## Nursing Care Management

On admission the nurse begins a thorough assessment by verifying that there are no contraindications to the version procedure. Maternal vital signs and a reactive NST are obtained. This initial assessment period provides an ideal time for educating the woman and her partner and for addressing their concerns. They can be encouraged to express their understanding and expectations of the procedure. At the same time, the possibility of failure of the ECV and slight risk of cesarean birth if the fetus becomes distressed should also be discussed. Explaining what will occur in either of these circumstances will better prepare the woman and her partner if intervention becomes necessary.

Throughout the procedure, the nurse continues to monitor maternal blood pressure, pulse, and comfort level frequently (because the mother may experience pain during the procedure). Fetal well-being is ascertained before, intermittently during, and for (at least) 30 minutes following the procedure, using electronic fetal monitoring (EFM), ultrasound, or both. The nurse also assesses maternal-fetal response to the tocolytic. Aftercare instructions, which may include maternal monitoring for contractions and fetal movement (fetal kick counts), are provided as well.

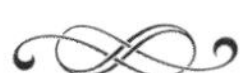

# Care of the Woman during Amniotomy

**Amniotomy** is the artificial rupture of the amniotic membranes (AROM). It is probably the most common operative procedure in obstetrics. Because the amniotomy requires that an instrument, called an *amnihook,* be inserted through the cervix, at least 2 cm of cervical dilatation is required. The amniotomy may be performed in hope of starting labor (inducing) or at any time during the first stage to augment labor (accelerate the progress). An amniotomy done after 3 cm of cervical dilatation will probably shorten the length of labor (Wolcott & Conry, 2000). Amniotomy may also be done during labor to apply an internal fetal heart monitoring electrode to the scalp, to insert an intrauterine pressure catheter, or to obtain a fetal scalp blood sample for acid-base determination and fetal pH monitoring. In addition, amniotomy allows assessment of the color and composition of amniotic fluid.

### AROM Procedure

While performing a vaginal examination, the physician or certified nurse-midwife (CNM) introduces an amnihook into the vagina and makes a small tear in the amniotic membrane, which allows amniotic fluid to escape.

## Nursing Care Management

The nurse explains the AROM procedure to the woman and then assesses fetal presentation, position, and station, because amniotomy is usually delayed until engagement has occurred. The woman is asked to assume a semireclining position and is draped to provide privacy. The FHR is assessed just before and immediately after the amniotomy, and the two FHR assessments are compared. If there are marked changes, the nurse should check for prolapse of the cord (see Chapter 19). The amniotic fluid is inspected for amount, color, odor, and the presence of meconium or blood. While wearing disposable gloves, the nurse cleanses and dries the perineal area and changes the underpads. Because there is now an open pathway for organisms to ascend into the uterus the number of vaginal exams must be kept to a minimum to reduce the chance of introducing an infection. In addition, the woman's temperature is monitored a minimum of every 2 hours. The nurse needs to provide information regarding the expected effects of the amniotomy. It is important for the woman to know that amniotic fluid is constantly produced, because some may worry that they will experience a "dry birth."

# Care of the Woman during Cervical Ripening

### Prostaglandin Gel

Prostaglandin $E_2$ ($PGE_2$) gel for **cervical ripening** (softening and effacing the cervix) may be used for the pregnant woman at or near term when there is a medical or obstetric indication for induction of labor. Two commonly used gels are Prepidil and Cervidil. These preparations have been demonstrated to cause cervical ripening and shorter labor and to lower requirements for oxytocin during labor induction. Vaginal birth is achieved within 24 hours for most women (Oei, Lidewijde, & Mol, 2000).

# DRUG GUIDE

## DINOPROSTONE (CERVIDIL) VAGINAL INSERT

### *Pregnancy Risk Category: C*

### *Overview of Maternal-Fetal Action*

Dinoprostone is a naturally occurring form of prostaglandin $E_2$. Dinoprostone can be used at term to ripen the cervix and can stimulate the smooth muscle of the uterus to enhance uterine contractions. A single vaginal insert may be used to ripen the cervix, and then oxytocin can be administered. (Forrest Pharmaceuticals, Inc. Drug Insert, 1995; Zatuchi & Slupik, 1996).

### *Route, Dosage, Frequency*

The vaginal insert contains 10 mg of dinoprostone. The insert is placed transversely in the posterior fornix of the vagina, and the client is kept supine for 2 hours but then may ambulate. The dinoprostone is released at approximately 0.3 mg/hr over a 12-hour period. The vaginal insert should be removed by pulling on the retrieval string upon onset of uterine contractions or after 12 hours (Forrest Pharmaceuticals, Inc. Drug Insert, 1995).

### *Contraindications*

- Client with known sensitivity to prostaglandins
- Presence of fetal distress
- Unexplained bleeding during pregnancy
- Strong suspicion of cephalopelvic disproportion
- Client already receiving oxytocin
- Client with six or more previous term pregnancies
- Client who is not anticipated to be able to give birth vaginally

Dinoprostone vaginal insert should be used with *caution* in clients with ruptured membranes, a fetus in breech presentation, presence of glaucoma, or history of asthma (Forrest Pharmaceuticals, Inc. Drug Insert, 1995).

### *Maternal Side Effects*

Uterine hyperstimulation with or without fetal distress has occurred in a very small number (2.8%–4.7%) of clients. Fewer than 1% of clients have experienced fever, nausea, vomiting, diarrhea, or abdominal pain (Forrest Pharmaceuticals, Inc. Drug Insert, 1995).

### *Effects on Fetus or Neonate*

Fetal distress (Zatuchi & Slupik, 1996).

### *Nursing Considerations*

- Assess for presence of contraindications.
- Monitor maternal vital signs, cervical dilatation, and effacement carefully.
- Monitor fetal status for presence of reassuring fetal heart rate pattern (baseline 120–160 bpm presence of short-term variability, average variability, presence of accelerations with fetal movement, absence of late or variable decelerations).
- Remove vaginal insert if uterine hyperstimulation, sustained uterine contractions, fetal distress, or any other maternal adverse actions occur.

Prostaglandin gel is best used only in a hospital birthing unit, and it is recommended that an obstetrician be readily available in case an emergency cesarean birth is needed (American College of Obstetricians and Gynecologists [ACOG], 1998b). See Drug Guide: Dinoprostone (Cervidil) for additional information.

## MISOPROSTOL (CYTOTEC)

Misoprostol (Cytotec) is a synthetic $PGE_1$ analogue that may also be used to ripen the cervix and induce labor. It is available in tablet form. Some contraindications for the use of misoprostol include the following (ACOG, 1999b):

- Presence of uterine contractions three times in 10 minutes
- Significant maternal asthma
- History of previous uterine scar or bleeding during the pregnancy
- Presence of placenta previa
- Nonreassuring fetal heart rate tracing

## NURSING CARE MANAGEMENT

Physicians, certified nurse-midwives (CNMs), and birthing room nurses who have had special education and training may administer $PGE_2$ products and misoprostol. The woman and her support person(s) are provided information about the procedure, and any questions are answered. Maternal vital signs are assessed for baseline, and an electronic fetal monitor is applied. The EFM tracing should indicate minimal or absent uterine activity, a reassuring FHR pattern, and a reactive NST. If uterine contractions are not occurring regularly, $PGE_2$ gel or a 25-μg misoprostol tablet is inserted into the vagina. The woman is requested to lie supine with a right hip wedge for a specified time (usually at least an hour). The woman can then assume any comfortable position. The nurse monitors the woman for uterine hyperstimulation and FHR abnormalities (changes in baseline rate, variability, presence of decelerations) for at least 2 hours following insertion (Schmidt, 1999).

During administration of $PGE_2$, if nausea and vomiting are present or contractions occur more frequently than every 2 minutes (and/or last >75 seconds) the gel is removed.

# Care of the Woman during Labor Induction

ACOG defines **labor induction** as the stimulation of uterine contractions before the spontaneous onset of labor, with or without ruptured fetal membranes, for the purpose of accomplishing birth. Induction may be indicated in the presence of the following (ACOG, 1999a):

- Diabetes mellitus
- Renal disease
- Pregnancy-induced hypertension (PIH)
- Premature rupture of membranes (PROM)
- History of rapid labor (precipitous labor and birth)
- Chorioamnionitis
- Postterm gestation
- Mild abruptio placentae with no fetal distress
- Intrauterine fetal demise (IUFD)
- Intrauterine fetal growth restriction (IUGR)
- Isoimmunization

All contraindications to spontaneous labor and vaginal birth are contraindications to the induction of labor. Relative maternal contraindications include but are not limited to the following (ACOG, 1999a):

- Client refusal
- Placenta previa or vasa previa
- Transverse fetal lie
- Prior classic uterine incision (vertical incision in the upper portion of the uterus)
- Active genital herpes infection
- Some instances of positive maternal human immunodeficiency virus (HIV) status

Before induction is attempted, appropriate assessment must indicate that both the woman and fetus are ready for the onset of labor. This includes evaluation of fetal maturity and cervical readiness.

## LABOR READINESS

### FETAL MATURITY

The gestational age of the fetus is best evaluated by accurate maternal menstrual dating and serial ultrasounds. Amniotic fluid studies also provide valuable information in assessing fetal lung maturity (see Chapter 14).

### CERVICAL READINESS

The findings on vaginal examination help determine whether cervical changes favorable for induction have occurred. Bishop (1964) developed a prelabor scoring system that is helpful in predicting the potential success of induction (Table 20–1). Components evaluated are cervical dilatation, effacement, consistency, and position, as well as the station of the fetal presenting part. A score of 0, 1, 2, or 3 is given to each assessed characteristic. The higher the total score for all the criteria, the more likely it is that labor will occur. The lower the total score, the higher the failure rate. A favorable cervix is the most important criterion for a successful induction (Cunningham, MacDonald, Gant, et al., 1997a). The presence of a cervix that is anterior, soft, 50% effaced, and dilated at least 2 cm, with the fetal head at −1 to +1 station or lower (Bishop score of 9) is favorable for successful induction (ACOG, 1995). If the cervix is unfavorable, a method of cervical ripening may be tried.

## INDUCTION BY OXYTOCIN INFUSION

Administration of oxytocin is an effective method of initiating uterine contractions to induce labor and may also be used to enhance ineffective contractions (**labor augmentation**). A primary line of 1000 mL of electrolyte

TABLE 20–1 Prelabor Status Evaluation Scoring System

| Factor | Assigned Value 0 | 1 | 2 | 3 |
|---|---|---|---|---|
| Cervical dilatation | Closed | 1–2 cm | 3–4 cm | 5 cm or more |
| Cervical effacement | 0%–30% | 40%–50% | 60%–70% | 80% or more |
| Fetal station | −3 | −2 | −1, 0 | +1, or lower |
| Cervical consistency | Firm | Moderate | Soft | |
| Cervical position | Posterior | Midposition | Anterior | |

*Source:* Bishop, E. H. (1964). Pelvic scoring for elective inductions. *Obstetrics and Gynecology, 24,* 266.

solution (eg, lactated Ringer's solution) is started intravenously. Ten units of oxytocin (Pitocin) are added to a secondary line of intravenous (IV) fluid so the resulting mixture will contain 10 mU/mL of oxytocin (1 mU/min, or 6 mL/h), and the prescribed dose can be calculated easily. After the primary infusion is started, the oxytocin solution is piggybacked into the primary tubing port closest to the catheter insertion. The infusion is then administered using an infusion pump to control the flow rate precisely. The rate of infusion is based on physician or CNM protocol and careful assessment of the contraction pattern. The goal for induction is to achieve stable contractions every 2 to 3 minutes that last 40 to 60 seconds. The uterus should relax to full baseline resting tone between each contraction. Progress is determined by changes in the effacement and dilatation of the cervix and station of the presenting part.

Oxytocin induction is not without some associated risks, including *hyperstimulation* of the uterus, resulting in uterine contractions that are too frequent or too intense, with an increased resting tone. Hypertonic contractions may lead to decreased placenta perfusion and fetal distress. Other risks include uterine rupture and water intoxication (Wilson, Shannon, & Stang, 2001).

### Induction by Misoprostol

During misoprostol induction, an IV is started to ensure access if needed later, and a 25-μg misoprostol tablet is inserted into the posterior vaginal fornix. The dose may be repeated every 3 to 4 hours until there are at least three uterine contractions in 10 minutes (ACOG, 1999b).

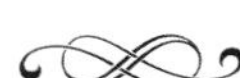

## Nursing Care Management

Aspects to address during client teaching about induction of labor include the purpose, the procedure itself, nursing care that will be provided, assessments, comfort measures, and a review of breathing techniques that may be used during labor. Regardless of the induction method used, close observation and accurate, ongoing assessments are mandatory to provide safe, optimal care for both woman and fetus. A qualified obstetrician should be readily accessible to manage any complications that may occur. As contractions are established, vaginal examinations are done to evaluate cervical dilatation, effacement, and station. The frequency of vaginal examinations primarily depends on the woman's parity, comfort level, and strength of her contractions. If evaluating the need for analgesia, a vaginal examination should be performed to avoid giving the medication too early and increasing the risk of prolonging labor and to identify advanced dilatation and imminent birth.

Although the use of misoprostol (Cytotec) for labor induction has been studied since 1993, universal protocols have not been established. One proposed protocol (Wilson, 2000) recommends the following:

- obtain baseline vital signs, then repeat blood pressure, pulse, and respiration every 30 minutes (×2), then lengthen time to 4 hour intervals (temperature every two hours if membranes are ruptured) after each administration of Cytotec
- perform vaginal exam to determine cervical status and fetal presentation
- apply fetal monitor and obtain non-stress test
- monitor uterine activity and FHR continuously for two hours; if reassuring, women may be permitted to ambulate until the next scheduled dose
- obtain IV access and administer IV fluids as ordered
- delay administration of additional doses for two hours (and monitor uterine activity) in the event of rupture of membranes.

## Critical Thinking in Practice

You are a birthing center nurse caring for Wendy Johnson, gravida 2, para 1, during an oxytocin infusion to induce her labor. Wendy has been receiving the medication via infusion pump for 4 hours and currently is receiving 6 mU/min (36 mL/hr). You have just completed your assessments and found the following: BP 120/80, pulse 80, respirations 16; contractions every 3 minutes lasting 60 seconds and of strong intensity; the FHR baseline is 144–150 with average long-term variability; and cervical dilatation is 6 cm. Will you continue the same infusion rate, increase the rate, or decrease the rate?

Answers can be found in Appendix I.

- oxytocin may be given 2 hours after last dose of misoprostol

Oxytocin induction protocols recommend obtaining baseline data (maternal temperature, pulse, respirations, blood pressure), a 20- to 30-minute EFM recording demonstrating a reassuring FHR, a reactive NST, and the contraction status before the induction is started. The fetal monitor is used to provide continuous data.

Before each increase of the oxytocin infusion rate the nurse assesses the following:

- Maternal blood pressure and pulse
- Contraction status including frequency, duration, intensity, and resting tone
- FHR baseline, variability, and reactivity, noting the presence of accelerations, any decelerations, or bradycardia

For additional information about nursing interventions during use of oxytocin, see Drug Guide: Oxytocin (Pitocin), on page 501, and Critical Pathway for Induction of Labor, on page 503.

### Holistic Methods for Cervical Ripening and Induction

In addition to the medical (allopathic) cervical ripening and induction methods previously discussed, a variety of more natural, noninvasive methods may also be used. These methods include sexual intercourse; self or partner nipple or breast stimulation; the use of herbs, castor oil, or enemas; acupuncture; stripping or sweeping the amniotic membranes; and mechanical dilatation of the cervix with balloon catheters (Summers, 1997). The cautions and contraindications are the same as those for medical induction of labor.

Although not frequently presented in medical (allopathic) or nursing texts, the natural methods are very effective (Summers, 1997). Many certified nurse midwives and their clients desire a less medical approach to birth and want to use natural methods whenever possible. It is important for basic nursing students, nurses, and consumers to be aware of all aspects of pregnancy care.

Sexual intercourse is a logical method of inducing cervical ripening and uterine contractions; female orgasm stimulates contractions, and male ejaculate contains a rich source of prostaglandins. In addition, breast and nipple stimulation, which are often part of lovemaking, cause the production of endogenous oxytocin, which in turn stimulates the uterus to contract (Summers, 1997).

Herbal preparations and other homeopathic solutions have not been scientifically studied to the same extent as other natural methods. The caregiver needs a thorough personal knowledge or ongoing consultation with a homeopathic physician to safely recommend the use of these approaches during late pregnancy (McFarlin, Gibson, O'Rear, et al., 1999).

Castor oil has been used for many years but has not been frequently studied as a method of labor induction. The mechanism by which castor oil stimulates uterine contractions is not understood. Some practitioners consider it to be an old-fashioned, nonuseful substance, whereas others have noted that it is especially effective for primigravidas (Summers, 1997).

## Care of the Woman during Amnioinfusion

**Amnioinfusion (AI)** is a technique by which warmed, sterile normal saline or Ringer's lactate solution is introduced into the uterus through an intrauterine pressure catheter (IUPC). Amnioinfusion can be used intrapartally to increase the volume of fluid in cases of oligohydramnios, in which cord compression causes FHR deceleration and fetal distress. It provides an extra cushion of fluid that relieves pressure on the umbilical cord and promotes increased perfusion to the fetus. AI is also implemented to dilute moderate to heavy meconium released in utero by a stressed fetus; when used for meconium dilution, amnioinfusion has resulted in a significant decrease of meconium below the cords after

# DRUG GUIDE

## OXYTOCIN (PITOCIN)

### *Overview of Obstetric Action*

Oxytocin (Pitocin) exerts a selective stimulatory effect on the smooth muscle of the uterus and blood vessels. It affects the myometrial cells of the uterus by increasing the excitability of the muscle cell, increasing the strength of the muscle contraction, and supporting propagation of the contraction (movement of the contraction from one myometrial cell to the next). Its effect on the uterine contraction depends on the dosage used and on the excitability of the myometrial cells. During the first half of gestation, there is little excitability of the myometrium, and the uterus is fairly resistant to the effects of oxytocin. However, from midgestation on, the uterus responds increasingly to exogenous intravenous oxytocin. Cautious use of diluted oxytocin administered intravenously at term results in a slow rise of uterine activity.

The circulatory half-life of oxytocin is 3 to 5 minutes. It takes approximately 40 minutes for a particular dose of oxytocin to reach a steady-state plasma concentration.

The effects of oxytocin on the cardiovascular system can be pronounced. Blood pressure initially may decrease but after prolonged administration increase by 30% above the baseline. Cardiac output and stroke volume increase. With doses of 20 mU/min or above, oxytocin exerts an antidiuretic effect, decreasing free water exchange in the kidney and markedly decreasing urine output.

Oxytocin is used to induce labor at term and to augment uterine contractions in the first and second stages of labor. It may also be used immediately after birth to stimulate uterine contraction and thereby control uterine atony.

### *Rodute, Dosage, Frequency*

For induction of labor: Add 10 units of Pitocin (1 mL) to 1000 mL of intravenous (IV) solution. (The resulting concentration is 10 mU oxytocin per 1 mL of intravenous fluid.) Using an infusion pump, administer IV, starting at 0.5–1 mU/min and increasing by 1–2 mU/min every 40–60 minutes. Alternatively, start at 1–2 mU/min and increase by 1 mU/min every 15 minutes until a good contraction pattern (every 2–3 minutes and lasting 40–60 seconds) is achieved.

### *Maternal Contraindications*

- Severe preeclampsia or eclampsia (pregnancy-induced hypertension [PIH])
- Predisposition to uterine rupture (in nullipara over 35 years of age, multigravida 4 or more, overdistention of the uterus, previous major surgery of the cervix or uterus)
- Cephalopelvic disproportion
- Malpresentation or malposition of the fetus, cord prolapse
- Preterm infant
- Rigid, unripe cervix; total placenta previa
- Presence of fetal distress

### *Maternal Side Effects*

Hyperstimulation of the uterus results in hypercontractility, which in turn may cause the following:

- Abruptio placentae
- Impaired uterine blood flow, leading to fetal hypoxia
- Rapid labor, leading to cervical lacerations
- Rapid labor and birth, leading to lacerations of cervix, vagina, or perineum; uterine atony; fetal trauma
- Uterine rupture
- Water intoxication (nausea, vomiting, hypotension, tachycardia, cardiac arrhythmia) if oxytocin is given in electrolyte-free solution or at a rate exceeding 20 mU/min; hypotension with rapid IV bolus administration postpartum

### *Effect on Fetus or Neonate*

- Primarily associated with the presence of hypercontractility of the maternal uterus, which decreases the oxygen supply to the fetus and is reflected by irregularities or decrease in fetal heart rate (FHR)
- Hyperbilirubinemia
- Trauma from rapid birth

### *Nursing Considerations*

- Explain induction or augmentation procedure to client.
- Apply fetal monitor and obtain 15- to 20-minute tracing and nonstress test (NST) to assess FHR before starting IV oxytocin.

## OXYTOCIN (PITOCIN) *continued*

- For induction or augmentation of labor, start with primary IV and piggyback secondary IV with oxytocin and infusion pump.
- Ensure continuous monitoring of the fetus and uterine contractions.
- The maximum rate is 40 mU/min (ACOG, 1999a). Not all protocols recommend a maximum dose. When indicated, the maximum dose is generally between 16 and 40 mU/min. Decrease oxytocin by similar increments once labor has progressed to 5–6 cm dilatation. Protocols may vary from one agency to another.

  0.5 mU/min = 3 mL/hr
  1.0 mU/min = 6 mL/hr
  1.5 mU/min = 9 mL/hr
  2 mU/min = 12 mL/hr
  4 mU/min = 24 mL/hr
  6 mU/min = 36 mL/hr
  8 mU/min = 48 mL/hr
  10 mU/min = 60 mL/hr
  12 mU/min = 72 mL/hr
  15 mU/min = 90 mL/hr
  18 mU/min = 108 mL/hr
  20 mU/min = 120 mL/hr

- Assess FHR, maternal blood pressure, pulse, frequency and duration of uterine contractions, and uterine resting tone before each increase in the oxytocin infusion rate.
- Record all assessments and IV rate on monitor strip and on client's chart.
- Record oxytocin infusion rate in milliunits per minute and milliliters per hour (eg, 0.5 mU/min [3 mL/hr]).
- Assess cervical dilatation as needed.
- Provide nursing comfort measures.
- Discontinue IV oxytocin infusion and infuse primary solution when (1) fetal distress is noted (bradycardia, late or variable decelerations), (2) uterine contractions are more frequent than every 2 minutes, (3) duration of contractions exceeds more than 60 seconds, or (4) insufficient relaxation of the uterus between contractions or a steady increase in resting tone is noted (ACOG, 1999a). In addition to discontinuing IV oxytocin infusion, turn client to side, and if fetal distress is present, administer oxygen by tight face mask at 7–10 L/min; notify physician.
- Maintain intake and output record.

### *For augmentation of labor:*

Prepare and administer IV Pitocin as for labor induction. Increase rate until labor contractions are of good quality. The flow rate is gradually increased at no less than every 30 minutes to a maximum of 10 mU/min (Cunningham et al., 1997a). In some settings or in a situation when limited fluids may be administered, a more concentrated solution may be used. When 10 U Pitocin are added to 500 mL IV solution, the resulting concentration is 1 mU/min = 3 mL/hr. If 10 U Pitocin are added to 250 mL IV solution, the concentration is 1 mU/min = 1.5 mL/hr.

### *For administration after delivery of placenta:*

- One dose of 10 U Pitocin (1 mL) is given intramuscularly or added to IV fluids for continuous infusion.
- Assess FHR, maternal blood pressure, pulse, frequency and duration of uterine contractions, and uterine resting tone before each increase in oxytocin infusion rate.
- Record all assessments and IV rate on monitor strip and on client's chart. Record oxytocin infusion rate in milliunits per minute and milliliters per hour (eg, 0.5 mU/min [3 mL/hr]).
- Record on monitor strip all client activities (such as change of position, vomiting), procedures done (amniotomy, sterile vaginal examination), and administration of analgesic agents to allow for interpretation and evaluation of tracing.
- Assess cervical dilatation as needed.
- Provide nursing comfort measures.
- Discontinue IV oxytocin infusion and infuse primary solution when (1) fetal stress or distress is noted (tachycardia or bradycardia, late or variable decelerations), (2) uterine contractions are more frequent than every 2 minutes, (3) duration of contractions exceeds 60 seconds, or (4) insufficient relaxation of the uterus between contractions or a steady increase in resting tone is noted (ACOG, 1999a). In addition to discontinuing IV oxytocin infusion, turn client to side, and if fetal distress is present, administer oxygen by tight face mask at 7–10 L/min; notify physician.
- Maintain intake and output record. Assess intake and output every hour.

# CRITICAL PATHWAY: *For Induction of Labor*

| Category | Immediate Care | Outcomes |
|---|---|---|
| **Referral** | Review prenatal record<br>Advise certified nurse-midwife (CNM) or physician of admission<br>Anesthesia | **Expected Outcomes**<br>Appropriate resources identified and utilized |
| **Assessments** | Previous pregnancies, present pregnancy, and childbirth preparation<br>Estimated gestational age of the fetus<br>Assess woman's feelings regarding induction as well as knowledge base regarding the induction process<br>Assess knowledge of breathing techniques; if woman does not have a method to use, teach breathing techniques before starting oxytocin infusion | **Expected Outcomes**<br>Potential and actual complications identified |
| **Teaching/psychosocial** | Provide emotional support through teaching and answering all questions | **Expected Outcomes**<br>Woman verbalizes or demonstrates understanding of information given |
| **Nursing care management and reports** | Examination of pregnant uterus (Leopold's maneuvers to determine fetal size and position)<br>Vaginal examination to evaluate cervical readiness:<br>• Ripe cervix feels soft to the examining finger, is located in a medial to anterior position, is more than 50% effaced, and is 2–3 cm dilated<br>• Unripe cervix feels firm to the examining finger, is long and thick, is perhaps in a posterior position, and is dilated little or not at all<br>Presence of contractions<br>Membranes intact or ruptured<br>Maternal vital signs and a 20-minute baseline fetal monitoring strip prior to induction to determine fetal well-being<br>Diagnostic studies:<br>• Fetal maturity tests (lecithin/sphingomyclin [L/S] ratio, creatinine concentrations, ultrasonography), NST, CST, BPP<br>• Maternal blood studies (complete blood count [CBC], hemoglobin, hematocrit, blood type, Rh factor)<br>• Urinalysis<br>Monitor for nausea, vomiting, hypotension, tachycardia, cardiac arrhythmias, headache, mental confusion, decreased urinary output<br>Monitor FHR by continuous electronic fetal monitoring; do not start infusion or advance rate (if induction has already begun) if FHR is not in range of 120–160 bpm, if decelerations are present, or if variability decreases<br>Evaluate and document maternal BP and pulse before beginning induction and then before each increase in infusion rate; do not advance infusion rate in presence of maternal hypertension or hypotension or radical changes in pulse rate<br>If the woman becomes hypotensive:<br>• Keep her on her side; may change to other side<br>• Discontinue oxytocin infusion<br>• Increase rate of primary IV line<br>• Monitor FHR<br>• Notify physician<br>• Assess for cause of hypotension<br>Evaluate and document contraction frequency, duration, and intensity prior to each increase in infusion rate<br>Discontinue oxytocin infusion if:<br>• Contractions are more frequent than every 2 minutes<br>• Contraction duration exceeds 90 seconds<br>• Uterus does not relax between contractions<br>Increase oxytocin IV infusion rate every 20 minutes until adequate contractions are achieved. Do not exceed an infusion rate of | **Expected Outcomes**<br>Progression of labor and birth without difficulty<br>Potential and actual complications minimized |

BP, blood pressure; bpm, beats per minute; BPP, biophysical profile; CBC, complete blood count; CST, contraction stress test; FHR, fetal heart rate; I&D, intake and output; IV, intravenous; NST, nonstress test; PRN, as needed; WNL, within normal limits

| Category | Immediate Care | Outcomes |
|---|---|---|
| **Nursing care management and reports *continued*** | 20–40 mL/min. (*Note:* Protocols directing how often oxytocin is increased may vary from 15 to 60 minutes. See ACOG, 1999a, for guidelines and refer to institutional protocols.)<br>Check infusion pump to ensure oxytocin is infusing. Check whether pump is on, chamber refills and empties, level of fluid in IV bottle becomes lower. If problem is found, correct and restart infusion at beginning dose. Check main IV site frequently. Check piggyback connection to primary tubing to ensure solution is not leaking.<br>Evaluate cervical dilatation by vaginal examination as indicated.<br>Monitor FHR continuously (normal range is 120–160 bpm). In episodes of bradycardia (<120 bpm) lasting for more than 30 seconds, administer oxygen by face mask at 7–10 L/min.<br>Stop oxytocin infusion. Position woman on left side if quick recovery of FHR does not occur.<br>Carefully evaluate fetal tachycardia (>160 bpm). Sustained tachycardia may necessitate discontinuation of oxytocin infusion. Assess for presence of meconium staining. Notify physician. | (previous page) |
| **Activity** | Ambulate until 5–10 cm then bed<br>Position woman in left lateral or semi-Fowler's position<br>Encourage her to avoid supine position | **Expected Outcomes**<br>Activity individualized for woman |
| **Comfort** | Provide support to woman as she uses breathing techniques<br>Encourage use of effleurage, back rub, and other supportive measures<br>Assess need for analgesia or anesthesia | **Expected Outcomes**<br>Optimal comfort level maintained |
| **Nutrition** | IV or lactated Ringer's solution<br>Ice chips, clear fluids | **Expected Outcomes**<br>Nutritional and hydration needs met |
| **Elimination** | Encourage voiding every 2 hours; monitor and record intake and output | **Expected Outcomes**<br>Intake and output WNL |
| **Medications** | Start primary IV as ordered<br>Administer oxytocin in electrolyte solution (piggyback oxytocin onto primary IV at closest site to IV needle insertion)<br>Pain medications prn | **Expected Outcomes**<br>Induction or augmentation of labor occurs within expected parameters |
| **Discharge planning/home care** | Photo packet<br>Birth certificate worksheet<br>Sibling visitation<br>Car seat | **Expected Outcomes**<br>Individualized discharge teaching completed |
| **Family involvement** | Family visitation policy per institutional protocol<br>Encourage significant other to stay close and assist with breathing of woman | **Expected Outcomes**<br>Family or support person involvement maximized |
| **Date** | | |

birth and a decrease in meconium aspiration. At birth, if the infant inhales any meconium present in the amniotic fluid, serious breathing problems and pneumonia may result. Amnioinfusion may also be indicated for preterm labor with premature rupture of membranes (Schmidt, 1997).

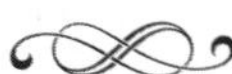

## Nursing Care Management

The nurse is often the first person to detect changes in fetal heart rate associated with cord compression or to observe meconium-stained amniotic fluid. When cord compression is suspected, the immediate intervention is to assist the laboring woman to another position. If this intervention is not successful in restoring the FHR, an amnioinfusion may be considered.

The nurse helps administer the AI, assesses the woman's vital signs and contraction status, and monitors the fetal heart rate by continuous EFM. It is important to provide ongoing information to the laboring woman and her partner and to answer questions as they arise. Comfort measures and positioning are vital because the woman is now on bed rest. Frequent changing of disposable underpads and perineal care are also needed because of the constant leakage of fluid from the vagina.

# Care of the Woman during an Episiotomy

An **episiotomy** is a surgical incision of the perineal body to enlarge the outlet. The second most common procedure in maternal-child care, the episiotomy has long been thought to minimize the risk of lacerations of the perineum and the overstretching of perineal tissues (Peleg, Kennedy, Merrill, et al., 1999). Though very common, the routine use of episiotomy is being seriously questioned. Research suggests that (1) rather than protecting the perineum from lacerations, the presence of an episiotomy makes it more likely that the woman will have deep perineal tears and (2) perineal lacerations heal more quickly than deep perineal tears (Keane, 1997). In clinical practice, research has shown that the incidence of major perineal trauma (extension to or through the anal sphincter) is four times more likely to happen if a midline episiotomy is done (Maier & Maloni, 1997) and that a repeat of the trauma is likely to occur with subsequent births (Peleg et al., 1999). Additional complications associated with episiotomy are blood loss, infection, pain and perineal discomfort that may continue for days or weeks past birth, including painful intercourse (Peleg et al., 1999).

## Factors That Predispose Women to Episiotomy

Overall factors that place a woman at increased risk for episiotomy are primigravida, large or macrosomic fetus, occiput-posterior position, use of forceps or vacuum extractor, and shoulder dystocia. Other factors that may be mitigated by nurses and physicians or CNMs include the following (Maier & Maloni, 1997):

- Use of lithotomy and other recumbent positions (causes excessive and uneven stretching of the perineum)
- Encouraging or requiring sustained breath holding during second-stage pushing (causes excessive and rapid perineal stretching, can adversely affect blood flow in mother and fetus, and requires woman to be responsive to caregiver directions rather than to her own urges to push spontaneously)
- Arbitrary time limit placed by the physician or CNM on the length of the second stage

## Preventative Measures

Following are some general tips to help reduce the incidence of routine episiotomies:

- Kegel exercises throughout pregnancy to improve vaginal tone
- Perineal massage during pregnancy (Labrecque, Eason, Marcoux, et al., 1999)
- Natural pushing during labor, and avoiding the lithotomy position or pulling back on legs (which tightens the perineum) (England & Horowitz, 1998)
- Side-lying position for pushing, which helps slow birth and diminish tears (England & Horowitz, 1998)
- Warm or hot compresses on the perineum and firm counterpressure

## Episiotomy Procedure

There are two types of episiotomy in current practice: midline and mediolateral (Figure 20–2♦). Just before birth, when approximately 3 to 4 cm of the fetal head is visible during a contraction, the episiotomy is performed using sharp scissors with rounded points (Cunningham, MacDonald, Gant, et al., 1997b). The incision begins at the bottom center of the perineal body and extends either straight down the midline or at a 45-degree angle in either mediolateral direction.

The episiotomy is usually performed with regional or local anesthesia but may be done without anesthesia in emergency situations. It is generally proposed that as crowning occurs, the distension of the tissues causes numbing. Repair of the episiotomy (episiorrhaphy) and any lacerations is completed either during the period between birth of the neonate and before expulsion of the placenta or after expulsion of the placenta. Adequate anesthesia must be given for the repair.

# Nursing Care Management

The woman needs to be supported during the episiotomy and the repair because she may feel some pressure

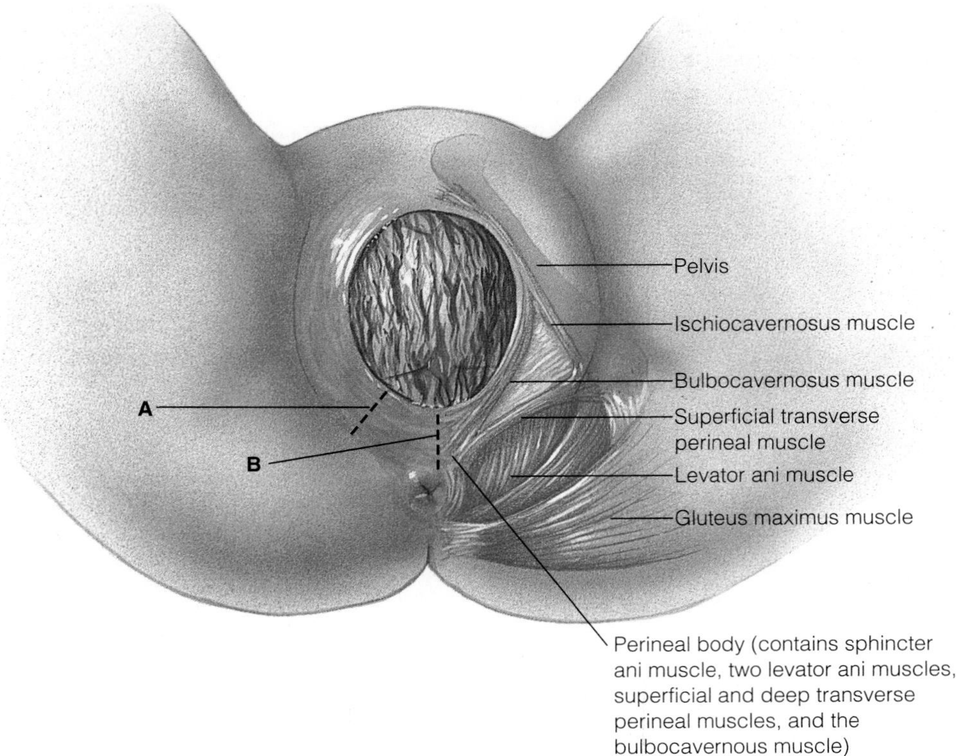


**FIGURE 20–2** ♦ The two most common types of episiotomy are midline and mediolateral. **A,** Right mediolateral. **B,** Midline.

sensations. In the absence of adequate anesthesia she may feel pain. Placing a hand on her shoulder and talking with her can provide comfort and distraction from the repair process. If the woman is having more discomfort than she can comfortably handle, the nurse needs to act as an advocate in communicating the woman's needs to the physician or CNM. At all times the woman needs to be the one who decides whether the amount of discomfort she is experiencing is tolerable. She should never be told, "This doesn't hurt." She is the person experiencing the discomfort, and her evaluation needs to be respected.

The type of episiotomy is recorded on the birth record. This information should also be included in a report to subsequent caregivers so that adequate assessments can be made and relief measures can be instituted.

Comfort measures may begin immediately after birth with the application of an ice pack to the perineum. For optimal effect the ice pack should be applied for 20 to 30 minutes and removed for at least 20 minutes before being reapplied. The nurse assesses the perineal tissues frequently to prevent injury from the ice pack. The episiotomy site should be inspected every 15 minutes during the first hour after the birth for redness, swelling, tenderness, and hematomas. As part of postpartum care the mother will need instruction in perineal hygiene care and comfort measures.

It is important for nurses to recognize that perineal pain continues for a period of time. Many women experience significant pain for a week after the birth, some continue to have pain at 8 weeks postpartum, and 10% of women have pain for a much longer period (Glazener 1997). This pain should not be discounted: Women who experience prolonged pain tend to have problems with breastfeeding and depression and are reluctant to reestablish sexual activity.

Nursing advocacy is needed to promote selective rather than routine episiotomy. It is imperative that each nurse stay current regarding new information and research in order to maintain current practice standards.

## Care of the Woman during Forceps-Assisted Birth

**Forceps** are surgical instruments designed to assist in the birth of a fetus by providing either traction or the means to rotate the fetal head to an occiput-anterior position. In medical literature and practice, *forceps-assisted birth* is also known as *instrumental delivery* or *operative vaginal delivery.* Three categories of forceps application exist:

1. *Outlet forceps* are applied when the fetal skull has reached the perineum, the fetal scalp is visible, and

the sagittal suture is not more than 45 degrees from the midline.

2. *Low forceps* are applied when the leading edge (presenting part) of the fetal skull is at a station of +2 or more.
3. *Midforceps* are applied when the fetal head is engaged.

Forceps may be indicated in the presence of any condition that threatens the mother or fetus and that can be relieved by birth. Conditions that put the woman at risk include heart disease, pulmonary edema, infection, and exhaustion. Fetal conditions include premature placental separation and fetal distress. Forceps may be used electively to shorten the second stage of labor and assist the woman's pushing effort or when regional anesthesia has affected the woman's motor innervation and she cannot push effectively.

Before forceps are used, the following conditions must be met (Charles, 1999):

- The cervix must be completely dilated and the exact position and station of the fetal head known.
- Membranes must be ruptured to allow a firm grasp on the fetal head, which must be engaged and in vertex or face presentation.
- The type of pelvis should be known, because certain pelvic types do not permit rotation.
- The maternal bladder should be empty and adequate anesthesia given.
- No degree of cephalopelvic disproportion can be present.

### Neonatal and Maternal Risks

Some neonates may develop a small area of ecchymosis and/or edema along the sides of the face as a result of forceps application. Caput succedaneum or cephalhematoma (with subsequent hyperbilirubinemia) may occur, as may transient facial paralysis.

Maternal risks include possible lacerations of the birth canal, extensions of a median episiotomy into the anus, increased bleeding, bruising, and perineal edema.

## Nursing Care Management

By using ongoing assessment, the nurse may note the variables that are associated with an increased rate of instrument-assisted or operative birth. Nursing care measures could then be directed toward variables that may reduce the incidence of these factors. For example, labor dystocia may be corrected by changing maternal position, ambulation, and frequent bladder emptying. FHR abnormalities may be improved by position changes, increased fluid intake, and/or adequate oxygen exchange.

If a forceps-assisted birth is required, the nurse explains the procedure briefly to the woman. With adequate regional anesthesia the woman should feel some pressure during the procedure but no pain. The nurse encourages the woman to use breathing techniques that help prevent her from pushing during application of the forceps (Figure 20–3♦). The nurse monitors contractions and advises the physician when one is present because traction is only applied with a contraction. With each contraction the physician provides traction on the forceps as the woman pushes. It is not uncommon to observe mild fetal bradycardia as traction is being applied to the forceps. This bradycardia results from head compression and is transient.

Immediately following birth, the newborn is assessed for facial edema, bruising, caput succedaneum, cephalhematoma, and any sign of cerebral edema. In the fourth stage the nurse assesses the woman for perineal swelling, bruising, hematoma, excessive bleeding, and hemorrhage. In the postpartum period it is important to assess for signs of infection if lacerations occurred during the procedure. The nurse provides an opportunity for questions and reiterates explanations provided. Nursing assessments of the woman and her newborn are also discussed.

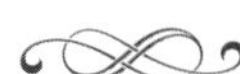

## Care of the Woman during Vacuum-Assisted Birth

**Vacuum-assisted birth** is an obstetric procedure used to facilitate the birth of a fetus by applying suction to the fetal head. The *vacuum extractor* is composed of a soft suction cup attached to a suction bottle (pump) by tubing. The suction cup, which comes in various sizes, is placed against the fetal occiput, and the pump is used to create negative pressure (suction) inside the cup. Traction is applied in coordination with uterine contractions, descent occurs, and the fetal head is born (Figure 20–4♦ on page 509). General recommendations include that there should be progressive descent with the first two pulls and that the procedure should not last longer than 30 minutes (Teng & Sayre, 1997).

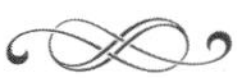

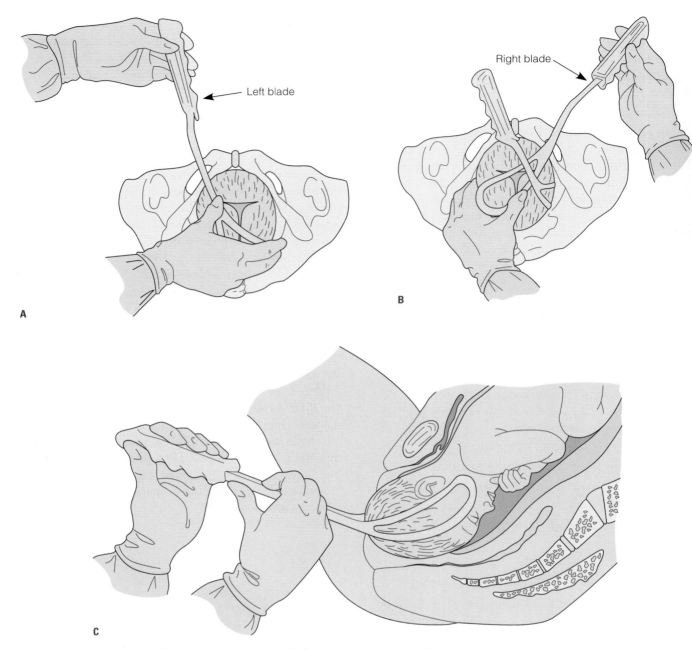

FIGURE 20–3 ♦ Application of forceps in occiput-anterior (OA) position. **A,** The left blade is inserted along the left side wall of the pelvis over the parietal bone. **B,** The right blade is inserted along the right side wall of the pelvis over the parietal bone. **C,** With correct placement of the blades, the handles lock easily. During uterine contractions traction is applied to the forceps in a downward and outward direction to follow the birth canal.

## Nursing Care Management

The nurse is responsible for keeping the woman and her partner informed about what is happening during the procedure. If adequate regional anesthesia has been administered, the woman feels only pressure during the procedure. The nurse assesses FHR by continuous EFM or by auscultation at least every 5 minutes. The parents need to be reassured that the caput (chignon) on the baby's head will disappear within 2 to 3 days. Assessment of the newborn should include inspection and continued observation for cephalhematomas, intracerebral hemorrhage, and retinal hemorrhages (Sachs, Kobelin, Castro, et al., 1999).

A

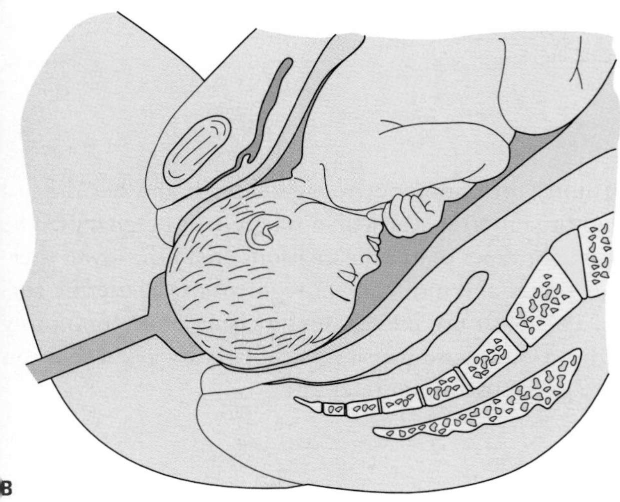

B

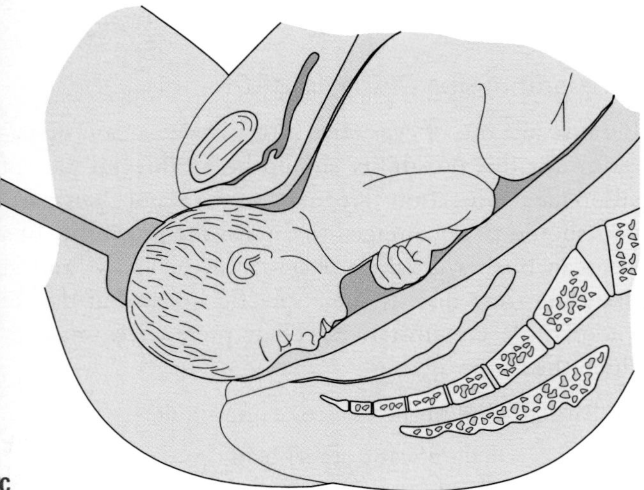

C

FIGURE 20–4 ♦ Vacuum extractor traction. **A,** The cup is placed on the fetal occiput and suction is created. Traction is applied in a downward and outward direction. **B,** Traction continues in a downward direction as the fetal head begins to emerge from the vagina. **C,** Traction is maintained to lift the fetal head out of the vagina.

# Care of the Family during Cesarean Birth

Cesarean birth is the birth of the infant through an abdominal and uterine incision. It is one of the oldest surgical procedures known. Until the 20th century cesarean procedures were primarily used in an attempt to save the fetus of a dying woman. As the maternal and perinatal morbidity and mortality rates associated with cesarean birth steadily decreased throughout the 20th century, the proportion of cesarean births increased. Beginning in the early 1970s the cesarean rate rose steadily for almost two decades, from 5.5% to nearly 25% of all births in the United States (Curtin & Kozak, 1997). Following this dramatic rise in surgical births, a steady decline began in 1989, primarily due to efforts to contain health care costs. In 1996 the total cesarean rate had decreased to 20.6% (Curtin & Mathews, 2000). However, in recent years the total percentage of cesarean births has again begun to rise and at the end of 1999 the rate was 22% (Cockey, 2000).

In an effort to generate and analyze data that can be used to help decrease the rising cesarean birth rate appropriately, the American College of Obstetricians and Gynecologists (ACOG) developed the *Evaluation of Cesarean Deliveries* document (ACOG, 2000). This resource is aimed at obtaining accurate statistics for clinicians and institutions using casemix adjusted data for two groups who have had cesareans: nulliparous women with a single, full-term fetus in vertex presentation (first-time cesareans) and multiparous women who have had one prior low-transverse cesarean birth for a single full-term fetus in a vertex presentation (repeat cesareans). These two groups were chosen because together they comprise two-thirds of cesarean births in the United States but represent the greatest variation in cesarean rates. ACOG recommends that physicians and hospitals monitor their cesarean rates for these two groups and then compare their rates with benchmark rates (Cockey, 2000). Other factors, such as the continuous presence of a nurse or trained support person, may also help lower cesarean birth rates and warrant further consideration (Sams, 2000).

## Indications

Cesarean births are performed in the presence of a variety of maternal and fetal conditions. Commonly accepted indications include complete placenta previa, cephalo pelvic disproportion, placental abruption, active genital herpes, umbilical cord prolapse, failure to progress in labor, proven fetal distress, benign and malignant tumors that obstruct the birth canal, and cervical cerclage (Keane, 1997). Indications that are more controversial include breech presentation, previous cesarean birth,

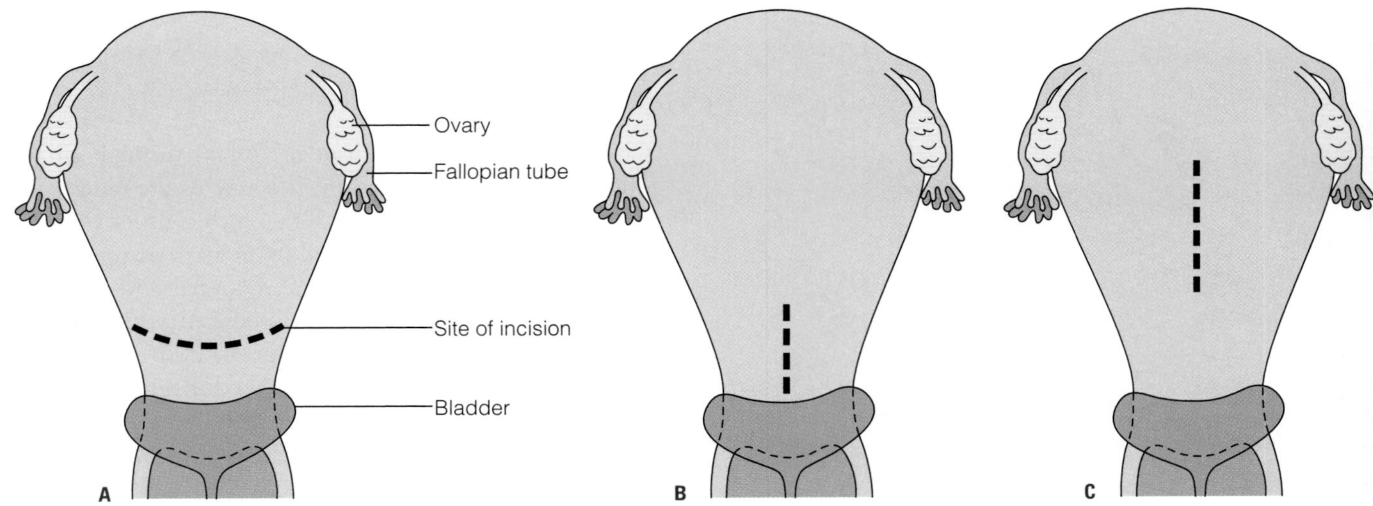


**FIGURE 20–5** ♦ Uterine incisions for a cesarean birth. **A,** This transverse incision in the lower uterine segment is called a Kerr incision. **B,** The Sellheim incision is a vertical incision in the lower uterine segment. **C,** This view illustrates the classic uterine incision that is done in the body (corpus) of the uterus. The classic incision was commonly used in the past but is associated with increased risk of uterine rupture in subsequent pregnancies and labor.

major congenital anomalies, and severe Rh isoimmunization. It should be noted that cesarean births have a higher maternal mortality rate than vaginal births and the morbidity factors associated with a surgical delivery are infection, reactions to anesthetic agents, blood clots, and bleeding (Bowes, 1999).

## Skin Incisions

The skin incision for a cesarean birth is either transverse (Pfannenstiel) or vertical and is not indicative of the type of incision made into the uterus. The transverse incision is made across the lowest and narrowest part of the abdomen. Since the incision is made just below the pubic hairline, it is almost invisible after healing. The limitation of this type of skin incision is that it does not allow for extension of the incision if needed. This incision is used when time is not of the essence (eg, with failure to progress and no fetal or maternal distress), because it usually requires more time to make and repair.

The vertical incision is made between the navel and the symphysis pubis. This type of incision is quicker and is therefore preferred in cases of fetal distress when rapid birth is indicated, with preterm or macrosomic infants, or when the woman is significantly obese (Cunningham et al., 1997b). Time factors, client preference, or physician preference determines the type of skin incision.

## Uterine Incisions

The type of uterine incision depends on the need for the cesarean. The choice of incision affects the woman's opportunity for a subsequent vaginal birth and her risks of a ruptured uterine scar with a subsequent pregnancy. The two major types of uterine incisions are in the lower uterine segment and in the upper segment of the uterine corpus. The lower uterine segment incision most commonly used is a transverse incision, although a vertical incision may also be used (Figure 20–5♦).

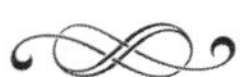

# Nursing Care Management

## Preparation for Cesarean Birth

Because one out of every five births is a cesarean, preparation for this possibility should be an integral part of all prenatal education. Pregnant women and their partners should be encouraged to discuss the possibility of a cesarean birth with their obstetrician or CNM and at the same time discuss their specific needs and desires under those circumstances. Their preferences may include the following:

- Participating in the choice of anesthetic
- Father (or significant other) being present during the procedures and/or birth
- Father (or significant other) being present in the recovery or postpartum room
- Audio recording and/or taking pictures of the birth

- Delayed instillation of eye drops to promote eye contact between parent and infant in the first hours after birth
- Physical contact or holding the infant while in the operating and/or recovery room (by the father if the mother cannot hold the newborn)
- Breastfeeding immediately after birth or in the recovery area

Information that couples need about cesarean birth includes the following:

- What preparatory procedures to expect
- Description or viewing of the delivery room
- Types of anesthesia for birth and analgesia available postpartum
- Sensations that may be experienced
- Roles of significant others
- Interaction with newborn
- Immediate recovery phase
- Postpartum phase

The context in which this information is relayed should be birth oriented rather than surgery oriented.

### Repeat Cesarean Birth

When a couple is anticipating a cesarean birth, they have time to analyze the information they are given and to prepare for the experience. Many hospitals and local groups provide preparation classes for cesarean birth. The instructor should impart factual information and a feeling of normality, which will allow a couple to make choices and participate in their birth experience. Couples who have had previous negative experiences need an opportunity to describe what they felt. They can be encouraged to identify what they would like to be different and to list options that would make the experience more positive. Those who have already had positive experiences need reassurance that their needs and desires will be met in a similar manner. In addition, an opportunity should be provided to discuss any fears or anxieties.

### Emergency Cesarean Birth

The period preceding surgery must be used to its greatest advantage. It is imperative that caregivers use their most effective communication skills in supporting the couple. The nurse describes what the couple may anticipate during the next few hours. Asking the couple "What questions or concerns do you have about the decision?" gives them an opportunity for clarification. The nurse can prepare the woman in stages, giving her information and the rationale for interventions before beginning any procedure. It is essential to tell the woman (1) what is going to happen, (2) why it is being done, and (3) what sensations she may experience. This allows the woman to be informed and to consent to the procedure, which gives her a sense of control and reduces her feelings of helplessness.

To reduce the likelihood of serious pulmonary damage if gastric contents are aspirated, antacids may be administered within 30 minutes of surgery. If epidural anesthesia is used, the nurse may assist with the procedure, monitor the woman's blood pressure and response, and continue EFM. An abdominal and perineal prep is done, and an indwelling catheter is inserted to prevent bladder distension. An intravenous line is started with a large-bore needle to permit blood administration if it becomes necessary. Preoperative medication may be ordered. The pediatrician should be notified and preparation made to receive the new baby. The nurse ensures that the infant warmer is working and that resuscitation equipment is available.

The nurse assists in positioning the woman on the operating table. Fetal heart rate is assessed before surgery and during preparation because fetal hypoxia can result from the supine position. A hip wedge (folded blanket or towels) is placed under the right hip to tip the uterus slightly and reduce compression of blood vessels A last-minute check is done to ensure that the fetal scalp electrode has been removed if the fetus was internally monitored.

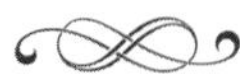

## Birth

Every effort should be made to include the father or partner in the birth experience. When attending the cesarean birth, the partner wears protective coverings similar to those worn by others in the operating suite. A stool can be placed beside the woman's head so that the partner can sit nearby to provide physical touch, visual contact, and verbal reassurance.

To promote the participation of the father who chooses not to be in the delivery room the nurse can

1. Allow the father to be near the delivery or operating room, where he can hear the newborn's first cry
2. Encourage the father to carry or accompany the infant to the nursery for the initial assessment
3. Involve the father in postpartum care in the recovery room

After birth the nurse assesses the Apgar score and completes the same initial assessment and identification procedures used for vaginal births. Every effort should be made to assist the parents in bonding with their infant. If the mother is awake, one of her arms can be freed to enable her to touch and stroke the infant. The newborn may be placed on the mother's chest or held in an *en face* position. If physical contact is not possible, the nurse can provide a running narrative so the mother knows what is happening with her baby. The nurse assists the anesthesiologist or nurse anesthetist with raising the mother's head so she can see her infant immediately after birth. The parents can be encouraged to talk to the baby, and the father can hold the baby until she or he is taken to the nursery.

### Analgesia and Anesthesia

There is no perfect anesthesia for cesarean birth. Each has its advantages, disadvantages, possible risks, and side effects. Goals for analgesia and anesthesia administration include safety, comfort, and emotional satisfaction for the client (see Chapter 18).

### Immediate Postpartal Recovery Period

The nurse caring for the postpartum woman assesses the mother's vital signs every 5 minutes until they are stable, then every 15 minutes for an hour, then every 30 minutes until she is discharged to the postpartum unit. The nurse should remain with the woman until she is stable.

The nurse evaluates the dressing and perineal pad every 15 minutes for at least an hour. The fundus should be gently palpated to determine whether it is remaining firm; it may be palpated by placing a hand to support the incision. Intravenous oxytocin is usually administered to promote the contractility of the uterine musculature. If the woman has been under general anesthesia, she should be positioned on her side to facilitate drainage of secretions, turned, and assisted with coughing and deep breathing every 2 hours for at least 24 hours. If she has received a spinal or epidural anesthetic, the level of anesthesia is checked every 15 minutes until full sensation has returned. It is important for the nurse to monitor intake and output and to observe the urine for bloody tinge, which could mean surgical trauma to the bladder. The physician prescribes medication to relieve the mother's pain and nausea, and it is administered as needed.

## Care of the Woman Undergoing Vaginal Birth after Cesarean (VBAC)

There is an increasing trend to have a trial of labor and **vaginal birth after cesarean (VBAC)** birth in cases of nonrecurring indications (such as umbilical cord accident, placenta previa, fetal distress). This trend has been influenced by consumer demand and studies that support VBAC as a viable alternative to repeat cesarean (Keane, 1997).

The ACOG (1998a) guidelines update states that the following aspects need to be considered for VBAC:

- A woman with one previous cesarean birth and a low transverse uterine incision should be counseled and encouraged to attempt VBAC.
- A woman with two or more previous cesareans may attempt VBAC.
- A classic uterine incision is a contraindication to VBAC.
- It must be possible to do a cesarean within 30 minutes.
- A physician who is able to do a cesarean needs to be available.

The most common risks associated with VBAC are hemorrhage and a less than 1% occurrence of uterine scar separation or rupture (Sachs et al., 1999).

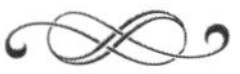

## Nursing Care Management

The nursing care of a woman undergoing VBAC varies according to institutional protocols. Generally, if the woman is at very low risk, a heplock is inserted for IV access if needed, continuous EFM is used, and clear fluids may be taken. A woman at higher risk may require additional precautionary measures. Care must be taken to ensure that the woman and her partner feel safe but not unduly restricted by the VBAC status.

Supportive and comfort measures are very important. The woman may be excited about this opportunity to experience labor and vaginal birth, or she may be hesitant and frightened about the possibility of complications. The presence of the nurse is important in providing information and encouragement for the laboring woman and her partner.

# Chapter Review

## CHAPTER HIGHLIGHTS

- An external (or cephalic) version may be done after 36 weeks' gestation to change a breech presentation to a cephalic presentation. The benefits of the version are that a lower-risk vaginal birth may be anticipated. The version is accomplished with the use of tocolytics to relax the uterus.
- Amniotomy (AROM) is performed to hasten labor. The risks are prolapse of the umbilical cord and infection.
- Prostaglandin $E_2$ may be used before an induction of labor to soften the cervix (called cervical ripening). The gel is inserted into the vagina and held in place with a diaphragm.
- Labor is induced for many reasons. The medical (allopathic) methods include amniotomy and intravenous oxytocin infusion. Nursing responsibilities are heightened during an induced labor.
- An episiotomy may be done just before birth of the fetus. Although very prevalent in the United States, its routine is questioned.
- Forceps-assisted birth can be accomplished using outlet, low, or midforceps. Outlet forceps are the most common and are associated with few maternal-fetal complications.
- A vacuum extractor is a soft, pliable cup attached to suction that can be applied to the fetal head and used in much the same way as forceps.
- At least one in five births is now accomplished by cesarean. The nurse has a vital role in providing information, support, and encouragement to the couple participating in a cesarean birth.
- Vaginal birth after cesarean (VBAC) is occurring more frequently now than in the past.

## CHAPTER REFERENCES


American College of Obstetricians and Gynecologists. (1995). *Dystocia and augmentation of labor* (Technical Bulletin No. 217). Washington, DC: Author.

American College of Obstetricians and Gynecologists. (1998a). *Guidelines for vaginal birth after previous cesarean birth* (ACOG Committee Opinion 64). Washington, DC: Author.

American College of Obstetricians and Gynecologists. (1998b). *Prostaglandin E gel for cervical ripening* (ACOG Committee Opinion 123). Washington, DC: Author.

American College of Obstetricians and Gynecologists. (1999a). *Induction of labor* (Practical Bulletin No. 10). Washington, DC: Author.

American College of Obstetricians and Gynecologists Committee on Practice. (1999b). *Induction of labor with misoprostol.* Washington, DC: Author.

American College of Obstetricians and Gynecologists (2000). *Evaluation of Cesarean Delivery.* Washington, DC: ACOG.

Bishop, E. H. (1964). Pelvic scoring for elective inductions. *Obstetrics and Gynecology, 24,* 266.

Bowes, W. A., Jr. (1999). Clinical aspects of normal and abnormal labor. In R. K. Creasy & R. Resnik (Eds.), *Maternal-fetal medicine* (4th ed., pp. 541–568). Philadelphia: Saunders.

Charles, A. G. (1999). Forceps delivery and vacuum extraction. In P. V. Dilts & J. J. Sciarri (Eds.), *Gynecology and Obstetrics (Vol. 2).* Philadelphia: Lippincott.

Cockey, C. D. (2000). Curbing cesarean rates; ACOG releases new comprehensive recommendations. AWHONN: Lifelines, 4(5), p. 17.

Cruikshank, D. P. (1999). Malpresentations and umbilical cord complications. In J. R. Scott, P. J. DiSaia, C. B. Hammond, & W. N. Spellacy (Eds.), *Danforth's obstetrics and gynecology* (8th ed., pp. 419–436). Philadelphia: Lippincott Williams & Wilkins.

Cunningham, F. G., MacDonald, P. C., Gant, N., Leveno, K. J., Gilstrap, L. C., Hankins, G. V., & Clark, S. L. (1997a). Cesarean delivery and cesarean hysterectomy. In *Williams obstetrics* (20th ed., pp. 509–533). Norwalk, CT: Appleton & Lange.

Cunningham, F. G., MacDonald, P. C., Gant, N. F., Leveno, K. J., Gilstrap, L. C., Hankins , G. V., & Clark, S. L. (1997b). Operative vaginal delivery. In *Williams obstetrics* (20th ed., pp. 473–494). Norwalk, CT: Appleton & Lange.

Curtin, S. C., & Kozak, L. J. (1997). Cesarean delivery rates in 1995 continue to decline in the United States. *Birth, 24,* 194–196.

Curtin, S. C., & Mathews, T. J. (2000). U.S. obstetric procedures, 1998. *Birth, 27*(2), 136–140.

England, P., & Horowitz, R. (1998). *Birthing from within* (pp. 136–140). Albuquerque, NM: Partera Press.

Forrest Pharmaceuticals, Inc. (1995). *Cervidil Sinoprostone 10mg. Vaginal insert.* Forrest Pharmaceuticals. St. Louis, MO. UAB Laboratories.

Glazener, C. M. A. (1997). Sexual function after childbirth: Women's experiences, persistent morbidity, and lack of professional recognition. *British Journal of Obstetrics and Gynecology, 104,* 330–335.

Keane, D. P. (1997). Operative procedures. In R. K. Creasy (Ed.), *Management of labor and delivery* (pp. 414–457). Malden, MA: Blackwell Science.

Labrecque, M., Eason, E., Marcoux, S., Lemieux, F., Pinault, J., Feldman, P., & Laperriere, L. (1999). Randomized controlled trial of prevention of perineal trauma by perineal massage during pregnancy. *American Journal of Obstetrics and Gynecology, 180*(3), 593–600.

Maier, J. S., & Maloni, J. A. (1997). Nurse advocacy for selective versus routine episiotomy. *Journal of Obstetric, Gynecologic, and Neonatal Nursing, 26,* 155–161.

McFarlin, B. L., Gibson, M. H., O'Rear, J., & Harman, P. (1999). A national survey of herbal preparation use by nurse-midwives for labor stimulation: Review of the literature and recommendations for practice. *Journal of Nurse-Midwifery, 44,* 205–216.

Oei, S. G., Lidewijde, J., & Mol, B. W. J. (2000). Randomized trial of administration of prostaglandin $E_2$ gel for induction of labor in the morning or the evening. *Journal of Perinatal Medicine, 28,* 20–25.

Peleg, D., Kennedy, C. M., Merrill, D., & Zlatnik, F. J. (1999). Risk of repetitions of a severe perineal laceration. *Obstetrics and Gynecology, 93,* 1021–1024.

Sachs, B. P., Kobelin, C., Castro, M. A., & Frigoletto, F. (1999). Sounding: The risks of lowering the cesarean-delivery rate. *New England Journal of Medicine, 340,* 54–57.

Sams, L. (2000). Evaluating cesarean deliveries: Exploring ACOG's recommendations to improve outcomes. *AWHONN: Lifelines,* 4(5), p. 15.

Schmidt, J. (1997). Fluid check: Making the case for intrapartum amnioinfusion. *AWHONN: Lifelines,* (1) pp. 47–51.

Schmidt, J. (1999). Prolonged pregnancy. In L. K. Mandeville & N. H. Troiano (Eds.), *AWHONN: High risk and critical care intrapartum nursing* (2nd ed., pp. 123–138). Philadelphia: Lippincott.

Summers, L. (1997). Methods of cervical ripening and labor induction. *Journal of Nurse-Midwifery, 42,* 71–82.

Teng, F. Y., & Sayre, J. W. (1997). Vacuum extraction: Does duration predict scalp injury? *Obstetrics and Gynecology, 89,* 281–285.

Wilson, B. A., Shannon, M. T., & Strang, C. L. (Eds.). (2001). *Nursing drug guide: 2001.* Upper Saddle River, NJ: Prentice-Hall.

Wilson, C. (2000). The nurse's role in misoprostol induction: A proposed protocol. *Journal of Obstretic, Gynecologic, and Neonatal Nursing,* 28(6), 574–583.

Wolcott, H. D., & Conry, J. A. (2000). Normal labor. In A. T. Evans & K. R. Niswander (Eds.), *Manual of obstetrics* (6th ed., pp. 392–424). Philadelphia: Lippincott Williams & Wilkins.

Zatuchi, G. L., & Slupik, R. I. (1996). *Obstetrics and gynecology drug handbook* (2nd ed.) St. Louis: Mosby.

## CONTEMPORARY MATERNAL-NEWBORN NURSING ON-LINE

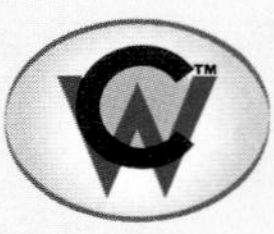

Additional interactive resources, including animations and video, for this chapter can be found on the Companion Website at http://www.prenhall.com/ladewig. Click on Chapter 20 and "Begin" to select the activities for this chapter.

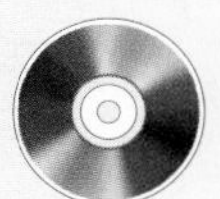

For NCLEX review questions and an audio glossary, access the accompanying CD-ROM in this book.

# Part Five

# The Newborn

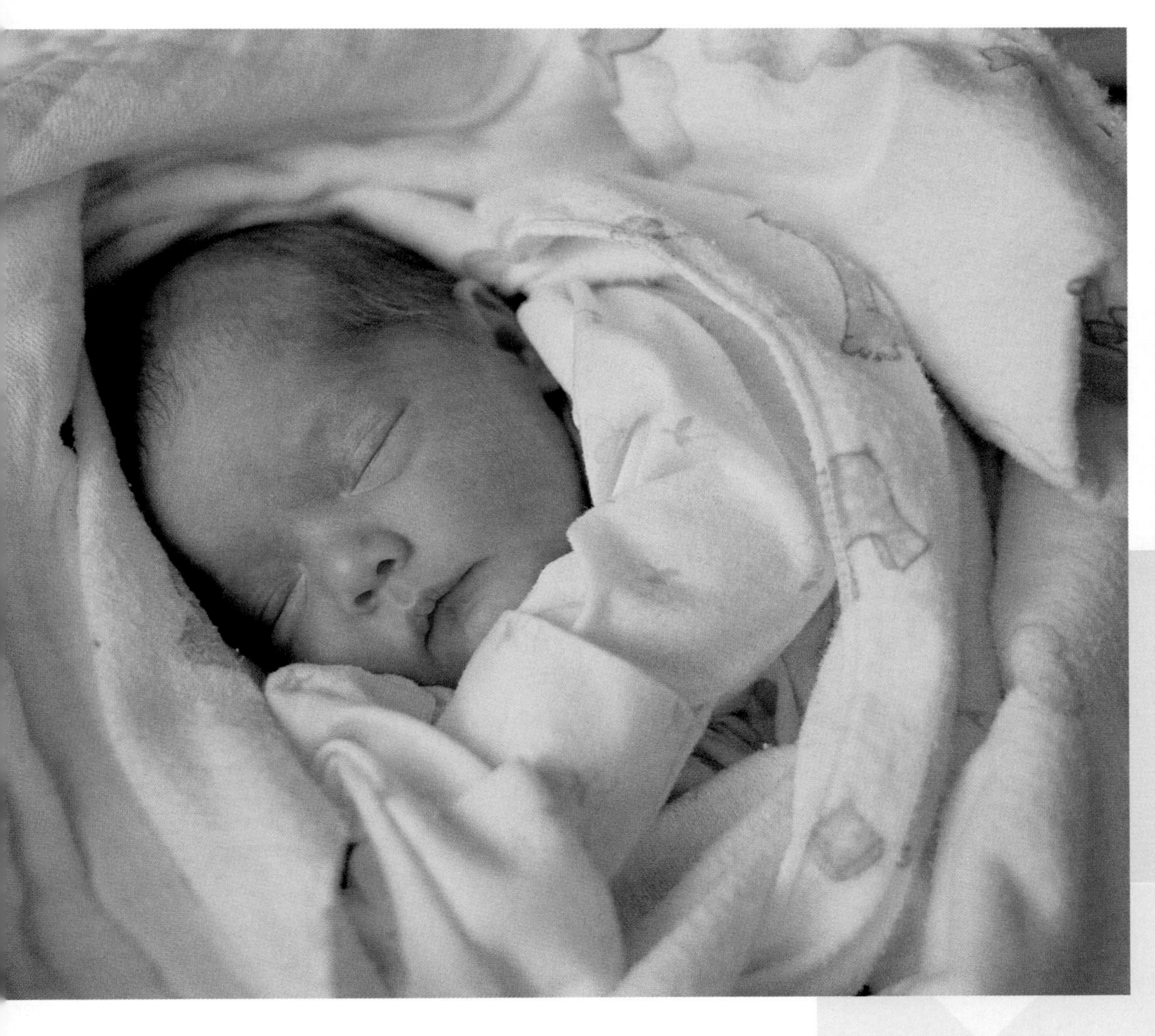

# Chapter 21

# The Physiologic Responses of the Newborn to Birth

*I had been a nurse for 9 years when my youngest sister asked me to be her labor coach. I thought I remembered my maternity nursing rotation, but it is so different when it is family. My sister was great, however, and my niece was active, beautiful, and full of life. I was struck by the reality that the transition babies must make to the world is simply staggering. You know, I love the work I do as a nurse, but this experience vividly reminded me that nursing is about life and death, joy and suffering, and everything in between.*

—Hospice Nurse

## KEY TERMS

| | |
|---|---|
| Active acquired immunity | 533 |
| Brown adipose tissue (BAT) | 526 |
| Cardiopulmonary adaptation | 519 |
| Conduction | 526 |
| Convection | 525 |
| Evaporation | 526 |
| Habituation | 536 |
| Meconium | 531 |
| Neonatal transition | 517 |
| Orientation | 536 |
| Passive acquired immunity | 533 |
| Periodic breathing | 520 |
| Periods of reactivity | 534 |
| Physiologic anemia of infancy | 523 |
| Physiologic jaundice | 529 |
| Radiation | 525 |
| Self-quieting ability | 536 |
| Surfactant | 517 |
| Thermal neutral zone (TNZ) | 524 |
| Total serum bilirubin | 528 |

## OBJECTIVES

- Summarize the respiratory and cardiovascular changes that occur during the transition to extrauterine life.
- Describe how various factors affect the newborn's blood values.
- Correlate the major mechanisms of heat loss in the newborn to the process of thermogenesis in the newborn.
- Explain the steps involved in conjugation and excretion of bilirubin in the newborn.
- Discuss the reasons a newborn may develop jaundice.
- Describe the functional abilities of the newborn's gastrointestinal tract and liver.
- Identify three reasons a newborn's kidneys have difficulty in maintaining fluid and electrolyte balance.
- List the immunologic responses available to the newborn.
- Explain the physiologic and behavioral responses of newborns during the periods of reactivity and identify possible interventions.
- Describe the normal sensory-perceptual abilities and behavioral states seen in the newborn period.

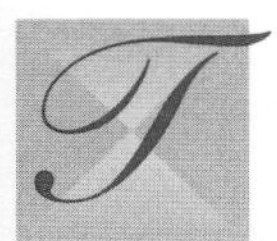he newborn period includes the time from birth through the 28th day of life. During this period, the newborn adjusts from intrauterine to extrauterine life. The nurse needs to be knowledgeable about a newborn's normal physiologic and behavioral adaptations and to be able to recognize alterations from normal.

To begin life as a separate being, the baby must immediately establish respiratory gas exchange in conjunction with marked circulatory changes. These radical and rapid changes are crucial to the maintenance of extrauterine life. The first few hours of life, in which the newborn stabilizes respiratory and circulatory functions, are called **neonatal transition.** All other newborn body systems change their level of functioning and become established over a longer period of time during the neonatal period.

# Respiratory Adaptations

Although significant respiratory events occur at birth, certain intrauterine factors also enhance the newborn's ability to breathe.

## Intrauterine Factors Supporting Respiratory Function

### Fetal Lung Development

The respiratory system is in an ongoing state of development during fetal life, and lung development continues into early childhood. During the first 20 weeks' gestation, development is limited to the differentiation of pulmonary, vascular, and lymphatic structures.

At 20 to 24 weeks, alveolar ducts begin to appear, followed by primitive alveoli at 24 to 28 weeks. During this time, the alveolar epithelial cells begin to differentiate into type I cells (structures necessary for gas exchange) and type II cells (structures that provide for the synthesis and storage of surfactant). **Surfactant** is a mixture of surface-active phospholipids that reduces surface tension of pulmonary fluids and contributes critically to the elasticity of pulmonary tissue.

At 28 to 32 weeks' gestation, the number of type II cells increases further, and surfactant is produced by a choline pathway within them. Surfactant production by this pathway peaks at about 35 weeks' gestation and remains high until term, paralleling late fetal lung development. At this time, the lungs are structurally developed enough to permit maintenance of lung expansion and adequate exchange of gases.

Clinically, the peak production of lecithin corresponds closely with a marked decrease in the incidence of respiratory distress syndrome for babies born after 35 weeks' gestation. Production of sphingomyelin (another component of surfactant) remains constant throughout gestation. The newborn born before the lecithin/sphingomyelin (L/S) ratio is 2:1 will have varying degrees of respiratory distress. (See discussion of L/S ratio in Chapter 26.)

### Fetal Breathing Movements

The newborn's ability to breathe air immediately when exposed to the extrauterine environment appears to be the consequence of weeks of intrauterine practice. In this respect, breathing can be perceived as a continuation of an intrauterine process as the lungs convert from a fluid-filled to a gas-filled organ. Fetal breathing movements (FBMs) occur as early as 11 weeks' gestation (see Chapter 14 for discussion). These breathing movements are essential for developing the chest wall muscles and the diaphragm and, to a lesser extent, for regulating lung fluid volume and resultant lung growth.

## Initiation of Breathing

To maintain life, the lungs must function immediately after birth. Two radical changes must take place for the lungs to function:

1. Pulmonary ventilation must be established through lung expansion following birth.
2. A marked increase in the pulmonary circulation must occur.

The first breath of life—the gasp in response to mechanical, chemical, thermal, and sensory changes associated with birth—initiates the serial opening of the alveoli. So begins the transition from a fluid-filled environment to an air-breathing, independent, extrauterine life. Figure 21–1♦ summarizes the initiation of respiration.

### Mechanical Events

During the latter half of gestation, the fetal lungs continuously produce fluid. This fluid expands the lungs almost completely, filling the air spaces. Some of the lung fluid moves up into the trachea and into the amniotic fluid and is then swallowed by the fetus.

Production of lung fluid diminishes 2 to 4 days before the onset of labor. However, approximately 80 to 110 mL of fluid remain in the respiratory passages of a normal full-term fetus at birth. This fluid must be removed from the lungs to permit adequate movement of air.

The primary mechanical events that initiate respiration involve the removal of fluid from the lungs as the fetus passes through the birth canal. During the birth process the fetal chest is compressed, increasing intrathoracic pressure, and approximately one-third of the fluid is squeezed out of the lungs. After the birth of the

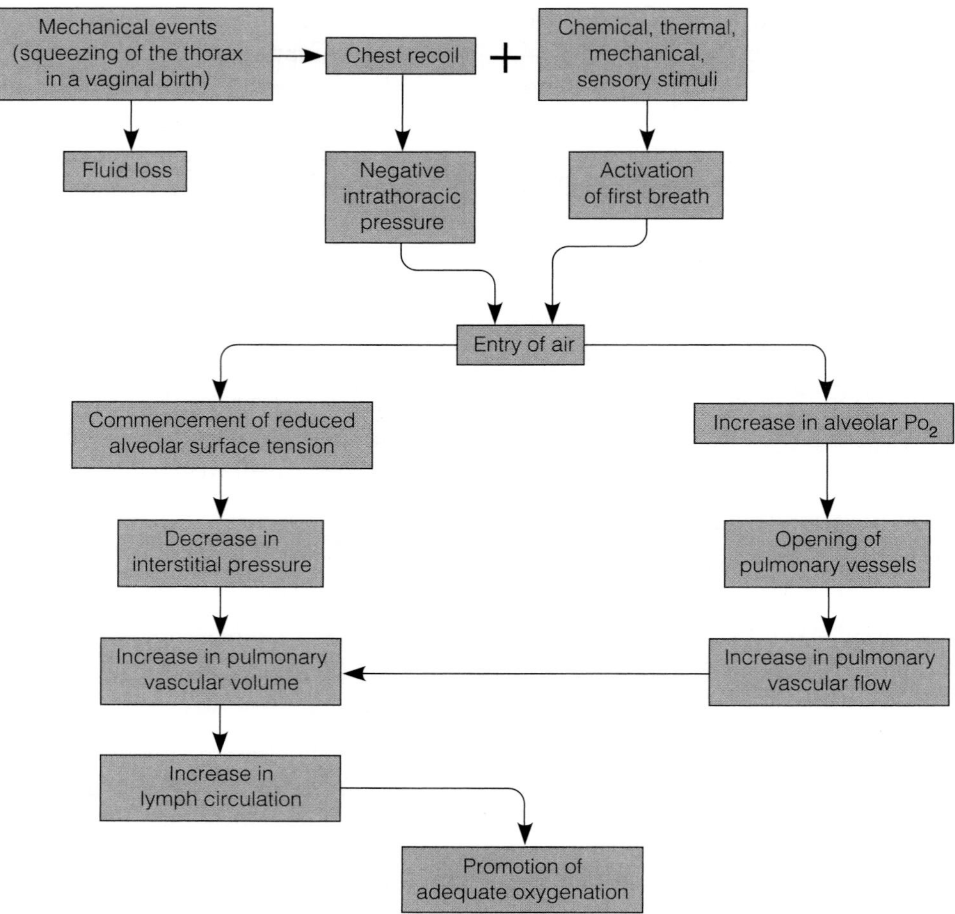


FIGURE 21–1 ♦ Initiation of respiration in the newborn.

newborn's trunk, the chest wall recoils. This chest recoil creates a negative intrathoracic pressure, which is thought to produce a small, passive inspiration of air that replaces the fluid that is squeezed out.

After this first inspiration, the newborn exhales, with crying, against a partially closed glottis, creating a positive intrathoracic pressure. The high positive intrathoracic pressure distributes the inspired air throughout the alveoli and begins the establishment of *functional residual capacity (FRC),* the air left in the lungs at the end of a normal expiration. The higher intrathoracic pressure also increases absorption of fluid via the capillaries and lymphatic system. The negative intrathoracic pressure resulting from downward movement of the diaphragm with inspiration causes lung fluid to flow from the alveoli across the alveolar membranes into the pulmonary interstitial tissue.

With each succeeding breath, the lungs expand. Because the protein concentration is higher in the pulmonary capillaries than in the interstitial tissue, oncotic pressure draws the interstitial fluid into the capillaries and lymphatic tissue. The expansion of the lung facilitates movement of the remaining lung fluid into the interstitial tissue. As pulmonary vascular resistance decreases, pulmonary blood flow increases, and more fluid is absorbed into the bloodstream. In the healthy term newborn, lung fluid moves rapidly into the interstitial tissue but may take several hours to move into the lymph and blood vessels. About 80% of the fluid is reabsorbed within 2 hours after birth, and it is completely absorbed within 12 to 24 hours after birth.

Although the initial chest compression and recoil generally clear the airways of accumulated fluid and permit further inspiration, some clinicians believe mucus and fluid should be suctioned from the newborn's mouth and oropharynx. They use a mucus trap attached to suction as soon as the newborn's head and shoulders are born and again as the newborn adapts to extrauterine life and stabilizes (see Procedure 17–1).

A variety of factors may cause problems associated with lung fluid clearance and initiation of respiratory activity. The lymphatic system may be underdeveloped, thus decreasing the rate at which the fluid is absorbed from the lungs. Complications that occur antenatally or during labor and birth can interfere with adequate lung expansion and cause failure to decrease pulmonary vascular resistance, resulting in decreased pulmonary blood flow.

These complications include inadequate compression of the chest wall in a very small newborn, the absence of chest wall compression in a newborn born by cesarean birth, respiratory depression due to maternal anesthesia, or aspiration of amniotic fluid or meconium.

### Chemical Stimuli

An important chemical stimulator that contributes to the onset of breathing is transitory asphyxia of the fetus and newborn. The first breath is an inspiratory gasp triggered by elevation in $PCO_2$ and decrease in pH and $PO_2$, which are the natural result of a normal vaginal birth with cessation of placental gas exchange when the cord is clamped. These changes, which are present in all newborns to some degree, stimulate the aortic and carotid chemoreceptors, initiating impulses that trigger the medulla's respiratory center. Although this brief period of asphyxia is a significant stimulator, prolonged asphyxia is abnormal and acts as a central nervous system (CNS) respiratory depressant.

### Thermal Stimuli

A significant decrease in environmental temperature after birth, 37°C to 21–23.9°C (98.6°F to 70–75°F), also stimulates the initiation of breathing. The cold stimulates skin nerve endings, and the newborn responds with rhythmic respirations. Normal temperature changes that occur at birth are apparently within acceptable physiologic limits. However, excessive cooling may result in profound depression and evidence of cold stress (see Chapter 26 for discussion of cold stress).

### Sensory Stimuli

As the fetus moves from a familiar, comfortable, quiet environment to one of sensory abundance, a number of physical and sensory influences help respiration begin. They include the numerous tactile, auditory, and visual stimuli of birth.

During intrauterine life, the fetus is in a dark, sound-dampened, fluid-filled environment and is nearly weightless. After birth the newborn experiences light, sounds, and the effects of gravity for the first time. Historically, vigorous stimulation was provided by slapping the buttocks or heels of the newborn, but the emphasis today is on gentle physical contact. Thoroughly drying the newborn and placing it in skin-to-skin contact with the mother's chest and abdomen provide ample stimulation in a far more comforting way and also decrease heat loss.

## Factors Opposing the First Breath

Three major factors may oppose the initiation of respiratory activity: (1) alveolar surface tension, (2) viscosity of lung fluid within the respiratory tract, and (3) degree of lung compliance.

The contracting force between the moist surfaces of the alveoli is called alveolar surface tension. This tension, which is necessary for healthy respiratory function, would nevertheless cause the small airways and alveoli to collapse between each inspiration were it not for the presence of surfactant. By reducing the attracting force between alveoli, surfactant prevents the alveoli from completely collapsing with each expiration and thus promotes lung expansion. Similarly, surfactant promotes lung compliance, the ability of the lung to fill with air easily. When surfactant decreases, compliance also decreases, and the pressure needed to expand the alveoli with air increases. Resistive forces of the fluid-filled lung, combined with the small radii of the airways, necessitate pressures of 30 to 40 cm of water to open the lung initially (Thureen, Deacon, O'Neill, et al., 1999). The first breath usually establishes FRC that is 30% to 40% of the fully expanded lung volume. This FRC allows alveolar sacs to remain partially expanded on expiration. Thus the air that remains in the lung after expiration (FRC) decreases the need for continuous high pressures for each of the following breaths. Subsequent breaths require only 6 to 8 cm $H_2O$ pressure to open alveoli during inspiration. Therefore, the first breath of life is usually the most difficult.

## Cardiopulmonary Physiology

The onset of respiration stimulates changes in the cardiovascular system that are necessary for successful transition to extrauterine life, hence the term **cardiopulmonary adaptation.** As air enters the lungs, $PO_2$ rises in the alveoli, which stimulates the relaxation of the pulmonary arteries and triggers a decrease in pulmonary vascular resistance. As pulmonary vascular resistance decreases, the vascular flow in the lung increases to 100% 24 hours after birth. This delivery of greater blood volume to the lungs contributes to the conversion from fetal circulation to newborn circulation. After pulmonary circulation is established, blood is distributed throughout the lung, although the alveoli may or may not be fully open. For adequate oxygenation to occur, the heart must deliver sufficient blood to functional, open alveoli. Shunting of blood is common in the early newborn period. Bidirectional blood flow, or right-to-left shunting through the ductus arteriosus, may divert a significant amount of blood away from the lungs, depending on the pressure changes of respiration, crying, and the cardiac cycle. This shunting in the newborn period is also responsible for the unstable transitional period in cardiopulmonary function.

## Oxygen Transport

The transportation of oxygen to the peripheral tissues depends on the type of hemoglobin in the red blood cells. In the fetus and newborn, a variety of hemoglobins exist, the most significant being fetal hemoglobin (Hb F) and adult hemoglobin (Hb A). Approximately 70% to 90% of the hemoglobin in the fetus and newborn is of the fetal variety. The greatest difference between Hb F and Hb A is related to the transport of oxygen.

Since Hb F has a greater affinity for oxygen than does Hb A, the oxygen saturation in the newborn's blood is greater than in the adult's, but the amount of oxygen available to the tissues is less. This situation is beneficial prenatally, because the fetus must maintain adequate oxygen uptake in the presence of very low oxygen tension (umbilical venous $PO_2$ cannot exceed the uterine venous $PO_2$). Because of this high concentration of oxygen in the blood, hypoxia in the newborn is particularly difficult to recognize. Clinical manifestations of cyanosis do not appear until low blood levels of oxygen are present. In addition, alkalosis (increased pH) and hypothermia can result in less oxygen being available to the body tissues, whereas acidosis, hypercarbia, and hyperthermia can result in less oxygen being bound to hemoglobin and more oxygen being released to the body tissues.

## Maintaining Respiratory Function

The lung's ability to maintain oxygenation and ventilation (the exchange of oxygen and carbon dioxide) is influenced by such factors as lung compliance and airway resistance. Anatomic differences in the newborn reduce elastic recoil of the lung tissue and thereby decrease lung compliance. The newborn has a relatively large heart and mediastinal structures that reduce available lung space. Also, the newborn chest is equipped with weak intercostal muscles and a rigid rib cage with horizontal ribs and a high diaphragm, which restricts the space available for lung expansion. The large abdomen further encroaches on the high diaphragm to decrease lung space. Another factor that limits ventilation is airway resistance, which depends on the radii, length, and number of airways.

## Characteristics of Newborn Respiration

The normal newborn respiratory rate is 30 to 60 breaths per minute. Initial respirations may be largely diaphragmatic and shallow and irregular in depth and rhythm. The abdomen's movements are synchronous with the chest movements. When the breathing pattern is characterized by pauses lasting 5 to 15 seconds, **periodic breathing** is occurring. Periodic breathing is rarely associated with differences in skin color or heart rate changes, and it has no prognostic significance. Tactile or other sensory stimulation increases the inspired oxygen and converts periodic breathing patterns to normal breathing patterns during neonatal transition. With deep sleep, the pattern is reasonably regular. Periodic breathing occurs with rapid-eye-movement (REM) sleep, and grossly irregular breathing is evident with motor activity, sucking, and crying. Cessation of breathing lasting more than 20 seconds is defined as apnea and is abnormal in term newborns. Apnea may or may not be associated with changes in skin color or heart rate (drop below 100 beats per minute). Apnea always needs to be further evaluated.

The newborn is an obligatory nose breather, and any obstruction will cause respiratory distress, so it is important to keep the nose and throat clear. Immediately after birth, and for about the next 2 hours after birth, respiratory rates of 60 to 70 breaths per minute are normal. Some cyanosis and acrocyanosis are normal for several hours; thereafter the infant's color improves steadily. If respirations drop below 30 or exceed 60 per minute when the infant is at rest, or if retractions, cyanosis, or nasal flaring and expiratory grunting occur, the clinician should be notified. Any increased use of the intercostal muscles (retractions) may indicate respiratory distress. (See Chapter 26 and Table 26–1 for signs of respiratory distress.)

# Cardiovascular Adaptations

As described earlier, the onset of respiration triggers increased blood flow to the lungs after birth. This greater blood volume contributes to the conversion from fetal circulation to neonatal circulation.

## Fetal-Newborn Transitional Physiology

During fetal life, blood with a higher oxygen content is diverted to the heart and brain. Blood in the descending aorta is less oxygenated and supplies the kidney and intestinal tract before it is returned to the placenta. Limited amounts of blood, pumped from the right ventricle toward the lungs, enter the pulmonary vessels. In the fetus, increased pulmonary resistance forces most of this blood through the ductus arteriosus into the descending aorta (see Table 21–1).

Marked changes occur in the cardiovascular system at birth. Expansion of the lungs with the first breath decreases pulmonary vascular resistance and increases pulmonary blood flow. Pressure in the left atrium increases as blood returns from the pulmonary veins. Pressure in the right atrium drops, and systematic vascular resistance increases as umbilical venous blood flow is halted when the cord is clamped. These physiologic mechanisms mark

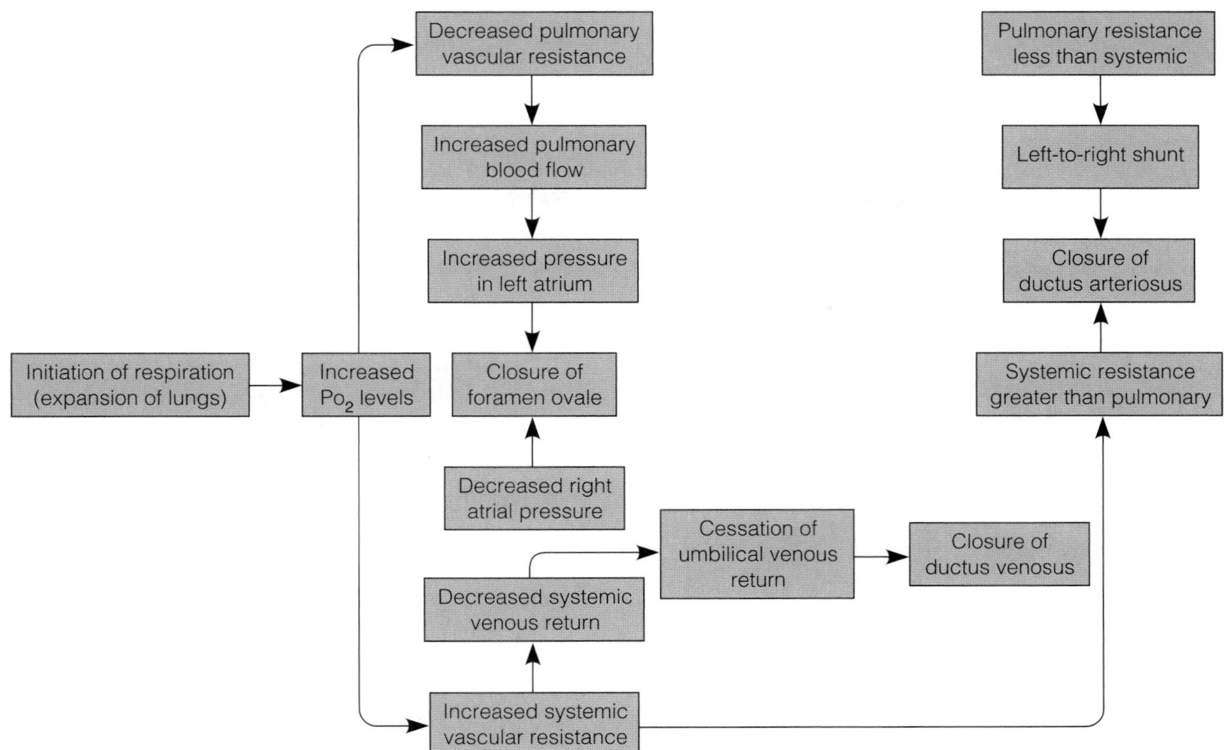


**FIGURE 21–2** ♦ Transitional circulation: conversion from fetal to neonatal circulation.

**TABLE 21–1 Fetal and Neonatal Circulation**

| *System* | *Fetal* | *Neonatal* |
|---|---|---|
| Pulmonary blood vessels | Constricted, with very little blood flow; lungs not expanded | Vasodilation and increased blood flow; lungs expanded; increased oxygen stimulates vasodilation. |
| Systemic blood vessels | Dilated, with low resistance; blood mostly in placenta | Arterial pressure rises due to loss of placenta; increased systemic blood volume and resistance. |
| Ductus arteriosus | Large, with no tone; blood flow from pulmonary artery to aorta | Reversal of blood flow; now from aorta to pulmonary artery because of increased left atrial pressure. Ductus is sensitive to increased oxygen and body chemicals and begins to constrict. |
| Foramen ovale | Patent, with increased blood flow from right atrium to left atrium | Increased pressure in left atrium attempts to reverse blood flow and shuts one-way valve. |

the transition from fetal to neonatal circulation and show the interplay of cardiovascular and respiratory systems (Figure 21–2♦). Five major areas of change occur in cardiopulmonary adaptation (Figure 21–3♦):

1. *Increased aortic pressure and decreased venous pressure.* Clamping of the umbilical cord eliminates the placental vascular bed and reduces the intravascular space. Consequently, aortic (systemic) blood pressure increases. At the same time, blood return via the inferior vena cava decreases, resulting in a decreased right atrial pressure and a small decrease in pressure within the venous circulation.
2. *Increased systemic pressure and decreased pulmonary artery pressure.* With the loss of the low-resistance placenta, systemic resistance pressure increases, resulting in greater systemic pressure. At the same time, lung expansion increases pulmonary blood flow, and the increased blood $PO_2$ associated with initiation of respirations dilates pulmonary blood vessels. The combination of vasodilation and increased pulmonary blood flow decreases pulmonary artery resistance. As the pulmonary vascular beds open, the systemic vascular pressure increases, enhancing perfusion of the other body systems.

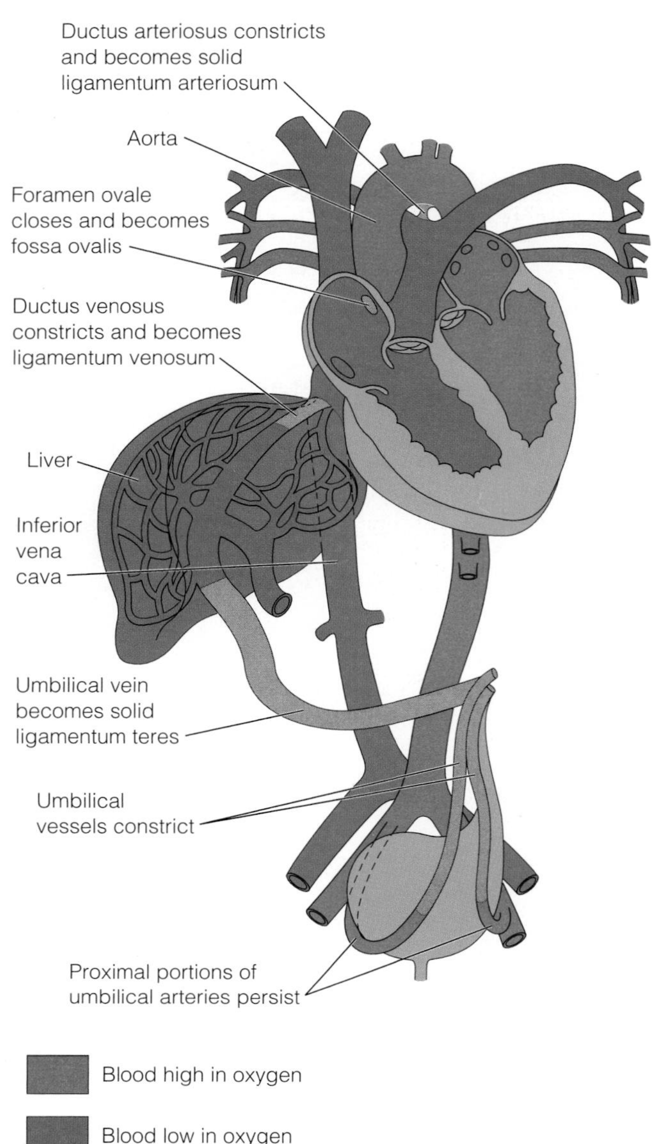


**FIGURE 21–3** ♦ Major changes that occur in the newborn's circulatory system. *Source:* Hole, J. W. (1993). *Human anatomy and physiology* (6th ed.). Dubuque, IA: W. C. Brown. 

3. *Closure of the foramen ovale.* Closure of the foramen ovale is a function of changing atrial pressures. In utero, pressure is greater in the right atrium, and the foramen ovale is open after birth. Decreased pulmonary resistance and increased pulmonary blood flow increase the pulmonary venous return into the left atrium, thereby increasing left atrial pressure slightly. The decreased pulmonary vascular resistance and the decreased umbilical venous return to the right atrium also decrease right atrial pressure. The pressure gradients across the atria are now reversed, left atrial pressure is greater, and the foramen ovale is functionally closed 1 to 2 hours after birth. However, a slight right-to-left shunting may occur in the early newborn period. Any increase in pulmonary resistance or right atrial pressure, such as occurs with crying, acidosis, or cold stress, may cause the foramen ovale to reopen, resulting in a right-to-left shunt. Permanent closure occurs within 6 months.
4. *Closure of the ductus arteriosus.* Initial elevation of the systemic vascular pressure above the pulmonary vascular pressure increases pulmonary blood flow by reversing the flow through the ductus arteriosus. Blood now flows from the aorta into the pulmonary artery. Furthermore, although the presence of oxygen causes the pulmonary arterioles to dilate, an increase in blood $PO_2$ triggers the opposite response in the ductus arteriosus—it constricts.

   In utero, the placenta provides prostaglandin $E_2$ ($PGE_2$), which causes ductus vasodilation. With the loss of the placenta and increased pulmonary blood flow, $PGE_2$ levels drop, leaving the active constriction by $PO_2$ unopposed. If the lungs fail to expand or if $PO_2$ levels drop, the ductus remains patent. Fibrosis of the ductus occurs within 3 weeks after birth, but functional closure is accomplished within 15 hours after birth (Nelson, 1999).
5. *Closure of the ductus venosus.* Although the mechanism initiating closure of the ductus venosus is not known, it appears to be related to mechanical pressure changes after severing of the cord, redistribution of blood, and cardiac output. Closure of the bypass forces perfusion of the liver. Fibrosis of the ductus venosus occurs within 2 months.

## Characteristics of Cardiac Function

### Heart Rate

Shortly after the first cry and the start of changes in cardiopulmonary circulation, the newborn heart rate accelerates to 175 to 180 beats per minute. The average resting heart rate in the first week of life is 125 to 130 beats per minute in a quiet, full-term newborn (Fanaroff & Martin, 1999). In the full-term newborn, the heart rate ranges from as low of 85 to 90 beats per minute while asleep to 120 to 160 beats per minute while awake. Apical pulse rates should be obtained by auscultation for a full minute, preferably when the newborn is asleep. Peripheral pulses of all extremities should also be evaluated to detect any inequalities or unusual characteristics. However, peripheral radial pulses are difficult to palpate in the newborn. They can be assessed when blood pressure is measured if blood pressure readings are taken on all four extremities.

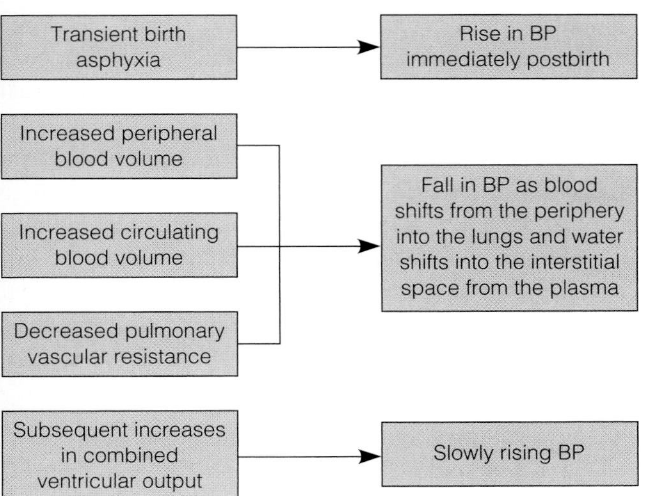


**FIGURE 21–4** ♦ Response of blood pressure (BP) to neonatal changes in blood volume.

### Blood Pressure

The blood pressure tends to be highest immediately after birth and then descends to its lowest level at about 3 hours of age. By days 4 to 6, the blood pressure rises and plateaus at a level approximately the same as the initial level. Blood pressure is sensitive to the changes in blood volume that occur in the transition to newborn circulation (Figure 21–4♦). Peripheral perfusion pressure is a particularly sensitive indicator of the newborn's ability to compensate for alterations in blood volume prior to changes in blood pressure. Capillary refill should be less than 2 to 3 seconds when the skin is blanched.

Blood pressure values during the first 12 hours of life vary with the birth weight. The average blood pressure is 72/47 mm Hg in the full-term, resting newborn and 64/39 mm Hg in the preterm newborn (Fanaroff & Martin, 1999). Crying may cause an elevation of 20 mm Hg in both the systolic and diastolic blood pressure. An accurate blood pressure is best obtained by using the Doppler technique or a 1- to 2-in cuff and a stethoscope over the brachial artery.

### Heart Murmurs

Murmurs are produced by turbulent blood flow. They may be heard when blood flows across an abnormal valve or across a stenosed valve, when there is an atrial or ventricular septal defect, or when there is increased flow across a normal valve. In newborns, 90% of all murmurs are transient and not associated with anomalies. Because of the current practice of early discharge, murmurs associated with ventricular septal defect and patent ductus arteriosus are not often picked up until the first well-baby checkup at 4 to 6 weeks of age. Murmurs are sometimes absent even in seriously malformed hearts (Johnston, 1998).

### Cardiac Workload

Before birth the right ventricle does approximately two-thirds of the cardiac work, resulting in increased size and thickness of the right ventricle at birth. After birth the left ventricle must assume a larger share of the cardiac workload, and it progressively increases in size and thickness. This may explain why right-sided heart defects are better tolerated than left-sided ones and why left-sided heart defects rapidly become symptomatic after birth.

## Hematopoietic System

Fetal erythrocytes are large but few in number. After birth, the red blood cell (RBC) count gradually increases as cell size decreases. Neonatal RBCs have a life span of 80 to 100 days, approximately two-thirds the life span of adult RBCs. In the first days of life, hematocrit may rise 1 to 2 g/dL above fetal levels as a result of placental transfusion, low oral fluid intake, and diminished extracellular fluid volume. By 1 week postnatally, peripheral hemoglobin is comparable to fetal blood counts. The hemoglobin level declines progressively over the first 2 to 3 months of life (Polin & Fox, 1998). This initial decline in hemoglobin creates a phenomenon known as **physiologic anemia of infancy.**

Leukocytosis is a normal finding, because the stress of birth stimulates increased production of neutrophils during the first few days of life. Neutrophils then decrease to 35% of the total leukocyte count by 2 weeks of age. Eventually, lymphocytes become the predominant type of leukocyte and the total white blood cell count falls.

Blood volume of the term infant is estimated to be 80 to 85 mL/kg of body weight. For example, an 8-lb (3.6-kg) newborn has a blood volume of 290 to 309 mL. Blood volume varies based on the amount of placental transfusion received during the delivery of the placenta, as well as other factors, including the following:

1. *Delayed cord clamping and the normal shift of plasma to the extravascular spaces.* Newborn hemoglobin and hematocrit values are higher when a placental transfusion occurs after birth. Placental vessels contain about 100 mL of blood at term, most of which can be transfused into the newborn by holding the newborn below the level of the placenta and delaying clamping of the cord. Blood volume increases by 50% with delayed cord clamping (Polin & Fox, 1998). The increase is reflected by a rise in hemoglobin level and an increase in the hematocrit to about 65% after birth (compared with 48% when the cord is clamped immediately). Although not a routine practice, for greatest accuracy, the initial hemoglobin and hematocrit levels should be measured in the cord blood.

2. *Gestational age.* There appears to be a positive association between gestational age, RBC numbers, and hemoglobin concentration.
3. *Prenatal and/or perinatal hemorrhage.* Significant prenatal or perinatal bleeding decreases the hematocrit level and causes hypovolemia.
4. *The site of the blood sample.* Hemoglobin and hematocrit levels are significantly higher in capillary blood than in venous blood. Sluggish peripheral blood flow creates RBC stasis, thereby increasing RBC concentration in the capillaries. Consequently, blood samples taken from venous blood sites are more accurate than those from capillary sites.

The concentration of serum electrolytes in the blood indicates the fluid and electrolyte status of the newborn. See Table 21–2 for normal term newborn electrolyte and blood values.

## Temperature Regulation

Temperature regulation is the maintenance of thermal balance by the loss of heat to the environment at a rate equal to the production of heat. Newborns are *homeothermic;* they attempt to stabilize their internal (core) body temperatures within a narrow range in spite of significant temperature variations in their environment.

Thermoregulation in the newborn is closely related to the rate of metabolism and oxygen consumption. Within a specific environmental temperature range, called the **thermal neutral zone (TNZ)**, the rates of oxygen consumption and metabolism are minimal, and internal body temperature is maintained because of thermal balance (Table 21–3). For an unclothed, full-term newborn, the TNZ is an ambient environmental temperature range of 32 to 34°C (89.6 to 93.2°F). The limits for an adult are 26 to 28°C (78.8 to 82.4°F) (Polin & Fox, 1998). Thus the normal newborn requires higher environmental temperatures to maintain a thermoneutral environment.

Several newborn characteristics affect the establishment of a TNZ:

- The newborn has decreased subcutaneous fat and a thin epidermis.
- Blood vessels are closer to the skin than those of an adult. Therefore, the circulating blood is influenced by changes in environmental temperature and in turn influences the hypothalamic temperature-regulating center.
- The flexed posture of the term newborn decreases the surface area exposed to the environment, thereby reducing heat loss.

Size and age may also affect the establishment of a TNZ. For example, the preterm or small-for-gestational-age (SGA) newborn has less adipose tissue and is hypoflexed and therefore requires higher environmental temperatures to achieve a thermal neutral environment. Larger, well-insulated newborns may be able to cope with lower environmental temperatures. If the environmental temperature falls below the lower limits of the TNZ, the newborn responds with increased oxygen consumption and metabolism, which results in greater heat production. Prolonged exposure to the cold may result in depleted glycogen stores and acidosis. Oxygen consumption also increases if the environmental temperature is above the TNZ.

**TABLE 21–2 Normal Term Newborn Blood Values**

| *Laboratory Data* | *Normal Range* |
|---|---|
| Hemoglobin | 15–20 g/dL |
| Hematocrit | 51%–56% |
| WBC | 10,000–30,000/mm³ |
| Neutrophils | 40%–80% |
| Immature WBC | 3%–10% |
| Platelets | 15,000–400,000/mm³ |
| Reticulocytes | 3%–6% |
| Blood volume | 82.3 mL/kg (third day after early cord clamping) |
| | 92.6 mL/kg (third day after delayed cord clamping) |
| Sodium | 135–147 mEq/L |
| Potassium | 4–6 mEq/L |
| Chloride | 90–114 mEq/L |
| Calcium | 7–10 mg/dL |
| Glucose | 40–80 mg/dL |

### Heat Loss

A newborn is at a distinct disadvantage in maintaining a normal temperature. With a large body surface in relation to mass and a limited amount of insulating subcutaneous fat, the full-term newborn loses about four times the heat an adult does. The newborn's poor thermal stability is primarily due to excessive heat loss rather than impaired heat production. Because of the risk of hypothermia and possible cold stress, minimizing heat loss in the newborn after birth is essential (see Chapters 17 and 23 for nursing measures).

Two major routes of heat loss are from the internal core of the body to the body surface and from the external surface to the environment. Usually the core temperature is higher than the skin temperature, resulting

## TABLE 21–3 Neutral Thermal Environmental Temperatures

| *Age and Weight* | *Range of Temperature (°C)* |
|---|---|
| **0–6 HOURS** | |
| Under 100 g | 34.0–35.4 |
| 1200–1500 g | 33.9–34.4 |
| 1501–2500 g | 32.8–33.8 |
| Over 2500 (and > 36 weeks) | 34.0–33.8 |
| **6–12 HOURS** | |
| Under 1200 g | 34.0–35.4 |
| 1200–1500 g | 33.5–34.4 |
| 1501–2500 g | 32.2–33.8 |
| Over 2500 (and > 36 weeks) | 31.4–33.8 |
| **12–24 HOURS** | |
| Under 1200 g | 34.0–35.4 |
| 1200–1500 g | 33.3–34.3 |
| 1501–2500 g | 31.8–33.8 |
| Over 2500 (and > 36 weeks) | 31.0–33.7 |
| **24–36 HOURS** | |
| Under 1200 g | 34.0–35.0 |
| 1200–1500 g | 33.1–34.2 |
| 1501–2500 g | 31.6–33.6 |
| Over 2500 (and > 36 weeks) | 30.7–33.5 |
| **36–48 HOURS** | |
| Under 1200 g | 34.0–35.0 |
| 1200–1500 g | 33.0–34.1 |
| 1501–2500 g | 31.4–33.5 |
| Over 2500 (and > 36 weeks) | 30.5–33.3 |
| **48–72 HOURS** | |
| Under 1200 g | 34.0–35.0 |
| 1200–1500 g | 33.0–34.0 |
| 1501–2500 g | 31.2–33.4 |
| Over 2500 (and > 36 weeks) | 30.1–33.2 |
| **72–96 HOURS** | |
| Under 1200 g | 34.0–35.0 |
| 1200–1500 g | 33.0–34.0 |
| 1501–2500 g | 31.1–33.2 |
| Over 2500 (and > 36 weeks) | 29.8–32.8 |
| **4–12 DAYS** | |
| Under 1500 g | 33.0–34.0 |
| 1501–2500 g | 31.0–33.2 |
| Over 2500 (and > 36 weeks) | |
| 4–5 days | 29.5–32.6 |
| 5–6 days | 29.4–32.3 |
| 6–8 days | 29.0–32.2 |
| 8–10 days | 29.0–31.8 |
| 10–12 days | 29.0–31.4 |
| **12–14 DAYS** | |
| Under 1500 g | 32.6–34.0 |
| 1500–2500 g | 31.0–33.2 |
| Over 2500 (and > 36 weeks) | 29.0–30.8 |
| **2–3 WEEKS** | |
| Under 1500 g | 32.2–34.0 |
| 1500–2500 g | 30.5–33.0 |
| **3–4 WEEKS** | |
| Under 1500 g | 31.6–33.6 |
| 1500–2500 g | 30.0–32.7 |
| **4–5 WEEKS** | |
| Under 1500 g | 31.2–13.0 |
| 1500–2500 g | 29.5–32.2 |
| **5–6 WEEKS** | |
| Under 1500 g | 30.6–32.3 |
| 1500–2500 g | 29.0–31.8 |

*Generally speaking, the smaller infants in each weight group will require a temperature in the higher portion of the temperature range. Within each time range, the younger the infant, the higher the temperature required.

*Source:* Adapted from Scopes and Ahmed (1966) (For his table Scopes had the walls of the incubator 1 to 2° warmer than the ambient air temperatures.) Reproduced, with permission, from Klaus, M. H., & Fanaroff, A. A. (1986). *Care of the high-risk neonate* (3rd ed., p. 103). Philadelphia: Saunders.

in continuous transfer of heat to the surface (Fanaroff & Martin, 1999). The greater the difference in temperature between core and skin, the more rapid the transfer. The transfer is accomplished through an increase in oxygen consumption, depletion of glycogen stores, and metabolizing of brown fat. Heat loss from the body surface to the environment takes place in four ways—by convection, radiation, evaporation, and conduction (Figure 21–5♦).

- **Convection** is the loss of heat from the warm body surface to the cooler air currents. Air-conditioned rooms, air currents with a temperature below the infant's skin temperature, oxygen by mask, and removal from an incubator for procedures increase convective heat loss in the newborn.
- **Radiation** losses occur when heat transfers from the heated body surface to cooler surfaces and objects not in direct contact with the body. The walls of a room or of an incubator are potential causes of heat loss by radiation, even if the ambient temperature of the incubator is within the thermal neutral range for that infant. Placing cold objects (such as ice for blood gases) onto the incubator or near the infant in the radiant warmer will increase radiant losses.

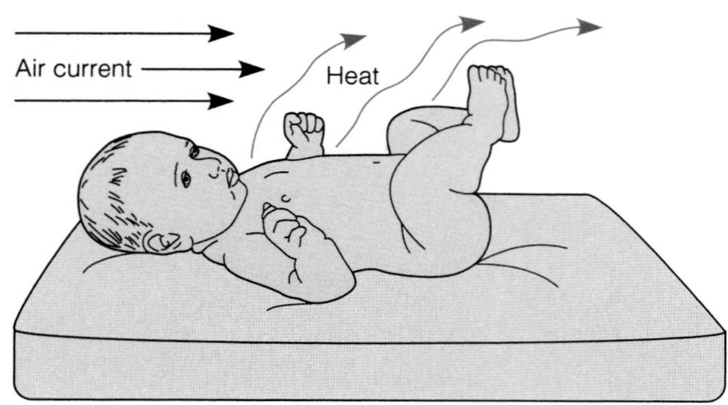


**A** **Convection**

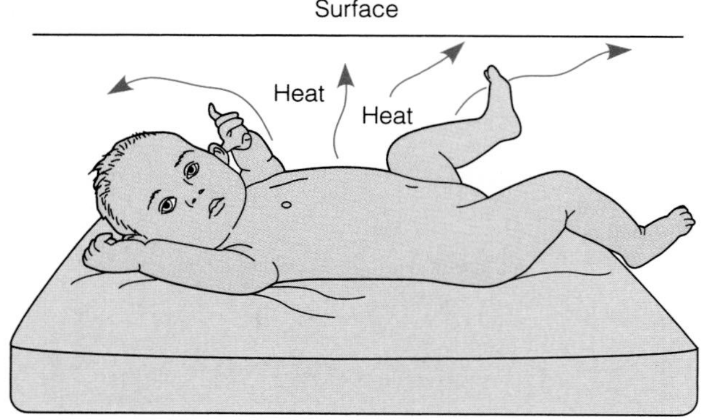


**B** **Radiation**

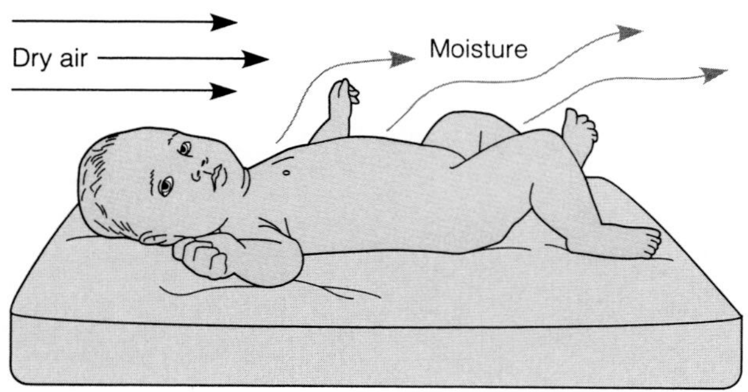


**C** **Evaporation**

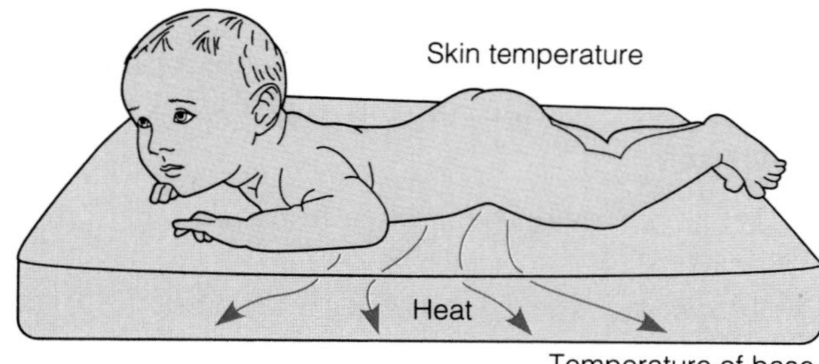


**D** **Conduction**

FIGURE 21–5 ♦ Methods of heat loss. **A**, Convection. **B**, Radiation. **C**, Evaporation. **D**, Conduction.

- **Evaporation** is the loss of heat incurred when water is converted to a vapor. The newborn is particularly prone to lose heat by evaporation immediately after birth (when wet with amniotic fluid), and during baths; therefore, drying the newborn is critical.
- **Conduction** is the loss of heat to a cooler surface by direct skin contact. Chilled hands, cool scales, cold examination tables, and cold stethoscopes can cause loss of heat by conduction. Even if objects are warmed to the incubator temperature, the temperature difference between the infant's core temperature and the ambient temperature may be significant. This difference results in heat transfer.

Once the infant has been dried after birth, the greatest losses of heat generally result from radiation and convection, because of the newborn's large body surface compared with weight, and from thermal conduction, because of the marked difference between core temperature and skin temperature. The newborn can respond to the cooler environmental temperature with adequate peripheral vasoconstriction, but this mechanism is not entirely effective because of the minimal amount of fat insulation present, the large body surface, and ongoing thermal conduction. Therefore minimizing the baby's heat loss and preventing hypothermia are imperative. (See Chapter 26 for nursing measures to prevent hypothermia and cold stress.)

## Heat Production (Thermogenesis)

When exposed to a cool environment, the newborn requires additional heat. The newborn has several physiologic mechanisms that increase heat production, or thermogenesis. These mechanisms include increased basal metabolic rate, muscular activity, and chemical thermogenesis (also called *nonshivering thermogenesis [NST]*) (Baumgart, Harrsch, & Touch, 1999).

NST, an important mechanism of heat production unique to the newborn, occurs when skin receptors perceive a drop in the environmental temperature and, in response, transmit sensations to stimulate the sympathetic nervous system. NST uses the infant's stores of **brown adipose tissue (BAT)** (also called brown fat) to provide heat in the cold-stressed newborn. It first appears in the fetus at about 26 to 30 weeks' gestation and continues to increase until 2 to 5 weeks after the birth of a term infant, unless the fat is depleted by cold stress. BAT is deposited in the midscapular area, around the neck, and in the axillas, with deeper placement around the trachea, esophagus, abdominal aorta, kidneys, and adrenal glands (Figure 21–6♦). BAT constitutes 2% to 6% of the newborn's

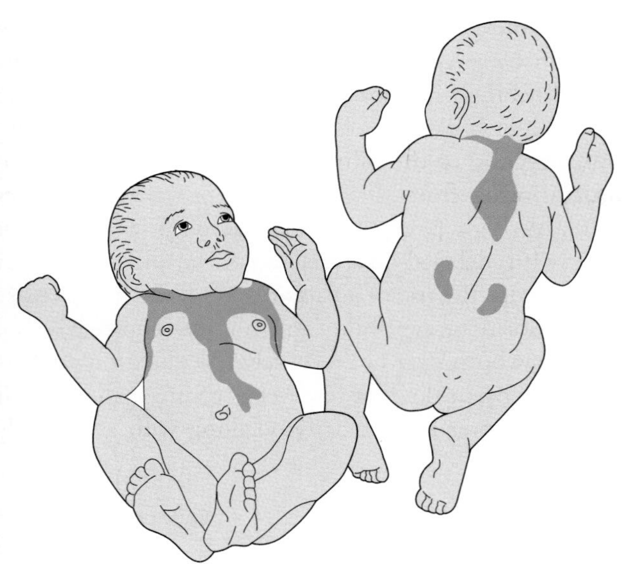

FIGURE 21–6 ♦ The distribution of brown adipose tissue (brown fat) in the newborn. *Source:* Adapted from Davis, V. (1980, November–December). Structure and function of brown adipose tissue in the neonate. *Journal of Obstetric, Gynecologic, and Neonatal Nursing, 9,* 364.

total body weight. Brown fat receives its name from the dark color caused by its enriched blood supply, dense cellular content, and abundant nerve endings. The large numbers of brown fat cells increase the speed with which triglycerides are metabolized to produce heat. These characteristics promote rapid metabolism, heat generation, and heat transfer to the peripheral circulation.

Shivering is rarely seen in the newborn, although it has been observed at ambient temperatures of 15°C (59°F) or less (Polin & Fox, 1998). If the newborn shivers, it means the newborn's metabolic rate has already doubled. The extra muscular activity does little to produce needed heat.

Thermographic studies of newborns exposed to cold show an increase in the skin heat produced over the newborn's brown fat deposits between 1 and 14 days of age. However, if the brown fat supply has been depleted, the metabolic response to cold is limited or lacking. The resulting hypothermia causes an increase in basal metabolism and an increase in oxygen consumption. A decrease in the environmental temperature of 2°C, from 33°C to 31°C, is a drop sufficient to double the oxygen consumption of a term newborn. Keeping the normal newborn warm promotes normal oxygen requirements, whereas chilling can cause the newborn to show signs of respiratory distress.

When exposed to cold, the normal term newborn is usually able to cope with the increase in oxygen requirements, but the preterm newborn may be unable to increase ventilation to the necessary level of oxygen consumption. (See Chapter 26 for discussion of cold stress.) Because oxidation of fatty acids depends on the availability of oxygen, glucose, and adenosine triphosphate (ATP), the newborn's ability to generate heat can be altered by pathologic events such as hypoxia, acidosis, and hypoglycemia or by medication that blocks the release of norepinephrine. The effect of certain drugs, such as meperidine (Demerol), may prevent metabolism of brown fat. Meperidine given to the laboring woman leads to a greater fall in the newborn's body temperature during the neonatal period. Newborn hypothermia prolongs as well as potentiates the effects of many analgesic and anesthetic drugs in the newborn.

### Response to Heat

Sweating is the usual initial response of the term newborn to hyperthermia. The newborn sweat glands have limited function until after the fourth week of extrauterine life; heat is lost through peripheral vasodilation and evaporation of insensible water loss. Oxygen consumption and metabolic rate also increase in response to hyperthermia. Severe hyperthermia can lead to death or to gross brain damage if the baby survives.

## Hepatic Adaptations

In the newborn, the liver is frequently palpable 2 to 3 cm below the right costal margin. It is relatively large and occupies about 40% of the abdominal cavity. The newborn liver plays a significant role in iron storage, carbohydrate metabolism, conjugation of bilirubin, and coagulation.

### Iron Storage and RBC Production

As RBCs are destroyed after birth, the iron is stored in the liver until needed for new RBC production. Newborn iron stores are determined by total body hemoglobin content and length of gestation. The term newborn has about 270 mg of iron at birth, and about 140 to 170 mg of this amount is in the hemoglobin. If the mother's iron intake has been adequate, enough iron will be stored to last until the infant is about 5 months of age. After about 6 months of age, foods containing iron or iron supplements must be given to prevent anemia.

### Carbohydrate Metabolism

At term, the newborn's cord blood glucose level is 70% to 80% of the maternal blood glucose level (Cornblath, Hawdon, Williams, et al., 2000). Newborn carbohydrate reserves are relatively low. One-third of this reserve is in the form of liver glycogen. Newborn glycogen stores are twice those of the adult. The newborn enters an energy crunch at the time of birth, with the removal of the maternal glucose supply and the increased energy expenditure associated with the birth process and extrauterine life. Fuel sources are consumed at a faster rate because of the work of breathing, loss of heat when exposed to cold, activity, and activation of muscle tone.

Glucose is the main source of energy in the first 4 to 6 hours after birth. During the first 2 hours of life, the serum blood glucose level declines, then rises, and finally reaches a steady state 2 to 3 hours after birth (Cornblath et al., 2000). Using a Chemstrip®, the nurse assesses the glucose level initially on admission to the newborn nursery and again 4 hours later. As stores of liver and muscle glycogen and blood glucose decrease, the newborn compensates by changing from a predominantly carbohydrate metabolism to fat metabolism. Energy can be derived from fat and protein, as well as from carbohydrates. The amount and availability of each of these "fuel substrates" depend on the ability of immature metabolic pathways (which lack specific enzymes or hormones) to function in the first few days of life.

## Conjugation of Bilirubin

*Conjugation* of bilirubin is the conversion of yellow lipid-soluble pigment into water-soluble pigment. Unconjugated (indirect) bilirubin is a breakdown product derived from hemoglobin released primarily from destroyed RBCs. Unconjugated bilirubin is not in excretable form and is a potential toxin. **Total serum bilirubin** is the sum of conjugated (direct) and unconjugated (indirect) bilirubin.

Fetal unconjugated bilirubin crosses the placenta to be excreted, so the fetus does not need to conjugate bilirubin. Total bilirubin at birth is usually less than 3 mg/dL unless an abnormal hemolytic process has been present in utero. After birth the newborn's liver must begin to conjugate bilirubin by itself. This produces a rise in serum bilirubin levels in the first few days of life.

The bilirubin formed after RBCs are destroyed is transported in the blood bound to albumin. The bilirubin is transferred into the hepatocytes and bound to two intracellular binding proteins. These two proteins determine the amount of bilirubin held in a liver cell for processing and consequently determine the amount of bilirubin uptake into the liver. The activity of glucuronyl transferase results in the attachment of unconjugated bilirubin to glucuronic acid (product of liver glycogen), producing conjugated (direct) bilirubin. Direct bilirubin is excreted into the common duct and duodenum. The conjugated (direct) bilirubin then progresses down the intestines, where bacteria transform it into urobilinogen. This product is not reabsorbed but is excreted as a yellow-brown pigment in the stools.

Even after the bilirubin has been conjugated and bound, it can be changed back to unconjugated bilirubin via the enterohepatic circulation. In the intestines β-glucuronidase enzyme acts to split off (deconjugate) the bilirubin from glucuronic acid if it has not first been acted on by gut bacteria to produce urobilinogen; the free bilirubin is reabsorbed through the intestinal wall and brought back to the liver via portal vein circulation. This recycling of the bilirubin and decreased ability to clear bilirubin from the system are prevalent in babies with very high β-glucuronidase activity levels and in those with delayed bacterial colonization of the gut (such as with the use of antibiotics) and further increase the newborn's susceptibility to jaundice (Figure 21–7♦).

The newborn liver has relatively less glucuronyl transferase activity in the first few weeks of life than an adult liver. This lower hepatic activity, along with a relatively

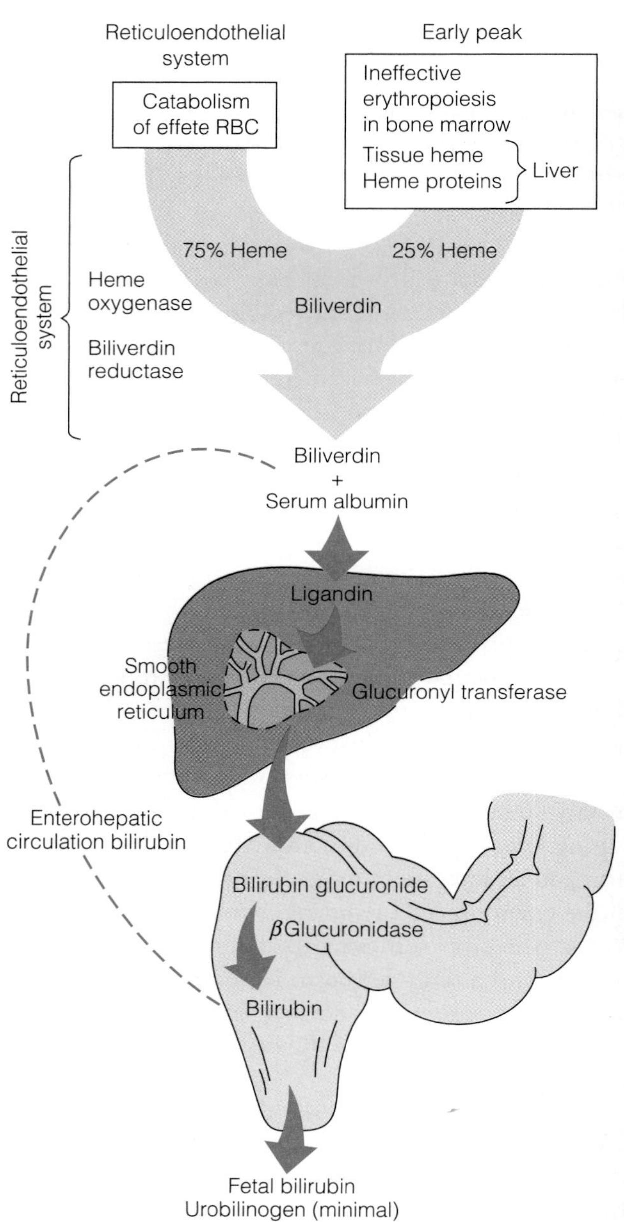


FIGURE 21–7 ♦ Conjugation of bilirubin in the newborn. *Source:* Avery, G. B., Fletcher, M. A., & MacDonald, M. G. (1994). *Neonatology: Pathophysiology and management of the newborn* (4th ed., p. 635). Philadelphia: Lippincott.

large bilirubin load, decreases the liver's ability to conjugate bilirubin and increases susceptibility to jaundice.

## Physiologic Jaundice

**Physiologic jaundice** is caused by accelerated destruction of fetal RBCs, impaired conjugation of bilirubin, and increased bilirubin reabsorption from the intestinal tract. This condition does not have a pathologic basis but is a normal biologic response of the newborn.

Maisels (1999) describes four factors, the interaction of which may give rise to physiologic jaundice:

1. *Increased amounts of bilirubin delivered to the liver.* The increased blood volume due to delayed cord clamping combined with faster RBC destruction in the newborn leads to an increased bilirubin level in the blood. A proportionately larger amount of nonerythrocyte bilirubin forms in the newborn. Therefore, newborns have two to three times greater production or breakdown of bilirubin than do adults. The use of forceps, which sometimes causes facial bruising or cephalhematoma (entrapped hemorrhage), can increase the amount of bilirubin to be handled by the liver. Decreased oxygen supplies to the liver associated with neonatal hypoxia or congenital heart disease lead to a rise in the bilirubin level. Reduced bowel motility, intestinal obstruction, or delayed passage of meconium increases the circulation of bilirubin in the enterohepatic pathway, thereby resulting in higher bilirubin values.
2. *Defective hepatic uptake of bilirubin from the plasma.* If the newborn does not ingest adequate calories, the formation of hepatic binding proteins diminishes, resulting in higher bilirubin levels.
3. *Defective conjugation of the bilirubin.* Decreased glucuronyl transferase activity, as in hypothyroidism, and inadequate caloric intake cause the intracellular binding proteins to remain saturated and result in greater unconjugated bilirubin levels in the blood. The fatty acids in breast milk are thought to compete with bilirubin for albumin-binding sites and therefore impede bilirubin processing.
4. *Defect in bilirubin excretion.* A congenital infection may cause impaired excretion. Delay in introduction of bacterial flora and decreased intestinal motility can also delay excretion and increase enterohepatic circulation of bilirubin.

About 50% of term and 80% of preterm newborns exhibit physiologic jaundice on about the second or third day after birth. The characteristic yellow color results from increased levels of unconjugated (indirect) bilirubin, which are a normal product of RBC breakdown and reflect the body's temporary inability to eliminate bilirubin. Serum levels of bilirubin are about 4 to 6 mg/dL before the yellow coloration of the skin and sclera appear. The signs of physiologic jaundice appear *after* the first 24 hours postnatally. This time frame differentiates physiologic jaundice from pathologic jaundice (see Chapter 26), which is clinically seen at birth or within the first 24 hours of postnatal life.

In the past, it was thought that during the first week unconjugated bilirubin levels in physiologic jaundice should not exceed 13 mg/dL in the term or preterm newborn. Peak bilirubin levels are reached between days 3 and 5 in the term infant and between days 5 and 7 in the preterm infant. These values are established for European and American Caucasian newborns. Chinese, Japanese, Korean, and Native American newborns have considerably higher bilirubin levels that are not as apparent and that persist for longer periods with no apparent ill effects (MacMahon, Stevenson, & Oski, 1998). Some studies propose levels up to 22 mg/dL (300 to 375 μmol/L) in well babies (Maisels, 1999).

The nursery or postpartum room environment, including lighting, may hinder the early detection of the degree and type of jaundice. Pink walls and artificial lights mask the beginning of jaundice in newborns. Daylight assists the observer in early recognition by eliminating distortions caused by artificial light.

If jaundice is suspected, the nurse can quickly assess the newborn's coloring by pressing the skin, generally on the forehead or nose, with a finger. As blanching occurs, the nurse can observe the icterus (yellow coloring).

Several newborn care procedures are designed to decrease the probability of high bilirubin levels; specifically, the nurse can

- Maintain the newborn's skin temperature at 36.5°C (97.8°F) or above, because cold stress results in acidosis. Acidosis in turn decreases available serum albumin–binding sites, weakens albumin-binding powers, and causes elevated unconjugated bilirubin levels.
- Monitor stool for amount and characteristics. Bilirubin is eliminated in the feces; inadequate stooling may result in reabsorption and recycling of bilirubin. Early breastfeeding should be encouraged because the laxative effect of colostrum increases excretion of stool.
- Encourage early feedings to promote intestinal elimination and bacterial colonization and provide caloric intake necessary for formation of hepatic binding proteins.

If jaundice becomes apparent, nursing care is directed toward keeping the newborn well hydrated and promoting intestinal elimination. (For specific nursing management and therapies, see the Critical Pathway for the Newborn with Hyperbilirubinemia in Chapter 26.)

Physiologic jaundice may be very upsetting to parents; they require emotional support and thorough explanation of the condition. If the baby is placed under phototherapy, additional days of hospitalization may be required, which may also be disturbing to parents. They can be encouraged to provide for the emotional needs of their newborn by continuing to feed, hold, and caress the infant. If the mother is discharged, the parents are encouraged to return for feedings and feel free to telephone or visit whenever possible. In many instances, the mother, especially if she is breastfeeding, may elect to remain hospitalized with her newborn; the nurse should support this decision. As an alternative to continued hospitalization, the newborn may be treated with home phototherapy.

## Breastfeeding Jaundice

Breastfeeding is implicated in prolonged jaundice in some newborns. From 1% to 5% of newborns being breastfed will develop breastfeeding jaundice. The bilirubin level of the newborn with breastfeeding jaundice begins to rise after the first week of life, when physiologic jaundice is waning after the mother's milk has come in. The level peaks at 2 to 3 weeks of age and may reach 20 to 25 mg/dL without intervention.

Some women's breast milk may contain several times the normal concentration of certain free fatty acids. These free fatty acids may compete with bilirubin for binding sites on albumin and inhibit the conjugation of bilirubin or increase lipase activity, which disrupts the RBC membrane. Increased lipase activity enhances absorption of bile across the gastrointestinal tract membrane, thereby increasing the enterohepatic circulation of bilirubin. In the past it was thought that the breast milk of women whose newborns have breastfeeding jaundice contained an enzyme that inhibited glucuronyl transferase, but this hypothesis is no longer believed to be true.

Newborns with breastfeeding jaundice appear well, and at present there is an absence of documented kernicterus with this type of jaundice. Temporary cessation of nursing may be advised if bilirubin reaches presumed toxic levels of approximately 20 mg/dL or if the interruption is necessary to establish the cause of the hyperbilirubinemia. Within 24 to 36 hours after breastfeeding is discontinued, the newborn's serum bilirubin levels begin to fall dramatically (Rebar, 1999).

Many physicians believe that breastfeeding may be resumed once other causes of jaundice have been ruled out. The bilirubin concentration may have a slight rise of 2 to 3 mg/dL, with a subsequent decline. Nursing mothers need encouragement and support in their desire to breastfeed their infants, assistance and instruction regarding pumping and expressing milk during the interrupted nursing period, and reassurance that nothing is wrong with their milk or mothering abilities. (See Key Facts to Remember: Jaundice.)

## Coagulation

The liver plays an important part in blood coagulation during fetal life and continues this function to some degree during the first few months after birth. Coagulation factors II, VII, IX, and X (synthesized in the liver) are activated under the influence of vitamin K and therefore are considered vitamin K dependent. The absence of normal flora needed to synthesize vitamin K in the newborn gut results in low levels of vitamin K and creates a transient blood coagulation alteration between the second and fifth day of life. From a low point at about 2 to 3 days after birth, these coagulation factors rise slowly, but they do not approach adult levels until 9 months of age or later. Other coagulation factors with low umbilical cord blood levels are XI, XII, and XIII. Fibrinogen and factors V and VII are near adult ranges.

Although newborn bleeding problems are rare, an injection of vitamin K (AquaMEPHYTON) is given prophylactically on the day of birth to combat potential clinical bleeding problems. (Chapter 26 discusses hemorrhagic disease of the newborn in greater depth.)

Platelet counts at birth are in the same range as for older children, but newborns may manifest mild transient difficulty in platelet aggregation functioning. This platelet problem is accentuated by phototherapy.

### KEY FACTS TO REMEMBER

*Jaundice*

**Physiologic Jaundice**

Physiologic jaundice occurs *after* the first 24 hours of life.

During the first week of life, bilirubin should not exceed 13 mg/dL. Some pediatricians allow levels up to 15 mg/dL.

Bilirubin levels peak at 3 to 5 days in term infants.

**Breast Milk Jaundice**

Bilirubin levels begin to rise about the fourth day after mature breast milk comes in.

Peak of 20–25 mg/dL is reached at 2 to 3 weeks of age.

It may be necessary to interrupt nursing for a short period when bilirubin reaches 20 mg/dL.

Prenatal maternal therapy with phenytoin sodium (Dilantin) or phenobarbital also causes abnormal clotting studies and newborn bleeding in the first 24 hours after birth. Infants born to mothers receiving warfarin sodium (Coumadin) may bleed, because these agents cross the placenta and accentuate existing vitamin K–dependent factor deficiencies.

## Gastrointestinal Adaptations

By 36 to 38 weeks' gestation, the gastrointestinal system is adequately mature, with enzymatic activity and the ability to transport nutrients. The full-term newborn has sufficient intestinal and pancreatic enzymes to digest most simple carbohydrates, proteins, and fats.

The carbohydrates requiring digestion in the newborn are usually disaccharides (lactose, maltose, sucrose). Lactose is the primary carbohydrate in the breastfeeding newborn and is generally easily digested and well absorbed. The only enzyme lacking is pancreatic amylase, which remains relatively deficient during the first few months of life. Newborns have trouble digesting starches (changing more complex carbohydrates into maltose). Therefore, starches should not be introduced into the diet until after the first few months of life.

Although proteins require more digestion than carbohydrates, they are well digested and absorbed from the newborn intestine. The newborn digests and absorbs fats less efficiently because of the minimal activity of the pancreatic enzyme lipase. The newborn excretes about 10% to 20% of the dietary fat intake, compared with 10% for the adult. The newborn absorbs the fat in breast milk more completely than the fat in cows' milk, because breast milk consists of more medium-chain triglycerides and contains lipase. (See Chapter 24 for further discussion of infant nutrition.)

By birth, the newborn has experienced swallowing, gastric emptying, and intestinal propulsion. In utero, fetal swallowing is accompanied by gastric emptying and peristalsis of the fetal intestinal tract. By the end of gestation, peristalsis becomes much more active in preparation for extrauterine life. Fetal peristalsis is also stimulated by anoxia, causing the expulsion of meconium into the amniotic fluid in more mature fetuses.

Air enters the stomach immediately after birth. The small intestine is filled with air within 2 to 12 hours and the large bowel within 24 hours. The salivary glands are immature at birth, and the newborn produces little saliva until about age 3 months. The newborn's stomach has a capacity of about 50 to 60 mL. It empties intermittently, starting within a few minutes of the beginning of a feeding and ending 2 to 4 hours after feeding. The newborn's gastric pH becomes less acidic about a week after birth and remains less acidic than that of adults for the next 2 to 3 months.

The cardiac sphincter is immature, as is neural control of the stomach, so some regurgitation may be noted in the newborn period. Regurgitation of the first few feedings during the first day or two of life can usually be lessened by avoiding overfeeding and by burping the newborn well during and after the feeding.

When no other signs and symptoms are evident, vomiting is limited and ceases within the first few days of life. Continuous vomiting or regurgitation should be observed closely. If the newborn has swallowed bloody or purulent amniotic fluid, lavage of the stomach may be indicated in the term newborn to relieve the problem. Bilious vomiting is abnormal and must be evaluated thoroughly because it might represent a condition that warrants prompt surgical intervention.

Adequate digestion and absorption are essential for newborn growth and development. If optimal nutritional support is available, postnatal growth should parallel intrauterine growth; that is, after 30 weeks' gestation, the fetus gains 30 g/day and adds 1.2 cm to body length daily. To gain weight at the intrauterine rate, the term newborn requires 120 cal/kg/day. After birth, caloric intake is often insufficient for weight gain until the newborn is 5 to 10 days old. During this time, there may be a weight loss of 5% to 10% in term newborns. A shift of intracellular water to extracellular space and insensible water loss account for the 5% to 10% weight loss; thus, failure to lose weight when caloric intake is inadequate may indicate fluid retention.

Term newborns usually pass meconium within 8 to 24 hours of life and almost always within 48 hours. **Meconium** is formed in utero from the amniotic fluid and its constituents, intestinal secretions, and shed mucosal cells. It is recognized by its thick, tarry black or dark-green appearance. Transitional (thin brown to green) stools consisting of part meconium and part fecal material are passed for the next day or two, and then the stools become entirely fecal. Generally the stools of a breastfed newborn are pale yellow (but may be pasty green); they are more liquid and more frequent than those of formula-fed newborns, whose stools are paler (Figure 21–8♦). Frequency of bowel movement varies but ranges from one every 2 to 3 days to as many as 10 daily. Totally breastfed infants often progress to stools that occur every 5 to 7 days. Mothers should be counseled that the newborn is not constipated as long as the bowel movement remains soft. (See Key Facts to Remember: Physiologic Adaptations to Extrauterine Life.)

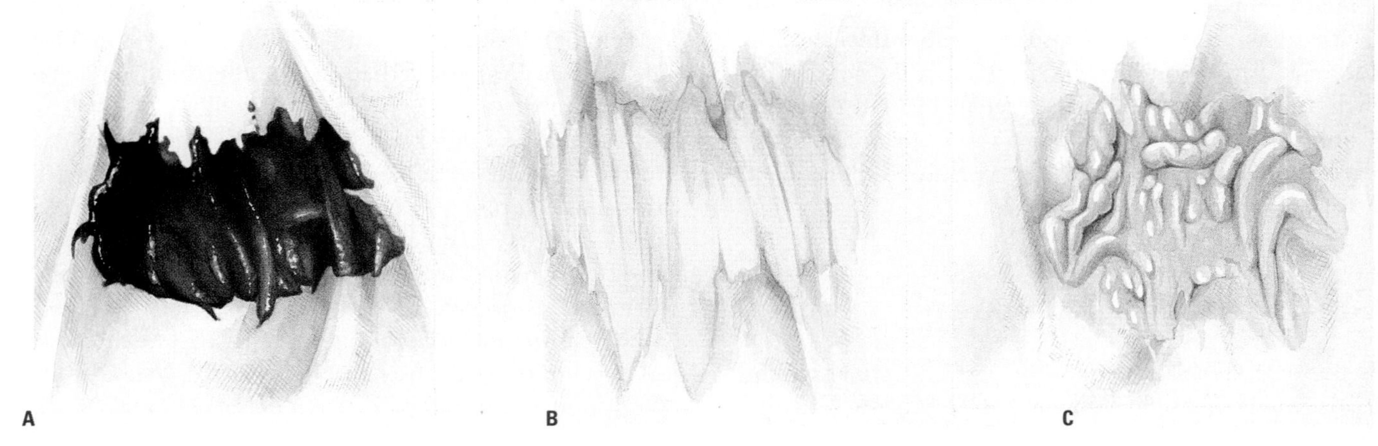


FIGURE 21–8 ♦ Newborn stool samples. A, Meconium stool. B, Breast milk stool. C, Cow's milk stool.

## KEY FACTS TO REMEMBER

*Physiologic Adaptations to Extrauterine Life*

Periodic breathing may be present.

Desired skin temperature 36–36.5°C (96.8–97.7°F) stabilizes 4 to 6 hours after birth.

Desired blood glucose level reaches 60–70 mg/dL by third postnatal day.

Stools (progress from):

- Meconium (thick, tarry, black)
- Transitional stools (thin, brown to green)
- Breastfed infants (yellow-gold, soft, or mushy)
- Bottle-fed infants (pale yellow, formed, and pasty)

# Urinary Adaptations

## Kidney Development and Function

Certain physiologic features of the newborn's kidneys influence the newborn's ability to handle body fluids and excrete urine:

1. The term newborn's kidneys have a full complement of functioning nephrons by 34 to 36 weeks' gestation.
2. The glomerular filtration rate of the newborn's kidney is low compared with the adult rate. Because of this physiologic inefficiency, the newborn's kidney is unable to dispose of water rapidly when necessary because it favors reabsorption of sodium.
3. The juxtamedullary portion of the nephron has limited capacity to reabsorb $HCO_3^-$ and $H^-$ and concentrate urine. The limitation of tubular reabsorption can lead to inappropriate loss of substances present in the glomerular filtrate, such as amino acids, bicarbonate, glucose, and sodium.

Full-term newborns are less able than adults to concentrate urine (reabsorb water back into the blood) because the tubules are short and narrow. There is a greater capacity for glomerular filtration than for tubular reabsorption and secretion. Although feeding practices may affect the osmolarity of the urine, the maximum concentrating ability of the newborn is a specific gravity of 1.025. The inability to concentrate urine is due to the limited excretion of solutes (principally sodium, potassium, chloride, bicarbonate, urea, and phosphate) in the growing newborn. The ability to concentrate urine fully is attained by 3 months of age.

Because the newborn has difficulty concentrating urine, the effect of excessive insensible water loss or restricted fluid intake is unpredictable. The newborn kidney is also limited in its dilutional capabilities. Maximal dilution ability is a specific gravity of 1.001. Concentrating and dilutional limitations of renal function are important considerations in monitoring fluid therapy to prevent dehydration or overhydration.

## Characteristics of Newborn Urinary Function

Many newborns void immediately after birth, and the voiding frequently goes unnoticed. Among normal newborns, 93% void by 24 hours after birth and 98% void by 48 hours after birth (Thureen et al., 1999). A newborn who has not voided by 48 hours should be assessed for adequacy of fluid intake, bladder distension, restlessness, and symptoms of pain. The appropriate clinical personnel should be notified if indicated.

The initial bladder volume is 6 to 44 mL of urine. Unless edema is present, normal urinary output is often limited, and the voidings are scanty until fluid intake increases. The fluid of edema is eliminated by the kidneys, so newborns with edema have a much higher urinary output. The first 2 days postnatally, the newborn voids two to six times daily, with a urine output of 15 mL/day. The newborn subsequently voids 5 to 25 times every 24 hours, with a volume of 25 mL/kg per day.

Following the first voiding, the newborn's urine frequently appears cloudy (due to mucus content) and has a high specific gravity, which decreases as fluid intake increases. Occasionally pink stains ("brick dust spots") appear on the diaper. These are caused by urates and are innocuous. Blood may occasionally be observed on the diapers of female newborns. This *pseudomenstruation* is related to the withdrawal of maternal hormones. Males may have bloody spotting from a circumcision if performed. In the absence of apparent causes for bleeding, the clinician should be notified. During early infancy, normal urine during early infancy is straw colored and almost odorless, although odor occurs when certain drugs are given, metabolic disorders exist, or infection is present. Table 21–4 contains urinalysis values for the normal newborn.

| TABLE 21–4 Newborn Urinalysis Values |
| --- |
| Protein < 5–10 mg/dL |
| WBC < 2–3 |
| RBC 0 |
| Casts 0 |
| Bacteria 0 |
| Specific gravity 1.00–1.025 |
| Color pale yellow |

## Immunologic Adaptations

The newborn's immune system is not fully activated until sometime after birth. The limitations in the newborn's inflammatory response result in failure to recognize, localize, and destroy invasive bacteria. Thus the signs and symptoms of infection are often subtle and nonspecific in the newborn. The newborn also has a poor hypothalamic response to pyrogens; therefore fever is not a reliable indicator of infection. In the neonatal period, hypothermia is a more reliable sign of infection.

The most common class of immune cells are immunoglobulins, a type of antibody secreted by lymphocytes and plasma cells into body fluids. Of the three major types of immunoglobulins primarily involved in immunity—IgG, IgA, and IgM—only IgG crosses the placenta. The pregnant woman forms antibodies in response to illness or immunization. This process is called **active acquired immunity.** When IgG antibodies are transferred to the fetus in utero, **passive acquired immunity** results, since the fetus does not produce the antibodies itself. IgG immunoglobulins are very active against bacterial toxins.

Because the maternal IgG is transferred primarily during the third trimester, preterm newborns (especially those born prior to 34 weeks gestation) may be more susceptible to infection. In general, newborns have immunity to tetanus, diphtheria, smallpox, measles, mumps, poliomyelitis, and a variety of other bacterial and viral diseases. The period of resistance varies: Immunity against common viral infections such as measles may last 4 to 8 months, whereas immunity to certain bacteria may disappear within 4 to 8 weeks.

The normal newborn produces antibodies in response to an antigen but not as effectively as an older child does. It is customary to begin immunization at 2 months of age; then the infant can develop active acquired immunity.

IgM immunoglobulins are produced in response to blood group antigens, gram-negative enteric organisms, and some viruses in the expectant mother. Because IgM does not normally cross the placenta, most or all is produced by the fetus beginning at 10 to 15 weeks' gestation. Elevated levels of IgM at birth may indicate placental leaks or, more commonly, antigenic stimulation in utero. Consequently elevations suggest that the newborn was exposed to an intrauterine infection such as syphilis or TORCH syndrome (toxoplasmosis, rubella, cytomegalovirus, herpesvirus hominis type 2 infection). (For further discussion, see Chapter 13.) The lack of available maternal IgM in the newborn also accounts for the susceptibility to gram-negative enteric organisms such as *Escherichia coli.*

The functions of IgA immunoglobulins are not fully understood. IgA appears to provide protection mainly on secreting surfaces such as the respiratory tract, gastrointestinal tract, and eyes. Serum IgA does not cross the placenta and is not normally produced by the fetus in utero. Unlike the other immunoglobulins, IgA is not affected by gastric action. Colostrum, the forerunner of breast milk, is very high in the secretory form of IgA. Consequently it may be of significance in providing some passive immunity to the infant of a breastfeeding mother. Newborns begin to produce secretory IgA in their intestinal mucosa about 4 weeks after birth.

## Neurologic and Sensory-Perceptual Functioning

The newborn's brain is about one-quarter the size of an adult's, and myelination of nerve fibers is incomplete.

Unlike the cardiovascular and respiratory systems, which undergo tremendous changes at birth, the nervous system is minimally influenced by the actual birth process.

Because many biochemical and histologic changes have yet to occur in the newborn's brain, the postnatal period is considered a time of risk with regard to the development of the brain and nervous system. For neurologic development—including development of intellect—to proceed, the brain and other nervous system structures must mature in an orderly, unhampered fashion. (For discussion of cranial nerves, see Chapter 22.)

## Intrauterine Factors Influencing Newborn Behavior

Newborns respond to and interact with the environment in a predictable pattern of behavior that is somewhat shaped by their intrauterine experience. This intrauterine experience is affected by intrinsic factors such as maternal nutrition and external factors such as the mother's physical environment. Depending on the newborn's intrauterine experience, neonatal behavioral responses to various stresses vary from dealing quietly with the stimulation, to becoming overreactive and tense, to a combination of the two.

Factors such as exposure to intense auditory stimuli in utero can eventually be manifested in the behavior of the newborn. For example, the fetal heart rate (FHR) initially increases when the pregnant woman is exposed to auditory stimuli, but repetition of the stimuli leads to decreased FHR. Thus the newborn who was exposed to intense noise during fetal life is significantly less reactive to loud sounds postnatally.

## Characteristics of Newborn Neurologic Function

Partially flexed extremities with the legs near the abdomen is the usual position of the normal newborn. When awake, the newborn may exhibit purposeless, uncoordinated bilateral movements of the extremities.

The organization and quality of the newborn's motor activity are influenced by a number of factors, including the following (Brazelton, 1984):

- Sleep-alert states
- Presence of environmental stimuli, such as heat, light, cold, and noise
- Conditions causing a chemical imbalance, such as hypoglycemia
- Hydration status
- State of health
- Recovery from the stress of labor and birth

Eye movements are observable during the first few days of life. An alert newborn is able to fixate on faces and geometric objects or patterns such as black-and-white stripes. A bright light shining in the newborn's eyes elicits the blinking reflex.

The cry of the newborn should be lusty and vigorous. High-pitched cries, weak cries, and no cries are all causes for concern.

Growth of the newborn's body progresses in a cephalocaudal (head-to-toe), proximal-distal fashion. The newborn is somewhat hypertonic; that is, there is resistance to extending the elbow and knee joints. Muscle tone should be symmetrical. Diminished muscle tone and flaccidity may indicate neurologic dysfunction.

Specific symmetrical deep tendon reflexes can be elicited in the newborn. Plantar flexion is present. The knee jerk is brisk; a normal ankle clonus may involve three to four beats. Other reflexes, including the Moro, grasping, Babinski, rooting, and sucking reflexes are characteristic of neurologic integrity (see Chapter 22).

Performance of complex behavioral patterns reflects the newborn's neurologic maturation and integration. Newborns who can bring a hand to their mouth may be demonstrating motor coordination as well as a self-quieting technique, thus increasing the complexity of the behavioral response. Newborns also possess complex, organized defensive motor patterns, as exhibited by the ability to remove an obstruction, such as a cloth across the face.

## Periods of Reactivity

The baby usually shows a predictable pattern of behavior during the first several hours after birth, characterized by two **periods of reactivity** separated by a sleep phase.

### First Period of Reactivity

The first period of reactivity lasts approximately 30 minutes after birth. During this period the newborn is awake and active and may appear hungry and have a strong sucking reflex. This is a natural opportunity to initiate breastfeeding if the mother has chosen it. Bursts of random, diffuse movements alternating with relative immobility may occur. Respirations are rapid, as high as 80 breaths per minute, and there may be retraction of the chest, transient flaring of the nares, and grunting. The heart rate is rapid, and the rhythm may be irregular. Bowel sounds are usually absent.

### Period of Inactivity to Sleep Phase

After approximately half an hour the newborn's activity gradually diminishes, and the heart rate and respirations decrease as the newborn enters the sleep phase. The sleep phase may last from a few minutes to 2 to 4 hours. During this period, the newborn will be difficult to awaken and will show no interest in sucking. Bowel sounds become audible, and cardiac and respiratory rates return to baseline values.

### Second Period of Reactivity

During the second period of reactivity, the newborn is again awake and alert. This period lasts 4 to 6 hours in the normal newborn. Physiologic responses are variable during this stage. The heart and respiratory rates increase; however, the nurse must be alert for apneic periods, which may cause a drop in the heart rate. The newborn is stimulated to continue breathing during such times. The newborn may develop rapid color changes and become mildly cyanotic or mottled during these fluctuations. Production of respiratory and gastric mucus increases, and the newborn responds by gagging, choking, and regurgitating.

Continued close observation and intervention may be required to maintain a clear airway during this period of reactivity. The gastrointestinal tract becomes more active. The first meconium stool is frequently passed during this second active stage, and the initial voiding may also occur at this time. The newborn will indicate readiness for feeding by such behaviors as sucking, rooting, and swallowing. If feeding was not initiated in the first period of reactivity, it is done at this time. (See Chapter 24 for further discussion of this first feeding.)

## Behavioral States of the Newborn

The behavior of the newborn can be divided into two categories, the sleep state and the alert state (Brazelton, 1999). These postnatal behavioral states are similar to those that have been identified during pregnancy. Subcategories are identified under each major category.

### Sleep States

The sleep states are as follows:

1. *Deep or quiet sleep.* Deep sleep is characterized by closed eyes with no eye movements; regular, even breathing; and jerky motions or startles at regular intervals. Behavioral responses to external stimuli are likely to be delayed. Startles are rapidly suppressed, and changes in state are not likely to occur. Heart rate may range from 100 to 120 beats per minute.
2. *Active rapid eye movement (REM).* Active REM sleep is characterized by irregular respirations; eyes closed, with rapid eye movements visible through the lids; irregular sucking motions; minimal activity; and irregular but smooth movement of the extremities. Environmental and internal stimuli may initiate a startle reaction and a change of state.

Sleep cycles in the newborn have been recognized and defined according to duration. The length of the cycle depends on the age of the newborn. At term, REM active sleep and quiet sleep occur in intervals of 45 to 50 minutes. About 45% to 50% of the total sleep of the newborn is active sleep, 35% to 45% is quiet sleep, and 10% is transitional between these two periods. It is hypothesized that REM sleep stimulates the growth of the neural system. Over a period of time, the newborn's sleep-wake patterns become diurnal; that is, the newborn sleeps at night and stays awake during the day. (See Chapter 22 for a short discussion of Brazelton's assessment of newborn states.)

### Alert States

In the first 30 to 60 minutes after birth, many newborns display a quiet alert state, characteristic of the first period of reactivity (Figure 21–9♦). Nurses should use these alert states to encourage bonding and breastfeeding. These periods of alertness tend to be short the first 2 days after birth to allow the baby to recover from the birth process. Subsequent alert states are of choice or of necessity (Brazelton, 1999). Increasing choice of wakefulness by the newborn indicates a maturing capacity to achieve and maintain consciousness. Heat, cold, and hunger are but a few of the stimuli that can cause wakefulness by necessity. Once the disturbing stimuli are removed, sleep tends to recur.

The following are subcategories of the alert state (Brazelton, 1999):

1. *Drowsy or semidozing.* The behaviors common to the drowsy state are open or closed eyes; fluttering eyelids; semidozing appearance; and slow, regular movements of the extremities. Mild startles may be noted from time to time. Although the reaction to a sensory stimulus is delayed, a change of state often results.
2. *Wide awake.* In the wide-awake state, the newborn is alert and follows and fixates on attractive objects, faces, or auditory stimuli. Motor activity is minimal, and the response to external stimuli is delayed.

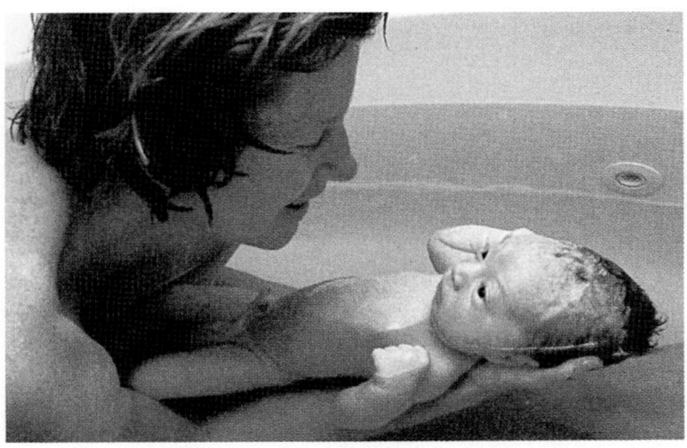

FIGURE 21–9 ♦ Mother and newborn gaze at each other. This quiet, alert state is the optimum state for interaction between baby and parents.

3. *Active awake.* In the active-awake state the newborn's eyes are open and motor activity is quite intense, with thrusting movements of the extremities. Environmental stimuli increase startles or motor activity, but individual reactions are difficult to distinguish because of the generally high activity level.
4. *Crying.* Intense crying is accompanied by jerky motor movements. Crying serves several purposes for the newborn. It may be a distraction from disturbing stimuli such as hunger and pain. Fussiness often allows the newborn to discharge energy and reorganize behavior. Most important, crying elicits an appropriate response of help from the parents.

## Behavioral-Sensory Capacities of the Newborn

**Habituation** is the newborn's ability to process and respond to visual and auditory stimulation. For example, when a bright light is flashed into the newborn's eyes, the initial response is blinking, constriction of the pupil, and perhaps a slight startle reaction. However, with repeated stimulation, the newborn's response repertoire gradually diminishes and disappears. The capacity to ignore repetitious disturbing stimuli is a newborn defense mechanism readily apparent in the noisy, well-lit nursery.

**Orientation** is the newborn's ability to be alert to, follow, and fixate on complex visual stimuli that are appealing and attractive. The newborn prefers the human face and eyes and bright shiny objects. As the face or object comes into the line of vision, the newborn responds with bright, wide eyes, still limbs, and fixed staring. This intense visual involvement may last several minutes, during which time the newborn is able to follow the stimulus from side to side. Figure 21–10♦ illustrates this response. The newborn uses this sensory capacity to become familiar with family, friends, and surroundings.

**Self-quieting ability** refers to newborns' ability to quiet and comfort themselves. Their repertoire includes hand-to-mouth movements, sucking on a fist or tongue, and attending to external stimuli. Neurologically impaired newborns are unable to use self-quieting activities and require more frequent comforting from caregivers when stimulated. For example, drug-positive newborns often exhibit abnormal sleep and feeding patterns and irritability.

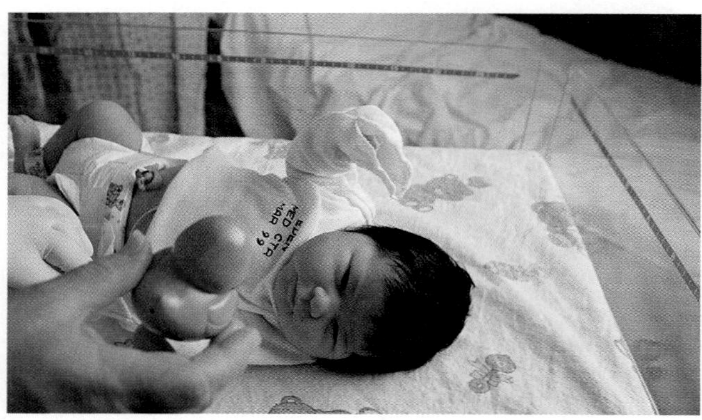

FIGURE 21–10 ♦ Head turning to follow movement.

### Auditory Capacity

The newborn responds to auditory stimulation with a definite, organized behavior repertoire. The stimulus used to assess auditory response should be selected to match the state of the newborn. A rattle is appropriate for light sleep, a voice for an awake state, and a clap for deep sleep. As the newborn hears the sound, the cardiac rate rises, and a minimal startle reflex may be observed. If the sound is appealing, the newborn will become alert and search for the site of the auditory stimulus.

### Olfactory Capacity

Newborns are apparently able to select people by smell. In one study, newborns were able to distinguish their mothers' breast pads from those of other mothers at just 5 days of age (Brazelton, 1999).

### Taste and Sucking

The newborn responds differently to varying tastes. Sugar, for example, increases sucking. Sucking pattern variations also exist in newborns fed with a rubber nipple versus the breast. When breastfeeding, the newborn sucks in bursts, with frequent regular pauses. The bottle-fed newborn tends to suck at a regular rate, with infrequent pauses.

When awake and hungry, the newborn displays rapid searching motions in response to the rooting reflex. Once feeding begins, the newborn establishes a sucking pattern according to the method of feeding. Finger sucking is present not only postnatally but also in utero. The newborn frequently uses nonnutritive sucking as a self-quieting activity, which assists in the development of self-regulation. Nonnutritive sucking with a pacifier should not be discouraged if the infant is bottle-fed. For breastfed infants pacifiers should be offered only after breastfeeding is well established. If the pacifier is offered too soon, a phenomenon called "nipple confusion" may occur in which the breastfed infant has difficulty learning to suck from the breast (see Chapter 24).

### Tactile Capacity

The newborn is very sensitive to being touched, cuddled, and held. Often a mother's first response to an upset or crying newborn is touching or holding. Swaddling, placing a hand on the abdomen, or holding the arms to prevent a startle reflex are other methods of soothing the newborn. The settled newborn is then able to attend to and interact with the environment.

# Chapter Review

## CHAPTER HIGHLIGHTS

- Newborn respiration is initiated primarily by chemical and mechanical events, in association with thermal and sensory stimulation.
- The production of surfactant is crucial to keeping the lungs expanded during expiration by reducing alveolar surface tension.
- The newborn is an obligatory nose breather. Respirations change from being primarily shallow, irregular, and diaphragmatic to synchronous abdominal and chest breathing. Normal respiratory rate is 30 to 60 beats per minute.
- Periodic breathing is normal, and newborn sleep states affect breathing patterns.
- The status of the cardiopulmonary system may be measured by evaluating the heart rate, blood pressure, and presence or absence of murmurs. The normal heart rate is 120 to 160 beats per minute.
- Oxygen transport in the newborn is significantly affected by the presence of greater amounts of Hb F (fetal hemoglobin) than Hb A (adult hemoglobin); Hb F holds oxygen easier but releases it to the body tissues only at low $PO_2$ levels.
- Blood values in the newborn are modified by several factors, such as site of the blood sample, gestational age, prenatal and/or perinatal hemorrhage, and the timing of the clamping of the umbilical cord.
- Blood glucose levels should reach a steady state by 4 hours of age.
- The newborn is considered to have established thermoregulation when oxygen consumption and metabolic activity are minimal.
- Evaporation is the primary heat loss mechanism in newborns who are wet from amniotic fluid or a bath. In addition, excessive heat loss occurs from radiation and convection, because of the newborn's larger surface area compared with weight, and from thermal conduction, because of the marked difference between core temperature and skin temperature.
- The primary source of heat in the cold-stressed newborn is brown adipose tissue.
- The normal newborn possesses the ability to digest and absorb nutrients necessary for newborn growth and development.
- The newborn's liver plays a crucial role in iron storage, carbohydrate metabolism, conjugation of bilirubin, and coagulation.
- Physiologic jaundice may be seen between 3 and 5 days of life in term infants.
- The newborn's stools change from meconium (thick, tarry, dark green) to transitional stools (thin, brown-to-green) and then to the distinct forms for either breastfed newborns (yellow-gold, soft, or mushy) or bottle-fed newborns (pale yellow, formed, and pasty). Most newborns pass their first stool within 24 hours of birth.
- The newborn's kidneys are characterized by a decreased rate of glomerular flow, limited tubular reabsorption, limited excretion of solutes, and limited ability to concentrate urine. Most newborns void within 24 hours of birth.
- The immune system in the newborn is not fully activated until sometime after birth, but the newborn possesses some immunologic abilities.
- Neurologic and sensory-perceptual functioning in the newborn are evident from the newborn's interaction with the environment, synchronized motor activity, and well-developed sensory capacities.
- The first period of reactivity lasts for 30 minutes after birth. The newborn is alert and hungry at this time, making this a natural opportunity to promote attachment.
- The second period of reactivity requires close monitoring by the nurse because apnea, decreased heart rate, gagging, choking, and regurgitation are likely to occur and require nursing intervention.
- The behavioral states in the newborn can be divided into sleep states and alert states.

## CHAPTER REFERENCES


Baumgart, S., Harrsch, S. C., & Touch, S. M. (1999). Thermoregulation. In G. B. Avery, M. A. Fletcher, & M. G. MacDonald (Eds.), *Neonatology: Pathophysiology and management of the newborn* (5th ed.). Philadelphia: Lippincott. Chap. 24 pp. 395–408.

Brazelton, T. B. (1984). *Neonatal behavioral assessment scale* (2nd ed.). London: Heineman.

Brazelton, T. B. (1999). Behavioral competence. In G. B. Avery, M. A. Fletcher, & M. G. MacDonald (Eds.), *Neonatology: Pathophysiology and management of the newborn* (5th ed.). Philadelphia: Lippincott. Chap. 20 pp. 321–332.

Cornblath, M., Hawdon, J. M., Williams, A. F., Aynseley-Green, A., Ward-Platt, M. P., Schwartz, R., & Kalhan, S. C. (2000). Controversies regarding definition of neonatal hypoglycemia: Suggested operational thresholds. *Pediatrics, 105*(5), 1141–1145.

Fanaroff, A. A., & Martin, R. J. (1999). *Neonatal-perinatal medicine* (7th ed.). St. Louis: Mosby.

Johnston, P. G. B. (1998). *The newborn child* (8th ed.). New York: Churchill.

MacMahon, J. R., Stevenson, D. K., & Oski, F. A. (1998). Physiologic jaundice. In H. W. Taeusch & R. A. Ballard (Eds.), *Avery's diseases of the newborn* (7th ed.). Philadelphia: Saunders. pp. 1003–1007 chap. 82.

Maisels, M. J. (1999). Jaundice. In G. B. Avery, M. A. Fletcher, & M. G. MacDonald (Eds.)., *Neonatology: Pathophysiology and management of the newborn* (5th ed.). Philadelphia: Lippincott. Chap. 38 pp. 765–819.

Nelson, N. M. (1999). The onset of respiration. In G. B. Avery, M. A. Fletcher, & M. G. MacDonald (Eds.), *Neonatology: Pathophysiology and management of the newborn,* (5th ed.). Philadelphia: Lippincott. Chap. 17 pp. 257–278.

Polin, R. A., & Fox, W. W. (1998). *Fetal and neonatal physiology* (2nd ed.). Philadelphia: Saunders.

Rebar, R. W. (1999). The breast and the physiology of lactation. In R. K. Creasy & R. Resnik (Eds.), *Maternal-fetal medicine.* (4th ed.). Philadelphia: Saunders. Chap. 8 pp. 106–121.

Thureen, P. J., Deacon, J., O'Neill, P., & Hernandez, J. (1999). *Assessment and care of the well newborn.* Philadelphia: Saunders.


## CONTEMPORARY MATERNAL-NEWBORN NURSING ON-LINE

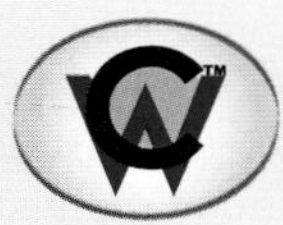

Additional interactive resources, including animations and video, for this chapter can be found on the Companion Website at http://www.prenhall.com/ladewig. Click on Chapter 21 and "Begin" to select the activities for this chapter.

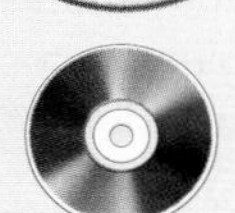

For NCLEX review questions and an audio glossary, access the accompanying CD-ROM in this book.

# A Day in the Life of a Nurse-Midwife

**TO ME, PREGNANCY IS A WONDERFUL,** normal experience—part of the cycle of life. That's why I love the fact that I can participate in all aspects of it, from pregnancy through birth and into the postpartal period. My practice enables me to ensure that a family's childbirth experience incorporates their personal beliefs and meets their expectations as much as possible. Come along with me for a day.

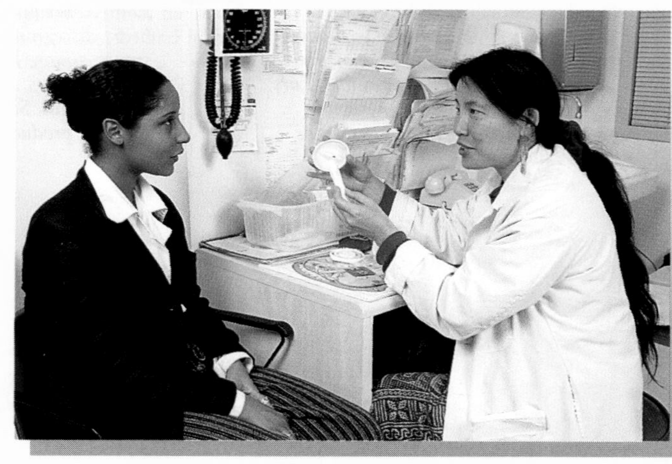

Cherrene has come for contraceptive information. I find it helpful to use models and examples during the discussion.

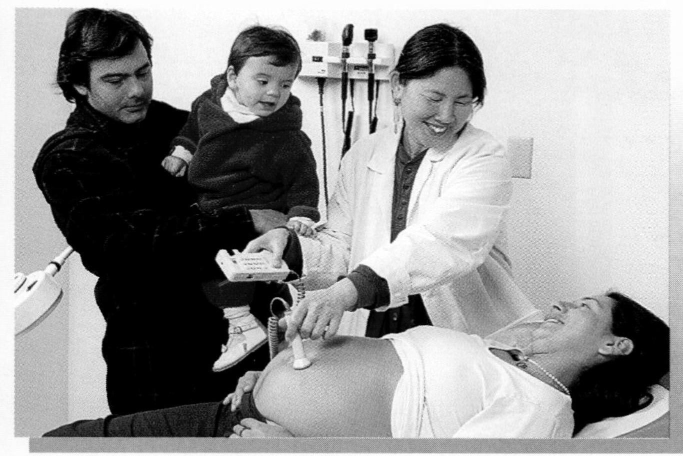

Dianne and her family come together for every appointment. We all enjoy listening to the fetal heartbeat.

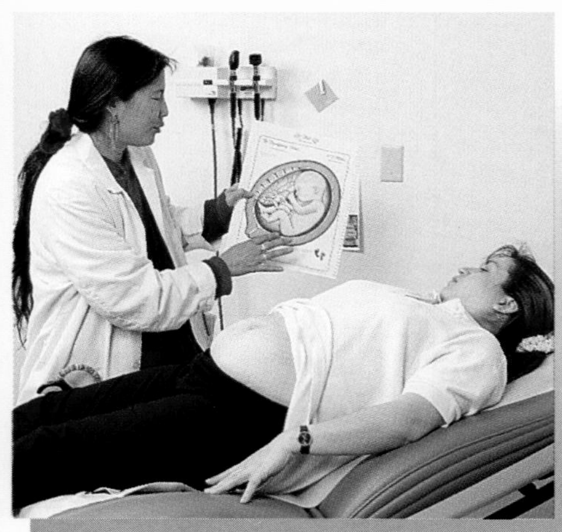

Gretchen's pregnancy is progressing well. She asks what her baby looks like now. I like to use a visual device as I talk with her about her baby's development.

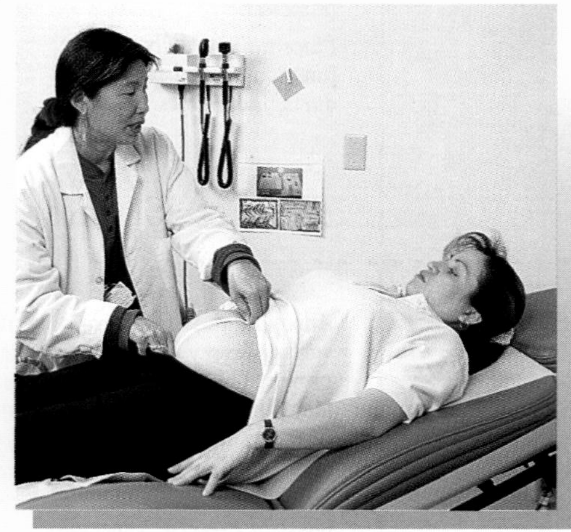

I measure the height of the fundus to determine if the baby is growing as expected. Gretchen and I talk about the impact of her nutrition, exercise, and healthy lifestyle habits on her baby and the outcome of her pregnancy.

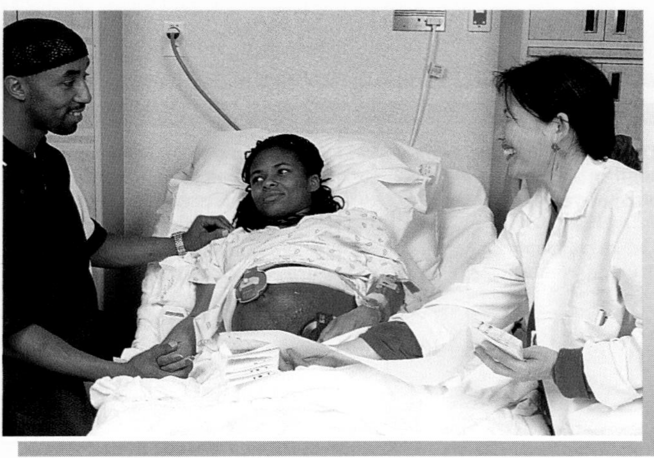

Darnell and Ayisha are expecting their first baby. Ayisha calls to tell me her labor has begun, and I meet them at the birth center. After the electronic fetal monitor is applied, we talk about the fetal heart tracing. I want to be sure they understand the monitor and have the opportunity to ask questions.

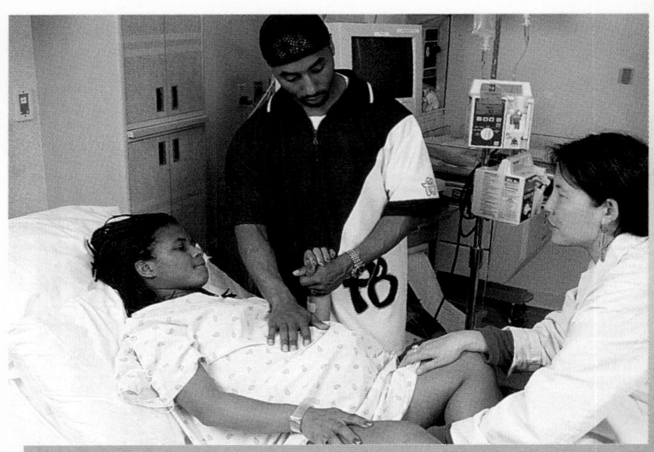

I do an exam to see how labor is progressing and share my findings with them.

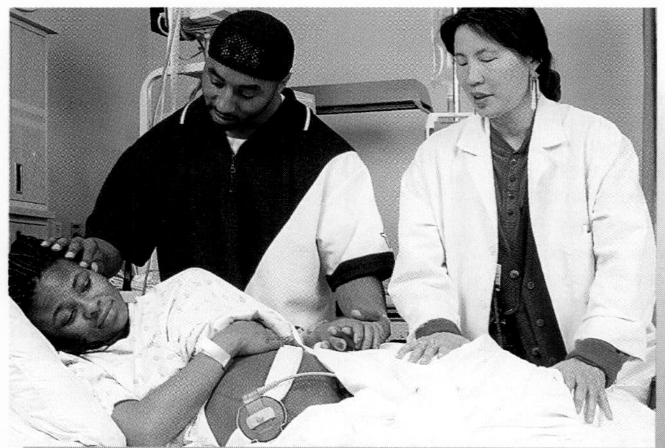

During the active phase of Ayisha's labor, Darnell lovingly provides comfort and support.

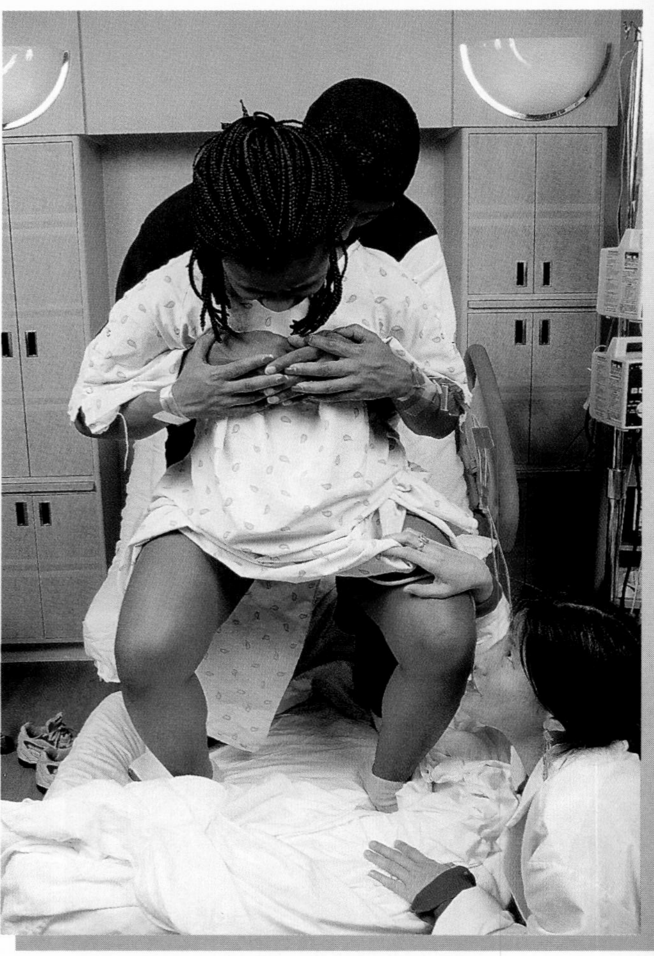

It's time to push. Ayisha wants to stand and is most comfortable on the bed. Darnell stands behind her and provides support. I continue to talk with them and provide encouragement. After an hour of pushing, baby Kinshasa is born.

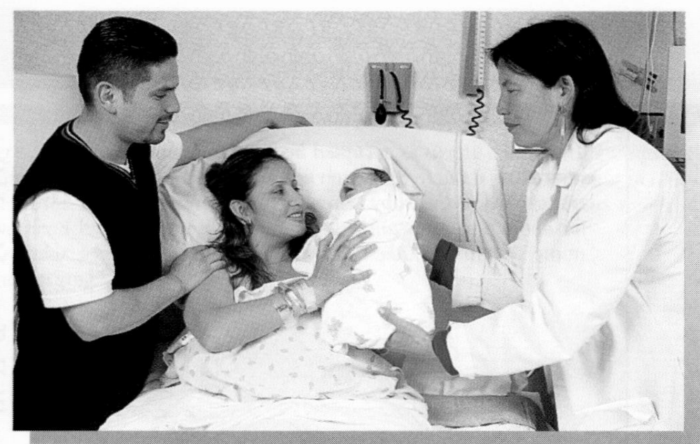

While I'm at the birth center, I check in on Alisa and Richard. Their baby, Lydia Rose, was born 6 hours ago. Alisa has asked for help with breast-feeding. Baby Lydia is a sleepy little one and needs encouragement to latch on and begin feeding.

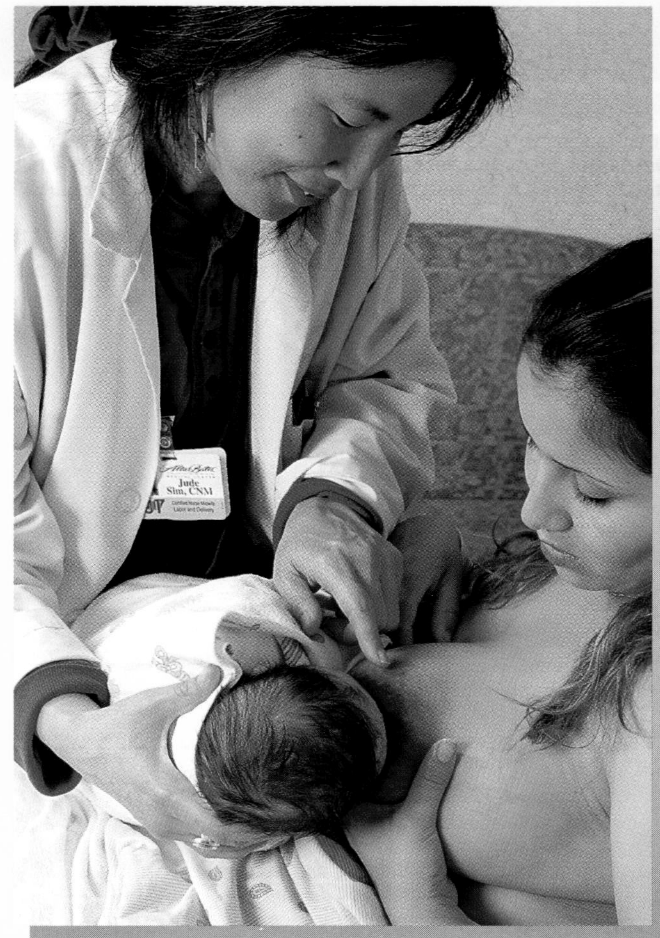


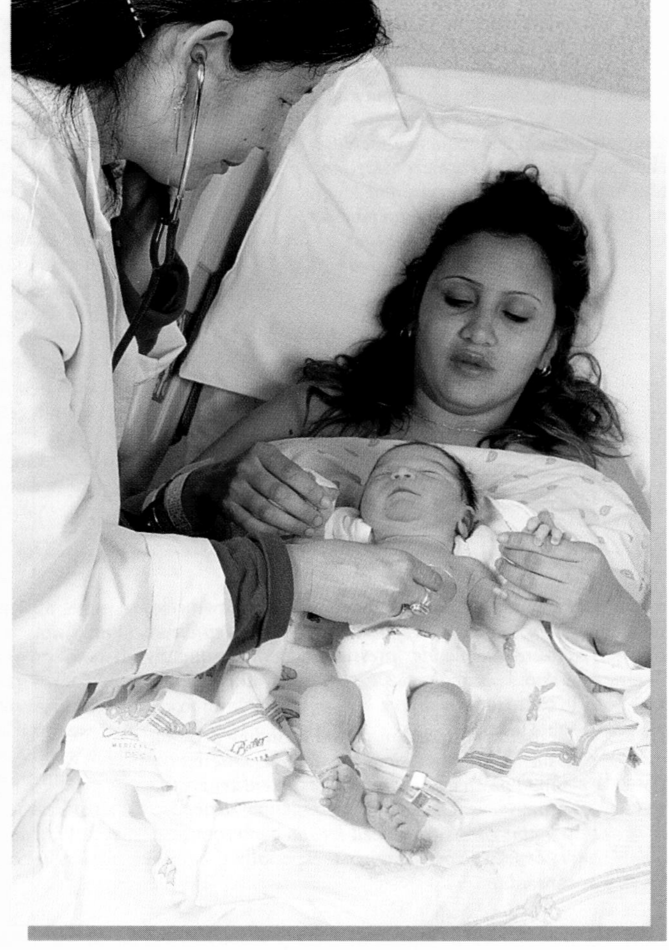

After baby Lydia has finished nursing, I do a physical assessment. I prefer to do an assessment in the room with the parents. It is such a wonderful opportunity for them to learn about their baby.

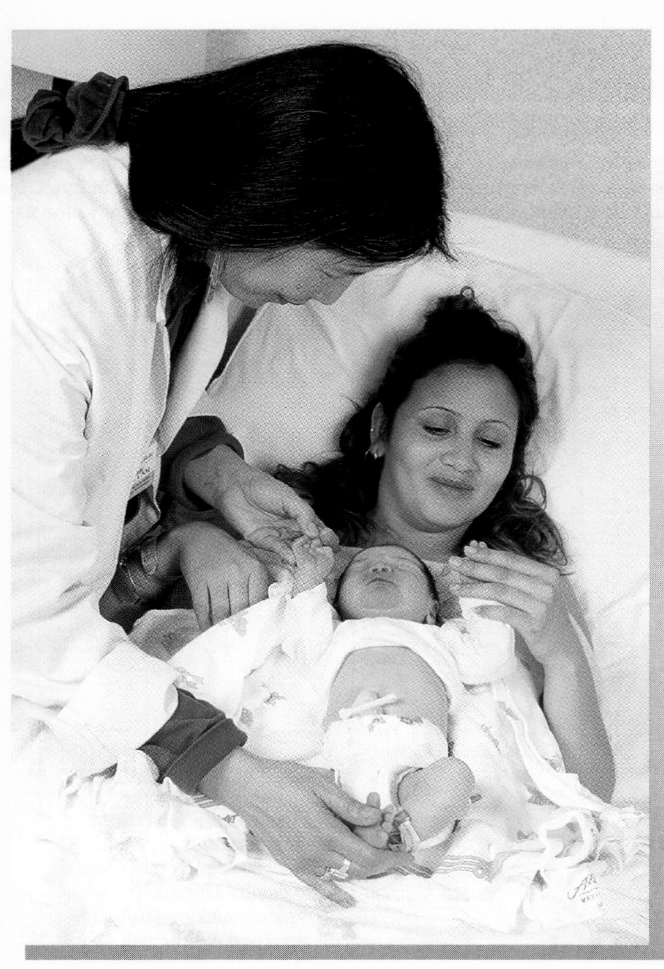

Alisa is fascinated with baby Lydia's tiny fingers and toes. I love being with parents as they explore their baby. Each new baby is such a wonder. . . such a miracle.

Now my attention turns to Alisa. As part of my assessment, I check the position and tone of her fundus. All is well. I head home after a busy, but rewarding, day.

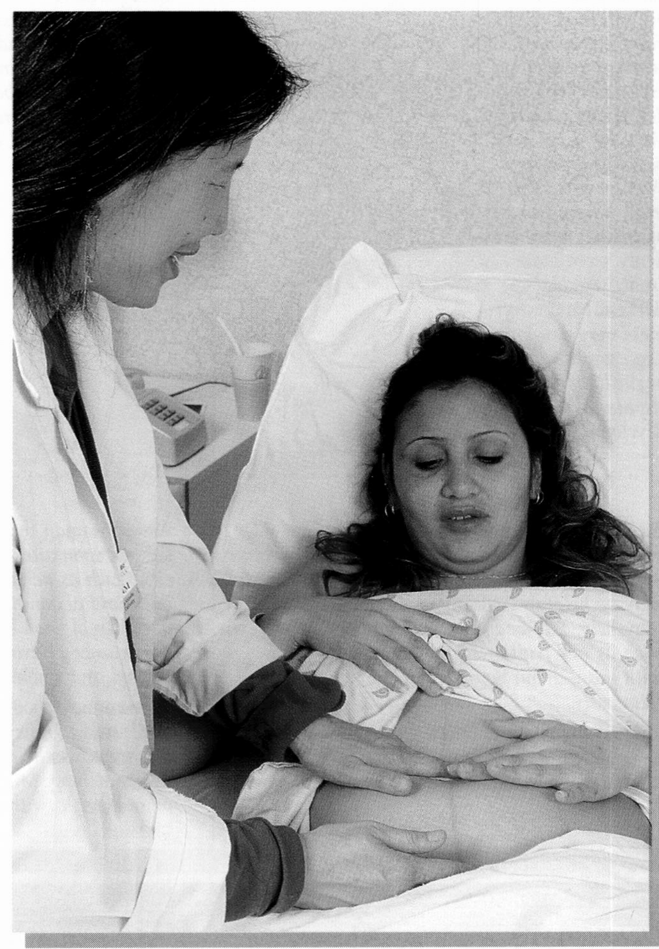

Chapter 22

# Nursing Assessment of the Newborn

*Each time I do a newborn's first bath I am struck anew by the magic of human life. It is one of my favorite parts of the day.*

—Newborn Nursery Nurse

## KEY TERMS

| | |
|---|---|
| Acrocyanosis | 553 |
| Babinski reflex | 566 |
| Barlow's maneuver | 564 |
| Brazelton Neonatal Behavioral Assessment Scale | 567 |
| Caput succedaneum | 556 |
| Cephalhematoma | 556 |
| Chemical conjunctivitis | 557 |
| Epstein's pearls | 559 |
| Erb-Duchenne paralysis (Erb's palsy) | 563 |
| Erythema toxicum | 553 |
| Forceps marks | 554 |
| Gestational age assessment tools | 541 |
| Grasping reflex | 565 |
| Harlequin sign | 553 |
| Jaundice | 553 |
| Milia | 554 |
| Molding | 555 |
| Mongolian spots | 554 |
| Moro reflex | 565 |
| Mottling | 553 |
| Nevus flammeus (port-wine stain) | 555 |
| Nevus vasculosus (strawberry mark) | 555 |
| Ortolani's maneuver | 563 |
| Pseudomenstruation | 562 |
| Rooting reflex | 565 |
| Skin turgor | 554 |
| Subconjunctival hemorrhage | 557 |
| Sucking reflex | 566 |
| Telangiectatic nevi (stork bites) | 554 |
| Thrush | 559 |
| Tonic neck reflex | 565 |
| Trunk incurvation (Galant reflex) | 566 |

## OBJECTIVES

- **Explain the various components of the gestational age assessment.**
- **Describe the normal physical and behavioral characteristics of the newborn.**
- **Summarize the components of a complete newborn assessment and the significance of normal variations and abnormal findings.**
- **Discuss the neurologic or neuromuscular characteristics of the newborn and the reflexes that may be present at birth.**
- **Describe the categories of the newborn behavioral assessment.**

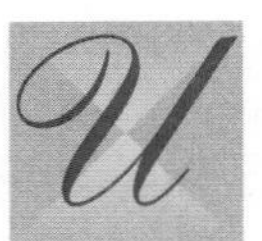

nlike the adult, the newborn communicates needs primarily by behavior. Because the nurse is the most consistent observer of the newborn, he or she can translate this behavior into information about the newborn's condition and respond with appropriate nursing interventions. This chapter focuses on the assessment of the newborn and the interpretation of the findings. Assessment of the newborn is a continuous process designed to evaluate development and adjustments to extrauterine life. In the birth setting, the Apgar scoring procedure (see Chapter 17 for discussion) and careful observation form the basis of assessment and are correlated with information such as the following:

- Maternal prenatal care history
- Birthing history
- Maternal analgesia and anesthesia
- Complications of labor or birth
- Treatment instituted immediately after birth, in conjunction with determination of clinical gestational age
- Consideration of the classification of newborns by weight and gestational age and by neonatal mortality risk
- Physical examination of the newborn

The nurse incorporates data from these sources with the assessment findings during the first 1 to 4 hours after birth to formulate a plan for nursing intervention. The various newborn assessments and the data obtained from them are only valuable to the degree to which they are shared with the parents. The parents must be included in the assessment process from the moment of their child's birth. The Apgar score and its meaning should be explained immediately to the family. As soon as possible, the parents should take part in the physical and behavioral assessments as well.

The nurse encourages the parents to identify the unique behavioral characteristics of their newborn. Attachment is promoted when parents have an opportunity to explore their newborn in private and identify individual physical and behavioral characteristics. The nurse's supportive responses to parents' questions and observations are essential throughout the assessment process. The newborn physical examination therefore is the beginning of newborn health surveillance and health education for the newborn's family that continues into the community setting.

## Timing of Newborn Assessments

The first 24 hours of life are significant because the newborn makes the critical transition from intrauterine to extrauterine life. The risk of mortality and morbidity is statistically high during this period. Assessment of the newborn is essential to ensure that the transition is proceeding successfully (Rinehart, Terrone, & Magann, 2000).

There are three major time frames for assessments of newborns while they are in the birth facility:

- The first assessment is done in the birthing area immediately after birth to determine the need for resuscitation or other interventions. The newborn who is stable can stay with the family after birth to initiate early attachment. The newborn who has complications is usually taken to the nursery for further evaluation and intervention.
- A second assessment is done within the first 4 hours after birth as part of routine admission procedures. During this assessment, the nurse carries out a brief physical examination to estimate gestational age and evaluate the newborn's adaptation to extrauterine life. No later than 2 hours after birth, the admitting nursery nurse should evaluate the newborn's status and any problems that place the newborn at risk (American Academy of Pediatrics [AAP] & American College of Obstetricians and Gynecologists [ACOG], 1997).
- Prior to discharge, a certified nurse-midwife, physician, or nurse practitioner carries out a behavioral assessment and a complete physical examination to detect any emerging or potential problems. A general assessment is also done at this time.

This chapter presents the procedures for estimating gestational age and performing the complete physical examination and behavioral assessment. See Key Facts to Remember: Timing and Types of Newborn Assessments. (Chapter 17 discusses the immediate postbirth assessment.)

## Estimation of Gestational Age

The nurse must establish the newborn's gestational age in the first 4 hours after birth so that careful attention can be given to age-related problems. Traditionally a newborn's gestational age was determined from the date of the pregnant woman's last menstrual period, but this method was accurate only 75% to 85% of the time. Because of the problems that develop with the preterm newborn or the newborn whose weight is inappropriate for gestational age, a more accurate system was developed to postnatally evaluate the newborn. Once learned, the procedure can be done in a few minutes. *It is essential*

## KEY FACTS TO REMEMBER

### *Timing and Types of Newborn Assessments*

Assess immediately after birth: need for resuscitation or if newborn is stable and can be placed with parents to initiate early attachment and bonding

Assessments within 1 to 4 hours after birth:

- Progress of newborn's adaptation to extrauterine life
- Determination of gestational age
- Ongoing assessment for high-risk problems

Assessment procedures within first 24 hours or prior to discharge:

- Complete physical examination (Depending on agency protocol, the nurse may complete some components independently, with the certified nurse-midwife, physician, or nurse practitioner completing the exam prior to discharge.)
- Nutritional status and ability to bottle-feed or breastfeed satisfactorily
- Behavioral state organization abilities

*that the nurse wear gloves when assessing the newborn in these early hours after birth and before the first bath.*

Clinical **gestational age assessment tools** have two components: external physical characteristics and neurologic or neuromuscular development. Physical characteristics generally include sole creases, amount of breast tissue, amount of lanugo, cartilaginous development of the ear, and testicular descent and scrotal rugae or labial development. These objective clinical criteria are not influenced by labor and birth and do not change significantly within the first 24 hours after birth. Optimal accuracy of gestational age takes place within 12 hours of birth.

Neurologic examination facilitates assessment of functional or physiologic maturation in addition to physical development. However, during the first 24 hours of life, the newborn's nervous system is unstable; thus neurologic findings based on reflexes or assessments dependent on the higher brain centers may not be reliable. If the neurologic findings drastically deviate from the gestational age derived by evaluation of external characteristics, a second assessment is done in 24 hours.

The neurologic assessment components (excluding reflexes) can aid in assessing the gestational age of newborns of less than 34 weeks' gestation. Between 26 and 34 weeks, neurologic changes are significant, whereas significant physical changes are less evident. One significant neurologic change consists of replacement of extensor tone by flexor tone in a *caudocephalad* (tail-to-head) progression.

Ballard, Khoury, Wedig, and coworkers' (1991) *estimation of gestational age by maturity* rating is a simplified version of the well-researched Dubowitz tool. Ballard's tool gives each physical and neuromuscular finding a value, and the total score is matched to a gestational age (Figure 22–1♦). The maximum score on Ballard's tool is 50, which corresponds to a gestational age of 44 weeks.

For example, on completion of a gestational assessment of a 1-hour-old newborn, the nurse gives a score of 3 to all the physical characteristics, for a total of 18, and gives a score of 3 to all neuromuscular assessments, for a total of 18. The physical characteristics score of 18 is added to the neurologic score of 18 for a total score of 36, which correlates with 38+ weeks' gestation. Because all newborns vary slightly in the development of physical characteristics and maturation of neurologic function, scores usually vary instead of all being 3, as in this example.

Current postnatal gestational age assessment tools can overestimate preterm gestational age and underestimate postterm gestational age. The tools have been shown to lose accuracy when newborns of fewer than 28 weeks' or more than 43 weeks' gestation are assessed. Also the assessments should be made within 12 hours of birth to optimize accuracy, especially in infants of less than 26 weeks' gestational age (Ballard et al., 1991). Current research still suggests a need for refinement of gestational age scoring scales when they are to be used for determining the care given extremely premature infants (Donovan, Tyson, Ehrenkranz, et al., 1999).

In carrying out gestational age assessments, the nurse keeps in mind that some maternal conditions, such as pregnancy-induced hypertension (PIH), diabetes, and maternal analgesia and anesthesia, may affect certain gestational assessment components and warrant further study. Maternal diabetes, although it appears to accelerate fetal physical growth, seems to retard maturation. Maternal hypertensive states, which retard fetal physical growth, seem to speed maturation.

Newborns of women with PIH have a poor correlation with the criteria involving active muscle tone and edema. Maternal analgesia and anesthesia may cause respiratory depression in the baby. Babies with respiratory distress syndrome (RDS) tend to be flaccid and edematous and to assume a "froglike" posture. These characteristics affect the scoring of the neuromuscular components of the assessment tool used.

## Assessment of Physical Characteristics

The nurse first evaluates observable characteristics without disturbing the baby (Rinehart et al., 2000). Selected

# NEWBORN MATURITY RATING & CLASSIFICATION

ESTIMATION OF GESTATIONAL AGE BY MATURITY RATING
Symbols: X - 1st Exam O - 2nd Exam

NEUROMUSCULAR MATURITY

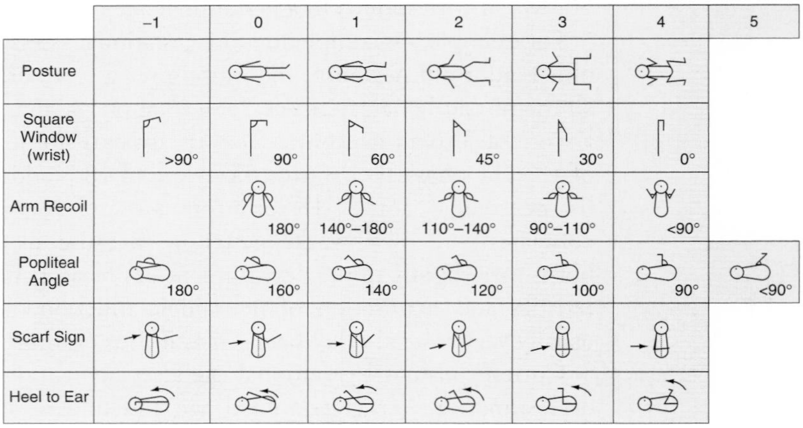

| | −1 | 0 | 1 | 2 | 3 | 4 | 5 |
|---|---|---|---|---|---|---|---|
| Posture | | | | | | | |
| Square Window (wrist) | >90° | 90° | 60° | 45° | 30° | 0° | |
| Arm Recoil | | 180° | 140°–180° | 110°–140° | 90°–110° | <90° | |
| Popliteal Angle | 180° | 160° | 140° | 120° | 100° | 90° | <90° |
| Scarf Sign | | | | | | | |
| Heel to Ear | | | | | | | |

Gestation by Dates ________ wks

Birth Date ________ Hour ________ am pm

APGAR ________ 1 min ________ 5 min

MATURITY RATING

| score | weeks |
|---|---|
| −10 | 20 |
| −5 | 22 |
| 0 | 24 |
| 5 | 26 |
| 10 | 28 |
| 15 | 30 |
| 20 | 32 |
| 25 | 34 |
| 30 | 36 |
| 35 | 38 |
| 40 | 40 |
| 45 | 42 |
| 50 | 44 |

PHYSICAL MATURITY

| | | | | | | | |
|---|---|---|---|---|---|---|---|
| Skin | sticky friable transparent | gelatinous red, translucent | smooth pink, visible veins | superficial peeling &/or rash, few veins | cracking pale areas rare veins | parchment deep cracking no vessels | leathery cracked wrinkled |
| Lanugo | none | sparse | abundant | thinning | bald areas | mostly bald | |
| Plantar Surface | heel-toe 40–50mm:–1 <40mm:–2 | >50mm no crease | faint red marks | anterior transverse crease only | creases ant. 2/3 | creases over entire sole | |
| Breast | imperceptible | barely perceptible | flat areola no bud | stippled areola 1–2mm bud | raised areola 3–4mm bud | full areola 5–10mm bud | |
| Eye/Ear | lids fused loosely:–1 tightly:–2 | lids open pinna flat stays folded | sl. curved pinna; soft; slow recoil | well curved pinna; soft but ready recoil | formed & firm instant recoil | thick cartilage ear stiff | |
| Genitals male | scrotum flat, smooth | scrotum empty faint rugae | testes in upper canal rare rugae | testes descending few rugae | testes down good rugae | testes pendulous deep rugae | |
| Genitals female | clitoris prominent labia flat | prominent clitoris small labia minora | prominent clitoris enlarging minora | majora & minora equally prominent | majora large minora small | majora cover clitoris & minora | |

SCORING SECTION

| | 1st Exam = X | 2nd Exam = 0 |
|---|---|---|
| Estimating Gest Age by Maturity Rating | ____Weeks | ____Weeks |
| Time of Exam | Date ____ Hour____ am pm | Date ____ Hour____ am pm |
| Age at Exam | ____ Hours | ____ Hours |
| Signature of Examiner | ____ M.D. | ____ M.D. |

FIGURE 22–1 ♦ Newborn maturity rating and classification. If a 1-hour-old newborn is given a score of 3 for each of the physical characteristics and neuromuscular assessments, the newborn's total score would be 36. A total score of 36 correlates with 38+ weeks' gestation.
*Source:* Ballard, J. L., Khoury, J. C., Wedig, K., Wang, L., Eilers-Walsmann, B. L., & Lipp, R. (1991) New Ballard score, expanded to include extremely premature infants. *Journal of Pediatrics, 119,* 417.

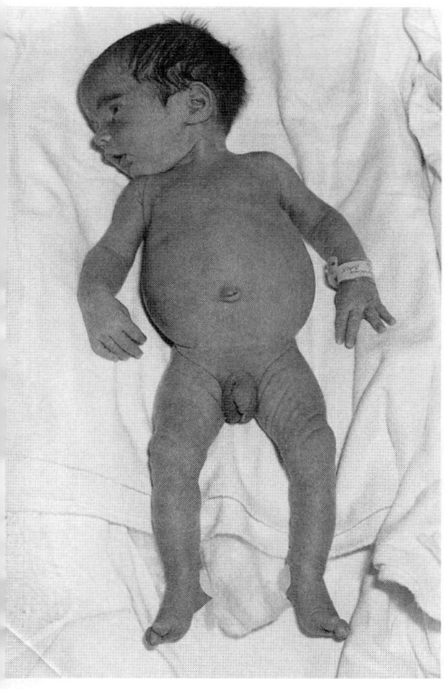
A

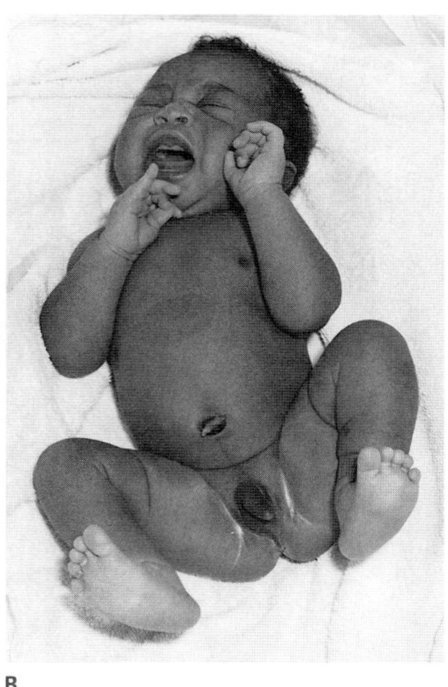
B

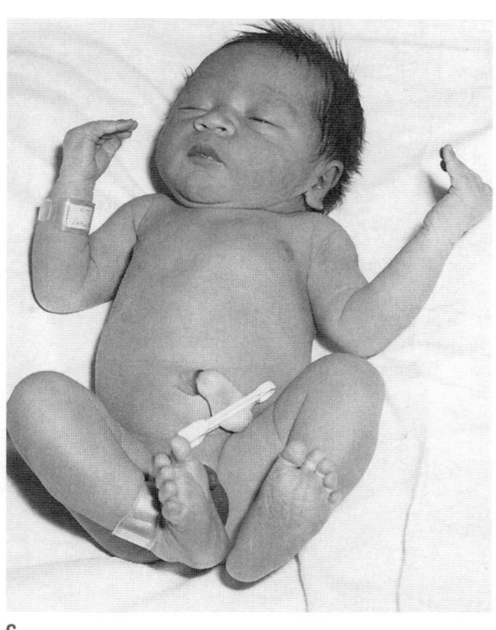
C

FIGURE 22–2 ♦ Resting posture. **A,** Newborn exhibits beginning of flexion of the thigh. The gestational age is approximately 31 weeks. Note the extension of the upper extremities. **B,** Newborn exhibits stronger flexion of the arms, hips, and thighs. The gestational age is approximately 35 weeks. **C,** The full-term newborn exhibits hypertonic flexion of all extremities. *Source:* Dubowitz, L., & Dubowitz, V. (1977). *The gestational age of the newborn.* Menlo Park, CA: Addison-Wesley. Reprinted by permission of V. Dubowitz, MD, Hammersmith Hospital, London, England.

physical characteristics common to all gestational assessment tools are presented here in the order in which they can be evaluated most effectively:

1. *Resting posture,* although a neuromuscular component, should be assessed as the baby lies undisturbed on a flat surface (Figure 22–2♦).
2. *Skin* in the preterm newborn appears thin and transparent, with veins prominent over the abdomen early in gestation. As term approaches, the skin appears opaque because of increased subcutaneous tissue. Disappearance of the protective vernix caseosa promotes skin desquamation and is commonly seen in postmature infants (infants of more than 42 weeks' gestational age and showing signs of placental insufficiency; see Chapter 25).
3. *Lanugo,* a fine hair covering, decreases as gestational age increases. The amount of lanugo is greatest at 28 to 30 weeks and then disappears, first from the face and then from the trunk and extremities.
4. *Sole (plantar) creases* are reliable indicators of gestational age in the first 12 hours of life. After this, the skin of the foot begins drying, and superficial creases appear. Development of sole creases begins at the top (anterior) portion of the sole and, as gestation progresses, proceeds to the heel (Figure 22–3♦). Peeling may also occur. Plantar creases vary with race. In newborns of African descent, sole creases may be less developed at term.
5. The *areola* and breast tissue are assessed for size. At term gestation, the tissue measures between 0.5 and 1 cm (5 and 10 mm). As gestation progresses, the breast tissue mass and areola enlarge. To assess size, the nurse gently palpates the *breast bud tissue* by applying the forefinger and middle finger to the breast area and measuring the tissue between them in centimeters or millimeters (Figure 22–4♦). During the assessment, the nipple is never grasped, because skin and subcutaneous tissue will prevent accurate estimation of size. The nurse must do this procedure gently to avoid causing trauma to the breast tissue. A large breast tissue mass can occur as a result of specific conditions other than advanced gestational age or the effects of maternal hormones on the baby. The newborn of a diabetic mother tends to be large for gestational age (LGA), and the accelerated development of breast tissue is a reflection of subcutaneous fat deposits. Small-for-gestational-age (SGA) term or postterm newborns may have used subcutaneous fat (which would have been deposited as breast tissue) to survive in utero; as a result, their lack of breast tissue may indicate a gestational age of 34 to 35 weeks, even though other factors indicate a term or postterm newborn.
6. *Ear form and cartilage distribution* develop with gestational age. The cartilage gives the ear its shape and substance (Figure 22–5♦). In a newborn of less than 34 weeks' gestation, the ear is relatively shapeless and

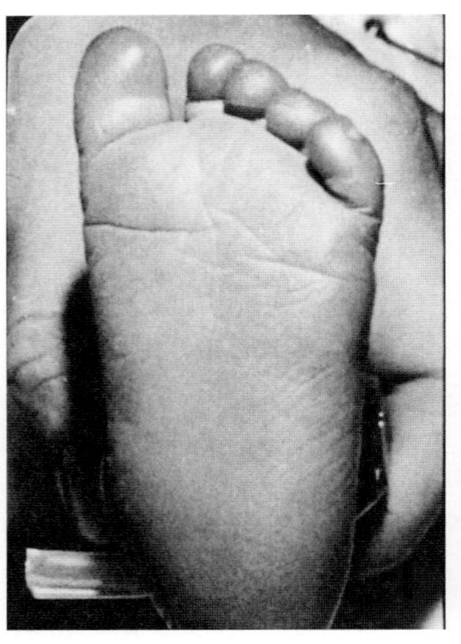

A

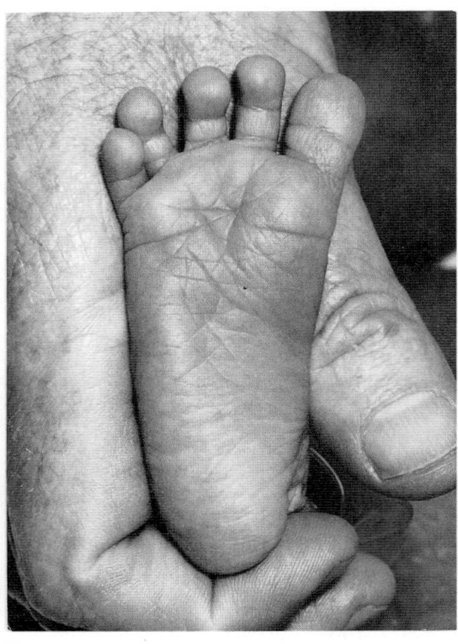

B

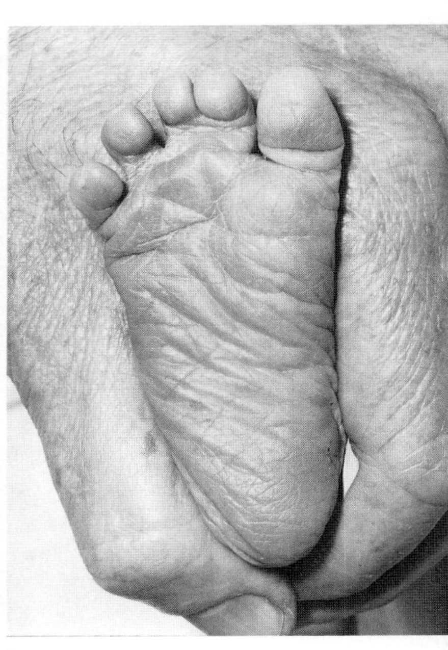

C

FIGURE 22–3 ♦ Sole creases. **A,** Newborn has a few sole creases on the anterior portion of the foot. Note the slick heel. The gestational age is approximately 35 weeks. **B,** Newborn has a deeper network of sole creases on the anterior two-thirds of the sole. Note the slick heel. The gestational age is approximately 37 weeks. **C,** The term newborn has deep sole creases down to and including the heel as the skin loses fluid and dries after birth. Sole (plantar) creases can be seen even in preterm newborns. *Source: B* and *C* from Dubowitz, L., & Dubowitz, V. (1977). *The gestational age of the newborn.* Menlo Park, CA: Addison-Wesley. Reprinted by permission of V. Dubowitz, MD, Hammersmith Hospital, London, England.

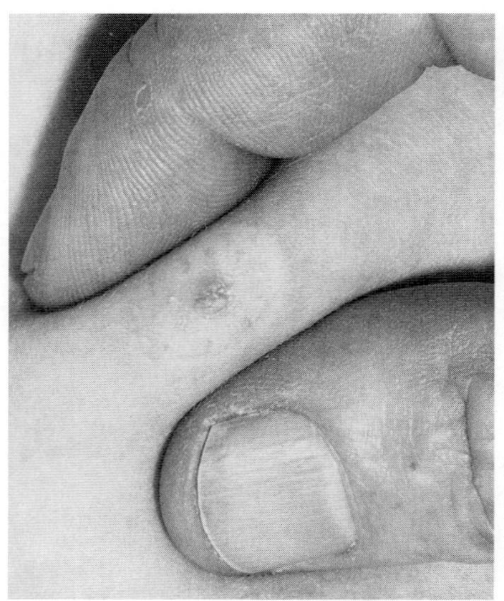

A

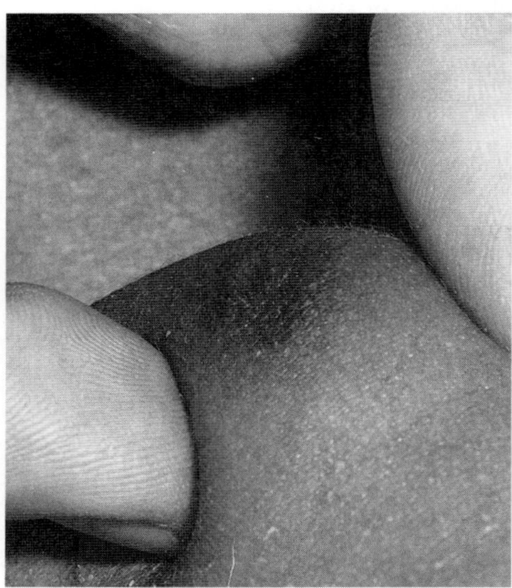

B

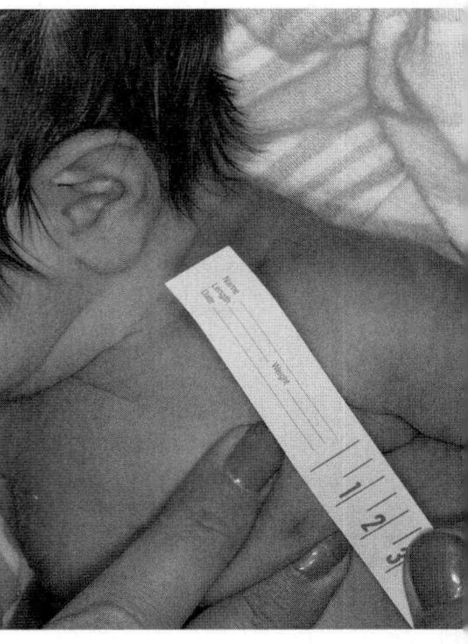

C

FIGURE 22–4 ♦ Breast tissue. **A,** Newborn has a visible raised area. On palpation the area is 4 mm. The gestational age is 38 weeks. **B,** Newborn has 10 mm breast tissue area. The gestational age is 40 to 44 weeks. **C,** Gently compress the tissue between the middle and index fingers and measure the tissue in centimeters or millimeters. Absence of or decreased breast tissue often indicates premature or small-for-gestational-age newborn. *Source: A* and *B* from Dubowitz, L., & Dubowitz, V. (1977). *The gestational age of the newborn.* Menlo Park, CA: Addison-Wesley. Reprinted by permission of V. Dubowitz, MD, Hammersmith Hospital, London, England.

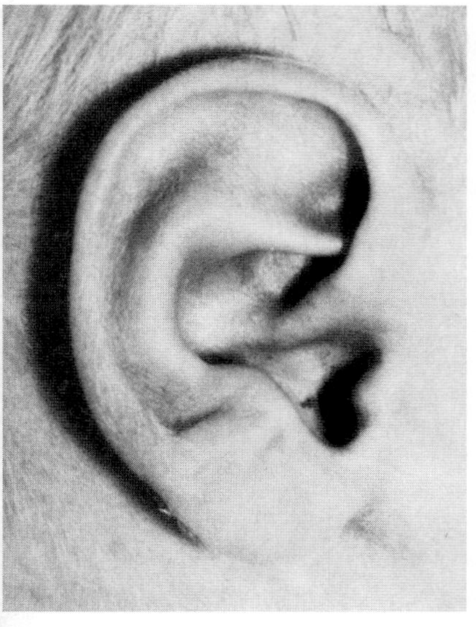

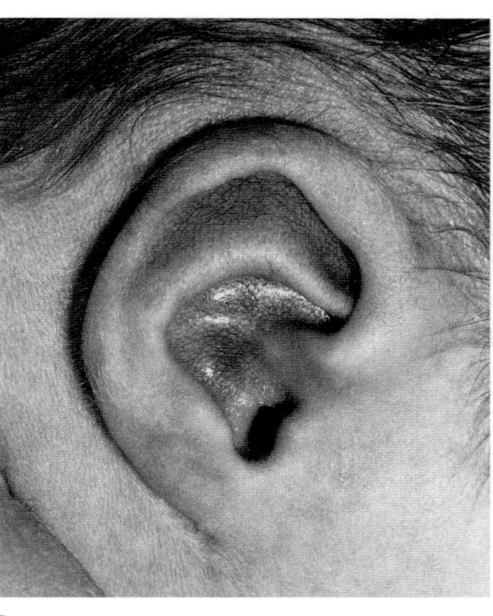

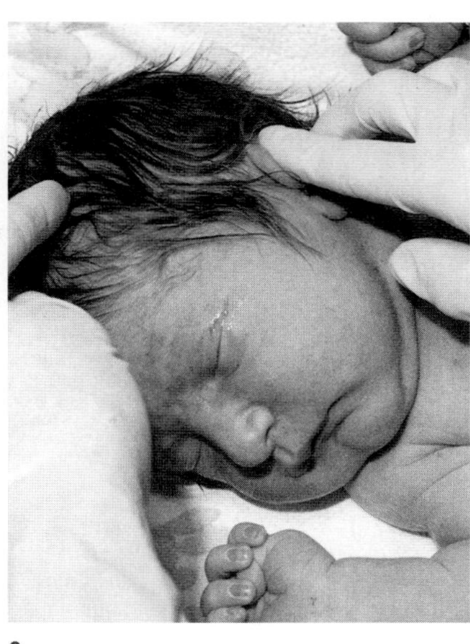

A B C

FIGURE 22–5 ♦ Ear form and cartilage. **A,** The ear of the infant at approximately 36 weeks' gestation shows incurving of the upper two-thirds of the pinna. **B,** Infant at term shows well-defined incurving of the entire pinna. **C,** If the auricle stays in the position in which it is pressed or returns slowly to its original position, it usually means the gestational age is less than 38 weeks. *Source: A* and *B* from Dubowitz, L., & Dubowitz, V. (1977). *The gestational age of the newborn.* Menlo Park, CA: Addison-Wesley. Reprinted by permission of V. Dubowitz, MD, Hammersmith Hospital, London, England.

flat; it has little cartilage, so the ear folds over on itself and remains folded. By approximately 36 weeks' gestation, some cartilage and slight incurving of the upper pinna are present, and the pinna springs back slowly when folded. (The nurse tests this response by holding the top and bottom of the pinna together with the forefinger and thumb and then releasing them or by folding the pinna of the ear forward against the side of the head, releasing it, and observing the response.) By term, the newborn's pinna is firm, stands away from the head, and springs back quickly from the folding.

7. *Male genitals* are evaluated for size of the scrotal sac, presence of rugae (wrinkles and ridges in the scrotum), and descent of the testes (Figure 22–6♦). Prior to 36 weeks, the scrotum has few rugae, and the testes are palpable in the inguinal canal. By 36 to 38 weeks, the testes are in the upper scrotum, and rugae have developed over the anterior portion of the scrotum. By term, the testes are generally in the lower scrotum, which is pendulous and covered with rugae.
8. The appearance of the *female genitals* depends in part on subcutaneous fat deposition and therefore relates to fetal nutritional status (Figure 22–7♦). The

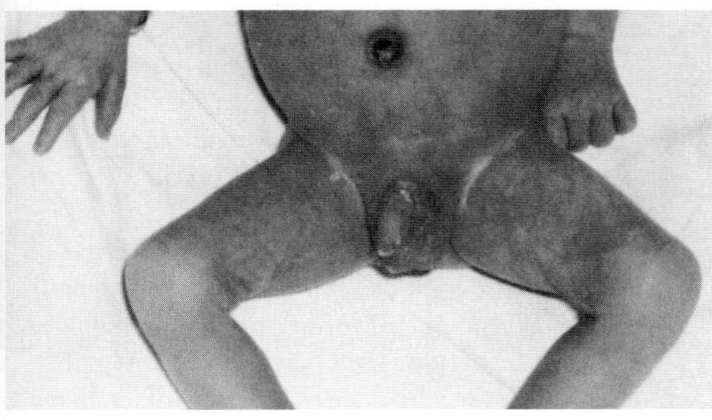

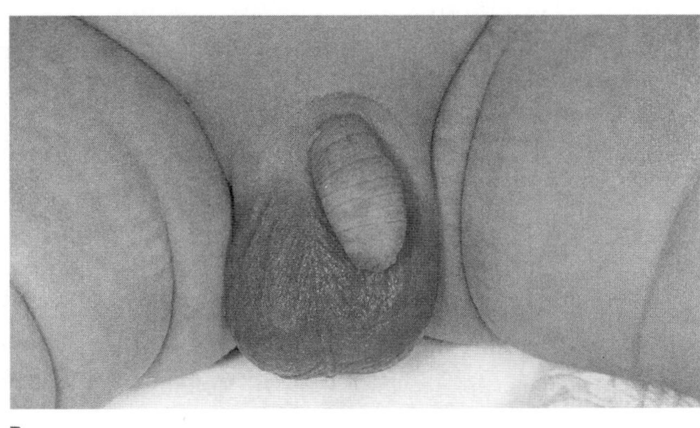

A B

FIGURE 22–6 ♦ Male genitals. **A,** Preterm newborn's testes are not within the scrotum. The scrotal surface has few rugae. **B,** Term newborn's testes are generally fully descended. The entire surface of the scrotum is covered by rugae. *Source: A* from Dubowitz, L., & Dubowitz, V. (1977). *The gestational age of the newborn.* Menlo Park, CA: Addison-Wesley. Reprinted by permission of V. Dubowitz, MD, Hammersmith Hospital, London, England.

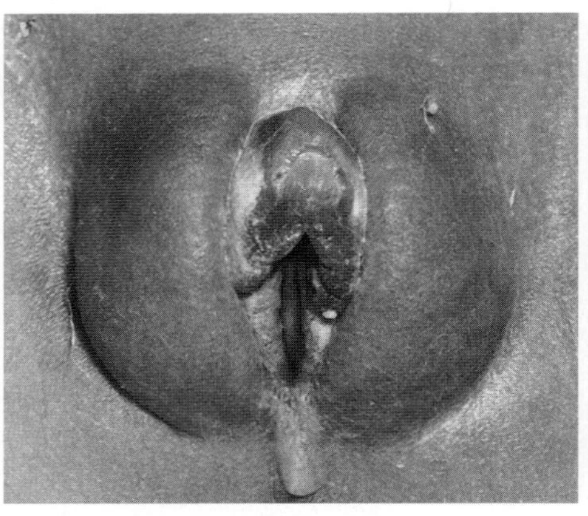

A

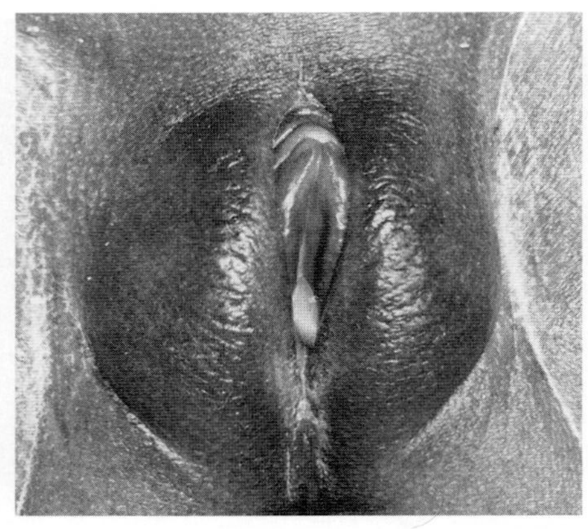

B

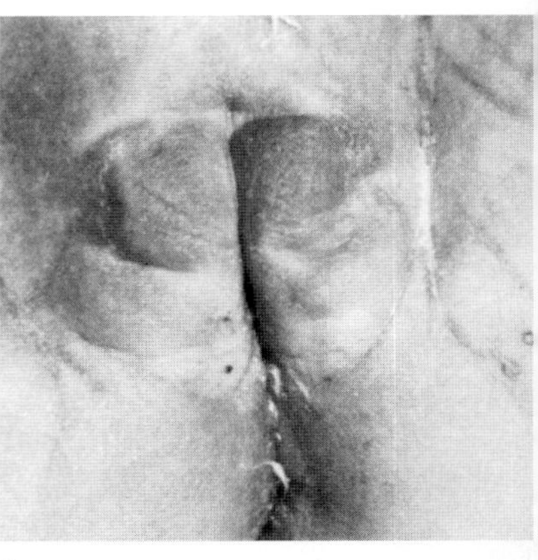

C

FIGURE 22–7 ♦ Female genitals. **A,** Newborn has a prominent clitoris. The labia majora are widely separated, and the labia minora, viewed laterally, would protrude beyond the labia majora. The gestational age is 30 to 36 weeks. **B,** The clitoris is still visible. The labia minora are now covered by the larger labia majora. The gestational age is 36 to 40 weeks. **C,** The term newborn has well-developed, large labia majora that cover both clitoris and labia minora. *Source:* Dubowitz, L., & Dubowitz, V. (1977). *The gestational age of the newborn.* Menlo Park, CA: Addison-Wesley. Reprinted by permission of V. Dubowitz, MD, Hammersmith Hospital, London, England.

clitoris varies in size, and occasionally is so swollen that it is difficult to identify the sex of the newborn. This swelling may be due to adrenogenital syndrome, which causes the adrenals to secrete excessive amounts of androgen and other hormones. At 30 to 32 weeks' gestation, the clitoris is prominent, and the labia majora are small and widely separated. As gestational age increases, the labia majora increase in size. At 36 to 40 weeks, they nearly cover the clitoris. At 40 weeks and beyond, the labia majora cover the labia minora and clitoris.

Other physical characteristics assessed by some gestational age scoring tools include the following:

1. Vernix covers the preterm newborn. The postterm newborn has little vernix. After noting vernix distribution, the birthing area nurse (wearing gloves) dries the newborn to prevent evaporative heat loss, thus disturbing the vernix and potentially altering this gestational age criterion. The birthing area nurse must communicate to the newborn nurse the amount of vernix and the areas of vernix coverage.
2. *Hair* of the preterm newborn has the consistency of matted wool or fur and lies in bunches rather than in the silky, single strands of the term newborn's hair.
3. *Skull firmness* increases as the fetus matures. In a term newborn the bones are hard, and the sutures are not easily displaced. The nurse should not attempt to displace the sutures forcibly.
4. *Nails* appear and cover the nail bed at about 20 weeks' gestation. Nails extending beyond the fingertips may indicate a postterm newborn.

## Assessment of Neuromuscular Maturity Characteristics

The central nervous system of the fetus matures at a fairly constant rate. Tests have been designed to evaluate neurologic status as manifested by neuromuscular tone development and correlated with gestational ages. In the fetus, neuromuscular tone develops from the lower to the upper extremities.

The neuromuscular evaluation requires more manipulation and disturbances than the physical evaluation of the newborn. The neuromuscular evaluation (see Figure 22–1♦) is best performed when the baby's condition has stabilized. The following characteristics are evaluated:

1. The *square window sign* is elicited by gently flexing the newborn's hand toward the ventral forearm until resistance is felt. The angle formed at the wrist is measured (Figure 22–8♦).
2. *Recoil* is a test of flexion development. Because flexion first develops in the lower extremities, recoil is first tested in the legs. The newborn is placed on its back on a flat surface. With a hand on the newborn's knees, the nurse places the baby's legs in flexion, then extends them parallel to each other and flat on the surface. The response to this maneuver is recoil of the newborn's legs. According to gestational age, they may not move or they may return slowly or quickly to the flexed position. Preterm infants have less muscle tone than term infants, so preterm infants have less recoil. Arm recoil is tested by flexion at the elbow and extension of the arms at the newborn's side. While the baby is in the supine position,

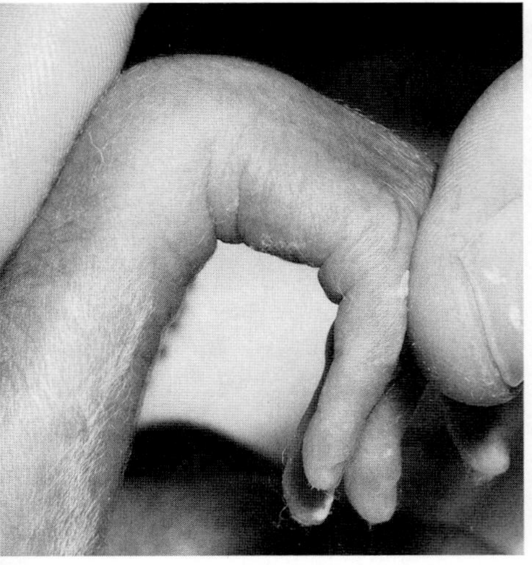

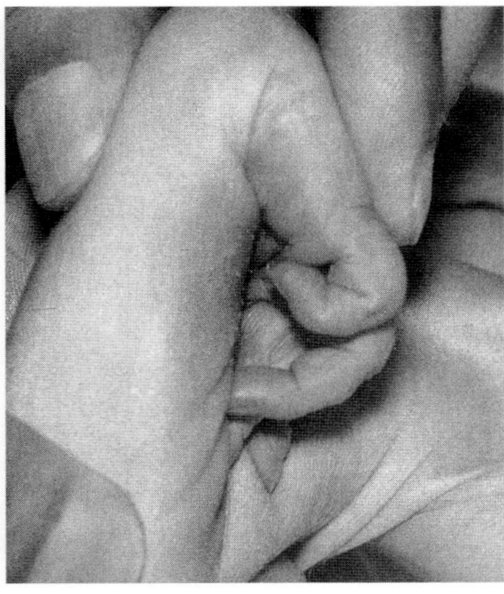

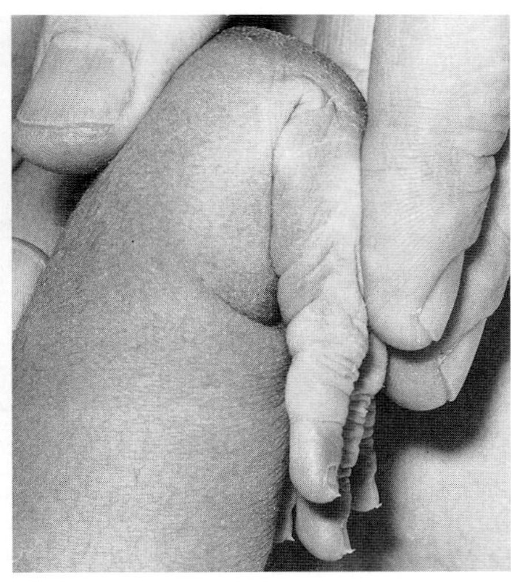

A B C

FIGURE 22–8 ♦ Square window sign. **A,** This angle is 90 degrees and suggests an immature newborn of 28 to 32 weeks' gestation. **B,** A 30-degree angle is commonly found from 39 to 40 weeks' gestation. **C,** A 0-degree angle can occur from 40 to 42 weeks. *Source:* Dubowitz, L., & Dubowitz, V. (1977). *The gestational age of the newborn.* Menlo Park, CA: Addison-Wesley. Reprinted by permission of V. Dubowitz, MD, Hammersmith Hospital, London, England.

the nurse completely flexes both elbows, holds them in this position for 5 seconds, extends the arms at the baby's side, and releases them. On release, the elbows of a full-term newborn form an angle of less than 90 degrees and rapidly recoil back to a flexed position. The elbows of a preterm newborn have slower recoil time and form an angle greater than 90 degrees. Arm recoil is also slower in healthy but fatigued newborns after birth; therefore arm recoil is best elicited after the first hour of birth, when the baby has had time to recover from the stress of the birth. Deep sleep state also decreases the arm recoil response. Assessment of arm recoil should be bilateral to rule out brachial palsy.

3. The *popliteal angle* (degree of knee flexion) is determined with the newborn flat on its back. The thigh is flexed on the abdomen and chest, and the nurse places the index finger of the other hand behind the newborn's ankle to extend the lower leg until resistance is met. The angle formed is then measured. Results vary from no resistance in the very immature newborn to an 80-degree angle in the term newborn.
4. The *scarf sign* is elicited by placing the newborn supine and drawing an arm across the chest toward the newborn's opposite shoulder until resistance is met. The location of the elbow is then noted in relation to the midline of the chest (Figure 22–9♦).

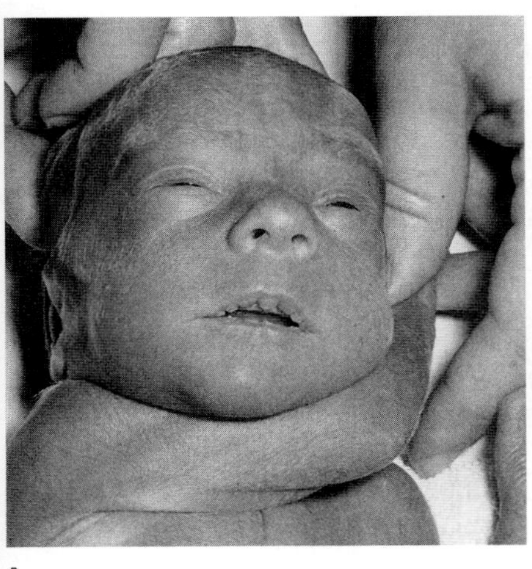

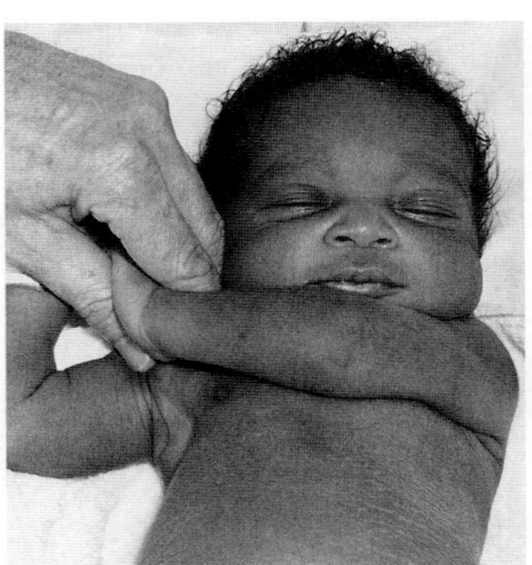

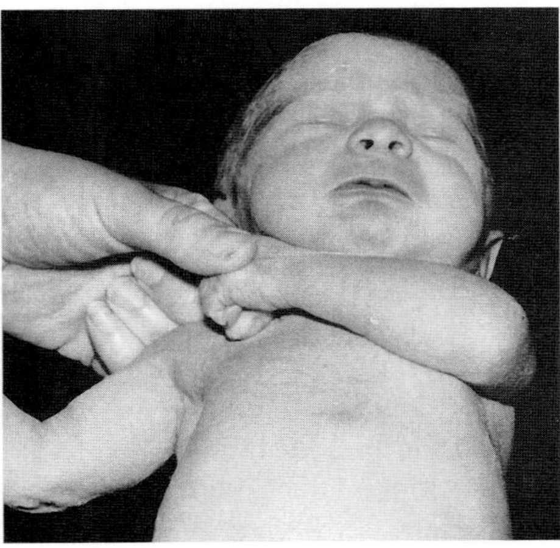

A B C

FIGURE 22–9 ♦ Scarf sign. **A,** No resistance is noted until after 30 weeks' gestation. The elbow moves readily past the midline. **B,** The elbow is at midline at 36 to 40 weeks' gestation. **C,** Beyond 40 weeks' gestation the elbow will not reach the midline. *Source:* Dubowitz, L., & Dubowitz V. (1977). *The gestational age of the newborn.* Menlo Park, CA: Addison-Wesley. Reprinted by permission of V. Dubowitz, MD, Hammersmith Hospital, London, England.

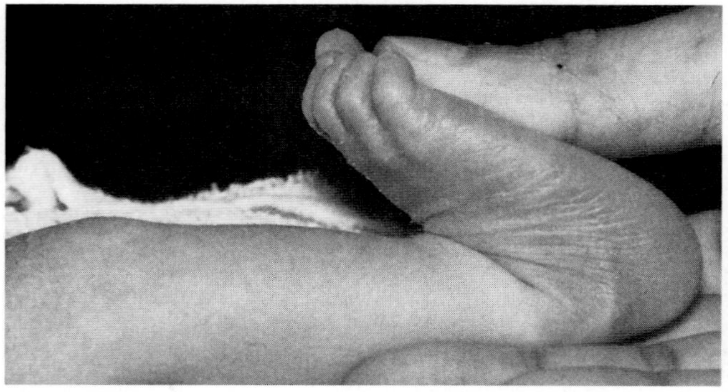

A

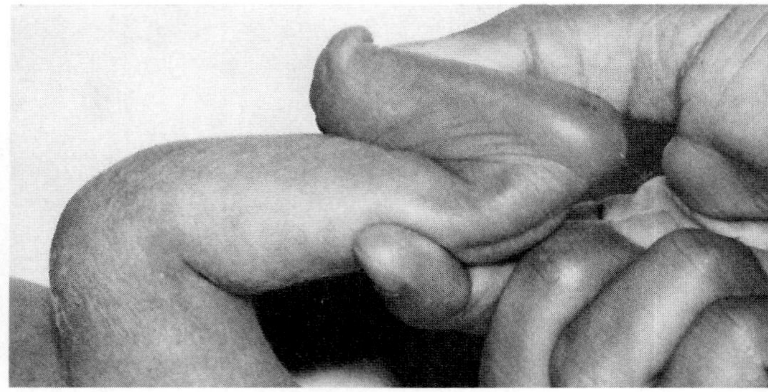

B

FIGURE 22–10 ♦ Ankle dorsiflexion. **A**, A 45-degree angle indicates 32 to 36 weeks' gestation. A 20-degree angle indicates 36 to 40 weeks' gestation. **B**, A 0-degree angle is common at 40 weeks' or more gestational age. *Source:* Dubowitz, L., & Dubowitz, V. (1977). *The gestational age of the newborn.* Menlo Park, CA: Addison-Wesley. Reprinted by permission of V. Dubowitz, MD, Hammersmith Hospital, London, England.

5. The *heel-to-ear extension* is performed by placing the newborn in a supine position and then gently drawing the foot toward the ear on the same side until resistance is felt. The nurse should allow the knee to bend during the test. It is important to hold the buttocks down to keep from rolling the baby. Both the proximity of foot to ear and the degree of knee extension are assessed. The leg of a preterm, immature newborn will remain straight and the foot will go to the ear or beyond. With advancing gestational age the newborn demonstrates increasing resistance to this maneuver. Maneuvers involving the lower extremities of newborns who had frank breech presentation should be delayed to allow for resolution of leg positioning.
6. *Ankle dorsiflexion* is determined by flexing the ankle on the shin. The nurse uses a thumb to push on the sole of the newborn's foot while the fingers support the back of the leg. Then the angle formed by the foot and the interior leg is measured (Figure 22–10♦). This sign can be influenced by intrauterine position and congenital deformities.
7. *Head lag* (neck flexor) is measured by pulling the newborn to a sitting position and noting the degree of head lag. Total lag is common in newborns up to 34 weeks' gestation, whereas postterm newborns (42+ weeks) hold their heads in front of their body lines. Full-term newborns can support their heads momentarily.
8. *Ventral suspension* (horizontal position) is evaluated by holding the newborn prone on the nurse's hand. The nurse then notes the position of the head and back and the degree of flexion in the arms and legs. Some flexion of arms and legs indicates 36 to 38 weeks' gestation; fully flexed extremities, with head and back even, are characteristic of a term newborn.
9. *Major reflexes* such as sucking, rooting, grasping, Moro, tonic neck, Babinski, and others are evaluated during the newborn exam. See discussion of reflexes on pages 565–566.

When the gestational age determination and birth weight are considered together, the newborn can be identified as *one whose growth is below the 10th percentile, or small for gestational age (SGA); appropriate for gestational age (AGA); or above the 90th percentile, or large for gestational age (LGA)* (Figure 22–11♦). This determination enables the nurse to anticipate possible physiologic problems and, in conjunction with a complete physical examination, to establish a plan of care appropriate for the individual newborn (Dodd, 1996). For example, an SGA newborn often requires frequent glucose monitoring and early feedings. (See Chapter 25 for more complete discussion of these categories and the potential problems associated with them).

The nurse also plots the gestational age against the newborn's length, head circumference, and weight on the appropriate growth chart to determine if these measurements fall within the average range—the 10th to 90th percentile for the corresponding gestational age (Figure 22–12♦). These correlations further document the level of maturity and appropriate category for the newborn. The comparison of the infant's weight-length ratio further facilitates identification of SGA infants as having symmetrical or asymmetrical growth restriction. (See Chapter 25 for further discussion.)

## Physical Assessment

After the initial determination of gestational age and related potential problems, a more extensive physical assessment is carried out. The nurse should choose a warm,

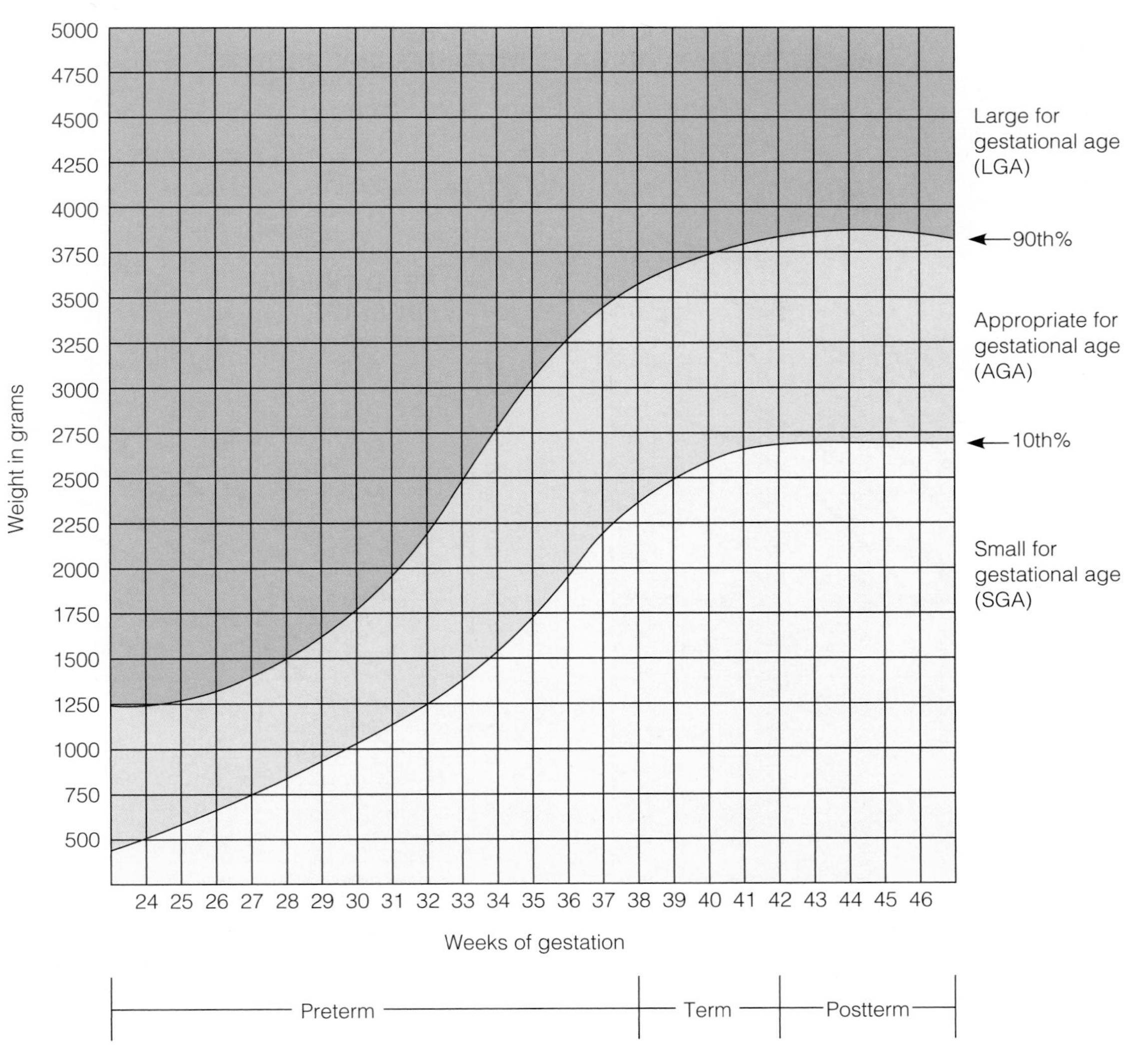


**FIGURE 22–11** ♦ Classification of newborns by birth weight and gestational age. The nurse places the newborn's birth weight and gestational age on the graph and classifies the newborn as large for gestational age (LGA), appropriate for gestational age (AGA), or small for gestational age (SGA). *Source:* Battaglia, F. C., & Lubchenco, L. O. (1967). A practical classification of newborn infants by weight and gestational age. *Journal of Pediatrics, 71,* 161.

well-lit area that is free of drafts. Completing the physical assessment in the presence of the parents provides an opportunity to acquaint them with their unique newborn. The examination is performed in a systematic, head-to-toe manner, and all findings are recorded. When assessing the physical and neurologic status of the newborn, the nurse should first consider general appearance and then proceed to specific areas.

A guide for systematically assessing the newborn appears on pages 568–581. Normal findings, alterations, and related causes are presented and correlated with suggested nursing responses. The findings are typical for a full-term newborn.

## General Appearance

The newborn's head is disproportionately large for its body. The center of the baby's body is the umbilicus rather than the symphysis pubis as in the adult. The body appears long and the extremities short. The flexed position that the newborn maintains contributes to the short appearance of the extremities. The hands are tightly clenched. The neck looks short because the chin rests on the chest. Newborns have a prominent abdomen, sloping shoulders, narrow hips, and rounded chests. They tend to stay in a flexed position similar to the one maintained in utero and will offer resistance when the extremities are straightened. After a breech birth, the feet are usually dorsiflexed, and it may take several weeks for the newborn to assume the typical newborn posture.

## Weight and Measurements

The normal full-term Caucasian newborn has an average birth weight of 3405 g (7 lb, 8 oz). Newborns of African-, Asian-, or Mexican-American descent are usually somewhat smaller at term (Brooks, Johnson, Steer, et al.,

## CLASSIFICATION OF NEWBORNS— BASED ON MATURITY AND INTRAUTERINE GROWTH

Symbols: X-1st Exam O-2nd Exam

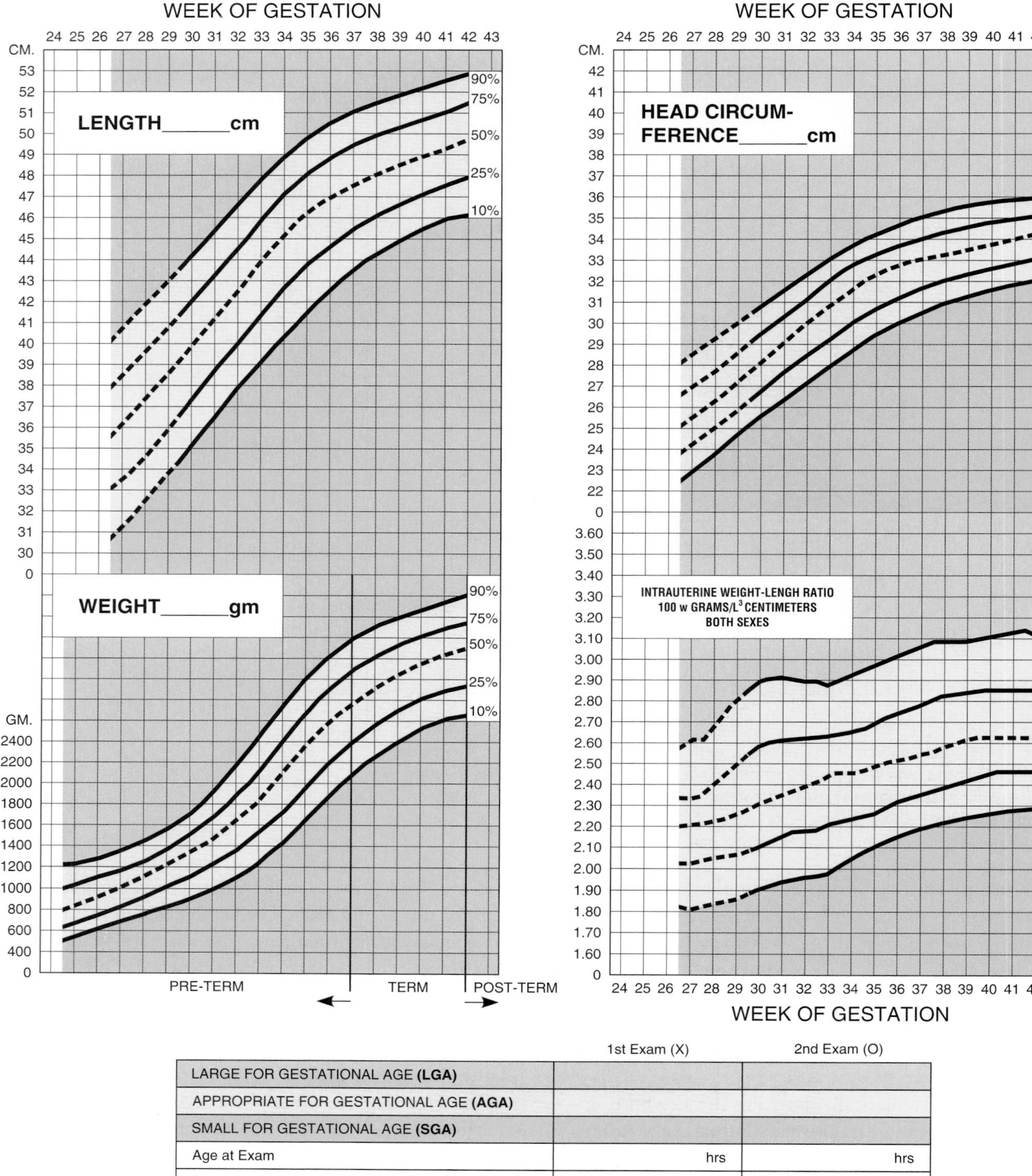


| | 1st Exam (X) | 2nd Exam (O) |
|---|---|---|
| LARGE FOR GESTATIONAL AGE **(LGA)** | | |
| APPROPRIATE FOR GESTATIONAL AGE **(AGA)** | | |
| SMALL FOR GESTATIONAL AGE **(SGA)** | | |
| Age at Exam | hrs | hrs |
| Signature of Examiner | M.D. | M.D. |

FIGURE 22–12 ♦ Classification of newborns based on maturity and intrauterine growth.

*Sources:* Adapted from Lubchenco, L. O., Hansman, C., & Boyd, E., (1966). Intrauterine growth in length and head circumference as estimated from live births at gestational ages from 26 to 42 weeks. *Pediatrics,* 37, 403–408; Battaglia, F. C., & Lubchenco, L. O. (1967). A practical classification of newborn infants by weight and gestational age. *Journal of Pediatrics, 71,* 159.

1995; Overpeck, Hediger, Zhang, et al., 1999). Other factors that influence weight are age and size of parents, health of mother (smoking and malnutrition decrease birth weight), and the interval between pregnancies (short intervals, such as every year, result in lower birth weight) (Basso, Olsen, Knudsen, et al., 1998). After the first week, and for the first 6 months, the newborn's weight increases about 198 g (7 oz) weekly.

Approximately 70% to 75% of the newborn's body weight is water. During the initial newborn period (the first 3 or 4 days), there is a physiologic weight loss of about 5% to 10% for term newborns because of fluid shifts. This weight loss may reach 15% for preterm newborns. Large babies also tend to lose more weight because of greater fluid loss in proportion to birth weight. If weight loss is greater than 10%, clinical reappraisal is indicated. Factors contributing to weight loss include small fluid intake resulting from delayed breastfeeding or a slow adjustment to the formula, increased volume of meconium excreted, and urination. Weight loss may be marked in the presence of temperature elevation (because of associated dehydration) or consistent chilling (because of nonshivering thermogenesis).

The length of the normal newborn is difficult to measure because the legs are flexed and tensed. To measure length, the nurse should place babies flat on their backs with their legs extended as much as possible (Figure 22–13♦). The average length is 50 cm (20 in), and the range is 48 to 52 cm (18 to 22 in). The newborn will grow approximately 1 in a month for the next 6 months. This is the period of most rapid growth.

At birth the newborn's head is one-third the size of an adult's head. The circumference (biparietal diameter) of the newborn's head is 32 to 37 cm (12.5 to 14.5 in). For accurate measurement, the tape is placed over the most prominent part of the occiput and brought just above the eyebrows (Figure 22–14A♦). The circumference of the newborn's head is approximately 2 cm greater than the circumference of the newborn's chest at birth, and the two parts will remain in this proportion for the next few months. (Factors that alter this measurement are discussed in the section titled "Head" later in this chapter.) It is best to take another head circumference on the second day if the newborn experienced significant head molding or developed a caput from the birth process.

At birth the average circumference of the chest is 32 cm (12.5 in) and ranges from 30 to 35 cm. (12–14 in.) Chest measurements are taken with the tape measure placed at the lower edge of the scapulas and brought around anteriorly, directly over the nipple line (Figure 22–14B♦). The abdominal circumference, or girth, may also be measured at this time, by placing the tape around the newborn's abdomen at the level of the umbilicus, with the bottom edge of the tape at the top edge of the umbilicus. (See Key Facts to Remember: Newborn Measurements.)

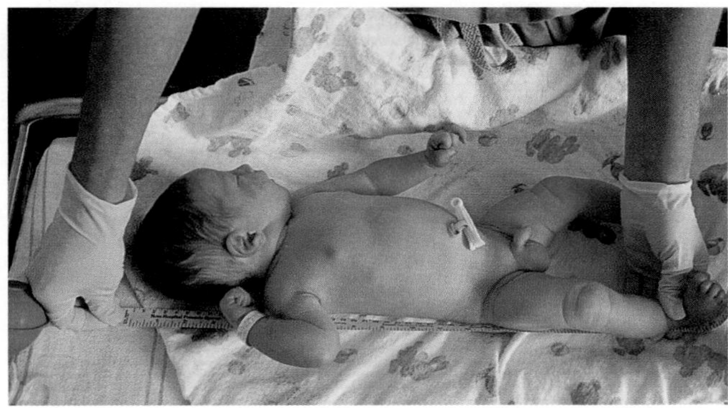

FIGURE 22–13 ♦ Measuring the length of the newborn.

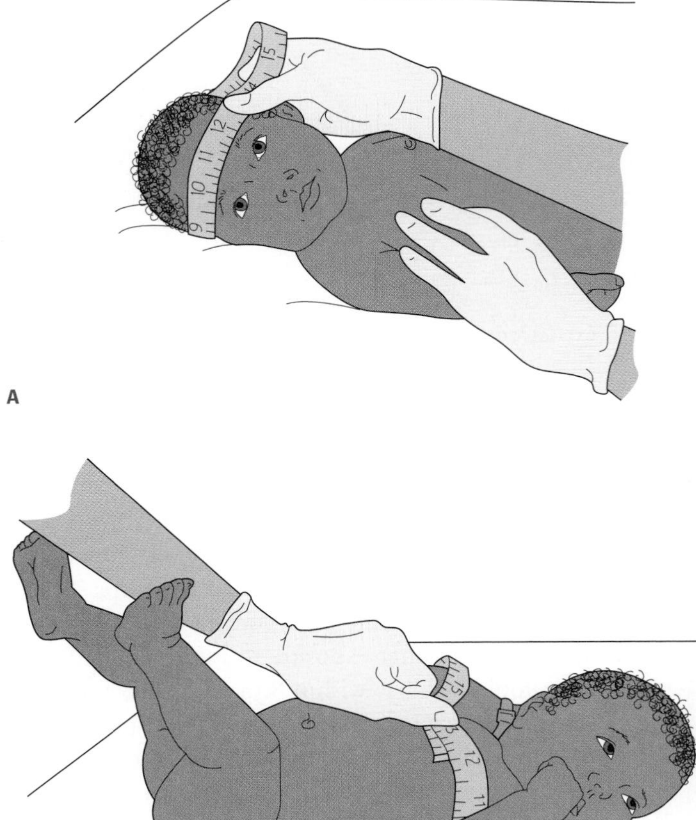


FIGURE 22–14 ♦ **A**, Measuring the head circumference of the newborn. **B**, Measuring the chest circumference of the newborn.

## Temperature

Initial assessment of the newborn's temperature is critical. In utero, the temperature of the fetus is about the same as, or slightly higher than, the expectant mother's. When babies enter the outside world, their temperature can suddenly drop as a result of exposure to cold drafts and the skin's heat loss mechanisms.

## KEY FACTS TO REMEMBER

### *Newborn Measurements*

**Weight**

Average: 3405 g (7 lb, 8 oz)

Range: 2500–4000 g (5 lb, 8 oz–8 lb, 13 oz)

Weight is influenced by racial origin and maternal age and size.

Physiologic weight loss: 5%–10% for term newborns, up to 15% for preterm newborns

Growth: 198 g (7 oz) per week for first 6 months

**Length**

Average: 50 cm (20 in)

Range: 48–52 cm (18–22 in)

Growth: 2.5 cm (1 in) per month for first 6 months

**Head Circumference**

32–37 cm (12.5–14.5 in)

Approximately 2 cm larger than chest circumference

**Chest Circumference**

Average: 32 cm (12.5 in)

Range: 30–35 cm (12–14 in)

If no heat conservation measures are started, the normal term newborn's deep body temperature falls 0.1°C (0.2°F) per minute; skin temperature drops 0.3°C (0.5°F) per minute. Skin temperature markedly decreases within 10 minutes after exposure to room air. The temperature should stabilize within 8 to 12 hours. Temperature is monitored when the newborn is admitted to the nursery and at least every 30 minutes until the newborn's status has remained stable for 2 hours. After that, the nurse should assess temperature at least once every 8 hours, or according to institutional policy (AAP & ACOG, 1997). (See Chapter 21 for a discussion of the physiology of temperature regulation.)

Temperature can be assessed by the axillary skin method, a continuous skin probe, the rectal route, or a tympanic thermometer. Axillary temperature reflects body (core) temperature and the body's compensatory response to the thermal environment. Axillary temperatures are the preferred method and are considered to be a close estimation of the rectal temperature. In preterm and term newborns, there is less than 0.1°C (0.2°F) difference between the two sites. With the axillary method, the thermometer must remain in place at least 3 minutes unless an electronic thermometer is used (Figure 22–15♦). Axillary temperature ranges from 36.5 to 37.0°C (97.7 to 98.6°F). The nurse should keep in mind that axillary temperatures can be misleading, because the friction caused by apposition of the inner arm skin and upper chest wall and the nearness of brown fat to the probe may elevate the temperature.

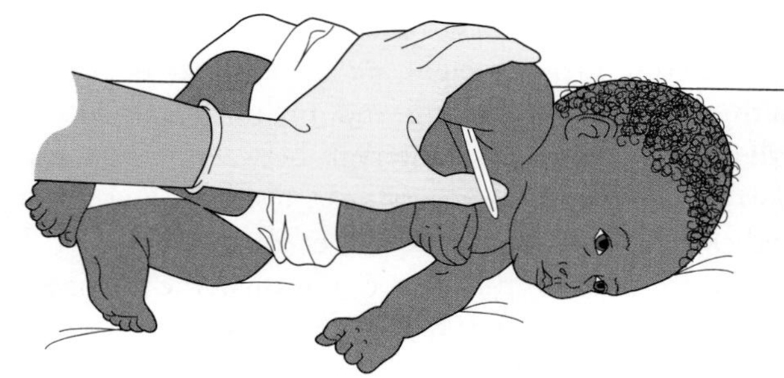

FIGURE 22–15 ♦ Axillary temperature measurement. The thermometer should remain in place for 3 minutes. The nurse presses the newborn's arm tightly but gently against the thermometer and the newborn's side, as illustrated.

Skin temperature is measured most accurately by means of continuous skin probe, especially for small newborns or newborns maintained in incubators or under radiant warmers. Normal skin temperature is 36 to 36.5°C (96.8 to 97.7°F). Continuous assessment of skin temperature allows time for initiation of interventions before a more serious fall in core temperature occurs (Figure 22–16♦).

Rectal temperature is assumed to be the closest approximation to core temperature, but the accuracy of this method depends on the depth to which the thermometer is inserted. Normal rectal temperature is 36.6 to 37.2°C (97.8 to 99°F). The rectal route is not recommended as a routine method, because it may irritate the rectal mucosa and increase chances of perforation.

Many institutions use tympanic thermometers. These are portable sensor probes with disposable covers that are placed in the auditory canal. The probe uses infrared

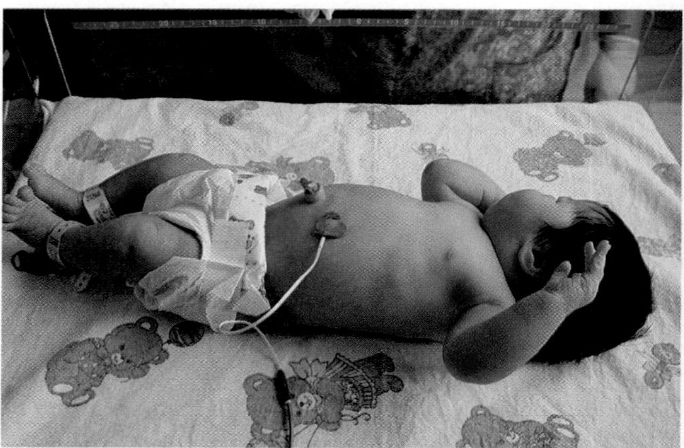

FIGURE 22–16 ♦ Temperature monitoring for the newborn. A skin thermal sensor is placed on the newborn's abdomen, upper thigh, or arm and secured with porous tape or a foil-covered foam pad.

technology to measure the temperature of the internal carotid artery blood flow within several seconds. Research suggests that tympanic and digital thermometer axillary temperatures are accurate estimations of body temperature in the *healthy* newborn (Sganga, Wallace, Kiehl, et al., 2000). Current research still questions the accuracy of tympanic thermometer readings from sick or potentially ill newborns (Sganga et al., 2000).

Temperature instability, a deviation of more than 1°C (2°F) from one reading to the next, or a subnormal temperature may indicate an infection. In contrast to an elevated temperature in older children, an increased temperature in a newborn may indicate reactions to too much covering, too hot a room, or dehydration. Dehydration, which tends to increase body temperature, occurs in newborns whose feedings have been delayed for any reason. Newborns may respond to overheating (a temperature greater than 37.5°C [99.5°F]) by increased restlessness and eventually by perspiration. The perspiration appears initially on the head and face and then on the chest. Many newborns initially cannot perspire, so they increase their respiratory and heart rates, which increases oxygen consumption.

## Skin Characteristics

Although the newborn's skin color varies with genetic background, all healthy newborns have a pink tinge to their skin. The ruddy hue results from increased red blood cell concentrations in the blood vessels and limited subcutaneous fat deposits.

Skin pigmentation is slight in the newborn period, so color changes may be seen even in darker-skinned babies. A newborn who is cyanotic at rest and pink only with crying may have *choanal atresia* (congenital blockage of the passageway between the nose and pharynx). If crying increases the cyanosis, heart or lung problems may be suspected. Very pale newborns may be anemic or have hypovolemia (low BP) and should be evaluated for these problems.

**Acrocyanosis** (bluish discoloration of the hands and feet) may be present in the first 2 to 6 hours after birth (Figure 22–17♦). This condition is caused by poor peripheral circulation, which results in vasomotor instability and capillary stasis, especially when the baby is exposed to cold. If the central circulation is adequate, the blood supply should return quickly when the skin is blanched with a finger. Blue hands and nails are a poor indicator of oxygenation in a newborn. The nurse should assess the face and mucous membranes for pinkness reflecting adequate oxygenation.

**Mottling** (lacy pattern of dilated blood vessels under the skin) occurs as a result of general circulation fluctuations. It may last several hours to several weeks or may come and go periodically. Mottling may be related to chilling or prolonged apnea.

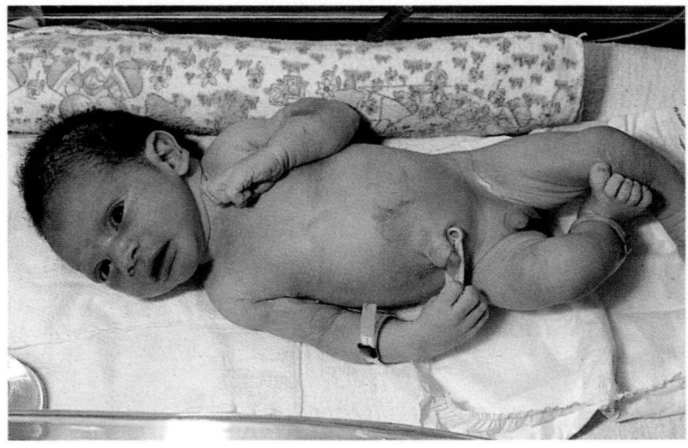

FIGURE 22–17 ♦ Acrocyanosis.

**Harlequin sign** (clown) color change is occasionally noted: A deep red color develops over one side of the newborn's body while the other side remains pale, so that the skin resembles a clown's suit. This color change results from a vasomotor disturbance in which blood vessels on one side dilate while the vessels on the other side constrict. It usually lasts from 1 to 20 minutes. Affected newborns may have single or multiple episodes, but they are transient and not of clinical significance.

**Jaundice** is first detectable on the face (where skin overlies cartilage) and the mucous membranes of the mouth and has a head-to-toe progression (Moyer, Ahn, & Sneed, 2000). It is evaluated by blanching the tip of the nose, the forehead, the sternum, or the gum line. This procedure must be carried out in appropriate lighting. If jaundice is present, the area will appear yellowish immediately after blanching. Another area to assess for jaundice is the sclera. Evaluation and determination of the cause of jaundice must be initiated immediately to prevent possibly serious sequelae. The jaundice may be related to breastfeeding (in a few cases), hematomas, immature liver function, or bruises from forceps, or it may be caused by blood incompatibility, oxytocin (Pitocin) augmentation or induction, or severe hemolysis process. Any jaundice noted before a newborn is 24 hours of age should be reported to the physician or nurse practitioner. (For detailed discussion of causes and assessment of jaundice, see Chapter 26.)

**Erythema toxicum** is a perifollicular eruption of lesions that are firm, vary in size from 1 to 3 mm, and consist of a white or pale yellow papule or pustule with an erythematous base. It is often called "newborn rash" or "flea bite" dermatitis. The rash may appear suddenly, usually over the trunk and diaper area, and is frequently widespread (Figure 22–18♦). The lesions do not appear on the palms of the hands or the soles of the feet. The peak incidence is at 24 to 48 hours of life. The condition rarely presents at birth or after 5 days of life. The cause is unknown, and no treatment is necessary. Some clinicians believe it may be caused

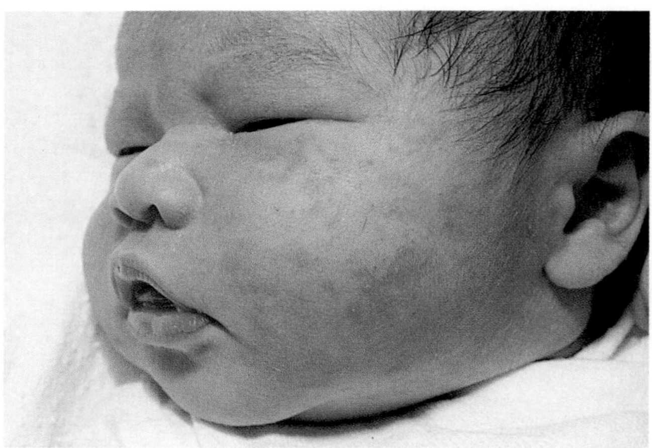

FIGURE 22–18 ♦ Erythema toxicum.

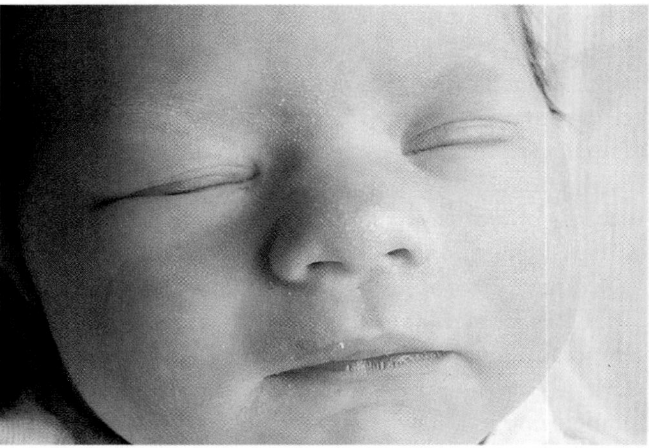

FIGURE 22–19 ♦ Facial milia.

by irritation from clothing. The lesions disappear in a few hours or days. If a maculopapular rash appears, a smear of the aspirated papule will show numerous eosinophils on staining; no bacteria will be cultured.

**Milia,** which are exposed sebaceous glands, appear as raised white spots on the face, especially across the nose (Figure 22–19♦). No treatment is necessary, because they will clear up spontaneously within the first month. Infants of African heritage have a similar condition called transient neonatal pustular melanosis.

**Skin turgor** is assessed to determine hydration status, the need to initiate early feedings, and the presence of any infectious processes. The usual place to assess skin turgor is over the abdomen or the thigh. Skin should be elastic and return to its original shape.

*Vernix caseosa,* a whitish, cheeselike substance, covers the fetus while in utero and lubricates the skin of the newborn. The skin of the term or postterm newborn has less vernix and is frequently dry; peeling is common, especially on the hands and feet.

**Forceps marks** may be present after a difficult forceps birth. The newborn may have reddened areas over the cheeks and jaws. It is important to reassure the parents that these marks will disappear, usually within 1 or 2 days. Transient facial paralysis resulting from the forceps pressure is a rare complication. Vacuum extractor suction marks on the vertex of the scalp are often seen when vacuum extractors are used to assist with the birth. These marks are benign and do not indicate any underlying brain lesions.

## BIRTHMARKS

**Telangiectatic nevi (stork bites)** appear as pale pink or red spots and are frequently found on the eyelids, nose, lower occipital bone, and nape of the neck (Figure 22–20♦). These lesions are common in newborns with light complexions and are more noticeable during periods of crying. These areas have no clinical significance and usually fade by the second birthday.

**Mongolian spots** are macular areas of bluish black or gray-blue pigmentation on the dorsal area and the buttocks (Figure 22–21♦). They are common in newborns of Asian and African descent and other dark-skinned races. They gradually fade during the first or second year of life. They may be mistaken for bruises and should be documented in the newborn's chart.

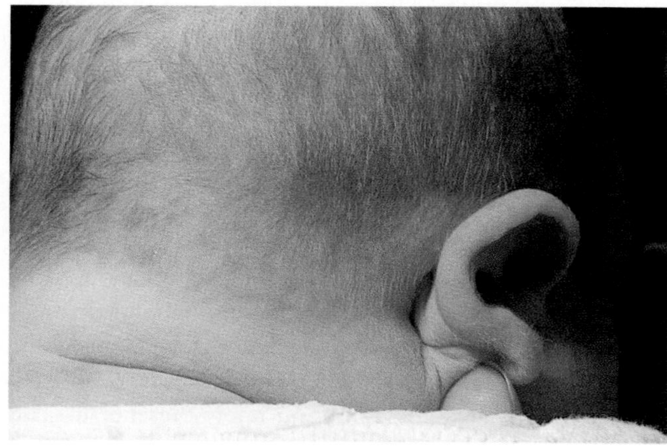

FIGURE 22–20 ♦ Stork bites.

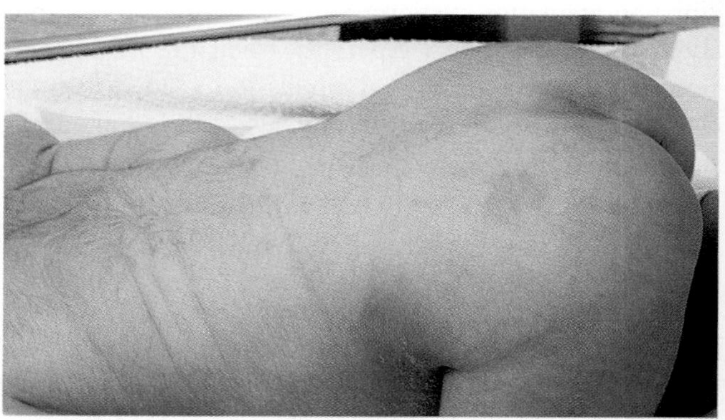

FIGURE 22–21 ♦ Mongolian spots.

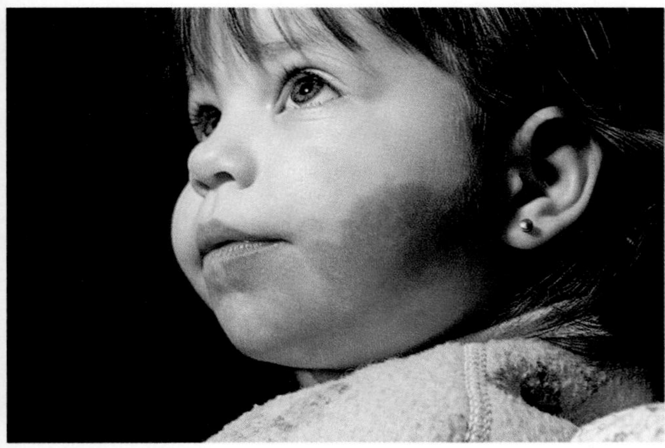

FIGURE 22–22 ♦ Port-wine stain.

**Nevus flammeus (port-wine stain),** a capillary angioma directly below the epidermis, is a nonelevated, sharply demarcated, red-to-purple area of dense capillaries (Figure 22–22♦). In infants of African descent, it may appear as a purple-black stain. The size and shape vary, but it commonly appears on the face. It does not grow in size, does not fade with time, and does not blanch as a rule. The birthmark may be concealed by using an opaque cosmetic cream. If convulsions and other neurologic problems accompany the nevus flammeus, the clinical picture is suggestive of *Sturge-Weber syndrome,* with involvement of the fifth cranial nerve (the ophthalmic branch of the trigeminal nerve).

**Nevus vasculosus (strawberry mark),** a capillary hemangioma, consists of newly formed and enlarged capillaries in the dermal and subdermal layers. It is a raised, clearly delineated, dark-red, rough-surfaced birthmark commonly found in the head region. Such marks usually grow (often rapidly) starting during the second or third week of life and may not reach their fullest size for 1 to 3 months (Rinehart et al., 2000). They begin to shrink and start to resolve spontaneously several weeks to months after they reach peak growth. Parents can be told that resolution is heralded by a pale purple or gray spot on the surface of the hemangioma. The best cosmetic effect is achieved when the lesions are allowed to resolve spontaneously.

Birthmarks are frequently a cause of concern for parents. The mother may be especially anxious, fearing that she is to blame ("Is my baby 'marked' because of something I did?"). Guilt feelings are common in the presence of misconceptions about the cause. Birthmarks should be identified and explained to the parents. By providing appropriate information about the cause and course of birthmarks, the nurse frequently relieves the fears and anxieties of the family. The nurse should note any bruises, abrasions, or birthmarks seen on admission to the nursery.

## HEAD

### GENERAL APPEARANCE

The newborn's head is large (approximately one-fourth of the body size), with soft, pliable skull bones. The head may appear asymmetrical in the newborn of a vertex birth. This asymmetry, called **molding,** is caused by overriding of the cranial bones during labor and birth (Figure 22–23♦). The degree of molding varies with the amount and length of pressure exerted on the head. Within a few days after birth, the overriding usually diminishes and the suture lines become palpable. Because head measurements are affected by molding, a second measurement is indicated a few days after birth. The heads of breech-born newborns and those born by elective cesarean are characteristically round and well shaped because no pressure was exerted on them during birth. Any extreme differences in head size may indicate microcephaly or hydrocephalus. Variations in the shape, size, or appearance of the head measurements may be due to *craniostenosis* (premature closure of the cranial sutures), which will need to be corrected through surgery to allow brain growth, and *plagiocephaly* (asymmetry caused by pressure on the fetal head during gestation).

Two *fontanelles* ("soft spots") may be palpated on the newborn's head. Fontanelles, which are openings at the juncture of the cranial bones, can be measured with the fingers. Accurate measurement necessitates that the examiner's finger be measured in centimeters. The assessment should be carried out with the newborn in a sitting position and not crying. The diamond-shaped *anterior fontanelle* is approximately 3 to 4 cm long by 2 to 3 cm

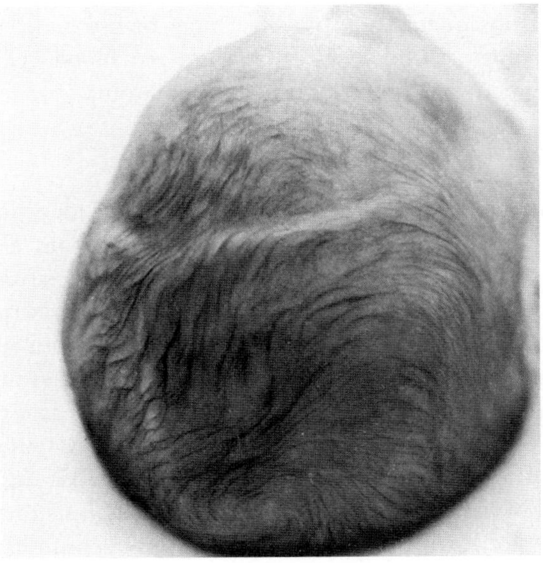

FIGURE 22–23 ♦ Overlapped cranial bones produce a visible ridge in a small, premature newborn. Easily visible overlapping does not occur often in term infants. *Source:* Korones, S. B. (1986). *High-risk newborn infants* (4th ed.). St. Louis: Mosby.

wide. It is located at the juncture of the frontal and parietal bones. The *posterior fontanelle,* smaller and triangular, is formed by the parietal bones and the occipital bone and is 0.5 by 1 cm. The fontanelles are smaller immediately after birth than several days later because of molding. The anterior fontanelle closes within 18 months, whereas the posterior fontanelle closes within 8 to 12 weeks.

The fontanelles are a useful indicator of the newborn's condition. The anterior fontanelle may swell when the newborn cries or passes a stool or may pulsate with the heartbeat, which is normal. A bulging fontanelle usually signifies increased intracranial pressure, and a depressed fontanelle indicates dehydration. The sutures between the cranial bones should be palpated for amount of overlapping. In newborns whose growth has been restricted the sutures may be wider than normal, and the fontanelles may also be larger due to impaired growth of the cranial bones. In addition to inspecting the newborn's head for degree of molding and size, the nurse should evaluate it for soft tissue edema and bruising.

### Cephalhematoma

**Cephalhematoma** is a collection of blood resulting from ruptured blood vessels between the surface of a cranial bone (usually parietal) and the periosteal membrane (Figure 22–24♦). The scalp in these areas feels loose and slightly edematous. These areas emerge as defined hematomas between the first and second day. Although external pressure may cause the mass to fluctuate, it does not increase in size when the newborn cries. Cephalhematomas may be unilateral or bilateral and do not cross suture lines. They are relatively common in vertex births and may disappear within 2 to 3 weeks or very slowly over subsequent months. They may be associated with physiologic jaundice, because extra red blood cells are being destroyed within the cephalhematoma.

### Caput Succedaneum

**Caput succedaneum** is a localized, easily identifiable, soft area of the scalp, generally resulting from a long and difficult labor or vacuum extraction. The sustained pressure of the presenting part against the cervix results in compression of local blood vessels, and venous return is slowed. Slowed venous return in turn causes an increase in tissue fluids, an edematous swelling, and occasional bleeding under the periosteum. The caput may vary from a small area to a severely elongated head. The fluid in the caput is reabsorbed within 12 hours to a few days after birth. Caputs resulting from vacuum extractors are sharply outlined, circular areas up to 2 cm thick. They disappear more slowly than naturally occurring edema. It is possible to distinguish between a cephalhematoma and a caput because the caput overrides suture lines (Figure 22–25♦), whereas the cephalhematoma, because of its location, never crosses a suture line. Also, caput succedaneum is present at birth, whereas cephalhematoma is not.

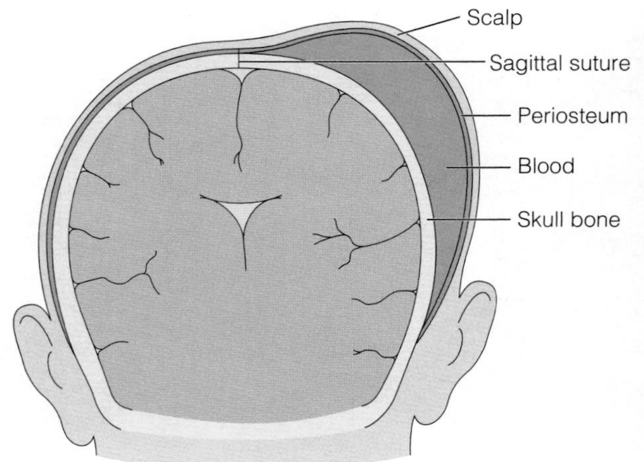


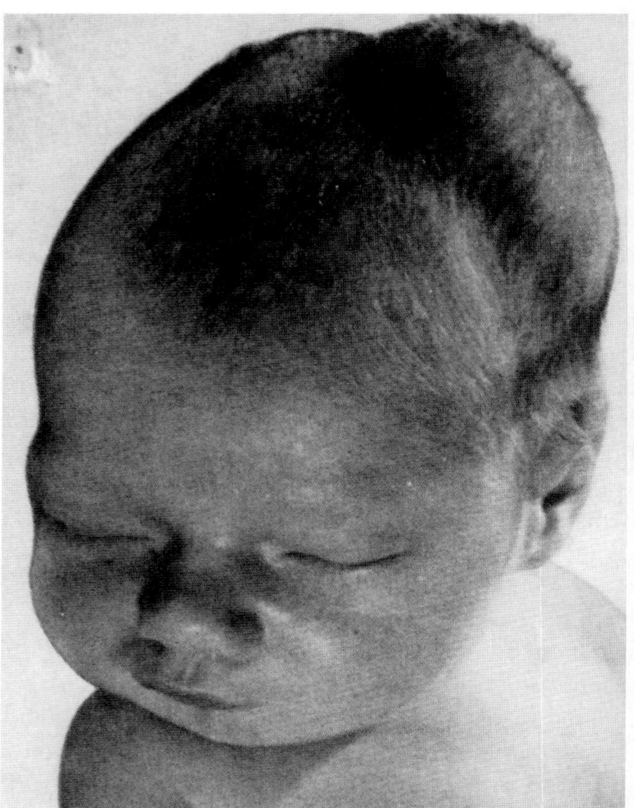

FIGURE 22–24 ♦ Cephalhematoma is a collection of blood between the surface of a cranial bone and the periosteal membrane. This is a cephalhematoma over the left parietal bone. *Source:* Potter, E. L., & Craig, J. M. (1975). *Pathology of the fetus and infant* (3rd ed.). Chicago: Year Book Medical Publishers. Reproduced with permission.

## Face

The newborn's face is well designed to help the newborn suckle. Sucking (fat) pads are located in the cheeks, and

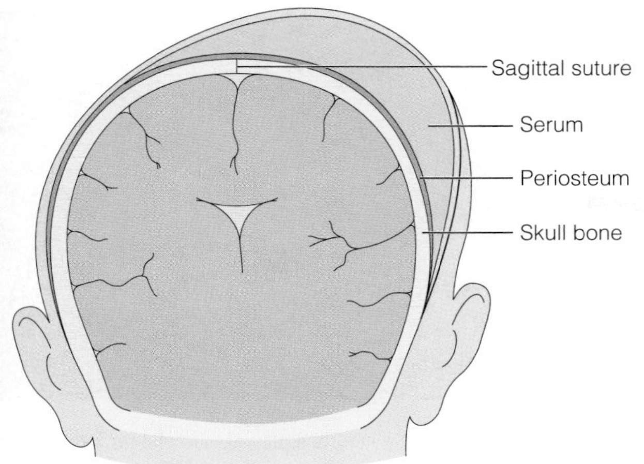


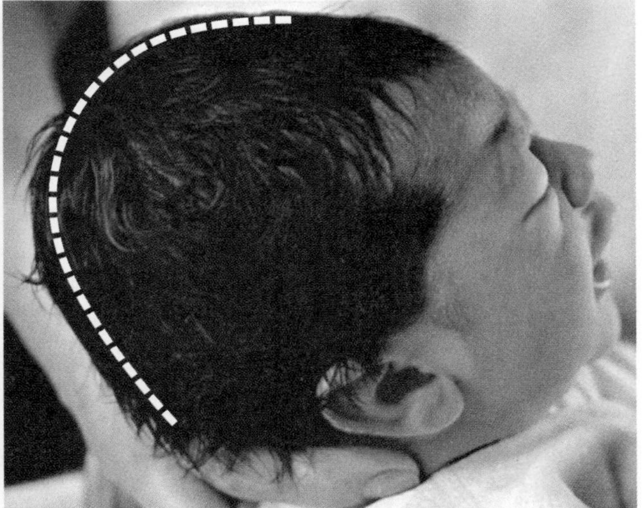

FIGURE 22–25 ♦ Caput succedaneum is a collection of fluid (serum) under the scalp. *Source:* Photo courtesy of Mead Johnson Laboratories, Evansville, IN.

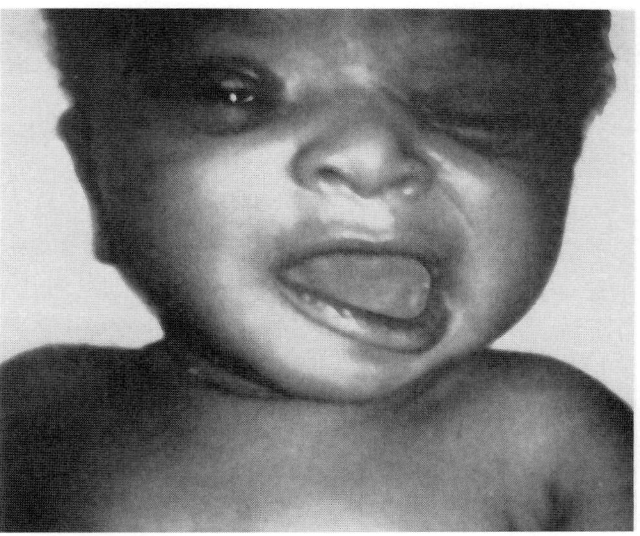

FIGURE 22–26 ♦ Facial paralysis. Paralysis of the right side of the face from injury to right facial nerve. *Source:* Courtesy of Dr. Ralph Platow. From Potter, E. L., & Craig, J. M. (1975). *Pathology of the fetus and infant* (3rd ed.). Chicago: Year Book Medical Publishers. Reproduced with permission.

a labial tubercle (sucking callus) is frequently found in the center of the upper lip. The chin is recessed, and the nose is flattened. The lips are sensitive to touch, and the sucking reflex is easily initiated.

Symmetry of the eyes, nose, and ears is evaluated. See the Newborn Physical Assessment Guide on pages 568–581 for deviations in symmetry and variations in size, shape, and spacing of facial features.

Facial movement symmetry should be assessed to determine the presence of facial palsy. Facial paralysis appears when the newborn cries; the affected side is immobile, and the palpebral (eyelid) fissure widens (Figure 22–26♦). Paralysis may result from forceps-assisted birth or pressure on the facial nerve from the maternal pelvis during birth. Facial paralysis usually disappears within a few days to 3 weeks, although in some cases it may be permanent.

## Eyes

The eyes of the newborn of northern European descent are a blue-gray or slate–blue–gray color. Scleral color tends to be bluish-white because of its relative thinness. A blue sclera is associated with osteogenesis imperfecta (Tappero & Honeyfield, 1996). The infant's eye color is usually established at approximately 3 months, although it may change any time up to 1 year. Dark-skinned newborns tend to have dark eyes at birth.

The eyes should be checked for size, equality of pupil size, reaction of pupils to light, blink reflex to light, and edema and inflammation of the eyelids. The eyelids are usually edematous during the first few days of life because of the pressure associated with birth.

Erythromycin and tetracycline are now frequently used prophylactically instead of silver nitrate and usually do not cause chemical irritation of the eye. The instillation of silver nitrate drops in the newborn's eyes may cause edema, and **chemical conjunctivitis** may appear a few hours after instillation, but it disappears in 1 to 2 days. If infectious conjunctivitis exists, the newborn has the same purulent (greenish yellow) discharge exudate as in chemical conjunctivitis, but it is caused by gonococcus, *Chlamydia,* staphylococci, or a variety of gram-negative bacteria and requires treatment with ophthalmic antibiotics. Onset is usually after the second day. Edema of the orbits or eyelids may persist for several days, until the newborn's kidneys can eliminate the fluid.

Small **subconjunctival hemorrhages** appear in about 10% of newborns and are commonly found on the sclera. These hemorrhages are caused by the changes in vascular tension or ocular pressure during birth. They will remain for a few weeks and are of no pathologic significance. Parents need reassurance that the newborn is not bleeding from within the eye and that vision will not be impaired.

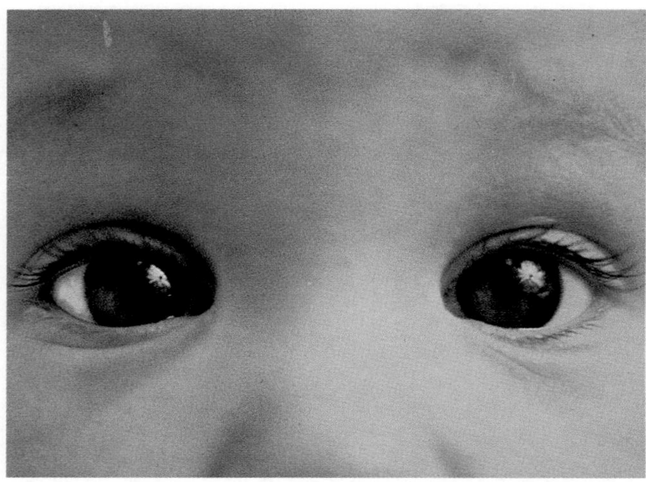

FIGURE 22–27 ♦ Transient strabismus may be present in the newborn due to poor neuromuscular control. *Source:* Photo courtesy of Mead Johnson Laboratories, Evansville, IN.

The newborn may demonstrate transient strabismus caused by poor neuromuscular control of eye muscles (Figure 22–27♦). It gradually regresses in 3 to 4 months. The "doll's eye" phenomenon is also present for about 10 days after birth. As the newborn's head position is changed to the left and then to the right, the eyes move to the opposite direction. This results from underdeveloped integration of head-eye coordination.

The nurse should observe the newborn's pupils for opacities or whiteness and for the absence of a normal red retinal reflex. Red retinal reflex is a red-orange flash of color observed when an ophthalmoscope light reflects off the retina. In a newborn with dark skin color, the retina may appear paler or more grayish. Absence of red reflex occurs with cataracts. Congenital cataracts should be suspected in newborns of mothers with a history of rubella, cytomegalic inclusion disease, or syphilis.

The cry of the newborn is commonly tearless because the lacrimal structures are immature at birth and are not usually fully functional until the second month of life. However, some babies produce tears during the newborn period. Poor oculomotor coordination and absence of accommodation limit visual abilities, but newborns have peripheral vision, can fixate on objects near (10 to 20 in.) their face for short periods, can accommodate to large objects (3 in. tall by 3 in. wide), and can seek out high-contrast geometric shapes. Newborns can perceive faces, shapes, and colors and begin to show visual preferences early. Visual acuity has been reported to be 20/400 (Reed & Davidhizar, 1997). Newborns generally blink in response to bright lights, to a tap on the bridge of the nose (glabellar reflex), or to a light touch on the eyelids. Pupillary light reflex is also present. Examination of the eye is best accomplished by rocking the newborn from an upright position to the horizontal a few times or by other methods, such as diminishing overhead lights, that elicit an opened-eye response.

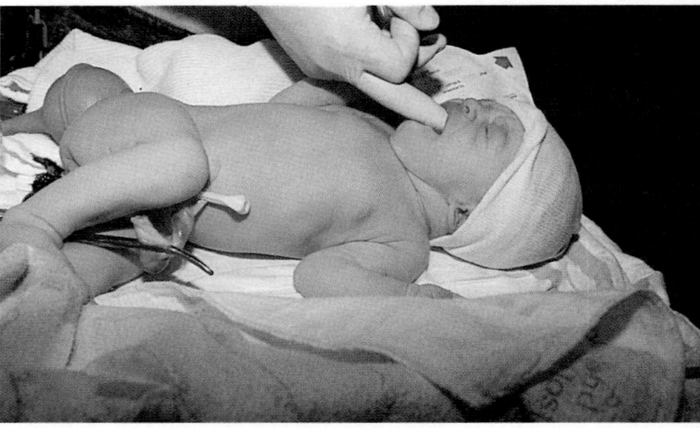

FIGURE 22–28 ♦ The nurse inserts a gloved index finger into the newborn's mouth and feels for any openings along the hard and soft palates. *Note:* Gloves or a finger cot are always worn to examine the palate.

## Nose

The newborn's nose is small and narrow. Infants are characteristically nose breathers for the first few months of life and generally remove obstructions by sneezing. Nasal patency is ensured if the newborn breathes easily with the mouth closed. If respiratory difficulty occurs, the nurse checks for choanal atresia.

The newborn has the ability to smell after the nasal passages are cleared of amniotic fluid and mucus. This ability is demonstrated by the search for milk. Newborns turn their heads toward a milk source, whether bottle or breast. Newborns react to strong odors, such as alcohol, by turning their heads away or blinking.

## Mouth

The lips of the newborn should be pink, and a touch on the lips should produce sucking motions. Saliva is normally scant. The taste buds develop before birth, and the newborn can easily discriminate between sweet and bitter flavors.

The easiest way to examine the mouth completely is to stimulate infants gently to cry by depressing their tongue, thereby causing them to open the mouth fully. It is extremely important to examine the entire mouth to check for a cleft palate, which can be present even in the absence of a cleft lip (Thurdeen, Deacon, O'Neill, et al., 1999) (Figure 22–28♦). Glove powder should always be removed before examining the newborn's mouth.

Occasionally, an examination of the gums will reveal *precocious teeth* over the area where the lower central incisor will erupt. If they appear loose, they should be removed to prevent aspiration. Gray-white lesions (inclusion cysts) on the gums may be confused with teeth. On

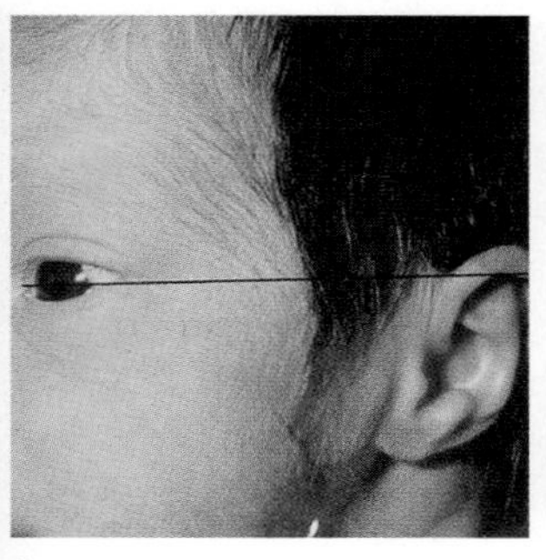
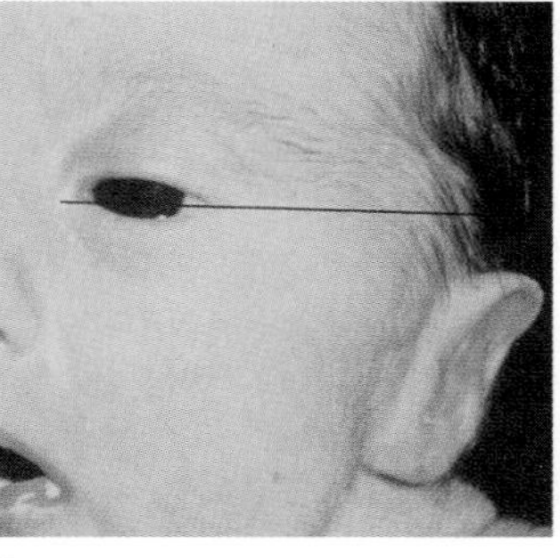

A B

FIGURE 22–29 ♦ The position of the external ear may be assessed by drawing a line across the inner and outer canthus of the eye to the insertion of the ear. **A**, Normal position. **B**, True low-set position.
*Source:* Photo courtesy of Mead Johnson Laboratories, Evansville, IN.

the hard palate and gum margins, **Epstein's pearls,** small glistening white specks (keratin-containing cysts) that feel hard to the touch, are often present. They usually disappear in a few weeks and are of no significance. **Thrush** may appear as white patches that look like milk curds adhering to the mucous membranes and cause bleeding when removed. Thrush is caused by *Candida albicans,* often acquired from an infected vaginal tract during birth or if the mother uses poor handwashing when handling her newborn. Thrush is treated with a preparation of nystatin (Mycostatin).

A newborn who is tongue-tied has a ridge of frenulum tissue attached to the underside of the tongue at varying lengths from its base, causing a heart shape at the tip of the tongue. "Clipping the tongue," or cutting the ridge of tissue, is not recommended. This ridge does not affect speech or eating, but cutting creates an entry for infection.

Transient nerve paralysis resulting from birth trauma may be manifested by asymmetrical mouth movements when the newborn cries or by difficulty with sucking and feeding.

## Ears

The ears of the newborn should be soft and pliable and should recoil readily when folded and released. In the normal newborn, the top of the ear (pinna) should be parallel to the outer and inner canthus of the eye. The ears should be inspected for shape, size, position, and firmness of cartilage. *Low-set ears* are characteristic of many syndromes and may indicate chromosomal abnormalities (especially trisomies 13 and 18), mental retardation, and internal organ abnormalities, especially bilateral renal agenesis as a result of embryologic developmental deviations (Figure 22–29♦). *Preauricular skin tags* may be present just in front of the ear.

Following the first cry, the newborn's hearing becomes acute as mucus from the middle ear is absorbed, the eustachian tube becomes aerated, and the tympanic membrane becomes visible. The nurse evaluates the newborn's hearing by noting the baby's response to loud or moderately loud noises unaccompanied by vibrations. The sleeping newborn should stir or awaken in response to nearby sounds. (This is not a very accurate test, but it may alert the examiner to a possible problem.) The newborn can discriminate the individual characteristics of the human voice and is especially sensitive to sound levels within the normal conversational range (Sininger, Doyle, & Moore, 1999). The newborn in a noisy nursery may habituate to the sounds and not stir unless the sound is sudden or much louder than usual.

## Neck

A short neck, creased with skin folds, is characteristic of the normal newborn. Because muscle tone is not well developed, the neck cannot support the full weight of the head, which rotates freely. The head lags considerably when the newborn is pulled from a supine to a sitting position, but the prone newborn is able to raise the head slightly. The neck is palpated for masses and the presence of lymph nodes and is inspected for webbing. Adequacy of range of motion and neck muscle function is determined by fully extending the head in all directions. Injury to the sternocleidomastoid muscle (congenital torticollis) must be considered in the presence of neck rigidity.

The nurse evaluates the clavicles for evidence of fractures, which occasionally occur during difficult births or in newborns with broad shoulders. The normal clavicle is straight. If fractured, a lump and a grating sensation (crepitus) during movements may be palpated along the course of the side of the break. The nurse also elicits Moro reflex (page 565) to evaluate bilateral equal movement of the arms. If the clavicle is fractured, the response will be demonstrated only on the unaffected side.

## Chest

The thorax is cylindrical at birth, and the ribs are flexible. The general appearance of the chest should be assessed. A protrusion at the lower end of the sternum, called the *xiphoid cartilage,* is frequently seen. It is under the skin and will become less apparent after several weeks as adipose tissue accumulates.

Engorged breasts occur frequently in both male and female newborns. This condition, which occurs by the third day, is a result of maternal hormonal influences and may last up to 2 weeks (Figure 22–30♦). A whitish secretion from the nipples may also be noted. The newborn's breast should not be massaged or squeezed, because this may cause a breast abscess. Extra nipples, or *supernumerary nipples,* are occasionally noted below and medial to

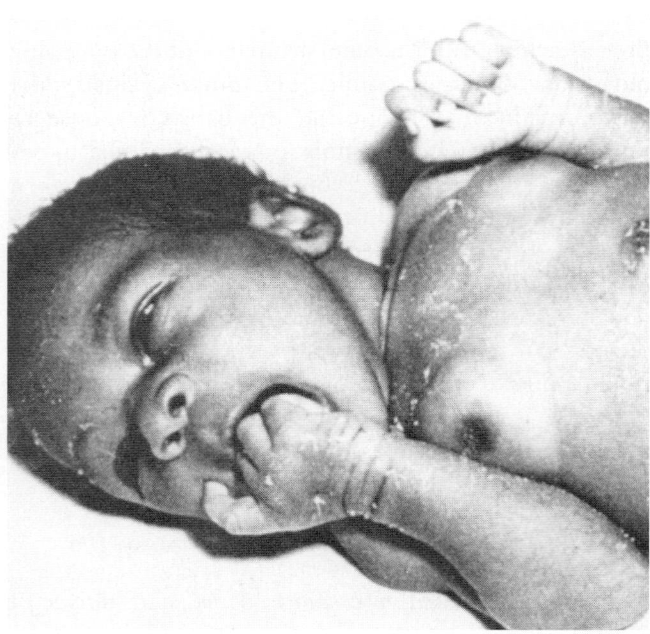

FIGURE 22–30 ♦ Breast hypertrophy. *Source:* Korones, S. B. (1986). *High-risk newborn infants,* (4th ed.). St. Louis: Mosby.

the true nipples. These harmless pink or brown (in darker-skinned newborns) spots vary in size and do not contain glandular tissue. Accessory nipples can be differentiated from a pigmented nevi (mole) by placing the fingertips alongside the accessory nipple and pulling the adjacent tissue laterally. The accessory nipple will appear dimpled. At puberty the accessory nipple may darken.

## Cry

The newborn's cry should be strong, lusty, and of medium pitch. A high-pitched, shrill cry is abnormal and may indicate neurologic disorders or hypoglycemia. Periods of crying usually vary in length after consoling measures are used. Babies' cries are an important method of communication and alert caregivers to changes in the baby's condition and needs.

## Respiration

Normal breathing for a term newborn is 30 to 60 respirations per minute and is predominantly diaphragmatic, with associated rising and falling of the abdomen during inspiration and expiration. The nurse should note any signs of respiratory distress, nasal flaring, intercostal or xiphoid retraction, expiratory grunt or sigh, seesaw respirations, or tachypnea (greater than 60 breaths per minute or sustained). Hyperextension (chest appears high) or hypoextension (chest appears low) of the anteroposterior diameter of the chest should also be noted. Both the anterior and posterior chest are auscultated. Some breath sounds are heard better when the newborn is crying, but localizing and identifying breath sounds are difficult in the newborn. Upper airway noises and bowel sounds may also be heard over the chest wall and make auscultation difficult. Because sounds may be transmitted from the unaffected lung to the affected lung, the absence of breath sounds may not be diagnosed. Air entry may be noisy in the first couple of hours until lung fluid resolves, especially after cesarean births. Brief periods of apnea (episodic breathing) occur, but no color or heart rate changes occur in healthy, term newborns.

## Heart

Heart rates can be as rapid as 180 beats per minute in newborns and fluctuate a great deal, especially if the baby moves or is startled. The normal range is 120 to 160 beats per minute. The heart is examined for rate and rhythm, position of the apical impulse, and heart sound intensity. Dysrhythmias should be reassessed by the physician.

The pulse rate is variable and is influenced by physical activity, crying, state of wakefulness, and body temperature. The examiner auscultates over the entire heart region (precordium), below the left axilla, and below the scapula. Apical pulse rates are obtained by auscultation for a full minute, preferably when the newborn is asleep.

The placement of the heart in the chest should be determined when the newborn is in a quiet state. The heart is relatively large at birth and is located high in the chest, with its apex somewhere between the fourth and fifth intercostal space. A shift of heart tones in the mediastinal area to either side may indicate pneumothorax, dextrocardia (heart placement on the right side of the chest), or a diaphragmatic hernia. The experienced nurse can diagnose these and many other problems early with a stethoscope.

Normally, the heart beat has a "toc tic" sound. A slur or slushing sound (usually after the first sound) may indicate a *murmur.* Although 90% of all murmurs are transient and are considered normal, they should be monitored closely by a physician. Many murmurs are related to a patent ductus arteriosus, which closes in about 1 to 2 days. In newborns, a low-pitched, musical murmur heard just to the right of the apex of the heart is fairly common. Occasionally, significant murmurs are heard, including the murmur of a patent ductus arteriosus, aortic or pulmonary stenosis, or small ventricular septal defect. (See Chapter 25 for a discussion of congenital heart defects.)

Peripheral pulses (brachial, femoral, pedal) are also evaluated to detect any lags or unusual characteristics. Brachial pulses are palpated bilaterally for equality and compared with the femoral pulses. Femoral pulses are palpated by applying gentle pressure with the middle finger over the femoral canal (Figure 22–31♦). Decreased or

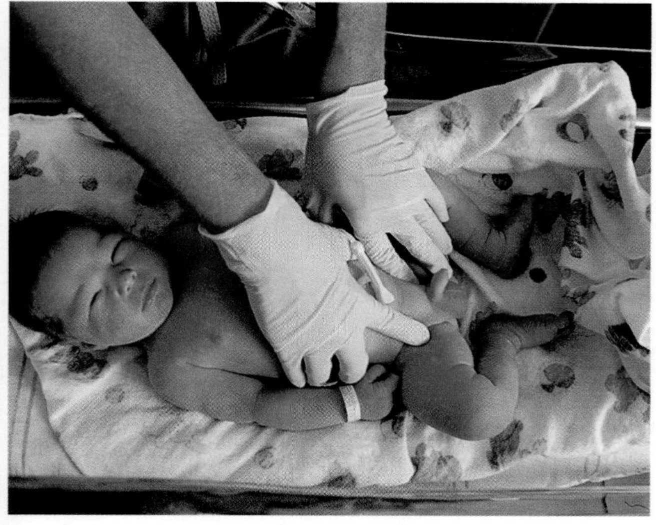

A

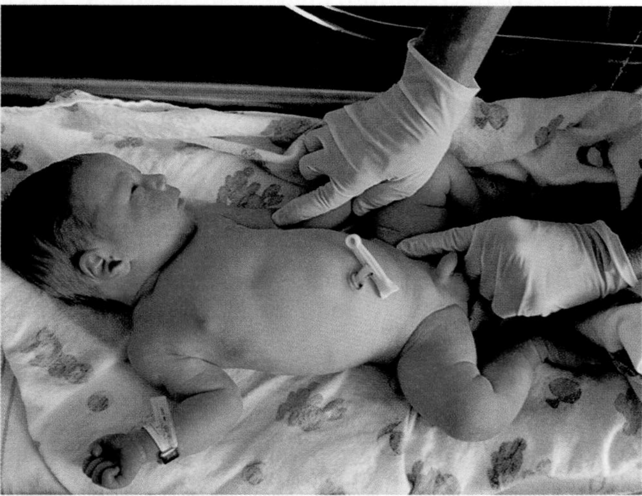

B

FIGURE 22–31 ♦ **A**, Bilaterally palpate the femoral arteries for rate and intensity of the pulses. Press fingertip gently at the groin as shown. **B**, Compare the femoral pulses to the brachial pulses by palpating the pulses simultaneously for comparison of rate and intensity.

absent femoral pulses indicate coarctation of the aorta and require additional investigation. A wide difference in blood pressure between the upper and lower extremities also indicates coarctation.

The measurement of blood pressure is best accomplished by using the Doppler technique or a 1- to 2-inch cuff and a stethoscope over the brachial artery (Figure 22–32♦). If a Doppler device is used, the newborn's extremities must be immobilized during the assessment, and the cuff should cover two-thirds of the upper arm or upper leg. Movement, crying, and inappropriate cuff size can give inaccurate measurements of the blood pressure.

Blood pressure may not be measured routinely on healthy newborns, but it is essential for newborns who are having distress, are premature, or are suspected of cardiac

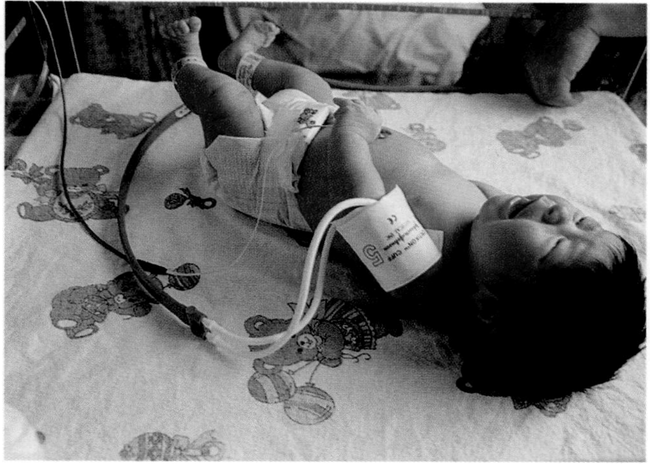

FIGURE 22–32 ♦ Blood pressure measurement using a Doppler device. The cuff can be applied to the upper arm or thigh.

anomaly (Taeusch & Sniderman, 1998). Infants who have birth asphyxia and are on ventilators have significantly lower systolic and diastolic blood pressures than healthy infants. If cardiac anomaly is suspected, blood pressure is measured in all four extremities (Key Facts to Remember: Newborn Vital Signs).

### KEY FACTS TO REMEMBER

*Newborn Vital Signs*

**Pulse**

120–160 bpm

During sleep as low as 100 bpm; if crying, up to 180 bpm

Apical pulse counted for 1 full minute

**Respirations**

30–60 respirations/minute

Predominantly diaphragmatic but synchronous with abdominal movements

Respirations are counted for 1 full minute

**Blood Pressure**

80–60/45–40 mm Hg at birth

100/50 mm Hg at day 10

**Temperature**

Normal range: 36.5–37.5°C (97.7–99.4°F)

Axillary: 36.4–37.2°C (97.5–99°F)

Skin: 36–36.5°C (96.8–97.7°F)

Rectal: 36.6–37.2°C (97.8–99°F)

## HINTS FOR PRACTICE

Vital sign assessments are most accurate if the newborn is at rest, so measure pulse and respirations first if the baby is quiet. To soothe a crying baby, try placing your moistened gloved finger in the baby's mouth and then complete your assessment while the baby suckles.

## ABDOMEN

The nurse can learn a great deal about the newborn's abdomen without disturbing the infant. The abdomen should be cylindrical and protrude slightly. A certain amount of laxness of the abdominal muscles is normal. A scaphoid (hollow-shaped) appearance suggests the absence of abdominal contents. No cyanosis should be present, and few if any blood vessels should be apparent to the eye. There should be no gross distension or bulging. The more distended the abdomen, the tighter the skin becomes, with engorged vessels appearing. Distension is the first sign of many of the abnormalities found in the gastrointestinal tract.

Before palpation of the abdomen, the nurse should auscultate for the presence or absence of bowel sounds in all four quadrants. Bowel sounds may be present by 1 hour after birth. Palpation can cause a transient decrease in intensity of the bowel sounds.

Abdominal palpation should be done systematically. The nurse palpates each of the four abdominal quadrants and moves in a clockwise direction until all four quadrants have been palpated for softness, tenderness, and the presence of masses.

## UMBILICAL CORD

Initially the umbilical cord is white and gelatinous in appearance, with the two umbilical arteries and one umbilical vein readily apparent. Because a single umbilical artery is frequently associated with congenital anomalies, the nurse should count the vessels during the newborn assessment. The cord begins drying within 1 or 2 hours of birth and is shriveled and blackened by the second or third day. Within 7 to 10 days it sloughs off, although a granulating area may remain for a few days longer.

Cord bleeding is abnormal and may result because the cord was inadvertently pulled or the cord clamp was loosened. Foul-smelling drainage is also abnormal and is generally caused by infection, which requires immediate treatment to prevent septicemia. If the newborn has a patent urachus (abnormal connection between the umbilicus and bladder), moistness or draining urine may be apparent at the base of the cord.

Serous or serosanguineous drainage that continues after the cord falls off may indicate a granuloma. It appears as a small red button deep in the umbilicus. Treatment involves cauterization by a physician with a silver nitrate stick (O'Donnell, Glick, & Cory, 1998).

## GENITALS

### FEMALE INFANTS

The nurse examines the labia majora, labia minora, and clitoris and notes the size of each as appropriate for gestational age. A vaginal tag or hymenal tag is often evident and will usually disappear in a few weeks. During the first week of life, the newborn may have a vaginal discharge composed of thick, whitish mucus. This discharge, which can become tinged with blood, is called **pseudomenstruation** and is caused by the withdrawal of maternal hormones. Smegma, a white, cheeselike substance, is often present between the labia. Removing it may traumatize tender tissue.

### MALE INFANTS

The nurse inspects the penis to determine whether the urinary orifice is correctly positioned. *Hypospadias* occurs when the urinary meatus is located on the ventral surface of the penis. It occurs most commonly among people of western European descent. *Phimosis* is a condition in which the opening of the foreskin (prepuce) is small and the foreskin cannot be pulled back over the glans at all. This condition may interfere with urination, so the adequacy of the urinary stream should be evaluated.

The nurse inspects the scrotum for size and symmetry, palpating to verify the presence of both testes and to rule out *cryptorchidism* (failure of testes to descend). The testes are palpated separately between the thumb and forefinger, with the thumb and forefinger of the other hand placed together over the inguinal canal. Scrotal edema and discoloration are common in breech births. *Hydrocele* (a collection of fluid surrounding the testes in the scrotum) is common in newborns and should be identified. It usually resolves without intervention. The presence of a discolored or dusky scrotum and solid testis should raise the suspicion of testicular torsion (Juretschke, 2000).

## ANUS

The nurse inspects the anal area to verify that it is patent and has no fissure. Imperforate anus and rectal atresia may be ruled out by observation. Digital examination, if necessary, is done by a physician or nurse practitioner. The

## HINTS FOR PRACTICE

Always examine more closely any infant who is reluctant to move an extremity. Fractures are often asymptomatic in the newborn; paralytic injuries are characterized by immobility of an extremity.

nurse also notes the passage of the first meconium stool. Atresia of the gastrointestinal tract or meconium ileus with resultant obstruction must be considered if the newborn does not pass meconium in the first 24 hours of life.

## EXTREMITIES

Extremities are examined for gross deformities, extra digits or webbing, clubfoot, and range of motion. Normal newborn extremities appear short, are generally flexible, and move symmetrically.

### ARMS AND HANDS

Nails extend beyond the fingertips in term newborns. The nurse should count fingers and toes. *Polydactyly* is the presence of extra digits on either the hands or the feet. *Syndactyly* refers to fusion (webbing) of fingers or toes. The hands are inspected for normal palmar creases. A single palmar crease, called *simian line* (see Figure 5–16♦), is frequently present in children with Down syndrome.

*Brachial palsy,* paralysis of portions of the arm, results from trauma to the brachial plexus during a difficult birth. It occurs commonly when strong traction is exerted on the head of the newborn in an attempt to deliver a shoulder lodged behind the symphysis pubis in the presence of shoulder dystocia. Brachial palsy may also occur during a breech birth if an arm becomes trapped over the head and traction is exerted.

The portion of the arm affected is determined by the nerves damaged. **Erb-Duchenne paralysis (Erb's palsy)** involves damage to the upper arm (fifth and sixth cervical nerves) and is the most common type. Injury to the eighth cervical and first thoracic nerve roots and the lower portion of the plexus produces the relatively rare *lower arm injury.* The *whole-arm type* results from damage to the entire plexus.

With Erb-Duchenne paralysis the newborn's arm lies limply at the side. The elbow is held in extension, with the forearm pronated. The newborn is unable to elevate the arm, and the Moro reflex cannot be elicited on the affected side (Figure 22–33♦). Lower arm injury causes paralysis of the hand and wrist; complete paralysis of the limb occurs with the whole-arm type.

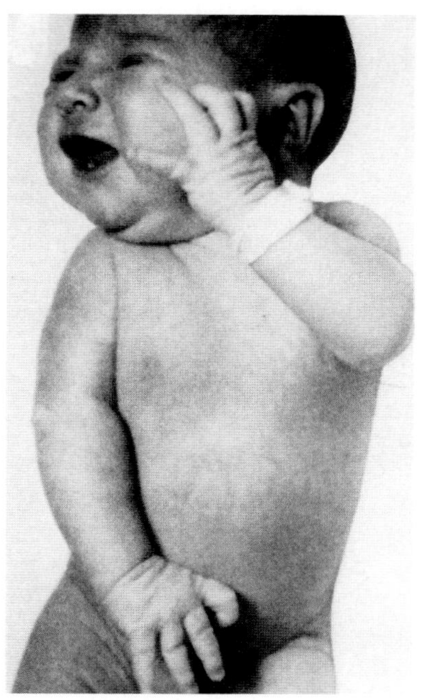

FIGURE 22–33 ♦ Right Erb's palsy resulting from injury to the fifth and sixth cervical roots of the brachial plexus. *Source:* Potter, E. L., & Craig, J. M. (1975). *Pathology of the fetus and infant* (3rd ed.). Chicago: Year Book Medical Publishers. Reproduced with permission.

The nurse carefully instructs the parents in the correct method of performing passive range of motion exercises (to prevent muscle contractures and restore function) and arranges supervised practice sessions. In more severe cases, splinting of the arm is indicated until the edema decreases. The arm is held in a position of abduction and external rotation with the elbow flexed 90 degrees.

Complete recovery occurs within a few months with minimal trauma (amount of nerve damage resulting from trauma and hemorrhage within the nerve sheath). Routine orthopedic follow-up should occur in all cases, because growth plate problems can occur years later. Moderate trauma may result in partial paralysis. Recovery is unlikely with severe trauma, and muscle wasting may develop.

### LEGS AND FEET

The legs of the newborn should be of equal length, with symmetrical skin folds. However, they may assume a "fetal posture" secondary to position in utero, and it may take several days for the legs to relax into a normal position. The nurse performs **Ortolani's maneuver** to rule out the possibility of congenital hip dysplasia (hip dislocation). With the newborn relaxed and quiet on a firm surface, with hips and knees flexed at a 90-degree angle, the nurse grasps the infant's thigh with the middle finger over the greater trochanter and lifts the thigh to bring the femoral head from its posterior position toward the acetabulum. With gentle abduction of the thigh, the

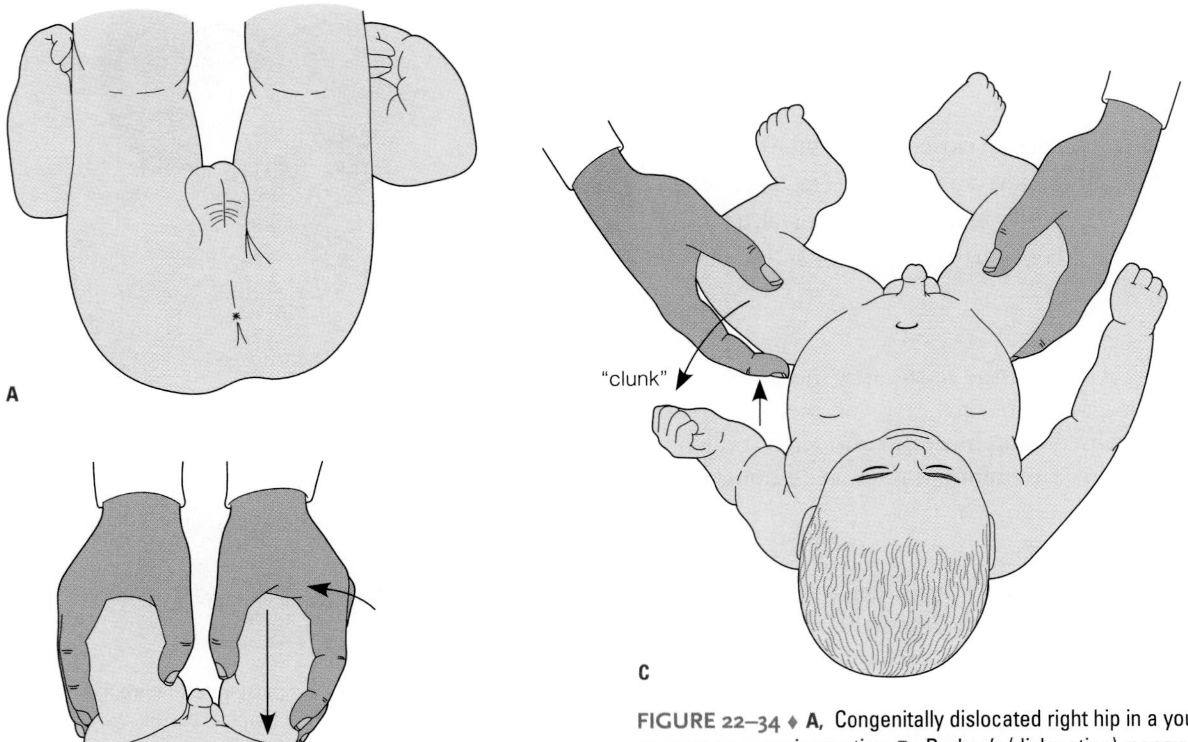


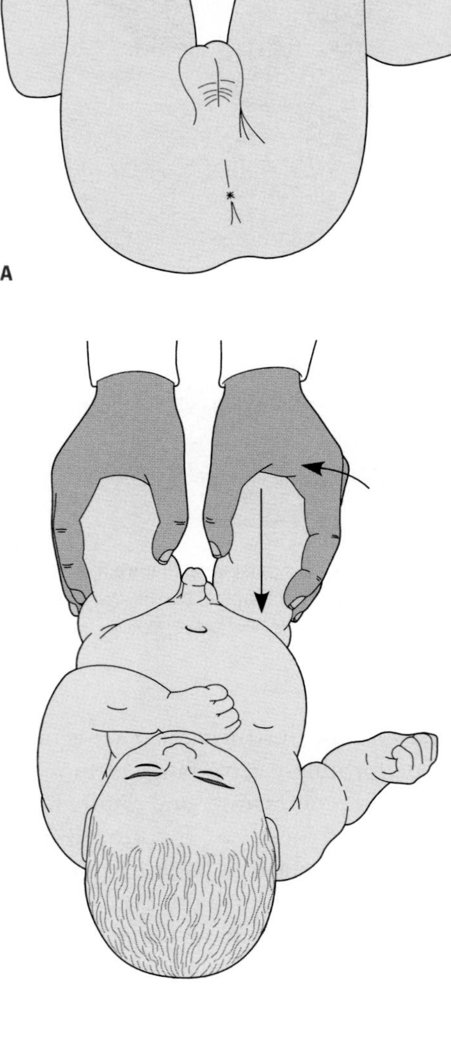

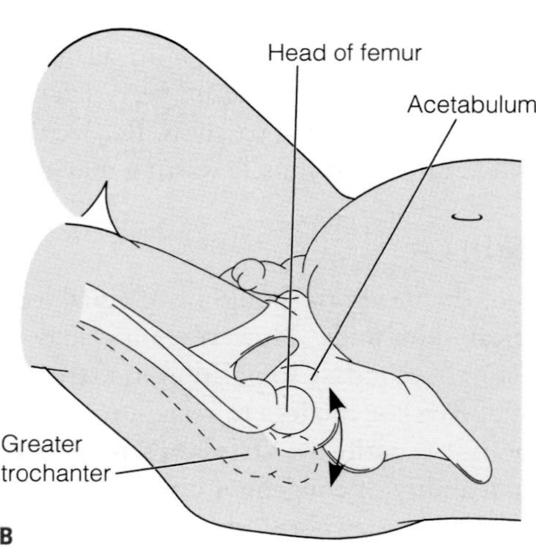


FIGURE 22–34 ♦ **A,** Congenitally dislocated right hip in a young infant as seen on gross inspection. **B,** Barlow's (dislocation) maneuver. Baby's thigh is grasped and adducted with gentle downward pressure. Dislocation is palpable as femoral head slips out of acetabulum. **C,** Ortolani's maneuver puts downward pressure on the hip and then inward rotation. If the hip is dislocated, this maneuver forces the femoral head over the acetabular rim with a noticeable “clunk.”

femoral head is returned to the acetabulum. Simultaneously, the examiner feels a sense of reduction or a “clunk” as the femoral head returns. This reduction is audible. With **Barlow's maneuver,** the nurse grasps and adducts the infant's thigh and applies gentle downward pressure. Dislocation is felt as the femoral head is then returned to the acetabulum using Ortolani's maneuver, confirming the diagnosis of an unstable or dislocated hip (Figure 22–34♦).

The nurse examines the feet for evidence of clubfoot. Intrauterine position frequently causes the feet to appear to turn inward (Figure 22–35♦). This finding is termed a “positional” clubfoot. If the feet can easily be returned to the midline by manipulation, no treatment is indicated and the nurse teaches range of motion exercises to the family. Further investigation is indicated when the foot will not turn to a midline position or align readily. This condition is a severe “true clubfoot,” or talipes equinovarus.

## Back

With the newborn prone, the nurse examines the back. The spine should appear straight and flat, since the lumbar and sacral curves do not develop until the newborn begins to sit. The nurse then examines the base of the spine for a dermal sinus. A nevus pilosus (“hairy nerve”) is only occasionally found at the base of the spine in newborns, but it is significant because it is frequently associated with spina bifida. A pilonidal dimple should be examined to ascertain that there is no connection to the spinal canal.

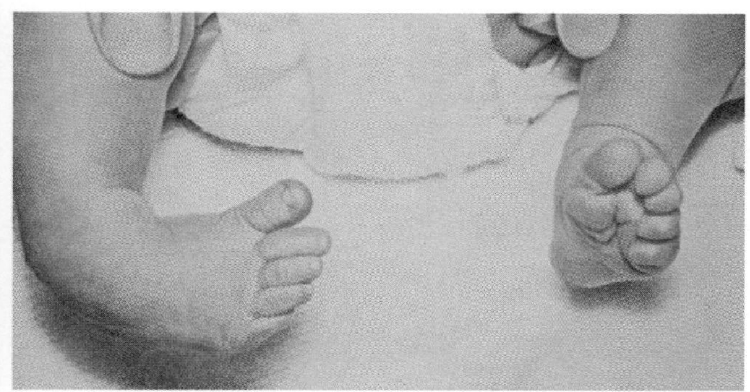

A

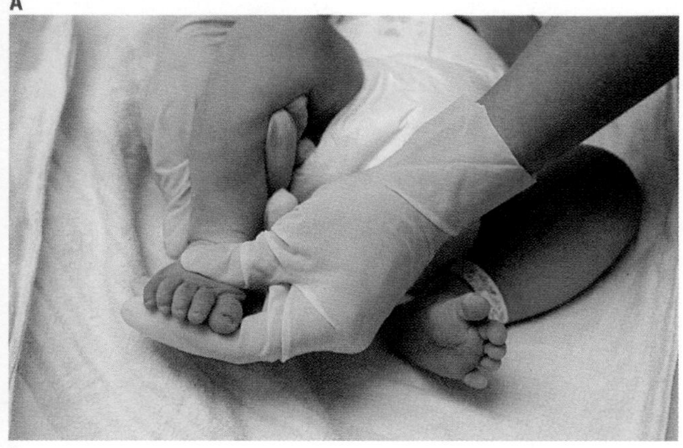

B

FIGURE 22–35 ♦ **A,** Unilateral talipes equinovarus (clubfoot). **B,** To determine the presence of clubfoot, the nurse moves the foot to the midline. Resistance indicates true clubfoot.

## Assessment of Neurologic Status

The neurologic examination should begin with a period of observation, noting the general physical characteristics and behaviors of the newborn. Important behaviors to assess are the *state of alertness, resting posture, cry,* and *quality of muscle tone* and *motor activity.*

The usual position of the newborn is with partially flexed extremities, with the legs abducted to the abdomen. When awake, the newborn may exhibit purposeless, uncoordinated bilateral movements of the extremities. If these movements are absent, minimal, or obviously asymmetrical, neurologic dysfunction should be suspected. Eye movements are observable during the first few days of life. An alert newborn is able to fixate on faces and brightly colored objects. A bright light shining in the newborn's eyes elicits the blinking response.

The nurse evaluates muscle tone by moving various parts of the body while the head of the newborn is in a neutral position. The newborn is somewhat hypertonic; that is, there should be resistance to extending the elbow and knee joints. Muscle tone should be symmetrical. Diminished muscle tone and flaccidity require further evaluation.

Tremors are common in the full-term newborn and must be evaluated to differentiate them from convulsions. A fine jumping of the muscle is likely to be a central nervous system (CNS) disorder and requires further evaluation. Tremors may also be related to hypoglycemia or hypocalcemia. Newborn seizures may consist of no more than chewing or swallowing movements, deviations of the eyes, rigidity, or flaccidity because of CNS immaturity.

The nurse can elicit specific deep tendon reflexes, but they have limited value unless they are obviously asymmetrical. The knee jerk is typically brisk; a normal ankle clonus may involve three or four beats. Plantar flexion is present.

The immature CNS of the newborn is characterized by a variety of reflexes. Because the newborn's movements are uncoordinated, methods of communication are limited, and control of bodily functions is drastically limited, the reflexes serve a variety of purposes. Some are protective (blink, gag, sneeze), some aid in feeding (rooting, sucking) and may not be very active if the infant has eaten recently, and some stimulate human interaction (grasping). Newborn reflex and general neurologic activity should be carefully assessed (Pressler & Hepworth, 1997).

The most common reflexes found in the normal newborn are the following:

- The **tonic neck reflex** (fencer position) is elicited when the newborn is supine and the head is turned to one side. In response, the extremities on the same side straighten, whereas on the opposite side they flex (Figure 22–36♦). This reflex may not be seen during the early newborn period, but once it appears it persists until about the third month.
- The **Moro reflex** is elicited when the newborn is startled by a loud noise or lifted slightly above the crib and then suddenly lowered. In response, the newborn straightens arms and hands outward while the knees flex. Slowly the arms return to the chest, as in an embrace. The fingers spread, forming a C, and the newborn may cry (Figure 22–37♦). This reflex may persist until about 6 months of age.
- The **grasping reflex** is elicited by stimulating the newborn's palm with a finger or object; the newborn grasps and holds the object or finger firmly enough to be lifted momentarily from the crib (Figure 22–38♦).
- The **rooting reflex** is elicited when the side of the newborn's mouth or cheek is touched. In response, the newborn turns toward that side and opens the lips to suck (if not fed recently) (Figure 22–39♦).

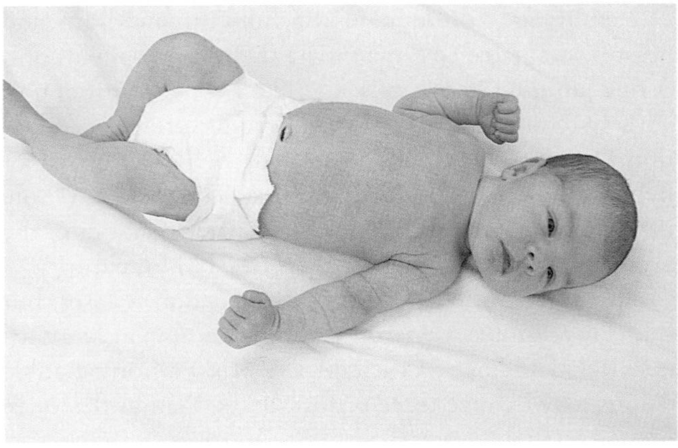

FIGURE 22–36 ♦ Tonic neck reflex.

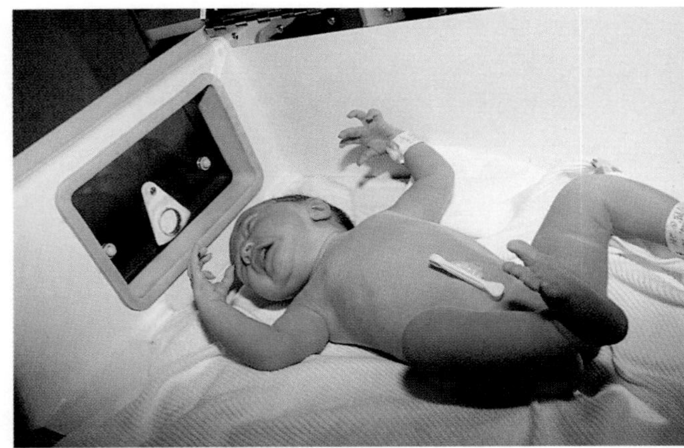

FIGURE 22–37 ♦ Moro reflex.

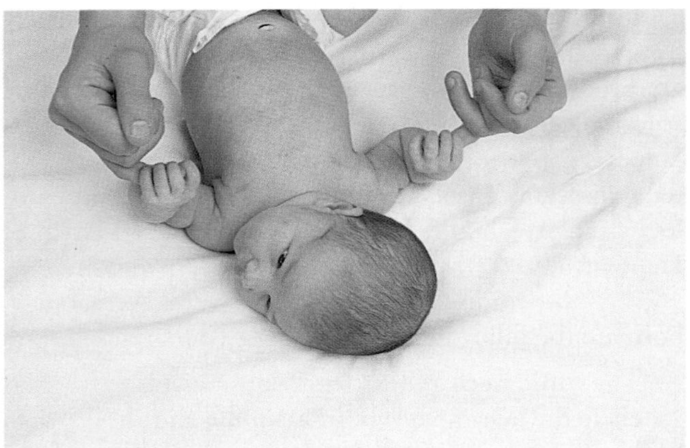

FIGURE 22–38 ♦ Grasping reflex.

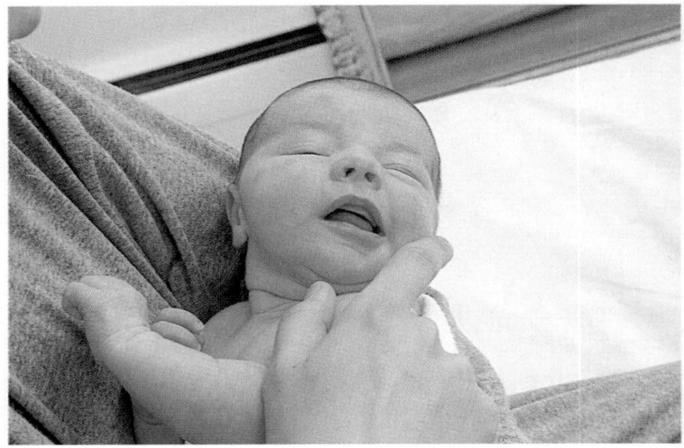

FIGURE 22–39 ♦ Rooting reflex.

- The **sucking reflex** is elicited when an object is placed in the newborn's mouth or anything touches the lips. Newborns suck even while sleeping; this is called nonnutritive sucking, and it can have a quieting effect on the baby.
- The **Babinski reflex,** or fanning and hyperextension of all toes, occurs when the lateral aspect of the sole is stroked from the heel upward across the ball of the foot. In adults, the toes flex.
- **Trunk incurvation (Galant reflex)** is seen when the newborn is prone. Stroking the spine causes the pelvis to turn to the stimulated side.

In addition to these reflexes, newborns can *blink, yawn, cough, sneeze,* and draw back from pain (protective reflexes). They can even move a little on their own. When placed on their stomachs, they push up and try to crawl (*prone crawl*). When held upright with one foot touching a flat surface, the newborn puts one foot in front of the other and "walks" (*stepping reflex*) (Figure 22–40♦). This reflex is more pronounced at birth and is lost in 4 to 5 months.

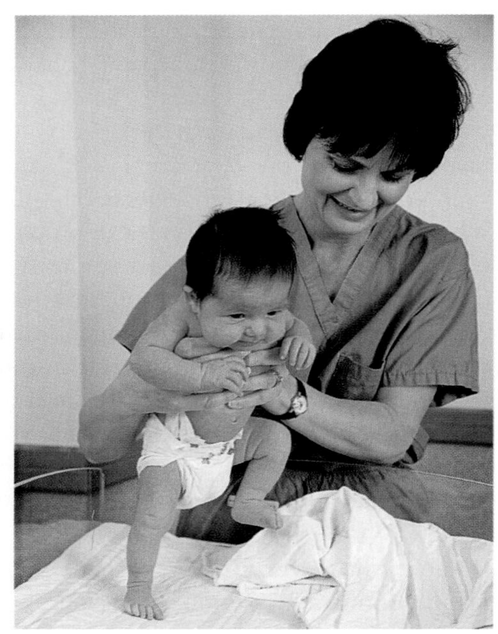

FIGURE 22–40 ♦ The stepping reflex disappears after about 4 to 5 months.

The following steps can be used as a means of assessing CNS integration:

1. Insert a gloved finger into the newborn's mouth to elicit a sucking reflex.
2. As soon as the newborn is sucking vigorously, assess hearing and vision responses by noting changes in sucking in the presence of a light, a rattle, and a voice.
3. The newborn should respond to such stimuli with a brief cessation of sucking, followed by continuous sucking with repetitious stimulation.

This examination demonstrates auditory and visual integrity as well as the capability of complex behavioral interactions (Pressler & Hepworth, 1997). The Newborn Physical Assessment Guide summarizes the stimulus for, and response of, the common newborn reflexes.

## Newborn Physical Assessment Guide

Following is a guide for systematically assessing the newborn (pages 568–581). Normal findings, alterations, and related causes are presented and correlated with suggested nursing responses. The findings are typical for a full-term newborn.

## Newborn Behavioral Assessment

Two conflicting forces influence parents' perceptions of their newborn. One is their preconceptions, based on hopes and fears, of what their newborn will be like. The other is their initial reaction to the baby's temperament, behaviors, and physical appearance. Nurses can assist parents in identifying their baby's specific behaviors.

The **Brazelton Neonatal Behavioral Assessment Scale** provides valuable guidelines for assessing the newborn's state changes, temperament, and individual behavior patterns. It provides a means by which the health care provider, in conjunction with the parents (primary caregivers), can identify and understand the individual newborn's states and capabilities. Families learn which responses, interventions, or activities best meet the special needs of their newborn, and this understanding fosters positive attachment experiences.

The assessment tool identifies the newborn's repertoire of behavioral responses to the environment and also documents the newborn's neurologic adequacy and capabilities. The examination usually takes 20 to 30 minutes and involves about 30 tests. Some items are scored according to the newborn's response to specific stimuli. Others, such as consolability and alertness, are scored as a result of continuous behavioral observations throughout the assessment. (For a complete discussion of all test items and maneuvers, see Brazelton & Nugent, 1995.)

## Critical Thinking in Practice

Maria Reyes, a 19-year-old G2 now P2 mother, delivered a 40-week-old female neonate 24 hours ago. The newborn exam was normal. Mrs. Reyes asks about the newborn's exam. She says she has noticed that the baby cries more than her first child did and seems to require holding for longer periods of time after feeding before "quieting down." She is concerned that there is something she is doing wrong and wants to know when her newborn will start to act like her first baby. What should you discuss with her about newborn behavior?

Answers can be found in Appendix I.

Assessment of the newborn should be carried out initially in a quiet, softly lit room, if possible. First the nurse determines the newborn's state of consciousness, because scoring and introduction of the test items are correlated with the sleep or waking state. The newborn's state depends on physiologic variables, such as the amount of time from the last feeding, positioning, environmental temperature, and health status; presence of such external stimuli as noises and bright lights; and the wake-sleep cycle of the newborn. An important characteristic of the newborn period is the pattern of states, as well as the transitions from one state to another. The pattern of states is a predictor of the newborn's receptivity and ability to respond to stimuli in a cognitive manner. Babies learn best in a quiet, alert state and in an environment that is supportive and protective and that provides appropriate stimuli.

The nurse should observe the newborn's sleep-wake patterns (as discussed in Chapter 23), including the rapidity with which the newborn moves from one state to another, ability to be consoled, and ability to diminish the impact of disturbing stimuli. The following questions may provide the nurse with a framework for assessment:

- Does the newborn's response style and ability to adapt to stimuli indicate a need for parental interventions that will alert the newborn to the environment so that he or she can grow socially and cognitively?
- Are parental interventions necessary to lessen the outside stimuli, as in the case of the baby who responds to sensory input with intensity?
- Can the baby control the amount of sensory input that he or she must deal with?

Text continues on page 581.

# NEWBORN PHYSICAL ASSESSMENT GUIDE

| Physical Assessment/ Normal Findings | Alterations and Possible Causes* | Nursing Responses to Data† |
|---|---|---|
| **Vital Signs** | | |
| *Blood pressure (BP)* | | |
| At birth: 80–60/45–40 mm Hg<br>Day 10: 100/50 mm Hg (may be unable to measure diastolic pressure with standard sphygmomanometer) | Low BP (hypovolemia, shock) | Monitor BP in all cases of distress, prematurity, or suspected anomaly.<br>Low BP: Refer to physician immediately so measures to improve circulation are begun. |
| *Pulse* | | |
| 120–160 bpm (if asleep, 100 bpm; if crying, up to 180 bpm) | Weak pulse (decreased cardiac output) | Assess skin perfusion by blanching (capillary refill test). |
| | Bradycardia (severe asphyxia, arrhythmia) | Correlate finding with BP assessments; refer to physician. |
| | Tachycardia (over 160 bpm at rest) (infection, central nervous system problems, arrhythmia) | Carry out neurologic and thermoregulation assessments. |
| *Respirations* | | |
| 30–60 breaths/minute<br>Synchronization of chest and abdominal movements<br>Diaphragmatic and abdominal breathing | Tachypnea (pneumonia, respiratory distress syndrome [RDS])<br>Rapid, shallow breathing (hypermagnesemia due to large doses given to mothers with PIH)<br>Respirations below 30 breaths/minute (maternal anesthesia or analgesia) | Identify sleep-wake state; correlate with respiratory pattern.<br>Evaluate for all signs of respiratory distress; report findings to physician. |
| Transient tachypnea | Expiratory grunting; subcostal and substernal retractions; flaring of nares (respiratory distress); apnea (cold stress, respiratory disorder) | Evaluate for cold stress.<br>Report findings to physician or nurse practitioner. |
| *Crying* | | |
| Strong and lusty<br>Moderate tone and pitch<br>Cries vary in length from 3 to 7 minutes after consoling measures are used | High pitched, shrill (neurologic disorder, hypoglycemia)<br>Weak or absent (CNS disorder, laryngeal problem) | Discuss newborn's use of cry for communication.<br>Assess and record abnormal cries.<br>Reduce environmental noises. |
| *Temperature* | | |
| Axilla 36.4–37.2°C (97.5–99°F)<br>Rectal 36.6–37.2°C (97.8–99°F); 36.8°C (98.8°F) desired<br>Heavier neonates tend to have higher body temperatures | Elevated temperature (room too warm, too much clothing or covers, dehydration, sepsis, brain damage)<br>Subnormal temperature (brain stem involvement, cold, sepsis)<br>Swings of more than 2°F from one reading to next or subnormal temperature (infection) | Notify physician of elevation or drop.<br>Counsel parents on possible causes of elevated or low temperatures, appropriate home care measures, when to call physician.<br>Teach parents how to take rectal and/or axillary temperature; assess parents' information regarding use of thermometer; provide teaching as needed. |
| *Weight* | | |
| 2500–4000 g (5 lb, 8 oz–8 lb, 13 oz) | $<$2748 g ($<$6 lb) = SGA or preterm infant<br>$>$4050 g ($>$9 lb) = LGA or infants of diabetic mothers | Plot weight and gestational age on growth chart to identify high-risk infants.<br>Ascertain body build of parents.<br>Counsel parents regarding appropriate caloric intake. |
| Within first 3 to 4 days, normal weight loss of 5%–10%<br>Large babies tend to lose more due to greater fluid loss in proportion to birth weight except infants of diabetic mothers | Loss greater than 15% (small fluid intake, loss of meconium and urine, feeding difficulties) | Notify physician of net losses or gains. Calculate fluid intake and losses from all sources (insensible water loss, radiant warmers, phototherapy lights). |

***Possible causes of alterations are placed in parentheses.**

**†This column provides guidelines for further assessment and initial nursing interventions.**

# NEWBORN PHYSICAL ASSESSMENT GUIDE *continued*

| Physical Assessment/ Normal Findings | Alterations and Possible Causes* | Nursing Responses to Data† |
|---|---|---|
| *Length* | | |
| 48–52 cm (18–22 in)<br>Grows 10 cm (3 in) during first 3 months | Less than 45 cm (congenital dwarf)<br>Short/long bones proximally (achondroplasia)<br>Short/long bones distally (Ellis–Van Creveld syndrome) | Assess for other signs of dwarfism.<br>Determine other signs of skeletal system adequacy.<br>Plot progress at subsequent well-baby visits. |
| **Posture** | | |
| Body usually flexed, hands may be tightly clenched, neck appears short because chin rests on chest<br>In breech births feet are usually dorsiflexed | Only extension noted, inability to move from midline (trauma, hypoxia, immaturity)<br>Constant motion (maternal caffeine intake) | Record spontaneity of motor activity and symmetry of movements.<br>If parents express concern about newborn's movement patterns, reassure and further evaluate if appropriate. |
| **Skin** | | |
| *Color* | | |
| Color consistent with genetic background<br>Newborns of European descent: pink-tinged or ruddy color over face, trunk, extremities<br>Newborns of African or Native American descent: pale pink with yellow or red tinge<br>Newborns of Asian descent: pink or rosy red to yellow tinge | Pallor of face, conjunctiva (anemia, hypothermia, anoxia)<br>Beefy red (hypoglycemia, immature vasomotor reflexes, polycythemia) | Discuss with parents common skin color variations to allay fears.<br>Document extent and time of occurrence of color change. |
| Common variations: acrocyanosis, circumoral cyanosis, or harlequin color change | Meconium staining (fetal distress)<br>Jaundice (hemolytic reaction from blood incompatibility within first 24 hours, sepsis) | Assess for respiratory difficulty.<br>Obtain Hb and hematocrit values; obtain bilirubin levels.<br>Differentiate between physiologic and pathologic jaundice. |
| Mottled when undressed | Cyanosis (choanal atresia, CNS damage or trauma, respiratory or cardiac problem, cold stress) | Assess degree of (central or peripheral) cyanosis and possible causes; refer to physician. |
| Minor bruising over buttocks in breech presentation and over eyes and forehead in facial presentations | | Discuss with parents cause and course of minor bruising related to labor and birth. |
| *Texture* | | |
| Smooth, soft, flexible; may have dry, peeling hands and feet | Generalized cracked or peeling skin (SGA or postterm; blood incompatibility; metabolic, kidney dysfunction)<br>Seborrheic-dermatitis (cradle cap)<br>Absence of vernix (postmature)<br>Yellow vernix (bilirubin staining) | Report to physician.<br>Instruct parents to shampoo the scalp and anterior fontanelle areas daily with soap; rinse well; avoid use of oil. |
| *Turgor* | | |
| Elastic, returns to normal shape after pinching | Maintains tent shape (dehydration) | Assess for other signs and symptoms of dehydration. |
| *Pigmentation* | | |
| Clear; milia across bridge of nose, forehead, or chin will disappear within a few weeks | | Advise parents not to pinch or prick these pimplelike areas. |
| Café-au-lait spots (one or two) | Six or more (neurologic disorder such as Von Recklinghausen disease, cutaneous neurofibromatosis) | If there are six or more café-au-lait spots, refer for genetic and neurologic consult. |
| Mongolian spots common over dorsal area and buttocks in dark-skinned infants | | Assure parents of normalcy of this pigmentation; it will fade in first year or two. |

***Possible causes of alterations are placed in parentheses.**

**†This column provides guidelines for further assessment and initial nursing interventions.**

## NEWBORN PHYSICAL ASSESSMENT GUIDE *continued*

| Physical Assessment/ Normal Findings | Alterations and Possible Causes* | Nursing Responses to Data† |
|---|---|---|
| Erythema toxicum | Impetigo (group A β-hemolytic streptococcus or *Staphylococcus aureus* infection) | If impetigo occurs, instruct parents about handwashing and linen precautions during home care. |
| Telangiectatic nevi | Hemangiomas:<br>Nevus flammeus (port-wine stain)<br>Nevus vasculosus (strawberry hemangioma)<br>Cavernous hemangiomas | Collaborate with physician.<br>Counsel parents about birthmark's progression to allay misconceptions.<br>Record size and shape of hemangiomas.<br>Refer for follow-up at well-baby clinic. |
| Rashes | Rashes (infection) | Assess location and type of rash (macular, papular, vesicular).<br>Obtain history of onset, prenatal history, and related signs and symptoms. |
| Petechiae of head or neck (breech presentation, cord around neck) | Generalized petechiae (clotting abnormalities) | Determine cause; advise parents if further health care is needed. |
| **Head** | | |
| General appearance, size, movement<br>Round, symmetric, and moves easily from left to right and up and down; soft and pliable | Asymmetric, flattened occiput on either side of the head (plagiocephaly)<br>Head held at angle (torticollis) | Instruct parents to change infant's sleeping positions frequently. |
| | Unable to move head side to side (neurologic trauma) | Determine adequacy of all neurologic signs. |
| Circumference: 32–37 cm (12.5–14.5 in); 2 cm greater than chest circumference<br>Head one-fourth of body size | Extreme differences in size may be due to microencephaly (Cornelia de Lange syndrome, cytomegalic inclusion disease [CID]), rubella, toxoplasmosis, chromosome abnormalities), hydrocephalus (meningomyelocele, achondroplasia), anencephaly (neural tube defect)<br>Head is 3 cm or more larger than chest circumference (preterm, hydrocephalus) | Measure circumference from occiput to frontal area using metal or paper tape.<br>Measure chest circumference using metal or paper tape and compare to head circumference.<br>Record measurements on growth chart.<br>Reevaluate at well-baby visits. |
| *Common variations* | | |
| Molding<br>Breech and cesarean newborns' heads are round and well shaped | Cephalhematoma (trauma during birth, persists up to 3 weeks)<br>Caput succedaneum (long labor and birth; disappears in 1 week) | Evaluate neurologic response.<br>Observe for hyperbilirubinemia.<br>Reassure parents regarding common manifestations due to birth process and when they should disappear. |
| *Fontanelles* | | |
| Palpation of juncture of cranial bones<br>Anterior fontanelle: 3–4 cm long by 2–3 cm wide, diamond shaped<br>Posterior fontanelle: 1–2 cm at birth, triangle shaped | Overlapping of anterior fontanelle (malnourished or preterm newborn)<br>Premature closure of sutures (craniostenosis)<br>Late closure (hydrocephalus) | Discuss normal closure times with parents and care of "soft spots" to allay misconceptions.<br>Refer to physician.<br>Observe for signs and symptoms of hydrocephalus. |
| Slight pulsation | Moderate to severe pulsation (vascular problems) | Refer to physician. |
| Moderate bulging noted with crying, stooling; pulsations with heartbeat | Bulging (increased intracranial pressure, meningitis)<br>Sunken (dehydration) | Evaluate hydration status.<br>Evaluate neurologic status.<br>Report to physician. |

***Possible causes of alterations are placed in parentheses.**

**†This column provides guidelines for further assessment and initial nursing interventions.**

## NEWBORN PHYSICAL ASSESSMENT GUIDE *continued*

| Physical Assessment/ Normal Findings | Alterations and Possible Causes* | Nursing Responses to Data† |
|---|---|---|
| **Hair** | | |
| *Texture* | | |
| Smooth with fine texture variations (*Note:* Variations depend on ethnic background.) | Coarse, brittle, dry hair ((hypothyroidism)<br>White forelock (Waardenburg syndrome) | Instruct parents regarding routine care of hair and scalp. |
| *Distribution* | | |
| Scalp hair high over eyebrows (Spanish-Mexican hairline begins midforehead and extends down back of neck.) | Low forehead and posterior hairlines may indicate chromosomal disorders. | Assess for other signs of chromosomal aberrations.<br>Refer to physician. |
| **Face** | | |
| Symmetric movement of all facial features, normal hairline, eyebrows and eyelashes present | | Assess and record symmetry of all parts, shape, regularity of features, sameness or differences in features. |
| *Spacing of features* | | |
| Eyes at same level, nostrils equal size, cheeks full, and sucking pads present | Eyes wide apart—ocular hypertelorism (Apert syndrome, cri-du-chat, Turner syndrome) | Observe for other signs and symptoms indicative of disease states or chromosomal aberrations. |
| Lips equal on both sides of midline | Abnormal face (Down syndrome, cretinism, gargoylism) | |
| Chin recedes when compared to other bones of face | Abnormally small jaw—micrognathia (Pierre Robin syndrome, Treacher Collins syndrome) | Maintain airway; do not position supine.<br>Initiate surgical consultation and referral. |
| *Movement* | | |
| Makes facial grimaces | Inability to suck, grimace, and close eyelids (cranial nerve injury) | Initiate neurologic assessment and consultation. |
| Symmetric when resting and crying | Asymmetry (paralysis of facial cranial nerve) | Assess and record symmetry of all parts, shape, regularity of features, and sameness or differences in features. |
| **Eyes** | | |
| *General placement and appearance* | | |
| Bright and clear; even placement; slight nystagmus (involuntary cyclical eye movements) | Gross nystagmus (damage to third, fourth, and sixth cranial nerves) | |
| Concomitant strabismus | Constant and fixed strabismus | Reassure parents that strabismus is considered normal up to 6 months. |
| Move in all directions | | |
| Blue- or slate-blue gray | Lack of pigmentation (albinism)<br>Brushfield spots may indicate Down syndrome (a light or white speckling of the outer two-thirds of the iris) | Discuss with parents any necessary eye precautions.<br>Assess for other signs of Down syndrome. |
| Brown color at birth in dark-skinned infants | | Discuss with parents that permanent eye color is usually established by 3 months of age. |
| | ***Possible causes of alterations are placed in parentheses.** | **†This column provides guidelines for further assessment and initial nursing interventions.** |

## NEWBORN PHYSICAL ASSESSMENT GUIDE *continued*

| Physical Assessment/ Normal Findings | Alterations and Possible Causes* | Nursing Responses to Data† |
|---|---|---|
| *Eyelids* | | |
| Position: above pupils but within iris, no drooping | Elevation or retraction of upper lid (hyperthyroidism) | Assess for signs of hydrocephalus and hyperthyroidism. |
| | "Sunset sign" lid retraction and downward gaze (hydrocephalus), ptosis (congenital or paralysis of oculomotor muscle) | Evaluate interference with vision in subsequent well-baby visits. |
| Eyes on parallel plane<br>Epicanthal folds in Asian and 20% of newborns of northern European descent | Upward slant in non-Asians (Down syndrome)<br>Epicanthal folds (Down syndrome, cri-du-chat syndrome) | Assess for other signs of Down syndrome. |
| *Movement* | | |
| Blink reflex in response to light stimulus<br>Eyes open wide in dimly lit room | Blink absent (CNS injury) | Evaluate neurologic status.<br>Refer to physician. |
| *Inspection* | | |
| Edematous for first few days of life, resulting from birth and instillation of silver nitrate (chemical conjunctivitis); no lumps or redness | Purulent drainage (infection); infectious conjunctivitis (gonococcus, chlamydia, staphylococcus, or gram-negative organisms)<br>Marginal blepharitis (lid edges red, crusted, scaly) | Initiate good handwashing.<br>Refer to physician.<br>Evaluate infant for seborrheic dermatitis; scales can be removed easily. |
| *Cornea* | | |
| Clear<br>Corneal reflex present | Ulceration (herpes infection); large cornea or corneas of unequal size (congenital glaucoma)<br>Clouding, opacity of lens (cataract) | Refer to ophthalmologist.<br>Assess for other manifestations of congenital herpes; institute nursing care measures. |
| *Sclera* | | |
| May appear bluish in newborn, then white; slightly brownish color frequent in newborns of African descent | True blue sclera (osteogenesis imperfecta) | Refer to physician. |
| *Pupils* | | |
| Pupils equal in size, round, and react to light by accommodation | Anisocoria—unequal pupils (CNS damage)<br>Dilation or constriction (intracranial damage, retinoblastoma, glaucoma)<br>Pupils nonreactive to light or accommodation (brain injury) | Refer for neurologic examination. |
| Slight nystagmus in newborn who has not learned to focus<br>Pupil light reflex demonstrated at birth or by 3 weeks of age | Nystagmus (labyrinthine disturbance, CNS disorder) | |
| *Conjunctiva* | | |
| Chemical conjunctivitis<br>Subconjunctival hemorrhage | Pale color (anemia) | Obtain hematocrit and hemoglobin.<br>Reassure parents that chemical conjunctivitis will subside in 1 to 2 days and subconjunctival hemorrhage disappears in a few weeks. |
| Palpebral conjunctiva (red but not hyperemic) | Inflammation or edema (infection, blocked tear duct) | |
| | ***Possible causes of alterations are placed in parentheses.** | **†This column provides guidelines for further assessment and initial nursing interventions.** |

## NEWBORN PHYSICAL ASSESSMENT GUIDE *continued*

| Physical Assessment/ Normal Findings | Alterations and Possible Causes* | Nursing Responses to Data† |
|---|---|---|
| *Vision* | | |
| 20/150<br>Tracks moving object to midline<br>Fixed focus on objects at a distance of about 10–20 in; may be difficult to evaluate in newborn<br>Prefers faces, geometric designs, and black and white to colors | Cataracts (congenital infection) | Record any questions about visual acuity and initiate follow-up evaluation at first well-baby checkup. |
| *Lashes and lacrimal glands* | | |
| Presence of lashes (lashes may be absent in preterm newborns) | No lashes on inner two-thirds of lid (Treacher Collins syndrome); bushy lashes (Hurler syndrome); long lashes (Cornelia de Lange syndrome) | |
| Cry commonly tearless | Excessive tearing (plugged lacrimal duct, natal narcotic withdrawal), glaucoma | Demonstrate to parents how to milk blocked tear duct.<br>Refer to ophthalmologist if tearing is excessive before third month of life. |
| **Nose** | | |
| *Appearance of external nasal aspects* | | |
| May appear flattened as a result of birth process | Continued flat or broad bridge of nose (Down syndrome) | Arrange consultation with specialist. |
| Small and narrow in midline, even placement in relationship to eyes and mouth | Low bridge of nose, beaklike nose (Apert syndrome, Treacher Collins syndrome)<br>Upturned (Cornelia de Lange syndrome) | Initiate evaluation of chromosomal abnormalities. |
| Patent nares bilaterally (nose breathers) | Blockage of nares (mucus and/or secretions), choanal atresia | Inspect for obstruction of nares.<br>Maintain oral airway until surgical correction is made. |
| Sneezing common to clear nasal passages | Flaring nares (respiratory distress) | |
| Responds to odors, may smell breast milk | No response to stimulating odors | Inspect for obstruction of nares. |
| **Mouth** | | |
| *Function of facial, hypoglossal, glossopharyngeal, and vagus nerves* | | |
| Symmetry of movement and strength | Mouth draws to one side (transient seventh cranial nerve paralysis due to pressure in utero or trauma during birth, congenital paralysis)<br>Fishlike shape (Treacher Collins syndrome) | Initiate neurologic consultation.<br>Administer eye care if eye on affected side of face is unable to close. |
| Presence of gag, swallowing, coordinated with sucking reflexes<br>Adequate salivation | Suppressed or absent reflexes | Evaluate other neurologic functions of these nerves. |

***Possible causes of alterations are placed in parentheses.**

**†This column provides guidelines for further assessment and initial nursing interventions.**

# NEWBORN PHYSICAL ASSESSMENT GUIDE *continued*

| Physical Assessment/ Normal Findings | Alterations and Possible Causes* | Nursing Responses to Data† |
|---|---|---|
| *Palate (soft and hard)* | | |
| Hard palate dome shaped<br>Uvula midline with symmetrical movement of soft palate | High-steepled palate (Treacher Collins syndrome), bivid uvula (congenital anomaly) | Assess for other congenital anomalies. |
| Palate intact, sucks well when stimulated | Clefts in either hard or soft palate (polygenic disorder) | Initiate a surgical consultation referral. |
| Epithelial (Epstein's) pearls appear on mucosa | | Assure parents that these are normal and will disappear at 2 or 3 months of age. |
| Esophagus patent, some drooling common in newborn | Excessive drooling or bubbling (esophageal atresia) | Test for patency of esophagus. |
| *Tongue* | | |
| Free moving in all directions, midline | Lack of movement or asymmetric movement (neurologic damage)<br>Tongue-tied | Further assess neurologic functions.<br>Test reflex elevation of tongue when depressed with tongue blade. |
| | Deviations from midline (cranial nerve damage) | Check for signs of weakness or deviation. |
| Pink color, smooth to rough texture, noncoated | White cheesy coating (thrush)<br>Tongue has deep ridges | Differentiate between thrush and milk curds.<br>Reassure parents that tongue pattern may change from day to day. |
| Tongue proportional to mouth | Large tongue with short frenulum (cretinism, Down syndrome, other syndromes) | Evaluate in well-baby clinic to assess development delays.<br>Initiate referrals. |
| **Ears** | | |
| *External ear* | | |
| Without lesions, cysts, or nodules | Nodules, cysts, or sinus tracts in front of ear<br>Adherent earlobes<br>Low set | Evaluate characteristics of lesions.<br>Counsel parents to clean external ear with washcloth only; discourage use of cotton-tip applicators. |
| | Preauricular skin tags | Refer to physician for ligation. |
| *Hearing* | | |
| Eustachian tubes are cleared with first cry<br>Absence of all risk factors | Presence of one or more risk factors | Assess history of risk factors for hearing loss. |
| Attends to sounds; sudden or loud noise elicits Moro reflex | No response to sound stimuli (deafness) | Test for Moro reflex. |
| **Neck** | | |
| *Appearance* | | |
| Short, straight, creased with skin folds | Abnormally short neck (Turner syndrome)<br>Arching or inability to flex neck (meningitis, congenital anomaly) | Report findings to physician. |
| Posterior neck lacks loose extra folds of skin | Webbing of neck (Turner syndrome, Down syndrome, trisomy 18) | Assess for other signs of the syndromes. |
| | ***Possible causes of alterations are placed in parentheses.** | **†This column provides guidelines for further assessment and initial nursing interventions.** |

## NEWBORN PHYSICAL ASSESSMENT GUIDE *continued*

| Physical Assessment/ Normal Findings | Alterations and Possible Causes* | Nursing Responses to Data† |
|---|---|---|
| *Clavicles* | | |
| Straight and intact | Knot or lump on clavicle (fracture during difficult birth) | Obtain detailed labor and birth history; apply figure-eight bandage. |
| Moro reflex elicitable | Unilateral Moro reflex response on unaffected side (fracture of clavicle, brachial palsy, Erb-Duchenne paralysis) | Collaborate with physician. |
| Symmetric shoulders | Hypoplasia | |
| **Chest** | | |
| *Appearance and size* | | |
| Circumference: 32.5 cm, 1–2 cm less than head<br>Wider than it is long | | Measure at level of nipples after exhalation. |
| Normal shape without depressed or prominent sternum<br>Lower end of sternum (xiphoid cartilage) may be protruding; less apparent after several weeks<br>Sternum 8 cm long | Funnel chest (congenital or associated with Marfan syndrome)<br>Continued protrusion of xiphoid cartilage (Marfan syndrome, "pigeon chest")<br>Barrel chest | Determine adequacy of other respiratory and circulatory signs.<br>Assess for other signs and symptoms of various syndromes. |
| *Expansion and retraction* | | |
| Bilateral expansion | Unequal chest expansion (pneumonia, pneumothorax, respiratory distress) | Assess respiratory effort regularity, flaring of nares, difficulty on both inspiration and expiration. |
| No intercostal, subcostal, or supracostal retractions | Retractions (respiratory distress)<br>See-saw respirations (respiratory distress) | Record and consult physician. |
| *Auscultation* | | |
| Breath sounds are louder in infants | Decreased breath sounds (decreased respiratory activity, atelectasis, pneumothorax) | Perform assessment and report to physician any positive findings. |
| Chest and axilla clear on crying | Increased breath sounds (resolving pneumonia or in cesarean births) | |
| Bronchial breath sounds (heard where trachea and bronchi closest to chest wall, above sternum and between scapulae):<br>Bronchial sounds bilaterally<br>Air entry clear<br>Rales may indicate normal newborn atelectasis<br>Cough reflex absent at birth, appears in 2 or more days | Adventitious or abnormal sounds (respiratory disease or distress) | Evaluate color for pallor or cyanosis.<br>Report to physician. |
| *Breasts* | | |
| Flat with symmetric nipples<br>Breast tissue diameter 5 cm or more at term<br>Distance between nipples 8 cm | Lack of breast tissue (preterm or SGA)<br>Discharge<br>Enlargement | Evaluate for infection. |
| Breast engorgement occurs on third day of life; liquid discharge may be expressed in term newborns | Breast abscesses | Reassure parents of normality of breast engorgement. |
| Nipples | Supernumerary nipples<br>Dark-colored nipples | No intervention is necessary. |

***Possible causes of alterations are placed in parentheses.**

**†This column provides guidelines for further assessment and initial nursing interventions.**

## NEWBORN PHYSICAL ASSESSMENT GUIDE *continued*

| Physical Assessment/ Normal Findings | Alterations and Possible Causes* | Nursing Responses to Data† |
|---|---|---|
| **Heart** | | |
| *Auscultation* | | |
| Location: lies horizontally, with left border extending to left of midclavicle | | |
| Regular rhythm and rate | Arrhythmia (anoxia), tachycardia, bradycardia | Refer all arrhythmia and gallop rhythms. |
| Determination of point of maximal impulse (PMI)<br>Usually lateral to midclavicular line at third or fourth intercostal space | Malpositioning (enlargement, abnormal placement, pneumothorax, dextrocardia, diaphragmatic hernia) | Initiate cardiac evaluation. |
| Functional murmurs<br>No thrills | Location of murmurs (possible congenital cardiac anomaly) | Evaluate murmur: location, timing, and duration; observe for accompanying cardiac pathology symptoms; ascertain family history. |
| Horizontal groove at diaphragm shows flaring of rib cage to mild degree | Marked rib flaring (vitamin D deficiency)<br>Inadequacy of respiratory movement | Initiate cardiopulmonary evaluation; assess pulses and blood pressures in all four extremities for equality and quality. |
| **Abdomen** | | |
| *Appearance* | | |
| Cylindrical, with some protrusion; appears large in relation to pelvis; some laxness of abdominal muscles<br>No cyanosis, few vessels seen<br>Diastasis recti—common in infants of African descent | Distension, shiny abdomen with engorged vessels (gastrointestinal abnormalities, infection, congenital megacolon)<br>Scaphoid abdominal appearance (diaphragmatic hernia)<br>Increased or decreased peristalsis (duodenal stenosis, small bowel obstruction)<br>Localized flank bulging (enlarged kidneys, ascites, absent abdominal muscles) | Examine abdomen thoroughly for mass or organomegaly.<br>Measure abdominal girth.<br>Report deviations of abdominal size.<br>Assess other signs and symptoms of obstruction.<br><br>Refer to physician. |
| *Umbilicus* | | |
| No protrusion of umbilicus (protrusion of umbilicus common in infants of African descent)<br>Bluish white color<br>Cutis navel (umbilical cord projects), granulation tissue present in navel | Umbilical hernia<br>Patent urachus (congenital malformation)<br>Omphalocele<br>Gastroschisis<br>Redness or exudate around cord (infection)<br>Yellow discoloration (hemolytic disease, meconium staining) | Measure umbilical hernia by palpating the opening and record; it should close by 1 year of age; if not, refer to physician.<br>Cover omphalocele with sterile, moist dressing.<br>Instruct parents on cord care and hygiene. |
| Two arteries and one vein apparent<br>Begins drying 1 to 2 hours after birth<br>No bleeding | Single umbilical artery (congenital anomalies)<br>Discharge or oozing of blood from the cord | Refer anomalies to physician. |
| Auscultation and percussion<br>Soft bowel sounds heard shortly after birth every 10–30 seconds | Bowel sounds in chest (diaphragmatic hernia)<br>Absence of bowel sounds<br>Hyperperistalsis (intestinal obstruction) | Collaborate with physician.<br><br>Assess for other signs of dehydration and/or infection. |
| *Femoral pulses* | | |
| Palpable, equal, bilateral | Absent or diminished femoral pulses (coarctation of aorta) | Monitor blood pressure in upper and lower extremities. |
| *Inguinal area* | | |
| No bulges along inguinal area<br>No inguinal lymph nodes felt | Inguinal hernia | Initiate referral.<br>Continue follow-up in well-baby clinic. |

***Possible causes of alterations are placed in parentheses.**

**†This column provides guidelines for further assessment and initial nursing interventions.**

# NEWBORN PHYSICAL ASSESSMENT GUIDE *continued*

| Physical Assessment/ Normal Findings | Alterations and Possible Causes* | Nursing Responses to Data† |
|---|---|---|
| *Bladder* | | |
| Percusses 1–4 cm above symphysis<br>Emptied about 3 hours after birth; if not, at time of birth<br>Urine—inoffensive, mild odor | Failure to void within 24–48 hours after birth<br>Exposure of bladder mucosa (exstrophy of bladder)<br>Foul odor (infection) | Check whether baby voided at birth.<br>Obtain urine specimen if infection is suspected.<br>Consult with clinician. |
| **Genitals** | | |
| Gender clearly delineated | Ambiguous genitals | Refer for genetic consultation. |
| **Male** | | |
| *Penis* | | |
| Slender in appearance, about 2.5 cm long, 1 cm wide at birth<br>Normal urinary orifice, urethral meatus at tip of penis | Micropenis (congenital anomaly)<br>Meatal atresia<br>Hypospadias, epispadias | Observe and record first voiding.<br>Collaborate with physician in presence of abnormality. Delay circumcision. |
| Noninflamed urethral opening | Urethritis (infection) | Palpate for enlarged inguinal lymph nodes and record painful urination. |
| Foreskin adheres to glans | Ulceration of meatal opening (infection, inflammation) | Evaluate whether ulcer is due to diaper rash; counsel regarding care. |
| Uncircumcised foreskin tight for 2 to 3 months | Phimosis—if still tight after 3 months | Instruct parents on how to care for uncircumcised penis. |
| Circumcised<br>Erectile tissue present | | Teach parents how to care for circumcision. |
| *Scrotum* | | |
| Skin loose and hanging or tight and small; extensive rugae and normal size<br>Normal skin color<br>Scrotal discoloration common in breech | Large scrotum containing fluid (hydrocele)<br>Red, shiny scrotal skin (orchitis)<br>Minimal rugae, small scrotum | Shine a light through scrotum (transilluminate) to verify diagnosis.<br>Assess for prematurity. |
| *Testes* | | |
| Descended by birth; not consistently found in scrotum | Undescended testes (cryptorchidism) | If testes cannot be felt in scrotum, gently palpate femoral, inguinal, perineal, and abdominal areas for presence. |
| Testes size 1.5–2 cm at birth | Enlarged testes (tumor)<br>Small testes (Klinefelter syndrome or adrenal hyperplasia) | Refer to and collaborate with physician for further diagnostic studies. |
| **Female** | | |
| *Mons* | | |
| Normal skin color, area pigmented in dark-skinned infants<br>Labia majora cover labia minora in term and postterm newborns; symmetric size appropriate for gestational age | Hematoma, lesions (trauma)<br>Labia minora prominent | Evaluate for recent trauma.<br>Assess for prematurity. |

***Possible causes of alterations are placed in parentheses.**

**†This column provides guidelines for further assessment and initial nursing interventions.**

## NEWBORN PHYSICAL ASSESSMENT GUIDE *continued*

| Physical Assessment/ Normal Findings | Alterations and Possible Causes* | Nursing Responses to Data† |
|---|---|---|
| *Clitoris* | | |
| Normally large in newborn<br>Edema and bruising in breech birth | Hypertrophy (hermaphroditism) | Refer to genetic workup. |
| *Vagina* | | |
| Urinary meatus and vaginal orifice visible (0.5 cm circumference)<br>Vaginal tag or hymenal tag disappears in a few weeks | Inflammation; erythema and discharge (urethritis)<br>Congenital absence of vagina | Collect urine specimen for laboratory examination.<br>Refer to physician. |
| Discharge; smegma under labia | Foul-smelling discharge (infection) | Collect data and further evaluate reason for discharge. |
| Bloody or mucoid discharge | Excessive vaginal bleeding (blood coagulation defect) | |
| **Buttocks and Anus** | | |
| Buttocks symmetric | Pilonidal dimple | Examine for possible sinus.<br>Instruct parents about cleansing this area. |
| Anus patent and passage of meconium within 24–48 hours after birth | Imperforate anus, rectal atresia (congenital gastrointestinal defect) | Evaluate extent of problems.<br>Initiate surgical consultation.<br>Perform digital examination to ascertain patency if patency uncertain. |
| No fissures, tears, or skin tags | Fissures | |
| **Extremities and Trunk** | | |
| Short and generally flexed; extremities move symmetrically through range of motion but lack full extension | Unilateral or absence of movement (spinal cord involvement)<br>Fetal position continued or limp (anoxia, CNS problems, hypoglycemia) | Review birth record to assess possible cause. |
| All joints move spontaneously; good muscle tone, of flexor type, birth to 2 months | Spasticity when infant begins using extensors (cerebral palsy, lack of muscle tone, "floppy baby" syndrome)<br>Hypotonia (Down syndrome) | Collaborate with physician. |
| *Arms* | | |
| Equal in length<br>Bilateral movement<br>Flexed when quiet | Brachial palsy (difficult birth)<br>Erb-Duchenne paralysis<br>Muscle weakness, fractured clavicle<br>Absence of limb or change of size (phocomelia, amelia) | Report to clinician. |
| *Hands* | | |
| Normal number of fingers | Polydactyly (Ellis–Van Creveld syndrome)<br>Syndactyly—one limb (developmental anomaly)<br>Syndactyly—both limbs (genetic component) | Report to clinician. |
| Normal palmar crease | Simian line on palm (Down syndrome) | Refer for genetic workup. |
| Normal-sized hands | Short fingers and broad hand (Hurler syndrome) | |

***Possible causes of alterations are placed in parentheses.**

**†This column provides guidelines for further assessment and initial nursing interventions.**

## NEWBORN PHYSICAL ASSESSMENT GUIDE *continued*

| Physical Assessment/ Normal Findings | Alterations and Possible Causes* | Nursing Responses to Data† |
|---|---|---|
| Nails present and extend beyond fingertips in term newborn | Cyanosis and clubbing (cardiac anomalies)<br>Nails long or yellow stained (postterm) | Evaluate for history of distress in utero. |
| *Spine* | | |
| C-shaped spine<br>Flat and straight when prone<br>Slight lumbar lordosis<br>Easily flexed and intact when palpated<br>At least half of back devoid of lanugo<br>Full-term infant in ventral suspension should hold head at 45-degree angle, back straight | Spina bifida occulta (nevus pilosus)<br>Dermal sinus<br>Myelomeningocele<br>Head lag, limp, floppy trunk (neurologic problems) | Evaluate extent of neurologic damage; initiate care of spinal opening. |
| *Hips* | | |
| No sign of instability | Sensation of abnormal movement, jerk, or snap of hip dislocation | Examine all newborn infants for dislocated hip prior to discharge from birthing center. |
| Hips abduct to more than 60 degrees | | If this is suspected, refer to orthopedist for further evaluation.<br>Reassess at well-baby visits. |
| *Inguinal and buttock skin creases* | | |
| Symmetric inguinal and buttock creases | Asymmetry (dislocated hips) | Refer to orthopedist for evaluation.<br>Counsel parents regarding symptoms of concern and discuss therapy. |
| *Legs* | | |
| Legs equal in length<br>Legs shorter than arms at birth | Shortened leg (dislocated hips)<br>Lack of leg movement (fractures, spinal defects) | Refer to orthopedist for evaluation.<br>Counsel parents regarding symptoms of concern and discuss therapy. |
| *Feet* | | |
| Foot is in straight line<br>Positional clubfoot—based on position in utero | Talipes equinovarus (true clubfoot) | Discuss differences between positional and true clubfoot with parents.<br>Teach parents passive manipulation of foot. |
| Fat pads and creases on soles of feet | Incomplete sole creases in first 24 hours of life (premature) | Refer to orthopedist if not corrected by 3 months of age. |
| Talipes planus (flat feet) normal under 3 years of age | | Reassure parents that flat feet are normal in infants. |
| **Neuromuscular** | | |
| *Motor function* | | |
| Symmetric movement and strength in all extremities | Limp, flaccid, or hypertonic (CNS disorders, infection, dehydration, fracture) | Appraise newborn's posture and motor functions by observing activities and motor characteristics. |
| May be jerky or have brief twitchings | Tremors (hypoglycemia, hypocalcemia, infection, neurologic damage) | Evaluate electrolyte imbalance, hypoglycemia, and neurologic functioning. |
| Head lag not over 45 degrees | Delayed or abnormal development (preterm, neurologic involvement) | |
| Neck control adequate to maintain head erect briefly | Asymmetry of tone or strength (neurologic damage) | Refer for genetic evaluation. |

***Possible causes of alterations are placed in parentheses.**

**†This column provides guidelines for further assessment and initial nursing interventions.**

## NEWBORN PHYSICAL ASSESSMENT GUIDE *continued*

| Physical Assessment/ Normal Findings | Alterations and Possible Causes* | Nursing Responses to Data† |
|---|---|---|
| **Reflexes** | | |
| *Blink* | | |
| Stimulated by flash of light; response is closure of eyelids | Lack of blink response (damage to cranial nerve, CNS injury) | Assess neurologic status. |
| *Pupillary reflex* | | |
| Stimulated by flash of light; response is constriction of pupil | Lack of reflex (damage to cranial nerve, CNS injury) | |
| *Moro* | | |
| Response to sudden movement or loud noise should be one of symmetric extension and abduction of arms with fingers extended; then return to normal relaxed flexion<br>Infant lying on back: slightly raised head suddenly released; infant held horizontally, lowered quickly about 6 in., and stopped abruptly<br>Fingers form a C<br>Present at birth; disappears by 6 months of age | Asymmetry of body response (fractured clavicle, injury to brachial plexus)<br>Consistent absence (brain damage) | Discuss normality of this reflex in response to loud noises and/or sudden movements.<br>Absence of reflex requires neurologic evaluation. |
| *Rooting and sucking* | | |
| Turns in direction of stimulus to cheek or mouth; opens mouth and begins to suck rhythmically when finger or nipple is inserted into mouth; difficult to elicit after feeding; disappears by 4 to 7 months of age<br>Sucking is adequate for nutritional intake and meeting oral stimulation needs; disappears by 12 months | Poor sucking or easily fatigable (preterm, breastfed infants of barbiturate-addicted mothers, possible cardiac problem)<br>Absence of response (preterm, neurologic involvement, depressed newborns) | Evaluate strength and coordination of sucking.<br>Observe newborn during feeding and counsel parents about mutuality of feeding experience and newborn's responses. |
| *Palmar grasp* | | |
| Fingers grasp adult finger when palm is stimulated and held momentarily; lessens at 3 to 4 months of age | Asymmetry of response (neurologic problems) | Evaluate other reflexes and general neurologic functioning. |
| *Plantar grasp* | | |
| Toes curl downward when sole of foot is stimulated; lessens by 8 months | Absent (defects of lower spinal column) | Assess for other lower extremity neurologic problems. |
| *Stepping* | | |
| When held upright and one foot touching a flat surface, will step alternately; disappears at 4 to 5 months of age | Asymmetry of stepping (neurologic abnormality) | Evaluate muscle tone and function on each side of body.<br>Refer to specialist. |
| *Babinski* | | |
| Fanning and extension of all toes when one side of sole is stroked from heel upward across ball of foot; disappears at about 12 months | Absence of response (low spinal cord defects) | Refer for further neurologic evaluation. |
| | ***Possible causes of alterations are placed in parentheses.** | **†This column provides guidelines for further assessment and initial nursing interventions.** |

## NEWBORN PHYSICAL ASSESSMENT GUIDE *continued*

| Physical Assessment/ Normal Findings | Alterations and Possible Causes* | Nursing Responses to Data† |
|---|---|---|
| *Tonic neck* | | |
| Fencer position—when head is turned to one side, extremities on same side extend and on opposite side flex; this reflex may not be evident during early neonatal period; disappears at 3 to 4 months of age<br>Response often more dominant in leg than in arm | Absent after 1 month of age or persistent asymmetry (cerebral lesion) | Assess neurologic functioning. |
| *Prone crawl* | | |
| While on abdomen, neonate pushes up and tries to crawl | Absence or variance of response (preterm, weak, or depressed newborns) | Evaluate motor functioning.<br>Refer to specialist. |
| *Trunk incurvation (Galant)* | | |
| In prone position stroking of spine causes pelvis to turn to stimulated side | Failure to rotate to stimulated side (neurologic damage) | |
| | ***Possible causes of alterations are placed in parentheses.** | **†This column provides guidelines for further assessment and initial nursing interventions.** |

The behaviors, and the sleep-wake states in which they are assessed, are categorized as follows:

1. *Habituation.* The nurse assesses the newborn's ability to diminish or shut down innate responses to specific repeated stimuli, such as a rattle, bell, light, or pinprick to heel.
2. *Orientation to inanimate and animate visual and auditory assessment stimuli.* The nurse observes how often and where the newborn attends to auditory and visual stimuli. Orientation to the environment is determined by an ability to respond to clues given by others and by a natural ability to fix on and follow a visual object horizontally and vertically. This capacity and parental appreciation of it are important for positive communication between infant and parents; the parents' visual (*en face*) and auditory (soft, continuous voice) presence stimulates their newborn to orient to them. Inability or lack of response may indicate visual or auditory problems. It is important for parents to know that their newborn can turn to voices soon after birth or by 3 days of age and can become alert at different times with a varying degree of intensity in response to sounds.
3. *Motor activity.* Several components are evaluated. Motor tone of the newborn is assessed in the most characteristic state of responsiveness. This summary assessment includes overall use of tone as the newborn responds to being handled—whether during spontaneous activity, prone placement, or horizontal holding—and overall assessment of body tone as the newborn reacts to all stimuli.
4. *Variations.* Frequency of alert states, state changes, color changes (throughout all states as examination progresses), activity, and peaks of excitement are assessed.
5. *Self-quieting activity.* This assessment is based on how often, how quickly, and how effectively newborns can use their resources to quiet and console themselves when upset or distressed. Considered in this assessment are such self-consolatory activities as putting hand to mouth, sucking on a fist or the tongue, and attuning to an object or sound. The newborn's need for outside consolation must also be considered (e.g., seeing a face; being rocked, held, or dressed; using a pacifier; being swaddled).
6. *Cuddliness or social behaviors.* This area encompasses the newborn's need for, and response to, being held. Also considered is how often the newborn smiles. These behaviors influence the couple's self-esteem and feelings of acceptance or rejection. Cuddling also appears to be an indicator of personality. Cuddlers appear to enjoy, accept, and seek physical contact; are easier to placate; sleep more; and form earlier and more intense attachments. Noncuddlers are active, restless, have accelerated motor development, and are intolerant of physical restraint. Smiling, even as a grimace reflex, greatly influences parent-newborn feedback. Parents identify this response as positive.

# Chapter Review

## CHAPTER HIGHLIGHTS

- A perinatal history, determination of gestational age, physical examination, and behavior assessment form the basis for a complete newborn assessment.
- The common physical characteristics included in the gestational age assessment are skin, lanugo, sole (plantar) creases, breast tissue and size, ear form and cartilage, and genitalia.
- The neuromuscular components of gestational age scoring tools are usually posture, square window sign, popliteal angle, arm recoil, heel-to-ear extension, and scarf sign.
- After determining the gestational age of the baby, the nurse can assess how the newborn will make the transition to extrauterine life and anticipate potential physiologic problems.
- The nurse identifies the newborn as SGA, AGA, or LGA and prioritizes individual needs.
- Normal ranges for vital signs assessed in the newborn are as follows: heart rate, 120 to 160 beats per minute; respirations, 30 to 60 respirations per minute; axillary temperature, 36.4 to 37.2°C (97.5 to 99°F); skin temperature, 36 to 36.5°C (96.8 to 97.7°F); rectal temperature, 36.6 to 37.2°C (97.8 to 99°F); and blood pressure at birth, 80–60/45–40 mm Hg.
- Normal newborn measurements are as follows: weight range, 2500 to 4000 g (5 lb, 8 oz, to 8 lb, 13 oz), with weight dependent on maternal size and age; length range, 45 to 55 cm (18 to 22 in); and head circumference range, 32 to 37 cm (12.5 to 14.5 in)—approximately 2 cm larger than the chest circumference.
- Commonly elicited newborn reflexes are tonic neck, Moro, grasp, rooting, sucking, and blink.
- Newborn behavioral abilities include habituation, orientation to visual and auditory stimuli, motor activity, cuddliness, and self-quieting activity.
- An important role of the nurse during the physical and behavioral assessments of the newborn is to teach parents about their newborn and involve them in their baby's care. This involvement facilitates the parents' identification of their newborn's uniqueness and allays their concerns.

## CHAPTER REFERENCES


American Academy of Pediatrics, Committee on Fetus and Newborn, & American College of Obstetricians and Gynecologists, Committee on Obstetrics. (1997). *Guidelines for perinatal care* (4th ed.). Evanston, IL: Author.

Ballard, J. L., Khoury, J. C., Wedig, K., Wang, L., Eilers-Walsmann, B. L., & Lipp, R. (1991). New Ballard score, expanded to include extremely premature infants. *Journal of Pediatrics, 119*(3), 417–423.

Basso, O., Olsen, J., Knudsen, L. B., & Christensen, K. (1998). Low birth weight and preterm birth after short interpregnancy intervals. *American Journal of Obstetrics and Gynecology, 178*(2), 259–263.

Brazelton, T. B., & Nugent, J. K. (1995). *The neonatal behavioral assessment scale.* (3rd ed.). London: MacKeith.

Brooks, A. A., Johnson, M. R., Steer, P. J., Pawson, M. E., & Abdella, H. I. (1995). Birth weight: Nature or nuture? *Early Human Development 42*(1), 29–35.

Dodd, V. (1996). Gestational age assessment. *Neonatal Network, 15*(1), 27.

Donovan, E. F., Tyson, J. E., Ehrenkranz, R. A., Verter, J., Wright, L. L., Korones, S. B., Bauer, C. R., Shankaran, S., Stoll, B. J., Fanaroff, A. A., Oh, W., Lemons, J. A., Stevenson, D. K., & Papile, L., (1999, August). Inaccuracy of Ballard scores before 28 weeks' gestation. *Journal of Pediatrics, 135,* 147–152.

Juretschke, L. J. (2000). Unilateral neonatal testicular torsion. *Journal of Obstretics, Gynecologie, and Neonatal Nursing, 29*(5), 451–456.

Moyer, V. A., Ahn, C., & Sneed, S. (2000, April). Accuracy of clinical judgment in neonatal jaundice. *Archives of Pediatric and Adolescent Medicine, 154* 391–394.

O'Donnell, K. A., Glick, P. L., & Cory, M. G. (1998). Pediatric umbilical problems. *Pediatric Clinics of North America, 45*(4), 791–799.

Overpeck, M. D., Hediger, M. L., Zhang, J., Trumble, A. C., & Klebanoff, M. A. (1999). Birth weight for gestational age of Mexican American infants born in the United States. *Obstetrics and Gynecology, 93*(6), 943–947.

Pressler, J. L., & Hepworth, J. T. (1997). Newborn neurologic screening using NBAS reflexes. *Neonatal Network, 16*(6), 33–46.

Reed, B., & Davidhizar, R. (1997, February). Setting their sights: Visual development in newborns. *Advances for Nurse Practitioner, 5*(2), pp. 67–68, 70.

Rinehart, T. T., Terrone, D. A., & Magann, E. (2000). The normal neonate: Assessment of early physical findings. In J. J. Sciarri & T. J. Watkins (Eds.), *Gynecology and obstetrics* (Vol. 2, Chap. 97, pp. 1–15). Philadelphia: Lippincott, Williams & Wilkins.

Sganga, A., Wallace, R., Kiehl, E., Irving, T., & Witter, L. (2000). A comparison of four methods of normal newborn temperature measurements. *American Journal of Maternal Child Nursing, 25*(2), 76–79.

Sininger, Y. S., Doyle, K. J., & Moore, J. K. (1999). The case for early identification of hearing loss in children. *Pediatric Clinics of North America, 46*(1), 1–14.

Tappero, E. P., & Honeyfield, M. E. (1996). *Physical assessment of the newborn* (2nd ed.). Petaluma, CA: NICU Ink.

Thurdeen, P. J., Deacon, J., O'Neill, P., & Hernandez, J. (1999). *Assessment and care of the well newborn.* Philadelphia: Saunders.

## CONTEMPORARY MATERNAL-NEWBORN NURSING ON-LINE

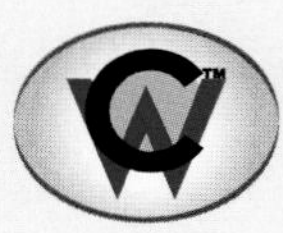

Additional interactive resources, including animations and video, for this chapter can be found on the Companion Website at http://www.prenhall.com/ladewig. Click on Chapter 22 and "Begin" to select the activities for this chapter.

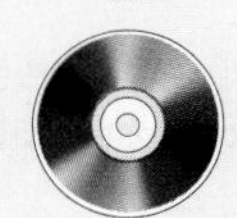

For NCLEX review questions and an audio glossary, access the accompanying CD-ROM in this book.

Chapter 23

# Normal Newborn: Needs and Care

*I've been a postpartum nurse for about 6 years. A large part of my job involves teaching or enhancing parenting skills. I get enormous satisfaction out of watching a hesitant dad change his newborn for the first time or helping a mother breastfeed this baby, when she wasn't able to with her last one. I only wish I had more time to spend with each family.*

—Mother-Baby Nurse

## OBJECTIVES

- **Summarize the essential areas of information to be obtained about a newborn's birth experience and immediate postnatal period.**
- **Relate the physiologic and behavioral responses of newborns to possible interventions needed.**
- **Discuss the major nursing considerations and activities to be carried out during the first 4 hours after birth (admission and transitional period) and subsequent daily care.**
- **Identify the activities that should be included in a daily care plan for a normal newborn.**
- **Determine common family concerns about their newborns.**
- **Describe the topics and related content to be included for parents' education on newborn and infant care.**
- **Identify opportunities to individualize parent teaching and enhance each parent's abilities and confidence while providing infant care in the birthing unit.**
- **Delineate the information to be included in discharge planning with the newborn's family.**

## KEY TERMS

At the moment of birth, numerous physiologic adaptations begin to take place in the newborn's body. Because of these dramatic changes, newborns require close observation to determine how smoothly they are making the transition to extrauterine life. Newborns also require specific care that enhances their chances of making the transition successfully.

The two broad goals of nursing care during this period are to promote the physical well-being of the newborn and to enhance the establishment of a well-functioning family unit. The nurse meets the first goal by providing comprehensive care to the newborn in the mother-baby unit. The nurse meets the second goal by teaching family members how to care for their new baby and by supporting their efforts so that they feel confident and competent. Thus the nurse must be knowledgeable about family adjustments that need to be made as well as the health care needs of the newborn. It is important that the family return home with the positive feeling that they have the support, information, and skills to care for their newborn. Equally important is the need for each member of the family to begin a unique relationship with the newborn. The cultural and social expectations of individual families and communities affect the way in which normal newborn care is carried out.

The previous two chapters presented an informational database of the physiologic and behavioral changes occurring in the newborn and the pertinent nursing assessments that are needed. This chapter discusses the nursing care management while the newborn is in the birthing unit. The Critical Pathway for Newborn Care starts on page 587.

# Nursing Care Management during Admission and the First 4 Hours of Life

## Nursing Assessment and Diagnosis

During the first 4 hours after birth, the nurse carries out a preliminary physical examination, including an assessment of the newborn's physiologic adaptations. In many birthing units, the nurse performs and documents the initial head-to-toe physical assessment during the first hour of transition. The nurse is responsible for notifying the physician or nurse practitioner of any deviation from normal. A complete physical examination is also performed later by the physician or nurse practitioner, within 24 hours after birth and within 24 hours before discharge. If timed correctly, only one physical examination may be necessary (American Academy of Pediatrics [AAP], 1997) (see Chapter 22 and Table 22–1).

Nursing diagnoses are based on an analysis of the assessment findings. Physiologic alterations of the newborn form the basis of many nursing diagnoses, as does the family members' incorporation of them in caring for their new baby. Nursing diagnoses that may apply to newborn include the following:

- ***Ineffective airway clearance*** related to presence of mucus and retained lung fluid
- ***Risk for altered body temperature*** related to evaporative, radiant, conductive, and convective heat losses
- ***Pain*** related to heel sticks for glucose or hematocrit tests or vitamin K injection

As discussed in Chapter 22, the newborn's physiologic adaptation to extrauterine life occurs rapidly. All body systems are affected. Therefore, many of these nursing diagnoses and associated interventions must be identified and implemented very quickly during this period. (See Key Facts to Remember: Signs of Newborn Transition.)

## Nursing Plan and Implementation

The nurse initiates newborn admission procedures and evaluates the newborn's need to remain under observation. The nurse monitors the newborn's ability to maintain a clear airway and stable vital signs, maintain body temperature, demonstrate normal neurologic status with no observable complications, and tolerate the first feeding. Satisfaction of these criteria indicates a successful beginning adaptation to extrauterine life, and the baby is moved to a regular nursery or back to the mother's room. This transfer usually takes place between 2 and 6 hours after birth.

### Initiation of Admission Procedures

After birth, the baby is formally admitted to the health care facility. The admission procedures include gestational age assessment and an assessment to ensure that the newborn's adaptation to extrauterine life is proceeding normally. This evaluation of the newborn's status and risk factors must be done within 2 hours after birth (AAP, 1997).

If the initial assessment indicates that the newborn is not at risk physiologically, the nurse performs many of the routine admission procedures in the presence of the parents in the birthing area. The care measures indicated by the assessment findings may be performed by the nurse or by the parents under the guidance of the nurse in an effort to educate and support the family.

## KEY FACTS TO REMEMBER

### *Signs of Newborn Transition*

Normal findings for the newborn during the first few days of life include the following:

Pulse: 120–160 beats/minute

- During sleep as low as 100 beats/minute
- If crying, up to 180 beats/minute
- Apical pulse is counted for 1 full minute because rate may fluctuate

Respirations: 30–60 respirations/minute

- Predominantly diaphragmatic but synchronous with abdominal movements
- Brief periods of apnea (5–10 seconds) with no color or heart rate changes

Temperature

- Axillary 36.5–37°C (97.5–98.6°F)
- Skin: 36–36.5°C (96.8–97.7°F)

Blood pressure: 80–60/45–40 mm Hg at birth; 100/50 mm Hg at day 10

Glucose > 40 mg%

Hematocrit: < 65%–70% central venous sample

Other interventions may be delayed until the newborn has been transferred to an observational nursery.

The nurse responsible for the newborn first checks and confirms the newborn's identification with the mother's identification and then obtains and records all significant information. The essential data to be recorded on the newborn's chart include the following:

1. *Condition of the newborn.* Pertinent information includes the newborn's Apgar scores at 1 and 5 minutes, resuscitative measures required in the birthing area, physical examination, vital signs, voidings, and passing of meconium. Complications to be noted are excessive mucus, delayed spontaneous respirations or responsiveness, abnormal number of cord vessels, and obvious physical abnormalities.
2. *Labor and birth record.* A copy of the labor and birth record should be placed in the newborn's chart or be accessible on computer. The record contains all the significant data about the birth, including duration, course, and status of mother and fetus throughout labor and birth and any analgesia or anesthesia administered to the mother. Particular care is taken to note any variation or difficulties, such as prolonged rupture of membranes, abnormal fetal position, meconium-stained amniotic fluid, signs of fetal distress during labor, nuchal cord (cord around the newborn's neck at birth), precipitous birth, use of forceps or vacuum-assisted device, maternal analgesics and anesthesia received within 1 hour before birth, and administration of antibiotics during labor.
3. *Antepartal history.* Any maternal problems that may have compromised the fetus in utero, such as pregnancy-induced hypertension (PIH), spotting, illness, recent infections, rubella status, serology results, hepatitis B screen results, exposure to group B streptococci, or a history of maternal substance abuse, are of immediate concern in newborn assessment (AAP, 1997). The chart should also include information about maternal age, estimated date of birth (EDB), previous pregnancies, and presence of any congenital anomalies. A human immunodeficiency virus (HIV) test result, if obtained, is also relevant. State statutes vary as to whom may have access to this information (AAP, 1997).
4. *Parent-newborn interaction information.* The nurse notes parents' interactions with their newborn and their desires regarding care, such as rooming-in, circumcision, and the type of feeding. Information about other children in the home, available support systems, and interactional patterns within each family unit assists the nurse in providing comprehensive care.

As part of the admission procedure, the nurse weighs the newborn in both grams and pounds. In the United States, parents understand weight best when it is stated in pounds and ounces (Figure 23–1♦). The nurse cleans and covers the scales each time a newborn is weighed to prevent cross infection and heat loss from conduction.

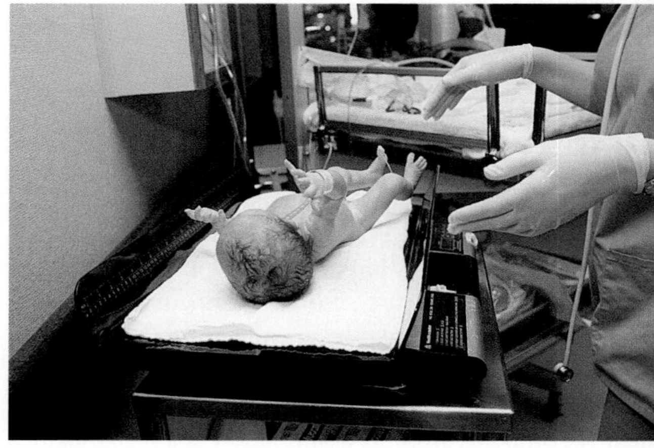

FIGURE 23–1 ♦ Weighing of newborns. The scale is balanced before each weighing, with the protective pad in place. The caregiver's hand is poised near the newborn as a safety measure.

# CRITICAL PATHWAY: *for Newborn Care*

| Category | First 4 Hours | 4–8 Hours Past Birth | 8–24 Hours Past Birth |
|---|---|---|---|
| **Referral** | Review labor/birth record<br>Review transitional nursing record<br>Check ID bands<br>Consult prn: orthopedics, genetics, infectious disease | Check ID bands<br>Transfer to mother-baby care at 4–6 hours of age if stable<br>As parents desire, obtain circumcision permit after their discussion with physician<br>Lactation consult prn | Check ID bands q shift<br>**Expected Outcomes**<br>Mother/baby ID bands correlate at time of discharge; consults completed prn |
| **Assessments** | Continue assessments begun first hour after birth<br>Vital sign: TPR, BP prn, q1h × 4 (skin temp 97.8–98.6°F, resp may be irregular but within 30–60 per min)<br>**Newborn Assessments**<br>• Respiratory status with resp distress scale × 1 then prn. If resp distress, assess q 5–15 min<br>• Cord: bluish white color, clamp in place<br>• Color: skin, mucous membranes, extremities, trunk pink with slight acrocyanosis of hands and feet<br>• Wt (5 lb, 8 oz–8 lb, 13 oz), length (18–22 in), HC (12.5–14.5 in), CC (32.5 cm, 1–2 in less than head)<br>• Extremity movement—may be jerky or brief twitches<br>• Gestational age classification—term AGA<br>• Anomalies (cong. anomalies can interfere with normal extrauterine adaptation) | Assess newborn's progress through periods of reactivity<br>Vital signs: TPR q8h and prn, BP prn<br>**Newborn Assessments**<br>• Skin color q4h prn (circulatory system stabilizing, acrocyanosis decreased)<br>• Eyes for drainage, redness, hemorrhage<br>• Ausculate lungs q4h (noisy, wet resp normal)<br>• Increased mucus production (normal in 2nd period of reactivity)<br>• Check apical pulse q4h<br>• Umbilical cord base for redness, drainage, foul odor, drying, clamp in place<br>• Extremity movement q4h<br>• Check for expected reflexes (suck, rooting, Moro, grasp, blink, yawn, sneeze, tonic neck, Babinski)<br>• Note common normal variations<br>• Assess such and swallow during feeding<br>• Note behavioral characteristics<br>• Temp before and after admission bath | VS q8h; normal ranges: T, 97.5–99°F; P, 120–160; R, 30–60; BP, 60–80/45–40 mm Hg<br>**Continue Newborn Assessments**<br>• Skin color q4h<br>• Signs of drying or infection in cord area<br>• Check out clamp in place until removed before discharge<br>• Check circ for bleeding after procedure, then q30min × 2, then q4h and prn<br>**Expected Outcomes**<br>Vital signs medically acceptable, color pink, assessments WNL, circ site without s/s infection, cord site without s/s infection and clamp removed; newborn behavior WNL |
| **Teaching/ psychosocial** | Admission activities performed at mother's bedside if possible, orient to nursery prn, handwashing, assess teaching needs<br>Teach parents use of bulb syringe, signs of choking, positioning, and when to call for assistance<br>Teach reasons for use of radiant warmer, infant hat, and warmed blankets when out of warmer<br>Discuss/teach infant security, identification | Reinforce teaching about choking, bulb syringe use, positioning, temperature maintenance with clothing and blankets<br>Teach infant positioning to facilitate breathing and digestion<br>Teach new parents holding and feeding skills<br>Teach parents soothing and calming techniques | Final discharge teaching: diapering, normal void and stool patterns, bathing, nail and cord care, circumcision/uncircumcised penis/genital care and normal characteristics, rashes, jaundice, sleep-wake cycles, soothing activities, taking temperatures, thermometer reading<br>Explain s/s of illness and when to call health care provider<br>Infant safety: car seats, immunizations, metabolic screening<br>**Expected Outcomes**<br>Mother/family verbalize comprehension of teaching; demonstrate care capabilities |
| **Nursing care management and reports** | Place under radiant warmer<br>Place hat on newborn (decreases convection heat loss)<br>Suction nares/mouth with bulb syringe prn<br>Keep bulb syringe with infant<br>Attach security sensor<br>Obtain lab tests: blood glucose; as needed<br>Obtain blood type, Rh, Coombs on cord blood, HSV culture if parental hx<br>Notify physician's office or exchange of infant's birth and status<br>Maintain Universal Precautions | Wean from radiant warmer (T98°F axillary)<br>Chemstrips prn; BP prn<br>Oxygen saturation prn<br>Bathe infant if temp > 97.8°F<br>Position on side<br>Suction nares prn (esp during 2nd period of reactivity)<br>Obtain peripheral Hct per protocol<br>Cord care per protocol<br>Fold diaper below cord (for plastic diapers, turn plastic layer away from skin) | Check for hearing test results<br>Weigh before discharge<br>Cord care q shift<br>DC cord clamp before discharge<br>Perform newborn metabolic screening blood tests before discharge<br>Circumcision if indicated; circumcision care: change diaper prn, noting ability to void; follow policy for circumcision clamp or Plastibell care<br>**Expected Outcomes**<br>Newborn maintains temp, lab test WNL, cord dry without s/s infection and clamp removed, screening tests accomplished, circ site without s/s infection or bleeding |

AGA, average for gestational age; Appt, appointment; CC, chest circumference; cong, congenital; esp, especially; HC, head circumference; Hct, hematocrit; Hx, history; ID, identification; OU, both eyes; s/s, signs and symptoms; temp, temperature; TPR, temperature, pulse, respirations; VS, vital signs; WNL, within normal limits.

| Category | First 4 Hours | 4–8 Hours Past Birth | 8–24 Hours Past Birth |
|---|---|---|---|
| **Activity and comfort** | Place under radiant warmer or wrap in pre–warmed blankets until stable<br>Soothe baby as needed with voice, touch, cuddling, nesting in warmer | Leave in warmer until stable, then swaddle<br>Position on side after each feeding | Place in open crib<br>Swaddle to allow movement of extremities in blanket, including hands to face<br>**Expected Outcomes**<br>Infant maintains temp WNL in open crib; infant attempts self calming |
| **Nutrition** | Assist newborn to breastfeed as soon as mother/baby condition allows<br>Supplement breast only when medically indicated or per agency policy<br>Initiate bottle-feeding within first hour<br>Gavage feed if necessary to prevent hypoglycemia | Breastfeed on demand, at least q3–4h<br>Teach positions, observe/assist with feeding, breast/nipple care, establishing milk supply, breaking suction, feeding cues, latching-on techniques, nutritive suck, burping<br>Bottle-feed on demand, at least q3–6hr<br>Determine readiness to feed and feeding tolerance | Continue breastfeeding or bottle-feeding pattern<br>Access feeding tolerance q4h<br>Discuss normal feeding requirements, signs of hunger and satiation, handing feeding problems, and when to seek help<br>**Expected Outcomes**<br>Mother verbalized knowledge of feeding information; breastfeeds on demand without supplement; bottle—tolerates formula feeding, nipples without problems |
| **Elimination** | Note first void and stool if not noted at birth | Note all voids, amount and color of stools q4h | Evaluate all voids and stool color q8h<br>**Expected Outcomes**<br>Voids qs; stools qs without difficulty; stool character WNL; diaper area without s/s skin breakdown or rashes |
| **Medication** | Prophylactic opthalmic ointment OU after baby makes eye contact with parents within 1 hr after birth<br>Administer AquaMEPHYTON IM, dosage according to infant weight per MD/NP order | Hepatitis B injection as ordered by physician after consent signed by parents | Hepatitis B vaccine before discharge<br>**Expected Outcomes**<br>Baby has received ophthalmic ointment and vitamin K injection; baby has received first Hep B vaccine if ordered and parental permission received |
| **Discharge planning/ home care** | Hepatitis B consent signed<br>Hearing screen consent signed<br>Plan discharge call with parent or guardian in 24 hrs to 2 days<br>Assess parents' discharge plans, needs, and support systems | Review/reinforce teaching with mother and significant other<br>Review home preparedness<br>Present birth certificate instructions | Initial newborn screening tests (hearing, blood tests, metabolic screen; ie, PKU) before discharge<br>Bath and feeding classes, videos, or written information given<br>Give written copy of discharge instructions<br>Newborn photographs<br>Set up appointment for follow-up PKU test<br>Have car seat available before discharge<br>All discharge referrals made, follow-up appt. scheduled<br>**Expected Outcomes**<br>Infant discharged home with family; mother verbalizes follow-up appt. time/date |
| **Family involvement** | Facilitate early investigation of baby's physical characteristics (maintain temp during unwrapping), hold infant *en face*<br>Dim lights to help infant keep eyes open | Assess parents' knowledge of newborn behaviors, such as alertness, suck and rooting, attention to human voice, response to calming techniques | Assess mother-baby bonding/interaction<br>Incorporate father and siblings in care<br>Enhance parent-infant interaction by sharing characteristics and behavioral assessment<br>Support positive parenting behaviors<br>Identify community referral needs and refer to community agencies<br>**Expected Outcome**<br>Demonstrates caring and family incorporation of infant |
| **Date** | | | |

The nurse then measures the newborn, recording the measurements in both centimeters and inches. The three routine measurements are length, circumference of the head, and circumference of the chest. In some facilities, abdominal girth may also be measured. The nurse rapidly assesses the baby's color, muscle tone, alertness, and general state. It is important to remember that the first period of reactivity may have concluded, and the baby may be in the sleep-inactive phase, which makes the infant hard to arouse. The nurse completes basic assessments for estimating gestational age and finishes the physical assessment (see Chapter 22).

In addition to obtaining vital signs, the nurse may perform a hematocrit and blood glucose evaluation on at-risk newborns or as clinically indicated (such as for small-for-gestational-age [SGA] or large-for-gestational-age [LGA] infants, or if the newborn is jittery). These procedures may be done on admission or within the first 4 hours after birth (AAP, 1997) (see Procedure 26–1.)

## Maintenance of a Clear Airway and Stable Vital Signs

The nurse positions the newborn on his or her side. If necessary, a bulb syringe or DeLee wall suction (Procedure 17–1) is used to remove mucus from the newborn's nasal passages and oral cavity. A DeLee catheter attached to suction may be used to remove mucus from the stomach to help prevent possible aspiration. This procedure also ensures that the esophagus is patent prior to the newborn's first feeding. Gastric suctioning can cause vagal nerve stimulation, which may result in bradycardia and apnea in the unstabilized newborn.

In the absence of any newborn distress, the nurse continues with the admission by taking the newborn's vital signs. The initial temperature is taken by the axillary method; a normal axillary temperature range is 36.5 to 37°C (97.7 to 98.6°F) (Merestein & Gardner, 1998).

Once the initial temperature is taken, the nurse monitors the core temperature either by obtaining axillary temperatures at intervals or by placing a skin sensor on the newborn for continuous reading. The usual skin sensor placement site is the newborn's abdomen, but placement on the upper thigh or arm can give a reading closely correlated with the mean body temperature. The vital signs for a healthy term newborn should be monitored at least every 30 minutes until the newborn's condition has remained stable for 2 hours (AAP, 1997). The newborn's respirations may be irregular yet still be normal. Brief periods of apnea, lasting only 5 to 10 seconds with no color or heart rate changes, are considered normal. The normal pulse range is 120 to 160 beats per minute, and the normal respiratory range is 30 to 60 respirations per minute.

## Maintenance of a Neutral Thermal Environment

A neutral thermal environment is essential to minimize the newborn's need for increased oxygen consumption and use of calories to maintain body heat in the optimal range of 36.4 to 37.2°C (97.5 to 99°F). If the newborn becomes hypothermic, the body's response can lead to metabolic acidosis, hypoxia, and shock.

A neutral thermal environment is best achieved by performing the newborn assessment and interventions with the newborn unclothed and under a radiant warmer. The thermostat of the radiant warmer is controlled by the thermal skin sensor taped to the newborn's abdomen, upper thigh, or arm. The sensor indicates when the newborn's temperature exceeds or falls below the acceptable temperature range. The nurse should be aware that leaning over the newborn may block the radiant heat waves from reaching the newborn.

It is common practice in some institutions to cover the newborn's head with a cap made of wool lined with gauze and cotton, Thinsulate, or cotton and polyester fill terry cloth to prevent further heat loss, in addition to placing the baby under a radiant warmer ("Neonatal Thermoregulation," 1997).

### HINTS FOR PRACTICE

A cap can be fashioned from a piece of stockinette to help reduce heat loss from the head.

When the newborn's temperature is normal and vital signs are stable (about 2 to 4 hours after birth), the baby may be given a sponge bath. However, this admission bath may be postponed for some hours if the newborn's condition dictates or the parents wish to give the first bath. In light of early discharge practices (12 to 48 hours), healthy term infants can be safely bathed immediately after the admission assessment is completed (Varda & Behnke, 2000). The baby is bathed while still under the radiant warmer; the bathing may be done in the parents' room. Bathing the newborn offers an excellent opportunity for teaching and welcoming parents' involvement in the care of their baby.

The nurse rechecks the baby's temperature after the bath and, if it is stable, dresses the newborn in a shirt, diaper, and cap; wraps the baby; and places the newborn in an open crib at room temperature or in the mother's arms. If the baby's axillary temperature is below 36.4°C (97.5°F), the baby returns to the radiant warmer for gradual rewarming and to prevent hypothermia. Once

## EVIDENCE-BASED PRACTICE

### The Newborn's First Bath

Your unit's current policy for newborn bathing stresses that the baby must be at least 2 hours old before bathing and also states that the bath must occur in the nursery. You have been asked to take the lead on a revision of this policy. You first look for a national guideline in which the evidence is reviewed and synthesized by a task force of experts. You find that there is a guideline on newborn skin care in development, but it is not yet available. Therefore you review the most recent nursing journals, a new edition of a maternal-newborn nursing textbook, and *Guidelines for Perinatal Care* (American Academy of Pediatrics & American College of Obstetricians and Gynecologists, 1997).

You find a study conducted by Varda and Behnke (2000) indicating that healthy full-term newborns with an axillary temperature of >36.8°C (98.2°F) can be bathed after 1 hour of life when appropriate care is taken to support thermal stability. This study and one by Penny-MacGillivary (1996) emphasize the importance of the newborn's temperature stability and maintaining the environment to minimize the potential for heat loss during bathing. After reading these studies, you recognize that assessment of the newborn's temperature is more important than rigid time frames for bathing or location of bathing.

Based on this evidence, your policy revision recommends three key elements:

- Stable temperature of at least 36.8°C
- Temperature monitoring
- Control of the environmental factors to minimize heat loss during bathing

You include the findings from the Varda and Behnke (2000) study, noting that bathing at 1 hour of age is reasonable if the infant's temperature is >36.8°C and the baby is protected from the factors that cause heat loss. However, this is only one study; thus your policy will not recommend this as routine practice at this time but will await further studies.

#### References

American Academy of Pediatrics & American College of Obstetricians and Gynecologists. (1997). *Guidelines for perinatal care* (4th ed.). Elk Grove Village, IL: Author.

Lund, C., Kuller, J., Lane, A., Wright-Lott, J., & Raines, D. (1999). Neonatal skin care. The scientific basis for practice. *Journal of Obstetric, Gynecologic, and Neonatal Nursing, 28* (3), 241–254.

Penny-MacGillivary, T. (1996). A newborn's first bath: When? *Journal of Obstetric, Gynecologic, and Neonatal Nursing, 25,* 481–487.

Varda, K., & Behnke, R. (2000). The effect of timing of initial bath on newborn's temperature. *Journal of Obstetric, Gynecologic, and Neonatal Nursing, 29*(1), 27–32.

the newborn is rewarmed, the nurse implements measures to prevent further heat loss, such as keeping the newborn away from cool surfaces or instruments, drafts, open windows or doors, and air conditioners. Blankets and clothing are stored in a warm place. (See the section "Temperature Regulation," in Chapter 21, and Procedure 23–1.)

### Prevention of Complications of Hemorrhagic Disease of Newborn

A prophylactic injection of vitamin $K_1$ (AquaMEPHYTON) is given to prevent hemorrhage, which can occur due to low prothrombin levels in the first few days of life (see Drug Guide: Vitamin $K_1$ Phytonadione [Aqua MEPHYTON] see pg. 594). The potential for hemorrhage is considered to result from the absence of gut bacterial flora, which influences the production of vitamin $K_1$ in the newborn (see Chapter 26 for further discussion). Newborns receive a single dose of 0.5 to 1.0 mg of natural vitamin $K_1$ (phytonadione) parenterally (preferred) or subcutaneously within 1 hour of birth (Zenk, Sills, & Koeppel, 1999).

The vitamin $K_1$ injection is given intramuscularly in the middle third of the vastus lateralis muscle, located in the lateral aspect of the thigh (Figure 23–2♦). An alternate site is the rectus femoris muscle in the anterior aspect of the thigh. However, this site is near the sciatic nerve and femoral artery and should be used with caution (Figure 23–3♦ on page 592).

# *Procedure 23–1* Thermoregulation of the Newborn

| *Nursing Action* | *Rationale* |
|---|---|
| **OBJECTIVE: PREPARE THE WARMING EQUIPMENT.** | |
| • Prewarm the incubator or radiant warmer. Make sure warmed towels and/or lightweight blankets are available. | *The change from a warm, moist intrauterine environment to a cool, dry, drafty environment stresses the newborn's immature thermoregulation mechanisms.* |
| • Maintain the birthing room at 22°C (71°F), with a relative humidity of 60%–65%. | |
| **OBJECTIVE: ESTABLISH A STABLE TEMPERATURE AFTER BIRTH.** | |
| • Wipe the newborn free of blood and excessive vernix, especially from the head, with prewarmed towels. | *This prevents loss of body heat from a large surface area through evaporation.* |
| • Place the newborn under the radiant warmer. | *The radiant warmer creates a heat-gaining environment.* |
| • Wrap the newborn in a prewarmed blanket and transfer the newborn to the mother. | *Use of the prewarmed blanket reduces convective heat loss and facilitates maternal-infant contact without compromising the newborn's thermoregulation.* |
| • Place the infant skin to skin on the mother's chest under a warmed blanket. | *Skin-to-skin contact with the mother or father helps maintain the newborn's temperature.* |
| **OBJECTIVE: MAINTAIN A STABLE INFANT TEMPERATURE.** | |
| • Diaper the newborn and place a stocking hat on his or her head. Place the newborn uncovered (except for diaper and hat) under the radiant warmer. | *Radiant heat warms the outer surface skin, so the skin needs to be exposed.* |
| • Tape a servocontrol probe on the newborn's anterior abdominal wall, with the metal side next to the skin, and cover the probe with an aluminum heat deflector patch. | *Do not place over ribs. The aluminum cover prevents heating of the probe directly and overheating the infant.* |
| • Turn the heater to servocontrol mode so that the abdominal skin is maintained at 36.5°C–37°C (97.5–98.6°F). | |
| • Monitor the newborn's axillary and skin probe temperature per institution's protocol. | *The temperature indicator on the radiant warmer continually displays the newborn's probe temperature, so the axillary temperature is checked to ensure that the machine accurately reports the newborn's temperature.* |
| • When the newborn's temperature reaches 37°C (98.6°F), remove the infant from the radiant warmer and place a T-shirt, diaper, and stocking hat on the newborn. | |
| • Double wrap (two blankets) the newborn and place the newborn in an open crib. | |
| • Recheck the newborn's axillary temperature in 1 hour. | *It is important to monitor the infant's ability to maintain its own thermoregulation.* |
| **OBJECTIVE: REWARM THE NEWBORN GRADUALLY IF TEMPERATURE DROPS BELOW 36.1°C (97°F).** | |
| • Access axillary temperature frequently, per agency routine, usually every 2–4 hours. | *Frequent assessment may detect hypothermia, which predisposes the newborn to cold stress.* |
| • If the newborn needs rewarming, place the newborn (unclothed except for diaper) under the radiant warmer with a servocontrol probe on the anterior abdominal wall. | |
| • Gradually rewarm back to normal temperature. | *Rapid heating can lead to hyperthermia, which is associated with apnea, increased insensible water loss, and increased metabolic rate.* |

| *Nursing Action* | *Rationale* |
|---|---|
| • Recheck the newborn's temperature in 30 minutes, then hourly. When the temperature reaches 37°C (98.6°F), remove the newborn from the radiant heater, dress the newborn, double wrap, and place in the open crib. Recheck the temperature in 1 hour. | |
| **OBJECTIVE: PREVENT DROPS IN THE NEWBORN'S TEMPERATURE.** | |
| The nurse carries out the following activities:<br>• Keep the newborn's clothing and bedding dry.<br>• Double wrap the newborn and put a stocking hat on him or her.<br>• Use the radiant warmer during procedures.<br>• Reduce the newborn's exposure to drafts.<br>• Warm objects that will come in contact with the newborn (eg, stethoscopes).<br>• Encourage the mother to snuggle with the newborn under blankets or breastfeed the newborn with hat and light cover on. | |

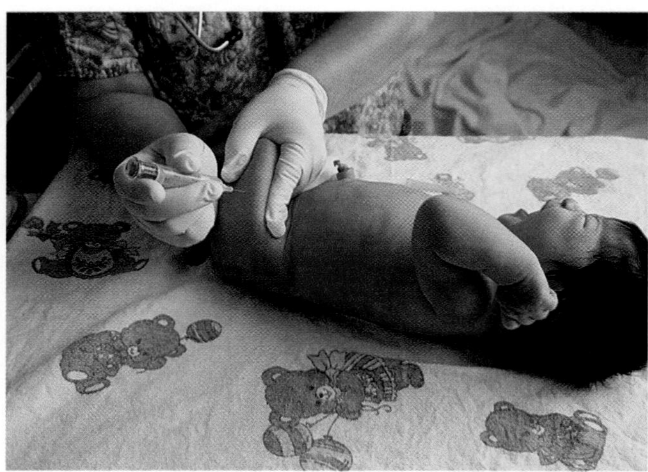

FIGURE 23–2 ♦ Procedure for vitamin K injection. Cleanse area thoroughly with alcohol swab and allow skin to dry. Bunch the tissue of the upper outer thigh (vastus lateralis muscle) and quickly insert a 25-gauge 5/8-in needle at a 90-degree angle to the thigh. Aspirate, then slowly inject the solution to distribute the medication evenly and minimize the baby's discomfort. Remove the needle and gently massage the site with an alcohol swab.

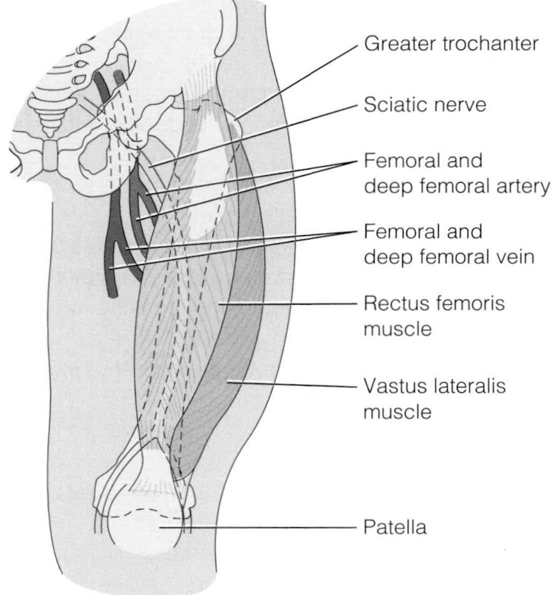


FIGURE 23–3 ♦ Injection sites. The middle third of the vastus lateralis muscle is the preferred site for intramuscular injection in the newborn. The middle third of the rectus femoris is an alternate site, but its proximity to major vessels and the sciatic nerve requires caution in using this site for injection.

Parents may request that vitamin K be given by mouth. Oral vitamin K has not been shown to be as effective as parenteral administration and is not currently recommended for use in the United States (AAP, 1997).

## Prevention of Eye Infection

The nurse is also responsible for giving the legally required prophylactic eye treatment for *Neisseria gonorrhoeae,* which may have infected the newborn of an infected mother during the birth process. A variety of topical agents appear to be equally effective. Ophthalmic ointments that are used include 1% silver nitrate, 0.5% erythromycin (Ilotycin Ophthalmic) (see Drug Guide: Erythromycin Ophthalmic Ointment [Ilotycin Ophthalmic]), on page 594 and 1% tetracycline. Erythromycin is also effective against chlamydia, which has a higher incidence rate than gonorrhea.

Successful eye prophylaxis requires that the medication be instilled into the lower conjunctival sac of each eye (Figure 23–4♦). The nurse massages the eyelid gently to distribute the ointment. Instillation may be delayed up to 1 hour after birth to allow eye contact during parent-newborn bonding (AAP, 1997).

Eye prophylaxis medications can cause chemical conjunctivitis, which gives the newborn some discomfort and may interfere with the ability to focus on the parents' faces. The resulting edema, inflammation, and discharge may cause concern if the parents have not been informed that the side effects will clear in 24 to 48 hours.

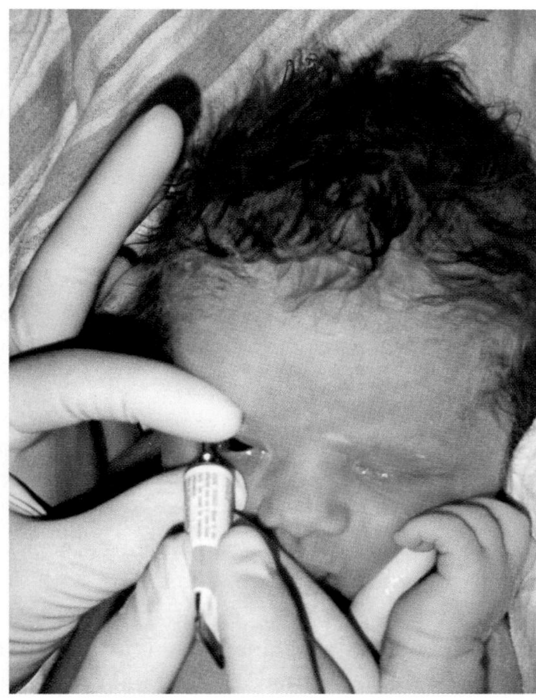

FIGURE 23–4 ♦ Ophthalmic ointment. Retract lower eyelid outward to instill 1/4-in-long strand of ointment from a single-dose tube along the lower conjunctival surface.

## Early Assessment of Neonatal Distress

During the first 24 hours of life, the nurse is constantly alert for signs of distress. If the newborn is with the parents during this period, the nurse must take extra care to teach them how to maintain their newborn's temperature, recognize the hallmarks of newborn distress, and respond immediately to signs of respiratory problems. The parents learn to observe the newborn for changes in color or activity, rapid breathing with chest retractions, or facial grimacing. Their interventions include nasal and oral suctioning with a bulb syringe, positioning, and vigorous fingertip stroking of the newborn's spine to stimulate respiratory activity if necessary. The nurse also must be available immediately if the newborn develops distress. (See Key Facts to Remember: Signs of Newborn Distress).

A common cause of neonatal distress is early-onset group B streptococcal (GBS) disease. Infected mothers transmit GBS infection to their infants during labor and birth; thus it is recommended that at-risk mothers receive intrapartum antimicrobial prophylaxis (IAP) for GBS disease. All infants of mothers identified as at risk should be assessed and observed for signs and symptoms of sepsis (bacteremia, pneumonia, or meningitis).

### KEY FACTS TO REMEMBER

#### *Signs of Newborn Distress*

- Increased respiratory rate (more than 60/minute) or difficult respirations
- Sternal retractions
- Nasal flaring
- Grunting
- Excessive mucus
- Facial grimacing
- Cyanosis (central: skin, lips, tongue)
- Abdominal distension or mass
- Vomiting of bile-stained material
- Absence of meconium elimination within 24 hours of birth
- Absence of urine elimination within 24 hours of birth
- Jaundice of the skin within 24 hours of birth or due to hemolytic process
- Temperature instability (hypothermia or hyperthermia)
- Jitteriness or blood glucose $< 40$ mg%

*Source:* Adapted from Tappero, E. P., & Honeyfield, M. E. (1996). *Physical assessment of the newborn* (2nd ed.). Petaluma, CA: NICU Ink.

# DRUG GUIDE

## VITAMIN $K_1$ PHYTONADIONE (AQUAMEPHYTON)

### *Overview of Neonatal Action*

Phytonadione is used in prophylaxis and treatment of hemorrhagic disease of the newborn. It promotes liver formation of the clotting factors, II, VII, IX, and X. At birth, the neonate does not have the bacteria in the colon that are necessary for synthesizing fat-soluble vitamin $K_1$, therefore, the newborn may have decreased levels of prothrombin during the first 5 to 8 days of life, reflected by a prolongation of prothrombin time.

### *Route, Dosage, Frequency*

Intramuscular injection is given in the vastus lateralis thigh muscle. A one-time-only prophylactic dose of 0.5 to 1 mg is given intramuscularly in the birthing area or within 1 hour of birth (Zenk, Sills, & Koeppel, 1999).

If the mother received anticoagulants during pregnancy, an additional dose may be ordered by the physician and is given at 6 to 8 hours after the first injection. IM/SC concentration: 1 mg/0.5 mL (neonatal strength); can use 10 mg/mL concentration to minimize volume injected.

### *Neonatal Side Effects*

Pain and edema may occur at injection site. Allergic reactions, such as rash and urticaria, may also occur.

### *Nursing Considerations*

- Protect drug from light.
- Give vitamin $K_1$ before circumcision procedure.
- Observe for signs of local inflammation.
- Observe for jaundice and severe hemolytic anemia especially in preterm infants.
- Observe for bleeding (usually occurs on second or third day). Bleeding may be seen as generalized ecchymoses or bleeding from umbilical cord, circumcision site, nose, or gastrointestinal tract. Results of serial PT and PTT should be assessed.

### Initiation of First Feeding

The timing of the first feeding varies depending on whether the newborn is to be breastfed or bottle-fed and whether there were any complications during pregnancy or birth, such as maternal diabetes, intrauterine growth restriction (IUGR), and so forth. Mothers who choose to breastfeed their newborns may seek to put their baby to the breast while in the birthing area. The nurse encourages this practice because successful, long-term breastfeeding during infancy appears to be related to beginning breastfeedings in the first few hours of life. Sleep-wake states affect feeding behavior and need to be considered when evaluating the newborn's sucking ability (MacMullen & Dulski, 2000). Formula-fed newborns usually begin the first feedings by 5 hours of age, during the second period of reactivity when they awaken and appear hungry. Signs indicating newborn readiness for the first feeding are active bowel sounds, absence of abdominal distension, and a lusty cry that quiets with rooting and sucking behaviors when a stimulus is placed near the lips.

### Facilitation of Parent-Newborn Attachment

Eye-to-eye contact between the parents and their newborn is extremely important during the early hours after birth, when the newborn is in the first period of reactivity. The newborn is alert during this time, the eyes are wide open, and the baby often makes direct eye contact with human faces within optimal range for visual acuity (7 to 8 in). It is theorized that this eye contact is an important foundation in establishing attachment in human relationships (Klaus & Klaus, 1985). Consequently, administration of the prophylactic eye medication is often delayed for the first hour after birth to provide an opportunity for a period of eye contact between parents and their newborn to facilitate the attachment process (AAP, 1997). Another situation that can facilitate attachment is the interactive bath. During the interactive bath experience, the newborn becomes an active participant and parents are drawn into an interaction with their newborn. The nurse can interpret the infant's behavior, model ways to respond to the behavior, and support parental strategies for doing so (Karl, 1999).

# DRUG GUIDE

## ERYTHROMYCIN OPHTHALMIC OINTMENT (ILOTYCIN OPHTHALMIC)

### *Overview of Neonatal Action*

Erythromycin (Ilotycin Ophthalmic) is used as prophylactic treatment of ophthalmia neonatorum, which is caused by the bacteria *Neisseria gonorrhoeae.* Preventive treatment of gonorrhea in the newborn is required by law. Erythromycin is also effective treatment against ophthalmic chlamydial infections. It is either bacteriostatic or bactericidal, depending on the organisms involved and the concentration of drug.

*Pregnancy risk category: C*

### *Route, Dosage, Frequency*

Ophthalmic ointment (0.5%) is instilled as a narrow ribbon or strand, 1/4 in long, along the lower conjunctival surface of each eye, starting at the inner canthus. It is instilled only once in each eye. The ointment may be administered in the birthing area or, alternatively, later in the nursery so that eye contact between infant and parent is facilitated and the bonding process immediately after birth is not interrupted.

### *Neonatal Side Effects*

Sensitivity reaction; such as edema, inflammation, or drainage may interfere with ability to focus and may cause edema and inflammation. Side effects usually disappear in 24 to 48 hours.

### *Nursing Considerations*

- Wash hands immediately prior to instillation to prevent introduction of bacteria.
- Clean the newborn's eyes to remove any drainage.
- Use new tube or single-use container for ophthalmic ointment administration shortly after birth.
- Massage eyelids gently to distribute the ointment (Zenk, Sills, & Koeppel, 1999).
- May wipe away excess after 1 minute (AAP, 1997).
- Do not irrigate the eyes after instillation.
- Observe for hypersensitivity.
- Teach parents about need for eye prophylaxis. Educate them regarding side effects and signs that need to be reported to the health care provider.

# Nursing Care Management for Newborn Care during Stay in Birthing Unit

## Nursing Diagnosis

Examples of nursing diagnoses that may apply during daily care of the newborn include the following:

- ***Altered nutrition: Less than body requirements*** related to limited nutritional and fluid intake and increased caloric expenditure
- ***Altered urinary elimination*** related to meatal edema secondary to circumcision
- ***Risk for infection*** related to umbilical cord healing, circumcision site, or immature immune system
- ***Health-seeking behaviors*** related to care needs of circumcised and uncircumcised newborns or pros and cons of breastfeeding and bottle-feeding
- ***Altered family processes*** related to integration of newborn into family unit or demands of newborn feeding schedule

## Nursing Plan and Implementation

### Maintenance of Cardiopulmonary Function

The nurse assesses vital signs every 6 to 8 hours or more, depending on the newborn's status. The newborn should always be in a propped, side-lying position when left unattended to prevent aspiration and facilitate drainage of mucus. A bulb syringe is kept within easy reach in case the baby needs oral-nasal suctioning. If the newborn has

## Critical Thinking in Practice

A mother calls you to her room. She sounds frightened and says her baby cannot breathe. You find the mother cradling her infant in her arms. The infant is mildly cyanotic, waving her arms, and has mucus coming from her nose and mouth. What would you do?

Answers can be found in Appendix I

respiratory difficulty, the nurse clears the airway. Vigorous fingertip stroking of the baby's spine will frequently stimulate respiratory activity. A cardiorespiratory monitor can be used on newborns who are not being observed at all times and are at risk for decreased respiratory or cardiac function. Indicators of risk are pallor, cyanosis, ruddy color, apnea, and other signs of instability. Changes in skin color may indicate the need for closer assessment of temperature, cardiopulmonary status, and hematocrit and bilirubin levels.

### Maintenance of Neutral Thermal Environment

The nurse makes every effort to maintain the newborn's temperature within the normal range. The nurse must make certain the newborn is dressed and exposed to the air as little as possible. A head covering should be used for the small newborn, who has less subcutaneous fat to act as insulation in maintaining body heat. The nurse should routinely monitor the ambient temperature of the room where the newborn is kept and carry out all nursing care activities as quickly as possible. A newborn whose temperature falls below optimal levels uses calories to maintain body heat rather than for growth. Chilling also decreases the affinity of serum albumin for bilirubin, thereby increasing the likelihood of newborn jaundice. In addition, it increases oxygen use and may cause respiratory distress.

On the other hand, an overheated newborn increases activity and respiratory rate in an attempt to cool the body. Both measures deplete caloric reserves, and the increased respiratory rate leads to increased insensible fluid loss ("Neonatal Thermoregulation," 1997).

### Promotion of Adequate Hydration and Nutrition

Newborn nutrition is addressed in depth in Chapter 24. The nurse records caloric and fluid intake and enhances adequate hydration by maintaining a neutral thermal environment and offering early and frequent feedings. Early feedings promote gastric emptying and increase peristalsis, thereby decreasing the potential for hyperbilirubinemia by decreasing the amount of time fecal material is in contact with beta glucuronidase in the small intestine. This enzyme frees the bilirubin from the feces, allowing it to be reabsorbed into the vascular system. The nurse records voiding and stooling patterns. The first voiding should occur within 24 hours and the first passage of stool within 48 hours. When they do not occur, the nurse continues the normal observation routine while assessing for abdominal distension, bowel sounds, hydration, fluid intake, and temperature stability.

The newborn is weighed at the same time each day for accurate comparisons. A weight loss of up to 10% for term newborns is considered within normal limits during the first week of life. This weight loss is the result of limited intake, loss of excess extracellular fluid, and passage of meconium. Parents should be told about the expected weight loss, the reason for it, and the expectations for regaining the birth weight. Birth weight is usually regained by 2 weeks if feedings are adequate.

Excessive handling can cause an increase in the newborn's metabolic rate and caloric use. The nurse should be alert to the newborn's subtle cues of fatigue, including a decrease in muscle tension and activity in the extremities and neck, as well as loss of eye contact, which may be manifested by fluttering or closure of the eyelids. The nurse quickly ceases stimulation when signs of fatigue appear and demonstrates to parents the need to be aware of newborn cues and to wait for periods of alertness for contact and stimulation. The nurse is also responsible for assessing the woman's comfort and latching-on techniques if breastfeeding, or bottle-feeding techniques.

### Promotion of Skin Integrity

Newborn skin care, including bathing, is important for the health and appearance of the individual newborn and for infection control within the nursery. Ongoing skin care involves cleansing the buttock and perianal areas with fresh water and cotton or a mild soap and water with diaper changes. The umbilical cord is assessed for signs of bleeding or infection, such as oozing and foul smell. Antimicrobial agents (triple-dye or bacitracin) may be applied to the normal newborn's cord if the baby is in a hospital nursery (World Health Organization [WHO], 1999). The nursery nurse is responsible for cord care per agency policy, which may be after the cord is cut only, once a day for the first 3 days of life, or each time the diaper is changed. In 24-hour rooming-in systems, in which the mother is the primary caregiver and clean cord care is practiced, application of an antiseptic to the stump is probably not needed because the risk of contaminating the cord is low (WHO, 1999). Clean cord care includes washing hands with clean water and soap before and after care. Alcohol is probably not effective in preventing microbial colonization of the cord and omphalitis and can delay drying of the cord.

## Promotion of Safety and Prevention of Complications

Safety of the newborn is paramount. It is essential that the nurse and other caregivers verify the identity of the newborn by comparing the numbers and names on the identification bracelets of mother and newborn before giving a baby to a parent. Another form of identification band has a built-in sensor unit that sounds an alarm if the baby is transported beyond set birthing unit boundaries. Individual birthing units should practice safety measures to prevent infant abduction and provide information to parents regarding their role in this area (Carroll, 2000). Parental measures to prevent abduction include the following:

- Checking that identification bands are in place as they care for their infant and if not have them replaced immediately
- Allowing only people with proper birthing unit identification to remove their baby from the parent's room
- Returning baby to nursery or having baby accompany the parent when leaving the room
- Reporting presence of any suspicious people on the birthing unit

Infection in the nursery is best prevented by requiring that all personnel who have direct contact with newborns scrub for 2 to 3 minutes from the fingertips to and including the elbows at the beginning of each shift. The hands must also be washed with soap and rubbed vigorously for 15 seconds ("Neonatal Skin Care," 1997) before and after contact with every newborn and after touching any soiled surface such as the floor or one's hair or face. Parents are often instructed to use an antiseptic hand cleaner before touching the baby. Anyone with an infection should refrain from working with newborns until the infection has cleared. A few agencies ask family members to wear gowns (preferably disposable) over their street clothes. Parents need to be taught that everyone handling the baby should always wash their hands before doing so, even after the baby is home.

Newborns are at continued risk for the complications of hemorrhage, late-onset cardiac symptoms, and infection. Pallor may be an early sign of hemorrhage and must be reported to the physician. The newborn is placed on a cardiorespiratory monitor to permit continuous assessment. Several newborn conditions put newborns at risk for hemorrhage. Cyanosis that is not relieved by oxygen administration requires emergency intervention, may indicate a congenital cardiac condition or shock, and requires ongoing assessment. The nurse assesses the circumcision for signs of hemorrhage and infection. The first voiding after a circumcision is also a significant assessment in evaluating for possible urinary obstruction due to trauma and edema. The nurse applies vaseline gauze to the circumcision site to prevent bleeding. The gauze is removed and replaced if it gets soiled.

## Circumcision

**Circumcision** is a surgical procedure in which the prepuce, an epithelial layer covering the penis, is separated from the glans penis and excised. This procedure supposedly permits exposure of the glans for easier cleaning.

The parents make the decision about circumcision for their newborn male child. In most cases the choice is based on cultural, social, and family tradition. Circumcision was originally a religious rite practiced by Jews and Muslims. The practice gained widespread cultural acceptance in the United States but is much less common in Europe. Many parents choose circumcision because they want their male child to have a physical appearance similar that of his father or the majority of other children. Other parents feel that it is expected by society. Another commonly cited reason for circumcising newborn males is to prevent the need for anesthesia, hospitalization, pain, and trauma if the procedure is needed later in life (AAP, Task Force on Circumcision, 1999). During the prenatal period, the nurse ensures that parents have clear and current information regarding the risks and benefits of circumcision.

### Current Recommendations

As in the past, recommendations regarding circumcision vary. The 1999 AAP policy statement does not recommend routine circumcision but acknowledges that medical indications for circumcision still exist. The organization recommends that analgesia (eg, EMLA cream, dorsal penile nerve block [DPNB], subcutaneous ring block) be used during circumcision to decrease procedural pain (AAP, Task Force on Circumcision, 1999). If a circumcision is to be performed, it should be done using the least painful method.

Circumcision should not be performed if the newborn is premature or compromised, has a known bleeding problem, or is born with a genitourinary defect such as hypospadias or epispadias, which may necessitate the use of the foreskin in future surgical repairs.

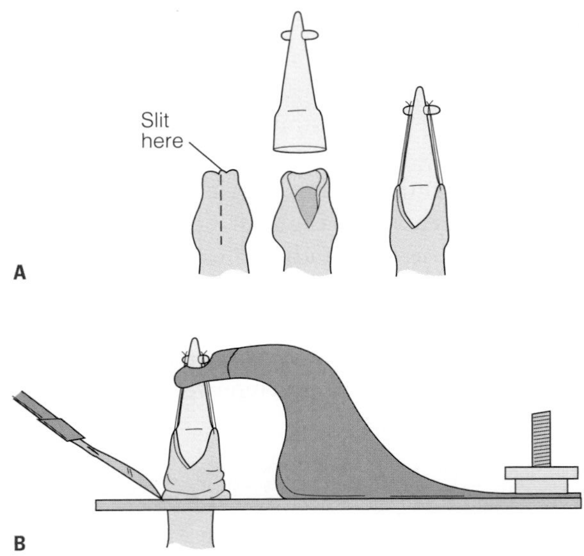


FIGURE 23–5 ♦ Circumcision using a circumcision clamp. **A,** The prepuce is drawn over the cone and **B,** the clamp is applied. Pressure is maintained for 3 to 4 minutes, and then excess prepuce is cut away.

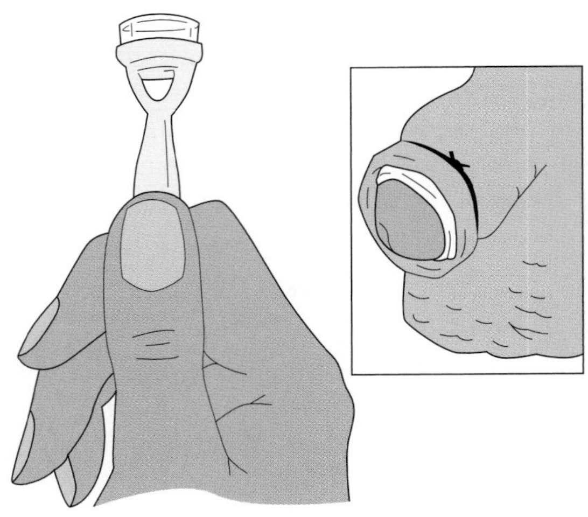

FIGURE 23–6 ♦ Circumcision using the Plastibell. The bell is fitted over the glans. A suture is tied around the bell's rim and the excess prepuce is cut away. The plastic rim remains in place for 3 to 4 days until healing occurs. The bell may be allowed to fall off; it is removed if still in place after 8 days.

### Nurse's Role

The nurse plays an essential role in providing parents with current information about circumcision. Nurses can facilitate parental informed consent because of their knowledge of the medical, social, and psychologic aspects of newborn circumcision. A well-informed nurse can allay parents' anxiety by sharing information and allowing them to express their concerns. Parents must be informed about potential risks and benefits of circumcision. Hemorrhage, infection, difficulty in voiding, separation of the edges of the circumcision, discomfort, and restlessness are early potential problems. Later there is a risk that the glans and urethral meatus may become irritated and inflamed from contact with the ammonia in urine. Adhesions and/or progressive stenosis, entrapment of the penis, and damage to the urethra are all potential complications that could require surgical correction (AAP, Task Force on Circumcision, 1999). Potential benefits include reduction in the risk of urinary tract infections (UTIs), sexually transmitted infections, and penile cancer.

The parents of an uncircumcised male infant require information from the nurse about hygienic practices. They are told that the foreskin and glans are two similar layers of cells that separate from each other. The separation process begins prenatally and is normally completed between 3 to 5 years of age. In the process of separation, sterile sloughed cells build up between the layers. This buildup looks similar to the smegma secreted after puberty, and it is harmless. Occasionally during the daily bath, the parent can gently test for retraction. If retraction has occurred, daily gentle washing of the glans with soap and water is sufficient to maintain adequate cleanliness. The parents should teach the child to incorporate this practice into his daily self-care activities.

If circumcision is desired, the procedure is performed when the newborn is well stabilized and has received his initial physical examination by a health care provider. The parents may also choose to have the circumcision done after discharge. However, they need to be advised that if the baby is older than 1 month, the current practice is to hospitalize him for the procedure.

Prior to a circumcision, the nurse ensures that the physician has explained the procedure and determines whether anesthesia is to be used, whether the parents have any further questions about the procedure, and that the circumcision permit is signed. The nurse gathers the equipment and prepares the newborn by removing the diaper and placing him on a circumcision board or some other type of restraint but restraining only the legs. In Jewish circumcision ceremonies, the infant is held by the father or godfather and given wine before the procedure (Reynolds, 1996).

A variety of techniques may be used for circumcision (Figures 23–5♦ and 23–6♦), and it is an almost bloodless procedure. However, the nurse should make special note of infants with a family history of bleeding disorders or with mothers who took anticoagulants, including aspirin, prenatally. During the procedure, the nurse assesses the newborn's response. One consideration is pain being experienced by the newborn. A DPNB using 1% lidocaine without epinephrine significantly minimizes the pain and the shifts in behavioral patterns such as crying, irritability, and erratic sleep cycles associated with circumcision.

Other studies are investigating the use of topical anesthetic applied 60 to 90 minutes before prepuce removal, acetaminophen, and cryoanalgesia (AAP, Task Force on Circumcision, 1999; Taddio, Pollock, Gilbert-MacLeod, et al., 2000). The nurse provides comfort measures such as lightly stroking the baby's head, providing a pacifier, and talking to him.

Following the circumcision, the infant should be held and comforted by a family member or the nurse. The nurse must be alert to any cues that these measures are overstimulating the newborn instead of comforting him. Such cues include turning away of the head, increased generalized body movement, skin color changes, hyperalertness, and hiccoughing. The nurse assesses the infant every hour for the first 12 hours or per agency protocol for any abnormal bleeding and applies gentle pressure as needed. A and D ointment, petroleum jelly, or antibiotic ointment is placed on the penis to keep the diaper from adhering to the site in all procedures except those using the Plastibell. New ointment is applied with each diaper change, or at least four to five times a day for 24 to 48 hours. The nurse checks that the newborn voids and for adequacy of the urine stream and presence of blood (Narchi & Kulaylat, 1998). The newborn may cry when he voids after circumcision because of the ammonia in the urine. He should be positioned on his back or side with the diaper fastened loosely to prevent undue pressure. He may remain fussy for several hours and be less interested in feedings than before the procedure.

Before discharge, the parents should be shown the appearance of a normal circumcised penis. Initially the glans penis is dark red and then becomes covered with whitish yellow exudate. The nurse discusses that the whitish yellow exudate around the glans is normal granulation tissue and not indicative of an infection. The exudate may be noted for about 2 or 3 days and should not be removed. Parents are instructed to squeeze warm water gently over the penis to remove urine and feces and pat it dry after each diaper change. Soap is used only after the circumcision is healed. The diaper is loosely fastened for 2 to 3 days, because the glans remains tender. Parents need to provide extra holding, feeding, and nonnutritive sucking opportunities for a day or two. The nurse instructs the family to look at the penis for bleeding or possible signs of infection (greenish discharge, swelling, redness). If bleeding occurs, they should apply light pressure intermittently to the site with a sterile gauze pad and notify the health care provider.

If the Plastibell is used, parents are informed that it may remain in place for up to 8 days and then fall off. If it is still in place after 8 days, it may require manual removal by the clinician.

### Enhancement of Parent-Infant Attachment and Parental Knowledge of Newborn Care

The nurse encourages **parent-newborn attachment** by involving both parents with the new family member. (For specific interventions see Chapters 17 and 28 and Teaching Guide: Enhancing Attachment.) Infant massage is a common child care practice in many parts of the world and has recently gained attention in the United States. Parents can be taught to use infant massage as a method to facilitate the bonding process and to reduce the stress and pain associated with colic, constipation, inoculations, and teething. Infant massage not only induces relaxation for the infant but also provides a calming and feel-good interaction for the parents, which fosters the development of warm, positive relationships. The nurse can discuss waking activities such as talking with the baby while making eye contact, holding the baby in an upright position (sitting or standing), gently bend the baby's back and forth while grasping under the knees and supporting the head and back with the other hand, or gently rubbing the baby's hands and feet. Quieting activities may include swaddling or bundling the baby to increase a sense of security; using slow, calming movements; and talking softly, singing, or humming to the baby. The nurse must also be aware of cultural variations in newborn care such as timing of naming the newborn, giving compliments about the baby, and needing good luck charms. The nurse plays a vital role in fostering parent-infant attachment (Figure 23–7♦). (See teaching card insert: Teaching techniques for waking and quieting newborns.)

## Nursing Plan and Implementation in Preparation for Discharge

### Parent Teaching

To meet parent's need for information, the nurse who is responsible for the care of the mother and newborn should assume the primary responsibility for education. Nearly every contact with the parents presents an opportunity for sharing information that can facilitate their sense of competence in newborn care. The nurse also needs to recognize and respect the many ways of providing safe care. Unless harmful to the newborn, the parents' methods of giving care should be reinforced rather than contradicted. In addition, the nurse needs to be sensitive to the cultural beliefs and values of the family (Table 23–1 on p. 602).

The information that follows is provided to increase the nurse's knowledge of newborn care and can also be

## TEACHING GUIDE *Enhancing Attachment*

### Assessment

The nurse provides maximum opportunity for parents to interact with their infant immediately after birth and while in the birthing unit. Observation and documentation of these interactions assist the nurse in determining the family's needs for teaching, support, or interventions.

### Nursing Diagnosis

The key nursing diagnosis will probably be altered family processes related to addition of a new baby to the family.

### Nursing Plan and Implementation

The teaching plan includes information about the infant's physical status and normal characteristics, comforting techniques, and the baby's emotional needs immediately after birth and during the newborn period. Encourage the parents to maintain continuous contact through rooming-in.

### Parent Goals

At the completion of the teaching the parents will be able to

1. Demonstrate appropriate nurturing behaviors such as touching, bonding, talking to, kissing, and holding their baby
2. Discuss normal characteristics and emotional needs of the newborn
3. List at least three comforting techniques

### *Teaching Plan*

| CONTENT | TEACHING METHOD |
|---|---|
| Present information on periods of reactivity and expected newborn responses. | Focus on open discussion. |
| Describe normal physical characteristics of newborn. | Present slides or pictures showing newborn characteristics. |
| Explain the bonding process, its gradual development, and the reciprocal interactive nature of the process. | |
| Discuss infant's capabilities for interaction, such as nonverbal communication abilities. The nonverbal communications include movement, gaze, touch, facial expressions, and vocalizations—including crying. Emphasize that eye contact is considered one of the cardinal factors in developing infant-parent attachment and will be integrated with touching and vocal behaviors. | Show a video on the interactive capabilities of newborns. Afterward, discuss woman's (couple's) response to the information. |
| Explain that touching, including stroking, patting, massaging, and kissing, will progress to interactive touch between parent and infant; discuss need to assimilate these behaviors into daily routine with baby. | Use a doll or the couple's infant to demonstrate behaviors. |
| Describe and demonstrate comforting techniques, including use of sound, swadding, rocking, stroking, and massage. | Demonstrate the techniques and ask for a return demonstration. |
| Discuss the progression of the infant's behaviors as the infant matures and the importance of parents' consistent response to their infant's cues and needs. | Allow time for questions. Provide written materials and handouts for future reference. |
| Provide information about available pamphlets, videos, and support groups in the community. | |

### Evaluation

Evaluate the learning by providing time for discussion, questions, and return demonstrations in the birthing unit, during postpartal return visit or home visit. Continue to observe the parents' positive interaction with their baby during remainder of their stay in birthing unit.

A Letter From Your Baby

Dear Parents:

I come to you a small, immature being with my own style and personality. I am yours for only a short time; enjoy me.

1. Please take time to find out who I am, how I differ from you and how much I can bring you joy.
2. Please feed me when I am hungry. I never knew hunger in the womb, and clocks and time mean little to me.
3. Please hold, cuddle, kiss, touch, stroke, and croon to me. I was always held closely in the womb and was never alone before.
4. Please don't be disappointed when I am not the perfect baby that you expected, nor disappointed with yourselves that you are not the perfect parents.
5. Please don't expect too much from me as your newborn baby, or too much from yourself as a parent. Give us both six weeks as a birthday present—six weeks for me to grow, develop, mature and become more stable and predictable, and six weeks for you to rest and relax and allow your body to get back to normal.
6. Please forgive me if I cry a lot. Bear with me and in a short time, as I mature, I will spend less and less time crying and more time socializing.
7. Please watch me carefully and I can tell you the things that soothe, console and please me. I am not a tyrant who was sent to make your life miserable, but the only way I can tell you that I am not happy is with my cry.
8. Please remember that I am resilient and can withstand the many natural mistakes you will make with me. As long as you make them with love, you cannot ruin me.
9. Please take care of yourself and eat a balanced diet, rest and exercise so that when we are together, you have the health and strength to take care of me.
10. Please take care of your relationship with others. Relationships that are good for you, support both you and me.

Although I may have turned your life upside down, please realize that things will be back to normal before long.

Thank you,

Your Loving Child

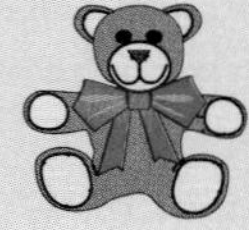

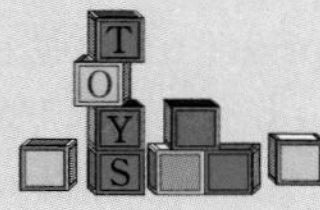


**FIGURE 23–7** ♦ A letter from your baby.

used to meet parents' needs for information. Parents may be familiar with handling and caring for infants, or this may be their first time to interact with a newborn. If they are new parents, the sensitive nurse gently teaches them by example and provides instructions geared to their needs and previous knowledge about the various aspects of newborn care.

The length of stay in the birthing unit for mother and baby after birth is often 48 hours or less. The challenge for the nurse is to use every opportunity to teach, guide, and support individual parents, fostering their capabilities and confidence in caring for their newborn. Including mother-baby care and home care instruction on the night shift assists with education needs for early-discharge parents.

The nurse observes how parents interact with their newborn during feeding and caregiving activities. Even during a short stay, there are opportunities for the nurse to provide information and observe whether the parents are comfortable with changing the diapers of, wrapping, handling, and feeding their newborn. Do both parents get involved in the newborn's care? Is the mother depending on someone else to help her at home? Does the mother give reasons (eg, "I'm too tired," "My stitches hurt," or "I'll learn later") for not wanting to be involved in her newborn's care? As the family provides care, the nurse can enhance parental confidence by giving them positive feedback. If the parents encounter problems, the nurse can express confidence in their abilities to master the new skill or information, suggest alternatives, and serve as a role model. All these factors need to be considered when evaluating the educational needs of the parents (Ruchala, 2000).

Several methods may be used to teach families about newborn care. Daily newborn care videos or classes are a nonthreatening way to convey general information. Individual instruction is helpful to answer specific questions or to clarify something that may have been confusing in class (Figure 23–8♦). (See Teaching Guide: What to Tell Parents about Infant Care (pg. 604) and Teaching Card: Teaching Infant Discharge Care Insert). Currently many birthing centers have 24-hour educational video channels or videos to be viewed in the mother's room on a variety of postpartum and newborn care issues. With shorter stays, most teaching unfortunately tends to focus on infant feeding and immediate physical care needs of the mothers, with limited anticipatory guidance provided in other areas (Cavendish & Jackson, 1999). One-to-one teaching while the nurse is in the mother's room is the most effective educational method. Both first-time and experienced postpartum mothers rated individual

## TABLE 23–1 Examples of Cultural Beliefs and Practices Regarding Baby Care*

### UMBILICAL CORD

People of Latin American or Filipino cultural background may use an abdominal binder or bellyband to protect against dirt, injury, and umbilical hernia. They may also apply oils to the stump of the cord or tape metal to the umbilicus to ward off evil spirits.

People of northern European ancestry may expect a sterile cutting of the cord at birth. They may allow the stump to air dry and discard the cord once it falls off.

Some Latin American cultures cauterize the stump with a hot flame, hot coal, or the like (WHO, 1999).

In Kenya women may express colostrum to the cord stump (WHO, 1999).

In Ecuador, the cord is left long in girls to prevent a small uterus and problems with childbirth (WHO, 1999).

### PARENT-INFANT CONTACT

People of Asian ancestry may pick up the baby as soon as it cries, or they may carry the baby at all times.

Some Native Americans, notably the Navajos, may use cradle boards.

Korean mothers may be reluctant to pick up or touch their infant, deferring infant care to the paternal grandmother (Schneiderman, 1996).

The Muslim father traditionally calls praise to Allah in the newborn's right ear and cleans the infant after birth (Hutchinson & Baqi-Aziz, 1994).

### FEEDING

Some people of Asian heritage may breastfeed their babies for the first 1 to 2 years of life.

Many Cambodian refugees practice breastfeeding on demand without restriction, or, if bottle-feeding, provide a "comfort bottle" in between feedings (Rasbridge & Kulig, 1995).

People of Iranian heritage may breastfeed female babies longer than male babies.

Some people of African ancestry may wean their babies after they begin to walk.

Most Korean mothers resist breastfeeding in the hospital, contending that they do not have "milk," and state that they will begin breastfeeding at home (Schneiderman, 1996).

Some Asians, Hispanics, Eastern Europeans, and Native Americans may delay breastfeeding because they believe colostrum is "bad" (Lipson, Dibble, & Minarik, 1996).

### CIRCUMCISION

People of Muslim and Jewish ancestry practice circumcision as a religious ritual (Hutchinson & Baqi-Aziz, 1994).

Many natives of Africa and Australia practice circumcision as a puberty rite.

Native Americans and people of Asian and Latin American cultures rarely perform circumcision.

Only 15% of the world's male population is circumcised.

### HEALTH AND ILLNESS

Some people from Latin American cultural backgrounds may believe that touching the face or head of an infant when admiring it will ward off the "evil eye." They may also neglect to cut the baby's nails to avoid nearsightedness and instead put mittens on the baby's hands to prevent scratching. They also may believe that fat babies are healthy.

Some people of Asian heritage may not allow anyone to touch the baby's head without asking permission.

Some Orthodox Jews believe that saying the baby's name before the formal naming ceremony will harm the baby.

Some Asians and Haitians delay naming their infants (Geissler, 1998).

Some people of Vietnamese ancestry believe that cutting a baby's hair or nails will cause illness.

**Note:* The information is meant only to provide examples of some of the behaviors that may be found within certain cultures. Not all members of a culture practice the behaviors described.

*Sources:* Adapted from Andrews, M. M. (1999). Transcultural perspectives in the nursing care of children and adolescents. In M. M. Andrews & J. S. Boyle (Eds.) (1999), *Transcultural concepts in nursing care* (3rd ed.). Philadelphia: Lippincott; Riordan, J., & Auerbach, K. G. (1999). *Breastfeeding and human lactation* (2nd ed.). Boston: Jones & Bartlett: World Health Organization. (1999). *Care of the umbilical cord: A review of the evidence* [On-line]. Available: www.who.int/rht/documents/MSM98-4

teaching as the most effective method of instruction (Beger & Loveland Cook, 1998). For the hearing-impaired parent, videotapes with the information in both spoken and signed formats will be most helpful.

## General Instructions for Newborn Care

Picking up a newborn is one of the first concerns of both student nurses and parents who have not had the experience. The newborn is easily picked up by sliding one hand under the neck and shoulders and the other hand under the buttocks or between the legs and then gently lifting the newborn. This technique provides security and support for the head (which the newborn is unable to support until 3 or 4 months of age).

The AAP (1997) recommends that healthy term infants be placed on their back or side to decrease the risk of sudden infant death syndrome. The nurse should demonstrate the proper positioning of the newborn and correct use of the bulb syringe. He or she can be an excellent role model for families in the area of safety. The baby should never be left alone anywhere but in the crib. The mother is reminded that while she and the newborn are together in the birthing unit, she should never leave

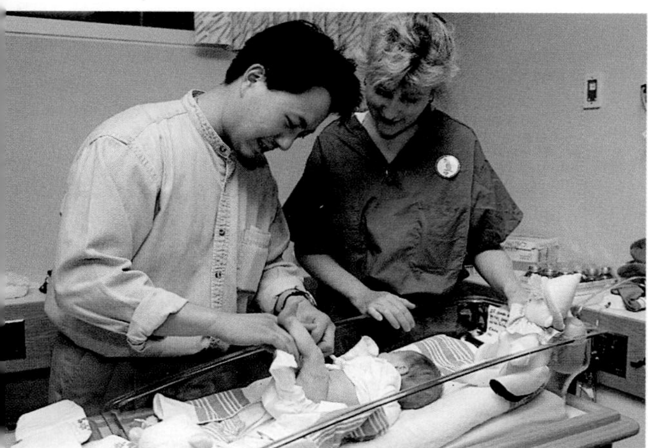

IGURE 23–8 ♦ Individualizing family education. Father returns
emonstration of diapering his son.

## HINTS FOR PRACTICE

Remember that left-handed people tend to hold the baby over their right-shoulder, and right-handed people do the opposite. This keeps the dominant hand free. However, most health personnel wear their name tags on the left side. To avoid scratching the baby's face, wear your name tag on the same side as your dominant hand.

he baby alone for security reasons and because newborns pit up frequently the first day or two after birth.

Information on newborn bathing, cord care, and temerature assessment is provided to the parents prior to ischarge. Current evidence does not support the routine pplication of topical antimicrobials to the drying umilical cord (Dore, Buchan, Coulas, et al., 1998; WHO, 999). Parents need to know the normal changes in the ord and possible problems that may occur such as right-red bleeding or greenish yellow drainage from the ord stump. If bleeding or drainage occurs, the parents re advised to call their health care provider. (See Teachng Guide: What to Tell Parents about Cord Care after Discharge, page 605.)

The nurse reviews with the family how to take axillary r tympanic temperatures and discusses the different ypes of thermometers. It is important that families unerstand the differences and know how to select a thernometer. The newborn's temperature needs to be taken nly when signs of illness are present. Parents are advised o call their physician or pediatric nurse practitioner imnediately if they observe any signs of illness.

## Critical Thinking in Practice

You are caring for a new mother who had her first child, a daughter, about 4 hours ago. She appears visibly upset when changing her infant's diaper and says she thinks something is wrong because her daughter has tissue protruding from her vagina and some blood in her diaper. What would you do?

Answers can be found in Appendix I

### Nasal and Oral Suctioning

Most newborns are obligatory nose breathers for the first months of life. They generally maintain air passage patency by coughing or sneezing. During the first few days of life, however, the newborn has increased mucus, and gentle suctioning with a bulb syringe may be indicated. The nurse can demonstrate the use of the bulb syringe in the mouth and nose and have the parents do a return demonstration. The parents should repeat this demonstration of suctioning and cleansing the bulb before discharge so they feel confident in performing the procedure. Care should be taken to apply only gentle suction to prevent nasal bleeding.

To suction the newborn, the bulb syringe is compressed *before* the tip is placed in the nostril. The nurse or parent must take care not to occlude the passageway. The bulb is permitted to reexpand slowly by releasing the compression on the bulb (Figure 23–9♦). The bulb syringe is removed from the nostril, and drainage is then compressed out of the bulb and onto a tissue. The bulb syringe may also be

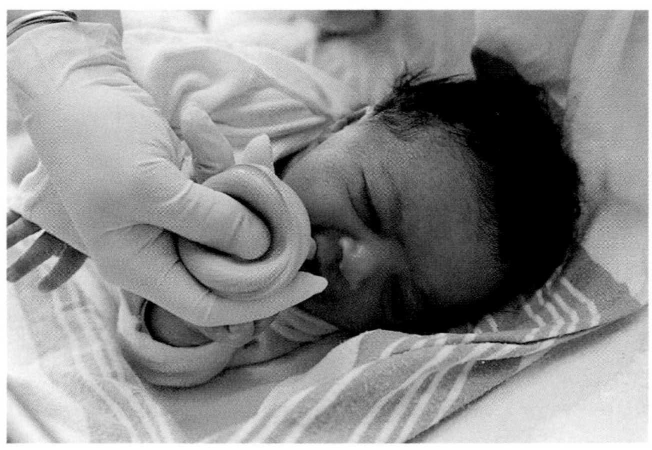

FIGURE 23–9 ♦ Nasal and oral suctioning. The bulb is compressed, the tip is placed in either the mouth or the nose, and the bulb is released.

## TEACHING GUIDE *What to Tell Parents about Infant Care*

### Assessment

The nurse determines parents' prior knowledge and experience with newborns and any concerns they may have about caring for their baby.

### Nursing Diagnosis

The key nursing diagnosis will probably be health-seeking behaviors: infant care information related to expressed parental desire to provide excellent care for the newborn.

### Nursing Plan and Implementation

The teaching plan includes information about sponge and tub baths, umbilical cord care, care of circumcised and uncircumcised infant, feeding techniques, positioning, elimination patterns, use of bulb syringe, signs and symptoms of illness, expected sleep patterns, comfort measures, and attachment behaviors.

### Parent Goals

At the completion of the teaching the parents will be able to

1. Demonstrate safe techniques of caring for their newborn, especially in use of bulb syringe, thermometer, cord cleaning, and comforting measures
2. List signs and symptoms of illness
3. Describe infant's sleep patterns and attachment behaviors
4. Demonstrate an emerging comfort level and confidence in their ability to care for their infant

### *Teaching Plan*

| CONTENT | TEACHING METHOD |
|---|---|
| Demonstrate sponge and tub bathing techniques, emphasizing safety and timing of cord separation. Review cord care to be carried out at home—see Teaching Guide: What to Tell Families about Cord Care after Discharge. | Focus on discussion and demonstration. Stress basic useful information that new parents need. Avoid patronizing tone. Provide opportunities for parents to practice. |
| Discuss care required for circumcision and uncircumcised infants. | Consider developing a demonstration video so that parents can review the content as often as they wish. |
| Discuss the signs of illness (see Key Facts to Remember: Signs of Neonatal Distress on page 593 and demonstrate use of thermometer and bulb syringe. | Discussion, handouts, pamphlets, and posters are helpful. Have handouts available in other languages for families who do not speak English. |
| Discuss normal newborn eating, sleep, and elimination patterns and behavioral characteristics. | Discuss and ask for return demonstration. |
| Review comfort measures for newborns. | Provide positive feedback to build confidence. |

### Evaluation

Evaluate the learning by asking parents to describe general newborn care and to demonstrate use of bulb syringe, taking temperature, umbilical cord care, and care of circumcision (if appropriate) prior to their newborn's discharge.

used in the mouth if the newborn is spitting up and unable to handle the excess secretions. The bulb is compressed, the tip of the bulb syringe is placed about 1 in to one side of the newborn's mouth, and compression is released. The resulting suction draws up the excess secretions. The procedure is repeated on the other side of the mouth. The roof of the mouth and back of the throat are avoided because suction in these areas might stimulate the gag reflex. The bulb syringe should be washed in warm, soapy water and rinsed in warm water daily and as needed after use. A bulb syringe should always be kept near the newborn. New parents and nurses who are inexperienced with newborns may fear that the baby will choke and are relieved to know how to take action if such an event occurs. They should be advised to turn the newborn's head to the side or down as soon as there is any indication of gagging or vomiting and to use the bulb syringe as needed.

### Swaddling the Newborn

Swaddling (wrapping) helps the newborn maintain body temperature, provides a feeling of closeness and security and may be effective in quieting a crying baby. A blanket is placed on the crib (or secure surface) in the shape of a diamond. The top corner of the blanket is folded down slightly, and the newborn's body is placed with the head at the upper edge of the blanket. The right corner of the

## TEACHING GUIDE *What to Tell Parents about Cord Care after Discharge*

### Assessment

The nurse focuses on the family's previous experience with newborns and their understanding of what the umbilical cord is and what naturally happens during the first few weeks after birth.

### Nursing Diagnosis

The key nursing diagnosis will probably be health-seeking behaviors: information on newborn cord care related to expressed parental desire to avoid infected umbilical cord in their newborn.

### Nursing Plan and Implementation

The teaching plan includes information about the need for daily cleansing, expected changes in the umbilical cord, and review of actual procedure for care of the umbilical cord.

### Parent Goals

At the completion of the teaching the parents will be able to

1. Describe the normal changes in the umbilical cord
2. List the signs of infection of the cord
3. Demonstrate proper cord care

### *Teaching Plan*

**CONTENT**

Clean cord care in the postnatal period includes washing hands with clean water and soap before and after care and keeping the cord dry and exposed to air or loosely covered with clean clothes. (If cultural custom demands binding of the abdomen, a sanitary method such as the use of a clean piece of gauze can be recommended.) The cord should be washed when necessary with clean water and soap (cleaning with alcohol seems to delay healing). Touching the cord, applying unclean substances to it, and applying bandages should be avoided.

Fold diapers below umbilical cord to air-dry the cord. Contact with wet or soiled diapers slows the drying process and increases the possibility of infection.

Check cord each day for any odor, oozing of greenish yellow material, or reddened areas around the cord. Area around cord may also be tender. Report to health care provider any signs of infection.

Normal changes in cord: Cord should look dark and dry up before falling off. A little drop of blood may appear on the diaper as the cord is about to fall off. Never pull the cord or attempt to loosen it.

**TEACHING METHOD**

Explain the rationale for regular umbilical cord care.

Use posters or a video describing the cleaning technique, warning signs of infection, and methods of diapering.

Review clean cord care and ask for return demonstration if questions exist.

### Evaluation

Evaluate the learning by asking parents to identify the signs of infection and normal changes seen in the cord prior to its falling off and to review proper cord care before their newborn's discharge.

blanket is wrapped around the newborn and tucked under the left side (not too tightly—the newborn needs a little room to move). The bottom corner is then pulled up to the chest, and the left corner wrapped around the newborn's right side (Figure 23–10♦). The nurse can show this wrapping technique to a new mother so she will feel more skilled in handling her baby.

### Sleep and Activity

Perhaps nothing is more individual to each newborn than the sleep-activity cycle. It is important for the nurse to recognize the individual variations of each newborn and to assist parents as they develop sensitivity to their newborn's communication signals and rhythms of activity and sleep. (See Chapter 22 for a more detailed discussion of sleep-wake activity.)

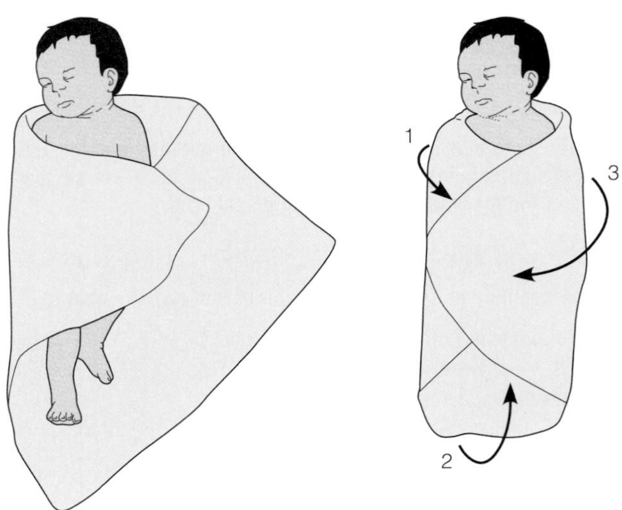


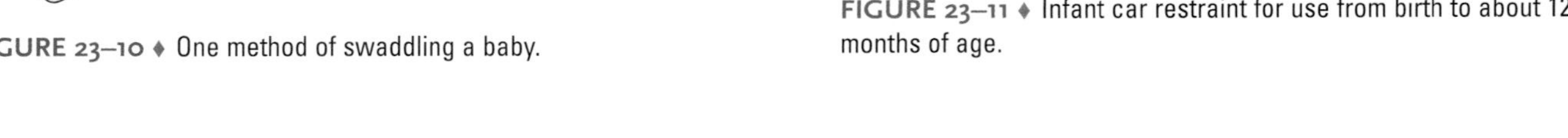

FIGURE 23–10 ♦ One method of swaddling a baby.

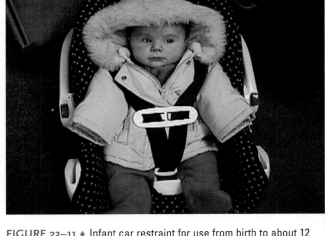

FIGURE 23–11 ♦ Infant car restraint for use from birth to about 12 months of age.

## Car Safety Considerations

Half of the children killed or injured in automobile accidents could have been protected by the use of federally approved car seats. Newborns should go home from the birthing unit in a car seat adapted to fit newborns (Figure 23–11♦). Babies should never be placed in the front seat of a car equipped with a passenger-side air bag. The car seat should be placed in the back seat and positioned to face the rear of the car until the baby is a year old or weighs 20 lb (9.09 kg). In many states, the use of car seats for children up to the age of 4 is mandatory. Nurses need to ensure that all parents are knowledgeable about the benefits of child safety seat use and proper installation (AAP, Committee on Injury and Poison Prevention, 1999).

## Newborn Screening and Immunization Program

Before the newborn and mother are discharged from the birthing unit, the nurse informs the parents about the normal **newborn screening tests** for newborns and tells them when to return to the birthing center or clinic if further tests are needed. The disorders that can be identified from a drop of blood obtained by a heel stick are cystic fibrosis, galactosemia, homocystinuria, hypothyroidism, maple syrup urine disease, phenylketonuria (PKU), and hemoglobinopathies. Early discharge puts infants at risk for delayed or even missed diagnosis of PKU and congenital hypothyroidism because of decreased sensitivity of screening; infants should be retested by 2 weeks of age if the first test was done prior to 24 hours of birth. The accuracy of the test for PKU is directly related to the newborn's age. The likelihood of detecting PKU increases as the infant grows older, so the infant needs to be at least 24 hours old for a valid test (Wallman, 1998).

The Centers for Disease Control and Prevention (CDC) and the AAP recommend immunization programs against the hepatitis B virus during early infancy (Selekman, 2000). As of July 1999, the recommendation for infants born to HbsAg-negative mothers is for receipt of the first dose of hepatitis B vaccine (thimerosal-free COMVAX™) by age 2 months. COMVAX™ also contains *Haemophilus b* (Hib) vaccine and is not approved for use in infants less than 6 weeks of age. If thimerosal-free vaccine is not available, hepatitis B virus vaccination should be initiated at 6 months of age (AAP, Committee on Infectious Diseases and Committee on Environmental Health, 1999). The recommendation for infants born to HbsAg-positive mothers remains unchanged. These infants should receive hepatitis B vaccine and 0.5 mL hepatitis B immune globulin (HBIG) within 12 hours of birth at separate injection sites. Parents need to be advised if their birthing center provides newborn hepatitis vaccinations so that an appropriate follow-up program can be set in motion. Now that sufficient quantities of thimerosal-free hepatitis B vaccine are becoming available, a return to the 1999 newborn immunization schedule, that all newborns receive their first Hepatitis B vaccine soon after birth, is recommended.

The nurse should teach the family all necessary caregiving methods before discharge. A checklist may be helpful to determine whether the teaching has been completed and to verify the parents' knowledge on leaving the birthing unit (Figure 23–12♦). The nurse needs to review

## NURSERY TEACHING CHECKLIST

Please read the *Mother/Baby* information booklet given to you after delivery. After reading it, please go through the following list and check whether you understand each topic or need to know more.

| | | I know this already | Doesn't apply to me | I need to know more | FOR NURSES ONLY: Taught/ reviewed/ demonstrated |
|---|---|---|---|---|---|
| Baby Care | What to do if baby is choking or gagging | | | | |
| | Safety | | | | |
| | How to do skin care/cord care | | | | |
| | How to take care of the circumcision or genital area | | | | |
| | How to know if my baby is sick and what to do | | | | |
| | What is jaundice and how to detect it | | | | |
| | Use of thermometer | | | | |
| | Use of bulb syringe | | | | |
| | How and when to burp baby | | | | |
| | Newborn behavior: crying/comforting | | | | |
| | How to position baby after feeding | | | | |
| | What does demand scheduling mean | | | | |
| Breastfeeding | I attended breastfeeding class/watched breastfeeding video | YES ☐ | NO ☐ | | |
| | How to position baby for feeding | | | | |
| | How to get baby to latch on to my nipple properly | | | | |
| | When and how long to nurse | | | | |
| | Removal of baby from my nipple | | | | |
| | What is the supply and demand concept | | | | |
| | What is the let down reflex | | | | |
| | When does breast milk come in | | | | |
| | Supplementing | | | | |
| | Proper diet for breastfeeding mothers | | | | |
| | Prevention and comfort measures for sore nipples | | | | |
| | Prevention and comfort measures for engorgement | | | | |
| | When and how to use a breast pump | | | | |
| | How to express milk by hand | | | | |
| | How to go back to work and continue to breastfeed | | | | |
| Bottle Feeding | How to feed my baby a bottle | | | | |
| | Reasons for NOT propping bottles | | | | |
| | How to clean nipple/bottle | | | | |
| | How to mix formula | | | | |
| | What formula should my baby drink | | | | |
| | **State Law requires use of infant car seat** | | | | |
| | I have a baby/infant car seat and know how to use it | YES ☐ | NO ☐ | | |

Other information:

______________________________

______________________________

______________________________

______________________________

______________________________

I have received and understand the instructions given on the above topics.

______________________________ ______________

MOTHER'S SIGNATURE DATE

Videos viewed/ Literature given:

______________________________

______________________________

______________________________

______________________________

Nurse's Signature(s):

______________________________

______________________________

______________________________

**FIGURE 23–12** ♦ Infant teaching checklist is completed by the time of discharge. *Source:* Adapted from Presbyterian/St. Luke's Medical Center, Denver, CO.

all areas with the mother and father, without rushing, and take time to answer all queries. Any concerns of the parents or nurse are noted.

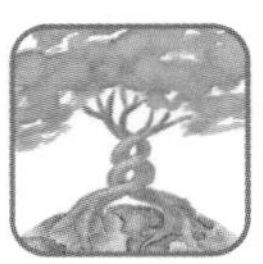

## Community-Based Nursing Care

By discussing with parents ways to meet their newborn's needs, ensure safety, and appreciate the newborn's unique characteristics and behaviors, and by assisting parents in establishing links with their community-based health care provider, the nurse can get the new family off to a good start. To assist parents in caring for their newborn at home, some physicians encourage pediatric prenatal visits so that this contact is established before birth. Public health nurses have long been involved in newborn care and parent education. In some programs the birthing unit staff nurses visit new families in their homes within a few hours or days of discharge to bridge the gap between early discharge and routine health care checkups (AAP, Council on Child and Adolescent Health, 1999). Parents need to know the signs of illness, how to reach the pediatrician or after-hours clinic, and the importance of follow-up after discharge. (See Key Facts to Remember: When Parents Should Call Their Health Care Provider and Teaching Card: Teaching Signs of Possible Illness during Newborn Period insert.) Parents should also check with their clinician for advice about over-the-counter medications to be kept in the medicine cabinet.

Education is a wonderful aspect of family-centered maternity care. The nurse who takes the time to get the family off to a good start can feel the satisfaction of providing optimal care.

### KEY FACTS TO REMEMBER

*When Parents Should Call Their Health Care Provider*

Temperature above 38.4°C (101°F) rectally or 38°C (100.4°F) axillary or below 36.1°C (97°F) rectally or 36.6°C (97.8°F) axillary

Continual rise in temperature

More than one episode of forceful vomiting or frequent vomiting (over 6 hours)

Refusal of two feedings in a row

Lethargy (listlessness), difficulty in awakening baby

Cyanosis with or without a feeding

Increasing jaundice (yellow tone) of the skin

Pustules, rashes, or blisters other than normal, newborn rash

Absence of breathing longer than 15 seconds

Inconsolable infant (quieting techniques are not effective) or continuous high-pitched cry

Discharge or bleeding from umbilical cord, circumcision, or any opening (except vaginal mucus or pseudomenstruation)

Two consecutive green or black watery stools or increased frequency of stools

Abdominal distension, crying when trying to pass stools, or absnece of stools after stool pattern is established

No wet diapers for 18 to 24 hours or fewer than six wet diapers per day after 4 days of age

Development of eye drainage

# Evaluation

Anticipated outcomes of nursing care include the following:

- The newborn's adaptation to extrauterine life is completed successfully.
- The newborn feeding pattern is satisfactorily established.
- The parents demonstrate safe techniques in caring for their newborn.
- The parents express understanding of the bonding process and display attachment behaviors.
- Parents verbalize developmentally appropriate behavioral expectations of their newborn and knowledge of community-based newborn follow-up care.

# Chapter Review

## CHAPTER HIGHLIGHTS

- The overall goal of newborn nursing care is to provide comprehensive care while promoting the establishment of the new family unit.
- In the period immediately after birth, during which adaptation to extrauterine life occurs, the newborn requires close monitoring to ensure normal transition.
- Nursing goals during the first 4 hours after birth (admission period) are to maintain a clear airway, maintain a neutral thermal environment, initiate oral feedings, facilitate attachment, and prevent hemorrhage and infection.
- The newborn is routinely given prophylactic vitamin K to prevent possible hemorrhagic disease of the newborn.
- Prophylactic eye treatment for *Neisseria gonorrhoeae* is legally required for all newborns.
- Nursing goals for ongoing newborn care include maintenance of cardiopulmonary function, maintenance of neutral thermal environment and skin integrity, promotion of adequate hydration and nutrition, promotion of safety, enhancement of attachment and family knowledge of child care, and prevention of complications.
- Following a circumcision, the newborn must be observed closely for signs of pain, bleeding, inability to void, and infection.
- Prior to discharge, the nurse provides parent teaching on nasal and oral suctioning, wrapping the newborn, sleep and activity, and safety considerations.
- Newborn screening for cystic fibrosis, galactosemia, homocystinuria, hypothyroidism, maple syrup urine disease, phenylketonuria, and hemoglobinopathies is done on all newborns in the first 1 to 3 days after birth.

## CHAPTER REFERENCES


American Academy of Pediatrics. (1997): *Guidelines for perinatal care* (4th ed.). Chicago: Author.

American Academy of Pediatrics, Council on Child and Adolescent Health. (1998). The role of home-visitation programs in improving health outcomes for children and families. *Pediatrics, 101*(3), 486–489.

American Academy of Pediatrics, Committee on Infectious Diseases and Committee on Environmental Health. (1999). Thimerosal in vaccines; An interim report to clinicians. *Pediatrics 104*(3), 570–574.

American Academy of Pediatrics, Committee on Injury and Poison Prevention. (1999). Safe transposition of newborns at hospital discharge. *Pediatrics 104*(4), 986–987.

American Academy of Pediatrics, Task Force on Circumcision. (1999). Circumcision policy statement. *Pediatrics 103*(3), 686–693.

Andrews, M. M. (1999). Transcultural perspectives in the nursing care of children and adolescents. In M. M. Andrews & J. S. Boyle (Eds.), *Transcultural concepts in nursing care* (3rd ed.), pp. 107–159. Philadelphia: Lippincott.

Beger, D., & Loveland Cook, C. A. (1998). Postpartum teaching priorities: The viewpoints of nurses and mothers. *Journal of Obstetric, Gynecologic, and Neonatal Nursing, 27*(2), 161–168.

Carroll, V. (2000). Infant abduction: Lowering the risk. AWHONN Lifelines, *3*(6), 25–27.

Cavendish, R., & Jackson, L. (1999). *Early discharge of the term newborn: Guideline for practice.* Des Plains, IL: NANN.

Dore, S., Buchan, D., Coulas, S., Hamber, L., Stewart, M., Cowan, D., & Jamieson, L. (1998). Alcohol versus natural drying for the newborn cord care. *Journal of Obstetric, Gynecologic, and Neonatal Nursing, 27*(6), 621–628.

Geissler, E. M. (1998). *Pocket guide to cultural assessment* (2nd ed.). St. Louis: Mosby.

Hutchinson, M. K., & Baqi-Aziz, M. (1994). Nursing care of the childbearing Muslim family. *Journal of Obstetric, Gynecologic, and Neonatal Nursing, 23* (9), 767–771.

Karl, D. J. (1999). The newborn bath: Using infant neurobehavior to connect parents and newborns. *American Journal of Maternal Child Nursing, 24*(6), 280–286.

Klaus, M., & Klaus, P. (1985). *The amazing newborn.* Menlo Park, CA: Addison-Wesley.

Lipson, J. G., Dibble, S. L., & Minarik, P. A. (1996). *Culture and nursing care; A pocket guide.* San Francisco, CA: University of California at San Francisco Nursing Press.

MacMullen, N. J., & Dulski, L. A. (2000). Factors related to sucking ability in healthy newborns. *Journal of Obstetric, Gynecologic, and Neonatal Nursing, 29*(4), 390–396.

Merestein, G. B., & Gardner, S. L. (1998). *Handbook of neonatal intensive care* (4th ed.). St Louis: Mosby.

Narchi, H., & Kulaylat, N. (1998). Neonatal circumcision: When can infants reliably be expected to void? *Pediatrics, 102*(10), 150–152.

Neonatal skin care. (1997). *NANN guidelines for practice.* Petaluma, CA: National Association of Neonatal Nurses.

Neonatal Thermoregulation. (1997). *NANN guidelines for practice.* Petaluma, CA: National Association of Neonatal Nurses.

Rasbridge, L. A., & Kulig, J. C. (1995). Infant feeding among Cambodian refugees. *American Journal of Maternal Child Nursing, 20*(4), 213–218.

Reynolds, R. D. (1996). Use of the Mogen clamp for neonatal circumcision. *American Family Physician 54*(1), 177–182.

Riordan, J., & Auerbach, K. G. (1999). *Breastfeeding and human lactation* (2nd ed.). Boston: Jones & Bartlett.

Ruchala, P. L. (2000). Teaching new mothers: Priorities of nurses and postpartum women. *Journal of Obstetric, Gynecologic, and Neonatal Nursing, 29*(3), 265–273.

Schneiderman, J. U. (1996). Postpartum nursing for Korean mothers. *American Journal of Maternal Child Nursing, 21*(3), 155–158.

Selekman, J. (2000). Immunization schedule 2000. *Pediatric Nursing, 26*(2), 209–210.

Taddio, A., Pollock, N., Gilbert-MacLeod, C., & Ohlsson, K. (2000). Combined analgesia and local anesthesia to minimize pain during circumcision. *Archives of Pediatric and Adolescent Medicine, 154,* 620–623.

Varda, K. E., & Behnke, R. S. (2000). The effect of timing of initial bath on newborn's temperature. *Journal of Obstetric, Gynecologic, and Neonatal Nursing, 29*(1), 27–32.

Wallman, C. M. (1998). Newborn genetic screening. *Neonatal Network, 17*(3), 55–60.

World Health Organization. (1999). *Care of the umbilical cord: A review of the evidence* [On-line]. Available: www.who.int/rht/documents/MSM98-4

Zenk, K. E., Sills, J. H., & Koeppel, R. M. (1999). *Neonatal medications and nutrition: A comprehensive guide.* Santa Rosa, CA: NICU Ink.

## CONTEMPORARY MATERNAL-NEWBORN NURSING ON-LINE

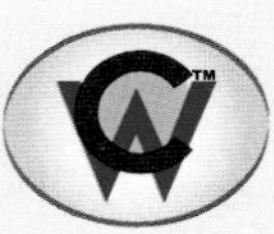

Additional interactive resources, including animations and video, for this chapter can be found on the Companion Website at http://www.prenhall.com/ladewig. Click on Chapter 23 and "Begin" to select the activities for this chapter.

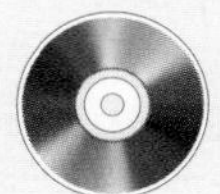

For NCLEX review questions and an audio glossary, access the accompanying CD-ROM in this book.

Chapter 24

# Newborn Nutrition

*As a lactation educator my goal is to ensure that breastfeeding is well established before the couplet (mom and baby) is discharged. I try to set the groundwork for trust and rapport, so that after they go home the family is not afraid to call me if questions arise. Sometimes I see the mom and baby weeks or even months later, and they will thank me for getting them off to a good start.*

—Hospital Lactation Nurse

## OBJECTIVES

- Compare the nutritional value and composition of breast milk and formula preparations.
- Discuss the advantages and disadvantages of breastfeeding and formula feeding for both mother and newborn.
- Develop guidelines for helping both breast- and formula-feeding mothers to feed their newborns successfully.
- Recognize the influence of cultural values on infant care, especially feeding practices.
- Delineate nursing responsibilities for client education about problems the breastfeeding mother may encounter at home.
- Incorporate knowledge of newborn nutrition and normal growth patterns into parent education and infant assessment.

## KEY TERMS

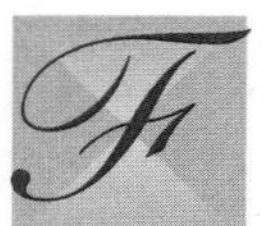

eeding their newborn is an exciting, satisfying, but often worrisome task for parents. Meeting this essential need of their new child helps parents strengthen their attachment to their child and fosters their self-images as nurturers and providers and yet carries great responsibility. Whether a woman chooses to breastfeed or formula feed, she can be reassured that she can adequately meet her infant's needs. As questions about feeding arise, the nurse works with the woman to help her develop skill in her chosen method. In every interaction, it is the nurse's responsibility to support the parents and promote the family's sense of confidence.

## KEY FACTS TO REMEMBER

### *Newborn Caloric and Fluid Needs*

- Caloric intake: 50–55 kcal/lb/day or 105–108 kcal/kg/day
- Fluid requirements: 64–73 mL/lb/day or 140–160 mL/kg/day
- Weight gain: First 6 months—1 oz/day
  Second 6 months—0.5 oz/day

# Nutritional Needs of the Newborn

The newborn's diet must supply nutrients to meet the rapid rate of physical growth and development. A neonatal diet should include protein, carbohydrate, fat, water, vitamins, and minerals. The recommended dietary allowances (RDAs) for birth through the first 6 months have been established. The calories (105 to 108 kcal/kg/day or 50 to 55 kcal/lb/day) in the newborn's diet are divided among protein, carbohydrate, and fat. Protein is needed for rapid cellular growth and maintenance. Carbohydrates provide energy. The fat portion of the diet provides calories, regulates fluid and electrolyte balance, and develops the newborn brain and neurologic system. Fluid requirements are high (140 to 160 mL/kg/day or 64 to 73 mL/lb/day) because of the newborn's inability to concentrate urine. Fluid needs increase further during illness or hot weather. (See Key Facts to Remember: Newborn Caloric and Fluid Needs.)

The infant's iron needs are affected by accumulation of iron stores during fetal life and the mother's iron and other food intake if she is breastfeeding. Ascorbic acid (usually in the form of fruit juices) and meat, poultry, and fish enhance absorption of iron in the mother, just as they do later in the infant. The newborn needs adequate minerals and vitamins to prevent deficiency states such as scurvy, cheilosis, and pellagra.

Formula-fed babies gain weight faster than breastfed babies because of the higher protein in commercially prepared formula and the larger volumes of formula that are needed to obtain the necessary nutrients. (Because breast milk is digested more easily than formula, the nutrients are more readily available.) Formula-fed infants tend to regain their birth weight by 10 days after birth and may gain 30 g (1 oz) or more per day, up to 6 months of age. Healthy breastfed babies tend to regain their birth weight about 14 days after birth and gain approximately 15 g (0.5 oz) per day in the first 6 months of life. Formula-fed infants generally double their weight within 3.5 to 4 months, whereas nursing infants double their weight at about 5 months of age.

## Breast Milk Feeding

The composition of human milk varies with the stage of lactation, the time of the day, the time during the feeding, maternal nutrition, and gestational age of the newborn at birth. During the establishment of lactation there are three stages of human milk: colostrum, transitional milk, and mature milk.

**Colostrum** is a yellowish or creamy-appearing fluid that is thicker than the mature milk and contains more protein, fat-soluble vitamins, and minerals (Kunz, Rodriguez-Palmero, Koletzko, et al., 1999). It also contains high levels of immunoglobulins (antibodies such as IgA) and can be a source of passive immunity for the newborn. Colostrum production begins early in pregnancy and may last for several days after birth. In most cases colostrum is replaced by transitional milk within 2 to 4 days after birth.

**Transitional milk** is produced from the end of colostrum production until approximately 2 weeks postpartum. This milk contains lactose, water-soluble vitamins, elevated levels of fat, and more calories than colostrum.

The final milk produced, **mature milk,** contains about 10% solids (carbohydrates, proteins, fats) for energy and growth; the rest is water, which is vital for maintaining hydration. The composition of mature milk varies according to the time during the feeding. **Foremilk** is the milk obtained at the beginning of the feeding. It is high in water content and contains vitamins and protein. **Hindmilk** is released after the initial letdown, or release of milk, and has a higher fat concentration. Although mature milk appears similar to skim milk (watery and somewhat bluish in color) and may cause mothers to question whether their milk is "rich enough," mature breast milk provides 20 kcal/oz, as do most prepared formulas. However, the percentage of calories derived from protein is lower in breast milk than in formulas, and a greater percentage of calories is derived from fat. In breastfed babies, protein metabolism produces less nitrogen waste, which has a positive effect on the infant's immature renal system.

The American Academy of Pediatrics (AAP) and American College of Obstetricians and Gynecologists (ACOG) (1997) recommend breast milk as the optimal food for the first 6 to 12 months of life. It is believed that breastfeeding provides newborns and infants with immunologic, nutritional, and psychosocial advantages.

### Immunologic Advantages

Immunologic advantages of breastfeeding include varying degrees of protection from respiratory and gastrointestinal infections, otitis media, meningitis, sepsis, and allergies (Kelleher & Duggan, 1999). This protection of the breastfed baby extends from the neonatal period through age 18 months, when the baby's own immunoglobulins become active. Secretory IgA, an immunoglobulin present in colostrum and breast milk, has antiviral, antibacterial, and antigenic-inhibiting properties. Secretory IgA plays a role in decreasing the permeability of the small intestine to antigenic macromolecules (Johnson & Reddick, 2000). Other properties in colostrum and breast milk that act to inhibit the growth of bacteria and viruses are *Lactobacillus bifidus,* lysozymes, lactoperoxidase, lactoferrin, transferrin, and various immunoglobulins. Immunoglobulins to the poliomyelitis virus are also present in the breast milk of mothers who have immunity to this virus. Because the presence of these immunoglobulins may inhibit the desired intestinal infection and immune response of the infant, some clinics suggest that breastfeeding be withheld for 30 to 60 minutes following the administration of the Sabin oral polio vaccine. In addition to its immunologic properties, breast milk is known to be nonallergenic.

### Nutritional Advantages

Breast milk is composed of lactose, lipids, polyunsaturated fatty acids, and amino acids, especially taurine, and has a whey-to-casein protein ratio that facilitates its digestion, absorption, and full use compared to formulas (Johnson & Riddick, 2000). Some researchers believe that the high concentration of cholesterol and the balance of amino acids in breast milk make it the best food for myelination and neurologic development (Johnson & Riddick, 2000). High cholesterol levels in breast milk may stimulate the production of enzymes that lead to efficient metabolism of cholesterol, thereby reducing its harmful long-term effects on the cardiovascular system.

Breast milk provides newborns with minerals in more appropriate doses than formulas do (Lawrence & Lawrence, 1999). Although the concentration of iron in breast milk is much lower than that in prepared formulas, it is much more readily and fully absorbed and appears sufficient to meet the infant's iron needs for the first 4 to 6 months. The AAP and ACOG (1997) state that breastfed newborns generally do not need supplemental iron before the age of 4 to 6 months. Furthermore, supplemental iron may decrease the ability of breast milk to protect the newborn by interfering with lactoferrin, an iron-binding protein that enhances the absorption of iron and has antiinfective properties.

Another advantage of breast milk is that all its components are delivered to the infant in an unchanged form, and vitamins are not lost through processing and heating. If the breastfeeding mother is taking daily multivitamins, her diet is adequate, and the baby is exposed to sunlight for 30 minutes a week if wearing a diaper or 2 hours a week if fully clothed, vitamin D supplements are not necessary for the exclusively breastfed infant (Lauwers & Shinski, 2000). If the mother's diet or vitamin intake is inadequate or questionable, caregivers may choose to prescribe additional vitamins for the infant.

### Psychosocial Advantages

The psychosocial advantages of breastfeeding are primarily those associated with maternal-infant attachment. The mother's level of oxytocin generally increases with breastfeeding, and studies indicate that this hormonal change coincides with more even mood responses and increased feelings of maternal well-being (Rogers, Golding, & Emmett, 1997). Breastfeeding enhances attachment by providing the opportunity for frequent, direct skin contact between the newborn and the mother. The newborn's sense of touch is highly developed at birth and is a primary means of communication. The tactile stimulation associated with breastfeeding can communicate warmth, closeness, and comfort. The increased closeness provides both newborn and mother with the opportunity to learn each other's behavioral cues and needs. The mother's sense of accomplishment in being able to satisfy her baby's needs for nourishment and comfort is enhanced when the newborn sucks vigorously and is satiated and calmed by the breastfeeding. Some mothers prefer breastfeeding as a means of extending the close, unique, nourishing relationship between mother and baby that existed before the baby's birth.

Breastfeeding twins not only is possible but can enhance the mother's individualization and attachment to each newborn. The fantasy of a single baby is replaced more readily with the reality of two individual babies when the mother has close and frequent contact with each. Fathers are encouraged to be a part of the feeding experience by offering fresh pumped or thawed (frozen) breast milk to the baby at one or more feedings daily.

### Contraindications and Disadvantages

There are some medical contraindications to breastfeeding. A mother with a diagnosis of breast cancer should not breastfeed so that she can begin treatment immediately. Women with the human immunodeficiency virus (HIV) or acquired immunodeficiency syndrome (AIDS) are counseled against breastfeeding except in countries where the risk of neonatal death from diarrhea and other disease (excluding AIDS) is high. Breastfeeding is also contraindicated for the infant suffering from galactosemia (Calamaro, 2000). Maternal medications may preclude breastfeeding, as discussed in Chapters 12 and 25. Medications such as metronidazole (Flagyl), used to treat trichomoniasis, pass into breast milk and may be harmful to the breastfeeding infant (Johnson & Riddick, 2000). Management of newborn jaundice may include a brief suspension of breastfeeding (see Chapter 26).

In the dominant Western culture, in which women actively pursue activities outside the home, being "tied down" to an infant for 9 to 12 feedings every day may be considered inconvenient and stressful. Another often-cited disadvantage of breastfeeding is the exclusion of the father from the nurturing involved in feeding the infant. However, since nurturing encompasses more than just feeding, the father can comfort and attend to the baby in many other ways (Figure 24–1♦).

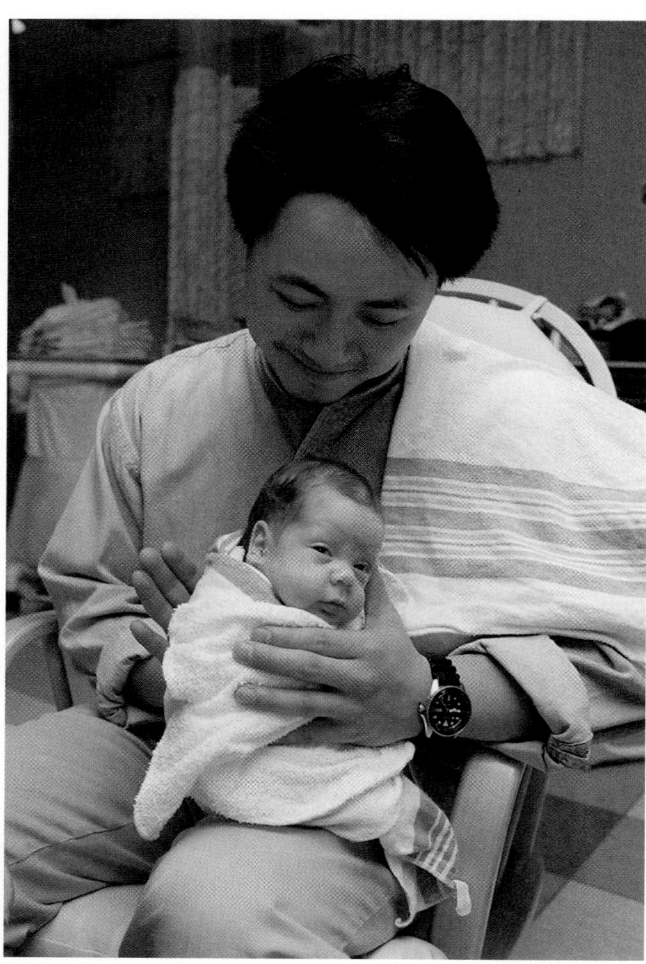

FIGURE 24–1 ♦ A father can nurture his baby in many ways.

Opinions vary on the advisability of continuing breastfeeding if the mother becomes pregnant with another child. Some believe the nutritional demands on the pregnant mother are too great and advocate gradual weaning. Others suggest that with adequate rest, a proper diet, and strong emotional support, continued breastfeeding during pregnancy is a valid choice. The practice of nursing one infant throughout pregnancy and then breastfeeding both infants after birth is called *tandem nursing.* When pregnancy occurs, the decision is best made on an individual basis after considering maternal health and motivation and the age of the first child.

Although many mothers obtain information about breastfeeding from written sources, family and friends, and **La Leche League** (an international lay support and information group), the nurse needs to be a ready source of information, encouragement, and support as well. The nurse can be helpful when parents are deciding whether to breastfeed, after the birth process when breastfeeding is just being established, and after the family returns home.

## Formula Feeding

Although breastfeeding is increasing in popularity, formula feeding is a viable and nurturing choice, particularly in developed countries, and meets the goal of successful growth of the baby. The closeness and warmth that can occur during breastfeeding is also an integral part of bottle-feeding. An advantage of bottle-feeding is that parents can share equally in this nurturing, caring experience with their baby. Numerous types of commercially prepared lactose formulas meet the nutritional needs of the infant. These formulas contain more tyrosine and phenylalanine and less taurine than breast milk does. Because many commercial formulas use a cow's milk base, they tend to have a high renal solute load, high protein and casein content, high proportion of saturated fats, low amounts of linoleic acid, poor mineral bioavailability, and increased risk for allergies to cow's milk proteins (Tigges, 1997).

Many companies make enriched formulas that are similar to breast milk. These formulas have sufficient levels of carbohydrate, protein, fat, vitamins, and minerals to meet the newborn's nutritional needs. Commercial formulas have been developed to minimize the harmful components of cow's milk. The formulas are enriched with carnitine and/or taurine and vitamins, particularly vitamin D; some of them are also enriched with long-chain polyunsaturated fatty acids. The three categories of infant formulas are formulas with cow's milk base, soy protein–based formulas, and specialized or therapeutic formulas. Soy protein–based formulas substitute soy protein supplemented with methionine for cow's milk protein and are used for primary lactase deficiency or galactosemia conditions. Specialized formulas such as casein-hydrolysated formulas (eg, Nutramigen, Pregestimil®, Alimentum®) are used when an infant has an allergy or intolerance to cow's milk protein. The AAP recommends hydrolysated formulas for infants with allergy or intolerance to cow's milk protein to avoid risk of concomitant allergy to soy protein (AAP, Committee on Nutrition, 2000). Whey-hydrolysated formulas, such as Carnation Good Start®, can also be used for infants with cow's milk allergy but not if the child has an IgE-mediated allergy to cow's milk.

### Potential Contraindications

If formula is prepared improperly (such as by adding too much powder), the excess salts (ie, sodium) may be detrimental to the newborn's kidneys and may lead to thirst in the formula-fed infant, causing overfeeding. If formula is overdiluted, the infant will not receive adequate nutrients.

Another potential problem with formulas is an allergic reaction in the newborn. The small intestine of the infant is permeable to macromolecules such as those found in cow's milk–based formulas. The introduction of a formula's foreign protein can cause an allergic reaction, with such signs as vomiting, colic, diarrhea, colitis, reluctance to feed, and eczema. (See Key Facts to Remember: Comparison of Breastfeeding and Formula Feeding)

Clinicians recommend that parents who bottle-feed use iron-fortified formulas or supplements because iron-deficiency anemia can occur (AAP, Committee on Nutrition, 1999). The RDA for iron is 6 mg/day from birth to 6 months. However, too much iron in the form of iron-fortified cereal may interfere with the infant's natural ability to defend against disease. Parents also need to be informed about the constipation that sometimes results from iron-enriched formula and about various methods of alleviating it.

The AAP and ACOG (1997) recommended that infants be given breast milk or iron-fortified formula rather than whole milk until 1 year of age. Neither unmodified cow's milk (ie, whole milk) nor skim milk is an acceptable alternative for infant feeding. The level of protein in unmodified cow's milk is much higher (50% to 75% greater) than in human milk, is poorly digested, and may cause bleeding of the gastrointestinal tract. It is also has higher levels of calcium, phosphorus, sodium, and potassium, which increase renal solute load and result in greater obligatory water loss. Skim milk lacks adequate calories, fat content, and essential fatty acids necessary for proper development of the infant's neurologic system. Nutritionists advise against giving cow's milk with decreased fat content (2% milk) or skim milk to children under 2 years of age.

## Newborn Feeding

### Initial Feeding

The physiologic and behavioral cues of the newborn determine the time of the first feeding. The nurse should assess for active bowel sounds, absence of abdominal distension, and a lusty cry that quiets and is replaced with rooting and sucking behaviors when a stimulus is placed near the lips. These signs indicate that the newborn is hungry and physically ready to tolerate the feeding.

The first feeding provides an opportunity for the nurse to assess the effectiveness of the newborn's suck, swallow, and gag reflexes. The mother who plans to breastfeed should be encouraged to nurse her newborn immediately after birth and allow the baby to nurse to satiety. Because colostrum is not irritating if aspirated (which may occur because of the newborn's initial uncoordinated sucking and swallowing abilities) and is readily absorbed by the respiratory system, breastfeeding can usually begin immediately after birth. Contraindications to immediate nursing include heavy sedation of the mother and physical compromise of either mother or baby. Bottle-feeding newborns are offered formula as soon as they show an interest.

Early breastfeeding benefits both mother and newborn because oxytocin helps expel the placenta and prevent excessive maternal blood loss, lactation is accelerated, and the infant receives the immunologic protection of colostrum. For both breastfed and formula-fed infants, early feeding stimulates peristalsis, facilitating elimination of the by-products of bilirubin conjugation (which decreases the risk of jaundice), and enhances maternal-infant attachment.

Throughout the first 2 hours after birth, especially during the first 20 to 30 minutes, the infant is usually alert and ready to nurse. However, newborn suckling patterns vary, and although many babies are eager to suckle at this time, some simply lick or nuzzle the nipple. This behavior is beneficial because the licking stimulates the release of oxytocin, which aids uterine involution and lactation (letdown). The nurse can assure the mother that this is a positive breastfeeding interaction (Riordan & Auerbach, 1999). Within minutes after birth the newborn shows early odor-based recognition of the mother's breasts. Maternal breast odors elicit preferential head orientation, which helps guide the newborn to the nipple (Porter & Winberg, 1999).

## KEY FACTS TO REMEMBER *Comparison of Breastfeeding and Formula Feeding*

| Breastfeeding | Iron-Enriched Formula Feeding |
|---|---|
| **Nutrition** | |
| Breast milk is species specific (ie, perfect balance of proteins, carbohydrates, fats, vitamins, and minerals for human infants). | Formula is as close to human milk as possible, but nutrients are not as efficiently utilized. |
| Breast milk contains higher levels of lactose, cystine, and cholesterol, which are necessary for brain and nerve growth. | Nutritional adequacy depends on proper preparation (overdilution results in decreased nutrients delivered to infant). |
| Proteins are easily digested and fats are well absorbed. | Some babies cannot tolerate the fats or carbohydrates found in regular formula. Companies offer alternative formulas. |
| Composition varies according to gestational age and stage of lactation, thereby meeting the changing nutritional requirements of individual infants as they grow. | |
| Infants determine the volume of milk consumed. | Pediatrician or caregiver determines the volume consumed. Overfeeding may occur if caregiver is determined that baby empty bottle. |
| Frequency of feeding is determined by infant cues. | Feeding is determined by infant's cues. |
| **Antiinfective and Antiallergic Properties** | |
| Breast milk contains immunoglobulins, enzymes, and leukocytes that protect against pathogens. | Formula is linked to an increased number of GI and respiratory infections. |
| Bacteriostatic properties permit storage at room temperature up to 6 hours, in refrigerator for 24 hours, and freezing for 6 months. | Potential for bacterial contamination exists during preparation and storage. |
| Breast milk decreases the incidence of allergy by eliminating exposure to potential antigens (cow and soy protein). | Some babies are allergic to cow or soy protein. Formula companies are offering alternative formulas suitable for babies who develop allergies. |
| **Psychosocial Aspects** | |
| Skin-to-skin contact enhances closeness. | Formula feeding provides an opportunity for positive parent-infant interaction. |
| Hormones of lactation promote maternal feelings and sense of well-being. | |
| The value system of an industrial society can create barriers to successful breastfeeding:<br>Mother may feel ashamed or embarrassed. | |
| Breastfeeding after return to work may be difficult. | |
| Father is not able to breastfeed, but he can feed expressed breast milk from a bottle and nurture the infant in ways other than feeding. | Father can feed the baby. |
| **Cost** | |
| Healthy diet for mother. | Formula is an expense. |
| Optional, but recommended, items include nursing pads, nursing bras. | Bottles or disposable nursers with plastic liners, nipples, and nipple caps must be purchased. |
| A breast pump may be needed. | |
| Refrigeration is necessary for storing expressed milk. | A refrigeration system is necessary if mixing formula for more than one feeding at a time or using large containers or ready-to-feed formula. |
| **Convenience** | |
| The milk is always the perfect temperature. | |
| No preparation time is needed. | Varying amounts of time are involved in formula preparation. |
| The mother must be available to feed or provide expressed milk to be given in her absence. | |
| If she misses a feeding, the mother must express milk to maintain lactation. | Anyone can feed the baby. |
| The mother may experience slight discomfort in the early days of lactation. | |
| Maternal medication may interrupt breastfeeding. | |

Assessment of the newborn's physiologic status is of primary and ongoing concern to the nurse throughout the first feeding. Extreme fatigue coupled with rapid respiration, circumoral cyanosis, and diaphoresis of the head and face may indicate cardiovascular complications and should be assessed further. The initial feeding also requires assessment of the infant for the rare congenital anomalies tracheoesophageal fistula and esophageal atresia (see Chapter 25). Findings associated with esophageal anomalies include maternal polyhydramnios and increased oral mucus in the infant. In cases of esophageal atresia, the feeding is taken well initially, but, as the esophageal pouch fills, the feeding is quickly regurgitated unchanged by stomach contents. If a fistula is present, the infant gags, chokes, regurgitates mucus, and may become cyanotic as fluid passes through the fistula and into the lungs.

It is not unusual for the newborn to regurgitate some mucus and water following a feeding, even if it was taken without difficulty. Consequently, the newborn is observed closely and positioned on the right side after a feeding to aid drainage and facilitate gastric emptying.

## Establishing a Feeding Pattern

An "on-demand" feeding program facilitates each baby's own rhythm and assists a new mother in establishing lactation. The newborn rapidly digests breast milk and may desire to nurse 8 to 10 times in a 24-hour period. After the initial period of alertness and eagerness to suckle, the infant progresses to light sleep, then deep sleep, followed by increased wakefulness and interest in nursing. As wakefulness and interest in nursing increase, the infant will often cluster 5 to 10 feeding episodes over 2 to 3 hours, followed by a 4- to 5-hour deep sleep. After this cluster of minifeeds and deep sleep, the infant will feed frequently but at more regular intervals. Maternal medications received during labor may affect newborn feeding behavior by delaying early cluster feedings. Delays in the normal feeding patterns depend on the specific drug and its half-life. Some newborns whose mothers received epidural analgesia have been noted to be irritable and demonstrate reduced motor organization, poor self-quieting skills, and decreased visual skills and alertness (Riordan & Auerbach, 1999).

Couplet care permits the mother to learn about and respond to her infant's early feeding cues. Early cues that indicate a newborn is interested in feeding include hand-to-mouth or hand-passing-mouth motion, whimpering, sucking, and rooting (Mulford, 1992). Crying is a late sign of hunger. When couplet care is not available, a supportive nursing staff and flexible nursery policies will allow the mother to feed her infant on cue. It is very frustrating to a new mother to attempt to feed a newborn who is sound asleep because he or she is either not hungry or exhausted from crying. Table 24–1 can be used to help parents identify their baby's cues for hunger and satiation.

Although people often accept crying as normal and healthy behavior for newborns, it may actually delay the transition to extrauterine life. Crying involves a Valsalva maneuver that increases pulmonary vascular pressure, which may cause unoxygenated blood to be shunted into systemic circulation through the foramen ovale and ductus arteriosus. Therefore, it may be advantageous for the baby to be in the room with the mother because she will respond to the baby's needs more quickly than the nursery staff may be able to, resulting in less infant crying.

**TABLE 24–1 Infant Feeding Behaviors**

| *Age* | *Hunger Behavior* | *Feeding Behavior* | *Satiety Behavior* |
|---|---|---|---|
| Birth to 13 weeks (0–3 months) | Cries; hands fisted; body tense | Rooting reflex; medial lip closure; strong suck reflex; suck-swallow pattern; tongue thrust and retraction; palmomental reflex, gags easily, needs burping | Withdraws head from nipple; falls asleep; hands relaxed; relief of body tension |
| 14–24 weeks (4–6 months) | Eagerly anticipates; grasps and draws bottle or breast to mouth; reaches with open mouth | Aware of hands; generalized reaching; intentional hand to mouth; tongue elevation; lips purse at corners—pucker; shifts food in mouth—prechewing; tongue protrudes in anticipation of nipple; tongue holds nipple firm; tongue projection strong; suck strength increases; coughs and chokes easily; preference for tastes | Tosses head back; fusses or cries; covers mouth with hands; ejects food; distracted by surroundings |

*Source:* Mott, S.R.; James, S.R.; Sperhac, A., (1990). *Nursing care of children and families* (2nd ed., p. 155). Redwood City, CA: Addison-Wesley Nursing.

Formula-fed newborns may awaken for feedings every 2 to 5 hours but are frequently satisfied with feedings every 3 to 4 hours. Because formula is digested more slowly, the bottle-fed infant may go longer between feedings but should not go longer than 4 hours. Babies may begin skipping the night feeding within about 8 to 12 weeks after birth (Riordan & Auerbach, 1999). The need for a night feeding is individual and depends on the size and development of the infant.

Both breastfed and bottle-fed infants experience growth spurts at certain times and require increased feeding. The mother of a breastfed infant may meet these increased demands by nursing more frequently to increase her milk supply. It will take about 24 hours for the milk supply to increase adequately to meet the new demand (Lawrence & Lawrence, 1999). A slight increase in feedings will meet the needs of the formula-fed infant.

## Community-Based Nursing Care

Providing nourishment for her newborn is a major concern of the new mother. Her feelings of success or failure may influence her self-concept as she assumes her maternal role. With proper instruction, support, and encouragement from professionals, feeding becomes a source of pleasure and satisfaction to both the parents and infant.

### Promotion of Successful Infant Feeding

Parents may see feeding their baby as the center of their relationship with this new family member. Whether the mother has chosen to formula feed or breastfeed, the nurse can be instrumental in assisting the mother to have a successful experience while in the birthing unit and during the early days at home. Feeding and caring for newborns may be routine tasks for the nurse, but the mother's success or failure during the first few times may determine her feelings about herself as an adequate mother.

The newborn's response to caring is an expression of personality but often has great significance for parents. A parent may interpret the newborn's behavior as rejection, which may alter the progress of parent-child relationships. A parent may also interpret the sleepy infant's refusal to suck or inability to retain formula as evidence of parental incompetence. The breastfeeding mother may deduce that the newborn does not like her if he or she fails to take her nipple readily. Conversely, infants pick up messages from the muscular tension of those holding them.

A nurse who is sensitive to the needs of the mother can form a relationship with her that permits sharing of knowledge about techniques and emotions connected with the feeding. Breastfeeding women frequently express disappointment in the help given to them by birthing unit nurses; they say they would like more encouragement, support, and practical information about feeding their newborn, especially with early discharge. Nonnursing mothers express similar concerns. Consistency in teaching by nurses is essential. A new mother becomes very frustrated if she is shown a number of different methods of feeding her newborn. With the technologic advances in formula production and the availability of knowledge about breastfeeding techniques, the mother should be confident that the choice she makes will promote normal growth and development of her newborn.

The mother's decision to breastfeed or formula feed is usually made by the sixth month of pregnancy and often even before conception. The final decision, however, may not be made until the mother's admission to the birth center. The decision is frequently influenced by relatives, especially the baby's father and maternal grandmother (Susin, Giugliani, Kummer, et al., 1999), by friends, and by social customs rather than being based on knowledge about the nutritional and psychologic needs of the mother and her newborn.

The goals of Healthy People 2010 continue to be 75% of infants breastfeeding in the early postpartal period and 50% taking in at least some human milk until age 6 months (Davis, Okuboye, & Ferguson, 2000). It is the health care provider's responsibility to provide the parents with accurate information about the distinct advantages of breastfeeding to the mother and infant. In times of short stays, the Baby-Friendly Hospital Initiative program promotes breastfeeding by designating hospitals as centers for breastfeeding education (Dodgson, Allard-Hale, Bramscher, et al., 1999). Unfortunately, as of 1998, only 17 hospitals in the United States had implemented the program (Davis et al., 2000). Parents have a right to hear about the data so they can make their own informed choices.

Once the parents have made an *informed choice* of feeding method, the nurse's primary responsibilities are to support the family's decision and to help the family achieve a positive result. No woman should be made to feel either inadequate or superior because of her choice in feeding. There are advantages and disadvantages to breastfeeding and bottle-feeding, but positive bonds in parent-child relationships can be developed with either method.

Before feeding, the mother should be as comfortable as possible. Preparations may include voiding, washing her hands, and assuming a position of comfort. The woman who has had a cesarean birth needs support so that the infant does not rest on her abdomen for long periods. When she is breastfeeding, she may be more comfortable lying on her side with a pillow behind her

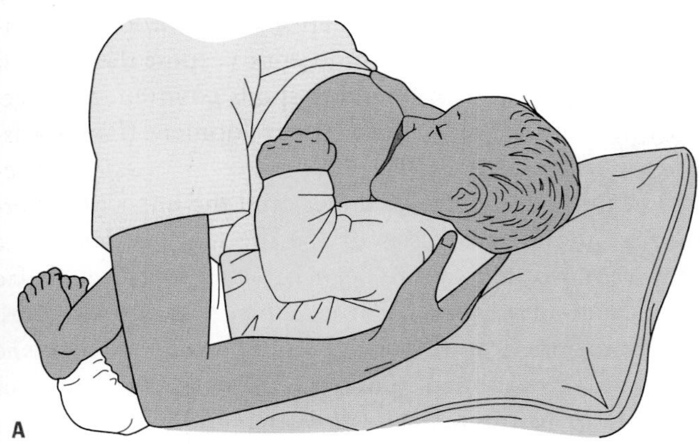
A

- Hold the baby's back and shoulders in the palm of your hand.
- Tuck the baby up under your arm, keeping the baby's ear, shoulder and hip in a straight line.
- Support the breast to touch baby's lips. Once the baby's mouth is open wide, pull the baby quickly to you.
- Hold your breast until the baby nurses easily.

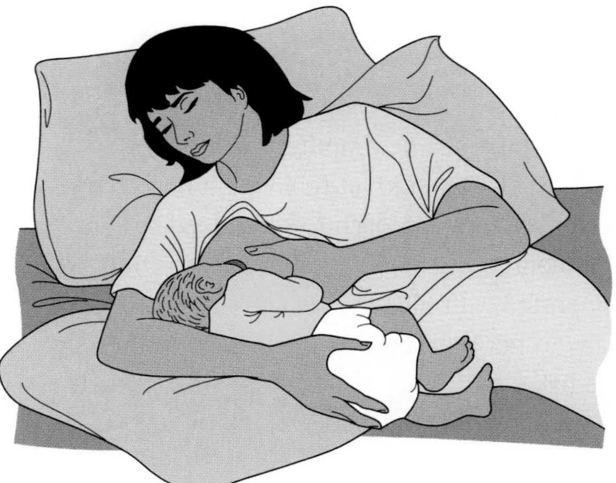
B

- Lie on your side with a pillow at your back and lay the baby so you are facing each other.
- To start, prop yourself up on your elbow and support your breast with that hand.
- Pull the baby close to you, lining up the baby's mouth with your nipple.
- Hold your breast with the opposite hand. Once the baby is nursing well, lie back down.

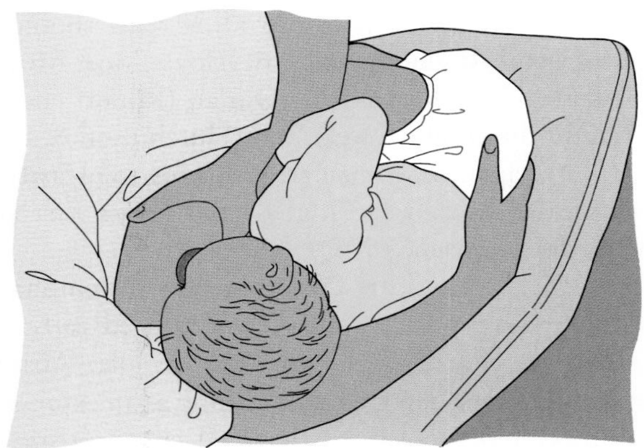
C

- Cradle the baby in the arm closest to the breast, with the baby's head in the crook of the arm.
- Have the baby's body facing you, tummy-to-tummy.
- Use your opposite hand to support the breast.

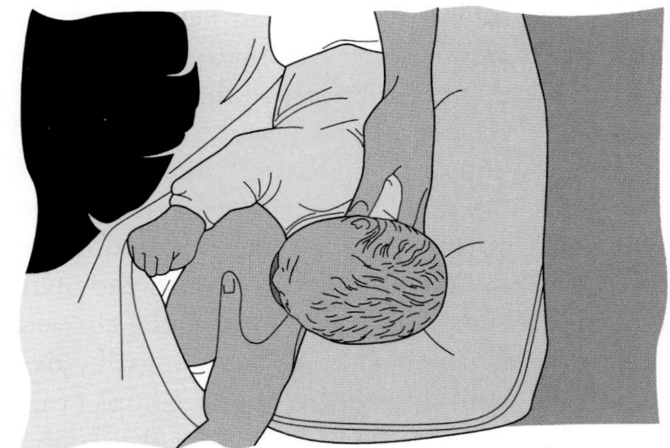
D

- Lay your baby on pillows across your lap.
- Turn the baby to face you.
- Reach across your lap to support the baby's back and shoulders with the palm of your hand.
- Support your breast from underneath. Once the baby's mouth is open wide, pull your baby quickly onto your breast.

FIGURE 24–2 ♦ Four common breastfeeding positions. **A**, Football hold. **B**, Lying down. **C**, Cradling. **D**, Across the lap. *Source: Breastfeeding: A Special Relationship.* Breastfeeding Education Resources, 1-800-869-7892, Raleigh, NC. Copyright Lactation Consultants of NC.

back and one between her legs. The nurse can position the newborn next to the woman's breast and place a rolled towel or small pillow behind the infant for support. At first the mother will need assistance in turning from side to side and burping the newborn. She may prefer to breastfeed sitting up with a pillow on her lap and the infant resting on the pillow rather than directly on her abdomen. It may be helpful to place a rolled pillow under the arm supporting the infant's head. An alternative position that prevents pressure on the incision while allowing for maximum visualization of the infant's face is the football hold. See Figure 24–2♦ for a variety of breastfeeding positions.

Mothers who have undergone cesarean birth frequently use the sitting position to bottle-feed. If incisional pain makes this position difficult, the mother may

## HINTS FOR PRACTICE

As you assist new mothers with breastfeeding, it is important to create a relaxed environment and approach to breastfeeding. Encourage mom to get into a comfortable position, well supported with pillows. Remind her to bring the baby to her breast rather than leaning forward to the baby.

find it helpful to assume the side-lying position. The infant can be moved to a semisitting position against a pillow close to the mother.

Depending on the newborn's level of hunger, the parents may want to use the time before feeding to get acquainted with their infant. The presence of the nurse during part of this time to answer questions and provide reinforcement of parenting skills will be helpful for the family. For the sleepy baby, a period of playful activity—such as gently rubbing the feet and hands or adjusting clothing and loosening coverings to expose the infant to room air—may increase alertness so that, when the feeding is initiated, the infant is ready and sucks eagerly. If an infant is overly hungry and upset, talking quietly and rocking gently may provide the baby with an opportunity to calm down so that he or she can find and grasp the nipple effectively. After the feeding, when the infant is satisfied and asleep, parents may explore the characteristics unique to their newborn. Routines must be flexible enough to allow this time for the family. Couplet care offers spontaneous, frequent encounters for the family and provides opportunities to practice handling skills, thereby increasing confidence in care after discharge. It also encourages feeding in response to the baby's cues rather than feeding by a fixed schedule. However, the nurse should understand and support the mother's choice to have her newborn cared for in the nursery so she can rest. This rest time is especially important if she must care for herself, the newborn, and other children without adult help at home.

## Cultural Considerations in Infant Feeding

It is important for the nurse to understand how culture and society influence infant feeding. Motherhood itself changes the woman's lifestyle. Perceptions of the mother's role and of breastfeeding as a biologic act also influence the mother's comfort with breastfeeding. Some mothers identify shame, modesty, and embarrassment as reasons they chose not to breastfeed. The amount of body contact considered acceptable also influences parental behaviors. North American and European societies sometimes consider it indecent to expose the breast, believe that too much handling spoils children, and regard weaning as a sign of infant development (Lawrence & Lawrence, 1999).

The nurse also needs to understand the impact of culture on the idiosyncrasies of specific feeding practices. How soon women want to begin breastfeeding after birth is culturally determined. For example, in many cultures (Mexican-American, Navajo, Filipino, and Vietnamese) and in some countries (Guinea, Pakistan) colostrum is not offered to the newborn (Geissler, 1998; Riordan & Auerbach, 1999). Breastfeeding begins only after the milk flow is established. In many Asian cultures, the newborn is given boiled water until the mother's milk flows. The newborn is fed on demand, and cries are responded to immediately. If the crying continues, evil spirits may be blamed and a priest's blessing may be sought. Although many of the Hmong women of Laos combine breastfeeding with some bottle-feeding, they usually find expressing their milk or pumping their breasts unacceptable. Thus other methods of providing relief should be suggested if breast engorgement develops. Most Muslim mothers breastfeed because the Qur'an (Koran) encourages it until the child is 2 years old (Hutchinson & Baqi-Aziz, 1994). Japanese women are returning to breastfeeding as the method of feeding for the baby's first year (Riordan & Auerbach, 1999).

The African-American culture tends to emphasize plentiful feeding. Solid foods are introduced early and may even be added to the infant's formula. African-American mothers view frequent feeding as an expression of hardiness and a positive behavioral characteristic for their children for the future (Vezeau, 1991). For the traditional Mexican, a fat baby is considered healthy and infants are fed on demand. "Spoiling" is encouraged.

These are but a few of the cultural practices related to feeding. When faced with an infant care practice different from the ones to which they are accustomed, nurses need to evaluate the effect of the practice. Different practices are not necessarily inferior. The nurse should intervene only if the practice is actually harmful to the mother and baby.

## Physiology of the Breasts and Lactation

The female breast is divided into 15 to 24 lobes separated from one another by fat and connective tissue. These lobes are subdivided into lobules, composed of small units called alveoli, where milk is synthesized by the alveolar secretory epithelium. The lobules have a system of lactiferous ductiles that join larger ducts and eventually open onto the nipple surface. During pregnancy, increased levels of estrogen stimulate breast development in preparation for lactation.

Birth results in a rapid drop in estrogen and progesterone with a concomitant increase in the secretion of **prolactin.** This hormone promotes milk production by stimulating the alveolar cells of the breast. Prolactin levels rise in response to the infant suckling. The newborn's suckling also stimulates the release of oxytocin from the posterior pituitary. This hormone increases the contractility of the myoepithelial cells lining the walls of the mammary ducts, and a flow of milk results. This is called the **letdown reflex,** or milk ejection reflex. Mothers have described the letdown reflex as a prickling or tingling sensation during which they feel the milk coming down. Other signs of letdown include increased uterine cramps and increased lochia (during the early postpartum period), milk leaking from the other breast, and a feeling of relaxation. It is not unusual for the breasts to leak some milk before feeding.

The letdown reflex can be stimulated by the newborn's sucking, presence, or cry, or even by maternal thoughts about her baby. It may also occur during sexual orgasm because oxytocin is released. Conversely, the mother's lack of self-confidence, fear of embarrassment, or pain connected with breastfeeding may prevent the milk from being ejected into the duct system.

Milk production decreases with repeated inhibition of the milk ejection reflex. Failure to empty the breasts frequently and completely also decreases production. As milk accumulates and is not withdrawn, the buildup of pressure in the alveoli suppresses secretion. Once lactation is established, prolactin production decreases. Oxytocin and sucking continue to facilitate milk production.

## Client Education for Breastfeeding Self-Care

The nurse caring for the breastfeeding mother should help the woman achieve independence and success in her feeding efforts (Figure 24–3♦). Prepared with a knowledge of the anatomy and physiology of the breast and lactation, the components and positive effects of breast milk, and techniques of breastfeeding, the nurse can help the woman and her family use their own resources to achieve a successful experience.

### Breastfeeding Process

The objectives involved in breastfeeding are (1) to provide adequate nutrition, (2) to facilitate maternal-infant attachment, and (3) to prevent trauma to the nipples. Information and support are aimed toward these goals. When assisting the mother with breastfeeding, the nurse should use disposable gloves because breast milk and newborn saliva are body substances that call for standard precautions.

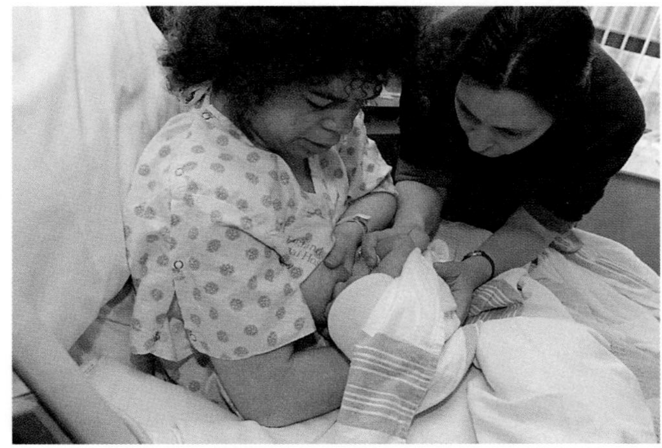

FIGURE 24–3 ♦ For many mothers, the nurse's support and knowledge are instrumental in establishing successful breastfeeding.

To facilitate successful breastfeeding, the nurse should arrange for privacy, help the mother find a comfortable position, and position the baby comfortably close to the mother. The mother should support her breast with her hand, using the C-hold or the scissors hold. In the C-hold the mother places her thumb well above the areola and the rest of her fingers below the areola and under the breast. The mother may also use the scissors hold, placing her index finger above the areola and her other three fingers below the areola and under the breast. Either method of presenting the breast to the infant is acceptable as long as the mother's hand is well away from the nipple so the baby can "latch on" to the breast (Figure 24–4♦).

The mother positions the baby so that her or his nose is at the level of the nipple. She lightly tickles the baby's lower lip with her nipple until the baby opens her or his mouth wide and then brings the baby to the breast. The baby needs to take the whole nipple into the mouth so that the gums are on the areola. This allows the jaws to compress the milk ducts directly beneath the areola when the baby suckles. The baby's nose and chin should touch the breast. If the breast occludes the baby's airway, simply lifting up on the breast will usually clear the nares. The baby's lips should be relaxed and flanged outward, with the tongue over the lower gum. At this point the baby should be facing the mother (tummy to tummy or chest to chest), with the ear, shoulder, and hip aligned (Figure 24–5♦).(See Teaching Card: Teaching Breastfeeding insert).

During early feedings the infant should be offered both breasts at each feeding to stimulate the supply-demand response. In some cases the newborn will suckle only one breast well before falling asleep. As long as each breast is

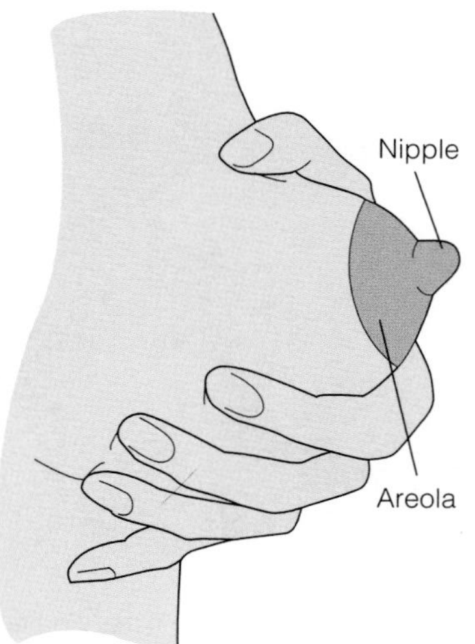


A

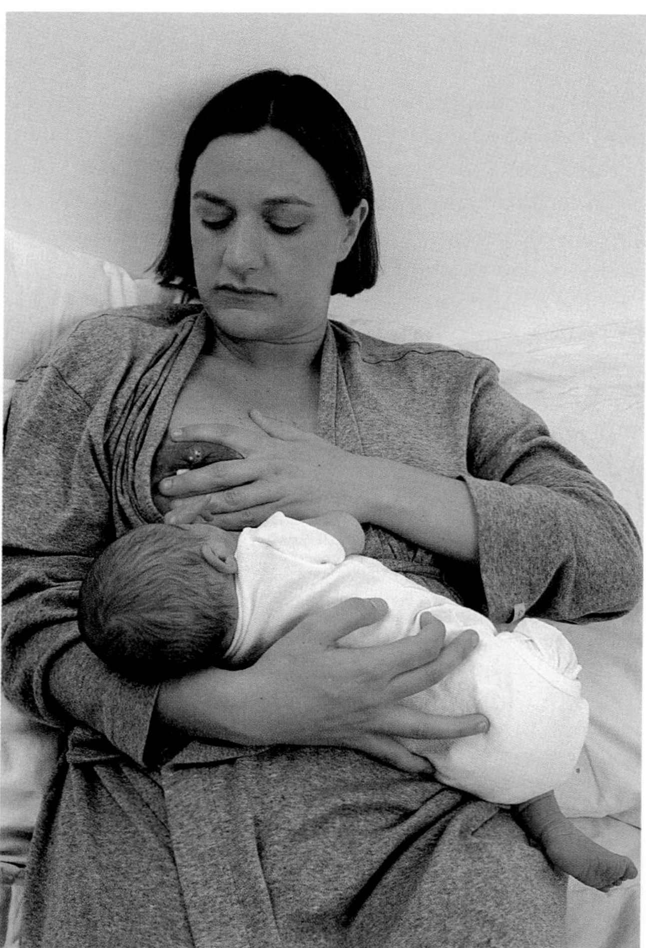

B

FIGURE 24–4 ♦ **A,** C-hold. **B,** Scissors hold. *Source:* A Courtesy Childbirth Graphics Ltd., Rochester, NY.

offered frequently (at least every 2 hours), single-breast feeds of whatever duration the baby wishes are appropriate until the baby shows a desire for both breasts. The mother should breastfeed until she becomes relaxed to the point of sleepiness—a delightful side effect of

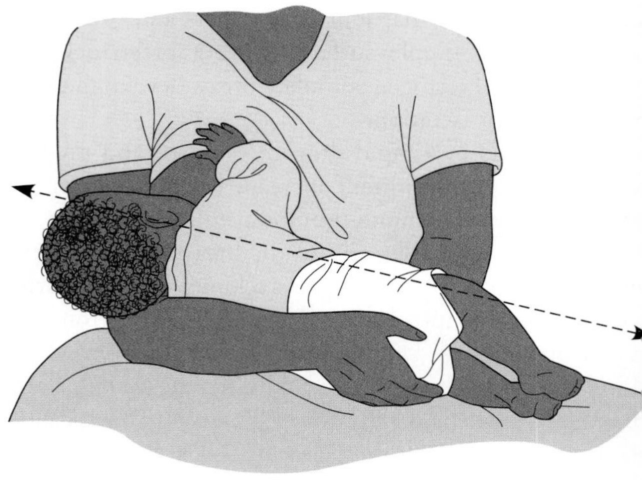

FIGURE 24–5 ♦ Infant in good breastfeeding position : tummy-to-tummy, with ear, shoulder, and hip aligned. *Source:* Adapted from Riordan, J., & Auerbach, K. (1993). *Breastfeeding and lactation.* (p. 248). Boston: Jones & Bartlett.

oxytocin secretion—or until she notes cues from the infant suggesting satiety (suckling activity ceases or the baby falls asleep). The length of the feedings is up to the mother; she need not watch a clock. Literature suggests that imposing time limits for breastfeeding does not prevent nipple soreness and in fact interferes with successful feeding. For example, the length of nursing time necessary to stimulate the milk ejection reflex varies with the individual. If the mother feeds according to the clock and disengages the baby before letdown, the baby will not get the hindmilk. Because the hindmilk is higher in fat and calories than the foremilk, the baby will be less satisfied, will need to nurse again sooner, and will gain less weight. The mother should learn to feed in response to her baby's cues and her body, not in accordance with an arbitrary time schedule. If the mother wishes to end the feeding before the infant falls asleep or detaches himself or herself, she should break the suction by gently inserting her fingers between the

## HINTS FOR PRACTICE

To encourage a sleepy baby to breastfeed, unwrap the baby and provide for lots of skin-to-skin contact between mom and baby; have mom rest with the baby near her breast so the baby can feel and smell the breast. Encourage mom to watch for feeding cues, such as hand-to-mouth activity, fluttering eyelids, vocalization but not necessarily crying, and mouthing activities.

| | 0 | 1 | 2 |
|---|---|---|---|
| **L**<br>Latch | Too sleepy or reluctant<br>No latch achieved | Repeated attempts<br>Hold nipple in mouth<br>Stimulate to suck | Grasps breast<br>Tongue down<br>Lips flanged<br>Rhythmic sucking |
| **A**<br>Audible swallowing | None | A few with stimulation | Spontaneous and intermittent <24 hours old<br>Spontaneous and frequent >24 hours old |
| **T**<br>Type of nipple | Inverted | Flat | Everted (after stimulation) |
| **C**<br>Comfort (breast/ nipple) | Engorged<br>Cracked, bleeding, large blisters or bruises<br>Severe discomfort | Filling<br>Reddened/small blisters or bruises<br>Mild/moderate discomfort | Soft<br>Tender |
| **H**<br>Hold (positioning) | Full assist (staff holds infant at breast) | Minimal assist (ie, elevate head of bed, place pillows for support)<br>Teach one side; mother does other<br>Staff holds and then mother takes over | No assist from staff<br>Mother able to position and hold infant |

FIGURE 24–6 ♦ LATCH: a breastfeeding charting and documentation tool. LATCH was created to provide a systematic method for breastfeeding assessment and charting. It can be used to assist the mother in establishing breastfeeding and define areas of needed intervention. *Source:* Jensen , D., Wallace, S., Kelsay, P. (1994). LATCH: A breastfeeding charting system and documentation tool. *Journal of Obstetric, Gynecologic, and Neonatal Nursing, 23*(1), 27–32.

baby's gums. Burping between feedings on each breast and at the end of the feeding continues to be necessary. If the infant has been crying, it is also advisable to burp before beginning feeding.

### Breastfeeding Assessment

During the birthing unit stay, the nurse carefully monitors the progress of the breastfeeding mother and child. A systematic assessment of several breastfeeding episodes provides the opportunity to teach the new mother about lactation and the breastfeeding process, provide anticipatory guidance, and evaluate the need for follow-up care after discharge. Criteria for evaluating a breastfeeding session include maternal and infant cues, latch-on, position, letdown, nipple condition, infant response, and maternal response. The literature provides various tools to guide the assessment and documentation of the breastfeeding efforts (Riordan & Koehn, 1997). The LATCH scoring table is one example (Figure 24–6♦).

### Leaking

Initially more milk is produced than the infant requires. During the first few weeks, infant needs and maternal responses are not yet well attuned, daily variabilities of feeding frequency and duration are greatest, and most women experience breast leaking. Stimuli that result in letdown or leaking breast milk include hearing a baby cry and even thinking about the baby. The nurse forewarns the mother about this possibility and recommends that breast pads be placed in her bra to absorb the secretions. The nurse also cautions the woman to remove wet pads frequently to prevent irritation to the nipples and infection. (Breast pads with plastic liners interfere with air circulation; the plastic should be removed before using them.) Once breastfeeding is well established—usually after the first month—the mother

## HINTS FOR PRACTICE

Digital suck training: If the baby is pulling the tongue back, humping the tongue, or thrusting the tongue, you can use digital suck training to bring the tongue down and forward. Place a finger in the baby's mouth, pad side up. When the baby starts sucking well, turn your finger so that the pad is down. If the baby is sucking correctly, the tongue will come forward and cup the finger, and the baby will continue to suckle. Performing this technique prior to feedings encourages the baby to use the tongue correctly.

may also be taught to apply direct pressure to the breast with her hand or forearm when leaking occurs.

## Supplementary Bottle-Feeding

Using supplementary bottle-feedings for the breastfeeding infant may weaken or confuse the sucking reflex or decrease the infant's interest in nursing. The newborn has to open her or his mouth wider to grasp the mother's nipple than to grasp a bottle nipple. The shape of the mouth and lips and the sucking mechanism are also different for sucking the breast and the bottle nipple. While suckling at the breast, the infant's tongue moves front to back, squeezing the milk from the nipple. While sucking on a rubber nipple, the tongue pushes forward against the nipple to control the milk flow. Some breastfeeding babies who are given supplementary bottles cannot adjust to these different techniques and push the mother's nipple out of their mouth in subsequent breastfeeding attempts. This can be frustrating for both mother and baby. Breastfeeding mothers should avoid introducing bottles until breastfeeding is well established. Parents are often concerned because they have no visual assurance about the amount of breast milk consumed. The mother can be taught the signs of milk transfer to the infant (ie, audible swallowing, milk appearing in the baby's mouth, her breast feeling soft after feeding, milk leaking from the opposite breast) (Mulford, 1992). In addition, if the infant gains weight and has six or more wet diapers per day without supplementary feedings of water or formula, he or she is receiving adequate amounts of milk. Parents should know that because breast milk is more easily digested than formula, the breastfed infant becomes hungry sooner. Thus the frequency of breastfeeding is greater than that of bottle-feeding. The parents may also expect the infant to demand more frequent nursing during growth spurts, such as ages 10 days to 2 weeks, 5 to 6 weeks, and 2.5 to 3 months.

## Expression of Milk

If the mother who desires to breastfeed is unable to nurse for medical or workplace reasons, she needs information about other means of stimulating milk production and storing the breast milk. The choice of method (manual or with breast pump) may depend on the mother's physiologic capabilities to produce the desired amount of milk and her personal preference. During the early postpartum period, if the baby cannot nurse at the breast (as in the case of some preterm or sick infants), the mother needs frequent breast stimulation to establish and increase her milk supply to prepare for later breastfeeding. She should use an electric breast pump at least eight times in each 24-hour period (Riordan & Auerbach, 1999). Research has shown that a pulsatile electric pump and double setup (allowing both breasts to be stimulated simultaneously) results in higher prolactin levels and a greater volume of milk than does manual expression (Lauwers & Shimski, 2000). After lactation is established, the mother may express the breast milk by the method that she finds most effective and convenient.

To express her milk manually, the woman washes her hands, then massages her breast to stimulate letdown. To massage her breast, the woman grasps the breast with both hands at the base of the breast near the chest wall. Using the palms of her hands, she firmly slides her hands toward her nipple. She repeats this process several times. Then she is ready to begin hand expression. The woman generally uses her left hand for her right breast and her right hand for her left breast. However, some women prefer to use the hand on the same side as the breast. The nurse should encourage the woman to use the method she finds most effective. The woman grasps the areola with her thumb on the top and her first two fingers on the lower portion (Figure 24–7♦). Without allowing her fingers to slide on her skin, she pushes inward toward the chest and then squeezes her fingers together while pulling

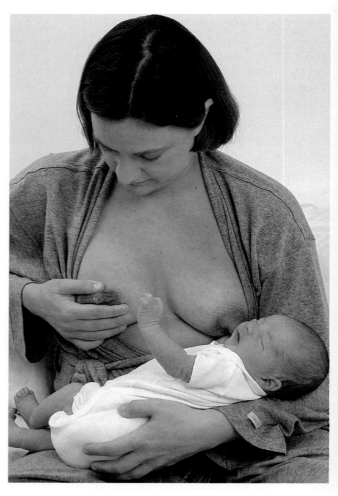

FIGURE 24–7 ♦ Hand position for manual expression of milk.

forward on the areola. She can use a container to catch any fluid that is squeezed out. She then repositions her hand by rotating it slightly so that she can repeat the process. She continues to reposition her hand and repeat the process to empty all the milk sinuses.

Breast pumps use suction to express milk. Some have collection systems to conveniently store the milk. Hand pumps are portable and inexpensive. Battery-operated pumps are more efficient than hand pumps but are also more expensive. Electric pumps are more efficient but are bulky and expensive; however, they can be rented in many areas. Many agencies have a variety of pumps available and provide instruction on correct use (Table 24–2). Videotapes and photographs are also useful in demonstrating the process to new mothers.

## Storing Breast Milk

Breast milk has bacteriostatic qualities because of the presence of IgA and IgG antibodies, which retard bacterial growth. Breast milk can be stored for up to 6 to 10 hours for mature milk and 12 to 24 hours for colostrum at room temperature or up to 8 days for mature milk in a refrigerator. If breast milk is to be refrigerated and then

### TABLE 24–2 Recommendations for the Nursing Mother Who Uses a Pump

***General Pumping Recommendations***

1. Read the instructions on the use and cleaning of a pump before expressing milk with any product.
2. Wash hands before each pumping session.
3. Frequency: For occasional pumping, pump during, after, or between feedings, whichever gives the best results. Most mothers tend to express more milk in the morning. Working mothers should use the pump on a regular basis for the number of nursings that are missed. For premature or ill babies who are not at breast, the number of pumpings should total eight or more in 24 hours. Initiation of pumping should be delayed no longer than 6 hours following birth unless medically indicated. This ensures appropriate development and sensitivity of prolactin receptors. More frequent pumping will avoid the buildup of excessive back pressure of milk during engorgement.
4. Duration: With single-sided pumping, optimal duration is 10 to 15 minutes with an electric pump and 10 to 20 minutes with a manual pump. If double pumping with an electric or two battery-operated pumps, 8 to 10 minutes is optimal. Encourage mothers to tailor these times to their own situation.
5. Technique:
   - Elicit the milk ejection reflex before using any pump.
   - Use only as much suction as is needed to maintain milk flow.
   - Massage the breast in quadrants during pumping to increase intramammary pressure.
   - Allow enough time for pumping to avoid anxiety.
   - Use inserts or different flanges if needed to obtain the best fit between pump and breast.
   - Avoid long periods of uninterrupted vacuum.
   - Stop pumping when the milk flow is minimal or has ceased

***Recommendations for Specific Types of Pumps***

1. Avoid pumps that use rubber bulbs to generate vacuum; they can cause bruising.
2. Cylinder pumps:
   - When 0-rings are used, they must be in place for proper suction.
   - Remove gaskets *after each use* for cleaning to avoid harboring bacteria in the pump.
   - Roll the gasket on the inner cylinder back and forth to restore it to its original shape.
   - The pump stroke may need to be shortened as the outer cylinder fills with milk.
   - The user may need to empty the outer cylinder once or twice during pumping.
   - Hand position should be palm up with the elbow held close to the body.
3. Battery-operated pumps:
   - Use alkaline batteries.
   - Replace batteries when cycles per minute decrease.
   - Interrupt vacuum frequently to avoid nipple pain and damage.
   - Use an AC adapter when possible, especially if the pump generates fewer than six cycles per minute.
   - Consider renting an electric pump for pumping that will continue for longer than 1 or 2 months.
   - Use two pumps simultaneously if pumping time is limited or to increase the quantity of milk obtained.
   - Choose a pump in which the vacuum can be regulated.
   - Massage the breast by quadrants during pumping.
4. Semiautomatic pumps:
   - Vacuum may be easier to control if the mother does not lift her finger completely off the hole but rolls it back and forth rhythmically so that the vacuum is efficient but not painful.
5. Automatic electric pumps:
   - Use the lowest pressure setting that is efficient.
   - Use a double setup (simultaneous pumping) when time is limited to increase the milk supply and for prematurity, maternal or infant illness, or other special situations.

*Source:* Riordan, J., & Auerbach, K. (1999). *Breastfeeding and human lactation* (2nd ed., p. 397). Boston: Jones & Bartlett.

fed to the infant, it should be stored in clean plastic containers because the white blood cells will adhere to glass, and their protective effect will be lost. Breast milk can be frozen in either glass or plastic because freezing destroys the white blood cells anyway. Breast milk can be stored in a freezer compartment inside the refrigerator for up to 2 weeks, in a self-contained freezer unit of a refrigerator for up to 3 to 4 months, and in a separate deep freeze unit at 0°F or less for up to 6 months. Frozen breast milk can be thawed by initially running cool water over the container, then gradually adding warm water until the milk is thawed. The container should then be gently shaken to return to suspension the fat molecules that separate during freezing. Breast milk should not be defrosted under hot running water or in boiling water. Breast milk should never be microwaved. Uneven heating patterns may alter the composition of the milk and can create hot spots that can burn the baby's mouth.

### External Supports

Nurses, dietitians, childbirth educators, certified nurse-midwives, lactation consultants, mother-to-mother support groups, and physicians must collaborate to provide consistent, timely information and support and to attend to the new mother's special needs. Breastfeeding mothers who work outside the home and are supported in their decision tend to breastfeed their infants for longer periods.

La Leche League International is an organized group of volunteers who work to provide education about breastfeeding and assistance to women who are breastfeeding infants. Through its small, neighborhood-based groups, it sponsors activities, provides printed materials, makes electric breast pumps available for rental, offers one-to-one counseling to mothers with questions or problems, and provides group support to breastfeeding mothers. Lactation consultants offer a variety of services through private practice and health care facilities.

Numerous books, pamphlets, and educational videos are also available to help the breastfeeding mother. The mother needs the support of all family members, her physician or certified nurse-midwife, pediatrician or certified nurse practitioner, and all nursing personnel, because it is often the attitudes of these people that ultimately lead the woman to success or failure.

### Drugs and Breastfeeding

It has long been recognized that certain medications taken by the mother may affect her infant. It should be noted that (1) most drugs pass into breast milk, (2) almost all medications appear in only small amounts in human milk (usually less than 1% of the maternal dosage), and (3) very few drugs are contraindicated for breastfeeding women.

The properties of a drug influence its passage into breast milk, as does the amount of the drug taken, the frequency and route of administration, and the timing of the dose in relationship to infant feeding. The drug's effects are influenced by the infant's age, the feeding frequency, the volume of milk taken, and the degree of absorption through the gastrointestinal tract.

Four adjustments should be made when administering drugs to a nursing mother to decrease the effects on the infant (Auerbach, 1999):

1. Long-acting forms of drugs should be avoided. The infant may have difficulty metabolizing and excreting them, and accumulation may be a problem.
2. Absorption rates and peak blood levels should be considered in scheduling the administration of the drugs. Less of the drug crosses into the milk if the medication is given immediately after the woman has nursed her baby.
3. The infant should be closely observed for any signs of drug reaction, including rash, fussiness, lethargy, or changes in sleeping or feeding patterns.
4. Whenever alternatives are available, the drug that shows the least tendency to pass into breast milk should be selected.

The mother should be informed about the potential of most drugs to cross into breast milk. She should also be advised to tell any physician who may prescribe medications for her that she is breastfeeding.

In counseling the nursing mother, the health care provider needs to weigh the benefits of the medication against the possible risk to the infant and its possible effect on the breastfeeding process. The potential risk to the infant must also be weighed against the effect of interrupting breastfeeding.

### Potential Problems in Breastfeeding

Because mothers are discharged from the birthing unit before breastfeeding is well established, they are frequently alone when they encounter changes in the breastfeeding process. Many women stop nursing if the situations they encounter seem problematic. The nurse can offer anticipatory guidance regarding common breastfeeding phenomena and provide resources for the woman's use after discharge. (See Chapter 29 for a detailed discussion of self-care measures the nurse can suggest to a woman with a breastfeeding problem after discharge from the birthing unit.)

## Client Education for Formula Feeding

With the great emphasis placed on successful breastfeeding, the teaching needs of the formula-feeding new mother may be overlooked. The mother who has chosen to bottle-feed her infant should be encouraged to assume a comfortable position with adequate arm support so that she can easily hold her infant. Most women cradle their infants in the crook of the arm close to the body, which provides the intimacy and cuddling so essential to an infant and offers the same benefits of closeness as breastfeeding. If the mother has had only limited experience in feeding infants, she may need some guidelines to feed her newborn successfully. The following information is helpful for parents to facilitate adequate nutrition and foster attachment:

1. Always hold bottles; never prop them. Positional otitis media may develop if the infant is fed horizontally, because milk and nasal mucus may block the eustachian tube. Holding the infant provides social and close physical contact for the baby and an opportunity for parent-child interaction and bonding (Figure 24–8♦).
2. The nipple should have a hole big enough to allow milk to flow in drops when the bottle is inverted. Too large an opening may cause overfeeding or regurgitation because of rapid feeding. If feeding is too fast, change the nipple and help the infant to eat more slowly by stopping the feeding frequently for burping and cuddling.
3. Point the nipple directly into the mouth, not toward the palate or tongue, and place it on top of the tongue. The nipple should be full of liquid at all times to prevent ingestion of extra air, which decreases the amount of feeding and increases discomfort. Nipples vary in shape, amount of energy needed to obtain the formula, and rate of formula flow through the nipple unit (Fadavi, Punwani, Jain, et al., 1997).
4. Burp the infant at intervals, preferably at the middle and end of the feeding. An infant who seems to swallow a great deal of air while sucking may need more frequent burping. If the infant has cried before being fed, air may have been swallowed; in such cases, the infant is burped before beginning to feed or after taking just enough to calm down. Burp the infant by holding him or her upright on the shoulder or in a sitting position on your lap with the infant's chin and chest supported on one hand. Then gently pat or stroke the infant's back with the other hand. Too-frequent burping may confuse a newborn who is attempting to coordinate sucking, swallowing, and breathing simultaneously.
5. Newborns frequently regurgitate small amounts of feedings. The amount may look large to the inexperienced parent, but it is normal. Initially it may be due to excessive mucus and gastric irritation from foreign substances such as aspirated blood in the stomach from birth. Later, regurgitation may result when the infant feeds too rapidly and swallows air. It may also occur when the infant is overfed and the cardiac sphincter allows the excess to be regurgitated. Because this is a common occurrence, experienced mothers and nurses generally keep a burp cloth available. Although regurgitation is normal, vomiting or a forceful expulsion of fluid is not. When forceful expulsion occurs, further evaluation may be indicated, especially if other symptoms are present.

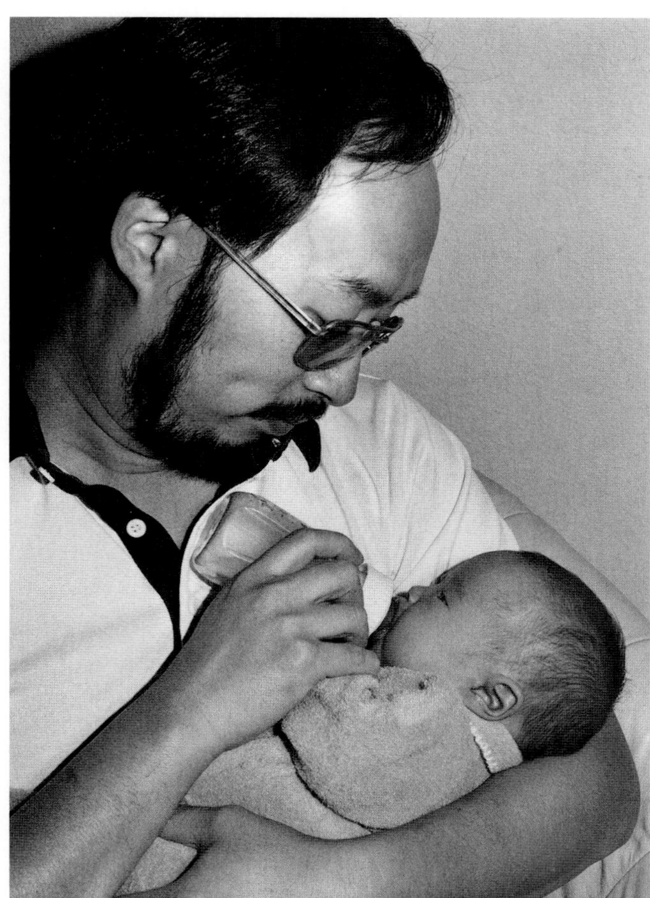

**FIGURE 24–8** ♦ An infant is supported comfortably during bottle-feeding.

6. A fat baby is not necessarily a healthy one. Avoid overfeeding or feeding infants every time they cry. Encourage but do not force the infant to feed and allow the infant to set the pace once feedings are established. Parents sometimes set artificial goals—"the baby must take all 5 oz"—and keep feeding the child until those goals are met, even though the infant may not be hungry. Overfeeding results in infant obesity. During early feedings, however, the infant may need simple tactile stimulation—such as gently rubbing feet and hands, adjusting clothing, and loosening coverings—to maintain adequate sucking for a sufficient time to complete a full feeding.

## HINTS FOR PRACTICE

When you help a mother bottle-feed her baby for the first time, you can help her avoid many potential frustrations. The first is often "flying arms" as the baby waves his or her arms in the air. The second is the "chin plunge," as the baby's head falls forward in the mother's tentative hold. To avoid the latter, assist the mother with positioning. A third frustration may arise when she tries to correctly place the nipple in the mouth. To ensure correct placement, put your index finger on the baby's chin and gently pull downward while quickly sliding the nipple in over the tongue.

The desirable amount and frequency of formula feeding vary with postnatal age of the infant. From birth to 2 months of age, the baby takes six to eight feedings of approximately 2 to 4 oz of formula at each feeding within a 24-hour period (Tigges, 1997). The three forms of formula are ready-to-feed, liquid concentrate, and powdered. (See Key Facts to Remember: Formula Preparation.)

The nurse is responsible for discussing formula preparation and sterilization techniques with families. Cleanliness is essential, but sterilization is necessary only if the water source is questionable. Bottles may be effectively prepared in the dishwasher or washed thoroughly in warm, soapy water and rinsed well. Nipples may be weakened by the temperature of dishwashers and therefore should be washed thoroughly by hand and rinsed well. Tap water, if from an uncontaminated source, may be used to mix powdered formulas, which are less expensive than the concentrated or ready-to-use formulas. Honey should not be used as a sugar source because of the danger of infant botulism.

Bottles may be prepared individually, or up to one day's supply of formula may be prepared at one time. Extra bottles can be stored in the refrigerator and warmed slightly before feeding. Ready-to-use disposable bottles of formula are convenient but expensive. Formula left in bottles after a feeding should be discarded. The Special Supplemental Food Program for Women, Infants, and Children (WIC) provides 8 lb of powdered formula or 403 oz of concentrated liquid formula per month. Individual states make provisions about when WIC nutritionists may distribute soy formulas and whether prescriptions are needed for special or therapeutic formulas. (See Teaching Card: Teaching Newborn Bottle-Feeding insert).

## KEY FACTS TO REMEMBER

### *Formula Preparation*

**Ready to Feed**

(20 kcal/oz; available in 32-oz cans or 4-oz bottles)

Use within 30 minutes to 1 hour once opened.

Do not dilute. Use directly from can, no mixing required.

Just add clean nipple to bottle.

Most expensive type of formula preparation.

**Formula Concentrate**

(available in 13-oz cans)

Mix equal amounts of concentrate and water from uncontaminated source. This provides a 20 kcal/30 mL (1 oz) dilution. For example, for a 4-oz feeding mix 2 oz of formula concentrate with 2 oz water.

Wash punch-type can opener and top of formula can before opening.

Prepare a single feeding by measuring water and liquid directly into nursing bottle.

Cover opened concentrate formula cans with foil or plastic wrap and refrigerate until next bottle is made up.

**Powdered Formula**

(52 scoops per can)

Mix one unpacked level scoop of powdered formula with each 60 mL (2 oz) of warm water.

Always pour water into bottle first; then add powder and stir well.

Make sure the powder and water are well mixed to ensure the formula composition is 20 kcal/30 mL (1 oz).

After opening, keep can tightly covered and use contents within 1 month to ensure freshness.

Will keep in refrigerator for up to 24 hours.

Least expensive type.

# Nutritional Assessment of the Infant

During the early months of life, the food offered to and consumed by infants will be instrumental in their proper growth and development. The infant's nutritional status is assessed at each well-baby visit. Assessment should include four components:

- Nutritional history from the parent
- Weight gain since the last visit
- Growth chart percentiles
- Physical examination

The nutritional history reports the type, amount, and frequency of milk, supplemental foods, vitamins, and minerals given to the infant on a daily basis. If the baby is taking formula, the history also includes how the formula is mixed (checking for under- or overdilution) and stored. Individual charts show the infant's growth with respect to height, weight, and head circumference. The important consideration is that infants continue to grow at their own individual rates. Healthy breastfed babies may fall within these weight-gain parameters but may also be normal while gaining 0.5 oz/day for the first 6 months.

For a mother who is concerned about whether her infant is getting adequate nutrition, the nurse can recommend looking for an appearance of weight gain and counting the number of wet and soiled diapers in a 24-hour period. Approximately six wet diapers or more and frequent stools in a day indicate adequate nutrition is being attained in the totally breastfed infant. If additional water is ingested, the diaper count should be higher. The presence of urine can most accurately be assessed when the diaper is free of feces. The diaper is most likely to be free of feces prior to feedings because the gastrocolic reflex often stimulates stooling after a feeding. For anxious parents, another means of reassurance of adequate intake and output is to keep a record of the frequency and duration of feedings, amount of swallowing, and the exact number of wet and/or soiled diapers. Keeping a record tends to give the worried parents a sense of control and a tangible basis for concern or relief. (See Key Facts to Remember: Successful Breastfeeding Evaluation.)

The physical examination will assist in identifying any nutritional disorders. Iron deficiency should be suspected in an obese infant who is pale, diaphoretic, and irritable.

By calculating the nutritional needs of infants, the nurse can recommend a diet that supplies appropriate nutrition for infant growth and development. The assessment is especially helpful in counseling mothers of infants under 6 months of age, because there is a tendency to add too many supplemental foods or offer too much formula to infants of this age. Clinicians generally advise that an infant not be given more than 32 oz/day of formula. If additional calories are needed, supplemental foods can be added to the diet. However, if the caloric intake is adequate or excessive, formula alone gives the infant enough calories and introduction of solid foods can be delayed.

When an infant's caloric intake and weight gain are found to be excessive, clinicians do not advise putting the infant on a weight-reduction diet, because tissue growth is rapid during this period and must be supported. The appropriate advice is to provide a maintenance caloric intake as a means of allowing the infant to maintain weight while maturing and growing in length.

Appropriate nutritional intake can be identified by comparing the infant's dietary intake with the desired caloric intake for the infant's weight and age. Most commercial formulas prescribed for the normal healthy newborn contain 20 kcal per 30 mL (1 oz). If the infant is eating solids, the caloric value of those foods must be determined and included in the calculation of nutritional intake. With knowledge of the amount of calories needed by the infant according to weight (108 kcal/kg/day [55 kcal/lb/day]), the nurse can counsel the parents about how many ounces of formula per day the infant needs to meet caloric requirements.

## KEY FACTS TO REMEMBER

### *Successful Breastfeeding Evaluation*

Babies are probably getting enough milk if

- They are nursing at least eight times in 24 hours.
- In a quiet room, their mothers can hear them swallow while nursing.
- Their mothers' breasts appear to soften after nursing.
- The number of wet diapers increases by the fourth or fifth day after birth, or there are at least six to eight wet diapers every 24 hours after day 5.
- The baby's stools are yellow or are beginning to lighten in color by the fourth or fifth day after birth.

Offering a supplemental bottle is not a reliable indicator because most babies will take a few ounces even if they are getting enough breast milk.

# Chapter Review

## CHAPTER HIGHLIGHTS

- The RDA for calories for the newborn is 105 to 108 kcal/kg/day (50 to 55 kcal/lb/day).
- The nurse must monitor the first feeding because this is when the newborn may initially manifest signs of cardiac complications or anomalies of the upper gastrointestinal tract.
- Breast milk has immunologic and nutritional properties that make it the optimal food for the first year of life.
- Signs indicating newborn readiness for the first feeding are active bowel sounds, absence of abdominal distension, and a lusty cry that quiets with rooting and sucking behaviors when a stimulus is placed near the lips.
- Mature breast milk and commercially prepared formulas (unless otherwise noted) provide 20 kcal/oz.
- Breastfed infants need supplements of iron after 6 months of age.
- Nurses must recognize that cultural values influence infant feeding practices, be sensitive to ethnic backgrounds of minority populations, and understand that the dominant culture in any society defines "normal" maternal-infant feeding interactions.
- Breastfed infants are getting adequate nutrition if they are gaining weight and have at least six wet diapers a day when they are not receiving additional water supplements.
- Breastfeeding mothers should be encouraged to ensure that the infant is correctly positioned at the breast, with a large portion of the areola in the infant's mouth. The mother is advised to rotate positions to ensure that all ducts are emptied.
- Most maternal medications are transmitted through breast milk. The effects on the infant and lactation depend on a variety of factors, including route of administration, timing of the dose with respect to feeding time, and multiple properties of the medication.
- Formula-fed infants regain their birth weight by 10 days of age and gain 1 oz/day for the first 6 months and 0.5 oz/day for the second 6 months; birth weight is doubled at 3.5 to 4 months of age. Healthy breastfed babies gain approximately 0.5 oz/day in the first 6 months of life, regain their birth weight by about 14 days of age, and double their birth weight at approximately 5 months of age.
- Formula-fed infants need no vitamin or mineral supplements other than iron, if it is not already in the formula, and fluoride, if it is not obtained in the water system.
- The bottle-feeding mother may require assistance with feeding and burping her infant. She will also benefit from information about feeding schedules and types of formula.
- The use of skim milk or cow's milk with lowered fat content is not recommended for children under 2 years of age.
- Nutritional assessment of the infant includes nutritional history from the parents, weight gain, growth chart percentiles, and physical examination.

## CHAPTER REFERENCES


American Academy of Pediatrics, Committee on Nutrition. (2000). Hypoallergenic infant formulas. *Pediatrics, 106*(2), 346–349.

American Academy of Pediatrics, Committee on Nutrition. (1999). Iron fortification of infant formulas. *Pediatrics, 104*(1), 119–123.

American Academy of Pediatrics & American College of Obstetricians and Gynecologists. (1997). *Guidelines for perinatal care* (4th ed.). Washington, DC: Author.

Auerbach, K. G. (1999). Breastfeeding and maternal medication use. *Journal of Obstetric, Gynecologic, and Neonatal Nursing, 28*(5), 554–562.

Calamaro, C. J. (2000). Infant nutrition in the first year of life: Tradition or science? *Pediatric Nursing, 26*(2), 211–215.

Davis, L. J., Okuboye, S., & Ferguson, S. L. (2000). Healthy People 2010: Examining a decade of maternal and infant health. *AWHONN Lifelines, 4*(3), 26–33

Dodgson, J. E., Allard-Hale, C. J., Bramscher, A., Brown, F., & Duckett, L. (1999). Adherence to the ten steps of the Baby-Friendly Hospital Initiative in Minnesota hospitals. *Birth, 26*(4), 239–246.

Fadavi, S., Punwani, I. C., Jain, L., & Vidyasagar, D. (1997). Mechanics and energetics of nutritive sucking: A functional comparison of commercially available nipples. *Journal of Pediatrics, 130*(5), 740–745.

Geissler, E. M. (1998). *Pocket guide to cultural assessment.* (2nd ed.). St. Louis: Mosby.

Hutchinson, M. K., & Baqi-Aziz, M. (1994). Nursing care of the childbearing Muslim family. *Journal of Obstetric, Gynecologic, and Neonatal Nursing, 23*(9), 767–771.

Johnson, J. V. & Riddick, D. H. (2000). The breast during pregnancy and lactation. In J. J. Sciarra & T. J. Watkins (Eds.), *Gynecology and obstetrics* (Vol. 5, chap. 31, pp. 1–12). Philadelphia: Lippencott Williams & Wilkins.

Kelleher, D. K., & Duggan, C. (1999). Breast milk and breastfeeding in the 1990s. *Current Opinion in Pediatrics, 11,* 275–280.

Kunz, C., Rodriguez-Palmero, M., Koletzko, B., & Jensen, R. (1999). Nutritional and biochemical properties of human milk, part I: General aspects, proteins, and carbohydrates. *Clinics in Perinatology, 26*(2), 307–333.

Lauwers, J., & Shinski, D. (2000). *Counseling the nursing mother: A lactation consultant's guide* (3rd ed.). Sudbury, MA: Jones & Bartlett.

Lawrence, R. A., & Lawrence, R. M. (1999). *Breastfeeding: A guide for the medical profession* (5th ed.). St Louis: Mosby.

Mulford, C. (1992). The mother-baby assessment (MBA): An "Apgar score" for breastfeeding. *Journal of Human Lactation, 8*(2), 79–82.

Porter, R. H., & Winberg, J. (1999). Unique salience of maternal breast odors for newborn infants. *Neuroscience and Biochemical Reviews, 23,* 439–449.

Riordan, J., & Auerbach, K. (1999). *Breastfeeding and human lactation* (2nd ed.). Boston: Jones & Bartlett.

Riordan, J. M., & Koehn, M. (1997). Reliability and validity testing of three breastfeeding assessment tools. *Journal of Obstetric, Gynecologic, and Neonatal Nursing, 26*(2), 181–187.

Rogers, I. S., Golding, J., & Emmett, P. M. (1997). The effects of lactation on the mother. *Early Human Development, 49* (Suppl.), S191–S203.

Susin, L. R. O., Giugliani, E. R. J., Kummer, S. C., Maciel, M., Simon, C., & da Silveira, L. C. (1999). Does parental breastfeeding knowledge increase breastfeeding rates? *Birth, 26*(3), 149–156.

Tigges, B. B. (1997). Infant formulas: Practical answers for common questions. *Nurse Practitioner, 22*(8), 70, 73, 77–80, 82–83, 86–87.

Vezeau, T. M. (1991). Investigating "greedy." *American Journal of Maternal Child Nursing 16*(6), 337–338.


## CONTEMPORARY MATERNAL-NEWBORN NURSING ON-LINE

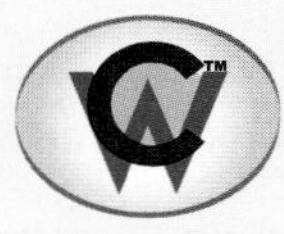

Additional interactive resources, including animations and video, for this chapter can be found on the Companion Website at http://www.prenhall.com/ladewig. Click on Chapter 24 and "Begin" to select the activities for this chapter.

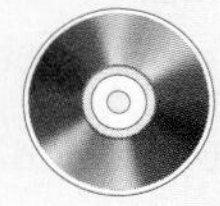

For NCLEX review questions and an audio glossary, access the accompanying CD-ROM in this book.

Chapter 25

# The Newborn at Risk: Conditions Present at Birth

*When a newborn is admitted into my unit, and into my care, there is an initial flurry of activity where my entire universe, everything that I am, constricts down to focus on this one little being. Gradually, as the situation stabilizes, I become aware again of the other team members working in concert around me. And I am reassured that this new life is getting the very best care available.*

—Neonatal Nurse Practitioner

## OBJECTIVES

- Identify factors present at birth that help identify an at-risk newborn.
- Compare the underlying etiologies of the physiologic complications of small-for-gestational-age (SGA) newborns and preterm appropriate-for-gestational-age (Pr AGA) newborns.
- Describe the impact of maternal diabetes mellitus on the newborn.
- Compare the characteristics and potential complications of the postterm newborn and the newborn with postmaturity syndrome.
- Discuss the physiologic characteristics of the preterm newborn that predispose each body system to various complications.
- Identify the information used in developing the nursing diagnoses required to plan interventions for the care of the preterm AGA newborn.
- Explain the special care needed by an alcohol- or drug-exposed newborn.
- Relate the consequences of maternal HIV/AIDS to the management of the newborn in the neonatal period.
- Identify the physical examination findings during the early newborn period that would make the nurse suspect a congenital cardiac defect.
- Summarize the nursing assessments of and initial interventions for a newborn born with selected congenital anomalies.
- Explain the special care needed by newborns with an inborn error of metabolism.

## KEY TERMS

Within the past 30 years, the field of neonatology has expanded greatly. Many levels of nursery care have evolved in response to increasing knowledge about at-risk newborns: special care, intensive care, and convalescent or transitional care. As a member of the multidisciplinary health care team, the nurse is a technically competent professional who contributes the high-touch human care necessary in the high-tech perinatal environment.

In addition to the availability of a high level of newborn care, various other factors influence the outcome of these at-risk infants, including the following:

- Birth weight
- Gestational age
- Type and length of newborn illness
- Environmental factors
- Maternal factors
- Maternal-infant separation

## Identification of At-Risk Newborns

An at-risk newborn is one susceptible to illness (morbidity) or even death because of dysmaturity, immaturity, physical disorders, or complications of birth. In most cases, the infant is the product of a pregnancy involving one or more predictable risk factors, including the following:

- Low socioeconomic level of the mother and limited access to health care
- Exposure to environmental dangers such as toxic chemicals and illicit drugs
- Preexisting maternal conditions such as heart disease, diabetes, hypertension, and renal disease
- Maternal factors such as age and parity
- Medical conditions related to pregnancy and their associated complications
- Pregnancy complications such as abruptio placentae

Various risk factors and their specific effects on the pregnancy outcome are listed in Table 8–1. Because these factors and the perinatal risks associated with them are known, the birth of at-risk newborns can often be anticipated. The pregnancy can be closely monitored, treatment can be started as necessary, and arrangements can be made for birth to occur at a facility with appropriate resources to care for both mother and baby.

At-risk infants cannot always be identified before the onset of labor, however, because the course of labor and birth and the infant's ability to withstand the stress of labor are not known before the actual birth process. Thus during labor, electronic fetal heart monitoring or fetal heart rate auscultation by fetoscope or Doppler by the nurse plays a significant role in detecting stress or distress in the fetus. Immediately after birth the Apgar score is a helpful tool for identifying the at-risk newborn, but it is not the only indicator of possible long-term outcome.

The newborn classification and neonatal mortality risk chart is another useful tool for identifying newborns at risk. Before this classification tool was developed, birth weight of less than 2500 g was the sole criterion for determining immaturity. Clinicians then recognized that a newborn could weigh more than 2500 g and still be immature. Conversely, an infant weighing less than 2500 g might be functionally at term or beyond. Thus birth weight and gestational age together are now the criteria used to assess neonatal maturity and mortality risk.

According to the newborn classification and neonatal mortality risk chart, gestation is divided as follows:

- Preterm: less than 37 (completed) weeks
- Term: 38 to 41 (completed) weeks
- Postterm: greater than 42 weeks

As shown in Figure 25–1♦, large-for-gestational-age (LGA) newborns are those above the 90th percentile curve. Appropriate-for-gestational-age (AGA) newborns are those that plot between the 10th percentile and 90th percentile curves. Small-for-gestational-age (SGA) newborns are those that plot below the 10th percentile curve. A newborn is assigned to a category depending on birth weight and gestational age. For example, a newborn classified as Pr SGA is preterm and small for gestational age. The full-term newborn whose weight is appropriate for gestational age is classified F AGA. It is important to remember that intrauterine growth charts are influenced by altitude and the ethnicity of the population the charts were based on. Also, the newborn classification may vary according to the intrauterine growth curve chart used; therefore, the chart used should correlate with the characteristics of the client population.

Neonatal mortality risk is the chance of death within the newborn period—that is, within the first 28 days of life. The neonatal mortality risk decreases as both gestational age and birth weight increase. Infants who are preterm and small for gestational age have the highest neonatal mortality risk. The previously high mortality rates for LGA newborns have decreased at most perinatal centers because of improved management of diabetes in pregnancy and increased recognition of potential problems of LGA newborns.

Newborn morbidity can be anticipated based on birth weight and gestational age. In Figure 25–2♦ the infant's birth weight is located on the vertical axis, and the gestational age in weeks is found along the horizontal axis. The area where the two meet on the graph identifies

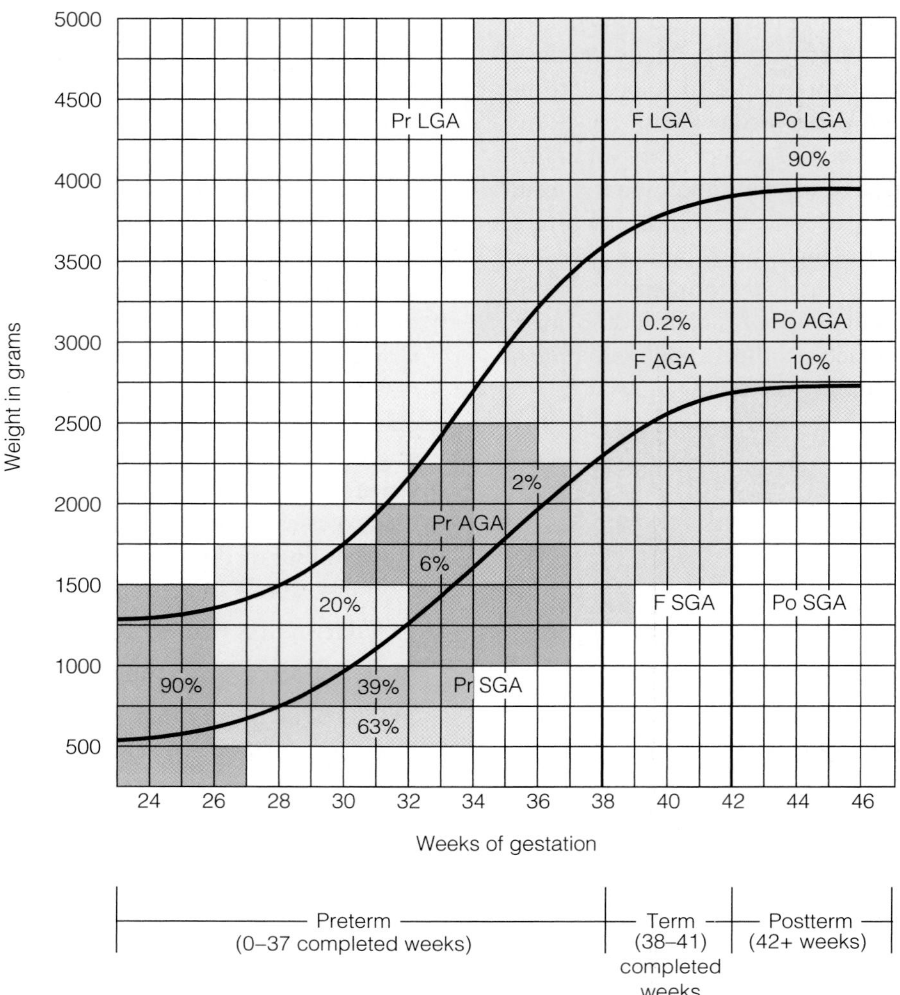


**FIGURE 25–1** ♦ Newborn classification and neonatal mortality risk chart. Infants are classified according to weight as small for gestational age (SGA), appropriate for gestational age (AGA), or large for gestational age (LGA) and by weeks of newborn as preterm (Pr), term (F), or postterm (Po). Corresponding neonatal mortality risks are indicated by the percentage in the various colored regions. *Source:* Koops, B. L., Morgan, L. P., & Battaglia, F. C. (1982). Neonatal mortality risk in relationship to birth weight and gestational age. *Journal of Pediatrics, 101*(6), 969.

common problems. This tool assists in determining the needs of particular infants for special observation and care. For example, an infant of 2000 g at 40 weeks' gestation should be carefully assessed for evidence of neonatal distress, hypoglycemia, congenital anomalies, congenital infection, and polycythemia.

Identifying the nursing care needs of the at-risk newborn depends on minute-to-minute observations of the changes in the newborn's physiologic status. The organization of nursing care must be directed toward the following:

- Decreasing physiologically stressful situations
- Constantly observing for subtle signs of change in clinical condition
- Interpreting laboratory data and coordinating interventions
- Conserving the infant's energy for healing and growth
- Providing for developmental stimulation and maintenance of sleep cycle
- Assisting the family in developing attachment behaviors
- Involving the family in planning and providing care

## Care of the Small-for-Gestational-Age (SGA) Newborn

Any newborn who at birth is at or below the 10th percentile for weight (intrauterine growth curves) on the newborn classification chart is considered **small for**

Weight in grams

5000
4750
4500
4250
4000
3750
3500
3250
3000
2750
2500
2250
2000
1750
1500
1250
1000
750
500

Increased mortality—cause undetermined

Congenital anomalies
Immaturity of all systems

Hypertension
Sepsis

Apnea
RDS
Inadequate calories
Gavage feeding
Jaundice
Bleeding
Hypoglycemia
Congenital anomalies

IDM
Hypoglycemia
RDS
Slow feeding
Increased jaundice
Hypothermia
Infection

Hypoglycemia
Congenital anomalies
Discordant twins
Small placenta

Birth trauma
Increased C-section rate
IDM
Hypoglycemia
Transposition of aorta

Morbidity due to intrapartum accidents and congenital anomalies

Fetal distress
Hypoglycemia
Congenital anomalies
Congenital infection
Polycythemia

Increased C-section rate
Birth trauma

Postmaturity syndrome

Fetal distress
Aspiration of meconium
Hypoglycemia
Congenital anomalies (trisomy 16 and 18)

24 25 26 27 28 29 30 31 32 33 34 35 36 37 38 39 40 41 42 43 44 45 46
Weeks of gestation

| Preterm | Term | Postterm |
|---|---|---|

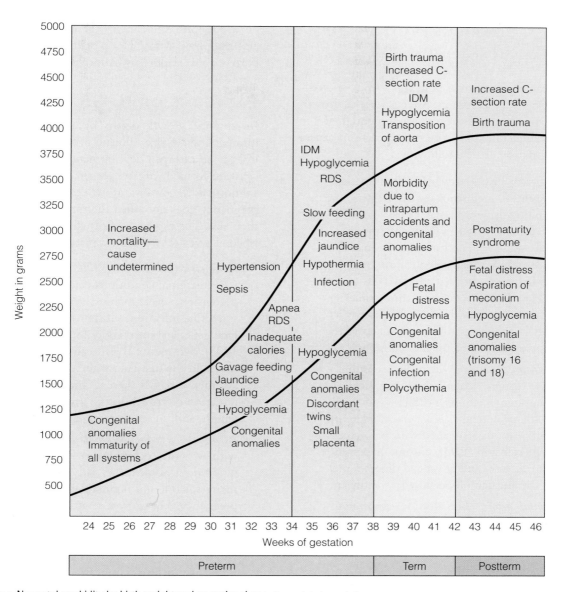

**FIGURE 25–2 ♦** Neonatal morbidity by birth weight and gestational age. *Source:* Lubchenco, L. O. (1976). *The high-risk infant* (p. 122). Philadelphia: Saunders.

**gestational age (SGA)** (Figure 25–3♦). For purposes of assigning the SGA classification to a newborn, birth weight charts should be based on the local population into which the newborn is born (Anderson & Hay, 1999). An SGA newborn may be preterm, term, or postterm. Other terms used to designate an undergrown newborn include **intrauterine growth restriction (IUGR),** which describes pregnancy circumstance of advanced gestation and limited fetal growth. The terms *SGA* and *IUGR* are used interchangeably.

SGA infants have an incidence of perinatal asphyxia five times that of AGA infants and a perinatal mortality rate eight times that of AGA infants (Sohl & Moore, 1998). The incidence of polycythemia and hypoglycemia is also higher in this group of infants.

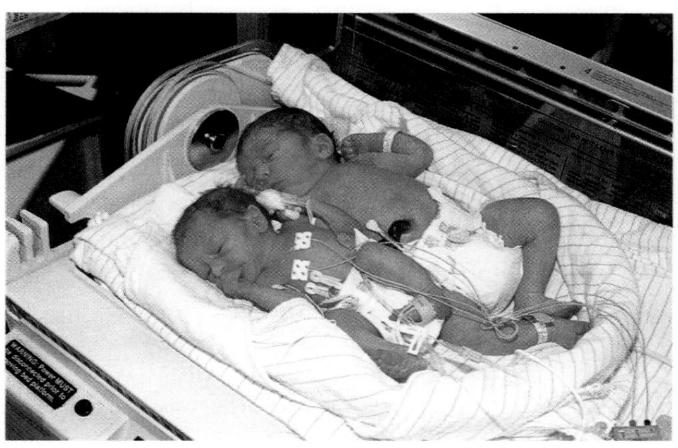

**FIGURE 25–3 ♦** Thirty-five-week gestational age twins. Twin B (on left) is SGA and weighs 1260 g and twin A (on right) is AGA and weighs 2605 g. Source: Courtesy of Carol Harrigan, RNC, MSN, NNP.

## Factors Contributing to IUGR

IUGR may be caused by maternal, placental, or fetal factors and may not be apparent antenatally. Intrauterine growth is linear in the normal pregnancy from approximately 28 to 38 weeks' gestation. After 38 weeks, growth is variable, depending on the growth potential of the fetus and placental function. The most common causes of growth retardation are the following:

- *Maternal factors.* Primiparity, grand multiparity, multiple-gestation pregnancy (twins, triplets, and so on), smoking, lack of prenatal care, age extremes (<16 years or >40 years), and low socioeconomic status (which can result in inadequate health care, inadequate education, and inadequate living conditions) affect IUGR (Anderson & Hay, 1999). Before the third trimester, the nutritional supply to the fetus far exceeds its needs. Only in the third trimester is maternal malnutrition a limiting factor in fetal growth.
- *Maternal disease.* Maternal heart disease, substance abuse (drugs, alcohol, smoking), sickle-cell anemia, phenylketonuria (PKU), and asymptomatic pyelonephritis are associated with SGA. Complications associated with pregnancy-induced hypertension (PIH), chronic hypertensive vascular disease, and advanced diabetes mellitus cause diminished blood flow to the uterus.
- *Environmental factors.* High altitude, exposure to x-rays, excessive exercise, work-related exposure to toxins, hyperthermia, and maternal use of drugs that have teratogenic effects, such as antimetabolites, anticonvulsants, and trimethadione, affect fetal growth (Anderson & Hay, 1999).
- *Placental factors.* Placental conditions such as small placenta, infarcted areas, abnormal cord insertions, placenta previa, and thrombosis may affect circulation to the fetus, which becomes more deficient with increasing gestational age.
- *Fetal factors.* Congenital infections (rubella, toxoplasmosis, syphilis, cytomegalic inclusion disease), congenital malformations, discordant twins (see Chapter 3), sex of the fetus (females tend to be smaller), chromosomal syndromes, and inborn errors of metabolism can predispose a fetus to fetal growth disturbances.

Antenatal identification of fetuses with IUGR is the first step in detecting common disorders associated with affected newborns. The perinatal history of maternal conditions, early dating of pregnancy by first-trimester ultrasound measurements, antepartal testing (nonstress test, contraction stress test, biophysical profile [see Chapter 14]), Doppler velocimetry, gestational age assessment, and the physical and neurologic assessment of the newborn are also important (Anderson & Hay, 1999).

## Patterns of IUGR

Intrauterine growth occurs by an increase in both cell number and cell size. If insult occurs early during the critical period of organ development in the fetus, fewer new cells are formed, organs are small, and organ weight is subnormal. In contrast, growth failure that begins later in pregnancy does not affect the total number of cells, only their size. The organs are normal, but their size is diminished. There are two clinical pictures of SGA newborns:

- *Symmetric (proportional) IUGR* is caused by long-term maternal conditions (such as chronic hypertension, severe malnutrition, chronic intrauterine infection, substance abuse, anemia) or fetal genetic abnormalities (Sohl & Moore, 1998). Symmetric IUGR can be noted by ultrasound in the first half of the second trimester. In symmetric IUGR there is chronic, prolonged retardation of growth in the size of organs, weight, length, and, in severe cases, head circumference.
- *Asymmetric (disproportional) IUGR* is associated with an acute compromise of uteroplacental blood flow. Some associated causes are placental infarcts, PIH, and poor weight gain in pregnancy. The growth retardation is usually not evident before the third trimester because, although weight is decreased, length and head circumference remain appropriate for that gestational age. An early indicator of asymmetric SGA is a decrease in the growth rate of the abdominal circumference, reflecting subnormal liver growth and a paucity of subcutaneous fat. Birth weight is below the 10th percentile, whereas head circumference and/or length may be between the 10th and 90th percentiles. Asymmetric SGA newborns are particularly at risk for perinatal asphyxia, pulmonary hemorrhage, hypocalcemia, and hypoglycemia in the newborn period.

Despite growth restriction, physiologic maturity develops according to gestational age. Therefore, the SGA newborn may be more physiologically mature than the preterm AGA newborn and less predisposed to complications of prematurity such as respiratory distress syndrome and hyperbilirubinemia. The SGA newborn's chances for survival are better than those of the preterm AGA newborn because of organ maturity, although this newborn still faces many other potential difficulties.

## Common Complications of the SGA Newborn

The complications occurring most frequently in the SGA newborn include the following:

- *Perinatal asphyxia.* The SGA newborn suffers chronic hypoxia in utero, which leaves little reserve to withstand the demands of normal labor and birth. Thus, intrauterine asphyxia, and its potential systemic problems, can occur. Cesarean birth may be necessary.
- *Aspiration syndrome.* In utero hypoxia can cause the fetus to gasp during birth, resulting in aspiration of amniotic fluid into the lower airways. It can also lead to relaxation of the anal sphincter and passage of meconium. This results in aspiration of the meconium with the first breaths after birth.
- *Heat loss.* Diminished subcutaneous fat (used for survival in utero), depletion of brown fat in utero, and a large surface area decrease the IUGR newborn's ability to conserve heat. The effect of surface area is diminished somewhat because of the flexed position assumed by the term SGA newborn.
- *Hypoglycemia.* An increase in metabolic rate in response to heat loss and poor hepatic glycogen stores causes hypoglycemia. In addition, the newborn is compromised by inadequate supplies of enzymes to activate gluconeogenesis (conversion of nonglucogen sources such as fatty acids and proteins to glucose).
- *Hypocalcemia.* Decreased calcium levels occur secondary to birth asphyxia and preterm birth.
- *Polycythemia.* The number of red blood cells is increased in the SGA newborn. This finding is considered a physiologic response to in utero chronic hypoxic stress.

Newborns with significant IUGR tend to have a poor prognosis, especially when born before 37 weeks' gestation. Factors contributing to poor outcome include the following:

- *Congenital malformations.* Congenital malformations occur 10 to 20 times more frequently in SGA infants than in AGA infants. The more severe the IUGR, the greater the chance for malformation as a result of impaired mitotic activity and cellular hypoplasia.
- *Intrauterine infections.* When fetuses are exposed to intrauterine infections such as rubella and cytomegalovirus, they are profoundly affected by direct invasion of the brain and other vital organs by the offending virus, resulting in IUGR.
- *Continued growth difficulties.* SGA newborns tend to be shorter than newborns of the same gestational age. Asymmetric IUGR infants can be expected to catch up in weight to normal-growth infants by 3 to 6 months of age. Symmetric SGA infants reportedly have varied growth potential but tend not to catch up to their peers (Anderson & Hay, 1999).
- *Learning difficulties.* Often SGA newborns who have poor brain development can exhibit subsequent failure to catch up and learning disabilities. The disabilities are characterized by hyperactivity, short attention span, and poor fine motor coordination (reading, writing, drawing). Some hearing loss and speech defects also occur.

## Clinical Therapy

The goal of clinical therapy is early recognition and implementation of the medical management of potential problems.

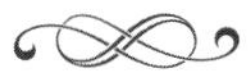

# Nursing Care Management

### Nursing Assessment and Diagnosis

The nurse is responsible for assessing gestational age and identifying signs of potential complications associated with SGA infants. All body parts of the symmetric IUGR infant are in proportion, but they are below normal size for the baby's gestational age. Therefore the head does not appear overly large or the length excessive in relation to the other body parts. These newborns are generally vigorous.

The asymmetric IUGR infant appears long, thin, and emaciated, with loss of subcutaneous fat tissue and muscle mass. The baby may have loose skin folds; dry, desquamating skin; and a thin and often meconium-stained cord. The head appears relatively large (although it approaches normal size) because the chest size and abdominal girth are decreased. The baby may have a vigorous cry and appear alert and wide eyed.

Nursing diagnoses that may apply to the SGA newborn include the following:

- ***Impaired gas exchange*** related to aspiration of meconium
- ***Hypothermia*** related to decreased subcutaneous fat
- ***Risk for injury*** to tissues related to decreased glycogen stores and impaired gluconeogenesis

- ***Risk for altered tissue perfusion*** related to increased blood viscosity

## Nursing Plan and Implementation

### *Hospital-Based Nursing Care*

Hypoglycemia, the most common metabolic complication of IUGR, produces such sequelae as CNS abnormalities and mental retardation. Conditions such as asphyxia, hyperviscosity, and cold stress may also affect the baby's outcome. Meticulous attention to physiologic parameters is essential for immediate nursing management and reduction of long-term disorders. (See Critical Pathway for Small-for-Gestational-Age Newborn, on pages 639–640.)

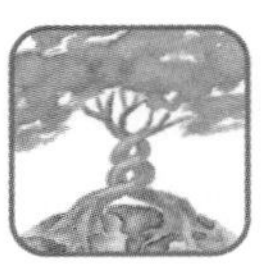

### COMMUNITY-BASED NURSING CARE

The long-term needs of the SGA newborn include careful follow-up evaluation of patterns of growth and possible disabilities that may later interfere with learning or motor functioning. Long-term follow-up care is essential for infants with congenital malformations, congenital infections, and obvious sequelae from physiologic problems. In addition, the parents of the IUGR newborn need support, because a positive atmosphere can enhance the baby's growth potential and the child's ultimate outcome.

## Evaluation

Anticipated outcomes of nursing care include the following:

- The SGA newborn is free from respiratory compromise.
- The SGA newborn maintains a stable temperature and glucose homeostasis.
- The SGA newborn gains weight and takes nipple feedings without developing physiologic distress or fatigue.
- The parents verbalize their concerns about their baby's health problems and understand the rationale behind management of their newborn.

# Care of the Large-for-Gestational-Age (LGA) Newborn

A newborn whose birth weight is at or above the 90th percentile on the intrauterine growth curve (at any week of gestation) is considered **large for gestational age (LGA).** Some AGA newborns have been incorrectly categorized as LGA because of miscalculation of the date of conception due to postconceptual bleeding. Careful gestational age assessment is essential to identify the potential needs and problems of such infants.

The most well-known condition associated with excessive fetal growth is maternal diabetes (White's classes A–C; see Table 12–3); however, only a minority of large newborns are born to diabetic mothers. The cause of the majority of cases of LGA newborns is unclear, but certain factors or situations have been found to correlate with their birth (Langer, 2000):

- Genetic predisposition is correlated proportionately to the mother's prepregnancy weight and to weight gain during pregnancy. Large parents tend to have large infants.
- Multiparous women have two to three times the number of LGA infants as primigravidas.
- Male infants are typically larger than female infants.
- Infants with erythroblastosis fetalis, Beckwith-Wiedemann syndrome (a genetic condition associated with omphalocele and neonatal hypoglycemia and hyperinsulinemia), or transposition of the great vessels are usually large.

The increase in the LGA infant's body size is characteristically proportional, although head circumference and body length are in the upper limits of intrauterine growth. The exception to this rule is the infant of the diabetic mother, whose body weight increases while length and head circumference may remain in the normal range. Macrosomic infants have poor motor skills and have difficulty in regulating behavioral states. LGA infants tend to be more difficult to arouse to a quiet alert state and may have feeding difficulties (Pressler & Hepworth,1997).

## COMMON COMPLICATIONS OF THE LGA NEWBORN

Disorders of the LGA newborn can include the following:

- *Birth trauma due to cephalopelvic disproportion (CPD).* Often LGA newborns have a biparietal diameter greater than 10 cm (4 in) or are associated with a maternal fundal height measurement greater than 42 cm (16 in) without the presence of hydramnios. Because of their excessive size, there are more breech presentations and shoulder dystocias. These complications may result in asphyxia, fractured clavicles, brachial palsy, facial paralysis, phrenic nerve palsy, depressed skull fractures, hematomas, and bleeding due to birth trauma.

Text continues on page 641.

# CRITICAL PATHWAY: *for Small-for-Gestational-Age Newborns*

| Category | Day of Birth—First 4 Hours | Remaining Day of Birth |
|---|---|---|
| **Referral** | Report from L&D, neonatal nurse practitioner<br>Check ID bands<br>Prn consults: high-risk peds, genetics | Check ID bands q shift<br>As parents desire, obtain circumcision permit after their discussion with MD<br>Lactation consult prn |
| **Assessments** | (Refer to Newborn Critical Pathway, pages 73 to 74)<br>• Complete set of VS<br>• Admission wt, length, HC<br>• Assess skin color<br>• Gestational age assessment<br>• Assess for s/s hypoglycemia. Chemstrip ASAP after birth, then follow SGA policy and procedure for blood glucose monitoring<br>• Assess for polycythemia: follow policy for treatment prn | Vital signs: T/P/R q4h and prn, BP prn<br>Newborn assessment q shift<br>(See Newborn Critical Pathway, pages 73 to 74)<br>Continue hypoglycemia assessments, chemstrips per SGA protocol<br>Assess mother-baby interaction |
| **Teaching/ psychosocial** | (See Newborn Critical Pathway, pages 000 to 000)<br>Admission activities performed at mother's bedside if possible, orient to nursery, handwashing, assess teaching needs<br>Teach parents rationale for SGA protocol | (See Newborn Critical Pathway, pages 73 to 74)<br>Reinforce previous teaching<br>Teach parent/guardian feeding methods, burping, diapering, calming techniques, s/s of stress, elimination norms |
| **Nursing care management and reports** | Diagnostic tests: blood type, Rh, Coombs' on cord blood when applicable, chemstrip within 1 h of birth and q1–2h until feedings initiated per protocol<br>Check chemstrip before at least two feedings or until condition stabilizes (chemstrip > 40 mg/dL × 2) | Femoral pulse or BP all four extremities if early DC<br>Hct per policy<br>Hearing screen<br>Cord care per policy<br>Bathe per policy |
| **Activity and comfort** | Place under radiant warmer, attach skin probe to maintain NTE<br>Soothe baby as needed with voice, touch, nesting in warmer | Leave in radiant warmer until stable, then swaddle in open crib<br>Incubator if temp instability; adjust incubator for infant size and gestation to maintain NTE |
| **Nutrition** | Initiate breast- or bottle-feeding as soon as mother and baby conditions allow<br>Lavage and gavage prn<br>Supplement breast when medically indicated or ordered by MD per policy<br>Feed SGA infants q3–4h<br>Monitor feeding tolerance, suck | Continue feeding schedule: small frequent feedings, high-calorie formula, nutritional fortifiers |
| **Elimination** | Note first void and stool if not at birth | Note all voids, amount and color of stools q4h |
| **Medication** | AquaMEPHYTON IM, dosage according to infant wt per MD orders, Ilotycin ophth ointment OU | Hep B vaccine as ordered by MD after consent signed by parent |
| **Discharge planning/ home care** | Hep B consent reviewed with parents<br>Plan DC with parent/guardian in 1–3 days<br>Evaluate for social services/home care/discharge planning needs | Hep B consent signed by parents<br>Birth certificate instructions/worksheet<br>Car seat for DC |
| **Family involvement** | Evaluate psychosocial needs<br>Evaluate parent teaching<br>Access community resources prn, ie, Teen "Healthy Starts" | Assess parents' knowledge of newborn behavior and reflexes<br>Encourage family involvement in infant's care as possible and as infant tolerates |
| **Date** | | |

ASAP, as soon as possible; C/S birth, cesarean birth; ID, identification; DC, discharge; HC, head circumference; Hct, hematocrit; LD, labor and delivery; NTE, neutral thermal environment; ophth, ophthalmic; OU, both eyes, q, every; SGA, small for gestational age; s/s signs and symptoms; vag, vaginal; VS, vital signs; wt, weight; WNL, within normal limits.

| Category | Day 1 | Day 2/3 (if applicable) |
|---|---|---|
| **Referral** | Check ID bands q shift | Check ID bands q shift<br>**Expected Outcomes**<br>Mother/baby ID bands correlate at time of discharge.<br>Consults completed prn. |
| **Assessments** | Assess thermoregulation<br>Assess for potential complications: perinatal asphyxia, aspiration syndrome, hypoglycemia, hypocalcemia, polycythemia<br>Assess mother-baby interaction | Assess color for jaundice<br>Assess for apnea<br>Assess mother-baby interaction<br>**Expected Outcomes**<br>Physical assessments, VS WNL; no complications of SGA noted |
| **Teaching/ psychosocial** | (See Newborn Critical Pathway, pages 73 to 74)<br>Reinforce previous teaching<br>Parent teaching: bathing, cord care, skin/nail care, use of thermometer, activity, sleep patterns, soothing, reflexes, jaundice, growth/feeding patterns | Final discharge teaching (see Newborn Critical Pathway, pages 73 to 74)<br>Review infant safety, s/s of illness, and when to call health care provider with parents<br>**Expected Outcomes**<br>Mother verbalizes comprehension of instructions, demonstrates care capabilities |
| **Nursing care management and reports** | Scalp treatment BID<br>Daily wt<br>Newborn assessment q shift<br>Check circumcision site q diaper change<br>Unclamp cord clamp<br>Cord care per policy<br>Total bilirubin level prn | Newborn assessment q shift<br>Daily wt<br>Check circumcision site<br>Cord care per policy<br>Note hearing test results<br>Femoral pulse or BP all four extremities<br>**Expected Outcomes**<br>Physical assessments WNL; cord unclamped and dry without s/s of infection; circ site unremarkable; gaining wt or wt stabilized to not >10% loss, labs WNL |
| **Activity and comfort** | Swaddled in open crib<br>Incubator if temp instability; adjust incubator for infant size and gestation to maintain NTE | **Expected Outcomes**<br>Maintains temp WNL swaddled in open crib |
| **Nutrition** | Continue enhanced feeding schedule, gavage prn per MD orders<br>Supplement breast only when medically indicated/policy or ordered by MD/NP<br>Encourage on-demand feeds, minimally q3–4h, breast or bottle | Continue enhanced feeding schedule, gavage prn per MD/NP orders<br>**Expected Outcomes**<br>Infant tolerates feedings, feeds on demand, breastfeeds without supplement, nipples without problems; regaining lost wt or wt stabilized |
| **Elimination** | Evaluate all voids and stool color q8h<br>**Expected Outcomes**<br>Voids and stools without difficulty | Note all voids and stool color q shift<br>**Expected Outcomes**<br>Voids qs, stools without difficulty and WNL |
| **Medication** | Hep B vaccine before discharge | **Expected Outcomes**<br>Infant has received ophth ointment OU and AquaMEPHYTON injection; received first Hep B vaccine if ordered and parental consent given |
| **Discharge planning/ home care** | Newborn photographs<br>Complete birth certificate packet<br>If vag birth, complete DC teaching | If C/S birth complete DC instructions (see Newborn Critical Pathway, pages 73 to 74)<br>**Expected Outcomes**<br>Infant DC home with mother; mother verbalizes follow-up appointment time/date |
| **Family involvement** | Bath, newborn care, and feeding classes<br>Newborn channel as available<br>Assess mother-baby bonding and interaction<br>Incorporate significant others and siblings in care<br>Support positive parenting behaviors<br>Evaluate mother/parent teaching | Assess mother-baby bonding and interaction<br>Identify community referral needs and refer to community agencies<br>**Expected Outcomes**<br>Demonstrates caring and family incorporation of infant |
| **Date** | | |

- *Increased incidence of cesarean births and oxytocin-induced births due to fetal size.* These births are accompanied by all the risk factors associated with cesarean births.
- *Hypoglycemia, polycythemia, and hyperviscosity.* These disorders are most often seen in infants with diabetic mothers, erythroblastosis fetalis, and Beckwith-Wiedemann syndrome.

## Nursing Care Management

The perinatal history, in conjunction with ultrasonic measurement of fetal skull and gestational age testing, is important in identifying an at-risk LGA newborn. Essential nursing care is directed toward monitoring vital signs, screening for hypoglycemia and polycythemia, and observing for signs and symptoms related to birth trauma. The nurse should address parental concerns about the visual signs of birth trauma and the potential for continuation of the overweight pattern. The nurse helps parents learn to arouse and console their newborn and facilitate attachment behaviors. Mothers of LGA infants with facial or head bruising may be reluctant to interact with their newborns because they fear causing their infant pain (Pressler & Hepworth, 1997). The nursing care involved in the complications associated with LGA newborns is similar to the care needed by the infant of a diabetic mother and will be discussed in the next section.

# Care of the Infant of a Diabetic Mother (IDM)

**Infants of diabetic mothers (IDMs)** are considered at risk and require close observation the first few hours to the first few days of life. Mothers with severe diabetes or diabetes of long duration (type I, or White's classes D–F, associated with vascular complications) may give birth to SGA infants. The typical IDM (type I, or White's classes A–C), however, is LGA. The infant is macrosomic, ruddy in color, and has excessive adipose fat tissue (Figure 25–4♦). The umbilical cord and placenta are large. There is a higher incidence of macrosomic infants born to certain ethnic groups (Native Americans, Mexican-Americans, African-Americans, Pacific Islanders).

IDMs have decreased total body water, particularly in the extracellular spaces, and are therefore not edematous.

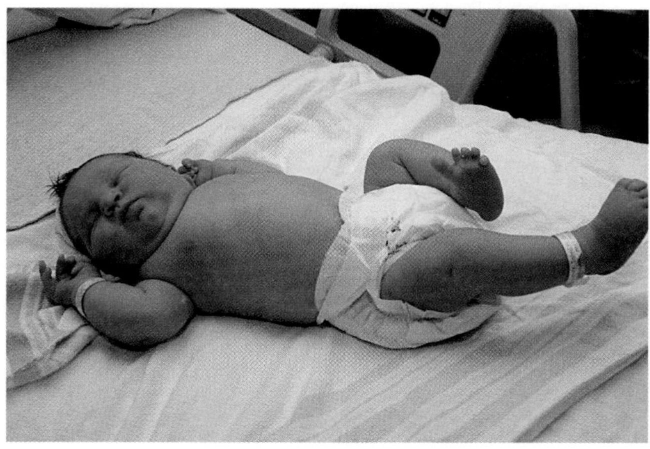

FIGURE 25–4 ♦ Macrosomic infant of diabetic mother. X-ray exam of this infant may reveal caudal regression of the spine.

Their excessive weight is due to increased weight of the visceral organs, cardiomegaly (hypertrophy), and increased body fat. The only organ not affected is the brain.

The excessive fetal growth of the IDM is caused by exposure to high levels of maternal glucose, which readily crosses the placenta. The fetus responds to these high glucose levels with increased insulin production and hyperplasia of the pancreatic beta cells. The main action of the insulin is to facilitate the entry of glucose into muscle and fat cells in a function similar to a cellular growth hormone. Once in the cells, glucose is converted to glycogen and stored. Insulin also inhibits the breakdown of fat to free fatty acids, thereby maintaining lipid synthesis, increasing the uptake of amino acids, and promoting protein synthesis. Insulin is an important regulator of fetal metabolism and has a "growth hormone" effect that results in increased linear growth. IDM has been associated with childhood obesity (Uvena-Celebrezze & Catalano, 2000).

### Common Complications of the IDM

Although IDMs are usually large, they are immature in physiologic functions and exhibit many of the problems of the preterm (premature) infant. The complications most often seen in an IDM are as follows:

- *Hypoglycemia.* Even though the high maternal blood supply is lost, this newborn continues to produce high levels of insulin, which deplete the blood glucose within hours after birth. IDMs also have less ability to release glucagon and catecholamines, which normally stimulate glucagon breakdown and glucose release. The incidence of hypoglycemia in IDMs varies from 30% to 50% (Uvena-Celebrezze & Catalano, 2000). The incidence of hypoglycemia varies according to the degree of success in controlling the maternal diabetes, the maternal blood sugar level at the time of birth, the length of labor, the class of maternal diabetes, and early versus late feedings of the newborn.

- *Hypocalcemia.* Tremors are the obvious clinical sign of hypocalcemia. They may be due to the IDM's increased incidence of prematurity and to the stresses of difficult pregnancy, labor, and birth, which predispose any infant to hypocalcemia. Diabetic women tend to have decreased serum magnesium levels at term secondary to increased urinary calcium excretion, which causes secondary hypoparathyroidism in their infants.

## HINTS FOR PRACTICE

When beginning fluids on an IDM, it is sometimes best to start at a higher concentration of dextrose to avoid hypoglycemia episodes.

- *Hyperbilirubinemia.* This condition may be seen at 48 to 72 hours after birth. It may be caused by slightly decreased extracellular fluid volume, which increases the hematocrit level, and the presence of hepatic immaturity. Enclosed hemorrhages resulting from complicated vaginal birth may also cause hyperbilirubinemia. There may also be an increase in the rate of bilirubin production in the presence of polycythemia.
- *Birth trauma.* Since most IDMs are LGA, trauma may occur during labor and birth.
- *Polycythemia.* This condition may be caused by the decreased extracellular volume in IDMs. Fetal hyperglycemia and hyperinsulinism result in increased oxygen consumption, leading to fetal hypoxia (Uvena-Celebrezze & Catalano, 2000). Hemoglobin $A_{1c}$ binds oxygen, which decreases the oxygen available to the fetal tissues. This tissue hypoxia stimulates increased erythropoietin production, which increases both the hematocrit level and the potential for hyperbilirubinemia.
- *Respiratory distress syndrome (RDS).* This complication occurs especially in newborns of diabetic mothers in White's classes A–C. Insulin antagonizes the cortisol-induced stimulation of lecithin synthesis that is necessary for lung maturation. Therefore, IDMs may have less mature lungs than expected for their gestational age. There is also a decrease in the phospholipid phosphatidylglycerol (PG), which stabilizes surfactant. The insufficiency of PG increases the incidence of RDS. RDS does not appear to be a problem for infants born of diabetic mothers in White's classes D–F; instead, the stresses of poor uterine blood supply may lead to increased production of steroids, which accelerates lung maturation. IDMs may also have a delay in closure of the ductus arteriosus and decreases in postnatal pulmonary artery pressure (Uvena-Celebrezze & Catalano, 2000).
- *Congenital birth defects.* These may include transposition of the great vessels, ventricular septal defect, patent ductus arteriosus, small left colon syndrome, and sacral agenesis (caudal regression) (Uvena-Celebrezze & Catalano, 2000). Early close control of maternal glucose levels before and during pregnancy decreases the risk of birth defects.

### CLINICAL THERAPY

Prenatal management is directed toward controlling maternal glucose levels, which minimizes the common complications of IDMs. Because the onset of hypoglycemia occurs between 1 and 3 hours after birth in IDMs (with a spontaneous rise to normal levels by 4 to 6 hours), blood glucose determinations should be done on cord blood hourly during the first 4 hours after birth and then at 4-hour intervals until the risk period (about 24 hours) has passed or per agency protocol.

IDMs whose serum glucose level falls below 40 mg/dL should have early feedings with formula or breast milk (colostrum). The infant may need to be gavage fed if lethargic. If normal glucose levels cannot be maintained with oral feedings or if seizures occur, an intravenous infusion of glucose will be necessary. Once the blood glucose level has been stable for 24 hours, the infusion rate can be decreased as oral feedings are increased. The newborn's blood glucose levels must be carefully monitored. Dextrose (25% to 50%) as a rapid infusion is contraindicated because it may lead to severe rebound hypoglycemia following an initial brief increase in glucose level.

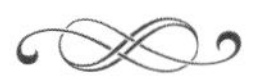

## NURSING CARE MANAGEMENT

### Nursing Assessment and Diagnosis

The nurse should not be lulled into thinking that a big baby is a mature baby. In almost every case, because of the infant's large size, the IDM will appear older than gestational age scoring indicates. The nurse must consider both the gestational age and whether the baby is AGA or LGA in planning and providing safe care. In caring for the IDM, the nurse assesses for signs of respiratory distress, hyperbilirubinemia, birth trauma, and congenital anomalies.

Nursing diagnoses that may apply to IDMs include the following:

- ***Altered nutrition: less than body requirements*** related to increased glucose metabolism secondary to hyperinsulinemia
- ***Impaired gas exchange*** related to respiratory distress secondary to impaired production of surfactant
- ***Ineffective family coping: compromise*** related to the illness of the baby

### Nursing Plan and Implementation

Nursing care of the IDM is directed toward early detection and ongoing monitoring of hypoglycemia (with glucose tests) and polycythemia (with central hematocrits), RDS, and hyperbilirubinemia. (These conditions are presented in Chapter 26.) The nurse also assesses for signs of birth trauma and congenital anomalies.

Parent teaching is directed toward preventing macrosomia and the resulting fetal-neonatal problems by instituting early and ongoing diabetic control. Parents are advised that with early identification and care most IDMs' neonatal problems have no significant sequelae.

### Evaluation

Expected outcomes of nursing care include the following:

- The IDM's respiratory distress and metabolic problems are minimized.
- The parents understand the effects of maternal diabetes on the baby and preventive steps they can initiate to decrease its impact on subsequent fetuses.
- The parents verbalize their concerns about their baby's health problems and understand the rationale behind management of their newborn.

# Care of the Postterm Newborn

The **postterm newborn** is any newborn born after 42 weeks' gestation. The term *postmature* applies only to the infant who is born after 42 completed weeks of gestation and who also demonstrates characteristics of the *postmaturity syndrome.*

Postterm, or prolonged, pregnancy occurs in approximately 3% to 12% of all pregnancies (Resnik & Calder, 1999). The cause of postterm pregnancy is not completely understood, but several factors are known to be associated with it. (See Chapter 19 for discussion of maternal factors.) Many pregnancies classified as prolonged are thought to be a result of inaccurate estimates of date of birth (EDB). A positive correlation exists between postterm pregnancy and Australian, Greek, and Italian ethnic groups. Most babies born as a result of prolonged pregnancy are of normal size and health; some keep on growing and are over 4000 g at birth, which supports the contention that the postterm fetus can remain well nourished. Potential intrapartal problems for these healthy but large fetuses are cephalopelvic disproportion (CPD) and shoulder dystocia.

Only about 5% of postterm newborns show signs of postmaturity syndrome. The major portion of the following discussion addresses the fetus who is not tolerating the prolonged pregnancy, is suffering from uteroplacental compromise to blood flow and resultant hypoxia, and is considered to have postmaturity syndrome.

## Common Complications of the Newborn with Postmaturity Syndrome

The truly postmature newborn is at high risk for morbidity and has a mortality rate two to three times greater than that of term infants. Although today the percentages are extremely low, the majority of postmature fetal deaths occur during labor, because the fetus uses up necessary body reserves. Decreased placental function impairs oxygenation and nutrition transport, leaving the fetus prone to hypoglycemia and asphyxia when the stresses of labor begin. The following are common disorders of the postmature newborn:

- *Hypoglycemia,* from nutritional deprivation and depleted glycogen stores.
- *Meconium aspiration* in response to in utero hypoxia. The presence of oligohydramnios increases the danger of aspirating thick meconium. Severe meconium aspiration syndrome increases the baby's chance of developing persistent pulmonary hypertension, pneumothorax, and pneumonia.
- *Polycythemia* due to increased production of red blood cells (RBCs) in response to hypoxia.
- *Congenital anomalies* of unknown cause.
- *Seizure activity* because of hypoxic insult.
- *Cold stress* because of loss or poor development of subcutaneous fat.

The long-term effects of postmaturity syndrome are unclear. At present, studies do not agree on the effect of postmaturity syndrome on weight gain and IQ scores (Resnik & Calder, 1999). Prolonged pregnancy itself is not solely responsible for the postmaturity syndrome. The characteristics of postmature newborns are primarily caused by a combination of advanced gestational age, placental aging and subsequent insufficiency, and continued exposure to amniotic fluid.

## Clinical Therapy

The aim of antenatal management is to differentiate the fetus who has postmaturity syndrome from the fetus who at birth is large, well nourished, alert, and tolerating the prolonged (postterm) pregnancy. (Antenatal and intrapartal tests that are done to evaluate fetal status and determine obstetric management and their use in postterm pregnancy are discussed in more depth in Chapters 14, 19.) If the amniotic fluid is meconium stained, an amnioinfusion may be done during labor. This procedure dilutes the meconium and thereby decreases the risk of meconium aspiration syndrome. (For detailed discussion of clinical management and care of the newborn at risk for meconium aspiration, see Chapter 26.) Hypoglycemia is monitored by serial glucose determinations per agency protocols. The baby may be placed on glucose infusions or given early feedings if respiratory distress is not present, but these measures must be instituted with caution because of the possibility of asphyxia.

As with SGA infants, peripheral and central hematocrits are tested to determine the presence of polycythemia. Fluid resuscitation can be initiated, and in extreme cases a partial exchange transfusion may be necessary to prevent polycythemia and adverse sequelae such as hyperviscosity. Oxygen is provided for respiratory distress. In addition, temperature instability and excessive loss of heat can result from decreased liver glycogen stores. (See Chapter 26 for thermoregulation techniques.)

# Nursing Care Management

## Nursing Assessment and Diagnosis

The nurse assesses the newborn for signs of postmaturity syndrome. The newborn with postmaturity syndrome appears alert; this wide-eyed, alert appearance is not necessarily a positive sign because it may indicate chronic intrauterine hypoxia. Postmature newborns are often voracious eaters.

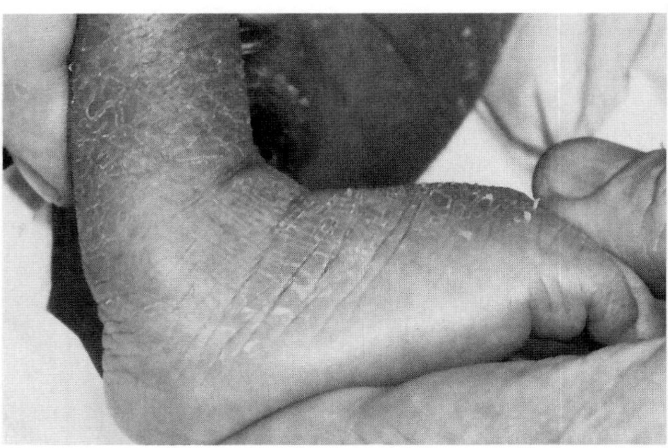

FIGURE 25–5 ♦ Postterm infant demonstrates deep cracking and peeling of skin. *Source:* Dubowitz, L., & Dubowitz, V. (1977). *The gestational age of the newborn.* Redwood City, CA: Addison-Wesley. Reprinted by permission of V. Dubowitz, MD, Hammersmith Hospital, London, England.

The infant typically has dry, cracking, parchmentlike skin without vernix or lanugo (Figure 25–5♦). Fingernails are long, and scalp hair is profuse. The infant's body appears long and thin. The wasting involves depletion of previously stored subcutaneous tissue, causing the skin to be loose. Fat layers are almost nonexistent.

Postmature newborns frequently have meconium staining, which colors the nails, skin, and umbilical cord. The varying shades (yellow to green) of meconium staining can give some clue as to whether the expulsion of meconium in utero was a recent or chronic problem. Green coloring indicates a more recent event.

Nursing diagnoses that may apply to the postmature newborn include the following:

- ***Hypothermia*** related to decreased liver glycogen and brown fat stores
- ***Altered nutrition: less than body requirements*** related to increased use of glucose secondary to in utero stress and decreased placenta perfusion
- ***Impaired gas exchange*** in the lungs and at the cellular level related to airway obstruction from meconium aspiration

## Nursing Plan and Implementation

### *Hospital-Based Nursing Care*

Nursing interventions are primarily supportive measures. The nurse needs to

- Monitor cardiopulmonary status because the stresses of labor are poorly tolerated and can result in hypoxemia in utero and possible asphyxia at birth
- Provide warmth to counterbalance the infant's poor response to cold stress and decreased liver glycogen and brown fat stores

- Frequently monitor blood glucose and initiate early feeding (at 1 or 2 hours of age) or intravenous glucose per physician order
- Obtain a central line hematocrit to determine accurately the presence of polycythemia

The nurse encourages parents to express their feelings and fears about the newborn's condition and potential long-term problems. The nurse gives careful explanations of procedures, includes the parents in the development of care plans for their baby, and encourages follow-up care as needed.

### Evaluation

Expected outcomes of nursing care include the following:

- The postterm newborn establishes effective respiratory function.
- The postmature baby is free of metabolic alterations (hypoglycemia) and maintains a stable temperature.

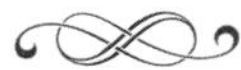

## Care of the Preterm (Premature) Newborn

With the help of modern technology, infants are surviving at younger gestational ages, but not without significant morbidity. The incidence of preterm births in the United States is approximately 8%. In socioeconomically deprived populations, it is 15% (American Academy of Pediatrics [AAP] & American College of Obstetricians and Gynecologists [ACOG], 1997). Prematurity and low birth weight are two common outcomes of pregnancy in single and young mothers. (See Chapter 19 for a discussion of preterm labor.)

A **preterm infant** is any infant born before the completion of 37 weeks' gestation. The length of gestation and thus the level of maturity vary even in the "premature" population. Figure 25–6♦ shows a preterm newborn.

The major problem of the preterm newborn is the variable immaturity of all systems, which depends on the length of gestation. The preterm newborn must traverse

## EVIDENCE-BASED PRACTICE

### Analgesia for Newborns Undergoing Painful Procedures

Bryan is born at 42 weeks' gestation. He has the wrinkled look of an old man, and his skin is very dry and cracked. Fortunately, however, he does not display signs of respiratory distress.

You will be conducting frequent heel sticks for blood glucose levels and you recognize that this is a painful procedure. Some of your colleagues offer newborns sucrose when they conduct a painful procedure because they say it soothes the baby. You are unclear about this practice and have asked if there is evidence to support its use.

In fact, there is evidence, you are told by the clinical specialist. The Cochrane Systematic Review on sucrose for analgesia in newborn infants examined 10 randomized trials to find that sucrose reduces two measures of pain, both heart rate and crying, following a painful procedure (Stevens & Ohlsson, 2000). The actual dose of sucrose varied across studies, however, so the ideal amount to administer remains unclear. In addition, the review cautions that repeated doses of sucrose and the use of sucrose with very-low-birth-weight and ventilated babies require further investigation.

Bryan is not in either group the review excluded, and you want to decrease his pain when you conduct the heel sticks. You ask the clinical specialist if you should gauge the amount of sucrose given by observation of the baby. She agrees and also suggests that you have the mother hold and comfort the baby during the procedure, then offer the bottle when the heel lance is completed. She advises that you continue to observe Bryan for signs of quieting and discontinue the sucrose at that time.

#### Reference

Stevens, B., & Ohlsson, A. (2000). Sucrose for analgesia in newborn infants undergoing painful procedures. (Cochrane Review). *Cochrane Library*, 2. Oxford: Update Software.

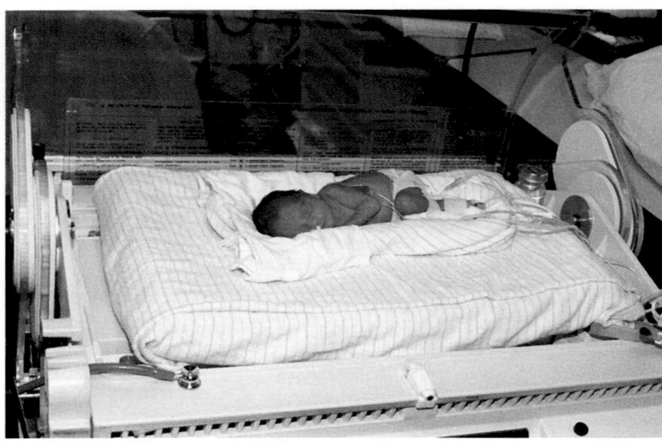

FIGURE 25–6 ♦ A 6-day-old, 28-week gestational age, 960-g preterm infant. *Source:* Courtesy of Carol Harrigan, RNC, MSN, NNP.

the same complex, interconnected pathways from intrauterine to extrauterine life as the term newborn. Because of immaturity, the premature newborn is ill equipped to make this transition smoothly. Maintenance of the preterm newborn falls within narrow physiologic parameters.

## Alteration in Respiratory and Cardiac Physiology

The preterm newborn is at risk for respiratory problems because the lungs are not fully mature and not fully ready to take over the process of oxygen and carbon dioxide exchange without assistance until 37 to 38 weeks' gestation. Critical factors in the development of respiratory distress include the following:

1. The preterm infant is unable to produce adequate amounts of surfactant. (See Chapter 21 for discussion of respiratory adaptation and development.) Inadequate surfactant lessens compliance (ability of the lung to fill with air easily), and the inspiratory pressure needed to expand the lungs with air increases. The collapsed (or atelectatic) alveoli will not facilitate an exchange of oxygen and carbon dioxide, resulting in hypoxia, inefficient pulmonary blood flow, and depletion of the preterm newborns' available energy.
2. The muscular coat of pulmonary blood vessels is incompletely developed. Consequently, the pulmonary arterioles do not constrict as well in response to decreased oxygen levels. Lower pulmonary vascular resistance leads to left-to-right shunting of blood through the ductus arteriosus back into the lungs.
3. The ductus arteriosus usually responds to increasing oxygen levels and prostaglandin E levels by vasoconstriction; in the preterm infant, who is more susceptible to hypoxia, the ductus may remain open. A patent ductus increases the blood volume to the lungs, causing pulmonary congestion, increased respiratory effort, carbon dioxide retention, and bounding femoral pulses.

The common complications of the cardiopulmonary system in preterm infants are discussed later in this chapter and in Chapter 26.

## Alteration in Thermoregulation

Heat loss is a major problem in preterm newborns that the nurse can do much to prevent. Two factors limiting heat production, however, are the availability of glycogen in the liver and the amount of brown fat available for metabolism. Both of these limiting factors appear in the third trimester. If the baby is chilled after birth, both glycogen and brown fat stores are metabolized rapidly for heat production, leaving the newborn with no reserves in the event of future stress. Since the muscle mass is small in preterm infants, and muscular activity is diminished (they are unable to shiver), little heat is produced.

Heat loss occurs as a result of five physiologic and anatomic factors:

1. The preterm baby has a higher ratio of body surface to body weight. This means that the baby's ability to produce heat (based on body weight) is much less than the potential for losing heat (based on surface area). The loss of heat in a preterm infant weighing 1500 g is five times greater per unit of body weight than in an adult.
2. The preterm baby has very little subcutaneous fat, which is the human body's insulation. Without adequate insulation, heat is easily conducted from the core of the body (warmer temperature) to the surface of the body (cooler temperature). Heat is lost from the body as the blood vessels, which lie close to the skin surface in the preterm infant, transport blood from the body core to the subcutaneous tissues.
3. The preterm baby has thinner, more permeable skin than the term infant. This increased permeability contributes to a greater insensible water loss as well as to heat loss.
4. The posture of the preterm baby is another important factor influencing heat loss. Flexion of the extremities decreases the amount of surface area exposed to the environment. Extension increases the surface area exposed to the environment and thus increases heat loss. The gestational age of the infant influences the amount of flexion, from completely hypotonic and extended at 28 weeks to strong flexion displayed by 36 weeks.
5. The preterm baby has a decreased ability to vasoconstrict superficial blood vessels and conserve heat in the body core.

In summary, gestational age is directly proportional to the ability to maintain thermoregulation; thus the more preterm the newborn, the less able the infant is to maintain heat balance. Preventing heat loss by providing a neutral thermal environment is one of the most important considerations in nursing management of the preterm infant. Cold stress, with its accompanying severe complications, can be prevented (see Chapter 26).

## Alteration in Gastrointestinal Physiology

The basic structure of the gastrointestinal (GI) tract is formed early in gestation. Maturation of the digestive and absorptive process is more variable, however, and occurs later in gestation. As a result of GI immaturity, the preterm newborn has the following ingestion, digestive, and absorption problems:

- A marked danger of aspiration and its associated complications due to the infant's poorly developed gag reflex, incompetent esophageal cardiac sphincter, and poor sucking and swallowing reflex.
- Difficulty in meeting high caloric and fluid needs for growth due to small stomach capacity.
- Limited ability to convert certain essential amino acids to nonessential amino acids. Certain amino acids, such as histidine, taurine, and cysteine, are essential to the preterm infant but not to the term infant.
- Inability to handle the increased osmolarity of formula protein due to kidney immaturity. The preterm infant requires a higher concentration of whey protein than of casein.
- Difficulty absorbing saturated fats because of decreased bile salts and pancreatic lipase. Severe illness of the newborn may also prevent intake of adequate nutrients.
- Difficulty with lactose digestion initially because processes may not be fully functional during the first few days of a preterm infant's life. The preterm newborn can digest and absorb most simple sugars.
- Deficiency of calcium and phosphorus since two-thirds of these minerals are deposited in the last trimester. Rickets and significant bone demineralization due to deficiency of calcium and phosphorus, which are deposited primarily in the last trimester.
- Increased basal metabolic rate and increased oxygen requirements due to fatigue associated with sucking.
- Feeding intolerance and necrotizing enterocolitis (NEC) as a result of diminished blood flow and tissue perfusion to the intestinal tract due to prolonged hypoxia and hypoxemia at birth.

## Alteration in Renal Physiology

The kidneys of the preterm infant are immature compared with those of the term infant. This situation poses clinical problems in the management of fluid and electrolyte balance. Specific characteristics of the preterm infant include the following:

- The glomerular filtration rate (GFR) is lower because of decreased renal blood flow. The GFR is directly related to lower gestational age, so the more preterm the newborn, the lower the GFR. The GFR is also decreased in the presence of diseases or conditions that decrease the renal blood flow and oxygen content, such as severe respiratory distress and perinatal asphyxia. Anuria and oliguria may be observed in the preterm infant after severe asphyxia with associated hypotension.
- The preterm infant's kidneys are limited in their ability to concentrate urine or to excrete excess amounts of fluid. This means that if excess fluid is administered, the infant is at risk for fluid retention and overhydration. If too little is administered, the infant will become dehydrated because of the inability to retain adequate fluid.
- The kidneys of the preterm infant begin excreting glucose (glycosuria) at a lower serum glucose level than those of the term infant. Therefore, glycosuria with hyperglycemia is common.
- The buffering capacity of the kidney is reduced, predisposing the infant to metabolic acidosis. Bicarbonate is excreted at a lower serum level, and acid is excreted more slowly. Therefore, after periods of hypoxia or insult, the preterm infants' kidneys require a longer time to excrete the lactic acid that accumulates. Sodium bicarbonate is frequently required to treat the metabolic acidosis.
- The immaturity of the renal system affects the preterm infant's ability to excrete drugs. Because excretion time is longer, many drugs are given over longer intervals in the preterm infant (ie, every 12 hours instead of every 8 hours). Urine output must be carefully monitored when the infant is receiving nephrotoxic drugs such as gentamicin, nafcillin, and others. If urine output is poor, drugs can become toxic in the infant much more quickly than in the adult.

## Alteration in Reactivity Periods and Behavioral States

The newborn infant's response to extrauterine life is characterized by two periods of reactivity (see Chapter 21). The preterm infant's periods of reactivity are delayed. In the very ill infant, these periods of reactivity may not be observed at all because the infant may be hypotonic and unreactive for several days after birth.

As the preterm newborn grows and the condition stabilizes, identifying behavioral states and traits unique to each infant becomes increasingly possible. In general, stable preterm infants do not demonstrate the same behavioral states as term infants. Preterm infants tend to be more disorganized in their sleep-wake cycles and are unable to attend as well to the human face and objects in the environment. Neurologically, their responses (sucking, muscle tone, states of arousal) are weaker than full-term infants' responses.

## Management of Nutrition and Fluid Requirements

Early feedings are extremely valuable in maintaining normal metabolism and lowering the possibility of such complications as hypoglycemia, hyperbilirubinemia, hyperkalemia, and azotemia. However, the preterm infant is at risk for complications that may develop because of immaturity of the digestive system.

The oral (enteral) caloric intake necessary for growth in an uncompromised healthy preterm newborn is 110 to 130 kcal/kg/day. In addition to these relatively high caloric needs, the preterm newborn requires more protein, 3 to 3.5 g/kg/day, as opposed to 2.0 to 2.5 g/kg/day for the full-term infant (Merenstein & Gardner, 1998). To meet these needs, many institutions use breast milk or special preterm formulas. Whether breast milk or formula is used, feeding regimens are established based on the infant's weight and estimated stomach capacity. Initial formula feedings are gradually increased as the infant tolerates them. In many institutions, it is necessary to supplement oral feedings with parenteral fluids to maintain adequate hydration and caloric intake until the baby is on full oral feedings.

In addition to a higher calorie and protein formula, preterm infants should receive supplemental multivitamins, including vitamin E and trace minerals. The requirement for vitamin E is increased by a diet high in polyunsaturated fats (which preterm infants tolerate best). Preterm infants fed iron-fortified formulas have higher red cell hemolysis and lower vitamin E concentrations and thus require additional vitamin E. Preterm formulas also need to contain medium-chain triglycerides (MCT) and additional amino acids such as cysteine, as well as calcium, phosphorus, and vitamin D supplements to increase mineralization of bones. Rickets and significant bone demineralization have been documented in very-low-birth-weight infants and otherwise healthy preterm infants.

Nutritional intake is considered adequate when there is consistent weight gain of 20 to 30 g/day. Initially, no weight gain may be noted for several days, but total weight loss should not exceed 15% of the total birth weight or more than 1% to 2% per day. Some institutions add the criteria of head circumference growth and increase in body length of 1 cm per week, once the newborn is stable.

Calculation of fluid requirements takes into account the infant's weight and postnatal age. Recommendations for fluid therapy in the preterm infant are approximately 80 to 100 mL/kg/day for day 1, 100 to 120 mL/kg/day for day 2, and 120 to 150 mL/kg/day by day 3 of life. These amounts may be increased up to 200 mL/kg/day if the infant is very small, receiving phototherapy, or under a radiant warmer because of increased insensible water losses. Fluid losses can be minimized through the use of heat shields and humidity, or "swamping."

## Common Complications of Preterm Newborns

The goals of medical and nursing care are to anticipate and manage the complications associated with prematurity and the preterm infant's growth and development needs. The most common of these complications are the following:

1. *Apnea. Apnea of prematurity* refers to cessation of breathing for 20 seconds or longer or for less than 20 seconds when associated with cyanosis and bradycardia. Apnea is a common problem in the preterm infant (less than 37 weeks' gestation) and is thought to be primarily a result of neuronal immaturity, a factor that contributes to the preterm infant's irregular breathing patterns. Factors that adversely affect brain nerve cells include hypoxia, acidosis, edema, intracranial bleeding, hyperbilirubinemia, hypoglycemia, hypocalcemia, and sepsis. Gastroesophageal reflux (GER) has been implicated in the production of apnea. It is believed that GER causes laryngospasm, which leads to bradycardia and apnea.
2. *Patent ductus arteriosus (PDA).* The ductus arteriosus fails to close because of decreased pulmonary arteriole musculature and hypoxemia. Symptomatic PDA is often seen around the time when premature infants are recovering from RDS. Patent ductus arteriosus often prolongs the course of illness in a preterm newborn and leads to chronic pulmonary dysfunction.

3. *Respiratory distress syndrome (RDS).* Respiratory distress results from inadequate surfactant production.
4. *Intraventricular hemorrhage (IVH).* Intraventricular hemorrhage is the most common type of intracranial hemorrhage in small preterm infants, especially those weighing less than 1500 g or of less than 34 weeks' gestation. Up to 35 weeks' gestation the preterm's brain ventricles are lined by the germinal matrix, which is highly susceptible to hypoxic events such as respiratory distress, birth trauma, and birth asphyxia. The germinal matrix is very vascular, and these blood vessels rupture in the presence of hypoxia.
5. *Anemia of prematurity.* The preterm infant is at risk for anemia because of the rapid rate of growth required, shorter red blood cell life, excessive blood sampling, decreased iron stores, and deficiency of vitamin E.

Other common problems of preterm infants such as hypocalcemia and NEC are discussed earlier in the physiologic sections. (For an in-depth discussion of RDS, hyperbilirubinemia, hypoglycemia, and sepsis see Chapter 26.)

## Long-Term Needs and Outcome

The care of preterm infants and their families does not stop on discharge from the nursery. Follow-up care is extremely important because many developmental problems are not noted until an infant is older and begins to demonstrate motor delays or sensory disability.

Within the first year of life, low-birth-weight preterm infants face higher mortality rates than term infants. Causes of death include sudden infant death syndrome (SIDS)—which occurs about five times more frequently in the preterm infant—respiratory infections, and neurologic defects. Morbidity is also much higher among preterm infants, with those weighing less than 1500 g at highest risk for long-term complications.

The most common long-term needs observed in preterm infants include the following:

- *Retinopathy of prematurity (ROP).* Premature newborns are particularly susceptible to characteristic retinal changes, known as ROP, which can result in visual impairment. The disease is now viewed as multifactorial in origin. Increased survival of very-low-birth-weight (VLBW) infants may be the most important factor in the increased incidence of ROP.
- *Bronchopulmonary dysplasia (BPD).* Long-term lung disease is a result of damage to the alveolar epithelium secondary to positive pressure respirator therapy and high oxygen concentration. These infants have long-term dependence on oxygen therapy and an increased incidence of respiratory infection during their first few years of life.
- *Speech defects.* The most frequently observed speech defects involve delayed development of receptive and expressive ability that may persist into the school-age years.
- *Neurologic defects.* The most common neurologic defects include cerebral palsy, hydrocephalus, seizure disorders, lower IQ, and learning disabilities. However, the socioeconomic climate and family support systems are extremely important influences on the child's ultimate school performance in the absence of major neurologic defects. Families can be reminded that risk does not equal injury, injury does not equal damage, and description of damage does not allow a precise prediction about recovery or outcome.
- *Auditory defects.* Preterm infants have a 1% to 4% incidence of moderate to profound hearing loss and should have a formal audiologic exam before discharge and at 3 to 6 months (corrected age). The test currently used to measure hearing functions of the newborn is the evoked otoacoustic emissions (EOAE) test. Any infant with repeated abnormal results should be referred to speech-and-language specialists.

When evaluating the infant's abilities and disabilities, it is important for parents to understand that developmental progress must be assessed from the expected date of birth, not from the actual date of birth. Developmental level cannot be evaluated based on chronologic age. In addition, the parents need the consistent support of health care professionals in the long-term management of their infant to promote the highest quality of life possible.

# Nursing Care Management

## Nursing Assessment and Diagnosis

The nurse needs to assess the physical characteristics and gestational age of the preterm newborn accurately to anticipate the special needs and problems of the baby. Physical characteristics vary greatly depending on gestational age, but the following characteristics are frequently present:

- Color is usually pink or ruddy but may be acrocyanotic. (Cyanosis, jaundice, and pallor are abnormal and should be noted.)

- Skin is reddened and translucent, blood vessels are readily apparent, there is little subcutaneous fat.
- Lanugo is plentiful and widely distributed.
- Head size appears large in relation to body.
- Skull bones are pliable; fontanelle is smooth and flat.
- Ears have minimal cartilage and are pliable, folded over.
- Nails are soft, short.
- Genitals are small; testes may not be descended.
- Resting position is flaccid, froglike.
- Cry is weak, feeble.
- Reflexes (sucking, swallowing, gag) are poor.
- Activity consists of jerky, generalized movements. (Seizure activity is abnormal.)

Determination of gestational age in preterm newborns requires knowledge and experience in administering gestational assessment tools. The tool used should be specific, reliable, and valid. (For a discussion of gestational age assessment tools, see Chapter 22.)

Nursing diagnoses that may apply to the preterm newborn include the following:

- ***Impaired gas exchange*** related to immature pulmonary vasculature and inadequate surfactant production
- ***Altered nutrition: less than body requirements*** related to weak suck and swallow reflexes and decreased ability to absorb nutrients
- ***Ineffective thermoregulation*** related to hypothermia secondary to decreased glycogen and brown fat stores
- ***Ineffective family coping*** related to anger or guilt at having delivered a premature baby

## Nursing Plan and Implementation

### *Maintenance of Respiratory Function*

There is increased danger of respiratory obstruction in preterm newborns because their bronchi and trachea are so narrow that mucus can obstruct the airway. The nurse must maintain patency through judicious suctioning, but only on an as-needed basis.

Positioning can also affect respiratory function, especially in the preterm newborn. If the baby is in the supine position, the nurse should slightly elevate the infant's head to maintain the airway, being careful to avoid hyperextension of the neck because the trachea will collapse. Also, because the newborn has weak neck muscles and cannot control head movement, the nurse should ensure that this head position is maintained by placing a small roll under the shoulders. Because the prone position splints the chest wall and decreases the amount of respiratory effort used to move the chest wall, it facilitates chest expansion and improves air entry and oxygenation. Weak or absent cough or gag reflexes increase the chance of aspiration in the premature newborn. The nurse should ensure that the infant's position facilitates drainage of mucus or regurgitated formula.

The nurse monitors heart and respiratory rates with cardiorespiratory monitors and observes the newborn to identify alterations in cardiopulmonary status. Signs of respiratory distress include the following:

- Cyanosis (serious sign when generalized)
- Tachypnea (sustained respiratory rate greater than 60/minute after first 4 hours of life)
- Retractions
- Expiratory grunting
- Flaring nostrils
- Apneic episodes
- Presence of rales or rhonchi on auscultation
- Diminished air entry

The nurse who observes any of these alterations records and reports them for further evaluation. If respiratory distress occurs, the nurse administers oxygen per physician or nurse practitioner order to relieve hypoxemia. If hypoxemia is not treated immediately, it may result in patent ductus arteriosus or metabolic acidosis. If oxygen is administered to the newborn, the nurse monitors the oxygen concentration with devices such as the transcutaneous oxygen monitor ($tcPO_2$) or the pulse oximeter. Monitoring of oxygen concentration in the baby's blood is essential since hyperoxemia may lead to ROP.

The nurse also needs to consider respiratory function during feeding. To prevent aspiration and increased energy expenditure and oxygen consumption, the nurse must ensure that the infant's gag and suck reflexes are intact before initiating oral feedings.

### *Maintenance of Neutral Thermal Environment*

Providing a neutral thermal environment minimizes the oxygen consumption required to maintain a normal core temperature; it also prevents cold stress and facilitates growth by decreasing the calories needed to maintain body temperature. The preterm infant's immature central nervous system provides poor temperature control, and stores of brown fat are decreased. A small infant (<1200 g) can lose 80 kcal/kg/day through radiation of body heat.

The nurse implements all the usual thermoregulation measures discussed in Chapter 23. In addition, to minimize heat loss and temperature instability effects the nurse should

1. Warm and humidify oxygen to minimize evaporative heat loss and decrease oxygen consumption.
2. Place the baby in a double-walled incubator or use a Plexiglas heat shield over small preterm infants in single-walled incubators to avoid radiative heat losses. Some institutions use radiant warmers and plastic wrap over the baby and pipe in humidity (swamping). Do not use Plexiglas shields on radiant warmer beds because they block the infrared heat.
3. Avoid placing the baby on cold surfaces such as metal treatment tables and cold x-ray plates, pad cold surfaces with diapers and use radiant warmers during procedures, place infant on prewarmed mattresses, and warm hands before handling the baby to prevent heat transfer via conduction.
4. Use warmed ambient humidity.
5. Keep the skin dry and place a cap on the baby's head to prevent heat loss via evaporation. (The head makes up 25% of the total body size.)
6. Keep radiant warmers, incubators, and cribs away from windows and cold external walls and out of drafts to prevent heat loss by radiation.
7. Use a skin probe to monitor the baby's skin temperature. Correlate ambient temperatures with the skin probe in the incubator using the servocontrol rather than the manual mode. The temperature should be 36 to 37°C (96.8 to 97.7°F). Temperature fluctuations indicate hypothermia or hyperthermia. Be careful not to place skin temperature probes over bony prominences, areas of brown fat, poorly vasoreactive areas such as extremities, or excoriated areas ("Neonatal Thermoregulation," 1997).
8. Warm formula or stored breast milk before feeding.
9. Use reflector patch over the skin temperature probe when using a radiant warmer bed so that the probe does not sense the higher infrared temperature as the baby's skin temperature and therefore decrease the heater output.

Once preterm infants are medically stable, they can be clothed with a double-thickness cap, cotton shirt, and diaper and, if possible, swaddled in a blanket. The nurse begins the process of weaning to a crib when the premature infant is medically stable, does not require assisted ventilation, weighs approximately 1500 g, has 5 days of consistent weight gain, and is taking oral feedings and when apnea and bradycardia episodes have stabilized. The nurse should be familiar with the individual institution's protocol for weaning to a crib.

### *Maintenance of Fluid and Electrolyte Status*

The nurse maintains hydration by providing adequate intake based on the newborn's weight, gestational age, chronologic age, and volume of sensible and insensible water losses. Adequate fluid intake should compensate for increased insensible losses and the amount needed for renal excretion of metabolic products. Insensible water losses can be minimized by providing high ambient humidity, humidifying oxygen, using heat shields, covering the skin with plastic wrap, and placing the infant in a double-walled incubator.

The nurse evaluates the hydration status of the baby by assessing and recording signs of dehydration. Signs of dehydration include sunken fontanelle, loss of weight, poor skin turgor (skin returns to position slowly when squeezed gently), dry oral mucous membranes, decreased urine output, and increased specific gravity (>1.013). The nurse must also identify signs of overhydration by observing the newborn for edema or excessive weight gain and by comparing urine output with fluid intake.

The nurse weighs the preterm infant at least once daily at the same time each day. Weight change is one of the most sensitive indicators of fluid balance. Weighing diapers is also important for accurate input and output measurement (1 mL = 1 g). A comparison of intake and output measurements over an 8- or 24-hour period provides important information about renal function and fluid balance. Assessment of patterns and whether they show a net gain or loss over several days is also essential to fluid management. In addition, the nurse monitors blood serum levels and pH to evaluate for electrolyte imbalances. Urine specific gravity and pH are obtained periodically. Urine osmolality provides an indication of hydration, although this factor must be correlated with other assessments (eg, serum sodium). Hydration is considered adequate when the urine output is 1 to 3 mL/kg/hr.

Accurate hourly intake calculations when administering intravenous fluids are essential to prevent overload. Accuracy can be ensured by using neonatal or pediatric infusion pumps. To prevent electrolyte imbalance and dehydration, the nurse takes care to give the correct intravenous (IV) solutions and volumes and concentrations of formulas.

### *Provision of Adequate Nutrition and Prevention of Fatigue during Feeding*

The preterm infant is fed by various methods depending on the infant's gestational age, health and physical condition, and neurologic status. The three most common oral feeding methods are bottle, breast, and gavage (discussed later in this section). Preterm infants who cannot tolerate any oral (enteral) feedings may be nourished by total parenteral nutrition (TPN). TPN uses hyperalimentation to provide calories, vitamins, minerals, protein, and glucose and intralipids to provide essential fatty acids.

**Inserting and Checking the Tube continued**

- If inserting the tube nasally, lubricate the tip in a cup of sterile water. Use water instead of an oil-based lubricant, in case the tube is inadvertently passed into a lung. Shake any excess drops to prevent aspiration.
- If inserting the tube orally, the oral secretions are enough to lubricate the tube adequately.
- Stabilize the infant's head with one hand and pass the tube via the mouth (or nose) into the stomach to the point previously marked. If the infant begins coughing or choking or becomes cyanotic or phonic, remove the tube immediately because the tube has probably entered the trachea.
- If no respiratory distress is apparent, lightly tape the tube in position, draw up 0.5–1.0 mL of air in the syringe, and connect the syringe to the tubing. Place the stethoscope over the epigastric area and briskly inject the air (Figure 25–9♦). You will hear a sudden rush as the air enters the stomach.

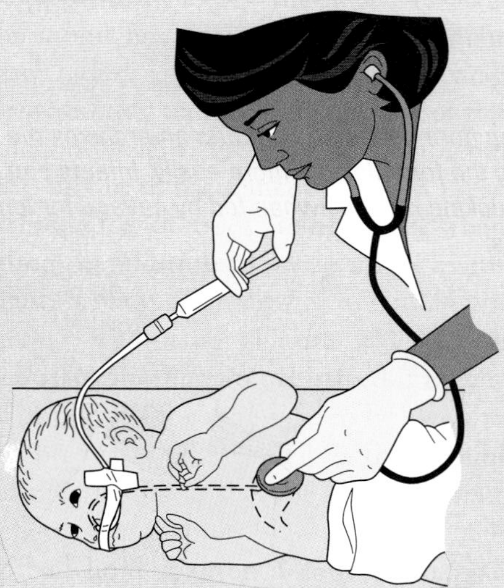

FIGURE 25–9 ♦ Auscultation for placement of gavage tube.

- *Aspirate the stomach contents with the syringe and note the amount, color, and consistency to evaluate the infant's feeding tolerance. Return the residual to the stomach unless you are asked to discard it. It is usually not discarded because of the potential for electrolyte imbalance.*
- *If the aspirated contents contain only a clear fluid or mucus and if it is unclear whether the tube is in the stomach, test the aspirate for pH. Stomach aspirate has a pH between 1 and 3.*

**Administering the Feeding**

- *Hold the infant for feeding or position the infant on the right side to decrease the risk of aspiration in case of emesis during feeding.*
- *Separate the syringe from the tube, remove the plunger from the barrel, reconnect the barrel to the tube, and pour the formula into the syringe.*
- *Elevate the syringe 6–8 in over the infant's head and allow the formula to flow by gravity at a slow, even rate. You may need to initiate the flow of formula by inserting the plunger of the syringe into the barrel just until you see formula enter the feeding tube. Do not use pressure.*
- *Regulate the rate to prevent sudden stomach distension, leading to vomiting and aspiration. Continue adding formula to the syringe until the infant has absorbed the desired volume.*

**Clearing and Removing the Tube**

- *Clear the tubing with 2–3 mL sterile water or with air. This ensures that the infant has received all of the formula. If the tube is going to be left in place, clearing it will decrease the risk of clogging and bacterial growth in the tube.*
- *To remove the tube, loosen the tape, fold the tube over on itself, and quickly withdraw the tube in one smooth motion to minimize the potential for fluid aspiration as the tube passes the epiglottis. If the tube is to be left in, position it so that the infant is unable to remove it. Replace the tube every 24 hours.*

is not intended to contribute to the total nutritional intake but rather to enhance gut metabolism. Trophic feedings may also help to encourage earlier advancement to full feedings, thereby decreasing the development of NEC and the complications of parenteral nutrition (Newell, 2000). Formula or breast milk (with or without fortifiers to increase caloric content) is incorporated into the feedings slowly. Initially, the feeding may be at quarter strength, then half strength, and so on.

Before each feeding, the nurse measures abdominal girth and auscultates the abdomen to determine the presence and quality of bowel sounds. Such assessments permit early detection of abdominal distension, visible bowel loops, and decreased peristaltic activity, which may indicate NEC or paralytic ileus. The nurse also checks for residual formula in the stomach before feeding when the newborn is fed by gavage. This procedure also can be performed when the nipple-fed newborn presents with abdominal distension. The presence of increasing residual formula is an indication of intolerance to the type or amount of feeding or the increase in amount of feeding. Residual formula is usually readministered because digestive processes have already been initiated and subtracted from the amount to be given at that feeding. The nurse should carefully watch for other signs of feeding intolerance including guaiac-positive stools (occult blood in stools), lactose in the stools (reducing substance in the stools), vomiting, and diarrhea.

## HINTS FOR PRACTICE

Residual feeding may indicate early NEC and should be called to the attention of the clinician.

Preterm newborns who are ill or who fatigue easily with nipple feedings are usually fed by gavage. The infant is essentially passive with these methods, thus conserving energy and calories. As the baby matures, gavage feedings are replaced with breast- or bottle-feedings to assist in strengthening the sucking reflex and in meeting oral and emotional needs. Signs that indicate readiness for oral feedings are a strong gag reflex, presence of nonnutritive sucking, rooting behavior, gestational age of 34 weeks or more, and weight over 1500 g. Both low-birth-weight and preterm infants nipple-feed more effectively in a quiet state. The nurse establishes a gradual nipple-feeding program, such as one nipple-feeding per day, then one nipple-feeding per shift, and then a nipple-feeding every other feeding. Daily weights are monitored because often there is a small weight loss when nipple-feedings are started. After feedings, the nurse places the baby on the right side (with support to maintain this position) to enhance gastric emptying and decrease the chance of aspiration if regurgitation occurs. Gastroesophageal reflux is not uncommon in preterm newborns.

## HINTS FOR PRACTICE

For an otherwise healthy, growing premature infant who is receiving total enteral intake and has started to experience apnea and bradycardia, one differential diagnosis to think about is reflux rather than sepsis, although sepsis may need to be ruled out.

The nurse involves the parents in feeding their preterm baby. This involvement is essential to the development of attachment between parents and infant. In addition, it increases parental knowledge about the care of their infant and helps them cope with the situation.

### *Prevention of Infection*

The preterm newborn is susceptible to infection because of an immature immune system and thin and permeable skin. Invasive procedures, techniques such as umbilical catheterization and mechanical ventilation, and prolonged hospitalization place the infant at greater risk for infection.

Strict handwashing, reverse isolation, and use of equipment for only one infant help minimize the preterm newborn's exposure to infectious agents. In addition, most nurseries have adopted the standard precautions recommended by the Centers for Disease Control and Prevention (CDC) of isolating every baby. Staff members are required to complete a 2- to 3-minute scrub using iodine-containing antibacterial solutions, which inhibit growth of gram-positive cocci and gram-negative rod organisms. Other specific nursing interventions include limiting visitors; requiring visitors to wash their hands; and maintaining strict aseptic practices when changing intravenous tubing and solutions (IV solutions and tubing should be changed every 24 hours), administering parenteral fluids, and assisting with sterile procedures. Incubators and radiant warmers should be changed weekly. The nurse prevents pressure-area breakdown by changing the baby's position regularly, doing range of motion exercises, and using a sheepskin (covered with a blanket or diapered beneath the infant's head) or a water bed. To avoid skin tears, a protective transparent covering can be applied over vulnerable joints but is used very sparingly (Siegfried, 1998). Chemical skin preps and tape may cause skin trauma and should be avoided as much as possible.

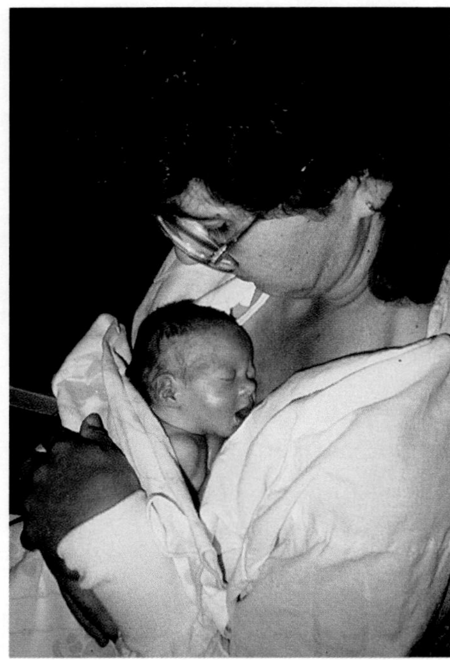

FIGURE 25–10 ♦ Kangaroo (skin-to-skin) care facilitates closeness and attachment between parents and their premature infant. *Source:* Courtesy of Kadlac Medical Center Kangaroo Care Study and Carol Thompson, RNC, MSN, NNP.

If infection (sepsis) occurs in the preterm newborn, the nurse may be the first to identify its subtle clinical signs. The nurse informs the clinician of the findings immediately and implements the treatment plan per clinician orders in the presence of infection. (For specific nursing care required for the newborn with an infection, see Chapter 26.)

### *Promotion of Parent-Infant Attachment*

Nurses need to take measures to promote positive parental feelings toward the preterm newborn. They can give photographs of the baby to parents to take home or to the mother if she is in a different hospital or too ill to come to the nursery and visit. The infant's first name is placed on the incubator as soon as it is known to help the parents feel that their infant is a unique and special person. A weekly card with the baby's footprint, weight, and length is also provided to promote bonding. Parents are given the telephone number of the nursery or intensive care unit and the names of staff members so that they have access to information about their baby at any time of the day or night.

Early parental involvement in the care of and decisions about their baby provides the parents with more realistic expectations for the future. The unique combination of personality characteristics of the infant and of the parents influences the bonding and interactive process for the family. By observing each infant's patterns of behavior and responses, especially sleep-wake states, the nurse can teach parents optimal times for interacting with their infant. The parents and nurse can plan nursing care around the times when the infant is alert and best able to attend. In addition, the more knowledge parents have about the meaning of their infant's responses, behaviors, and cues for interaction, the better prepared they will be to meet their newborn's needs and form a positive attachment with their child. Parents need education to develop caregiving skills. Their daily participation (if possible) is encouraged, as are early and frequent visits. The nurse provides opportunities for parents to touch, hold, talk to, and care for the baby. Skin-to-skin (kangaroo care) helps parents feel close to their small infants (Figure 25–10♦). Kangaroo care has been shown to improve sleep periods and parents' perception of their caregiving ability (Moran et al., 1999).

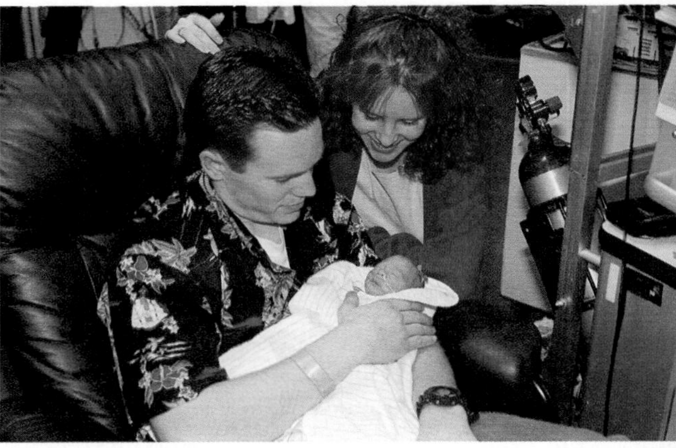

FIGURE 25–11 ♦ Family bonding occurs when parents have opportunities to spend time with their infant. *Source:* Courtesy of Carol Harrigan, RNC, MSN, NNP.

Some parents may progress easily to touching and cuddling their infant; others will not. Parents need to know that their feelings are normal and that the progression of acquaintanceship is slow. Rooming-in can provide another opportunity for the stable preterm infant and family to get acquainted; it offers both privacy and readily available help (Figure 25–11♦).

### *Promotion of Developmentally Supportive Care*

Prolonged separation and the neonatal intensive care unit (NICU) environment necessitate individualized baby sensory stimulation programs. The nurse plays a key role in determining the appropriate type and amount of visual, tactile, and auditory stimulation (Horns, 1998).

Some preterm infants are not developmentally able to deal with more than one sensory input at a time. The Assessment of Preterm Infant Behavior (APIB) scale (Als, Lester, Tronick, et al., 1982) identifies individual preterm newborn behaviors according to five areas of development. The preterm baby's behavioral reactions to stimulation are observed, and developmental interventions are then based on reducing detrimental environmental stimuli to the lowest possible level and providing appropriate opportunities for development (Als, 1998).

The NICU environment contains many detrimental stimuli that the nurse can help reduce. Noise levels can be lowered by replacing alarms with lights or silencing them quickly and keeping conversations away from the baby's bedside. Dimmer switches should be used to shield the baby's eyes from bright lights, and blankets may be placed over the top portion of the incubator. Dimming the lights may encourage infants to open their eyes and be more responsive to their parents. Nursing care should be planned to decrease the number of times the baby is disturbed. Signs (ie, "Quiet Please") can be placed near the bedside to allow the baby some periods of uninterrupted sleep (Blackburn, 1998). Some other suggested developmentally supportive interventions include the following:

- Facilitate handling by using containment measures when turning or moving the infant or doing procedures such as suctioning. Use the hands to hold the infant's arms and legs, flexed, close to the midline of the body. Containment measures help stabilize the infant's motor and physiologic subsystems during stressful activities.
- Touch the infant gently and avoid sudden postural changes.
- Promote self-consoling and soothing activities, such as placing blanket rolls or approved manufactured devices next to the infant's sides and against the feet to provide "nesting." Swaddle the infant with the extremities in a flexed position and ensure that the hands can reach the face for hand-to-mouth activities, which can be consoling (Figure 25–12♦).
- Simulate the kinesthetic advantages (decreased motor activity, improved sleep, fewer behavior state changes) of the intrauterine environment by using sheepskin or approved water beds.
- Provide opportunities for nonnutritive sucking with a pacifier. Nonnutritive sucking improves oxygen saturation; decreases body movements; improves sleep, especially after feedings; and increases weight gain (Engebretson & Wardell, 1997).
- Provide objects for the infant to grasp (eg, a piece of blanket, oxygen tubing, a finger) during caregiving. Grasping may comfort the baby.

Teaching the parents to read behavioral cues will help them move at their infant's own pace when providing stimulation. Parents are ideally equipped to meet the baby's need for stimulation. Stroking, rocking, cuddling, quiet singing, and talking to the baby can all be integral parts of the baby's care. Visual stimulation in the form of *en face* interaction with caregivers and mobiles is also important.

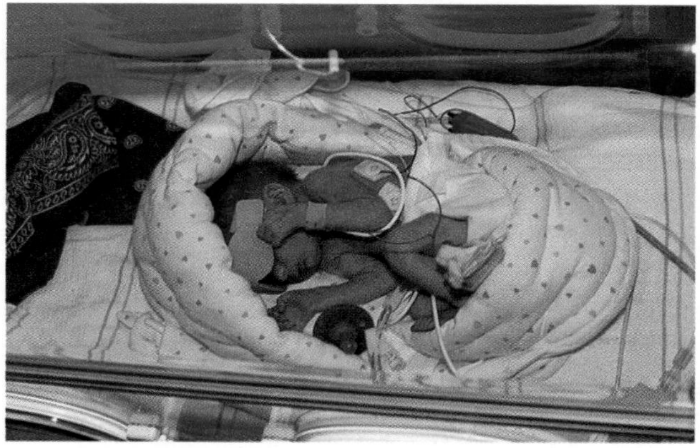

**FIGURE 25–12 ♦** Infant is "nested." Hand-to-mouth behavior facilitates self-consoling and soothing activities. *Source:* Courtesy of Theresa Kledzik, RN, Developmental Nurse, Memorial Hospital, Colorado.

### *Preparation for Home Care*

Parents are often anxious when their premature infant is transferred out of the NICU or is discharged home. Parents of preterm babies should receive the same postpartal teaching as any parent taking a new infant home. In preparing for discharge, the nurse encourages the parents to spend time caring directly for their baby. Direct caregiving familiarizes them with their baby's behavior patterns and helps them establish realistic expectations about the infant. Some NICUs have a special room near the nursery where parents can spend the night with their baby prior to discharge.

Discharge instruction includes breast- and bottle-feeding techniques, formula preparation, and vitamin administration. If the mother wishes to breastfeed, the nurse teaches her to pump her breasts to keep the milk flowing and provide milk even before discharge. The nurse gives information on bathing, diapering, hygiene, and normal elimination patterns and prepares the parents to expect changes in the color of the baby's stool, number of bowel movements, and timing of elimination when the infant is switched from bottle- to breastfeeding. This information can prevent unnecessary concern by the parents. The nurse also discusses normal growth and development patterns, reflexes, and activity for preterm infants. In these discussions, the nurse should emphasize ways to promote bonding behaviors and deal with newborn crying. Care of the preterm infant with complications, preventing infections, recognizing signs of a sick baby, and the need for continued medical follow-up are other key issues.

Families with preterm infants usually do not need to be referred to community agencies, such as visiting nurse assistance. However, referral may be necessary if the infant has severe congenital abnormalities, feeding problems, or complications with infections or respiratory problems or if the parents seem unable to cope with an at-risk baby. Parents of preterm infants can benefit from meeting with others in a similar situation to share common experiences and concerns. Nurses can refer parents to support groups sponsored by the hospital or by others in the community and make connections for parents with early education intervention centers.

#### Evaluation

Expected outcomes of nursing care include the following:

- The preterm newborn is free of respiratory distress and establishes effective respiratory function.
- The preterm newborn gains weight and shows no signs of fatigue or aspiration during feedings.
- The parents are able to verbalize their anger and guilt feelings about the birth of a preterm baby and show attachment behavior such as frequent visits and growing confidence in their participatory care activities.

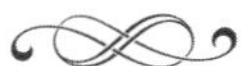

## Care of the Newborn of a Substance-Abusing Mother

An **infant of a substance-abusing mother (ISAM)** was formerly called an infant of an addicted mother. This terminology changed because abuse without addiction can provoke the same outcomes for the newborn. The newborn of an alcoholic or drug-addicted woman may also be alcohol or drug dependent. After birth, when an infant's connection with the maternal blood supply is severed, the newborn may suffer withdrawal. In addition, the drugs ingested by the mother may be teratogenic, resulting in congenital anomalies.

### Alcohol Dependence

The **fetal alcohol syndrome (FAS)** includes a series of malformations frequently found in infants exposed to alcohol in utero. It has been estimated that the complete FAS syndrome occurs in 2 live births per 1000 (Ostrea, Posecion, & Villanueva, 1999). FAS rates are higher among Native Americans, Alaska natives, African-Americans, and those of low socioeconomic status. **Fetal alcohol effects (FAE),** or **alcohol-related birth defects (ARBD),** are usually determined only by a positive maternal drinking history and cognitive difficulties (Gardner, 2000). The new diagnostic categories for FAS take into consideration the various clinical manifestations of FAS, the social and family environment, and, if available, the maternal alcohol history (Hess & Kenner, 1998).

Although it is known that ethanol freely crosses the placenta to the fetus, it is still not known whether the alcohol alone or the breakdown products of alcohol cause the damage. (Chapter 12 discusses alcohol abuse in pregnancy.) The effects of other substances often combined with alcohol, such as nicotine, diazepam (Valium), marijuana, and caffeine, as well as poor diet, enhance the likelihood of FAS.

#### Long-Term Complications for the Infant with FAS

The long-term prognosis for the FAS newborn is less than favorable. Many FAS infants are evaluated for organic and inorganic failure to thrive. These infants have a delay in oral feeding development but have a normal progression of oral motor function. Many FAS infants nurse poorly and have persistent vomiting until 6 to 7 months of age. They have difficulty adjusting to solid foods and show little spontaneous interest in food.

Central nervous system dysfunctions are the most common and serious problem associated with FAS. Hypotonicity and increased placidity are seen in these infants. They also have a decreased ability to block out repetitive stimuli. Children exhibiting FAS can be severely mentally retarded or have normal intelligence. Generally the more abnormal the facial features, the lower the IQ scores. Often there is little improvement in intelligence (as measured by IQ) despite positive environmental and educational factors (Hess & Kenner, 1998). These children show impulsivity, cognitive impairment, and speech and language abnormalities indicative of CNS involvement (Ostrea et al., 1999).

## Nursing Care Management

#### Nursing Assessment and Diagnosis

The nurse assesses the newborn for the following characteristics typical of FAS:

- ***Abnormal structural development and CNS dysfunction,*** including mental retardation, microcephaly, and hyperactivity.

- ***Growth deficiencies.*** The growth of infants with FAS, are often growth retarded with weight, length, and head circumference, being affected. These infants continue to show a persistent postnatal growth deficiency, with head circumference and linear growth most affected.
- ***Distinctive facial abnormalities.*** These include short palpebral fissures; epicanthal folds; broad nasal bridge; flattened midfacies; short, upturned, or beaklike nose; micrognathia (abnormally small lower jaw); hypoplastic maxilla; thin upper lip or vermilion border; and smooth philtrum (groove on upper lip) (Malanga & Kosofsky, 1999).
- ***Associated anomalies.*** Abnormalities affecting cardiac (primarily septal and valvular defects), ocular, renal, and skeletal (especially involving joints, such as congenital dislocated hips) systems are often noted.

An alcohol-exposed newborn in the first week of life may show symptoms that include sleeplessness, excessive arousal states, unconsolable crying, abnormal reflexes, hyperactivity with little ability to maintain alertness and attentiveness to environment, jitteriness, abdominal distension, and exaggerated mouthing behaviors such as hyperactive rooting and increased nonnutritive sucking. These symptoms commonly persist throughout the first month of life but may continue longer (Ostrea et al., 1999). Alcohol dependence in the infant is physiologic, not psychologic. Signs and symptoms of withdrawal often appear within 6 to 12 hours and at least within the first 3 days of life. Seizures after the neonatal period are rare.

### Nursing Plan and Implementation

#### *Hospital-Based Nursing Care*

The nurse's awareness of the signs and symptoms of FAEs is important in planning and delivering nursing care. Nursing care of the FAS newborn is aimed at avoiding heat loss, providing adequate nutrition, and reducing environmental stimuli. The FAS baby is most comfortable in a quiet, dimly lit environment. Because of their feeding problems, these infants require extra time and patience during feedings. It is important to provide consistency in the staff working with the baby and parents and to keep personnel and visitors to a minimum at any one time.

The nurse should inform the alcohol-dependent mother that breastfeeding is not contraindicated but that excessive alcohol consumption may intoxicate the newborn and inhibit the letdown reflex. The nurse should monitor the newborn's vital signs closely and observe for evidence of seizure activity and respiratory distress.

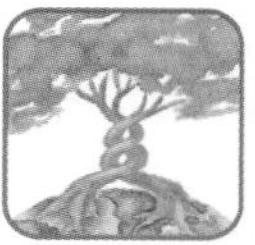

#### Community-Based Nursing Care

Infants affected by maternal alcohol abuse are also at risk psychologically. Restlessness, sleeplessness, agitation, resistance to cuddling or holding, and frequent crying can be frustrating to parents because their efforts to relieve the distress are unrewarded. Feeding difficulties can also result in frustrations for the caregiver and digestive upsets for the infant. Frustration may cause the parents to punish the baby or result in the unconscious desire to stay away from the infant. Either outcome may create an unstable family environment and result in failure to thrive.

The nurse should focus on providing support for the parents and reinforcing positive parenting activity. Prior to discharge, parents should be given opportunities to provide baby care so that they can feel confident in their interpretations of their baby's cues and ability to meet the baby's needs. Referring the family to social services and visiting nurse or public health nurse associations is essential for the well-being of the infant. Follow-up care and teaching can strengthen the parents' skill and coping abilities and help them create a stable, healthy environment for their family. The infant with FAS or ARBD should be involved in intervention programs that monitor the child's developmental progress, health, and home environment.

### Evaluation

Expected outcomes of nursing care include the following:

- The FAS newborn is able to tolerate feedings and gain weight.
- The FAS infant's hyperirritability or seizures are controlled, and the baby has suffered no physical injuries.
- The parents are able to identify the special needs of their newborn and accept outside assistance as needed.

## Drug Dependency

Drugs of abuse by the pregnant woman can include the following substances, used singularly or in combination: tobacco, cocaine, phencyclidine (PCP), methamphetamines, inhalants, marijuana, heroin, and methadone.

Drug-dependent infants are predisposed to a number of problems. Since almost all drugs cross the placenta and enter the fetal circulation, the fetus can develop problems in utero or soon after birth.

The greatest risks to the fetus of the drug-abusing mother are as follows:

- *Intrauterine asphyxia.* Asphyxia is often a direct result of fetal withdrawal secondary to maternal withdrawal. Fetal withdrawal is accompanied by hyperactivity, with increased oxygen consumption. Insufficiency of oxygen can lead to fetal asphyxia. Moreover, women addicted to narcotics tend to have a higher incidence of PIH, abruptio placentae, and placenta previa, resulting in placental insufficiency and fetal asphyxia.
- *Intrauterine infection.* Sexually transmitted infection, HIV infection, and hepatitis are often connected with the pregnant addict's lifestyle. Such infections can involve the fetus.
- *Alterations in birth weight.* These alterations may depend on the type of drug the mother uses. Women using predominantly heroin have infants of lower birth weight who are SGA. Women maintained on methadone have higher-birth-weight infants, some of whom are LGA.
- *Low Apgar scores.* These low scores may be related to the intrauterine asphyxia or the medication the woman received during labor. The use of a narcotic antagonist (nalorphine or naloxone) to reverse respiratory depression is contraindicated because it may precipitate acute withdrawal in the infant.

Patterns of abuse of alcohol, marijuana, and heroin in childbearing women have changed very little, but the incidence of cocaine (especially crack) use has risen dramatically (see Chapter 12 for more discussion of maternal substance abuse). Marijuana, alcohol, and nicotine are sometimes used in conjunction with cocaine.

## Common Complications of the Drug-Dependent Newborn

The newborn of a woman who abused drugs during her pregnancy is predisposed to the following problems:

- *Respiratory distress.* The heroin-addicted newborn frequently suffers respiratory stress, mainly meconium-aspiration pneumonia and transient tachypnea. Meconium aspiration is usually secondary to increased oxygen consumption and activity experienced by the fetus during intrauterine withdrawal. Transient tachypnea may develop secondary to the inhibitory effects of narcotics on the reflex responsible for clearing the lungs. Respiratory distress syndrome, however, occurs less often in heroin-addicted newborns, even in those who are premature, because they have tissue-oxygen-unloading capabilities comparable to those of a 6-week-old term infant. In addition, heroin stimulates production of glucocorticoids via the anterior pituitary gland.
- *Jaundice.* Newborns of methadone-addicted women may develop jaundice due to prematurity. By contrast, infants of mothers addicted to heroin or cocaine have a lower incidence of hyperbilirubinemia because these substances contribute to early maturity of the liver.
- *Congenital anomalies and growth retardation.* The incidence of anomalies of the genitourinary and cardiovascular systems is slightly increased in infants of heroin- and cocaine-addicted mothers. Infants of cocaine-addicted mothers exhibit congenital malformations involving bony skull defects, such as microencephaly, and symmetric intrauterine growth retardation, cardiac defects, and genitourinary defects. Congenital anomalies, however, are rare (Bauer, 1999).
- *Behavioral abnormalities.* Babies exposed to cocaine have poor state organization. They exhibit decreased interactive behaviors when tested with the Brazelton Neonatal Behavioral Assessment Scale (Bauer, 1999). These infants also have difficulty moving through the various sleep and awake states and have problems attending to and actively engaging in auditory and visual stimuli.
- *Withdrawal.* The most significant postnatal problem of the drug-exposed newborn is opiate withdrawal (usually from heroin or methadone). The onset of the withdrawal manifestations often occurs after discharge, especially with short birthing unit stays. See the section "Nursing Assessment and Diagnosis" for a discussion of withdrawal symptoms.

## Long-Term Effects

During the first 2 years of life, many cocaine-exposed infants demonstrate susceptibility to behavior lability and the inability to express strong feelings such as pleasure, anger, or distress, or even a strong reaction to being separated from their parents. Cocaine-exposed infants are at higher risk for motor development problems, delays in expressive language skills, and feeding difficulties because of swallowing problems (Eyler & Behnke, 1999).

Infants of drug-addicted mothers often demonstrate a higher incidence of gastrointestinal and respiratory illnesses. These illnesses can be related not to drug exposure but to the mother's lack of education regarding proper infant care, feeding, and hygiene.

Another important long-term complication is the high rate (15 to 20 per 1000 births) of SIDS in heroin- or methadone-exposed infants in comparison to those in the general population. After birth the infant born to a drug-dependent mother may also be subject to neglect, abuse, or both (Ostrea et al., 1999).

### Clinical Therapy

For optimal fetal and neonatal outcome, the opiate-addicted woman should receive complete prenatal care as early as possible (Chapter 12) and pharmacologic management of neonatal withdrawal. She should be started on a methadone program, with the aim being to prevent heroin use (Buchi, 1998). The maintenance dose of methadone should be sufficient to ensure this goal (Kandall, Doberczak, Jantunen, et al., 1999). It is not recommended that the woman be withdrawn completely from narcotics while pregnant because it induces fetal withdrawal with poor newborn outcomes.

Newborn treatment may include management of newborn complications; serologic tests for syphilis, HIV, and hepatitis B; urine or hair drug screen and/or meconium analysis; and social service referral (Smeriglio & Wilcox, 1999). Drugs used to control withdrawal symptoms vary and may be regionally based. They include phenobarbital, paregoric, oral morphine sulfate solution, Donnatal® elixir, and simethicone (Mylicon) drops. Nutritional support is important in light of the increase in energy expenditure that withdrawal may entail.

# Nursing Care Management

## Nursing Assessment and Diagnosis

Early identification of the newborn needing medical or pharmacologic interventions because of maternal substance abuse decreases the incidence of neonatal mortality and morbidity. During the newborn period, nursing assessment focuses on the following:

- Discovering the mother's last drug intake and dosage level. This is accomplished through the perinatal history and laboratory tests. Women may be reluctant to disclose this information; therefore, a nonjudgmental interview technique is essential (Smeriglio & Wilcox, 1999).
- Assessing for congenital malformations and the complications related to intrauterine withdrawal such as SGA, intrauterine asphyxia, meconium aspiration, and prematurity.
- Identifying the signs and symptoms of newborn withdrawal or neonatal abstinence syndrome.

Signs and symptoms of newborn withdrawal can be classified in five groups:

1. Central nervous system signs
    - Hyperactivity
    - Hyperirritability (persistent shrill cry)
    - Increased muscle tone
    - Exaggerated reflexes
    - Tremors and myoclonic jerks
    - Sneezing, hiccups, yawning
    - Short, unquiet sleep
    - Fever (accompanies the increased neuromuscular activities)
2. Respiratory signs
    - Tachypnea (> 60 breaths per minute when quiet)
    - Excessive secretions
3. Gastrointestinal signs
    - Disorganized, vigorous suck
    - Vomiting
    - Drooling
    - Sensitive gag reflex
    - Hyperphagia
    - Diarrhea
    - Abdominal cramping
    - Poor feeding (<15 mL on first day of life; takes longer than 30 minutes per feeding)
4. Vasomotor signs
    - Stuffy nose, yawning, sneezing
    - Flushing
    - Sweating
    - Sudden, circumoral pallor
5. Cutaneous signs
    - Excoriated buttocks, knees, elbows
    - Facial scratches
    - Pressure-point abrasions

Although many of the signs and symptoms of drug withdrawal are similar to those seen with hypoglycemia and hypocalcemia, glucose and calcium values are reported to be within normal limits for these infants.

The severity of withdrawal can be assessed by a scoring system based on clinical manifestations. The system evaluates the infant on potentially life-threatening signs such as vomiting, diarrhea, weight loss, irritability, tremors, and tachypnea (Table 25–1).

Nursing diagnoses that may apply to drug-dependent newborns include the following:

- ***Altered nutrition: less than body requirements*** related to vomiting and diarrhea, uncoordinated

| TABLE 25–1 | Assessment of the Clinical Severity of Neonatal Narcotic Withdrawal | | |
|---|---|---|---|
| *Symptom* | *Mild* | *Moderate* | *Severe* |
| Vomiting | Spitting up | Extensive vomiting for three successive feedings | Vomiting associated with imbalance of serum electrolytes |
| Diarrhea | Watery stools < four times per day | Watery stools five to six times per day for 3 days; no electrolyte imbalance | Diarrhea associated with imbalance of serum electrolytes |
| Weight loss | <10% of birth weight | 10%–15% of birth weight | >15% |
| Irritability | Minimal | Marked but relieved by cuddling or feeding | Unrelieved by cuddling or feeding |
| Tremors or twitching | Mild tremors when stimulated | Marked tremors or twitching when stimulated | Convulsions |
| Tachypnea | 60–80 breaths/minute | 80–100 breaths/minute | >100 breaths/minute; associated with respiratory alkalosis |

*Source:* Ostrea, E. M., Chavez, C. J., & Stryker, J. S. (1978). *The care of the drug dependent woman and her infant* (p. 33). Lansing, MI: Michigan Department of Public Health.

suck and swallow reflex, and hypertonia secondary to withdrawal

- ***Sleep pattern disturbance*** related to CNS excitation secondary to drug withdrawal
- ***Altered parenting*** related to hyperirritable behavior of the infant
- ***Ineffective family coping: disabling*** related to drug abuse, poverty, and lack of education

## Nursing Plan and Implementation

### *Hospital-Based Nursing Care*

Care of the drug-dependent newborn is based on reducing withdrawal symptoms and promoting adequate respiration, temperature, and nutrition. See Critical Pathway for Newborn of a Substance-Abusing Mother on pages 663–665 for specific nursing measures. General nursery care measures include the following:

- Temperature regulation
- Careful monitoring of pulse and respirations every 15 minutes until stable; stimulation if apnea occurs
- Small, frequent feedings, especially in the presence of vomiting, regurgitation, and diarrhea
- Intravenous therapy as needed
- Medications as ordered, such as phenobarbital and paregoric (but not methadone because of possible neonatal addiction to it); use of paregoric is controversial because it contains alcohol and camphor (AAP, Committee on Drugs, 1998)
- Positioning on the right side to avoid possible aspiration of vomitus or secretions
- Monitoring frequency of diarrhea and vomiting and weighing infant every 8 hours during withdrawal
- Observation for problems of SGA or LGA newborns
- Swaddling with hands near mouth to minimize injury and help achieve more organized behavioral state; gentle, vertical rocking can be successful in calming an infant who is out of control
- Placing newborn in quiet, dimly lit area of nursery

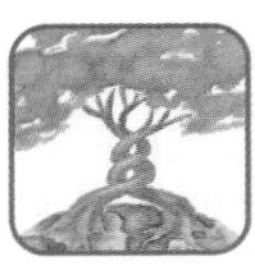

## Community-Based Nursing Care

Parents need assistance to prepare for what they can expect for the first few months at home. At the time of discharge, the mother should be instructed to anticipate mild jitteriness and irritability in the newborn, which may persist from 8 to 16 weeks, depending on the initial severity of the withdrawal. The nurse should help the mother learn feeding techniques, comforting measures, how to recognize newborn cues, and appropriate parenting responses (French, Pituch, Brandt, et al., 1998). Parents are to be counseled regarding available resources, such as support groups, and signs and symptoms that indicate the need for further care. Ongoing evaluation is necessary because of the potential for long-term problems. Follow-up on missed appointments can bring parents back into the health care system, thereby improving parent and infant outcomes and promoting a positive, interactive environment after birth.

## Evaluation

Expected outcomes of nursing care include the following:

- The newborn tolerates feedings, gains weight, and has a decreased number of stools.
- The parents learn ways to comfort their newborn.
- The parents are able to cope with their frustrations and begin to use outside resources as needed.

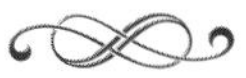

# CRITICAL PATHWAY: *For Newborn of a Substance-Abusing Mother*

| Category | Day of Birth—First 4 Hours | Remainder of Birth Day |
|---|---|---|
| **Referral** | Report from L&D, neonatal nurse practitioner<br>Check ID bands<br>High-risk peds/neonatology consults prn | Check ID bands q shift<br>As parents request, obtain circumcision permit after their discussion with MD |
| **Assessments** | Complete set of VS<br>Admission wt, length, HC<br>Assess skin color, skin integrity for rashes, breakdown<br>Gestational age assessment<br>Monitor activity (lethargy, character of cry, exaggerated startle responses)<br>Maternal hx of drugs consumed during each month of pregnancy<br>Obtain prior hx of addiction and treatment<br>Withdrawl s/s: hyperactivity, jitteriness, irritability, shrill high-pitched cry, vomiting, diarrhea, weak suck, stuffy nose, frequent sneezing, yawning, tachycardia, hypertension, apnea, seizure activity<br>Cocaine withdrawal pattern may be unpredictable or may be asymptomatic with only subtle behavioral state organization problems | Vital signs: T/P/R q4h and prn, BP prn<br>Newborn assessment q shift<br>Assess for hypothermia<br>Assess mother-baby interaction |
| **Teaching/ psychosocial** | (See Newborn Critical Pathway, pages 73 to 74)<br>Admission activities performed at mother's bedside if possible; orient parents to NSY, handwashing; assess teaching needs and readiness for learning<br>Evaluate additional psychosocial needs (provide time for verbalizing concerns, determine parental understanding of substance abuse)<br>Provide information including:<br>• s/s of baby's withdrawal, current condition, and rationale for treatment<br>• Newborn capabilities and developmental behaviors, cues<br>• Newborn's need for appropriate stimulation as well as rest, depending on cues<br>• Physical care needs (feeding, bathing, clothing, holding)<br>• Safety-bulb syringe, choking, positioning | Reinforce previous teaching<br>Discuss/teach infant security, identification<br>Discuss/teach temperature maintenance with clothing/blankets<br>Teach parents/guardian feeding methods, burping, diapering, and elimination norms<br>Teach parents calming techniques, s/s of stress and infant cues to stress |
| **Nursing care management and reports** | • Serum electrolytes to detect losses from vomiting/diarrhea<br>• Blood type, Rh, Coombs' on cord blood when applicable<br>• Chemstrip prn; BP prn<br>• Baer hearing test<br>• Maintain standard precautions<br>• Bathe ASAP if foul-smelling amniotic fluid/cord care per policy<br>• Hep B form reviewed and/or signed by parent; administer if ordered after bath<br>• Peripheral hematocrit per protocol<br>• Toxicology screen to identify drugs and drug levels in infant<br>• CBC and blood cultures to detect sepsis<br>• Intravenous access for meds, hydration, nutritional support | • Check for Baer hearing test results<br>• Femoral pulse or BP all four extremities if early DC<br>• Vital signs: q4h, T/P/R<br>• Daily wt<br>• Assess color q shift and prn<br>• Cord care per policy q diaper change<br>• Monitor for s/s of substance withdrawal, seizure activity; notify NP/MD prn, offer supportive care<br>• Maintain intravenous access prn |
| **Activity and comfort** | • Adjust and monitor radiant warmer to maintain skin temp until stable<br>• Provide calming techniques:<br>Swaddle infant tightly in side-lying or prone position with blanket roll to back, nest<br>Provide quiet, dim environment for rest<br>Hold, rock, and cuddle infant. Use touching, petting, smiling, talking. Use infant snuggly for closeness, carrying infant. Provide pacifier or swaddle to allow infant hand-to-mouth movement | Leave in radiant warmer until stable, then swaddle in open crib<br>Continue calming/soothing techniques prn<br>Cluster care, provide care on infant's schedule<br>Avoid overstimulation |

ASAP, as soon as possible; DC, discharge; HC, head circumference; hx, history; ID, identification; L&D, Labor and delivery; NTE, neutral thermal environment; NSY, nursery; OU, both eyes; s/s, signs and symptoms; vag, vaginal; VS, vital signs; WIC, Women, Infants and Children program; WNL, within normal limits; wt, weight.

| Category | Day of Birth—First 4 Hours | Remainder of Birth Day |
|---|---|---|
| **Nutrition** | Initiate bottle-feeding<br>Initiate breastfeeding as soon as mother and baby conditions allow lavage and gavage prn<br>Supplement breast only when medically indicated or ordered by MD per protocol<br>Assess for increased nutritional needs because of gestational age, weight, uncoordinated suck and swallow, vomiting, diarrhea, and regurgitation | Continue feeding schedule<br>Encourage frequent feedings at least q3–4h during day<br>Feed on demand breast or bottle<br>Consider breast milk evaluation to r/o active or residual drug presence |
| **Elimination** | Note first void and stool color<br>Urine specific gravity to detect dehydration | Monitor stools for amount, type, consistency, and pattern changes<br>Monitor all voids q shift |
| **Medication** | Administer medications for withdrawal as ordered, such as paregoric, chlorpromazine, phenobarbital, Donnatal® elixir, observe for effectiveness and side effects<br>AquaMEPHYTON IM, dosage according to infant wt and protocol after bath<br>Ilotycin ophth ointment OU—after bath | Continue medications as ordered and necessary to alleviate s/s substance withdrawal, to allow newborn rest and ability to suck/maintain nutritional status |
| **Discharge planning/ home care** | Evaluate for social services, visiting nurses service, and DC planning needs<br>Plan DC with parent/guardian in 1–3 days | Present birth certificate instructions/worksheet<br>Car seat available for DC<br>Newborn photographs |
| **Family involvement** | Evaluate parent teaching<br>Access community resources prn, ie, Teen "Healthy Starts"<br>Encourage/support positive mothering/parenting behaviors with infant | Evaluate parent teaching<br>Assess parents' knowledge of newborn behavior and reflexes<br>Encourage family involvement in infant's care as soon as possible and as infant tolerates |
| **Date** | | |

| Category | Day 1 | Day 2/3 (if applicable) |
|---|---|---|
| **Referral** | Check ID bands when baby leaves nursery<br>Lactation consult prn | Check ID bands q shift<br>**Expected Outcomes**<br>Mother/baby ID bands correlate at time of DC<br>Consults completed prn |
| **Assessments** | Assess mother-baby interaction<br>Continue newborn assessments q shift<br>Assess thermoregulation/VS q shift and prn<br>Assess abdominal distention, gastric residuals<br>Assess altered sleep-wake cycle and rhythm at 24–48h | Assess mother-baby interaction<br>Assess abdominal distension, gastric residuals, wt gain, s/s drug withdrawal and complications<br>**Expected Outcomes**<br>Physical assessments, VS WNL; no complications of newborn of substance-abusing mother noted |
| **Teaching/ psychosocial** | (See Newborn Critical Pathway, pages 73 to 74)<br>Reinforce previous teaching<br>Parental teaching: bathing, cord care, skin/nail care, use of thermometer, activity, sleep patterns, calming activities, reflexes, s/s jaundice, growth/feeding patterns, special nutritional needs, report feeding intolerance, circumcision care<br>Evaluate mother/parent teaching; provide information about HIV s/s, group support and community resources for persons with substance abuse issues | Final discharge teaching (see Newborn Critical Pathway, pages 73 to 74): Review with parents/guardian infant safety, s/s illness, and when to call health care provider<br>**Expected Outcomes**<br>Mother verbalizes comprehension of instructions, demonstrates care capabilities |
| **Nursing care and management and reports** | Newborn assessment q shift<br>Daily wt<br>Circumcision care q diaper change<br>Femoral pulse or BP all four extremities before DC or first 48h<br>Unclamp cord clamp, cord care q diaper change<br>HSV culture per parental hx of HSV<br>Maintain NTE<br>Newborn screen<br>Continue to monitor for s/s of drug withdrawal, seizure activity<br>Administer meds for withdrawal s/s as ordered; monitor infant response, report to NP/MD prn | Newborn assessment and VS q shift<br>Daily wt<br>Cord care per policy<br>Note Baer hearing test results<br>Cord care, circumcision care q diaper change<br>**Expected Outcomes**<br>Physical assessments WNL; cord unclamped and dry without s/s infection; circ site unremarkable; gaining wt or stabilized to not >10% loss; labs WNL; without s/s of substance withdrawal or infection; infant not requiring medication for relief of s/s of drug withdrawal |

| Category | Day 1 | Day 2/3 (if applicable) |
|---|---|---|
| **Activity and comfort** | Swaddled in open crib<br>Incubator if temp instability; adjust incubator for infant size, gestation, layers of clothing to maintain NTE | Swaddle to allow movement of hands to face<br>**Expected Outcomes**<br>Maintains temp WNL swaddled in open crib |
| **Nutrition** | • Supplement oral or gavage feedings with intravenous intake per orders; evaluate necessity prn<br>• Give small, frequent feedings q3–4h breast milk or formula as ordered, increasing strength of feeding as tolerated and as ordered (may start with half-strength breast milk/formula)<br>• Feed calorically enhanced breast milk/formula as ordered; monitor infant's tolerance to feedings<br>• Check for gastric residuals before q feeding; adjust volume of feeding prn with high or increasing residuals; notify NP/MD of increasing residuals<br>• Increase feeding volume as tolerated and as hyperactivity decreases<br>• Supplement breast only when medically indicated and ordered by NP/MD<br>• Feed on demand, minimally q3–4h | Feed on demand, minimally q3–4h<br>Gavage feed prn, as ordered to maintain nutrition<br>Supplement breast only when medically indicated and ordered by NP/MD<br>Encourage frequent feedings during day<br>Monitor infant for s/s of active or residual presence of drugs with breast milk feedings versus normal satiation after feeding; consider toxicology screen of breast milk, fresh or frozen, prn<br>**Expected Outcomes**<br>Infant tolerates feedings, feeds on demand; breastfeeds without supplement, nipples without problems; regaining lost wt or wt stabilized |
| **Elimination** | Monitor stools for amount, consistency, pattern changes, occult blood, reducing substances<br>Monitor voids q8h | Continue monitoring of all voids and stools q shift, noting changes<br>**Expected Outcomes**<br>Voids qs; stools without difficulty qs with stool character WNL; diaper area without s/s breakdown |
| **Medication** | Hep B vaccine before DC<br>Administer meds for withdrawal or seizure activity prn as ordered; observe for s/s of effectiveness and side effects | **Expected Outcomes**<br>Infant has received ophth ointment OU and AquaMEPHYTON injection; received first Hep B vaccine if ordered and parental consent received; infant not requiring meds for s/s withdrawal or seizure activity |
| **Discharge planning/ home care** | Newborn photographs<br>Complete birth certificate packet<br>If vag birth, complete DC teaching<br>Access community referrals, support groups for mother/family prn (ie, drug rehab, developmental, occupational and physical therapy, WIC, financial resources, public health nursing for home visits) | If cesarean birth, complete DC teaching<br>Complete DC summary<br>(See Newborn Critical Pathway, pages 73 to 74)<br>**Expected Outcomes**<br>Infant DC home with mother; mother verbalizes follow-up appointment times, dates, referral sources |
| **Family involvement** | Bath, newborn care, and feeding class<br>Newborn channel as available<br>Assess mother-baby bonding/interaction<br>Incorporate significant other/siblings in infant care<br>Support positive parenting behaviors<br>Evaluate mother/parent teaching | Assess mother-baby interaction<br>Identify community referral needs and refer to community agencies<br>Evaluate mother/parent teaching<br>Encourage questions<br>**Expected Outcomes**<br>Mother/family demonstrates caring and family incorporation of infant |
| **Date** | | |

## Care of the Newborn at Risk for HIV/AIDS

An increasing number of newborns are being born infected with HIV or at risk for acquiring it in the newborn period or early infancy. Transmission during the perinatal and neonatal periods can occur across the placenta or through breast milk or contaminated blood. Maternal-to-newborn vertical transmission rates are about 25% to 30% in the United States; the majority of infants who are born to an infected mother ultimately remain uninfected (Freij & Sever, 1999). The risk of vertical transmission can be decreased by two-thirds in mothers taking zidovudine during gestation. (For discussion of maternal and fetal HIV/AIDS, see Chapter 12.)

Early identification of babies with or at risk for HIV/AIDS is essential during the newborn period but difficult. The currently available HIV serologic tests (enzyme-linked immunosorbent assay [ELISA] and Western blot test) cannot distinguish between maternal and infant antibodies; therefore, they are inappropriate for infants up to 15 months of age. It may take up to 15 months for infected infants to form their own antibodies to the HIV (Bellanti, Zeligs, & Pung, 1999). Testing by HIV DNA polymerase chain reaction (PCR) or viral culture should be performed at birth and again at 1 to 2 months of age (AAP, Committee on Pediatric AIDS, 2000). Umbilical cord blood should not be used for HIV testing. Opportunistic diseases such as gram-negative sepsis and problems associated with prematurity are the primary causes of mortality in HIV-infected babies. Some infants infected by maternal-fetal transmission suffer from severe immunodeficiency, with HIV progressing more rapidly during the first year of life. For infants who have two or more negative HIV antibody tests, the National Pediatric HIV Resource Center recommends a final HIV antibody test at 24 months of age for HIV-exposed infants whose previous testings have been negative. (AAP, Committee on Pediatric AIDS, 2000).

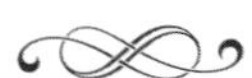

# Nursing Care Management

### Nursing Assessment and Diagnosis

Many newborns with HIV/AIDS are premature, SGA, or both and show evidence of failure to thrive during neonatal and infant periods. They can also show signs and symptoms of disease within days of birth. Signs that may be seen in the early infancy period include enlarged spleen and liver, swollen glands, recurrent respiratory infections, rhinorrhea, interstitial pneumonia (rarely seen in adults), recurrent GI (diarrhea and weight loss) and urinary system infections, persistent or recurrent oral candidiasis infections, and loss of developmental milestones (Freij & Sever, 1999). Some cranial and facial stigmas have been associated with HIV/AIDS contracted in utero. However, these findings do not establish a diagnosis of HIV infection at birth.

Nursing diagnoses that may apply to an infant exposed to HIV/AIDS include the following:

- ***Altered nutrition: less than body requirements*** related to formula intolerance and inadequate intake
- ***Risk for infection*** related to perinatal exposure and immunoregulation suppression secondary to HIV/AIDS
- ***Altered parenting*** related to diagnosis of HIV/AIDS and fear of future outcome

### Nursing Plan and Implementation

*Hospital-Based Nursing Care*

Nursing care of the newborn exposed to HIV/AIDS includes all the care normally given to any newborn in a nursery. In addition, the nurse must include care for a newborn suspected of having a blood-borne infection, as with hepatitis B. Standard precautions should be used when caring for the newborn immediately after birth and when obtaining blood samples via vein puncture or heel stick. (The blood of all newborns must be considered potentially infectious because the status of the infant's blood is often not known until after the infant is discharged. There is a window of time before seroconversion occurs when the baby is still considered infectious.) Nursing care involves providing for comfort; keeping the newborn well nourished and protected from opportunistic infections; and facilitating growth, development, and attachment. Most institutions recommend that their caregivers wear gloves during all diaper changes and examination of babies. Disposable gloves are worn when changing diapers or cleaning the diaper area, especially in the presence of diarrhea, because blood may be found in the stool (AAP, Committee on Pediatric AIDS and Committee on Infectious Diseases, 1999). Good skin care is essential to prevent skin rashes (see Table 25–2).

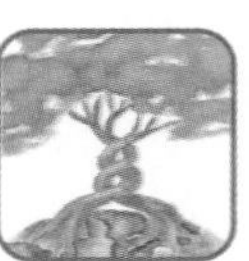

### Community-Based Nursing Care

Handwashing is crucial when caring for newborns with HIV/AIDS. Parents should be taught proper handwashing technique. Nutrition is essential because failure to thrive and weight loss are common. Small, frequent feedings and food supplementation are helpful. The nurse discusses with parents sanitary techniques for preparing formula. The nurse also informs the parents that the baby should not be put to bed with juice or formula because of potential bacteria growth. Parents need to be alert to the signs of feeding intolerance, such as increasing regurgitation, abdominal distention, and loose stools. The newborn is weighed three times a week.

The baby has his or her own skin care items, towels, and washcloths. Most clothing and linens can be washed with other household laundry. Linen that is visibly soiled with blood or body fluids should be kept and washed separately in hot, sudsy water with household bleach. Prompt diaper changing and perineal care can prevent or minimize diaper rash and promote comfort. Soiled diapers should be placed in plastic bags, sealed, and disposed of daily. The diaper-changing area in the home should be separate from food preparation and serving areas. Diaper-changing areas should be cleaned with a 1:10 dilution of household bleach after each diaper change. In addition, toys should be kept as clean as possible, not shared with other children, and checked for sharp edges to prevent scratches.

## Critical Thinking in Practice

Mrs. Jean Corrigan, a 23-year-old GIPI, positive for HIV, has just given birth to a 7 lb, 1 oz, baby girl. As she watches you assessing her daughter in the birthing room, she asks why you are wearing gloves and whether her daughter will have to be in isolation. What will your response be?

Answers can be found in Appendix I.

The nurse instructs the parents about signs of infection to be alert to and when to call their health care provider. The inability to feed without pain may indicate esophageal yeast infection and may require administration of Nystatin (Mycostatin) for the oral thrush. If

**TABLE 25–2 Issues for Caregivers of Infants at Risk for HIV/AIDS**

| Issue | Guideline |
|---|---|
| Resuscitation | For suctioning use a bulb syringe, mucus extractor, or meconium aspirator with wall suction on low setting. Use masks, goggles, and gloves. |
| Admission care | To remove blood from baby's skin, give warm water–mild soap bath using gloves as soon as possible after admission. |
| Handwashing | Thorough handwashing is indicated before and after caring for infant. Hands must be washed immediately if contaminated with blood or body fluids. Wash hands after removal of gloves. |
| Gloves | Gloves are indicated with touching blood or other high-risk fluids. Gloves should also be worn when handling newborns before and during their initial baths, cord care, eye prophylactics, and vitamin K administration. |
| Mask, goggle, and gown | Not routinely needed unless coming in contact with placenta or the blood and amniotic fluid on the skin of the newborn. |
| Needles and syringes | Used needles should not be recapped or bent; they should be disposed of in a puncture-resistant plastic container belonging specifically to that baby. After the newborn is discharged the container is discarded. |
| Specimens | Blood and other specimens should be double-bagged and/or sealed in an impervious container and labeled according to agency protocol. |
| Equipment and linen | Articles contaminated with blood or body fluids should be discarded or bagged according to isolation or institution protocol. |
| Body fluid spills | Blood and body fluids should be cleaned promptly with a solution of 5.25% sodium hypochlorite (household bleach) diluted 1:10 with water. Apply for at least 30 seconds then wipe after the minimum contact time. |
| Education and support | Provide education and psychologic support for family and staff. Caregivers who avoid contact with baby at risk or who overdress in unnecessary isolation garb subtly exacerbate an already difficult family situation. Information resources include the National AIDS Hotline (1-800-342-2437). |
| Exempted personnel | Immunologically compromised staff (pregnant women may be included in this group) and possibly infectious staff members should not care for these infants. |

*Sources:* Adapted from American Academy of Pediatrics, Committee on Pediatric AIDS and Committee on Infectious Diseases. (1999). Issues related to human immunodeficiency virus transmission in schools, child care, medical settings, the home, and community. *Pediatrics, 104*(2), 318–324; Mendez, H., & Jule, J. E. (1990). Care of the infant born exposed to HIV. *Obstetric and Gynecologic Clinics of North America, 17*(3), 637.

diarrhea occurs, the baby needs frequent perineal care, fluid replacements, and topical Mycostatin or Desitin ointment for the diaper rashes. Antidiarrheal medications are often ineffective. Taking rectal temperature should be avoided, because it may stimulate diarrhea. Irritability may be the first sign of fever. Fluids, antipyretics, and sponging with tepid water are of use in managing fever.

Parents and family members need to be reassured that there are no documented cases of people contracting HIV/AIDS from routine care of infected babies. Emotional support for family members is essential because of the stress and social isolation they may face. In addition, they may have concerns about their own health and their ability to meet the baby's long-term needs. Because of these stresses, parents may not bond with the baby or they may fail to provide the baby with enough sensory and tactile stimulation. The nurse encourages the parents to hold the baby during feedings because the infant benefits from frequent, gentle touch. Auditory stimulation may also be provided by using music or tapes of parents' voices. The nurse offers families information about support groups, available counseling, and information resources. Current therapeutic information about HIV is available to both health care providers and families through the AIDS Clinical Trials Information Service (1-800-TRIALS-A). The CDC recommends that HIV-infected women in developed countries not breastfeed because HIV has been found to be transmitted via breast milk. Therefore, if possible, a viable alternative feeding method should be used (AAP, Committee on Pediatric AIDS and Committee on Infectious Diseases, 1999).

All infants born to HIV-positive mothers require regular clinical, immunologic, and virologic monitoring. Preventive care for exposed infants is the same as for other infants and includes routine immunizations, with the exclusion of the live polio vaccine. At 1 month of age the baby's physical exam should include a developmental assessment and complete blood count, including differential blood count, CD4+ count, and platelet. Prophylaxis for *Pneumocystis carinii* pneumonia (PCP) for all infants born to HIV-infected women should be initiated at 4 to 6 weeks of age, regardless of the infant's CD4+ lymphocyte count. Pediatric HIV disease raises many health care issues for the family. The parents, depending on their health status, may or may not be able to care for their infant, and they must deal with many psychosocial and economic issues.

#### Evaluation

Expected outcomes of nursing care include the following:

- The parents are able to bond with their infant and have realistic expectations about the baby.
- Potential opportunistic infections are identified early and treated promptly.
- The parents verbalize their concerns about their baby's existing and potential health problems and long-term care needs and accept outside assistance as needed.

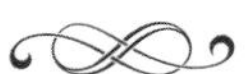

## Care of the Newborn with Congenital Anomalies

The birth of a baby with a congenital defect places both newborn and family at risk. Many congenital anomalies can be life threatening if not corrected within hours after birth; others are very visible and cause the families emotional distress. When one congenital anomaly is found, health care providers should look for other ones, particularly in body systems that develop at the same time during gestation. Table 25–3 identifies some common anomalies and their early management and nursing care in the neonatal period.

## Care of the Newborn with Congenital Heart Defect

The incidence of congenital heart defects is 4 to 5 per 1000 live births. They account for one-third of the deaths caused by congenital defects in the first year of life. Because accurate diagnosis and surgical treatment are now available, many such deaths can be prevented. Corrective cardiac surgery is being done at earlier ages; for example, more than half the children undergoing surgery are less than 1 year of age, and one-fourth are less than 1 month old. It is crucial for the nurse to have comprehensive knowledge of congenital heart disease to detect deviations from normal and initiate interventions.

### Overview of Congenital Heart Defects

Factors that might influence development of congenital heart malformation can be classified as environmental and genetic or chro vironmental factors are quite varied. For example, infections of the pregnant woman, such as rubella, cytomegalovirus, coxsackie B, and influenza, have been implicated. Steroids, alcohol, lithium, and some anticonvulsants have been shown to cause malformations of the heart. Seasonal spraying of pesticides has also been linked to an increase in congenital heart defects.

Text continues on page 671.

**TABLE 25–3 Congenital Anomalies: Identification and Care in Newborn Period**

| *Congenital Anomaly* | *Nursing Assessments* | *Nursing Goals and Interventions* |
|---|---|---|
| Congenital hydrocephalus | Enlarged head<br>Enlarged or full fontanelles<br>Split or widened sutures<br>"Setting sun" eyes<br>Head circumference >90% on growth chart | Assess presence of hydrocephalus; Measure and plot occipital-frontal baseline measurements; then measure head circumference once a day.<br>Check fontanelle for bulging and sutures for widening.<br>Assist with head ultrasound and transillumination.<br>Maintain skin integrity: Change position frequently.<br>Clean skin creases after feeding or vomiting.<br>Use sheepskin pillow under head.<br>Postoperatively, position head off operative site.<br>Watch for signs of infection. |
| Choanal atresia | Occlusion of posterior nares<br>Cyanosis and retractions at rest<br>Snorting respirations<br>Difficulty breathing during feeding<br>Obstruction by thick mucus | Assess patency of nares: Listen for breath sounds while holding baby's mouth closed and alternately compressing each nostril.<br>Assist with passing feeding tube to confirm diagnosis.<br>Maintain respiratory function: Assist with taping airway in mouth to prevent respiratory distress.<br>Position with head elevated to improve air exchange. |
| Cleft lip | Unilateral or bilateral visible defect<br>May involve external nares, nasal cartilage, nasal septum, and alveolar process<br>Flattening or depression of midfacial contour | Provide nutrition: Feed with special nipple.<br>Burp frequently (increased tendency to swallow air and reflex vomiting).<br>Clean cleft with sterile water (to prevent crusting on cleft prior to repair).<br>Support parental coping: Assist parents with grief over loss of idealized baby.<br>Encourage verbalization of their feelings about visible defect.<br>Provide role model in interacting with infant.<br>(Parents internalize others' responses to their newborn.)<br><br>(At left) Unilateral cleft lip with cleft abnormally involving both hard and soft palates. |
| Cleft palate | Fissure connecting oral and nasal cavity<br>May involve uvula and soft palate<br>May extend forward to nostril involving hard palate and maxillary alveolar ridge<br>Difficulty in sucking<br>Expulsion of formula through nose | Prevent aspiration/infection: Place prone or in side-lying position to facilitate drainage.<br>Suction nasopharyngeal cavity (to prevent aspiration or airway obstruction).<br>During newborn period feed in upright position with head and chest tilted slightly backward (to aid swallowing and discourage aspiration).<br>Provide nutrition: Feed with special nipple that fills cleft and allows sucking. Also decreases chance of aspiration through nasal cavity.<br>Clean mouth with water after feedings.<br>Burp after each ounce (tend to swallow large amounts of air).<br>Thicken formula to provide extra calories.<br>Plot weight gain patterns to assess adequacy of diet.<br>Provide parental support: Refer parents to community agencies and support groups.<br>Encourage verbalization of frustrations because feeding process is long and frustrating.<br>Praise all parental efforts.<br>Encourage parents to seek prompt treatment for upper respiratory infection (URI) and teach them ways to decrease URI. |

## TABLE 25–3 Congenital Anomalies: Identification and Care in Newborn Period *continued*

| *Congenital Anomaly* | *Nursing Assessments* | *Nursing Goals and Interventions* |
|---|---|---|
| Tracheoesophageal fistula (type 3) | History of maternal hydramnios<br>Excessive mucous secretions<br>Constant drooling<br>Abdominal distention beginning soon after birth<br>Periodic choking and cyanotic episodes<br>Immediate regurgitation of feeding<br>Clinical symptoms of aspiration pneumonia (tachypnea, retractions, rhonchi, decreased breath sounds, cyanotic spells)<br>Failure to pass nasogastric tube | Maintain respiratory status and prevent aspiration:<br>Withhold feeding until esophageal patency is determined.<br>Quickly assess patency before putting to breast in birth area.<br>Place on low intermittent suction to control saliva and mucus (to prevent aspiration pneumonia).<br>Place in warmed, humidified incubator (liquefies secretions, facilitating removal).<br>Elevate head of bed 20–40 degrees (to prevent reflux of gastric juices).<br>Keep quiet (crying causes air to pass through fistula and to distend intestines, causing respiratory embarrassment).<br>Maintain fluid and electrolyte balance. Give fluids to replace esophageal drainage and maintain hydration.<br>Provide parent education: Explain staged repair—provision of gastrostomy and ligation of fistula, then repair of atresia.<br>Keep parents informed; clarify and reinforce physician's explanations regarding malformation, surgical repair, pre- and postoperative care, and prognosis (knowledge is ego strengthening).<br>Involve parents in care of infant and in planning for future; facilitate touch and eye contact (to dispel feelings of inadequacy, increase self-esteem and self-worth, and promote incorporation of infant into family). |
| Diaphragmatic hernia | Difficulty initiating respirations<br>Gasping respirations with nasal flaring and chest retraction<br>Barrel chest and scaphoid abdomen<br>Asymmetric chest expansion<br>Breath sounds may be absent, usually on left side<br>Heart sounds displaced to right<br>Spasmodic attacks of cyanosis and difficulty in feeding<br>Bowel sounds may be heard in thoracic cavity | Nurse should never ventilate with bag and mask $O_2$ because the stomach will inflate, further compressing the lungs.<br>Maintain respiratory status: Immediately administer oxygen.<br>Initiate gastric decompression.<br>Place in high semi-Fowler's position (to use gravity to keep abdominal organs' pressure off diaphragm).<br>Turn to affected side to allow unaffected lung expansion.<br>Carry out interventions to alleviate respiratory and metabolic acidosis.<br>Assess for increased secretions around suction tube (denotes possible obstruction).<br>Aspirate and irrigate tube with air or sterile water. |

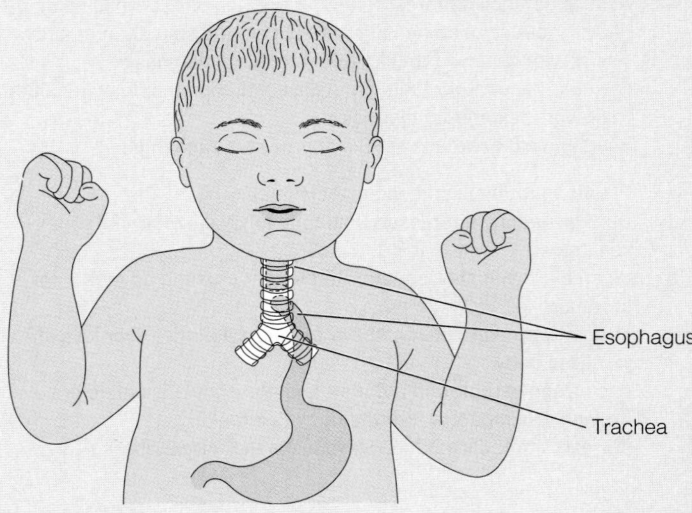


(At left) The most frequently seen type of congenital tracheoesophageal fistula and esophageal atresia.

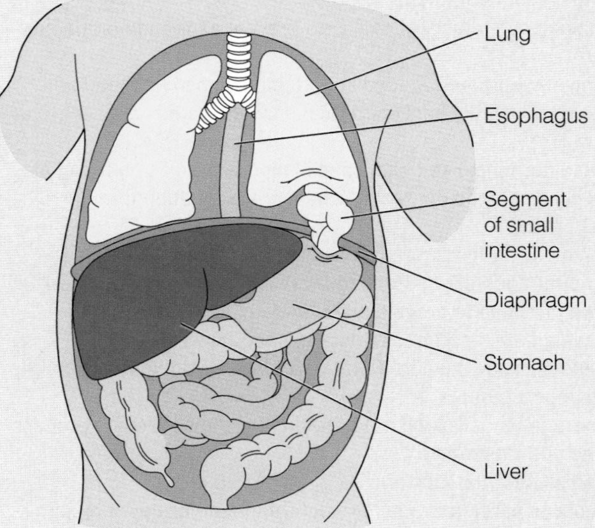


(At left) Diaphragmatic hernia. Note compression of the lung by the intestine on the affected side.

| TABLE 25–3 Congenital Anomalies: Identification and Care in Newborn Period *continued* | | |
|---|---|---|
| ***Congenital Anomaly*** | ***Nursing Assessments*** | ***Nursing Goals and Interventions*** |
| Myelomeningocele | Saclike cyst containing meninges, spinal cord, and nerve roots in thoracic and/or lumbar area<br>Myelomeningocele directly connects to subarachnoid space so hydrocephalus often associated<br>No response or varying response to sensation below level of sac<br>May have constant dribbling of urine<br>Incontinence or retention of stool<br>Anal opening may be flaccid<br>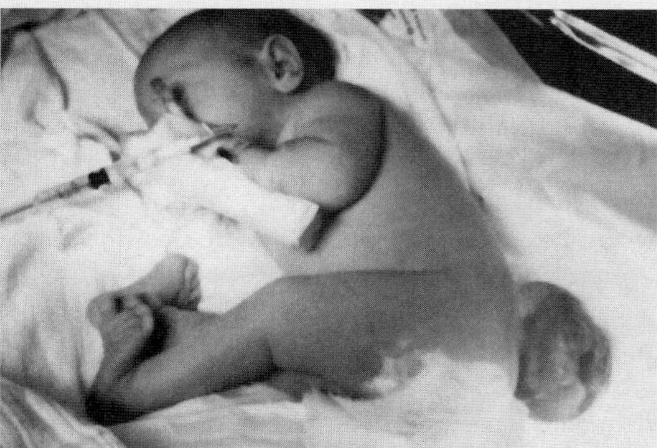 | Prevent trauma and infection.<br>Position on abdomen or on side and restrain (to prevent pressure and trauma to sac).<br>Meticulously clean buttocks and genitals after each voiding and defecation (to prevent contamination of sac and decrease possibility of infection).<br>May put protective covering over sac (to prevent rupture and drying).<br>Observe sac for oozing of fluid or pus.<br>Credé bladder (apply downward pressure on bladder with thumbs, moving urine toward the urethra) as ordered to prevent urinary stasis.<br>Assess amount of sensation and movement below defect.<br>Observe for complications.<br>Obtain occipital-frontal circumference baseline measurements; then measure head circumference once a day (to detect hydrocephalus).<br>Check fontanelle for bulging.<br>(At left) Newborn with lumbar myelomeningocele.<br>*Source:* Courtesy of Dr. Paul Winchester. |
| Omphalocele | Herniation of abdominal contents into base of umbilical cord<br>May have an enclosed transparent sac covering | Maintain hydration and temperature:<br>Provide $D_5LR$ and albumin for hypovolemia.<br>Place infant in sterile bag up to and covering defect.<br>Cover sac with moistened sterile gauze, and place plastic wrap over dressing (to prevent rupture of sac and infection).<br>Initiate gastric decompression by insertion of nasogastric tube attached to low suction (to prevent distension of lower bowel and impairment of blood flow).<br>Prevent infection and trauma to defect.<br>Position to prevent trauma to defect.<br>Administer broad-spectrum antibiotics. |
| Imperforate anus, congenital dislocated hip, and clubfoot | See discussion in Chapter 22, Anus and Extremities | Identify defect and initiate appropriate referral early. |

Clinicians are also beginning to see cardiac defects in infants of mothers with PKU who do not follow their diets. Chromosomal factors may include infants with Down syndrome and trisomy 13/15 and 16/18 infants with heart lesions. Increased incidence and risk of recurrence of specific defects occur in families.

It is customary to describe congenital malformations of the heart as either *acyanotic* (those that do not present with cyanosis) or *cyanotic* (those that do present with cyanosis). If an opening exists between the right and left sides of the heart, blood will normally flow from the area of greater pressure (left side) to the area of lesser pressure (right side). This process is known as left-to-right shunt and does not produce cyanosis because oxygenated blood is being pumped out to the systemic circulation. If pressure in the right side of the heart, due to obstruction of normal flow, exceeds that in the left side, unoxygenated blood will flow from the right side to the left side of the heart and out into the systemic circulation. This right-to-left shunt causes cyanosis. If the opening is large, there may be a bidirectional shunt with mixing of blood in both sides of the heart, which also produces cyanosis.

The most common cardiac defects seen in the first 6 days of life are left ventricular outflow obstructions (mitral stenosis, aortic stenosis or atresia), hypoplastic left heart, coarctation of the aorta, patent ductus arteriosus (PDA, the most common defect, especially in premature infants), transposition of the great vessels, tetralogy of Fallot, and large ventricular septal defect or atrial septal defects. Many cardiac defects may not manifest themselves until after discharge from the birthing unit.

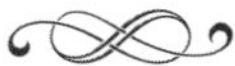

## Nursing Care Management

The primary goal of the neonatal nurse is to identify cardiac defects early and initiate referral to the physician. The three most common manifestations of cardiac defect are cyanosis, detectable heart murmur, and congestive heart failure signs (tachycardia, tachypnea, diaphoresis, hepatomegaly, cardiomegaly). Table 25–4 presents the clinical manifestations and medical-surgical management of these specific cardiac defects.

Initial repair of heart defects in the newborn period is becoming more commonplace. The staff of the NICUs are involved in both the preoperative and postoperative care of newborns. The benefits for the cardiac infant of being cared for by NICU staff include the staff's knowledge of neonatal anatomy and physiology, experience in supporting the family, and an awareness of the developmental needs of the newborn.

After the baby is stabilized, decisions are made about ongoing care. The parents need careful and complete explanations and the opportunity to take part in decision making. They also require ongoing emotional support. Families with any baby born with a congenital anomaly also need genetic counseling about future conception. Parents need opportunities to verbalize their concerns about their baby's health maintenance and understand the rationale for follow-up care.

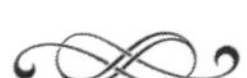

# Care of the Newborn with Inborn Errors of Metabolism

**Inborn errors of metabolism** are a group of hereditary disorders transmitted by mutant genes. Each causes an enzyme defect that blocks a metabolic pathway and leads to an accumulation of toxic metabolites. Most of the disorders are transmitted by an autosomal recessive gene, requiring two heterozygous parents to produce a homozygous infant with the disorder. Heterozygous parents carrying some inborn errors of metabolism disorders can be identified by special tests, and some inborn errors of metabolism can be detected in utero. Many inborn errors of metabolism are now detected neonatally through newborn screening programs. These programs principally test for disorders associated with mental retardation.

**Phenylketonuria (PKU)** is the most common of the amino acid disorders. Newborn screening has revealed its incidence to be about 1 in 11,000 live births in the United States; however, the incidence varies considerably among ethnic groups (Kenner & Dreyer, 2000). The highest incidence is noted in white populations from northern Europe and the United States. It is rarely observed in people of African, Chinese, or Japanese descent.

Phenylalanine is an essential amino acid the body uses for growth, and in the normal individual any excess is converted to tyrosine. The newborn with PKU lacks this converting ability, which results in an accumulation of phenylalanine in the blood. Phenylalanine produces two abnormal metabolites, phenylpyruvic acid and phenylacetic acid, which are eliminated in the urine, producing a musty odor. Excessive accumulation of phenylalanine and its abnormal metabolites in the brain tissue leads to progressive mental retardation.

*Maple syrup urine disease (MSUD)* is an inborn error of metabolism that, when untreated, is a rapidly progressing and often fatal disease caused by an enzymatic defect in the metabolism of the branched-chain amino acids leucine, isoleucine, and valine. Diagnosis of MSUD is made by analyzing blood levels of leucine, isoleucine, and valine. Confirmation of the diagnosis depends on blood assay for the enzyme oxidative decarboxylase.

*Galactosemia* is an inborn error of carbohydrate metabolism in which the body is unable to use the sugars galactose and lactose. Enzyme pathways in liver cells normally convert galactose and lactose to glucose. In galactosemia, one step in that conversion pathway is absent, either because of the lack of the enzyme galactose-1-phosphate uridyl transferase or because of the lack of the enzyme galactokinase. High levels of unusable galactose circulate in the blood, which causes cataracts, brain damage, and liver damage. There appear to be ethnic differences in age at onset of symptoms and in severity of course. Caucasians have more severe symptoms and earlier onset (3 to 14 days) than people of African descent (14 to 28 days).

Another disorder frequently included in mandatory newborn screening blood tests is *congenital hypothyroidism.* An inborn enzymatic defect, lack of maternal dietary iodine, or maternal ingestion of drugs that depress or destroy thyroid tissue can cause congenital hypothyroidism.

The incidence of metabolic errors is relatively low, but these disorders pose a threat to survival for affected infants and they frequently require lifelong treatment.

Text continues on page 675.

## TABLE 25–4 Cardiac Defects of the Early Newborn Period

| *Congenital Heart Defect* | *Clinical Findings* | *Medical-Surgical Management* |
|---|---|---|
| ACYANOTIC | | |
| **Patent ductus arteriosus (PDA)**<br>↑ in females, maternal rubella, RDS, <1500 g preterm newborns, high-altitude births<br>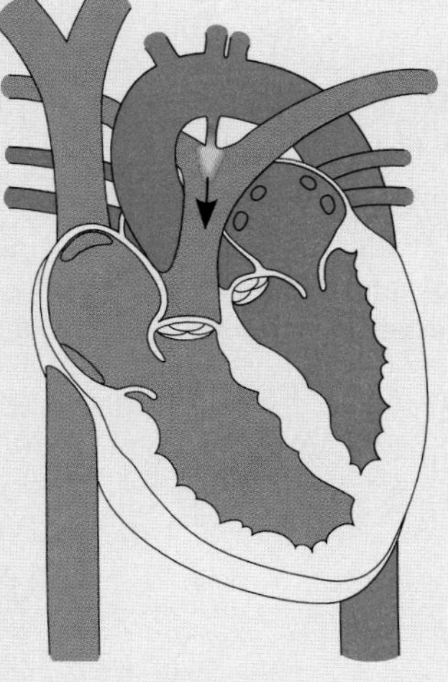 | Harsh grade 2–3 machinery murmur upper left sternal border (LSB) just beneath clavicle<br>↑ difference between systolic and diastolic pulse pressure<br>Can lead to right heart failure and pulmonary congestion<br>↑ left atrial (LA) and left ventricular (LV) enlargement, dilated ascending aorta<br>↑ pulmonary vascularity | Indomethacin—0.2 mg/kg orally (prostaglandin inhibitor)<br>Surgical ligation<br>Use of $O_2$ therapy and blood transfusion to improve tissue oxygenation and perfusion<br>Fluid restriction and diuretics |
| | The patent ductus arteriosus is a vascular connection that, during fetal life, short-circuits the pulmonary vascular bed and directs blood from the pulmonary artery to the aorta. Postnatally, blood shunts through the ductus from the aorta to the pulmonary artery. | |
| **Atrial septal defect (ASD)**<br>↑ in females and Down syndrome | Initially frequently asymptomatic<br>Systolic murmur second left intercostal space (LICS)<br>With large ASD, diastolic rumbling murmur lower left sternal (LLS) border<br>Failure to thrive, upper respiratory infection (URI), poor exercise tolerance | Surgical closure with patch or suture |
| **Ventricular septal defect (VSD)**<br>↑ in males | Initially asymptomatic until end of first month or large enough to cause pulmonary edema<br>Loud, blowing systolic murmur at third to fourth intercostal space (ICS) Inc. pulmonary blood flow<br>Right ventricular hypertrophy<br>Rapid respirations, growth failure, feeding difficulties<br>CHF at 6 weeks to 2 months of age | Follow medically—some spontaneously close<br>Use of lanoxin and diuretics in right congestive heart failure (CHF)<br>Surgical closure with Dacron patch |
| **Coarctation of aorta**<br>Can be preductal or postductal<br>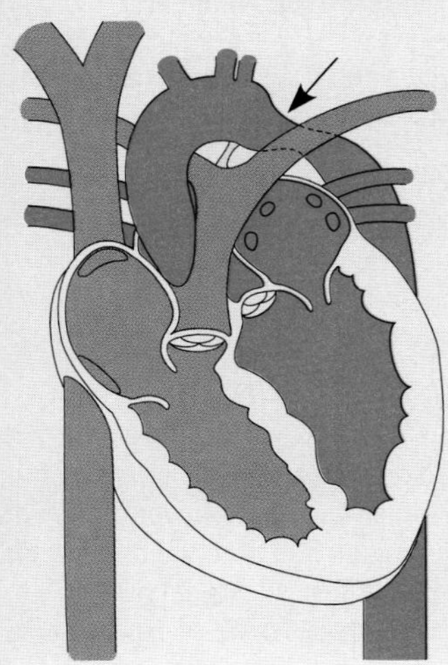 | Absent or diminished femoral pulses<br>Increased brachial pulses<br>Late systolic murmur left intrascapular area<br>Systolic BP in lower extremities<br>Enlarged left ventricle<br>Can present in CHF at 7–21 days of life | Surgical resection of narrowed portion of aorta<br>Prostaglandin $E_1$ to maintain peripheral perfusion<br>No afterload reducer drugs |
| | Coarctation of the aorta is characterized by a narrowed aortic lumen. The lesion produces an obstruction to the flow of blood through the aorta, causing an increased left ventricular pressure and workload. | |

## TABLE 25–4 Cardiac Defects of the Early Newborn Period *continued*

| *Congenital Heart Defect* | *Clinical Findings* | *Medical-Surgical Management* |
|---|---|---|
| **Hypoplastic left heart syndrome** | Normal at birth—cyanosis and shocklike congestive heart failure develop within a few hours to days<br>Soft systolic murmur just left of the sternum<br>Diminished pulses<br>Aortic and/or mitral atresia<br>Tiny, thick-walled left ventricle<br>Large, dilated, hypertrophied right ventricle<br>X-ray, cardiac enlargement and pulmonary venous congestion | $PGE_1$ until decision made<br>Transplant<br>Currently no effective corrective treatment |
| **CYANOTIC** | | |
| **Tetralogy of Fallot**<br>(Most common cyanotic heart defect)<br>Pulmonary stenosis<br>Ventricular septal defect (VSD)<br>Overriding aorta<br>Right ventricular hypertrophy | May be cyanotic at birth or within first few months of life<br>Harsh systolic murmur LSB<br>Crying or feeding increases cyanosis and respiratory distress<br>X-ray: boot-shaped appearance secondary to small pulmonary artery<br>Right ventricular enlargement | Prevention of dehydration, intercurrent infections<br>Alleviation of paroxysmal dyspneic attacks<br>Palliative surgery to increase blood flow to the lungs<br>Corrective surgery—resection of pulmonic stenosis, closure of VSD with Dacron patch |

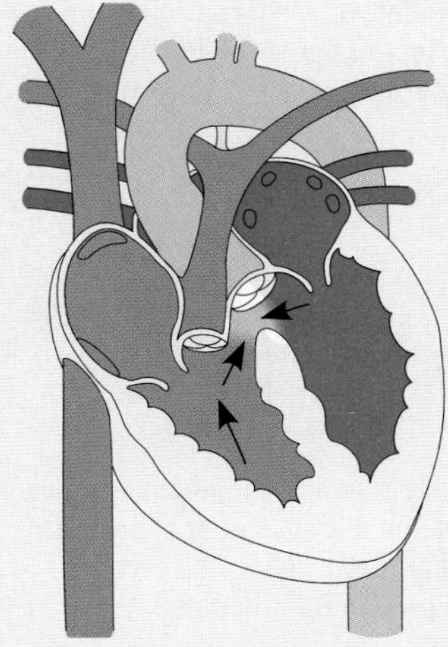

In tetralogy of Fallot, the severity of symptoms depends on the degree of pulmonary stenosis, the size of the ventricular septal defect, and the degree to which the aorta overrides the septal defect.

| *Congenital Heart Defect* | *Clinical Findings* | *Medical-Surgical Management* |
|---|---|---|
| **Transposition of great vessels (TGA)**<br>(↑ females, IDMs, LGAs) | Cyanosis at birth or within 3 days<br>Possible pulmonic stenosis murmur<br>Right ventricular hypertrophy<br>Polycythemia<br>"Egg on its side" x-ray | Prostaglandin E to vasodilate ductus to keep it open<br>Inotropic support<br>Initial surgery to create opening between right and left side of heart if none exists<br>Total surgical repair—usually the arterial switch procedure—done within first few days of life |

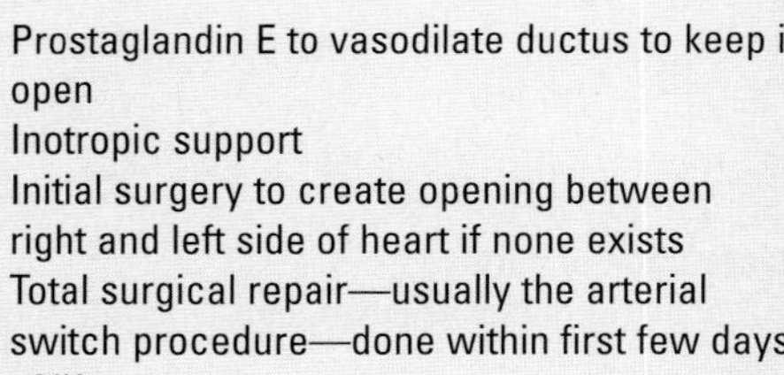

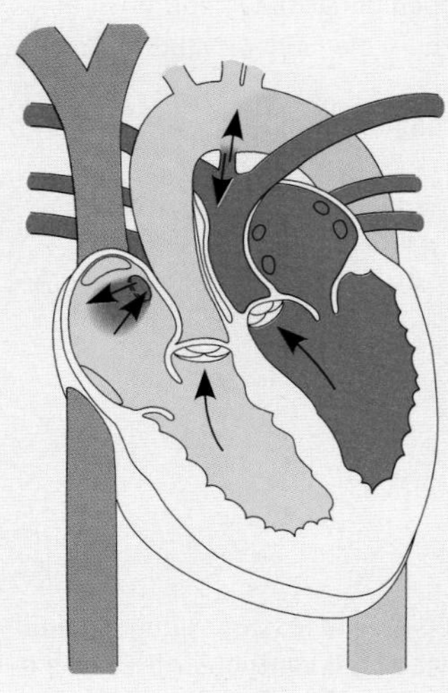

Complete transposition of great vessels is an embryonic defect caused by a straight division of the bulbar trunk without normal spiraling. As a result, the aorta originates from the right ventricle, and the pulmonary artery from the left ventricle. An abnormal communication between the two circulations must be present to sustain life.

## Clinical Therapy

All states require screening of newborns for PKU and congenital hypothyroidism (AAP, Newborn Screening Task Force, 2000). Mandatory newborn screening for other inborn errors of metabolism varies among states. Some states simultaneously test all newborns for galactosemia, MSUD, homocystinuria, biotinidase deficiency, and PKU. Identification via newborn screening and early clinical intervention for inborn errors of metabolism have become more difficult with the advent of early discharge of newborns. If the initial specimen is obtained before the newborn is 24 hours of age, then a second specimen should be obtained at 1 to 2 weeks of age (Kirby, 1999). Newborns in NICUs who required interhospital transfers and healthy newborns discharged early are at risk for nonscreening (Burton, 1999). The first filter paper test screens for PKU, homocystinuria, MSUD, galactosemia, and sickle-cell anemia. A second blood specimen is often required and tests only for PKU.

In several states newborn screening includes an enzyme assay for galactose-1-phosphate uridyl transferase; however, this test does not detect galactosemia if it is caused by a deficiency of the enzyme galactokinase.

# Nursing Care Management

The nurse assesses the newborn for signs of inborn errors of metabolism and carries out state-mandated newborn screening tests. Typically, a PKU baby is a normal-appearing newborn, most often with blond hair, blue eyes, and fair complexion. Decreased pigmentation may be related to the competition between phenylalanine and tyrosine for the available enzyme tyrosinase. Tyrosine is needed for the formation of melanin pigment and the hormones epinephrine and thyroxine. Without treatment, the infant fails to thrive and develops vomiting and eczematous rashes. By about 6 months of age, the infant exhibits behaviors indicative of mental retardation and other CNS involvement, including seizures and abnormal electroencephalogram (EEG) patterns.

Newborns with MSUD have feeding problems and neurologic signs (seizures, spasticity, opisthotonus) during the first week of life. Often the parents report a maple syrup odor of the urine; when ferric chloride is added to the urine, its color changes to gray-green (Burton, 1999).

Clinical manifestations of galactosemia include vomiting soon after ingestion of milk-based formula or breast milk, diarrhea, poor weight gain, jaundice, and mental retardation. The condition is frequently associated with *Escherichia coli* sepsis and cataracts in the neonatal period (Burton, 1999). Except for cataracts and mental retardation, those findings are reversible when galactose is excluded from the diet. Mental retardation can be prevented by early diagnosis and careful dietary management.

A large tongue, umbilical hernia, cool and mottled skin, low hairline, hypotonia, and large fontanelles are frequently associated with congenital hypothyroidism. Early symptoms include prolonged neonatal jaundice, poor feeding, constipation, low-pitched cry, poor weight gain, inactivity, and delayed motor development. In addition, premature infants of less than 30 weeks' gestation frequently have lower $T_4$ and thyroid-stimulating hormone (TSH) values than those of term infants. This difference may reflect the premature infant's inability to bind thyroid and a risk for hypothyroidism.

### PKU Screening

The Guthrie blood test for PKU, required for all newborns before discharge, uses a drop of blood collected from a heel stick and placed on filter paper. It should be done at least 24 hours after the initiation of feedings containing the usual amounts of breast milk or formula so phenylalanine metabolites can begin to build up in the PKU baby. High-risk newborns should receive a 60% milk intake, with no more than 40% of their total intake from nonprotein intravenous fluids. The PKU testing of high-risk newborns should be deferred for at least 48 hours after hyperalimentation is initiated. It is vital that the parents understand the need for the screening procedure, and a follow-up check is necessary to confirm that the test was done.

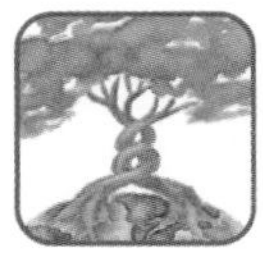

## Community-Based Nursing Care

Some states routinely request a repeat PKU test when an infant is 1 to 2 weeks of age because of early newborn discharge (Kirby, 1999). The nurse advises parents that once identified, an afflicted PKU infant can be treated by a special diet that limits ingestion of phenylalanine. Special formulas low in phenylalanine, such as Lofenalac®, Minafen, and Albumaid XP, are available. Special food lists are helpful for parents of a PKU child (Kirby, 1999). If treatment is begun before 1 month of age, CNS damage can be minimized. There is an increased risk of producing a child with mental retardation if the mother with PKU is not on a low-phenylalanine diet during pregnancy. It is recommended that the woman reinstate her low-phenylalanine diet before becoming pregnant (Kirby, 1999).

Newborns with MSUD must be given a formula that is low in the branched-chain amino acids leucine, isoleucine, and valine, which is continued indefinitely. Dietary treatment prior to 12 days of life has been reported to result in normal intelligence (AAP, Committee on Genetics, 1996).

A baby with galactosemia is placed on a galactose-free diet. Galactose-free formulas include Nutramigen® (a protein hydrolysate process formula), meat-based formulas, and soybean formulas. As the infant grows, parents must be educated to avoid giving their child milk and milk products and to read all labels carefully and avoid any foods containing dry milk products. Even with early treatment, children may have learning disabilities, speech problems, and ovarian failure (Burton, 1999).

Babies with hypothyroidism need frequent follow-up laboratory monitoring and adjustment of thyroid medication to accommodate growth and development of the child. With adequate treatment, children remain free of symptoms, but if the condition is left untreated, stunted growth and mental retardation occur.

Infants with homocystinuria are placed on a diet that is low in methionine but supplemented with cystine and pyridoxine (vitamin $B_6$). With early diagnosis and careful management, mental retardation may be prevented.

Parents of affected newborns should be referred to support groups. The nurse should also ensure that parents are informed about centers that can provide them with information about biochemical genetics and dietary management.

### Evaluation

Expected outcomes of nursing care include the following:

- The risk of inborn errors of metabolism is promptly identified, and early intervention is initiated.
- The parents verbalize their concerns about their baby's health problems, long-term care needs, and potential outcomes.
- The parents are aware of available community health resources and use them as indicated.

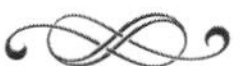

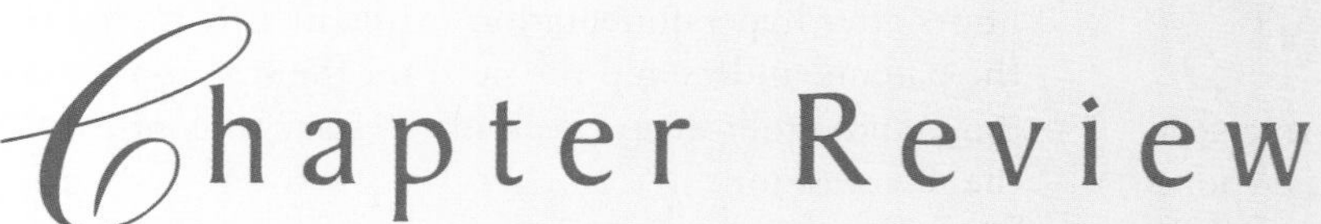

# Chapter Review

## CHAPTER HIGHLIGHTS

- Early identification of potential high-risk fetuses through assessment of prepregnant, prenatal, and intrapartal factors facilitates strategically timed nursing observations and interventions.
- High-risk newborns, whether premature, SGA, LGA, postterm, IDM, or ISAM, have many similar problems, although their problems are based on different physiologic processes.
- SGA newborns are at risk for perinatal asphyxia and resulting aspiration syndrome, hypothermia, hypoglycemia, hypocalcemia, polycythemia, congenital anomalies, and intrauterine infections. Long-term problems include continued growth and learning difficulties.
- LGA newborns are at risk for birth trauma as a result of CPD, hypoglycemia, polycythemia, and hyperviscosity.
- IDMs are at risk for hypoglycemia, hypocalcemia, hyperbilirubinemia, polycythemia, and respiratory distress due to delayed maturation of their lungs.
- Postterm newborns frequently encounter the following problems: CPD (shoulder dystocia) and birth traumas, hypoglycemia, polycythemia, meconium aspiration, cold stress, and possible seizure activity. Long-term complications may involve poor weight gain and low IQ scores.
- The common problems of the preterm newborn are a result of the baby's immature body

systems. Potential problems include RDS, patent ductus arteriosus, hypothermia and cold stress, feeding difficulties and NEC, marked insensible water loss and loss of buffering agents through the kidneys, infection, anemia of prematurity, apnea and intraventricular hemorrhage, retinopathy of prematurity, and behavioral state disorganization. Long-term needs and problems include bronchopulmonary dysplasia, speech defects, sensorineural hearing loss, and neurologic defects.

- Newborns of alcohol-dependent mothers are at risk for physical characteristic alterations and the long-term complications of feeding problems; CNS dysfunction, including low IQ, hyperactivity, and language abnormalities; and congenital anomalies.
- Newborns born to drug-dependent mothers experience drug withdrawal as well as respiratory distress, jaundice, congenital anomalies, and behavioral abnormalities. With early recognition and intervention, the potential long-term physiologic and emotional consequences of these difficulties can be avoided or at least minimized.
- Newborns exposed to HIV/AIDS require early recognition and treatment to lessen the severity of the physiologic and emotional consequences and to implement CDC guidelines.
- Cardiac defects are a significant cause of morbidity and mortality in the newborn period. Early identification and nursing and medical care of newborns with cardiac defects are essential to improve the outcome of these infants. Care is directed toward lessening the workload of the heart and decreasing oxygen and energy consumption.
- Inborn errors of metabolism such as galactosemia, PKU, and MSUD are often included in a newborn screening program designed to prevent mental retardation through dietary management and medication.
- The nursing care of the newborn with special problems involves the understanding of normal physiology, the pathophysiology of the disease process, clinical manifestations, and supportive or corrective therapies. Only with this theoretical background can the nurse make appropriate observations about responses to therapy and development of complications.
- The nurse facilitates interdisciplinary communication with the parents.
- Parents of at-risk newborns need support from nurses and health care providers to understand the special needs of their baby and feel confident in their ability to care for their children at home.

## CHAPTER REFERENCES


Als, H. (1998). Developmental care in the newborn intensive care unit. *Current Opinion in Pediatrics, 10,* 138–142.

Als, H., Lester, B. M., Tronick, E., & Brazelton, T. B. (1982). Assessment of preterm infant behavior (APIB). In B. M. Fitzgerald Lester & M. W. Yogman (Eds.), *Theory and research in behavioral pediatrics* (Vol. 1). New York: Plenum. pp. 35–82.

American Academy of Pediatrics, Committee on Drugs. (1998). Neonatal drug withdrawal. *Pediatrics, 101*(6), 1079–1088.

American Academy of Pediatrics, Committee on Genetics. (1996). Newborn screening fact sheets. *Pediatrics, 98*(3), 473–501.

American Academy of Pediatrics, Committee on Pediatric AIDS. (2000). Identification and care of HIV-exposed and HIV-infected infants, children, and adolescents in foster care. *Pediatrics, 102*(1), 149–153.

American Academy of Pediatrics, Committee on Pediatric AIDS and Committee on Infectious Diseases. (1999). Issues related to human immunodeficiency virus transmission in schools, child care, medical settings, the home, and community. *Pediatrics, 104*(2), 318–324.

American Academy of Pediatrics, Newborn Screening Task Force (2000). Newborn screening: A blueprint for the future. *Pediatrics, 106*(2), 389–427.

American Academy of Pediatrics & American College of Obstetricians and Gynecologists. (1997). *Guidelines for perinatal care* (4th ed.). Elk Grove Village, IL: Author

Anderson, M. S., & Hay, W. W. (1999). Intrauterine growth restriction and the small-for-gestational-age infant. In G. B. Avery, M. A. Fletcher, & M. G. MacDonald (Eds.), *Neonatology: Pathophysiology and management of the newborn* (5th ed.). Philadelphia: Lippincott Williams & Wilkins. Chap. 25 pp. 411–444.

Bauer, C. R. (1999). Perinatal effects of prenatal drug exposure. *Clinics in Perinatology,. 26*(1), 87–106.

Bellanti, J. A., Zeligs, B. J., & Pung, Y. (1999). Immunology of the fetus and newborn. In G. B. Avery, M. A. Fletcher, & M. G. MacDonald (Eds.), *Neonatology: Pathophysiology and management of the newborn* (5th ed.). Philadelphia: Lippincott Williams & Wilkins. Chap. 46 pp. 1093–1122.

Blackburn, S. (1998). Environmental impact of the NICU on developmental outcomes. *Journal of Pediatric Nursing, 13*(5), 279–289.

Buchi, K. F. (1998). The drug-exposed infant in the well-baby nursery. *Clinics in Perinatology, 25*(2), 335–350.

Burton, B. K. (1999). Inherited metabolic disorders. In G. B. Avery, M. A. Fletcher, & M. G. MacDonald (Eds.), *Neonatology: Pathophysiology and management of the newborn* (5th ed.). Philadelphia: Lippincott Williams & Wilkins. Chap. 39 pp. 821–838.

Engebretson, J. C., & Wardell, D. W. (1997). Developing of a pacifier for low-birth-weight infants' nonnutritive sucking. *Journal of Obstetric, Gynecologic, and Neonatal Nursing, 26*(6), 660–664.

Eyler, F. D., & Behnke, M. (1999). Early development of infants exposed to drugs prenatally. *Clinics in Perinatology, 26*(1), 107–150.

Freij, B. J., & Sever, J. L. (1999). Chronic infections. In G. B. Avery, M. A. Fletcher, & M. G. MacDonald (Eds.), *Neonatology: Pathophysiology and management of the newborn* (5th ed.). Philadelphia: Lippincott Williams & Wilkins. Chap. 48. pp. 1123–1188.

French, E. D., Pituch, M., Brandt, J., & Pohorecki, S. (1998). Improving interactions between substance-abusing mothers and their substance-exposed newborns. *Journal of Obstetric, Gynecologic, and Neonatal Nursing, 27*(3), 262–269.

Gardner, J. (2000). Fetal alcohol syndrome. *American Journal of Maternal Child Nursing, 25*(5), 252–257.

Hess, D. J., & Kenner, C. (1998). Families caring for children with fetal alcohol syndrome: The nurse's role in early identification and intervention. *Holistic Nursing Practice, 12*(3), 47–54.

Horns, K. M. (1998). Being-in-tune caregiving. *Journal of Perinatal Neonatal Nursing, 12*(3), 38–49.

Kandall, S. R., Doberczak, T. M., Jantunen, M., & Stein, J. (1999). The methadone-maintained pregnancy. *Clinics in Perinatology, 26*(1), 173–183.

Kenner, C., & Dreyer, L. A. (2000). Prenatal and neonatal testing and screening: A double-edged sword. *Nursing Clinics of North America, 35*(3), 627–641.

Kirby, R. B. (1999). Maternal phenylketonuria: A new cause for concern. *Journal of Obstetric, Gynecologic, and Neonatal Nursing, 28*(30), 227–234.

Langer, O. (2000). Fetal macrosomia: Etiologic factors. *Clinical Obstetrics and Gynecology, 43*(2), 283–297.

Malanga, C. J., & Kosofsky, B. E. (1999). Mechanisms of action of drugs of abuse on the developing fetal brain. *Clinics in Perinatology, 26*(1), 17–37.

Merenstein, G. B., & Gardner, S. L. (1998). *Handbook of neonatal intensive care* (4th ed.). St. Louis: Mosby.

Moran, M., Radzyminski, S. G., Higgins, K. R., Dowling, D. A., Miller, M. J., & Cranston Anderson, G. (1999). Maternal kangaroo (skin-to-skin) care in the NICU beginning 4 hours postbirth. *Journal of Maternal Child Nursing, 24*(2), 74–79.

Neonatal thermoregulation. (1997). In *NANN guidelines for practice.* Petaluma, CA: National Association of Neonatal Nurses. pp. 1–15

Newell, S. J. (2000). Enteral feeding of the micropremie. *Clinics in Perinatology, 27*(1), 221–234.

Ostrea, E. M., Posecion, E. C., & Villanueva, M. E. T. (1999). The infant of the drug-dependent mother. In G. B. Avery, M. A. Fletcher, & M. G. MacDonald (Eds.), *Neonatology: Pathophysiology and management of the newborn* (5th ed.). Philadelphia: Lippincott Williams & Wilkins. Chap 56. pp. 1407–1446.

Pressler, J. L., & Hepworth, J. T. (1997). Behavior of macrosomic and appropriate-for-gestational-age newborns. *Journal of Obstetric, Gynecologic, and Neonatal Nursing, 26*(2), 198–205.

Resnik, R., & Calder, A. (1999). Post-term pregnancy. In R. K. Creasy & R. Resnik (Eds.), *Maternal-fetal medicine* (4th ed.). Philadelphia: Saunders. Chap 33. pp. 532–540.

Siegfried, E. C. (1998). Neonatal skin and skin care. *Dermatologic Clinics, 16*(3), 437–446.

Smeriglio, V. L., & Wilcox, H. C. (1999). Prenatal drug exposure and child outcome: Past, present, future. *Clinics in Perinatology, 26*(1), 1–16.

Sohl, B., & Moore, T. R. (1998). Abnormalities of fetal growth. In H. W. Taeusch & R. A. Ballard (Eds.), *Avery's diseases of the newborn* (7th ed.). Philadelphia: Saunders. Chap 9. pp. 90–102.

Uvena-Celebrezze, J., & Catalano, P. M. (2000). The infant of the woman with gestational diabetes mellitus. *Clinical Obstetrics and Gynecology, 43*(1), 127–139.


## CONTEMPORARY MATERNAL-NEWBORN NURSING ON-LINE

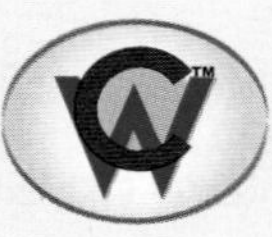

Additional interactive resources, including animations and video, for this chapter can be found on the Companion Website at http://www.prenhall.com/ladewig. Click on Chapter 25 and "Begin" to select the activities for this chapter.

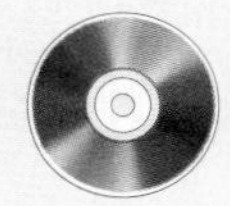

For NCLEX review questions and an audio glossary, access the accompanying CD-ROM in this book.

Chapter 26

# The Newborn at Risk: Birth-Related Stressors

*I work primarily in what our system calls the "high-risk transition nursery." When I am called to attend a delivery it is usually because the labor and delivery team has detected a potential problem and they think the newborn will need some additional care at birth. The Neonatal Nurse Practitioner (NNP) and I work together to anticipate and respond to whatever is needed at the time. Each situation is unique and deserves our complete attention. But it is also essential that the parents be kept informed and comforted as much as possible. With each infant that I care for, I ask myself "if this were my baby, how would I be feeling right now, and what would I want to know?"*

—High-Risk Nursery Nurse

## OBJECTIVES

- Discuss how to identify infants in need of resuscitation and the appropriate method of resuscitation based on the labor record and observable physiologic indicators.
- Based on clinical manifestations, differentiate between the various types of respiratory distress (respiratory distress syndrome, transient tachypnea of the newborn, and meconium aspiration syndrome) in the newborn and their related nursing care.
- Discuss selected metabolic abnormalities (including cold stress and hypoglycemia), their effects on the newborn, and the nursing implications.
- Differentiate between physiologic and pathologic jaundice based on onset, cause, possible sequelae, and specific management.
- Explain how Rh incompatibility or ABO incompatibility can lead to the development of hyperbilirubinemia.
- Summarize the nurse's role in the care of an infant with hemolytic disease.
- Identify nursing responsibilities in caring for the newborn receiving phototherapy.
- Discuss selected hematologic problems such as anemia and polycythemia and the nursing implications associated with them.
- Describe the nursing assessment that would lead the nurse to suspect newborn sepsis.
- Relate the consequences of selected maternally transmitted infections, such as maternal syphilis, gonorrhea, herpesvirus, and chlamydia, to the management of the infant in the neonatal period.
- Identify the special initial and long-term needs of parents of at-risk infants.

## KEY TERMS

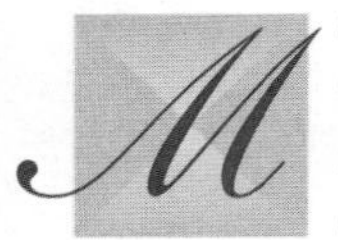

arked homeostatic changes occur during the transition from fetal to neonatal life. The most rapid anatomic and physiologic changes of this period occur in the cardiopulmonary system. Thus the major problems of the newborn are usually related to this system. These problems include asphyxia, respiratory distress, cold stress, jaundice, hemolytic disease, and anemia. Ideally, problems are anticipated and identified prenatally, and appropriate intervention measures are begun at or immediately after birth.

# Care of the Newborn at Risk Due to Asphyxia

Neonatal asphyxia results in circulatory, respiratory, and biochemical changes. Circulatory patterns that accompany asphyxia indicate an inability of the newborn to make the transition to extrauterine circulation—in effect, a return to fetal circulatory patterns. Failure of lung expansion and establishment of respiration rapidly produces hypoxia (decreased $PaO_2$), acidosis (decreased pH), and hypercarbia (increased $PCO_2$). These biochemical changes cause pulmonary vasoconstriction, with retention of high pulmonary vascular resistance, hypoperfusion of the lungs, and a large right-to-left shunt through the ductus arteriosus. The foramen ovale opens (as right atrial pressure exceeds left atrial pressure), and blood now flows from right to left. (See Chapter 21 for a review of normal newborn cardiopulmonary adaptation.)

Biochemical changes that occur in asphyxia contribute to these circulatory changes. The most serious biochemical abnormality is a change from aerobic to anaerobic metabolism in the presence of hypoxia. This change results in the accumulation of lactate and the development of metabolic acidosis. Simultaneous respiratory acidosis may also occur due to a rapid increase in $PCO_2$ during asphyxia. In response to hypoxia and anaerobic metabolism, the amounts of free fatty acids (FFAs) and glycerol in the blood increase. Glycogen stores are also mobilized to provide a continuous glucose source for the brain. Hepatic and cardiac stores of glycogen may be used up rapidly during an asphyxial attack.

The newborn is supplied with several protective mechanisms against hypoxic insults. These include a relatively immature brain and a resting metabolic rate lower than that of adults, an ability to mobilize substances within the body for anaerobic metabolism and to use energy more efficiently, and an intact circulatory system able to redistribute lactate and hydrogen ions in tissues still being perfused. Unfortunately, severe, prolonged hypoxia overcomes these protective mechanisms, resulting in brain damage or death of the newborn.

The newborn who is apneic at birth requires immediate resuscitative efforts. The need for resuscitation can be anticipated if specific risk factors are present during the pregnancy or labor and birth.

## Risk Factors Predisposing to Asphyxia

The need for resuscitation may be anticipated if the mother demonstrates the antepartal and intrapartal risk factors described in Tables 7–1 and 16–1. Neonatal risk factors for resuscitation are as follows:

- Nonreassuring fetal heart rate pattern
- Difficult birth
- Fetal blood loss
- Apneic episode unresponsive to tactile stimulation
- Inadequate ventilation
- Prematurity
- Structural lung abnormality (congenital diaphragmatic hernia, lung hypoplasia)
- Cardiac arrest

At times no risk factors may be apparent prenatally. Particular attention must be paid to all at-risk pregnancies during the intrapartal period. Certain aspects of labor and birth challenge the oxygen supply to the fetus, and often the at-risk fetus has less tolerance for the stress of labor and birth.

## Clinical Therapy

The initial goal of medical management is to identify the fetus at risk for asphyxia, so that resuscitative efforts can begin at birth. Fetal biophysical assessment (see Chapter 14), combined with monitoring of fetal and maternal pH and blood gases and fetal heart rates during the intrapartal period, may help identify fetal distress. If fetal distress is present, appropriate measures can be taken to deliver the fetus immediately, before major damage occurs, and to treat the asphyxiated newborn.

In addition to the fetal biophysical profile, fetal scalp blood sampling may indicate asphyxic insult and the degree of fetal acidosis, when considered in relation to the stage of labor, uterine contractions, and the presence of nonreassuring fetal heart rate (FHR) patterns. The stress of labor causes an intermittent decrease in exchange of gases in the placental intervillous space, which causes the fall in pH and fetal acidosis. The acidosis is primarily metabolic.

During labor, a fetal pH of 7.20 or higher is considered normal. A pH value of 7.20 or less is considered an ominous sign. However, low fetal pH without associated hypoxia can be caused by maternal acidosis secondary to prolonged labor, dehydration, and maternal lactate production.

The treatment of fetal or newborn asphyxia is resuscitation. The goals of resuscitation are to provide an adequate airway with expansion of the lungs, to decrease the $Pco_2$ and increase the $Po_2$, to support adequate cardiac output, and to minimize oxygen consumption by reducing heat loss.

Initial resuscitative management of the newborn is extremely important. Caregivers should keep the infant in a head-down position before the first gasp to avoid aspiration of the oropharyngeal secretions and must suction the oropharynx and nasopharynx immediately. Clearing the nasal and oral passages of fluid that may obstruct the airway establishes a patent airway. Suctioning is always performed before resuscitation so that mucus, blood, or meconium is not aspirated into the lungs.

After the first few breaths, the nurse places the newborn in a level position under a radiant heat source and dries the baby quickly with towels to maintain skin temperature at about 36.5°C (97.7°F). Drying is also a good stimulation to breathing. Heat loss through evaporation is tremendous during the first few minutes of life. The temperature of a wet, 1500-g baby in a cold (16°C [62°F]) birthing room drops 1°C (33.8°F) every 3 minutes. Hypothermia increases oxygen consumption. In an asphyxiated infant, it increases the hypoxic insult and may lead to severe acidosis and development of respiratory distress.

Assessment of the newborn's need for resuscitation begins at the time of birth. The nurse should note the time of the first gasp, first cry, and onset of sustained respirations in the order of occurrence. The Apgar score (see Chapter 17) may be helpful in determining the severity of the neonatal depression, but interventions should never be delayed pending the 1-minute Apgar score.

Breathing is established by employing the simplest form of resuscitative measures initially, with progression to more complicated methods as required:

1. Simple stimulation is provided by rubbing the newborn's back or flicking the feet.
2. If respirations have not been initiated or are inadequate (gasping or occasional respirations), the lungs must be inflated with positive pressure. The mask is positioned securely on the face (over nose and mouth, avoiding the eyes), with the infant's head in a "sniffing" or neutral position (Figure 26–1♦). Hyperextension of the infant's neck obstructs the trachea. An airtight connection is made between the baby's face and the mask (thus allowing the bag to inflate). The lungs are inflated rhythmically by squeezing the bag. Oxygen can be delivered at 100% with an anesthesia bag with manometer or modified self-inflating bag and adequate liter flow. The self-inflating (Ambu or Hope) bag delivers only 40% oxygen unless it has been adapted, and it may not be possible to maintain adequate inspiratory pressure. In a crisis situation, it is crucial that 100% oxygen be delivered with adequate pressure.

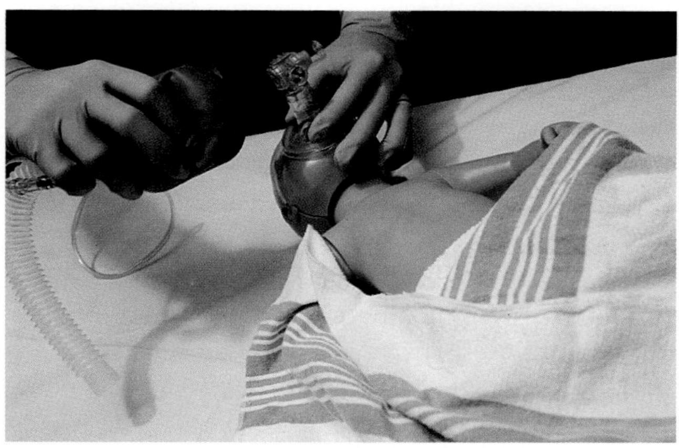

FIGURE 26–1 ♦ Demonstration of resuscitation of an infant with bag and mask. Note that the mask covers the nose and mouth, and the head is in a neutral position. The resuscitating bag is placed to the side of the baby so that chest movement can be seen.

3. The rise and fall of the chest are observed for proper ventilation. Air entry and heart rate are checked by auscultation. Manual resuscitation is coordinated with any voluntary efforts. The rate of ventilation should be between 40 and 60 breaths per minute. Pressure should be adequate to move the chest wall. The pressure gauge (manometer) must be in place to avoid overdistension of the newborn's lungs and other problems such as pneumothorax or abdominal distension. In newborns with normal lungs, 15 to 25 cm $H_2O$ may be adequate. If the newborn has lung disease, 20 to 40 cm $H_2O$ may be necessary. If the newborn has not taken a first breath after birth, pressures of $>$ 30 cm $H_2O$ may be transiently required to expand collapsed alveoli. If ventilation is adequate, the chest moves with each inspiration, bilateral breath sounds are audible, and the lips and mucous membranes become pink. Distension of the stomach is controlled by inserting a nasogastric tube for decompression.
4. Endotracheal intubation may be needed. However, most newborns, except for very-low-birth-weight (VLBW) infants, can be resuscitated by bag and mask ventilation. If the baby is intubated and the color and heart rate fail to respond to ventilatory efforts, poor or improper placement of an endotracheal tube may be the cause. If the baby is intubated properly, pneumothorax, diaphragmatic hernia, or hypoplastic lungs (Potter's association) may exist.

Once breathing has been established, the heart rate should increase to over 100 beats per minute. If the heart rate is less than 60 beats per minute 30 seconds of effective positive pressure ventilation with 100% oxygen, external cardiac massage (chest compression) is begun. Chest compressions are started immediately if there is no detectable heartbeat. Following is the procedure for performing chest compressions:

1. The infant is positioned properly on a firm surface.
2. The resuscitator may use the two-finger method (Figure 26–2♦) or may stand at the foot of the infant and place both thumbs over the lower third of the sternum (just below an imaginary line drawn between the nipples), with the fingers wrapped around and supporting the back.
3. The sternum is depressed approximately one-third of the distance to the vertebral column at a rate of 90 compressions per minute (AAP & AHA, 2000). Use a 3:1 ratio of heartbeat to assisted ventilation.

Drugs that should be available in the birthing area include those needed in the treatment of shock, cardiac arrest, and narcosis. Oxygen, because of its effective use in ventilation, is the drug most often used.

If, after 30 seconds of ventilation and cardiac compression, the newborn has not responded with spontaneous respirations and a heart rate above 60 beats per minute, resuscitative medications are necessary (AAP & AHA, 2000). The most accessible route for administering medications is the umbilical vein. If bradycardia is present, epinephrine (0.1 to 0.3 mL/kg of a 1:10,000 solution) is given through the umbilical vein catheter, the peripheral IV setup, or the endotracheal tube (if an IV has not yet been started). When epinephrine is administered by endotracheal tube, two to three times the IV dose of epinephrine is given, followed immediately by 1 mL of normal saline (Young & Mangum, 2000). In a severely asphyxiated newborn, sodium bicarbonate (1 to 2 mEq/kg of 4.2% solution) is given slowly over at least 2 minutes, at a rate of 1 mEq/kg/min, to correct metabolic acidosis, but only after effective ventilation is established. Dextrose is given to prevent progression of hypoglycemia. A 10% dextrose in water intravenous solution is usually sufficient to prevent or treat hypoglycemia in the birthing area. Naloxone hydrochloride (0.1 mg/kg), a narcotic antagonist, is used to reverse narcotic depression (Young & Mangum, 2000). (See Drug Guide: Naloxone Hydrochloride [Narcan].)

If shock develops (low blood pressure or poor peripheral perfusion), the baby may be given a volume expander such as 5% albumin or lactated Ringer's solution in a dose of 10 mL/kg. Whole blood, fresh frozen plasma, plasminate, and packed red blood cells can also be used for volume expansion and treatment of shock. In some instances of prolonged resuscitation associated with shock and poor response to resuscitation, dopamine (5 mg/kg/min) may be necessary.

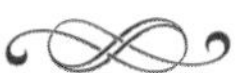

# Nursing Care Management

## Nursing Assessment and Diagnosis

Communication between the obstetric office or clinic and the birthing area nurse facilitates the identification of newborns who may need resuscitation. When the woman arrives in the birthing area, the nurse should have the antepartal

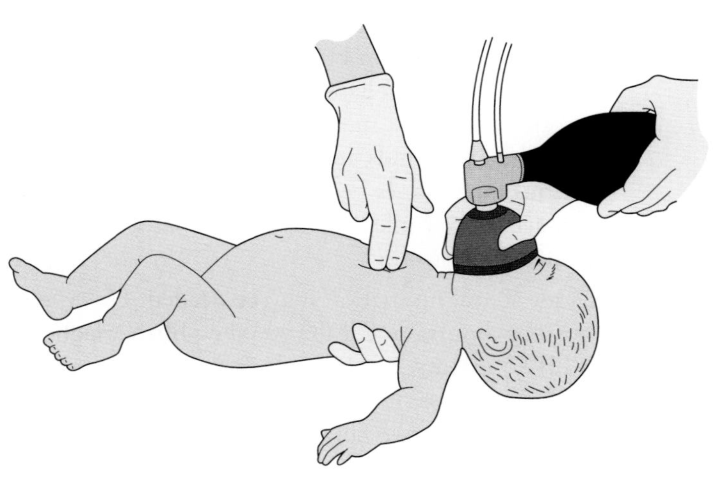


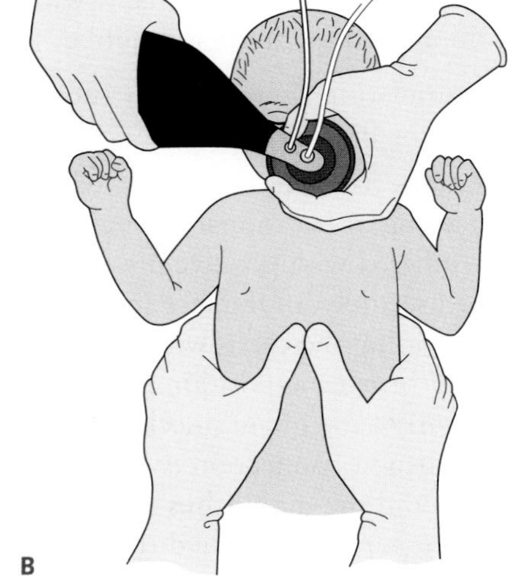


FIGURE 26–2 ♦ External cardiac massage. The lower third of the sternum is compressed with two fingertips or thumbs at a rate of 90 beats per minute. **A,** The two-fingers method uses the tips of two fingers of one hand to compress the sternum and the other hand or a firm surface to support the infant's back. **B,** The thumb method uses the fingers to support the infant's back and uses both thumbs to compress the sternum.

# DRUG GUIDE

## NALOXONE HYDROCHLORIDE (NARCAN)

### *Overview of Neonatal Action*

Naloxone hydrochloride (Narcan) is used to reverse respiratory depression due to acute narcotic toxicity. It displaces morphinelike drugs from receptor sites on the neurons; therefore the narcotics can no longer exert their depressive effects. Naloxone reverses narcotic-induced respiratory depression, analgesia, sedation, hypotension, and pupillary constriction.

### *Route, Dosage, Frequency*

Intravenous dose is 0.1 to 0.2 mg/kg (0.25 to 0.5 mL/kg of 0.4 mg/mL preparation) concentration at birth, including premature infants. This drug is usually given through the umbilical vein or endotracheal tube, although naloxone can be given intramuscularly or subcutaneously. The use of "neonatal" naloxone (Narcan 0.02 mg/mL) is discouraged because of the extremely large fluid volumes that are needed.

Reversal of drug depression occurs within 1–2 minutes after IV administration. The duration of action is variable (minutes to hours) and depends on the amount of the drug present and the rate of excretion. Dose may be repeated in 3–5 minutes. If there is no improvement after two or three doses, discontinue naloxone administration. If initial reversal occurs, repeat dose as needed.

### *Neonatal Contraindications*

Naloxone should not be administered to infants of narcotic-addicted mothers because it may precipitate acute withdrawal syndrome (increased HR and BP, vomiting, tremors).

Respiratory depression may result from nonmorphine drugs, such as sedatives, hypnotics, anesthetics, or other nonnarcotic CNS depressants.

### *Neonatal Side Effects*

Excessive doses may result in irritability, increased crying, and possible prolongation of partial thromboplastin time (PTT).

Tachycardia may occur.

### *Nursing Considerations*

- Monitor respirations closely—rate and depth.
- Assess for return of respiratory depression when naloxone effects wear off and effects of longer-acting narcotics reappear.
- Have resuscitative equipment, $O_2$, and ventilatory equipment available.
- Monitor bleeding studies.
- Note that naloxone is incompatible with alkaline solutions.
- Store at room temperature and protect from light.
- Compatible with heparin.

record and should note any contributory perinatal history factors and assess present fetal status. As labor progresses, nursing assessments include ongoing monitoring of fetal heartbeat and its response to contractions, assisting with fetal scalp blood sampling, and observing for the presence of meconium in the amniotic fluid to assess for fetal asphyxia. In addition, the nurse should alert the resuscitation team and the practitioner responsible for care of the newborn of any potential high-risk laboring women.

Nursing diagnoses that may apply to the newborn with asphyxia include the following:

- ***Ineffective breathing pattern*** related to lack of spontaneous respirations at birth secondary to in utero asphyxia
- ***Decreased cardiac output*** related to impaired oxygenation
- ***Ineffective family coping*** related to baby's lack of spontaneous respirations at birth and fear of losing their newborn

## Nursing Plan and Implementation

### *Hospital-Based Nursing Care*

Following identification of possible high-risk situations, the next step in effective resuscitation is to assemble the necessary equipment and ensure proper functioning. It is desirable to provide for pH and blood gas determination as well. Necessary equipment includes a radiant warmer that provides an overhead radiant heat source (a thermostatic mechanism taped to the infant's abdomen triggers the radiant warmer to turn on or off to maintain a level of thermoneutrality) and an open bed for easy access to the newborn. It is essential that the nurse keep the newborn warm. To do so the nurse dries the newborn quickly with warmed towels or blankets to prevent evaporative heat loss and places him or her under the radiant warmer with the servocontrol set at 36.5°C. (97.7°F).

Resuscitative equipment in the birthing room must be sterilized after each use. In the high-risk nursery resuscitation may be needed at any time. Equipment reliability must be maintained at all times. The nurse inspects all equipment—bag and mask, oxygen and flow meter, laryngoscope, and suction machine—for damaged or nonfunctioning parts before a birth or when setting up an admission bed. A systematic check of the emergency cart and equipment is a routine responsibility of each shift.

Training and knowledge about resuscitation are vital to personnel in the birth setting for both normal and at-risk births. Since resuscitation is at least a two-person effort, the nurse calls for additional support as needed. Resuscitative efforts are recorded on the newborn's chart so that all members of the health care team have access to the information.

### *Parent Teaching*

Birthing room resuscitation is particularly distressing for parents. If the need for resuscitation is anticipated, the parents should be assured that a team will be present at the birth to care specifically for their newborn. As soon as the infant's condition has stabilized, a member of the interdisciplinary team needs to discuss the newborn's condition with the parents. The parents may have many fears about the reasons for resuscitation and the condition of their baby after resuscitation.

## Evaluation

Expected outcomes of nursing care include the following:

- The risk of asphyxia is promptly identified, and intervention is started early.
- The newborn's metabolic and physiologic processes are stabilized, and recovery is proceeding without complications.
- The parents can verbalize the reason for resuscitation and what was done to resuscitate their newborn.
- The parents can verbalize their fears about the resuscitation process and potential implications for their baby's future.

# Care of the Newborn with Respiratory Distress

One of the severest conditions to which the newborn may fall victim is respiratory distress—an inappropriate respiratory adaptation to extrauterine life. The nursing care of a baby with respiratory distress needs to understand the normal pulmonary and circulatory physiology (Chapter 21), the pathophysiology of the disease process, clinical manifestations, and supportive and corrective therapies. Only with this knowledge can the nurse make appropriate observations about responses to therapy and development of complications. Unlike the verbalizing adult client, the newborn communicates needs only by behavior. The neonatal nurse interprets this behavior as clues about the baby's condition.

**Respiratory distress syndrome (RDS),** also referred to as *hyaline membrane disease (HMD),* is the result of a primary absence, deficiency, or alteration in the production of pulmonary surfactant. It is a complex disease that affects approximately 20,000 to 30,000 infants a year in the United States, most of whom are preterm infants. Nearly 50% of these infants are born at gestational ages of 26 to 28 weeks (Whitsett, Pryhuber, Rice, et al., 1999). The syndrome occurs more frequently in premature Caucasian infants than in infants of African descent and almost twice as often in males as in females.

All the factors precipitating the pathologic changes of RDS have not been determined, but two main factors are associated with its development:

1. *Prematurity.* All preterm newborns—whether AGA, SGA, or LGA—and especially (IDMs) are at risk for RDS. The incidence of RDS increases with the degree of prematurity, and most deaths occur in newborns weighing less than 1500 g. The maternal and fetal factors resulting in preterm labor and birth, complications of pregnancy, cesarean birth (and its indications), and familial tendency are all associated with RDS.
2. *Surfactant deficiency disease.* Normal pulmonary adaptation requires adequate surfactant, a lipoprotein that coats the inner surfaces of the alveoli. Surfactant provides alveolar stability by decreasing the alveoli's surface tension and tendency to collapse. Surfactant is produced by type II alveolar cells starting at about 24 weeks' gestation. In the normal or mature newborn lung, it is continuously synthesized, oxidized during breathing, and replenished. Adequate surfactant levels lead to better lung compliance and permit breathing with less work. RDS is due to alterations in surfactant quantity, composition, function, or production.

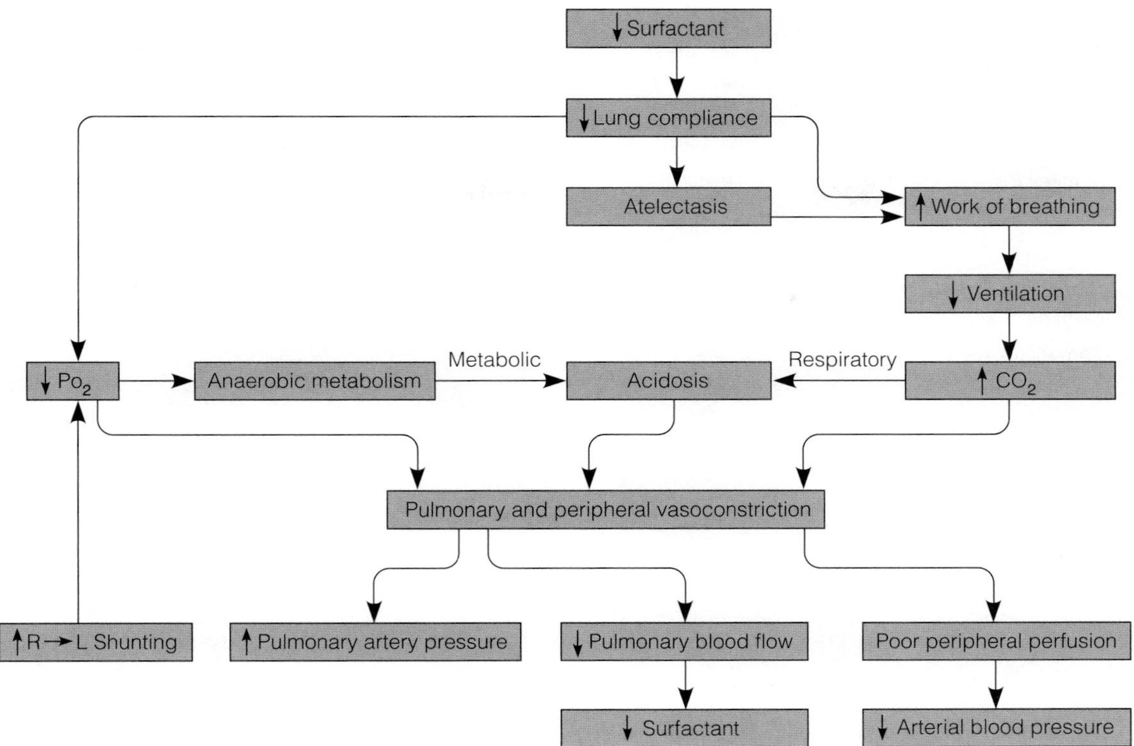


**FIGURE 26–3** ♦ Cycle of events of RDS leading to eventual respiratory failure. *Source:* Modified from Gluck, L., & Kulovich, M. V. (1973). Fetal lung development. *Pediatric Clinics of North America, 20,* 375.

Development of RDS indicates a failure to synthesize surfactant, which is required to maintain alveolar stability (see Chapter 21). On expiration this instability increases atelectasis, which causes hypoxia and acidosis because of the lack of gas exchange. These conditions further inhibit surfactant production and cause pulmonary vasoconstriction. The resulting lung instability causes the biochemical problems of hypoxemia (decreased $PO_2$), hypercarbia (increased $PCO_2$), and acidemia (decreased pH), primarily metabolic, which further increases pulmonary vasoconstriction and hypoperfusion. The cycle of events of RDS leading to eventual respiratory failure is diagrammed in Figure 26–3♦.

Because of these pathophysiologic conditions, the newborn must expend increasing amounts of energy to reopen the collapsed alveoli with every breath, so that each breath becomes as difficult as the first. The progressive expiratory atelectasis upsets the physiologic homeostasis of the pulmonary and cardiovascular systems and prevents adequate gas exchange. Lung compliance decreases, which accounts for the difficulty of inflation, labored respirations, and increased work of breathing.

The physiologic alterations of RDS produce the following complications:

1. *Hypoxia.* As a result of hypoxia, the pulmonary vasculature constricts, pulmonary vascular resistance increases, and pulmonary blood flow is reduced. Increased pulmonary vascular resistance may precipitate a return to fetal circulation as the ductus opens and blood flow is shunted around the lungs. This shunting increases the hypoxia and further decreases pulmonary perfusion. Hypoxia also causes impairment or absence of metabolic response to cold; reversion to anaerobic metabolism, resulting in lactate accumulation (acidosis); and impaired cardiac output, which decreases perfusion to vital organs.
2. *Respiratory acidosis.* Increased $PCO_2$ and decreased pH are results of alveolar hypoventilation, whereas persistently rising $PCO_2$ and decrease in pH are poor prognostic signs of pulmonary function and adequacy.
3. *Metabolic acidosis.* Because of the lack of oxygen at the cellular level, the newborn begins an anaerobic pathway of metabolism, with an increase in lactate levels and a resulting base deficit (loss of bicarbonate). As the lactate levels increase, the pH decreases in an attempt to maintain acid-base homeostasis.

The classic radiologic picture of RDS is diffuse reticulogranular density that occurs bilaterally, with portions of the air-filled tracheobronchial tree (air bronchogram) outlined by the opaque ("white-out") lungs and widespread atelectasis (Hansen, Cooper, & Weisman, 1998) (Figure 26–4♦). The progression of x-ray findings parallels the pattern of resolution, which usually occurs in 4 to 7 days, and the time of surfactant reappearance, unless

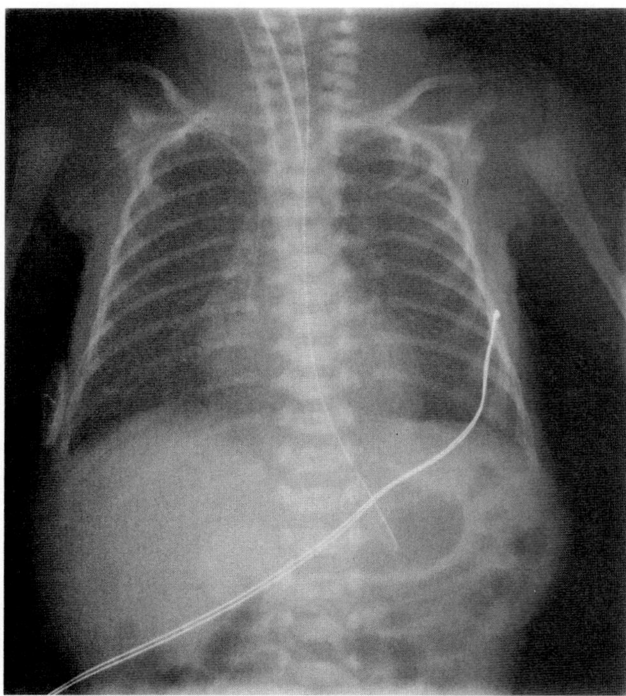

**FIGURE 26–4** ♦ RDS chest x-ray. Chest radiograph of respiratory distress syndrome characterized by a reticulogranular pattern with areas of microatelectasis of uniform opacity and air bronchograms. *Source:* Courtesy of Carol Harrigan, RNC, MSN, NNP.

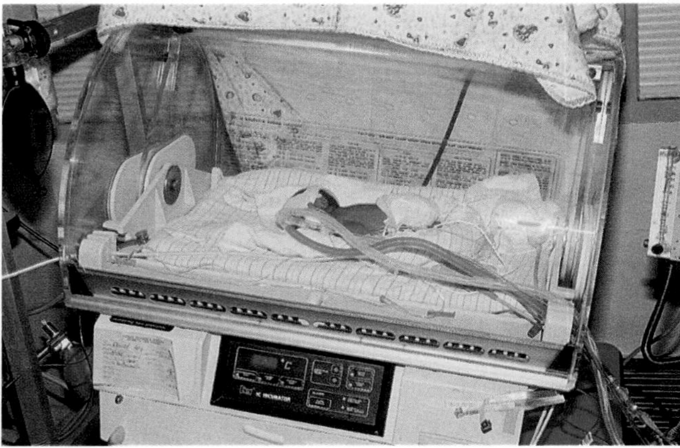

**FIGURE 26–5** ♦ One-day-old, 29 weeks' gestational age, 1450-g baby on respirator and in isolette. *Source:* Courtesy of Carol Harrigan, RNC, MSN, NNP.

surfactant replacement therapy has been used. Echocardiography is a valuable tool in diagnosing vascular shunts that move blood either away from or toward the lungs.

## Clinical Therapy

The antenatal treatment goal for respiratory distress due to preterm labor is the use of antenatal therapies to enhance fetal lung development (see Chapter 13). The goals of postnatal therapy are to maintain adequate oxygenation and ventilation, correct acid-base imbalance, and provide the supportive care required to maintain homeostasis.

Supportive medical management consists of ventilation therapy, transcutaneous oxygen and carbon dioxide monitoring, blood gas monitoring, correction of acid-base imbalance, environmental temperature regulation, adequate nutrition, and protection from infection. Ventilation therapy is directed toward preventing hypoventilation and hypoxia. Mild cases of RDS may require only increased humidified oxygen concentrations. Use of continuous positive airway pressure (CPAP) may be required in moderately afflicted infants. Babies with severe RDS require mechanical ventilatory assistance from a respirator (Figure 26–5♦). High-frequency or jet ventilation has been tried when conventional ventilator therapy has not been successful (Whitsett et al., 1999). Nitric oxide inhalation therapy may also be a useful adjunctive therapy for infants with RDS (Gomez, Hansen, & Corbet, 1998). Other therapies used to improve respiratory function are short-term and long-term steroids and bronchodilators. Morphine or fentanyl for analgesic and sedation may be indicated for infants who have air leak respiratory problems. Concurrent use of the ventilator and pancuronium (Pavulon) for muscle relaxation is controversial.

Surfactant replacement therapy is available for infants to decrease the severity of RDS in low-birth-weight newborns. Surfactant replacement therapy is delivered through an endotracheal tube and may be given in either the birthing room or the nursery and as indicated by the severity of RDS. Repeat doses are often required. The most frequent reported response to treatment is rapidly improved oxygenation and decreased need for ventilatory support (American Academy of Pediatrics [AAP], Committee on Fetus and Newborn, 1999).

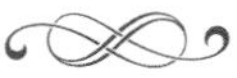

# Nursing Care Management

## Nursing Assessment and Diagnosis

The nurse should look for characteristics of RDS such as increasing cyanosis, tachypnea, grunting respirations, nasal flaring, significant retractions, and apnea. Table 26–1 on page 688 reviews clinical findings associated with respiratory distress in general. The Silverman-Andersen index (Figure 26–6♦) may be helpful in evaluating the signs of respiratory distress used in the birthing area.

Nursing diagnoses that may apply to the newborn with RDS include the following:

- ***Impaired gas exchange*** related to inadequate lung surfactant

- ***Altered nutrition: less than body requirements*** related to increased metabolic needs of the stressed infant
- ***Risk for infection*** related to invasive procedures

## Nursing Plan and Implementation

### *Hospital-Based Nursing Care*

Based on clinical parameters, the neonatal nurse implements therapeutic approaches to maintain physiologic homeostasis and provides supportive care to the newborn with RDS. (See Critical Pathway for Care of a Newborn with Respiratory Distress, on pages 692–695.)

Nursing interventions and criteria for instituting mechanical ventilation depend on institutional protocol. Methods of oxygen monitoring and nursing interventions are included in Table 26–2 on page 691. The nursing care of infants on ventilators or with umbilical artery catheters is not discussed here. These infants have severe respiratory distress and are cared for in neonatal intensive care units by nurses with advanced knowledge and training. The parents of a baby with respiratory distress should be provided with a very supportive environment.

## Critical Thinking in Practice

You are caring for baby girl Linn, who is a 39-week, AGA female born by repeat cesarean birth to a 34-year-old G3 now P3 mother. Baby Linn's Apgar scores were 7 and 9 at 1 and 5 minutes. At 2 hours of age, an elevated respiratory rate of 70 to 80 and mild cyanosis were noted. She is now receiving 30% oxygen and has a respiratory rate of 100 to 120. The baby's clinical course, chest x-ray examination, and lab work are all consistent with transient tachypnea of the newborn. Her mother calls you to ask about her baby. She tells you that her last child was born at 30 weeks' gestation, had respiratory distress syndrome requiring ventilator support, and was hospitalized for 6 weeks. She asks you, "Is this the same respiratory distress?" What will you tell her?

Answers can be found in Appendix I.

## EVIDENCE-BASED PRACTICE

### Early Surfactant Treatment

You have just finished a difficult 12-hour shift during which you cared for a mother who delivered a baby boy at 30 2/7 weeks gestation despite many efforts to stop her preterm labor. The baby was flaccid at birth and immediately intubated by the neonatal team. On your way out of the hospital, you stop by the NICU.

The baby is receiving surfactant prior to developing an established case of RDS. The nurse practitioner tells you that the evidence from four randomized controlled trials has demonstrated that early selective surfactant administration decreases the risk of acute pulmonary injury through such complications as pneumothorax and pulmonary interstitial emphysema. Research also indicates a decrease in neonatal mortality and chronic lung disease with this intervention (Yost & Soll, 2000).

The studies compared early with delayed selective surfactant therapy in newborns intubated for RDS within the first 2 hours of life. The risk for pulmonary complications was reduced significantly with the early treatment groups.

You recognize this effect is also significant emotionally for the baby's family. A newborn who can avoid protracted complications is likely to achieve outcomes for successful discharge more readily.

#### Reference

Yost, C. C. & Soll, R. F. (2000). Early versus delayed selective surfactant treatment for neonatal respiratory distress syndrome. *Cochrane Library*, 2. Oxford: Update Software.

## TABLE 26–1 Clinical Assessments Associated with Respiratory Distress

| *Clinical Picture* | *Significance* |
|---|---|
| **SKIN COLOR** | |
| Pallor or mottling | These represent poor peripheral circulation due to systemic hypotension and vasoconstriction and pooling of independent areas (usually in conjunction with severe hypoxia). |
| Cyanosis (bluish tint) | Depending on hemoglobin concentration, peripheral circulation, intensity and quality of viewing light, and acuity of observer's color vision, this is frankly visible in advanced hypoxia. Central cyanosis is most easily detected by examination of mucous membranes and tongue. |
| Jaundice (yellow discoloration of skin and mucous membranes due to presence of unconjugated [indirect] bilirubin) | Metabolic alterations (acidosis, hypercarbia, asphyxia) of respiratory distress predispose a newborn to dissociation of bilirubin from albumin-binding sites and deposition in the skin and central nervous system. |
| Edema (presents as slick, shiny skin) | This is characteristic of preterm infants because of low total protein concentration, with a decrease in colloidal osmotic pressure and transudation of fluid. Edema of hands and feet is frequently seen within first 24 hours and resolved by fifth day in infants with severe RDS. |
| **RESPIRATORY SYSTEM** | |
| Tachypnea (normal respiratory rate 30–60/minute, elevated respiratory rate 60+/minute) | Increased respiratory rate is the most frequent and easily detectable sign of respiratory distress after birth. This compensatory mechanism attempts to increase respiratory dead space to maintain alveolar ventilation and gas exchange in the face of an increase in mechanical resistance. As a decompensatory mechanism it increases workload and energy output by increasing respiratory rate, which causes increased metabolic demand for oxygen and thus increases alveolar ventilation on an already overstressed system. During shallow, rapid respirations, there is an increase in dead space ventilation, thus decreasing alveolar ventilation. |
| Apnea (episode of nonbreathing for more than 20 seconds; periodic breathing, a common "normal" occurrence in preterm infants, is defined as apnea of 5–10 seconds alternating with 10–15 seconds of ventilation) | This poor prognostic sign indicates cardiorespiratory disease, CNS disease, metabolic alterations, intracranial hemorrhage, sepsis, or immaturity. Physiologic alterations include decreased oxygen saturation, respiratory acidosis, and bradycardia. |
| Chest | Inspection of the thoracic cage includes shape, size, and symmetry of movement. Respiratory movements should be symmetrical and diaphragmatic; asymmetry reflects pathology (pneumothorax, diaphragmatic hernia). Increased anteroposterior diameter indicates air trapping (meconium aspiration syndrome). |
| Labored respirations (Silverman-Anderson index in Figure 26–6 indicates severity of retractions, grunting, and nasal flaring, which are signs of labored respirations) | Indicates marked increase in the work of breathing. |
| Retractions (inward pulling of soft parts of the chest cage—suprasternal, substernal, intercostal, subcostal—at inspiration) | These reflect the significant increase in negative intrathoracic pressure necessary to inflate stiff, noncompliant lungs. Infants attempt to increase lung compliance by using accessory muscles. Lung expansion markedly decreases. Seesaw respirations are seen when the chest flattens with inspiration and the abdomen bulges. Retractions increase the work of breathing and $O_2$ need so that assisted ventilation may be necessary due to exhaustion. |
| Flaring nares (inspiratory dilation of nostrils) | This compensatory mechanism attempts to lessen the resistance of the narrow nasal passage. |

| TABLE 26–1 Clinical Assessments Associated with Respiratory Distress *continued* | |
|---|---|
| ***Clinical Picture*** | ***Significance*** |
| Expiratory grunt (Valsalva maneuver in which the infant exhales against a closed glottis, thus producing an audible moan) | This increases transpulmonary pressure, which decreases or prevents atelectasis, thus improving oxygenation and alveolar ventilation. Intubation should not be attempted unless the infant's condition is rapidly deteriorating, because it prevents this maneuver and allows the alveoli to collapse. |
| Rhythmic body movement with labored respirations (chin tug, head bobbing, retractions of anal area) | This is a result of using abdominal and other respiratory accessory muscles during prolonged forced respirations. |
| Auscultation of chest reveals decreased air exchange, with harsh breath sounds or fine inspiratory rales; rhonchi may be present | Decrease in breath sounds and distant quality may indicate interstitial or intrapleural air or fluid. |
| **CARDIOVASCULAR SYSTEM** | |
| Continuous systolic murmur may be audible | Patent ductus arteriosus is a common occurrence with hypoxia, pulmonary vasoconstriction, right-to-left shunting, and congestive heart failure. |
| Heart rate usually within normal limits (fixed heart rate may occur with a rate of 110–120/minute) | A fixed heart rate indicates a decrease in vagal control. |
| Point of maximal impulse usually located at fourth to fifth intercostal space, left sternal border | Displacement may reflect dextrocardia, pneumothorax, or diaphragmatic hernia. |
| **HYPOTHERMIA** | This is inadequate functioning of metabolic processes that require oxygen to produce necessary body heat. |
| **MUSCLE TONE** | |
| Flaccid, hypotonic, unresponsive to stimuli<br>Hypertonia and/or seizure activity | These may indicate deterioration in the newborn's condition and possible CNS damage due to hypoxia, acidemia, or hemorrhage. |

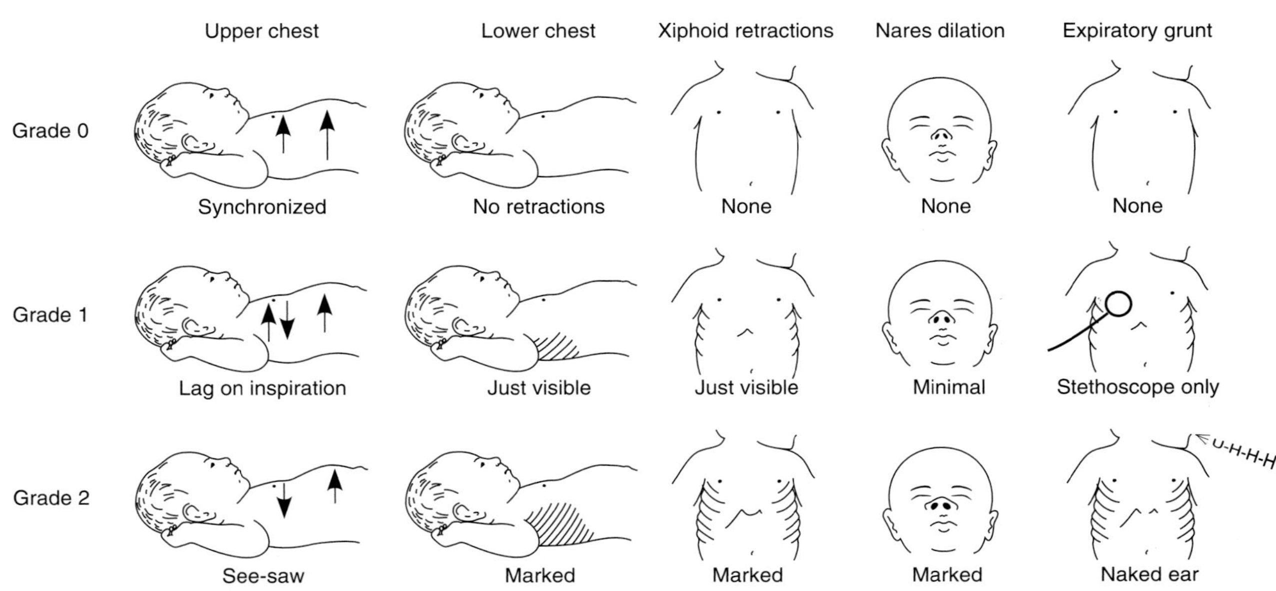


**FIGURE 26–6** ♦ Evaluation of respiratory status using the Silverman-Andersen index. The baby's respiratory status is assessed. A grade of 0, 1, or 2 is determined for each area, and a total score is charted in the baby's record or on a copy of this tool and placed in the chart.
*Source:* Ross Laboratories, Nursing Aid No. 2. Columbus, OH; Silverman, W. A., & Andersen, D. H. (1956). *Pediatrics, 17,* 1–10. Copyright 1956, American Academy of Pediatrics.

## HINTS FOR PRACTICE

In babies with RDS who are on ventilators, increased urination (determined by weighing diapers) may be an early clue that the baby's condition is improving. As fluid moves out of the lungs and into the bloodstream, alveoli open and kidney perfusion increases, which results in increased voiding. At this point, the nurse must monitor chest expansion closely. If chest expansion is increasing, ventilator settings may have to be decreased. Too high a ventilator may "blow the lung," resulting in pneumothorax.

### Evaluation

Expected outcomes of nursing care include the following:

- The risk of RDS is promptly identified and early intervention is initiated.
- The newborn is free of respiratory distress and metabolic alterations.
- The parents verbalize their concerns about their baby's health problem and survival and understand the rationale behind the management of their newborn.

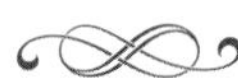

## Transient Tachypnea of the Newborn

Some AGA preterm and near-term infants may develop progressive respiratory distress that can resemble classic RDS. They may have had intrauterine or intrapartal asphyxia due to maternal oversedation, maternal bleeding, prolapsed cord, breech birth, or maternal diabetes. The resultant effect on the newborn is failure to clear the airway of lung fluid, mucus, and other debris or an excess of fluid in the lungs due to aspiration of amniotic or tracheal fluid. Transient tachypnea is also more prevalent in cesarean birth newborns who have not had the thoracic squeeze that occurs during vaginal birth and removes some of the lung fluid.

Usually the newborn experiences little or no difficulty at the onset of breathing. However, shortly after birth, expiratory grunting, flaring of the nares, and mild cyanosis may be noted in the newborn breathing room air. Tachypnea is usually present by 6 hours of

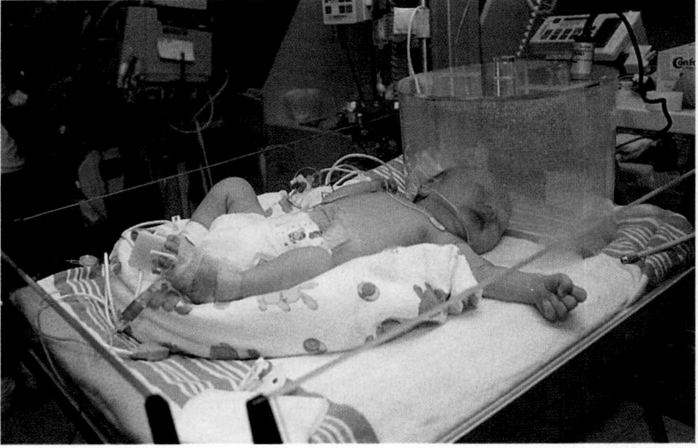

**FIGURE 26–7** ♦ An infant under an oxyhood.

age, with respiratory rates as high as 100 to 140 breaths per minute.

### Clinical Therapy

Initial x-ray findings may be identical to those showing RDS within the first 3 hours. However, radiographs of infants with transient tachypnea usually reveal a generalized overexpansion of the lungs (hyperaeration of alveoli), which is identified principally by flattened contours of the diaphragm. Dense streaks (increased vascularity) radiate from the hilar region and represent engorgement of the lymphatic vessels, which clear alveolar fluid on initiation of air breathing. Within 48 to 72 hours, the chest x-ray examination is normal (Hansen et al., 1998).

Ambient oxygen concentrations of 30% to 50%, usually under an oxyhood, may be required to correct the hypoxemia (Figure 26–7♦). Fluid and electrolyte requirements should be met with intravenous fluids during the acute phase of the disease. Oral feedings are contraindicated because of rapid respiratory rates. The infant should be improving by 8 to 24 hours. The duration of the clinical course of transient tachypnea is approximately 72 hours. Mild respiratory and metabolic acidosis may be present at 2 to 6 hours.

When hypoxemia is severe and tachypnea continues, persistent pulmonary hypertension must be considered and treatment measures initiated. If pneumonia is suspected initially, antibiotics may be administered prophylactically.

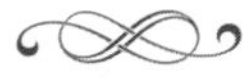

## Nursing Care Management

For nursing actions, see the Critical Pathway for Care of a Newborn with Respiratory Distress on pages 692–695.

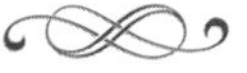

## TABLE 26–2 Oxygen Monitors

| *Type* | *Function and Rationale* | *Nursing Interventions* |
|---|---|---|
| **PULSE OXIMETRY—$SP_{O_2}$** | | |
| Estimates beat-to-beat arterial oxygen saturation. | Calibration is automatic. | Understand and use oxyhemoglobin dissociation curve. |
| Microprocessor measures saturation by the absorption of red and infrared light as it passes through tissue. | Less dependent on perfusion than $TcP_{O_2}$ and $TcP_{CO_2}$, however, functions poorly if peripheral perfusion is decreased due to low cardiac output. | Monitor trends over time and correlate with arterial blood gases (Merenstein & Gardner, 1998).<br>Check disposable sensor at least q8h. |
| Changes in absorption related to blood pulsation through vessel determine saturation and pulse rate (Merenstein & Gardner, 1998). | Much more rapid response time than $TcP_{O_2}$—offers real-time readings.<br>Can be located on extremity, digit, or palm of hand, leaving chest free; not affected by skin characteristics.<br>Requires understanding of oxyhemoglobin dissociation curve.<br>Pulse oximeter reading of 85% to 95% reflects clinically safe range of saturation.<br>Extreme sensitivity to movement; decreases if average of 7th or 14th beat is selected rather than beat to beat.<br>Poor correlation with extreme hyperoxia. | Use disposable cuffs (reusable cuffs allow too much ambient light to enter, and readings may be inaccurate). |
| **TRANSCUTANEOUS OXYGEN MONITOR—$TCP_{O_2}$** | | |
| Measures oxygen diffusion across the skin.<br>Clark electrode is heated to 43°C (preterm) or 44°C (term) to warm the skin beneath the electrode and promote diffusion of oxygen across the skin surface. $P_{O_2}$ is measured when oxygen diffuses across the capillary membrane, skin, and electrode membrane (Merenstein & Gardner, 1998). | When transcutaneous monitors are properly calibrated and electrodes are appropriately positioned, they will provide reliable, continuous, noninvasive measurements of $P_{O_2}$, $P_{CO_2}$, and oxygen saturation.<br>Readings vary when skin perfusion is decreased.<br>Reliable as trend monitor.<br>Frequent calibration necessary to overcome mechanical drift.<br>Following membrane change, machine must "warm up" 1 hour prior to initial calibration; otherwise, after turning it on, it must equilibrate for 30 minutes prior to calibration.<br>When placed on infant, values will be low until skin is heated; approximately 15 minutes required to stabilize. | Use $TcP_{O_2}$ to monitor trends of oxygenation with routine nursing care procedures.<br>Clean electrode surface to remove electrolyte deposits; change solution and membrane once a week.<br>Allow machine to stabilize before drawing arterial gases; note reading when gases are drawn and use values to correlate.<br>Ensure airtight seal between skin surface and electrode; place electrodes on clean, dry skin on upper chest, abdomen, or inner aspect of thigh; avoid bony prominences. |
| | Second-degree burns are rare but can occur if electrodes remain in place too long.<br>Decreased correlations noted with older infants (related to skin thickness), with infants with low cardiac output (decreased skin perfusion), and with hyperoxic infants. | Change skin site and recalibrate at least every 4 hours; inspect skin for burns; if burns occur, use lowest temperature setting and change position of electrode more frequently. |
| | The adhesive that attaches the electrode may abrade the fragile skin of the preterm infant.<br>May be used for both preductal and postductal monitoring of oxygenation for observations of shunting. | Adhesive disks may be cut to a smaller size, or skin prep may be used under the adhesive circle only; allow membrane to touch skin surface at center. |

# CRITICAL PATHWAY: *Care of a Newborn with Respiratory Distress*

| Category | Day of Birth—First 4 Hours | Remainder of Birth Day |
|---|---|---|
| **Referral** | Report from L&D, neonatal nurse practitioner<br>Check ID bands<br>Consults prn: high-risk peds, neonatology | Check ID bands q shift<br>Lactation consult prn |
| **Assessments** | Assess development of s/s respiratory distress:<br>• Tachypnea (>60 respirations/min)<br>• Expiratory grunting (audible), subcostal/intercostal/suprasternal retractions, nasal flaring on inspiration<br>• Cyanosis and pallor<br>• Signs of increased air hunger (apnea, hypotonus), labored respirations<br>• Arterial blood gases (indicating respiratory failure): $Pa_{O_2}$ less than 50 mm Hg, and $Pc_{O_2}$ above 60 mm Hg<br>Auscultation:<br>• Initially breath sounds may be normal, then decreased air exchange occurs with harsh breath sounds and, upon deep inspiration, rales<br>• Later, a low-pitched systolic murmur indicates patent ductus arteriosus<br>Determine baseline of respiratory effort and ventilator adequacy:<br>• Observe chest wall movement<br>• Assess skin, mucous membranes color, capillary refill<br>• Auscultate quality of air entry bilaterally<br>• Assess arterial blood gases and pH<br>Increasing oxygen concentration requirements to maintain adequate $P_{O_2}$ levels<br>VS: temp (ax), pulse, respirations, BP<br>Admission wt, length, HC, peripheral pulses × 4<br>Monitor pulse oximeter<br>Gestational age assessment (only as tolerated without increasing infant's work of breathing, or defer)<br>Gestational history: recent episodes of fetal or intrapartal stress (maternal hypotension, bleeding, maternal and resultant fetal oversedation), fetal lung circulation compromise<br>Lung maturity assessment: amniotic, tracheal, and/or gastric aspirates as available for PG<br>Newborn Hx: birth asphyxia resulting in acute hypoxia, hypothermia, low Apgar scores, bag/mask resuscitation<br>Monitor activity (increasing lethargy, s/s seizure activity) | Continue previous assessments q2–4h and prn<br>Assess color, respiratory status<br>Assess mother-baby interaction as appropriate<br>Observe infant for temperature instability, signs of increased oxygen consumption, and metabolic acidosis<br>Observe infant for s/s sepsis: apnea, lethargy, cyanosis, temp instability |
| **Teaching/psychosocial** | Admission activities performed at mother's bedside as possible; orient parents to nursery, handwashing; assess teaching needs and readiness for learning<br>Provide parents information on infant's condition, minimal handling rationale, equipment and monitoring devices prn | Reinforce previous teaching; keep parents apprised of infant's status<br>Discuss/teach infant security, identification<br>Teach parents s/s respiratory distress, calming techniques, bulb syringe, positioning, when to call for assistance |
| **Nursing care management and reports** | Admit directly to special care nursery prn<br>Labs as ordered: blood type, Rh, Coombs' on cord blood prn, tracheal or gastric aspirate for PG, chemstrip, peripheral hct, blood cultures, CBC, electrolytes, arterial or capillary blood gas<br>Administer IV antibiotics as ordered<br>Intravenous access for meds, hydration, nutritional support<br>Assist MD/NP with placement of umbilical or arterial lines prn<br>Attach servo probe to infant's skin, radiant warmer bed on servo control<br>Attach three-lead EKG for continuous cardiac, resp monitoring prn<br>Attach pulse oximeter to infant extremity<br>Set up, monitor oxygen administration prn (or assist respiratory therapist prn), nasal cannula, oxygen hood | Vital signs: q4h and prn, use monitoring devices to decrease infant stimulation; daily wt using bed scale as necessary<br>Monitor antibiotic drug levels<br>Continue assessments q4h and prn<br>Cord care per policy (q diaper change after infant stable and possibility of placing umbilical lines remote)<br>Rotate pulse oximetry sites q8h and prn; TCOM sites q4h and prn depending on infant's skin integrity |

BP, blood pressure; DC, discharge; EKG, electrocardiograph; f/u, follow-up; HC, head circumference; Hx, history; ID, identification; IM, intramuscular; IV, intravenous; L&D, labor and delivery; meds, medications; MD, medical doctor; MD/NP, medical doctor/nurse practitioner; NTE, neutral thermal environment; OU, both eyes; $O_2$, oxygen; peds, pediatrics; PG, phosphotidylglycerol; prn, as needed; RDS, respiratory distress syndrome; resp, respirators; s/s, signs and symptoms; temp, temperature; TCOM, transcutaneous oxygen monitor; TPN, total parenteral nutrition; via, by way of; VS, vital signs; WIC, Women, Infants, and Children; WNL, within normal limits; WOB, work of breathing.

| Category | Day of Birth—First 4 Hours | Remainder of Birth Day |
|---|---|---|
| **Activity and comfort** | Adjust and monitor radiant warmer to maintain skin temp and NTE<br>Provide calming techniques<br>Cluster care procedures (allow recovery time between procedures), nest<br>Minimal stimulation, quiet and dim environment<br>Provide pacifier for nonnutritive sucking | Leave in radiant warmer until stable, then swaddle and move to isolette or open crib as condition allows<br>Encourage parent interaction/holding as soon as infant tolerates<br>Avoid overstimulation, cluster care procedures, assess on infant's schedule<br>Reposition for comfort q4h, prn; position on surfboard while prone |
| **Nutrition** | Provide total parenteral nutrition (TPN) as ordered and indicated<br>Provide adequate caloric intake: consider amount of intake, route of administration, need for supplementation of intake by other routes, type of feeding (breast/formula)<br>Gavage feeding prn<br>Maintain IV rate via infusion pump (usually 60–80 mL/kg/day dependent on gestational age and organ efficiency)<br>• Record intake hourly (oral, parenteral type and amount)<br>• Monitor vital signs, lung auscultation, heart sounds for s/s fluid overload | Advance intake as tolerated from parenteral to gastrointestinal.<br>Gavage or nipple feed, supplementing with IV prn, discontinue IV when oral intake sufficient<br>Initiate breastfeeding as soon as mother/baby condition allows<br>Supplement breastfeeding only when medically indicated and ordered by MD/NP<br>Initiate bottle-feeding as applicable |
| **Elimination** | Note first void and stool<br>Record hourly output<br>Monitor urine specific gravity | Continue accurate hourly output monitoring (1–3 mL/kg/hr)<br>Monitor stools for amt, type, pattern changes<br>Continue specific gravity monitoring |
| **Medication** | AquaMEPHYTON IM, dosage according to infant wt per MD order<br>Ilotycin ophth ointment OU after retinal assessment by MD/NP<br>Antibiotic therapy as ordered | Continue antibiotic therapy as ordered |
| **Discharge planning/ home care** | Plan DC with parent/guardian<br>Evaluate for social services/home care/DC planning needs | Birth certificate instructions/worksheet<br>Car seat available for DC |
| **Family involvement** | Evaluate psychosocial needs: provide time for expressions of concerns, determine parents' understanding of respiratory distress syndrome (RDS)<br>Evaluate parent teaching | Encourage family involvement in infant's care as possible and as infant tolerates<br>Keep family apprised of infant's progress and current status<br>Evaluate parent teaching |
| **Date** | | |

| Category | Day 1 after Birth | Day 2/3 (as applicable) after Birth |
|---|---|---|
| **Referral** | Check ID bands q shift | **Expected Outcomes**<br>Mother/baby ID band correlate at time of DC<br>Consults completed prn<br>Assess respiratory effort and level of distress |
| **Assessments** | Continue high-risk assessment for RDS q4h<br>Assess respiratory effort and ventilatory adequacy<br>Assess mother-baby interaction<br>Assess thermoregulation<br>Assess abdominal distension, gastric residuals<br>Monitor blood gases, capillary refill, O2 saturation, pulses all four extremities | Continue high-risk assessment for resp distress q4h as needed<br>Assess mother-baby interaction<br>Continue monitoring blood gases, capillary refill, $O_2$ saturation, pulses all four extremities q4h prn, wean to q8h as infant recovers<br>**Expected Outcomes**<br>Physical assessments, VS WNL; no complications or residual respiratory distress noted |

| Category | Day 1 after Birth | Day 2/3 (as applicable) after Birth |
|---|---|---|
| **Teaching/psychosocial** | (See Newborn Critical Pathway, pages 73 to 74)<br>Reinforce previous teaching<br>Parental teaching: bathing, cord care, skin/nail care, use of thermometer, activity, sleep patterns, calming methods, reflexes, jaundice, growth/feeding patterns, burping, diapering, elimination norms<br>Provide information including<br>• Newborn capabilities and developmental behaviors, cues<br>• Temperature maintenance with clothing and blankets<br>• Safety (choking, positioning, use of bulb syringe) | Final discharge teaching (see Newborn Critical Pathway, pages 73 to 74)<br>Review infant safety, s/s illness and when to call health care provider with parents<br>**Expected Outcomes**<br>Mother verbalizes comprehension of instructions, demonstrates care capabilities |
| **Nursing care management and reports** | Maintain on respiratory and cardiac monitors:<br>• Check and calibrate all monitoring and measuring devices q8h<br>• Calibrate oxygen devices to 21% and 100% $O_2$ concentrations<br>Provide warmed air and humidified oxygen<br>Monitor oxygen concentrations at least q1h<br>Femoral pulses or BPs all four extremities before DC or at 48 hours<br>VS q4h<br>Daily wt<br>Continue high-risk assessments for resp distress q4h, wean to q8h as infant stabilizes and recovers<br>Isolette if temp instability: adjust and monitor to maintain skin temp and NTE<br>Use servo control to maintain constant temp regulation<br>Monitor activity<br>Administer meds as ordered<br>Newborn screen, monitor therapeutic drug levels, blood gases prn | Newborn/high-risk assessment q8h if resp status WNL and stable<br>Baer hearing test<br>Daily wt<br>VS q8h and prn<br>Continue oxygen administration as warranted (oxyhood, nasal cannula)<br>Monitor $_{0}2$ concentrations q1–2h<br>Prepare infant for/assist with circumcision as applicable<br>Cord care per policy<br>Administer antibiotics/monitor levels as ordered<br>Continue universal precautions<br>HSV culture per parental hx HSV<br>Wean from radiant warmer or isolette to open crib if VS WNL, stable<br>**Expected Outcomes**<br>Physical assessments WNL; cord unclamped and dry without s/s infection; circ site unremarkable; no s/s respiratory distress; labs WNL; wt stabilized to not >10% loss |
| **Activity and comfort** | Change position q4h and prn<br>Swaddled in open crib as condition permits<br>Isolette if temp instability; adjust temp for infant size, gestation, layers of clothing to maintain NTE | Swaddled in open crib as condition permits<br>Allow movement of hands to face<br>**Expected Outcomes**<br>Maintains temp WNL swaddled in open crib |
| **Nutrition** | Supplement breast only when medically indicated/ordered<br>Gavage feed prn<br>Encourage on-demand feedings as tolerated, minimally q3–4h<br>Bottle-feed q3–4 on demand<br>Decrease parenteral support as oral feedings increase | Continue feeding schedule<br>Feed on demand breast or bottle<br>Supplement breast only when medically indicated/ordered<br>**Expected Outcomes**<br>Infant tolerates feedings, feeds on demand; breastfeeds without supplement, nipples without problems or s/s increased WOB; regaining lost wt or wt stabilized after birth |
| **Elimination** | Monitor stools for amount, consistency, pattern changes, occult blood, reducing substances<br>Monitor voids q8h<br>Continue accurate intake and output as warranted | Continue monitoring of all voids and stools q shift, noting changes<br>Accurate intake output as warranted<br>**Expected Outcomes**<br>Voids qs, stools without difficulty qs, stool character WNL |
| **Medication** | Hep B vaccine as ordered by MD/NP after consent signed by parent | Hep B vaccine before DC<br>**Expected Outcomes**<br>Infant has received ophthalmic ointment OU and AquaMEPHYTON injection; received first Hep B vaccine if ordered and parental consent given; antibiotics regimen completed with resolution RDS |
| **Discharge planning/ home care** | Newborn photographs<br>Complete birth certificate packet<br>Continue DC teaching<br>Access community referrals, support groups for mother/family prn (ie, WIC, financial resources, public health nursing) | Complete DC teaching<br>Complete DC summary, give written copy DC instructions (see Newborn Critical Pathway, pages 73 to 74<br>Set up appointment for follow-up newborn screening blood test<br>All discharge referrals made, follow-up appointments scheduled |

| Category | Day 1 after Birth | Day 2/3 (as applicable) after Birth |
|---|---|---|
| Discharge planning/ home care | | **Expected Outcomes**<br>Infant discharged home with family; mother verbalizes f/u appointment times and dates; mother verbalizes comprehension of DC instructions and available resources (ie, lactation, new parents support groups) |
| Family involvement | Bath and feeding class<br>Newborn channel as available<br>Assess mother-baby bonding/interaction<br>Incorporate significant other/siblings in care<br>Support positive parenting behaviors<br>Evaluate mother/parent teaching<br>Encourage significant other's presence during MD visits with mother on infant's progress, current status, and plan formation | Assess mother-baby bonding/interaction<br>Identify community referral needs and refer to community agencies<br>**Expected Outcomes**<br>Demonstrates caring and family incorporation of infant |
| Date | | |

# Care of the Newborn with Meconium Aspiration Syndrome

The presence of meconium in amniotic fluid indicates an asphyxial insult to the fetus before or during labor. The physiologic response to asphyxia is increased intestinal peristalsis, relaxation of the anal sphincter, and passage of meconium into the amniotic fluid. However, passage of meconium in a breech position does not necessarily indicate asphyxia.

Approximately 13% of live-born infants are born through meconium-stained amniotic fluid (MSAF). Of the newborns born through MSAF, 5% to 12% develop **meconium aspiration syndrome (MAS)** (Wiswell, Gannon, Jacob, et al., 2000). This fluid may be aspirated into the tracheobronchial tree in utero or during the first few breaths taken by the newborn. This syndrome primarily affects term, SGA, and postterm newborns and those who have experienced a long labor.

Presence of meconium in the lungs produces a ball-valve action (air is allowed in but not exhaled), so that alveoli overdistend; rupture with pneumomediastinum or pneumothorax is a common occurrence. The meconium also initiates a chemical pneumonitis in the lung, with oxygen and carbon dioxide trapping and hyperinflation. Secondary bacterial pneumonia can occur.

Clinical manifestations of MAS include (1) fetal hypoxia in utero a few days or a few minutes prior to birth, indicated by a sudden increase in fetal activity followed by diminished activity, slowing of FHR or weak and irregular heartbeat, loss of beat-to-beat variability, and meconium staining of amniotic fluid; and (2) presence of signs of distress at birth, such as pallor, cyanosis, apnea, slow heartbeat, and low Apgar scores (below 6) at 1 and 5 minutes. As the victims of intrauterine asphyxia, meconium-stained newborns, or newborns who have aspirated meconium, are depressed at birth and require resuscitation to establish adequate respiratory effort.

After the initial resuscitation, the severity of clinical symptoms correlates with the extent of aspiration. Many infants require mechanical ventilation at birth because of immediate signs of distress (generalized cyanosis, tachypnea, and severe retractions). An overdistended, barrel-shaped chest with increased anteroposterior diameter is common. Auscultation reveals diminished air movement, with prominent rales and rhonchi. Abdominal palpation may reveal a displaced liver caused by diaphragmatic depression resulting from the overexpansion of the lungs. Yellowish staining of the skin, nails, and umbilical cord is usually present.

The chest x-ray film reveals nonuniform, coarse, patchy densities and hyperinflation (9 to 11 rib expansion). Evidence of pulmonary air leak is frequently present. Extreme hypoxia is also caused by the cardiopulmonary shunting and resultant failure to oxygenate and can lead to *persistent pulmonary hypertension of the newborn (PPHN).*

## Clinical Therapy

The combined efforts of the maternity and pediatric team are needed to prevent MAS. The most effective form of preventive management is as follows:

1. After the head of the newborn is born and while the shoulders and chest are still in the birth canal, the baby's oropharynx and then nasopharynx are

suctioned. (The same procedure is followed with a cesarean birth.) To decrease the possibility of human immunodeficiency virus (HIV) transmission, low-pressure wall suction is used.

2. If the infant is vigorous and there is thick meconium in the amniotic fluid, the glottis is visualized and meconium is suctioned from the trachea.
3. If the infant is vigorous and there is only thin meconium in the amniotic fluid, no subsequent special resuscitation is indicated.
4. For any depressed infant (heart rate less than 100 beats per minute or poor respiratory effort with meconium staining), the glottis is visualized and the trachea suctioned (Wiswell et al., 2000).

If the newborn's head is not adequately suctioned on the perineum (at the time the head is born but the shoulder and chest are still in the vagina), respiratory or resuscitative efforts will push meconium into the airway and into the lungs. Stimulation of the newborn should be avoided to minimize respiratory movements. Further resuscitative efforts are undertaken as indicated, following the same principles of clinical therapy used for asphyxia (discussed earlier in this chapter). Resuscitated newborns should be transferred immediately to the nursery for closer observation. An umbilical arterial line may be used for direct monitoring of arterial blood pressures; blood sampling for pH and blood gases; and infusion of intravenous fluids, blood, or medications.

Treatment usually involves delivery of high levels of oxygen and ventilation. Ventilation with low positive end-expiratory pressure (PEEP) is preferred to avoid air leaks. Unfortunately, high pressures may be needed to cause sufficient expiratory expansion of obstructed airways or to stabilize airways that are weakened by inflammation so that the most distal atelectatic alveoli are ventilated.

Surfactant replacement therapy is most effective when used prophylactically. It improves oxygenation and decreases the incidence of air leaks. Systemic blood pressure and pulmonary blood flow must be maintained; this may be accomplished using dopamine or dobutamine and/or volume expanders.

Full-term newborns over 3.17 kg (7 lb) with respiratory failure who are not responding to ventilator therapy may require treatment with high-frequency ventilation and/or nitric oxide therapy or extracorporeal membrane oxygenation (ECMO). ECMO treatment, a form of heart-lung bypass, has proved successful for newborns with meconium aspiration, pneumonia, and PPHN who are not responding to traditional treatment modalities.

Treatment includes chest physiotherapy (chest percussion, vibration, and drainage) to remove debris. Prophylactic intravenous antibiotics are frequently given. Bicarbonate may be necessary for several days for severely ill newborns. Mortality in term or postterm infants is very high, because the cycle of hypoxemia and acidemia is difficult to break.

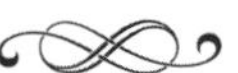

# Nursing Care Management

## Nursing Assessment and Diagnosis

During the intrapartal period, the nurse should observe for signs of fetal hypoxia and meconium staining of amniotic fluid. At birth, the nurse assesses the newborn for signs of distress. She or he carefully observes for complications such as pulmonary air leaks; anoxic cerebral injury manifested by cerebral edema and/or convulsions; anoxic myocardial injury evidenced by congestive heart failure or cardiomegaly; disseminated intravascular coagulation (DIC) resulting from hypoxic hepatic damage with depression of liver-dependent clotting factors; anoxic renal damage demonstrated by hematuria, oliguria, or anuria; fluid overload; sepsis secondary to bacterial pneumonia; and any signs of intestinal necrosis from ischemia, including gastrointestinal obstruction or hemorrhage.

Nursing diagnoses that may apply to the newborn with MAS and the infants' parents include the following:

- ***Ineffective gas exchange*** related to aspiration of meconium and amniotic fluid during birth
- ***Altered nutrition: less than body requirements*** related to respiratory distress and increased energy requirements
- ***Ineffective family coping: compromised*** related to life-threatening illness in term newborn

## Nursing Plan and Implementation

### *Hospital-Based Nursing Care*

Initial interventions are aimed at prevention of the aspiration by assisting with the removal of the meconium from the infant's oropharynx and nasopharynx prior to the first extrauterine breath. When significant aspiration occurs, the primary goals of therapy are to maintain appropriate gas exchange and minimize complications. Nursing interventions after resuscitation should include maintaining adequate oxygenation and ventilation, regulating temperature, performing glucose testing by glucometer at 2 hours of age to check for hypoglycemia, observing intravenous fluids administration, calculating necessary fluids (which may be restricted in the first 48 to 72 hours due to cerebral edema), providing caloric requirements, and monitoring intravenous antibiotic therapy.

## Evaluation

Expected outcomes of nursing care include the following:

- The risk of MAS is promptly identified and early intervention is initiated.
- The newborn is free of respiratory distress and metabolic alterations.
- The parents verbalize their concerns about their baby's health problem and survival and understand the rationale behind the management of their newborn.

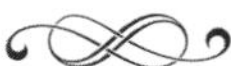

# Care of the Newborn with Cold Stress

**Cold stress** is excessive heat loss resulting in the use of compensatory mechanisms (such as increased respirations and nonshivering thermogenesis) to maintain core body temperature. Heat loss that results in cold stress occurs in the newborn through the mechanisms of evaporation, convection, conduction, and radiation. (See Chapter 21 for types of thermoregulation.) Heat loss at birth that leads to cold stress can play a significant role in the severity of RDS and the ultimate outcome for the infant.

The amount of heat an infant loses depends to a large extent on the actions of the nurse or caregiver. Both preterm and SGA newborns are at risk for cold stress because they have decreased adipose tissue, brown fat stores, and glycogen available for metabolism.

As discussed in Chapter 21, the newborn infant's major source of heat production in nonshivering thermogenesis (NST) is brown fat metabolism. The ability of an infant to respond to cold stress by NST is impaired in the presence of several conditions:

- Hypoxemia ($PO_2$ less than 50 torr)
- Intracranial hemorrhage or any CNS abnormality
- Hypoglycemia (blood glucose level <40 mg/dL)

When these conditions occur, the infant's temperature should be monitored closely and the neutral thermal environment conscientiously maintained. It is important for the nurse to recognize these conditions and treat them as soon as possible. The metabolic consequences of cold stress can be devastating and potentially fatal to an infant. Oxygen requirements rise, glucose use increases, acids are released into the bloodstream, and surfactant production decreases. The effects are graphically depicted in Figure 26–8♦.

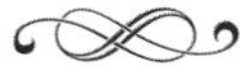

## Nursing Care Management

The nurse observes the baby for signs of cold stress, including increased movement and respirations, decreased skin temperature and peripheral perfusion, development of hypoglycemia, and possibly development of metabolic acidosis.

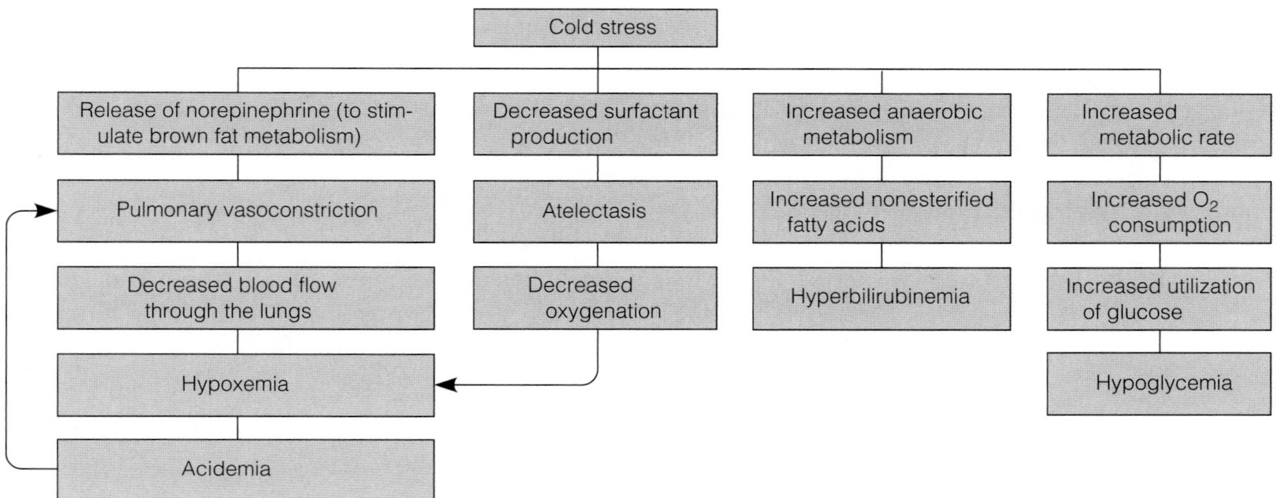


**FIGURE 26–8** ♦ Cold stress chain of events. The hypothermic, or cold-stressed, newborn attempts to compensate by conserving heat and increasing heat production. These physiologic compensatory mechanisms initiate a series of metabolic events that result in hypoxemia and altered surfactant production, metabolic acidosis, hypoglycemia, and hyperbilirubinemia.

Skin temperature assessments are used because initial response to cold stress is vasoconstriction, resulting in a decrease in skin temperature. Therefore, monitoring rectal temperature is not satisfactory. A decrease in rectal temperature means that the infant has long-standing cold stress, with decompensation in the newborn's ability to maintain core body temperature.

If a decrease in skin temperature is noted, the nurse determines whether hypoglycemia is present. Hypoglycemia is a result of the metabolic effects of cold stress and is suggested by glucometer values below 45 mg/dL, tremors, irritability or lethargy, apnea, or seizure activity.

If hypothermia occurs, the nurse initiates the following care plan ("Neonatal Thermoregulation," 1997):

- Keep the ambient air temperature 1 to 1.5°C higher than the infant's temperature.
- Warm the newborn slowly because rapid temperature elevation may cause hypotension and apnea.
- Increase the air temperature in hourly increments of 1°C until infant's temperature is stable.
- Monitor skin temperature every 15 to 30 minutes to determine if the newborn's temperature is increasing.
- Remove plastic wrap, caps, and heat shields while rewarming the infant so that cool air is not trapped along with the warm air.
- Warm intravenous fluids prior to infusion.
- Initiate efforts to block heat loss by evaporation, radiation, convection, and conduction and maintain the newborn in a neutral thermal environment.

The nurse assesses for the presence of anaerobic metabolism and initiates interventions for the resulting metabolic acidosis. Attempts to burn brown fat increase oxygen consumption, lactic acid levels, and metabolic acidosis. Hypoglycemia may be reversed by adequate glucose intake, as described in the following section.

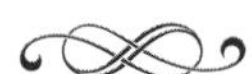

# Care of the Newborn with Hypoglycemia

A widely used cutoff point or threshold for intervention in newborn **hypoglycemia** is a *plasma glucose concentration* of 40 mg/dL (Cornblath, Hawdon, Williams, et al., 2000). Plasma glucose values <20 to 25 mg/dL should be treated with parenteral glucose, regardless of the age or gestation. Hypoglycemia is the most common metabolic disorder occurring in IDMs, SGA infants, and preterm AGA infants. The pathophysiology of hypoglycemia differs for each classification.

AGA preterm infants have not been in utero a sufficient time to store glycogen and fat. As a result, they have decreased ability to carry out gluconeogenesis. This situation is further aggravated by increased use of glucose by the tissues (especially the brain and heart) during stress and illness (chilling, asphyxia, sepsis, RDS).

Infants of White's Classes A–C or type I diabetic mothers have increased stores of glycogen and fat (see Chapter 25) and higher circulating insulin and insulin responsiveness levels than other newborns. Because the high in utero glucose loads stop at birth, the newborn experiences rapid and profound hypoglycemia (Ogata, 1999). The SGA infant has used up glycogen and fat stores because of intrauterine malnutrition and has a blunted hepatic enzymatic response with which to produce and use glucose. Any newborn who is stressed at birth (from asphyxia or cold) also quickly uses up available glucose stores and becomes hypoglycemic. In addition, epidural anesthesia may alter maternal-fetal glucose homeostasis, resulting in hypoglycemia.

## Clinical Therapy

The goal of management includes early identification of hypoglycemia through observation and screening of newborns at risk. The newborn may be asymptomatic, or any of the following may occur:

- Lethargy, jitteriness
- Poor feeding
- Vomiting
- Pallor
- Apnea, irregular respirations, respiratory distress, cyanosis
- Hypotonia, possible loss of swallowing reflex
- Tremors, jerkiness, seizure activity
- High-pitched cry

Differential diagnosis of a newborn with nonspecific hypoglycemic symptoms includes determining if the newborn has any of the following:

- (CNS) disease
- Sepsis
- Metabolic aberrations
- Polycythemia
- Congenital heart disease
- Drug withdrawal
- Temperature instability
- Hypocalcemia

Aggressive treatment is recommended after a single low blood glucose value if the infant shows any of these symptoms. In at-risk infants, routine screening should be done frequently during the first 4 hours of life and then at 4-hour intervals until the risk period has passed (Ogata, 1999) or whenever any of the noted clinical manifestations appear.

Hypoglycemia may also be defined as a glucose oxidase reagent strip below 45 mg/dL, but only when corroborated with laboratory plasma glucose testing (see Procedure 26–1). Bedside glucose oxidase strip tests may be used for screening for hypoglycemia, but laboratory determinations must confirm the results before a diagnosis of hypoglycemia can be made. Glucose reagent strips should not be used by themselves to screen for and diagnose hypoglycemia, because their results depend on the baby's hematocrit and there is a wide variance (5 to 15 mg/dL) between their results and laboratory plasma determinations.

## HINTS FOR PRACTICE

Wrapping the foot in a warm washcloth or disposable diaper is a simple way to create adequate vasodilation for obtaining a blood specimen.

Blood glucose sampling techniques can significantly affect the accuracy of the blood glucose value. Common bedside methods use *whole* blood, an enzymatic reagent strip, and a reflectance meter or color chart. It is important to note that whole blood glucose concentrations are 10% to 15% lower than plasma glucose concentrations. The higher the hematocrit, the greater the difference between whole blood and plasma values. Also, venous blood glucose concentrations are approximately 15% to 19% lower than arterial blood glucose concentrations because the tissues extract some glucose before the blood enters the venous system ("Neonatal Hypoglycemia," 2000). Newer techniques, such as using a glucose oxidase analyzer or an optical bedside glucose analyzer, are more reliable for bedside screening but must also be validated with laboratory chemical analysis.

Adequate caloric intake is important. Early formula feeding or breastfeeding is one of the major preventive approaches. If early feeding meets the recommended fluid and caloric needs, the blood glucose concentration is likely to remain above the hypoglycemic level. During the first hours after birth, asymptomatic newborns may also be given oral glucose. Another plasma glucose measurement is then obtained within 30 to 60 minutes after feeding. For at-risk newborns who are feeding, blood sampling should be done before feeding.

## HINTS FOR PRACTICE

Blood samples for the laboratory should be placed on ice and analyzed within 30 minutes of drawing to prevent continued metabolism of glucose by the red blood cells.

Intravenous infusions of a dextrose solution (5% to 10%) begun immediately after birth also should prevent hypoglycemia. Plasma glucose levels are obtained when the parenteral infusion is started. However, in the very small AGA infant, infusions of 10% dextrose solution may cause *hyperglycemia* to develop, requiring an alteration in the glucose concentration. Infants require 6 to 8 mg/kg/min of glucose to maintain normal glucose concentrations. Therefore, an intravenous glucose solution should be calculated based on the infant's body weight, with blood glucose tests to determine adequacy of the infusion treatment.

A rapid infusion of 25% to 50% dextrose is contraindicated because it may lead to profound rebound hypoglycemia following an initial brief increase. In prolonged hypoglycemic periods, corticosteroids may be administered. It is thought that steroids enhance gluconeogenesis from noncarbohydrate protein sources (Ogata, 1999). The untreated hypoglycemia may result in permanent, untreatable CNS damage or death.

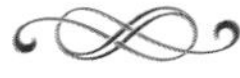

## NURSING CARE MANAGEMENT

### Nursing Assessment and Diagnosis

The objectives of nursing assessment are to identify newborns at risk and to screen symptomatic infants. For newborns diagnosed with hypoglycemia, assessment is ongoing and includes careful monitoring of glucose values. In addition, urine dipstick and urine volume tests (monitor only if above 1 to 3 mL/kg/hr) may be evaluated frequently for osmotic diuresis and glycosuria. Nursing diagnoses that may apply to the newborn with hypoglycemia include the following:

- ***Altered nutrition: less than body requirements*** related to increased glucose use secondary to physiologic stress

# Procedure 26–1 Performing a Heel Stick on a Newborn

| *Nursing Action* | *Rationale* |
|---|---|
| **Objective: Assemble the equipment.**<br>• Microlancet (do not use a needle)<br>• Alcohol swabs<br>• 2 × 2 sterile gauze squares<br>• Small bandage<br>• Transfer pipette<br>• Glucose reagent strips or reflectance meters | *Equipment organization facilitates the procedure. A needle may nick the periosteum.* |
| • Gloves | *Gloves are used to implement universal precautions and prevent nosocomial infections.* |
| **Objective: Prepare the infant's heel for the procedure.**<br>• Use a warm, wet wrap or specially designed chemical heat pad to warm the infant's heel for 5–10 seconds to facilitate blood flow. | |
| • Select a clear, previously unpunctured site.<br>• Clean the site by rubbing vigorously with 70% isopropyl alcohol swab, followed by a dry gauze square.<br>• Blot the site dry completely before lancing. | *The selection of a previously unpunctured site minimizes the risk of infection and excessive scar formation. Friction produces local heat, which aids vasodilation. Alcohol is irritating to injured tissue, and it may also produce hemolysis.* |
| **Objective: Lance the infant's heel and ensure accurate blood sampling. See the step-by-step instructions that follow.** | |
| **Objective: Prevent excessive bleeding.**<br>• Apply a folded gauze square to the puncture site and secure it firmly with a bandage.<br>• Check the puncture site frequently for the first hour after sampling. | |
| **Objective: Record the findings on the infant's chart.**<br>Report immediately any results under 45 mg/dL or over 175 mg/dL for glucose. | *Recording the results helps identify possible complications.* |

**Performing the Heel Stick**

The infant's lateral heel is the site of choice because it precludes damaging the posterior tibial nerve and artery, plantar artery, and the important longitudinally oriented fat pad of the heel, which in later years could impede walking (Figure 26–9♦). This is especially important for infants undergoing multiple heel stick procedures. Toes are acceptable sites if necessary.

Lancing the Heel

- Grasp the infant's lower leg and foot so as to impede venous return slightly. This will facilitate extraction of the blood sample.
- With a quick, piercing motion, puncture the lateral heel with a microlancet. Be careful not to puncture too deeply. Optimal penetration is 4 mm (Figure 26–10♦).

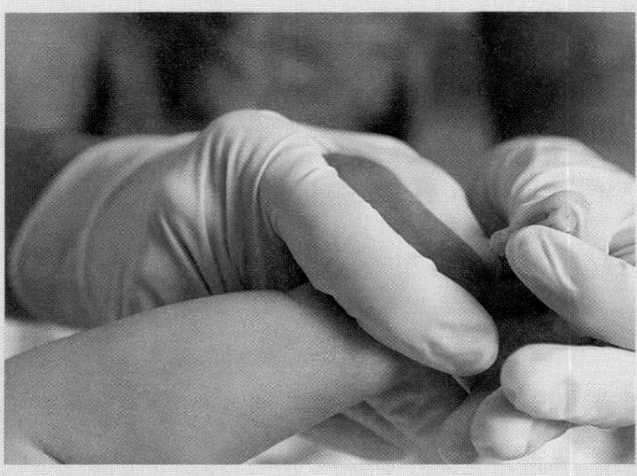

FIGURE 26–9 ♦ Heel sticks.

# Procedure 26–1 Performing a Heel Stick on a Newborn

*continued*

*Collecting the Blood Sample*

- Use transfer pipette to place drop of blood on glucose reflectance meter.
- Use capillary tube for hematocrit testing.

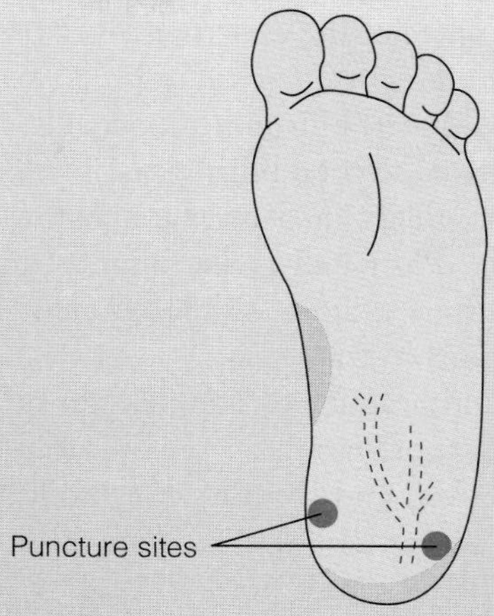


FIGURE 26–10 ♦ Potential sites for heel sticks. Avoid shaded areas to prevent injury to arteries and nerves in the foot.

- ***Ineffective breathing pattern*** related to tachypnea and apnea
- ***Pain*** related to frequent heel sticks secondary to glucose monitoring

## Nursing Plan and Implementation

Infants in at-risk groups should be monitored no later than 2 hours after birth and before feedings or whenever there are abnormal signs (Cornblath et al., 2000). The IDM should be monitored within 30 minutes of birth. Once an at-risk infant's blood sugar level is stable, glucose testing every 2 to 4 hours (or per agency protocol), or prior to feedings, adequately monitors glucose levels.

Calculating glucose requirements and maintaining intravenous glucose are necessary for any symptomatic infant with low serum glucose levels. Careful attention to glucose monitoring is again required during the transition from intravenous to oral feedings. Titration of intravenous glucose may be required until the infant is able to take adequate amounts of formula or breast milk to maintain a normal blood sugar level. This titration is accomplished by decreasing the concentration of parenteral glucose gradually to 5%, then reducing the rate of infusion to 6 mg/kg/min, then to 4 mg/kg/min, and slowly discontinuing it over 4 to 6 hours.

The method of feeding greatly influences glucose and energy requirements. In addition, the therapeutic nursing measure of nonnutritive sucking during gavage feedings has been reported to increase the baby's daily weight gain and lead to earlier bottle-feeding or breastfeeding and discharge. Nonnutritive sucking may also lower activity levels, which allows newborns to conserve their energy stores. Activity can increase energy requirements; crying alone can double the baby's metabolic rate. Establishment and maintenance of a neutral thermal environment have a potent influence on the newborn's metabolism. The nurse pays careful attention to environmental conditions, physical activity, and organization of care and integrates these factors into delivery of nursing care. The nurse identifies any discrepancies between the baby's caloric requirements and received calories and weighs the newborn daily at consistent times, preferably before a feeding. Only then can findings of unusual losses or gains, as well as the pattern of weight gain, be considered reliable.

## Evaluation

Expected outcomes of nursing care include the following:

- The risk of hypoglycemia is promptly identified, and intervention is started early.
- The newborn's metabolic and physiologic processes are stabilized, and recovery is proceeding without sequelae.

## Care of the Newborn with Jaundice

The most common abnormal physical finding in newborns is **jaundice.** Jaundice is a yellowish coloration of the skin and sclera of the eyes that develops from deposit of the yellow pigment *bilirubin* in lipid tissues. Fetal unconjugated (indirect) bilirubin is normally cleared by the placenta in utero, so total bilirubin at birth is usually less than 3 mg/dL unless an abnormal hemolytic process has been present. Postnatally, the infant must conjugate bilirubin (convert a lipid-soluble pigment into a water-soluble pigment) in the liver.

The rate and amount of conjugation of bilirubin depend on the rate of hemolysis, the bilirubin load, the maturity of the liver, and the presence of albumin-binding sites. (See Chapter 21 for discussion of conjugation of bilirubin.) The liver of a normal, healthy term infant is usually mature enough and producing enough glucuronyl transferase that the total serum bilirubin does not reach a pathologic level. However, physiologic jaundice remains a common problem for the term newborn and may require treatment with phototherapy. Physiologic jaundice is due to the newborn's shorter red cell life span, slower uptake by the liver, lack of intestinal bacteria, and poorly established hydration.

### Pathophysiology

Serum albumin-binding sites are usually sufficient to meet the normal demands of the newborn. However, certain conditions tend to decrease the sites available. Fetal or neonatal asphyxia and neonatal drugs such as indomethacin decrease the binding affinity of bilirubin to albumin, because acidosis impairs the capacity of albumin to hold bilirubin. Hypothermia and hypoglycemia release free fatty acids that dislocate bilirubin from albumin. Also, premature infants have less albumin available for binding with bilirubin. Maternal use of sulfa drugs or salicylates interferes with conjugation or with serum albumin-binding sites by competing with bilirubin for these sites.

Although the exact mechanism of bilirubin-produced neuronal injury is uncertain, it is known that high concentrations of total bilirubin can be neurotoxic. Unconjugated bilirubin has a high affinity for extravascular tissue, such as fatty tissue (subcutaneous tissue) and the brain. Bilirubin not bound to albumin can cross the blood-brain barrier, damage cells of the CNS, and produce kernicterus or bilirubin encephalopathy. **Kernicterus** (meaning "yellow nucleus") refers to the deposition of indirect or unconjugated bilirubin in the basal ganglia of the brain and to the permanent neurologic sequelae of untreated hyperbilirubinemia. The classic bilirubin encephalopathy of kernicterus most commonly found with Rh and ABO blood group incompatibility is less common today due to aggressive treatment with phototherapy and exchange transfusions. But cases of kernicterus are reappearing as a result of early discharge and the increased incidence of dehydration (as a result of discharge before the mother's milk is established).

### Causes of Hyperbilirubinemia

A primary cause of **hyperbilirubinemia** (elevation of bilirubin level) is **hemolytic disease of the newborn** secondary to Rh incompatibility. All pregnant women who are Rh negative or who have blood type O (possible ABO blood incompatibility) should be asked about outcomes of any previous pregnancies and history of blood transfusion. Prenatal amniocentesis with spectrophotographic examination may be indicated in some cases. Cord blood from newborns is evaluated for bilirubin level, which should not exceed 5 mg/dL. Newborns of Rh-negative and O blood type mothers are carefully assessed for appearance of jaundice and levels of serum bilirubin.

Isoimmune hemolytic disease, also known as **erythroblastosis fetalis,** occurs when an Rh-negative mother is pregnant with an Rh-positive fetus and transplacental passage of maternal antibodies takes place. Maternal antibodies enter the fetal circulation, then attach to and destroy the fetal red blood cells (RBCs). The fetal system responds by increasing RBC production. Jaundice, anemia, and compensatory erythropoiesis result. A marked increase in immature RBCs (erythroblasts) also occurs, hence the designation erythroblastosis fetalis.

**Hydrops fetalis,** the most severe form of erythroblastosis fetalis, occurs when maternal antibodies attach to the Rh site on the fetal RBCs, making them susceptible to destruction; severe anemia and multiorgan system failure result. Cardiomegaly with severe cardiac decompensation and hepatosplenomegaly occurs. Severe generalized massive edema (*anasarca*) and generalized fluid effusion into the pleural cavity (hydrothorax), pericardial sac, and peritoneal cavity (ascites) develop. Jaundice is not present initially because the bilirubin pigments are excreted through the placenta into the maternal circulation. The hydropic hemolytic disease process is also characterized by hyperplasia of the pancreatic islets, which predisposes the infant to neonatal hypoglycemia similar to that of IDMs. In addition, these infants have increased bleeding tendencies due to associated thrombocytopenia and hypoxic damage to the capillaries. Hydrops is a frequent cause of intrauterine death among infants with Rh disease.

ABO incompatibility (the mother is blood type O and the baby is blood type A or B) may result in jaundice, although it rarely results in hemolytic disease severe enough to be clinically diagnosed and treated. Hepatosplenomegaly may be found occasionally in newborns with ABO incompatibility, but hydrops fetalis and stillbirth are rare.

Certain prenatal and perinatal factors predispose the newborn to hyperbilirubinemia. During pregnancy, maternal conditions that predispose the fetus to neonatal hyperbilirubinemia include hereditary spherocytosis, diabetes, intrauterine infections, and gram-negative bacilli infections that stimulate production of maternal isoimmune antibodies, drug ingestion (such as sulfas, salicylates, novobiocin, diazepam), and oxytocin.

In addition to Rh or ABO incompatibility, other conditions predispose the newborn to hyperbilirubinemia: polycythemia (central hematocrit 65% or more), pyloric stenosis, obstruction or atresia of the biliary duct or of the lower bowel, low-grade urinary tract infection, sepsis, hypothyroidism, enclosed hemorrhage (cephalhematoma, large bruises), asphyxia neonatorum, hypothermia, acidemia, and hypoglycemia. Neonatal hepatitis, atresia of the bile ducts, and gastrointestinal atresia all can alter bilirubin metabolism and excretion.

The prognosis for a newborn with hyperbilirubinemia depends on the extent of the hemolytic process and the underlying cause. Severe hemolytic disease results in fetal and early neonatal death from the effects of severe anemia—cardiac decompensation, edema, ascites, and hydrothorax. Hyperbilirubinemia that is not aggressively treated may lead to kernicterus. The resultant neurologic damage is responsible for death, cerebral palsy, possible mental retardation, or hearing loss or, to a lesser degree, perceptual impairment, delayed speech development, hyperactivity, muscle incoordination, or learning difficulties.

## Clinical Therapy

Early prenatal identification of the fetus at risk for Rh or ABO incompatibility allows prompt treatment. (See Chapter 13 for discussion of in utero management of this condition.) When one or more of the predisposing factors for jaundice is present, the maternal and neonatal blood types should be tested in the laboratory for Rh or ABO incompatibility. Other necessary laboratory evaluations are Coombs' test, serum bilirubin levels (direct and total), hemoglobin, reticulocyte percentage, white cell count, and positive smear for cellular morphology.

Neonatal hyperbilirubinemia must be considered pathologic if any of the following criteria are met (MacMahon, Stevenson, & Oski, 1998):

1. Clinically evident jaundice in the first 24 hours of life, or after the fourth day of life, unless the infant is premature
2. Serum bilirubin concentration rising by more than 5 mg/dL/day
3. Total serum bilirubin concentrations exceeding 12.9 mg/dL in term infants or 15 mg/dL in preterm babies (because preterm newborns have less subcutaneous fat, bilirubin may reach higher levels before it is visible)
4. Conjugated bilirubin concentrations greater than 2 mg/dL
5. Persistence of clinical jaundice beyond 7 days in term infants or beyond 14 days in preterm infants

Initial diagnostic procedures are aimed at differentiating jaundice resulting from increased bilirubin production, impaired conjugation or excretion, increased intestinal reabsorption, or a combination of these factors. The Coombs' test is performed to determine whether jaundice is due to Rh or ABO incompatibility.

If the hemolytic process is due to Rh sensitization, laboratory findings reveal the following: (1) an Rh-positive neonate with a positive Coombs' test; (2) increased erythropoiesis with many immature circulating red blood cells (nucleated blastocysts); (3) anemia, in most cases; (4) elevated levels (5 mg/dL or more) of bilirubin in cord blood; and (5) a reduction in albumin-binding capacity. Maternal data may include an elevated anti-Rh titer and spectrophotometric evidence of a fetal hemolytic process.

The indirect Coombs' test measures the amount of Rh-positive antibodies in the mother's blood. Rh-positive red blood cells are added to the maternal blood sample. If the mother's serum contains antibodies, the Rh-positive red blood cells will agglutinate (clump) when rabbit immune antiglobulin is added, which is a positive test result.

The direct Coombs' test reveals the presence of antibody-coated (sensitized) Rh-positive red blood cells in the newborn. Rabbit immune antiglobulin is added to the specimen of neonatal blood cells. If the neonatal red blood cells agglutinate, they have been coated with maternal antibodies, a positive result.

If the hemolytic process is due to ABO incompatibility, laboratory findings reveal an increase in reticulocytes. The resulting anemia is usually not significant during the newborn period and is rare later on. The direct Coombs' test may be negative or mildly positive, whereas the indirect Coombs' test may be strongly positive. Infants with a positive direct Coombs' test have increased incidence of jaundice, with bilirubin levels in excess of 10 mg/dL. Increased numbers of spherocytes (spherical, plump, mature erythrocytes) are seen on a peripheral blood smear. Increased numbers of spherocytes are not seen on blood smears from infants with Rh disease.

Regardless of the cause of hyperbilirubinemia, treatment is directed toward preventing bilirubin toxic effects. Although kernicterus is rare, there is evidence that healthy term infants are at risk. Early discharge of newborns from birthing centers has significantly influenced the diagnosis and management of neonatal jaundice, increasing the emphasis on outpatient and home care management. All infants discharged before 48 hours after birth should be followed up by a health care practitioner within 2 to 3 days of discharge for assessment of jaundice (AAP, Provisional Committee for Quality Improvement and Subcommittee on Hyperbilirubinemia, 1994).

Therapeutic management of hyperbilirubinemia includes phototherapy, exchange transfusion, infusion of albumin, and drug therapy. If hemolytic disease is present, it may be treated with phototherapy, exchange transfusion, and drug therapy. When determining the appropriate management of hyperbilirubinemia due to hemolytic disease, the three relevant variables are the newborn's (1) serum bilirubin level, (2) birth weight, and (3) age in hours. If a newborn has hemolysis with an unconjugated bilirubin level of 14 mg/dL, weighs less than 2500 g (birth weight), and is 24 hours old or less, an exchange transfusion may be the best management. However, if that same newborn is over 24 hours of age, which is past the time during which an increase in bilirubin would occur due to pathologic causes, phototherapy may be the treatment of choice to prevent the possible complication of kernicterus.

## PHOTOTHERAPY

**Phototherapy** is the exposure of the newborn to high-intensity light. It may be used alone or in conjunction with exchange transfusion to reduce serum bilirubin levels. Exposure of the newborn to high-intensity light (a bank of fluorescent lightbulbs or bulbs in the blue-light spectrum) decreases serum bilirubin levels in the skin by facilitating biliary excretion of unconjugated bilirubin. When the light is absorbed by the tissue, unconjugated bilirubin is converted into two isomers, called photobilirubin. The photobilirubin moves from the tissues to the blood by a diffusion mechanism. In the blood it is bound to albumin and transported to the liver. It moves into the bile and is excreted into the duodenum for removal with feces without requiring conjugation by the liver. In addition, the photodegradation products formed when light oxidizes bilirubin can be excreted in the urine.

Phototherapy plays an important role in preventing a rise in bilirubin levels but does not alter the underlying cause of jaundice, and hemolysis may continue to produce anemia. It is generally accepted that phototherapy should be started at 4 to 5 mg/dL below the calculated exchange level for each infant (see Table 26–3). Sick newborns of less than 1000 g should have phototherapy instituted at a bilirubin concentration of 5 mg/dL. Many authors have recommended initiating phototherapy "prophylactically" in the first 24 hours of life in high-risk, very-low-birth-weight infants. Sick preterm infants who are at least 1500 g should have phototherapy instituted when the bilirubin level is 10 mg/dL. Any newborn with a bilirubin level of 20 mg/dL or above may need an exchange transfusion if illness or associated conditions are present (Maisels, 1999).

Phototherapy can be provided by banks of phototherapy lights, by a fiber-optic blanket attached to a halogen light source around the trunk of the newborn, or by a combination of both delivery methods (AAP, Provisional Committee for Quality Improvement and Subcommittee on Hyperbilirubinemia, 1994).

**TABLE 26–3 American Academy of Pediatric Guidelines for the Management of Hyperbilirubinemia in the Healthy Term Newborn**

| | Total Serum Bilirubin Level, mg/dL (μmol/L) | | | |
|---|---|---|---|---|
| *Age (hours)* | *Consider Phototherapy** | *Phototherapy* | *Exchange Transfusion if Intensive Phototherapy Fails†* | *Exchange Transfusion and Intensive Phototherapy* |
| 25–48‡ | ≥12 (170) | ≥15 (260) | ≥20 (340) | ≥25 (430) |
| 49–72 | ≥15 (260) | ≥18 (310) | ≥25 (430) | ≥30 (510) |
| >72 | ≥17 (290) | ≥20 (340) | ≥25 (430) | ≥30 (510) |

*Phototherapy at these total serum bilirubin (TSB) levels is a clinical option, meaning that the intervention is available and may be used on the basis of individual clinical judgment.

†Intensive phototherapy should produce a decline of TSB of 1 to 2 mg/dL within 4 to 6 hours, and the TSB level should continue to decline and remain below the threshold level for exchange transfusion. If this does not occur, phototherapy has failed. Intensive phototherapy includes the use of more than one bank of lamps containing "special blue" bulbs, maximizing the surface area illuminated by using a phototherapy blanket or other means, and providing phototherapy on a continuous, noninterrupted schedule.

‡Term infants who are clinically jaundiced at ≤24 hours old are not considered healthy and require further evaluation.

*Source:* Used with permission of the American Academy of Pediatrics. (1994). Practice parameter: Management of hyperbilirubinemia in the healthy term newborn. *Pediatrics, 94,* 560.

With the fiber-optic blanket, the light stays on at all times, and the newborn is accessible for care, feeding, and diaper changes. The eyes are not covered. The babies do not get overheated, and fluid and weight loss are not complications of this system. Furthermore, it makes the infant accessible to the parents and is less alarming to parents than standard phototherapy (Thureen, Deacon, O'Neill, et al., 1999). Many institutions and pediatricians use fiber-optic blankets for home care. A combination of a fiber-optic light source in the mattress under the baby and a standard light source above has also been recommended (MacMahon et al., 1998).

#### Exchange Transfusion

Exchange transfusion is the withdrawal and replacement of the newborn's blood with donor blood. It is used to treat anemia with red blood cells that are susceptible to maternal antibodies, remove sensitized red blood cells that would by lysed soon, remove serum bilirubin, and provide bilirubin-free albumin and increase the binding sites for bilirubin. Concerns about exchange transfusion are related to the use of blood products and associated potential for HIV infection and hepatitis.

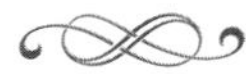

## Nursing Care Management

### Nursing Assessment and Diagnosis

Assessment is aimed at identifying prenatal and perinatal factors that predispose the newborn to the development of jaundice and at recognizing the jaundice as soon as it is apparent. Clinically, ABO incompatibility presents as jaundice and occasionally as hepatosplenomegaly. Fetal hydrops or erythroblastosis is rare (see Chapter 13). Hemolytic disease of the newborn is suspected if the placenta is enlarged; if the newborn is edematous, with pleural and pericardial effusion plus ascites; if pallor or jaundice is noted during the first 24 to 36 hours; if hemolytic anemia is diagnosed; or if the spleen and liver are enlarged. The nurse carefully notes changes in behavior and observes for evidence of bleeding. If laboratory tests indicate elevated bilirubin levels, the nurse checks the newborn for jaundice about every 2 hours and records observations.

To check for jaundice in lighter-skinned babies, the nurse blanches the skin over a bony prominence (forehead, nose, sternum) by pressing firmly with the thumb. After pressure is released, if jaundice is present, the area appears yellow before normal color returns. The nurse checks oral mucosa and the posterior portion of the hard palate and conjunctival sacs for yellow pigmentation in darker-skinned babies. Assessment in daylight gives the best results, because pink walls and surroundings may mask yellowish tints and yellow light makes differentiation of jaundice difficult. The time at onset of jaundice is recorded and reported. If jaundice appears, careful observation of the increase in depth of color and of the newborn's behavior is mandatory.

The nurse assesses the newborn's behavior for neurologic signs associated with hyperbilirubinemia, which are rare but may include hypotonia, diminished reflexes, lethargy, or seizures.

Nursing diagnoses that may apply to care of a newborn with jaundice include the following:

- ***Fluid volume deficit*** related to increased insensible water loss and frequent loose stools
- ***Sensory-perceptual alterations*** related to neurologic damage secondary to kernicterus
- ***Risk for altered parenting*** related to parenting a newborn with jaundice

### Nursing Plan and Implementation

#### *Hospital-Based Nursing Care*

Hospital-based care is described in the Critical Pathway for Care of a Newborn with Hyperbilirubinemia, on pages 707–708. If phototherapy lights are used, the nurse exposes the entire skin surface of the newborn to the light. Minimal covering may be applied over the genitals and buttocks to expose maximum skin surface while still protecting the bedding from soiling. Phototherapy success is measured every 12 hours or with daily serum bilirubin levels. The nurse must turn lights off while blood is drawn to ensure accurate serum bilirubin levels. Because it is not known if phototherapy injures the delicate eye structures, particularly the retina, the nurse applies eye patches over the newborn's closed eyes during exposure to banks of phototherapy lights (see Figure 26–11♦). Phototherapy is discontinued and the eye patches are removed at least once per shift to assess the eyes for conjunctivitis. Patches are also removed to allow eye contact during feeding (social stimulation) or when parents are visiting (to promote parental attachment).

### Hints for Practice

If the area of jaundice around the eyes begins to disappear, then the eye patches are allowing light to enter and better eye protection is needed.

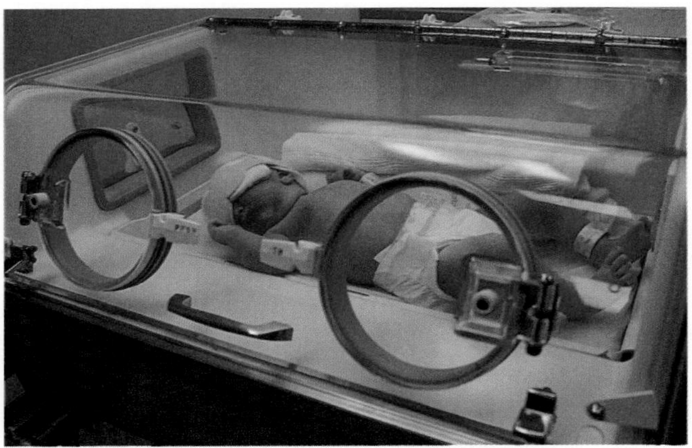

**FIGURE 26–11** ♦ Infant receiving phototherapy. The phototherapy light is positioned over the incubator. Bilateral eye patches are always used to protect the baby's eyes during phototherapy.

**TABLE 26–4 Instructional Checklist for In-Room Phototherapy**

Explain and demonstrate the placement of eye patches and explain that they must be in place when the infant is under the lights.

Explain the clothing to be worn (diaper under lights, dress and wrap when away from the lights).

Explain the importance of taking the infant's temperature regularly.

Explain the importance of adequate fluid intake.

Explain the charting flow sheet (intake, output, eyes covered).

Explain how to position the lights at a proper distance.

Explain the need to keep the infant under phototherapy except during feeding and diaper changes.

Most phototherapy units provide the desired level of irradiance with the infant 45 to 50 cm below the lamps. The nurse uses a photometer to measure and maintain desired irradiance levels. Disadvantages of lights are that they create a difficult environment in which to work and can distort an infant's color.

The nurse monitors the newborn's temperature to prevent hyperthermia and hypothermia. The newborn requires additional fluids to compensate for the increased water lost through the skin and loose stools. Loose stools and increased urine output are the results of increased bilirubin excretion. The infant is observed for signs of dehydration and perianal excoriation.

A benign transient bronze discoloration of the skin may occur with phototherapy when the infant has elevated direct serum bilirubin levels or liver disease. As a side effect of phototherapy, some newborns develop a maculopapular rash. In addition to assessing the newborn's skin color for jaundice and bronzing, the nurse examines the skin for developing pressure areas. The newborn should be repositioned at least every 2 hours to permit the light to reach all skin surfaces, to prevent pressure areas, and to vary the stimulation to the infant. The nurse keeps track of the number of hours each lamp is used so that it can be replaced before its effectiveness is lost. The nurse must be careful about using ointment under bilirubin lights because this combination may cause burns.

The terms *jaundice, hyperbilirubinemia, exchange transfusion,* and *phototherapy* may sound frightening and threatening. Some parents may feel guilty about their baby's condition and think they have caused the problem. Under stress, parents may not be able to understand the physician's first explanations. The nurse anticipates that the parents will need explanations repeated and clarified and that they may need help in voicing their questions and fears. Eye and tactile contact with the newborn is encouraged. The nurse can coach parents when they visit with the baby. After the mother's discharge, parents are kept informed of their infant's condition and are encouraged to return to the hospital or telephone at any time so that they can be fully involved in the care of their infant. Parents are advised that after discontinuation of phototherapy, a rebound of 1 to 2 mg/dL can be expected and a follow-up bilirubin test may be done.

While the mother is still hospitalized, phototherapy can also be carried out in the parents' room if the only problem is hyperbilirubinemia. The parents must be willing to keep the baby in the room for 24 hours a day, be able to take emergency action (eg, for choking) if necessary, and complete instruction checklists. Some institutions require that parents sign a consent form. The nurse instruct the parents but also continues to monitor the infant's temperature, activity, intake and output, and positioning of eye patches at regular intervals (Table 26–4).

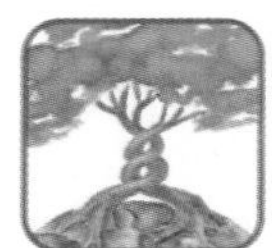

## Community-Based Nursing Care

If the baby is to receive phototherapy at home, the nurse teaches the parents to record the infant's temperature, weight, fluid intake and output, stools, and feedings and to use the phototherapy equipment. In addition, if phototherapy lights are being used, parents must agree that the baby will be exposed to the lights for long periods of time; that they will hold the baby for only short periods for feeding, comforting, and cleansing of the perineal area; and that the room temperature will be regulated to minimize heat loss. Fiber-optic phototherapy blankets eliminate the need for eye patches, decrease heat loss because the baby is clothed, and provide more opportunities for interaction between the baby and parents. The best method of home

# CRITICAL PATHWAY: *For Care of a Newborn with Hyperbilirubinemia*

| Category | Day 1 | Day 2/Discharge |
|---|---|---|
| **Referral** | Refer to lactation consultant | **Expected Outcomes**<br>Consults completed |
| **Assessments** | Lab work (CBC, Rh, Coombs' direct, retic count, bilirubin level, both direct and indirect)<br>Hearing test if bilirubin >18<br>Obtain maternal/paternal history<br>Obtain birth and newborn history<br>Assess sclera and skin color for jaundice; assess mucous membranes for jaundice with dark pigmented skin<br>Continue routine newborn assessments (see Newborn Critical Pathway, pages 73 to 74) | Bilirubin levels as ordered BID<br>Assess for s/s dehydration<br>Assess sclera and skin color for progression of jaundice<br>**Expected Outcomes**<br>Physical assessments, VS WNL; skin/mucous membranes pink, sclera clear of jaundice color; laboratory work WNL, total bilirubin level stabilized or decreasing |
| **Teaching/ psychosocial** | Evaluate additional psychosocial needs of parents/family<br>Orient family to nursery, equipment, patient room if rooming-in<br>Instruct parents on s/s of hyperbilirubinemia (slight lethargy, irritability)<br>Discuss possible side effects of phototherapy (stool character changes, increased fluid loss, temp changes, rash, altered sleep-wake patterns)<br>Instruct parents on care and treatment of hyperbilirubinemia:<br>• Phototherapy rationale, indications, and precautions<br>• Placement of bili mask over closed eyes<br>• Lab draws: rationale, frequency<br>• Accurate intake and output to monitor for s/s dehydration<br>Review cord care, skin care, care of genitalia (circumcision care as applicable)<br>Review role of pumping breasts if necessary and offering formula for limited period of time | Teach/encourage parents to provide cuddling, tactile stimulation, and eye contact during diaper changes and feedings, talk to baby frequently<br>Reinforce previous teaching; evaluate parental comprehension<br>Provide opportunities for parents to express concerns/feelings<br>**Expected Outcomes**<br>Parents verbalize comprehension of care of infant with hyperbilirubinemia and potential sequelae of no treatment; parents verbalize comprehension of the risks/benefits of phototherapy as treatment; parents demonstrate developmentally appropriate care for infant during diaper changes and feedings; parents verbalize concerns, ask appropriate questions prn |
| **Nursing care management and reports** | Vital signs q4h with axillary temps<br>Monitor thermoregulation<br>Daily wt<br>Initiate phototherapy as indicated and ordered<br>• Maintain bili mask over eyes<br>• Keep genitalia covered per policy<br>• Check eyes for discharge, excessive pressure, corneal abrasions<br>• Expose as much skin surface as possible to bili lights<br>• Bilimeter reading q shift<br>• No lotion or ointment on infant skin<br>• Turn bili lights off during lab draws<br>Continue infant assessments including<br>• Note and document skin color q shift<br>• Thorough skin care with diaper changes; note s/s breakdown, rash<br>• Assess neuro status for s/s abnormality q interaction (hypotonia, lethargy, poor sucking reflex) | VS q4h with axillary temps<br>Monitor thermoregulation, maintain NTE<br>Daily wt<br>Continue phototherapy as indicated<br>• Maintain bili mask over eyes<br>• Cover genitalia per policy<br>• Check eyes for discharge, conjunctivitis, corneal abrasions<br>• Expose as much skin surface as possible to bili lights<br>• Bilimeter reading q shift<br>• No lotion or ointment on infant skin<br>• Turn bili lights off during lab draws<br>Continue infant assessments as per day 1<br>**Expected Outcomes**<br>VS WNL; wt stabilized or gaining wt; no s/s kernicterus; skin integrity intact; skin and mucous membranes pink; eyes without drainage, sclera clear; labs WNL, with stabilized or decreasing bilirubin level |
| **Activity and comfort** | Nest in open crib if infant able to maintain temp beneath bili lights<br>Isolette if infant unable to maintain temp beneath bili lights<br>Reposition q2–4h<br>Remove bili mask, swaddle, and cuddle during feedings<br>Cluster care procedures, remove from lights for feedings | Nest in open crib if infant's temp stable beneath bili lights<br>Isolette if infant unable to maintain temp beneath bili lights<br>**Expected Outcomes**<br>Infant's temp WNL; infant able to rest with nested boundaries; infant cuddled, has eye contact with caregiver during care procedures and feedings |

bili, bilirubin; CPR, cardiopulmonary resuscitation; DC, discharge; info, information; IV, intravenous; lab draws, laboratory blood withdrawal; MD/NP, medical doctor/nurse practitioner; NSY, nursery; NTE, neutral thermal environment; prn, as needed; s/s, signs and symptoms; VS, vital signs; WNL, within normal limits; wt, weight.

| Category | Day 1 | Day 2/Discharge |
|---|---|---|
| **Nutrition** | Breast- or bottle-feed q2–4h<br>Monitor for dehydration, supplement with oral/IV fluid as indicated<br>Remove newborn from bili lights, remove mask for feedings | Continue to feed q2–4h, monitor for dehydration, cuddle for feeding<br>**Expected Outcomes**<br>Infant tolerating feedings q2–4h without sequelae |
| **Elimination** | Record urine color and frequency<br>Specific gravity each void<br>Record quantity and characteristics each stool<br>Strict intake and output (weight diapers before discarding) | Continue noting urine and stool quanity and characteristics<br>**Expected Outcomes**<br>Voids qs, stools qs without difficulty, stool characteristics WNL for resolving hyperbilirubinemia; specific gravity WNL, no s/s dehydration |
| **Medication** | Evaluate routine meds<br>Evaluate need for IV fluids | **Expected Outcomes**<br>Routine meds given; IV fluids administered prn, IV fluids tapered as oral intake adequate to prevent dehydration |
| **Discharge planning/home care** | Evaluate social services/visiting nurse/DC planning needs<br>Possible home phototherapy<br>Schedule follow-up bili levels as outpatient; follow-up with MD/NP | Offer info on CPR classes and/or film, give CPR booklet<br>**Expected Outcomes**<br>Infant DC home with parent(s); mother verbalizes follow-up appointments |
| **Family involvement** | Evaluate additional psychosocial needs<br>Orient family to NSY, equipment, room<br>Discuss rationale for treatment and possible side effects of phototherapy with family (stool changes, increased fluid loss, possible temp instability, slight lethargy, rash, altered sleep-wake patterns)<br>Instruct family on infant's care while undergoing phototherapy:<br>• Safety precautions—bili mask, isolette door closed and latched, covering genitalia per policy<br>• Skin care, cord care, circ care as appropriate<br>• Lab draws, rationale for intake and output<br>As necessary, review role of pumping breasts and offering formula for limited time<br>Encourage parent/significant other/sibling involvement in infant care as possible<br>Evaluate family's understanding of information | Encourage parents to provide tactile stimulation during feeding and diaper changes<br>Encourage cuddling and eye contact during feedings<br>Offer suggestions to comfort restless infant:<br>• Nesting beneath bili lights<br>• Talking softly/singing quietly to infant<br>• Taped music or tape recording of evening activities from home<br>• Rhythmic patting of infant's buttocks<br>• Firm, nonstroking touch, assisting with control of extremities<br>• Pacifier for nonnutritive sucking<br>Encourage family/friend support of mother/parents (ie., meals, rest, child care for siblings, allow expression of concerns/feelings)<br>**Expected Outcomes**<br>Parents verbalize understanding of rationale and possible side effects of phototherapy; parents/family demonstrate safety precautions when caring for infant; parents getting meals, rest, verbalize support given |
| **Date** | | |

phototherapy depends on the cause of the hyperbilirubinemia and the rate of progression of the jaundice.

### Evaluation

Expected outcomes of nursing care include the following:

- The risks for development of hyperbilirubinemia are identified, and action is taken to minimize the potential impact of hyperbilirubinemia.
- The baby does not have any corneal irritation or drainage, skin breakdown, or major fluctuations in temperature.
- Parents understand the rationale for, goal of, and expected outcome of therapy.
- Parents verbalize their concerns about their baby's condition and identify how they can facilitate their baby's improvement.

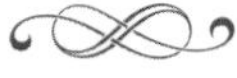

## Care of the Newborn with Anemia

Neonatal anemia is often difficult to recognize by clinical evaluation alone. The hemoglobin concentration in a term newborn is 15 to 20 g/dL, slightly higher than that in premature newborns, in whom the mean hemoglobin is 14 to 18 g/dL. Infants with hemoglobin values of less than 14 g/dL (term) and 13 g/dL (preterm) are usually considered anemic. The most common causes of neonatal anemia are blood loss, hemolysis, and impaired red blood cell production.

Blood loss (hypovolemia) occurs in utero from placental bleeding (placenta previa or abruptio placentae). Intrapartal blood loss may be fetomaternal, fetofetal, or the result of umbilical cord bleeding. Birth trauma to abdominal organs or the cranium may produce significant blood loss, and cerebral bleeding may occur because of hypoxia.

Excessive hemolysis of red blood cells is usually a result of blood group incompatibilities but may be due to infections. The most common cause of impaired red blood cell production is a deficiency in G-6-PD, which is genetically transmitted. Anemia and jaundice are the presenting signs.

A condition known as **physiologic anemia** exists as a result of the normal gradual drop in hemoglobin for the first 6 to 12 weeks of life. Theoretically, the bone marrow stops production of red blood cells as a response to the elevated oxygenation of extrauterine respirations. When the amount of hemoglobin decreases, reaching levels of 10 to 11 g/dL at about 8 to 12 weeks of age in term newborns, the bone marrow begins production of RBCs again, and the anemia disappears.

Anemia in preterm newborns is seen earlier than in term newborns, and increased production of red blood cells does not start until hemoglobin is 7 to 10 g/dL. The preterm baby's hemoglobin reaches a low sooner (by 6 weeks after birth) than does a term newborn's (8 to 12 weeks) because a preterm infant's red blood cell survival time is shorter than that of a term newborn (Doyle, Schmidt, & Zipursky, 1999). This difference is due to several factors: the preterm infant's rapid growth rate, decreased iron stores, and an inadequate production of erythropoietin (EPO) (Juul, 1999).

### Clinical Therapy

Hematologic problems can be anticipated based on the pregnancy history and clinical manifestations. The age at which anemia is first noted is also of diagnostic value. Clinically, light-skinned anemic infants are very pale in the absence of other symptoms of shock and usually have abnormally low red blood cell counts. In acute blood loss, symptoms of shock, such as pallor, low arterial blood pressure, and a decreasing hematocrit value, may be present. The initial laboratory workup should include hemoglobin and hematocrit measurements, reticulocyte count, ferritin concentrations, examination of peripheral blood smear, bilirubin determinations, direct Coombs' test of infant's blood, and examination of maternal blood smear for fetal erythrocytes (Kleihauer-Betke test). Clinical management depends on the severity of the anemia and on whether blood loss is acute or chronic. The baby should be placed on constant cardiac and respiratory monitoring. Mild or slow chronic anemia may be treated adequately with iron supplements alone or with iron-fortified formulas. Frequent determinations of hemoglobin, hematocrit, and bilirubin levels (in hemolytic disease) are essential. In severe cases of anemia, transfusions are the treatment of choice. Management of anemia of prematurity includes recombinant human erythropoietin (rEPO) and supplemental iron. Blood transfusions (dedicated units of blood) are kept to a minimum (Juul, 1999).

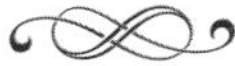

### Nursing Care Management

The nurse assesses the newborn for symptoms of anemia (pallor). If the blood loss is acute, the baby may exhibit signs of shock (a capillary filling time greater than 3 seconds, decreased pulses, tachycardia, low blood pressure). Continued observation is necessary to identify physiologic anemia as the preterm newborn grows. Signs of compromise include poor weight gain, tachycardia, tachypnea, and apneic episodes. The nurse promptly reports any symptoms indicating anemia or shock. The amount of blood drawn for all laboratory tests should be recorded so that total blood removed can be assessed and replaced by transfusion when necessary. If the newborn exhibits signs of shock, the nurse may need to initiate interventions.

## Care of the Newborn with Polycythemia

**Polycythemia,** a condition in which blood volume and hematocrit values are increased, is more common in SGA and full-term infants with delayed cord clamping, maternal-fetal and twin-to-twin transfusions, or chronic intrauterine hypoxia than in other newborns (Doyle et al., 1999). An infant is considered polycythemic when the central venous hematocrit value is greater than 65% to 70% or the venous hemoglobin level is greater than 22 g/dL during the first week of life. Other conditions that present with polycythemia are chromosomal anomalies such as trisomy 21, 18, and 13; endocrine disorders such as hypoglycemia and hypocalcemia; and births at altitudes over 5000 feet.

## Clinical Therapy

The goal of therapy is to reduce the central venous hematocrit value to a range of 55% to 60% in symptomatic infants (Doyle et al., 1999). To decrease the red blood cell mass, the symptomatic infant receives a partial exchange transfusion in which blood is removed from the infant and replaced millimeter for millimeter with fresh frozen plasma or 5% albumin. Supportive treatment of presenting symptoms is required until resolution which usually occurs spontaneously following the partial exchange transfusion.

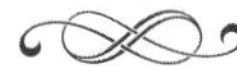

## Nursing Care Management

The nurse assesses for, records, and reports symptoms of polycythemia. The nurse also does an initial screening of the newborn's hematocrit value on admission to the nursery. If a capillary hematocrit is done, warming the heel prior to obtaining the blood helps to decrease falsely high values (Procedure 26–1). Peripheral venous hematocrit samples are usually obtained from the antecubital fossa.

Many infants are asymptomatic, but as symptoms develop, they are related to the increased blood volume, hyperviscosity (thickness) of the blood, and decreased deformability of red blood cells, all of which result in poor perfusion of tissues. The infants have a characteristic plethoric (ruddy) appearance. The most common symptoms observed include the following:

- Tachycardia and congestive heart failure due to the increased blood volume
- Respiratory distress with grunting, tachypnea, and cyanosis; increased oxygen need; or respiratory hemorrhage due to pulmonary venous congestion, edema, and hypoxemia
- Hyperbilirubinemia due to increased numbers of red blood cells breaking down
- Decrease in peripheral pulses, discoloration of extremities, alteration in activity or neurologic depression, renal vein thrombosis with decreased urine output, hematuria, or proteinuria due to thromboembolism
- Jitteriness, decreased activity and tone, and seizures due to decreased perfusion of the brain and increased vascular resistance secondary to sluggish blood flow, which can result in neurologic or developmental problems

The nurse observes closely for the signs of distress or change in vital signs during the partial exchange. The nurse assesses carefully for exchange transfusion complications such as transfusion overload (which may result in congestive heart failure), irregular cardiac rhythm, bacterial infection, hypovolemia, and anemia. The newborn needs to be reunited with the parents as soon as the baby's status permits.

# Care of the Newborn with Infection

Newborns up to 1 month of age are particularly susceptible to an infection, referred to as **sepsis neonatorum,** caused by organisms that do not cause significant disease in older children. Once any infection occurs in the newborn, it can spread rapidly through the bloodstream, regardless of its primary site. The incidence of primary neonatal sepsis is 1 to 10 per 1000 live births (0.1% to 1%) (Wolach, 1997). Nosocomial infection frequency ranges from 0.6% to 1.7% in normal newborn infants and from 0.9% to 18.2% in infants in the neonatal intensive care unit (NICU) (Payne, Schilling, & Steinberg, 1994).

One predisposing factor is prematurity. Prematurity and low birth weight are associated with nosocomial infection rates up to 15 times higher than average (Payne et al., 1994). The general debilitation and underlying illnesses often associated with prematurity necessitate invasive procedures such as umbilical catheterization, intubation, resuscitation, ventilator support, monitoring, parenteral alimentation (especially lipid emulsions), and prior broad-spectrum antibiotic therapy. However, even full-term infants are susceptible, because their immunologic systems are immature. They lack the complex factors involved in effective phagocytosis and the ability to localize infection or to respond with a well-defined, recognizable inflammatory response. In addition, newborns lack IgM immunoglobin, which is necessary to protect against bacteria, because it does not cross the placenta (refer to Chapter 21 for immunologic adaptations in the newborn period).

Most nosocomial infections in the NICU present as bacteremia or sepsis, urinary tract infections, meningitis, or pneumonia. Maternal antepartal infections such as rubella, toxoplasmosis, cytomegalic inclusion disease, and herpes may cause congenital infections and resulting disorders in the newborn. Intrapartal maternal infections, such as amnionitis and those resulting from premature rupture of membranes and precipitous birth, are sources of neonatal infection (see Chapter 13 for more detailed information). Passage through the birth canal and contact with the vaginal flora (β-hemolytic streptococci, herpes, listeria, gonococci) expose the infant to infection (Table 26–5). With

TABLE 26–5 Maternally Transmitted Newborn Infections

| *Infection* | *Nursing Assessment* | *Nursing Plan and Implementation* |
|---|---|---|
| **GROUP B STREPTOCOCCUS**<br>1%–2% colonized, with 1 in 10 developing disease<br>Early onset—usually within hours of birth or within first week<br>Late onset—1 week to 3 months | Severe respiratory distress (grunting and cyanosis).<br>May become apneic or demonstrate symptoms of shock.<br>Meconium-stained amniotic fluid seen at birth | Early assessment of clinical signs necessary.<br>Assist with x-ray examination—shows aspiration pneumonia or hyaline membrane disease.<br>Immediately obtain blood, gastric aspirate, external ear canal, and nasopharynx cultures.<br>Administer antibiotics, usually aqueous penicillin or ampicillin combined with gentamicin, as soon as cultures are obtained.<br>Early assessment and intervention are essential to survival.<br>Initiate referral to evaluate for blindness, deafness, learning or behavioral problems. |
| **SYPHILIS**<br>Spirochetes cross placenta after 16th–18th week of gestation | Check perinatal history for positive maternal serology<br>Assess infant for<br>Elevated cord serum IgM and FTA-ABS IgM<br>Rhinitis (snuffles)<br>Fissures on mouth corners and excoriated upper lip<br>Red rash around mouth and anus<br>Copper-colored rash over face, palms, and soles<br>Irritability<br>Generalized edema, particularly over joints; bone lesions; painful extremities<br>Hepatosplenomegaly, jaundice<br>Congenital cataracts<br>SGA and failure to thrive | Initiate isolation techniques until infants have been on antibiotics for 48 hours.<br>Administer penicillin.<br>Provide emotional support for parents because of their feelings about mode of transmission and potential long-term sequelae. |
| **GONORRHEA**<br>Approximately 30%–35% of newborns born vaginally to infected mothers acquire the infection | Assess for<br>Ophthalmia neonatorum (conjunctivitis)<br>Purulent discharge and corneal ulcerations<br>Neonatal sepsis with temperature instability, poor feeding response, and/or hypotonia, jaundice | Administer 1% silver nitrate solution or ophthalmic antibiotic ointment (see Drug Guide: Erythromycin [Ilotycin] Ophthalmic Ointment in Chapter 23) or, in lieu of silver nitrate, penicillin.<br>Initiate follow-up referral to evaluate any loss of vision. |
| **HERPES TYPE 2**<br>1 in 7500 births.<br>Usually transmitted during vaginal birth; a few cases of in utero transmission have been reported | Small cluster vesicular skin lesions over all the body<br>Check perinatal history for active herpes genital lesions<br>Disseminated form—DIC, pneumonia, hepatitis with jaundice, hepatosplenomegaly, and neurologic abnormalities. Without skin lesions, assess for fever or subnormal temperature, respiratory congestion, tachypnea, and tachycardia | Carry out careful handwashing and gown and glove isolation with linen precautions.<br>Administer intravenous vidarabine (Vira A) or acyclovir (Zovirax).<br>Initiate follow-up referral to evaluate potential sequelae of microcephaly, spasticity, seizures, deafness, or blindness.<br>Encourage parental rooming-in and touching of their newborn.<br>Show parents appropriate handwashing procedures and precautions to be used at home if mother's lesions are active.<br>Obtain throat, conjunctiva, cerebral spinal fluid (CSF), blood, urine, and lesion cultures to identify herpesvirus type 2 antibiotics in serum IgM fraction. Cultures positive in 24–48 hours. |
| **ORAL CANDIDAL INFECTION (THRUSH)**<br>Acquired during passage through birth canal | Assess newborn's buccal mucosa, tongue, gums, and inside the cheeks for white plaques (seen 5 to 7 days of age)<br>Check diaper area for bright-red, well-demarcated eruptions<br>Assess for thrush periodically when newborn is on long-term antibiotic therapy | Differentiate white plaque areas from milk curds by using cotton tip applicator (if it is thrush, removal of white areas causes raw, bleeding areas).<br>Maintain cleanliness of hands, linen, clothing, diapers, and feeding apparatus.<br>Instruct breastfeeding mothers on treating their nipples with nystatin.<br>Administer gentian violet (1%–2%) swabbed on oral lesions 1 hour after feeding or nystatin instilled in baby's oral cavity and on mucosa.<br>Swab skin lesions with topical nystatin.<br>Discuss with parents that gentian violet stains mouth and clothing.<br>Avoid placing gentian violet on normal mucosa; it causes irritation. |
| **CHLAMYDIA TRACHOMATIS**<br>Acquired during passage through birth canal | Assess for perinatal history of preterm birth.<br>Symptomatic newborns present with pneumonia—conjunctivitis after 3–4 days<br>Chronic follicular conjunctivitis (corneal neovascularization and conjunctival scarring) | Instill ophthalmic erythromycin (see Drug Guide: Erythromycin [Ilotycin] Ophthalmic Ointment, in Chapter 23).<br>Initiate follow-up referral for eye complications and late development of pneumonia at 4–11 weeks postnatally. |

infection anywhere in the fetus or newborn, the adjacent tissues or organs are very easily penetrated, and the blood-brain barrier is ineffective. Septicemia is more common in males, except for infections caused by group B β-hemolytic streptococcus.

At present, gram-negative organisms (especially *Escherichia coli, Enterobacter, Proteus,* and *Klebsiella*) and the gram-positive organism β-hemolytic streptococcus are the most common causative agents. *Pseudomonas* is a common fomite contaminant of ventilator support and oxygen therapy equipment. Gram-positive bacteria, especially coagulase-negative staphylococci, are common pathogens in nosocomial bacteremias, pneumonias, and urinary tract infections. Other gram-positive bacteria frequently isolated are enterococci and *Staphylococcus aureus* (Gaynes, Edwards, Jarvis, et al., 1996).

Protection of the newborn from infections starts prenatally and continues throughout pregnancy and birth. Prenatal prevention should include maternal screening for sexually transmitted infections and monitoring of rubella titers in women who test negative. Intrapartally, sterile technique is essential. Smears from genital lesions are taken, and placenta and amniotic fluid cultures are obtained if amnionitis is suspected. If genital herpes is present toward term, cesarean birth may be indicated. All newborns' eyes should be treated with silver nitrate or an antibiotic ophthalmic ointment to prevent damage from gonococcal infection. Prophylactic antibiotic therapy, for asymptomatic (group B *streptococcus*) GBS-culture-positive women during the intrapartum period, has been shown to be beneficial in preventing early-onset sepsis (Schuchat, 1998).

## Clinical Therapy

Cultures should be taken as soon after birth as possible for infants with a history of possible exposure to infection in utero (eg, premature rupture of membranes [PROM] more than 24 hours before birth or questionable maternal history of infection). They are obtained before antibiotic therapy is begun.

1. Two blood cultures are obtained from different peripheral sites. They are taken from a peripheral rather than an umbilical vessel, because catheters have yielded false-positive results due to contamination. The skin is prepared by cleaning with an antiseptic solution, such as one containing iodine, and allowed to dry; the specimen is obtained with a sterile needle and syringe.
2. Spinal fluid culture is done following a spinal tap.
3. The specimen for urine culture is best obtained by a suprapubic bladder aspiration.
4. Skin cultures are taken of any lesions or drainage from lesions or reddened areas.
5. Nasopharyngeal, rectal, ear canal, and gastric aspirate cultures may be obtained.

Other laboratory investigations include a complete blood count, chest x-ray examination, serology, and gram stains of cerebrospinal fluid, urine, skin exudate, and umbilicus. White blood cell (WBC) count with differential may indicate the presence or absence of sepsis. A level of 30,000 WBCs may be normal in the first 24 hours of life, and a low WBC count may be indicative of sepsis. A low neutrophil count and a high band (immature white blood cells) count indicate that an infection is present. Stomach aspirate should be sent for culture and smear if a gonococcal infection or amnionitis is suspected. The C-reactive protein level may or may not be elevated. Serum IgM levels are elevated (normal level less than 20 mg/dL) in response to transplacental infections. If available, counterimmunoelectrophoresis tests for specific bacterial antigens are performed.

Evidence of congenital infections may be seen on skull x-ray films for cerebral calcifications (cytomegalovirus, toxoplasmosis), on bone x-ray films (syphilis, cytomegalovirus), and in serum-specific IgM levels (rubella). Cytomegalovirus infection is best diagnosed by urine culture.

Because neonatal infection causes high mortality, therapy is instituted before results of the septic workup are obtained. A combination of two broad-spectrum antibiotics, such as ampicillin and gentamicin, is given in large doses until a culture with sensitivities is obtained.

After the pathogen and its sensitivities are determined, appropriate specific antibiotic therapy is begun. Combinations of penicillin or ampicillin and kanamycin have been used in the past, but new kanamycin-resistant enterobacteria and penicillin-resistant staphylococcus necessitate increasing use of gentamicin.

Rotating aminoglycosides has been suggested to prevent development of resistance. Use of cephalosporins and, in particular, cefotaxime has emerged as an alternative to aminoglycoside therapy in the treatment of neonatal infections. Duration of therapy varies from 7 to 14 days (Table 26–6). If cultures are negative and symptoms subside, antibiotics may be discontinued after 3 days. Supportive physiologic care may be required to maintain respiratory, hemodynamic, nutritional, and metabolic homeostasis.

# Nursing Care Management

## Nursing Assessment and Diagnosis

Symptoms of infection are most often noticed by the nurse during daily care of the newborn. The infant may deteriorate rapidly in the first 12 to 24 hours after birth

| TABLE 26–6 Neonatal Sepsis Antibiotic Therapy | | | | |
|---|---|---|---|---|
| *Drug* | *Dose (mg/kg) Total Daily Dose* | *Schedule for Divided Doses* | *Route* | *Comments* |
| Ampicillin | 50–100 mg/kg | Every 12 hours*<br>Every 8 hours† | IM or IV | Effective against gram-positive microorganisms, *Haemophilus influenzae,* and majority of *Escherichia coli* strains. Higher doses indicated for meningitis. Used with aminoglycoside for synergy. |
| Cefotaxime | 50 mg/kg<br>100–150 mg/kg/day | Every 12 hours*<br>Every 8 hours† | IM or IV | Active against most major pathogens in infants; effective against aminoglycoside-resistant organisms; achieves CSF bactericidal activity; lack of ototoxicity and nephrotoxicity; wide therapeutic index (levels not required); resistant organisms can develop rapidly if used extensively; ineffective against pseudomonas, listeria. |
| Gentamicin | 2.5–3 mg/kg<br>5.0–7.5 mg/kg/day | Every 12–24 hours*†<br>Every 8–24 hours† | IM or IV | Effective against gram-negative rods and staphylococci; may be used instead of kanamycin against penicillin-resistant staphylococci and *E. coli* strains and *Pseudomonas aeruginosa.* May cause ototoxicity and nephrotoxicity. Need to follow serum levels. Must never be given as IV push. Must be given over at least 30–60 minutes. In presence of oliguria or anuria, dose must be decreased or discontinued. In infants less than 1000 g or 29 weeks, lower dosage 2.5–3.0 mg/kg/day. Monitor serum levels before administration of second dose.<br>Peak 5–10 μg/mL<br>Trough 1–2 μg/mL |
| Methicillin | 25–50 mg/dose<br>50–100 mg/kg/day | Every 12 hours*<br>Every 6–8 hours† | IM or IV | Effective against penicillinase-resistant staphylococci. Monitor CBC and UA.<br>Slow IV push. |
| Nafcillin | 25–50 mg/kg<br>50–100 mg/kg/day | Every 8–12 hours*<br>Every 6–8 hours† | IM or IV | Effective against penicillinase-resistant staphylococci. Caution in presence of jaundice. |
| Penicillin G (aqueous crystalline) | 25,000–50,000 IU/kg<br>50,000–125,000 IU/kg/day | Every 12 hours*<br>Every 8 hours† | IM or IV | Initial sepsis therapy effective against most gram-positive microorganisms except resistant staphylococci; can cause heart block in infants. |
| Vancomycin | 10–20 mg/kg<br>30 mg/kg/day | Every 12–24 hours*‡<br>Every 8 hours† | IV | Effective for methicillin-resistant strains (*Staphylococcus epidermidis*); must be administered by slow intravenous infusion to avoid prolonged cutaneous eruption. For smaller infants <1200 g, <29 weeks, smaller dosages and longer intervals between doses. Nephrotoxic, especially when given in combination with aminoglycosides. Slow IV infusion over at least 60 minutes.<br>Peak 25–40 μg/mL<br>Trough 5–10 μg/mL |

*Up to 7 days of age.
†Greater than 7 days of age.
‡Dependent on GA.

if β-hemolytic streptococcal infection is present, with signs and symptoms mimicking RDS. In other cases, the onset of sepsis may be gradual, with more subtle signs and symptoms. The most common signs observed include the following:

1. Subtle behavioral changes; the infant "is not doing well" and is often lethargic or irritable (especially after the first 24 hours) and hypotonic; color changes may include pallor, duskiness, cyanosis, or a "shocky" appearance; skin is cool and clammy
2. Temperature instability, manifested by either hypothermia (recognized by a decrease in skin temperature) or, rarely in newborns, hyperthermia (elevation of skin temperature) necessitating a corresponding increase or decrease in incubator temperature to maintain a neutral thermal environment

3. Feeding intolerance, as evidenced by a decrease in total intake, abdominal distension, vomiting, poor sucking, lack of interest in feeding, and diarrhea
4. Hyperbilirubinemia
5. Tachycardia initially, followed by spells of apnea or bradycardia

Signs and symptoms may suggest CNS disease (jitteriness, tremors, seizure activity), respiratory system disease (tachypnea, labored respirations, apnea, cyanosis), hematologic disease (jaundice, petechial hemorrhages, hepatosplenomegaly), or gastrointestinal disease (diarrhea, vomiting, bile-stained aspirate, hepatomegaly). A differential diagnosis is necessary because of the similarity of symptoms to other more specific conditions.

Nursing diagnoses that may apply to the infant with sepsis neonatorum and the family include the following:

- ***Risk for infection*** related to immature immunologic system
- ***Fluid volume deficit*** related to feeding intolerance
- ***Ineffective family coping*** related to present illness resulting in prolonged hospital stay for the newborn

## Nursing Plan and Implementation

In the nursery, environmental control and prevention of acquired infection are the responsibilities of the neonatal nurse. The nurse must promote strict handwashing technique for all who enter the nursery, including nursing colleagues; physicians; laboratory, x-ray, and respiratory therapists; and parents. The nurse must be prepared to assist in the aseptic collection of specimens for laboratory investigations. Scrupulous care of equipment—changing and cleaning of incubators at least every 7 days, removing and sterilizing wet equipment every 24 hours, preventing cross use of linen and equipment, cleaning sink-side equipment such as soap containers periodically, and taking special care with the open radiant warmers (access without prior handwashing is much more likely than with the closed incubator)—will prevent fomite contamination or contamination through improper handwashing. An infected newborn can be effectively isolated in an incubator and receive close observation. Visits to the nursery area by unnecessary personnel should be discouraged.

The nurse administers antibiotics as ordered by the nurse practitioner or physician. In addition to the five rights of drug administration, it is the nurse's responsibility to be knowledgeable about the following:

- The proper dose to be administered, based on the weight of the newborn and desired peak and trough levels
- The appropriate route of administration, because some antibiotics cannot be given intravenously
- Admixture incompatibilities, because some antibiotics are precipitated by intravenous solutions or by other antibiotics
- Side effects and toxicity

In the case of term infants who are being treated for infections, neonatal home infusion of antibiotics should be considered as a viable alternative to continued hospitalization. The infusion of antibiotics at home by skilled RNs facilitates parent-infant bonding while meeting the ongoing health care needs of the infant (Anastasi, 1998).

In addition to antibiotic therapy, physiologic supportive care is essential in caring for a septic infant (Askin, 1995). Following are responsibilities of the nurse:

- Observe for resolution of symptoms or development of other symptoms of sepsis
- Maintain neutral thermal environment with accurate regulation of humidity and oxygen administration
- Provide respiratory support: administer oxygen and observe and monitor respiratory effort
- Provide cardiovascular support: observe and monitor pulse and blood pressure; observe for hyperbilirubinemia, anemia, and hemorrhagic symptoms
- Provide adequate calories, because oral feedings may be discontinued due to increased mucus, abdominal distension, vomiting, and aspiration
- Provide fluids and electrolytes to maintain homeostasis; monitor weight changes, urine output, and urine specific gravity
- Observe for the development of hypoglycemia, hyperglycemia, acidosis, hyponatremia, and hypocalcemia

Restricting parental visits has not been shown to have any effect on the rate of infection and may be harmful for the newborn's psychologic development. With instruction and guidance from the nurse, both parents should be allowed to handle the baby and participate in daily care. Support of the parents is crucial. They need to be informed of the newborn's prognosis as treatment continues and to be involved in care as much as possible (Figure 26–12♦). They also need to understand how infection is transmitted.

## Evaluation

Expected outcomes of nursing care include the following:

- The risks for development of sepsis are identified early, and immediate action is taken to minimize the development of the illness.

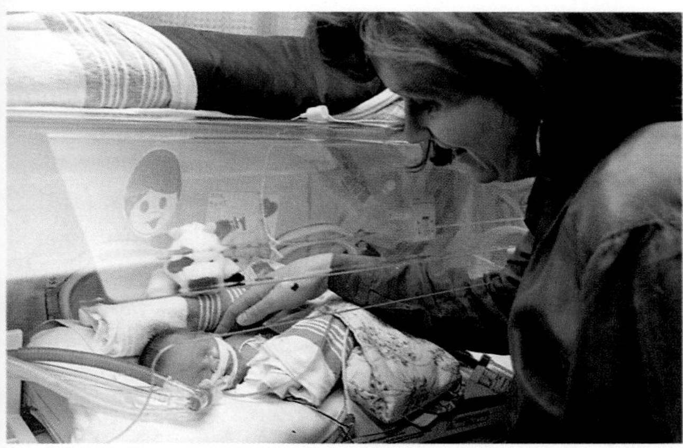

FIGURE 26–12 ♦ When parents participate in their baby's care, they tend to have realistic expectations about the child's long-term developmental needs.

- Appropriate use of aseptic technique protects the newborn from further exposure to illness.
- The baby's symptoms are relieved, and the infection is treated.
- The parents verbalize their concerns about their baby's illness and understand the rationale behind the management of their newborn.

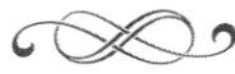

## Care of Family with Birth of an At-Risk Newborn

The birth of a preterm or ill infant or an infant with a congenital anomaly is a serious crisis for a family. Acute grief reactions follow the loss of the idealized baby family members have envisioned. In the case of a preterm birth, the mother is denied the last few weeks of pregnancy that seem to prepare her psychologically for the stress of birth and the attachment process. Attachment at this time is fragile, and interruption of the process by separation can affect the future mother-child relationship. Feelings of guilt and failure often plague mothers of preterm newborns. They may question themselves: "Why did labor start?" or "What did I do (or not do)?" A woman may have guilt fantasies and wonder: "Was it because I had sexual intercourse with my husband [a week, 3 days, a day] ago?" "Was it because I carried three loads of wash up from the basement?" or "Am I being punished for something done in the past—even in childhood?"

The birth of the newborn with an illness or congenital abnormalities also engenders feelings of guilt and failure. As in the birth of a preterm infant, the woman may entertain ideas of personal guilt: "What did I do (or not do) to cause this?" or "Am I being punished for something?"

The birth of an at-risk newborn alters parental reactions and steps of attachment. Parents must recognize and deal with a variety of new feelings, reactions, and stresses before they can work toward the establishment of a healthy parent-infant relationship.

Although reactions and steps of attachment are altered by the birth of these infants, a healthy parent-child relationship can occur. Kaplan and Mason (1974) have identified four psychologic tasks as essential for coping with the stress of an at-risk newborn and for providing a basis for the maternal-infant relationship:

1. Anticipatory grief as a psychologic preparation for possible loss of the child while still hoping for his or her survival
2. Acknowledgment of maternal failure to produce a term or perfect newborn expressed as anticipatory grief and depression and lasting until the chances of survival seem secure
3. Resumption of the process of relating to the infant, which was interrupted by the threat of nonsurvival; this task may be impaired by continuous threat of death or abnormality, and the mother may be slow in her response of hope for the infant's survival
4. Understanding of the special needs and growth patterns of the at-risk newborn, which are temporary and yield to normal patterns

Most authorities agree that the birth of a preterm infant or an infant with a problem requires major adjustments as the parents are forced to surrender the image they had nurtured for so long of their ideal child. *Grief work,* the emotional reaction to a significant loss, must occur before adequate attachment to the actual child is possible. Parental detachment precedes parental attachment.

Solnit and Stark (1961) postulate that grief and mourning over the loss of the loved object—the idealized child—mark parental reactions to a child with abnormalities. Simultaneously, they must adopt the imperfect child as the new love object. Parental responses to a child with health problems may be viewed as a five-stage process (Klaus & Kennell, 1982):

1. *Shock* is felt at the reality of the birth of this child. This stage may be characterized by forgetfulness, amnesia about the situation, and a feeling of desperation.
2. There is disbelief (*denial*) of the reality of the situation, characterized by a refusal to believe the child is defective. This stage is exemplified by assertions that "It didn't really happen!" or "There has been a mistake; it's someone else's baby."
3. *Depression* over the reality of the situation and a corresponding grief reaction follows acceptance of the

situation. This stage is characterized by much crying and sadness. Anger may also emerge at this stage. A projection of blame on others or on self and feelings of "not me" are characteristic of this stage.

4. *Equilibrium and acceptance* are characteristic of a decrease in the emotional reactions of the parents. This stage is variable and may be prolonged by a continuing threat to the infant's survival. Some parents experience chronic sorrow in relation to their child.
5. *Reorganization* of the family is necessary to deal with the child's problems. Mutual support of the parents facilitates this process, but the crisis of the situation may precipitate alienation between the mother and father.

# Nursing Care Management

## Nursing Assessment and Diagnosis

Development of a positive nurse-family relationship facilitates information gathering in areas of concern. A concurrent illness of the mother or other family members or other concurrent stress (lack of hospitalization insurance, loss of job, age of parents) may alter the family response to the baby. Feelings of apprehension, guilt, failure, and grief expressed verbally or nonverbally are important aspects of the nursing history. These observations enable all professionals to be aware of the parental state, coping behaviors, and readiness for attachment, bonding, and caretaking. Appropriate nursing observations during interviewing and relating to the family include the nurse's assessment of the following:

1. *Level of understanding:* observations concerning the ability to assimilate the information given and to ask appropriate questions; the need for constant repetition of information
2. *Behavioral responses:* appropriateness of behavior in relation to information given; lack of response; flat affect
3. *Difficulties with communication:* deafness (reads lips only); blindness; dysphagia; understanding only of foreign language
4. *Paternal and maternal education level:* parents unable to read or write; parents with eighth-grade-level education; parents with a graduate-level degree or health care background; and so on

Documentation of such information, which the nurse obtains through continuing contact and development of a therapeutic relationship with the family, enables all professionals to understand and use the nursing history to provide continuous individual care.

Visiting and caregiving patterns give an indication of the level or lack of parental attachment. A record of visits, caretaking procedures, affect (in relating to the newborn), and telephone calls is essential. It is important that the nurse note serial observations rather than just isolated observations that cause concern. Grant (1978) has developed a conceptual framework depicting adaptive and maladaptive responses to parenting of an infant with an actual or potential problem (Figure 26–13♦).

If a pattern of distancing behaviors evolves, the nurse should institute appropriate intervention. Follow-up studies have found that a statistically significant number of preterm, sick, and congenitally defective infants suffer from failure to thrive, battering, or other parenting disorders. Early detection and intervention will prevent these aberrations in parenting behaviors from leading to irreparable damage or death.

Nursing diagnoses that may apply to the family of a newborn at risk include the following:

- ***Dysfunctional grieving*** related to loss of idealized newborn
- ***Fear*** related to emotional involvement with an at-risk newborn
- ***Altered parenting*** related to impaired bonding secondary to feelings of inadequacy about caretaking activities

## Nursing Plan and Implementation

### *Hospital-Based Nursing Care*

#### Support of Parents for Initial Visit to the Newborn

Before parents see their child, the nurse must prepare them for the visit. It is important to maintain a positive, realistic attitude regarding the infant. An overly negative, fatalistic attitude further alienates the parents from their infant and retards attachment behaviors. Instead of beginning to bond with their child, the parents will anticipate their loss and begin the process of grieving. Once started, the grieving process is difficult to reverse.

Before preparing parents for the first view of their infant, the nurse should observe the baby. All infants exhibit strengths as well as deficiencies, and the nurse should prepare the parents to see both the deviations and the normal aspects of their infant. The nurse may say, "Your baby is small, about the length of my two hands. She weighs 2 lb, 3 oz, but is very active and cries when we disturb her. She is having some difficulty breathing but is breathing without assistance and in only 35% oxygen."

The equipment being used for the at-risk newborn and its purpose should be described before the parents

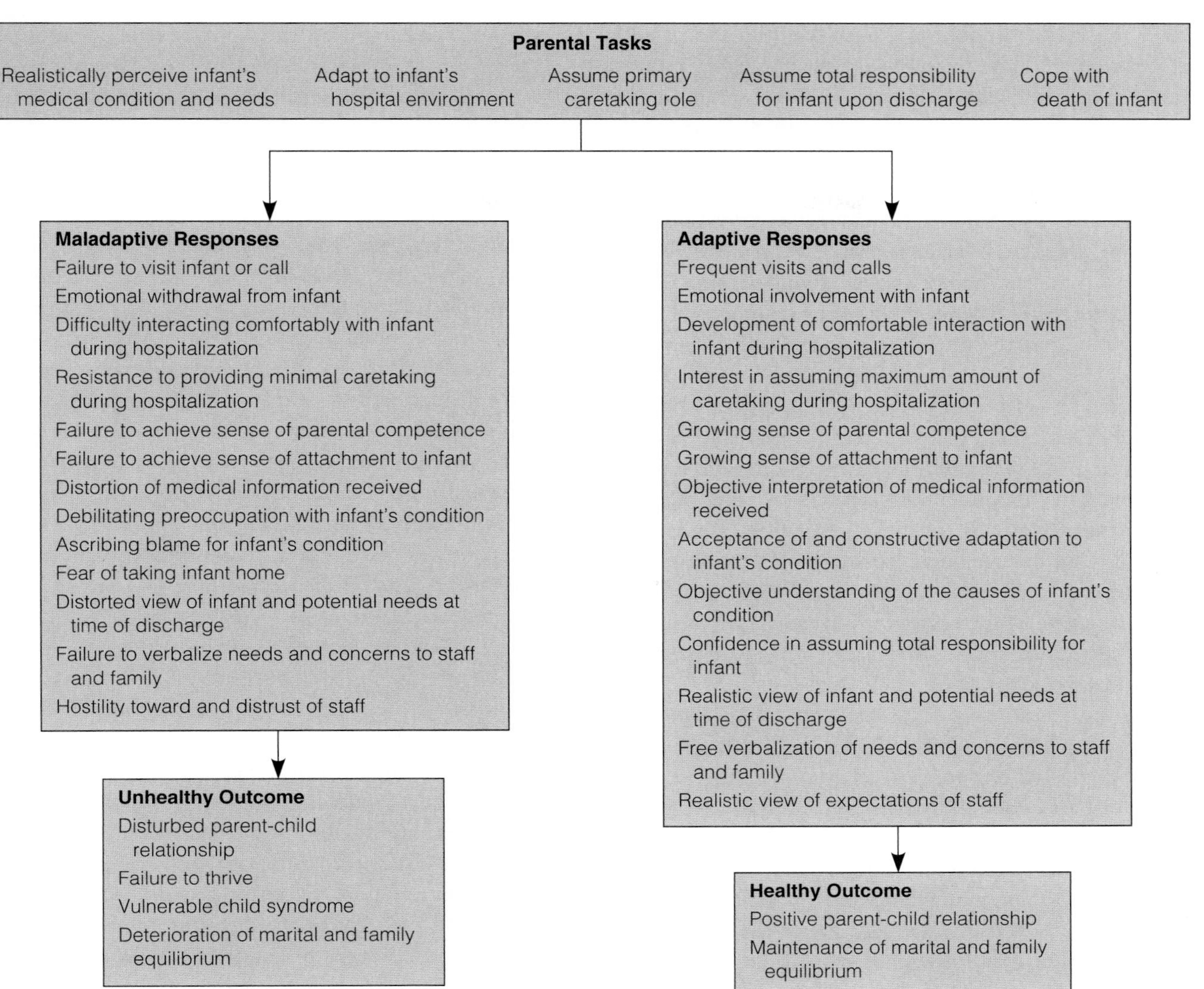

Parental Tasks
Realistically perceive infant's medical condition and needs
Adapt to infant's hospital environment
Assume primary caretaking role
Assume total responsibility for infant upon discharge
Cope with death of infant
Maladaptive Responses
Failure to visit infant or call
Emotional withdrawal from infant
Difficulty interacting comfortably with infant during hospitalization
Resistance to providing minimal caretaking during hospitalization
Failure to achieve sense of parental competence
Failure to achieve sense of attachment to infant
Distortion of medical information received
Debilitating preoccupation with infant's condition
Ascribing blame for infant's condition
Fear of taking infant home
Distorted view of infant and potential needs at time of discharge
Failure to verbalize needs and concerns to staff and family
Hostility toward and distrust of staff
Unhealthy Outcome
Disturbed parent-child relationship
Failure to thrive
Vulnerable child syndrome
Deterioration of marital and family equilibrium
Adaptive Responses
Frequent visits and calls
Emotional involvement with infant
Development of comfortable interaction with infant during hospitalization
Interest in assuming maximum amount of caretaking during hospitalization
Growing sense of parental competence
Growing sense of attachment to infant
Objective interpretation of medical information received
Acceptance of and constructive adaptation to infant's condition
Objective understanding of the causes of infant's condition
Confidence in assuming total responsibility for infant
Realistic view of infant and potential needs at time of discharge
Free verbalization of needs and concerns to staff and family
Realistic view of expectations of staff
Healthy Outcome
Positive parent-child relationship
Maintenance of marital and family equilibrium


**FIGURE 26–13 ♦** Maladaptive and adaptive parental responses during crisis period, showing unhealthy and healthy outcomes. *Source:* Grant, P. (1978). Psychological needs of families of high-risk infants. *Family and Community Health, 1*(3), 93; with permission of Aspen Publisher, Inc., © 1978.

enter the intensive care unit. Many NICUs have booklets for parents to read before entering the units. Through explanations and pictures, the parents are better prepared to deal with the feelings they may experience when they see their infant for the first time.

Upon entering the unit, parents may be overwhelmed by the sounds of monitors, alarms, and respirators, as well as by the unfamiliar language and "foreign" atmosphere. Preparing the parents by having the same health care professionals accompany them to the unit can be reassuring. The primary nurse and physician caring for the newborn need to be with the parents when they first visit their baby. Parental reactions vary, but initially there is usually an element of shock. Providing them with chairs and time to regain composure assists the parents. Slow, complete, and simple explanations—first about the infant and then about the equipment—allay fear and anxiety.

As parents attempt to deal with the initial stages of shock and grief, they may fail to grasp new information. They may need repeated explanations to accept the reality of the situation, procedures, equipment, and the infant's condition on subsequent visits.

Misconceptions about equipment and its placement on the infant and about its potential harm are common. Such questions as "Does the fluid go into the brain?" "Does the white wire on the abdomen go into the stomach?" and "Does the monitor make the baby's heart beat?" reveal fear for the infant's safety and misconception about the machines. The nurse can alleviate these worries by simple explanations of all equipment being used.

Concern about the infant's physical appearance is common yet may remain unvoiced. Parents may express such concerns as "He looks so small and red—like a drowned rat," "Why do her genitals look so abnormal?"

and "Will that awful-looking mouth [cleft lip and palate] ever be normal?" The nurse needs to anticipate and address such questions. Use of pictures, such as of an infant after cleft lip repair, may be reassuring to doubting parents. Knowledge of the development of a "normal" preterm infant allows the nurse to make reassuring statements such as "The baby's labia may look very abnormal to you, but they are normal for her level of maturity. As she grows, the outer lips of the labia will become larger and the clitoris will be covered, and the genitals will then look as you expect them to. She is normal for her level of maturity."

The nursing staff set the tone of the NICU. Nurses foster the development of a safe, trusting environment by viewing the parents as essential caregivers, not as visitors or nuisances in the unit. Providing privacy when needed and offering easy access to staff and facilities are important in developing an open, comfortable environment. An uncrowded and welcoming atmosphere lets parents know they are welcome there. However, even in crowded physical surroundings, the nurses can convey an attitude of openness and trust.

A trusting relationship is essential for collaborative efforts in caring for the infant. Nurses need to therapeutically use their own responses to relate to the parents on a one-to-one basis. Each individual has different needs, different ways of adapting to crisis, and different means of support. Nurses can use techniques that are real and spontaneous to them and avoid words or actions that are foreign to them. Nurses must also gauge their interventions so that they match the parents' pace and needs.

#### Facilitation of Attachment if Neonatal Transport Occurs

Transport to a regional referral center that may be some distance from the parents' community may be necessary. It is essential that the mother see and touch her infant before the infant is transported. The nurse can bring the mother to the nursery or take the infant in a warmed transport incubator to the mother's bedside to allow her to see the infant before transportation to the center. When the infant reaches the referral center, a staff member should call the parents with information about the infant's condition during transport, safe arrival at the center, and present condition.

Occasionally the mother may be unable to see the infant before transport (eg, if she is still under general anesthesia or experiencing complications such as shock, hemorrhage, or seizures). In these cases, before the infant is transported, the nurse can take a photograph of the infant to give to the mother, along with an explanation of the infant's condition and problems and a detailed description of the infant's characteristics. An additional photograph is also helpful for the father to share with siblings or extended family. With the increased attention on improved fetal outcome, prenatal maternal transports, rather than neonatal transports, are occurring more frequently. This practice gives the mother of an at-risk infant the opportunity to visit and care for her infant during the early postpartal period.

#### Promotion of Touching and Parental Caretaking

Parents visiting a small or sick infant may need several visits to become comfortable and confident in their ability to touch the infant without injuring her or him. Barriers such as incubators, incisions, monitor electrodes, and tubes may delay the mother's development of comfort in touching the newborn. Knowledge of this normal delay in touching behavior will help the nurse understand parental behavior.

Klaus and Kennell (1982) have demonstrated a significant difference in the amount of eye contact and touching behaviors of mothers of normal newborns and mothers of preterm infants. Whereas mothers of normal newborns progress within minutes to palm contact of the infant's trunk, mothers of preterm infants are slower to progress from fingertip to palm contact and from the extremities to the trunk. The progression to palm contact with the infant's trunk may take several visits to the nursery.

Through support, reassurance, and encouragement, the nurse can facilitate the mother's positive feelings about her ability and her importance to her infant. Touching facilitates familiarity with the infant and thus establishes a bond between mother and infant. Touching and seeing the infant help the mother realize the normal aspects and potential of her baby (Figure 26–14♦).

The nurse can also encourage parents to meet their newborn's need for stimulation. Stroking, rocking, cuddling, singing, and talking should be an integral part of the parents' caretaking responsibilities. The nurse can promote bonding by encouraging parents to visit and become involved in their baby's care (Figure 26–15♦). When visiting is impossible, the parents should feel free to phone whenever they wish to receive information about their baby. A nurse's warm, receptive attitude provides support. Nurses can also facilitate parenting by personalizing a baby to the parents, by referring to the infant by name or by relating personal behavioral characteristics. Remarks such as "Jenny loves her pacifier" help make the infant seem individual and unique.

Caretaking may be delayed for the mother of a preterm, at-risk, or sick infant. The variety of equipment needed for life support is hardly conducive to anxiety-free caretaking by the parents. However, even the sickest infant may be cared for, if only in a small way, by the parents. As a facilitator of parental caretaking, the nurse can promote the parents' success. Demonstration and explanation, followed by support of the parents in initial caretaking behaviors, positively reinforce this behavior.

STAGE I: Touching
Uses fingertips
Uses whole hand
Strokes child
Holds and studies child "*en face*"
Spontaneously lowers crib rails to fondle, hold, or talk to child

↓

STAGE II: Caretaking
Provides clean clothing, toys, grooming aids
Performs activities of daily living (bathing, diapering, feeding, dressing)
Performs caretaking tasks with proficiency and expresses pleasure in meeting infant's needs
Able to comfort child when distressed or crying
Able to meet child's special health needs (suctioning, cleaning stoma sites, treatments)

↓

STAGE III: Identity
Brings linens from home
Takes photographs
Brings individualized toys
Can make personalized observations about child
Offers suggestions and makes demands for personalized care
Demonstrates "advocacy" behavior
Feels he or she can care for child better than anyone else
Demonstrates consistent visiting and/or calling pattern
Questions focus on total child, not only physiologic parameters

FIGURE 26–14 ♦ Stages of parenting behavior toward infants in intensive care. *Source:* Adapted from work of Rubin, Schaeffer, Jay, and Schraeder by Schraeder, B. D. (1980). Attachment and parenting despite lengthy intensive care. *Journal of Maternal Child Nursing 5,* 38. Reprinted with permission from the American Journal of Nursing Company, 1980.

Changing their infant's diaper, providing skin or oral care, or helping the nurse turn the infant may at first provoke anxiety, but the parents will become more comfortable and confident in caretaking and feel satisfied by the baby's reactions and their ability "to do something." Complimenting the parents' competence in caretaking also increases their self-esteem, which may have been damaged by feelings of guilt and failure. It is vitally important that the nurse never give the parents a task that they might not be able to accomplish.

Often parents of high-risk infants have ambivalent feelings toward the nurse. As they watch the nurse competently perform caretaking tasks, they may feel both grateful for the nurse's abilities and expertise and jealous of the nurse's ability to care for their infant. These feelings may take the form of criticism of the care of the infant, manipulation of staff, or personal guilt. Instead of fostering (by silence) these inferiority feelings of parents, nurses need to recognize that such feelings are needed to intervene appropriately to enhance parent-infant attachment. For example, the nurse should avoid making unfavorable comparisons between the baby's responses to parental and nursing caretaking. During a quiet time it may help for the nurse to encourage the parents to talk about their hopes and fears and to facilitate their involvement in parent groups (Raines, 1998).

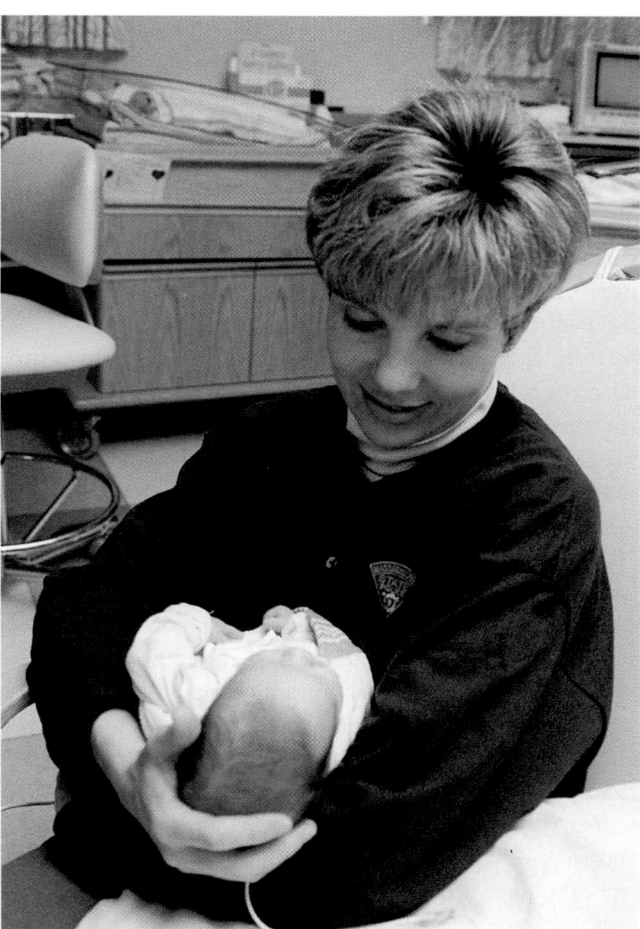

FIGURE 26–15 ♦ It is important that the parents of high-risk infants be given the opportunity to get acquainted with their children. Physical contact is extremely important in the bonding process and should be encouraged whenever possible.

Nurses who are understanding and secure are able to support the parents' egos instead of collecting rewards for themselves. To reinforce positive parenting behaviors, professionals must first believe in the importance of the parents. The nurse can hardly convince doubting parents of their importance to the infant if she or he does not really believe it. Both attitudes and words must convey that they are good parents and have an important contribution to make in the care of their infant. Unless as much care is taken in facilitating parental attachment as in providing physiologic care, the outcome may not be a healthy family.

Verbalizations by the nurse that improve parental self-esteem are essential and easily shared. For example, the nurse can point out that, in addition to physiologic use, breast milk is important because of the emotional investment of the mother. Pumping, storing, labeling, and delivering quantities of breast milk is a time-consuming labor of love for mothers. Positive remarks about breast milk reinforce the maternal behavior of caretaking and providing for her infant: "Breast milk is something that only you can give your baby," "You really have brought a lot of milk today," "Look how rich this breast milk is," or "Even small amounts of milk are important, and look how rich it is." If the infant begins to gain weight while being fed breast milk, it is important that the nurse point this correlation out to the mother. The nurse also needs to advise the parents that initial weight loss with beginning nipple-feedings is common because of the increased energy expended when the infant begins active rather than passive nutritional intake.

Provision of care by the parents is appropriate even for very sick or defective infants who are likely to die. It has been found that detachment is easier after attachment, because the parents are comforted by the knowledge that they did all they could for their child while he or she was alive.

#### Facilitation of Family Adjustment

During crisis, it is difficult to maintain interpersonal relationships. Yet in a newborn intensive care area, the parents are expected to relate to many different care providers. It is important that parents have as few professionals as possible relaying information to them. A primary nurse should coordinate care and provide continuity for parents. Care providers are individuals and thus will use different terms, inflections, and attitudes. These subtle differences are monumental to parents and may confuse, confound, and produce anxiety. The transfer of the baby from NICU to a step-down unit or transport back to the home hospital provokes parental anxiety because they must now deal with new health care professionals. The nurse not only functions as a liaison between the parents and the various professionals interacting with the infant and parents but also offers clarification, explanation, interpretation of information, and support to the parents.

The nurse encourages parents to deal with the crisis with help from their support system. The support system attempts to meet the emotional needs and to provide support for the family members in crisis and stress situations. Biologic kinship is not the only valid criterion for a support system; an emotional kinship is the most important factor. In our mobile society of isolated nuclear families, the support system may be a next-door neighbor, a best friend, or perhaps a schoolmate. The nurse needs to search out the significant others in the lives of the parents and help them understand the problems so that they can support the parents.

The impact of the crisis on the family is individual and varied. The nurse obtains information about the family's ability to adapt to the situation through interaction with the family. To institute appropriate interventions, the nurse should view the birth of the infant (normal newborn, preterm infant, infant with congenital anomaly) as it is defined by the family.

It is important for the nurse to encourage open intrafamily communication. The nurse should discourage the family from keeping secrets from one another, especially between spouses, because secrets undermine the trust of relationships. Well-meaning rationales such as "I want to protect her," "I don't want him to worry about it," and so on can be destructive to open communication and to the basic element of a relationship—trust.

Open communication is especially important when the mother is hospitalized apart from the infant. The first person to visit the infant relays information regarding the infant's care and condition to the mother and family. In this situation, the mother has had minimal contact, if any, with her infant. Because of her anxiety and isolation, she may mistrust all those who provide information (the father, nurse, physician, or extended family) until she sees the infant for herself. This can put tremendous stress on the relationship between spouses. The parents (and family) should be given information together. This practice helps overcome misunderstandings and misinterpretations and promotes cooperative working through of problems.

The nurse should encourage the entire family—siblings as well as other relatives—to visit and obtain information about the baby. Methods of intervention in helping the family cope with the situation include providing support, confronting the crisis, and understanding the reality. Support, explanations, and the helping role must extend to the kin network, as well as to the nuclear family, to aid the extended family in communication and support ties with the nuclear family.

The needs of siblings should not be overlooked. Siblings have been looking forward to the new baby, and they, too, suffer a degree of loss. Young children may react with hostility and older ones with shame at the birth of an infant with an anomaly. Both reactions may make them feel guilty. Parents, who may be preoccupied with working through their own feelings, often cannot give the other children the attention and support they need. Sometimes another child becomes the focus of family tension. Anxiety thus directed can take the form of finding fault or of overconcern. This is a form of denial; the parents cannot face the real worry—the infant at risk. After assessing the situation, the observant nurse can ensure that another family member or friend steps in to support the siblings of the affected baby.

The nurse must respect and seek to meet the desires and needs of the individuals involved and understand that differences can exist side by side. The nurse can often elicit the parents' feelings about the experience by asking "How are *you* doing?" The emphasis is on *you,* and the interest must be sincere.

Families with children in the NICU may become friends and support one another. To encourage the development of these friendships and to provide support, many units have established parent groups. The core of the groups consists of parents whose infants were once in the intensive care unit. Most groups make contact with families within a day or two of the infant's admission to the unit, through either phone calls or visits to the hospital. Early one-on-one parent contacts are more effective than discussion groups in helping families work through their feelings. This personalized method gives the grieving parents an opportunity to express personal feelings about the pregnancy, labor, and birth and their different-than-expected infant with others who have experienced the same feelings and with whom they can identify.

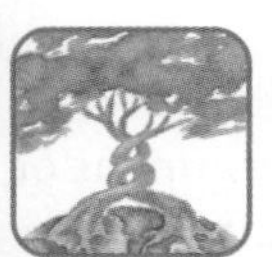

## Community-Based Nursing Care

Predischarge planning begins once the infant's condition becomes stable and it seems likely the newborn will survive (AAP, Hospital Discharge of the High-Risk Neonate, 1998). Adequate predischarge teaching helps parents transform any feelings of inadequacy they may have into feelings of self-assurance and attachment. From the beginning the parents should be taught about their infant's special needs and growth patterns (Bracht, Ardal, Bot, et al., 1998). This teaching and involvement are best facilitated by a nurse who is familiar with the infant and his or her family over a period of time and who has developed a comfortable and supportive relationship with them.

The nurse's responsibility is to provide home care instructions in an optimal environment for parental learning. Learning should take place over time, to avoid bombarding the parents with instructions in the day or hour before discharge. Parents often enjoy performing minimal caretaking tasks, with gradual expansion of their role. Many NICUs provide facilities for parents to room-in with their infants for a few days before discharge. This practice allows parents a degree of independence in the care of their infant with the security of nursing help nearby. It is particularly helpful for anxious parents, parents who have not had the opportunity to spend extended time with their infant, or parents who will be giving complex physical care at home, such as tracheostomy care (Costello & Chapman, 1998; Dracup, Doering, Moser, et al., 1998).

In addressing the basic elements of home care instruction the nurse needs to do the following:

1. Teach the parents routine well-baby care, such as bathing, taking a temperature, preparing formula, and breastfeeding.
2. Help parents learn to do special procedures as needed by the newborn, such as gavage or gastrostomy feedings, tracheostomy or enterostomy care, medication administration, cardiopulmonary resuscitation (CPR), and operation of the apnea monitor. Before discharge, the parents should be as comfortable as possible with these tasks and should demonstrate independence. Written instructions are useful for parents to refer to once they are home with the infant, but they should not replace actual participation in the infant's care.
3. Refer parents to community health and support organizations. The Visiting Nurses' Association, public health nurses, or social services can assist the parents in the stressful transition from hospital to home by providing the necessary home teaching and support. Some NICUs have their own parent support groups to help bridge the gap between hospital and home care. Parents can also find support from a variety of community organizations, such as mothers-of-twins groups, trisomy 13 clubs, the March of Dimes Birth Defects Foundation, handicapped children services, and teen mother and child programs. Each community has numerous agencies capable of assisting the family in adapting emotionally, physically, and financially to the chronically ill infant. The nurse should be familiar with community resources and help the parents identify which agencies may benefit them.
4. Help parents recognize the growth and development needs of their infant. A development program begun in the hospital can be continued at home, or parents may be referred to an infant development program in the community.
5. Arrange medical follow-up care before discharge. A family pediatrician, a well-baby clinic, or a specialty clinic may provide follow-up care for the infant. The first appointment should be made before the infant is discharged from the hospital (Hussey-Gardner, Wachtel, & Viscardi, 1998).
6. Evaluate the need for special equipment for infant care (such as a respirator, oxygen, apnea monitor) in the home. Any equipment or supplies should be placed in the home before the infant's discharge.

Further evaluation after the infant has gone home is useful in determining whether the crisis has been resolved satisfactorily. The parents are usually given the intensive care nursery's telephone number to call for support and advice. It is suggested that staff follow up with each family with visits or telephone calls at intervals for several weeks to assess and evaluate the infant's (and parents') progress.

### Evaluation

Expected outcomes of nursing care include the following:

- The parents are able to verbalize their feelings of grief and loss.
- The parents verbalize their concerns about their baby's health problems, care needs, and potential outcome.
- The parents participate in their infant's care and show attachment behaviors.

## Considerations for the Nurse Who Works with At-Risk Newborns

The birth of a baby with a problem is a traumatic event with the potential for either disruption or growth of the involved family. Throughout the pregnancy, both parents, together and separately, have felt excitement, experienced thoughts of acceptance, and pictured what their baby would look like. Both parents have wished for a perfect baby and feared an unhealthy one. Each parent and family member must accept and adjust when the fantasized fears become reality.

The period of waiting between suspicion and confirmation of abnormality or dysfunction is a very anxious one for parents because it is difficult, if not impossible, to begin attachment to the infant if the newborn's future is questionable. During the waiting period parents need support and acknowledgment that this is an anxious time and they must be kept informed about efforts to gather additional data and to maintain the infant's viability. It is helpful to tell both parents about the problem at the same time, with the baby present. An honest discussion of the problem and anticipatory management at the earliest possible time by health professionals help the parents (1) maintain trust in the physician and nurse, (2) appreciate the reality of the situation by dispelling fantasy and misconception, (3) begin the grieving process, and (4) mobilize internal and external support.

In their sensitive and vulnerable state, parents are acutely perceptive of others' responses and reactions (particularly nonverbal) to the child. Parents can be expected to identify with the responses of others. Therefore, it is imperative that medical and nursing staff be fully aware of and come to terms with their feelings so they are comfortable and at ease with the baby and grieving family.

Nurses may feel uncomfortable, may not know what to say to parents, or may fear confronting their own feelings as well as those of the parents. Each nurse must work out personal reactions with instructors, peers, clergy, parents, or significant others. It is helpful to have a stockpile of therapeutic questions and statements to initiate meaningful dialogue with parents. Opening statements might include the following: "You must be wondering what could have caused this," "Are you thinking that you (or someone else) may have done something?" "How can I help?" and "Are you wondering how you are going to manage?" Statements such as "It could have been worse," "It's God's will," "You have other children," "You are still young and can have more," and "I understand how you feel" should be avoided. This child is important now. The entire multidisciplinary team may need to pool its resources and expertise to help the parents of children born with problems or disorders so that both parents and children thrive.

Nurses cannot provide support unless they themselves are supported. Working in an emotional environment of life-and-death situations takes its toll on staff. NICUs are among the most stressful areas in health care for patients, families, and nurses. Nurses bear most of the stress and largely determine the atmosphere of the NICU. The nurse's ability to cope with stress is the key to creating an emotionally healthy environment and a positive working atmosphere. The emotional needs and feelings of the staff must be recognized and dealt with so that staff can support the parents. An environment of openness to feelings and support in dealing with their human needs and emotions is essential for personnel. As caregivers, nurses may be unaware of their need to grieve for their own losses in the NICU. Nurses must also go through the grief work that parents experience. Techniques such as group meetings, individual support, and primary care nursing may assist in maintaining staff mental health. The staff NICU nurses may never see the long-term results of the specialized, sensitive care they give to parents and their newborns. Their only immediate evidence of effective care may be the beginning of resolution of parental grief, discharge of a recovered, thriving infant to the care of happy parents, and the beginning of reintegration of family life.

# Chapter Review

## CHAPTER HIGHLIGHTS

- The sick newborn—whether preterm, term, or postterm—must be managed within narrow physiologic parameters.
- These parameters (respiratory and thermal regulation) maintain physiologic homeostasis and prevent introduction of iatrogenic stress to the already stressed infant.
- The nursing care of the newborn with special problems involves the understanding of normal physiology, the pathophysiology of the disease process, clinical manifestations, and supportive or corrective therapies. Only with this theoretical background can the nurse caring for newborns make appropriate observations concerning responses to therapy and development of complications.
- Asphyxia results in significant circulatory, respiratory, and biochemical changes in the newborn that make the successful transition to extrauterine life difficult. Asphyxia requires early identification and resuscitative management.
- Newborn conditions that commonly present with respiratory distress and require oxygen and ventilator assistance are respiratory distress syndrome, meconium aspiration syndrome, and transient tachypnea of the newborn.
- Cold stress sets up the chain of physiologic events of hypoglycemia, pulmonary vasoconstriction, hyperbilirubinemia, respiratory distress, and metabolic acidosis. Nurses are responsible for early detection and initiation of treatment for hypoglycemia.
- Differentiation between pathologic and physiologic jaundice is the key to early and successful intervention.
- Anemia (decreased red blood cell volume) and polycythemia (increased volume) place the newborn at risk for alterations in blood flow and the oxygen-carrying capacity of the blood.
- Nursing assessment of the septic newborn involves identification of very subtle clinical signs that are also seen in other clinical disease states.
- The nurse is the facilitator for interdisciplinary communication with the parents and identifies their understanding of their infant's care and their needs for emotional support.
- Parents of at-risk newborns need support from nurses and health care providers to understand the special needs of their baby and to feel comfortable in an overwhelming and often unfamiliar environment.

## CHAPTER REFERENCES


American Academy of Pediatrics, American Heart Association. Kattwinkel, J., Short, J. Eds (2000). *Textbook of neonatal resuscitation.* 4th ed. Elk Grove Village, Il: American Academy of Pediatrics, American Heart Association.

American Academy of Pediatrics, Committee on Fetus and Newborn. (1999). Surfactant replacement therapy for respiratory distress syndrome. *Pediatrics, 103*(3), 684–685.

American Academy of Pediatrics, Provisional Committee for Quality Improvement and Subcommittee on Hyperbilirubinemia. (1994). Practice parameter: Management of hyperbilirubinemia in the healthy term newborn. *Pediatrics, 94*(4, Pt. 1), 558–565. (Published erratum appears in 1995 *Pediatrics, 95*[3], 458–461.

American Academy of Pediatrics Committee on Fetus and Newborn (1998). Hospital discharge of the high-risk neonate—proposed guidelines. *Pediatries,* 102(2), 411–417.

Anastasi, J. M. (1998). Innovations in care: Neonatal home antibiotic infusion therapy. *Neonatal Network, 17*(4), 33–38.

Askin, D. F. (1995). Bacterial and fungal infections in the neonate. *Journal of Obstetric, Gynecologic, and Neonatal Nursing, 24*(7), 635–643.

Bracht, M., Ardal, F., Bot, A., & Cheng, C. M. (1998). Initiation and maintenance of a hospital-based parent group for parents of premature infants: Key factors for success. *Neonatal Network, 17*(3), 33–37.

Cornblath, M., Hawdon, J. M., Williams, A. F., Aynsley-Green, A., Ward-Platt, M. P., Schwartz, R., & Kalhan, S. C. (2000). Controversies regarding definition of neonatal hypoglycemia: Suggested operational thresholds. *Pediatrics, 105*(5), 1141–1145.

Costello, A., & Chapman, J. (1998). Mother's perception of the care-by-parent program prior to hospital discharge of their preterm infants. *Neonatal Network, 17*(4), 37–42.

Doyle, J. J., Schmidt, V., & Zipursky, A. (1999). Hematology. In G. B. Avery, M. A. Fletcher, & M. G. MacDonald (Eds.), *Neonatology: Pathophysiology and management of the newborn* (5th ed.). Philadelphia: Lippincott Williams & Wilkins. Chap. 45, pp. 1045–1092.

Dracup, K., Doering, L. V., Moser, D. K., & Evangelista, L. (1998). Retention and use of cardiopulmonary resuscitation skills in parents of infants at risk for cardiopulmonary arrest. *Pediatric Nursing, 24*(3), 219–225.

Gaynes, R. P., Edwards, J. R., Jarvis, W. R., Culver, D. H., Tolson, J. S., & Martone, W. J. (1996). Nosocomial infections among neonates in high risk nurseries in the United States. National Nosocomial Infections Surveillance System. *Pediatrics, 98*(3, Pt. 1), 357–361.

Gomez, M., Hansen, T., & Corbet, A. (1998). Therapies for intractable respiratory failure. In H. W. Taeusch & R. A. Ballard (Eds.), *Avery's diseases of the newborn* (7th ed.). Philadelphia: Saunders. Chap. 51 pp. 576–594.

Grant, P. (1978). Psychological needs of families of high-risk infants. *Families and Community Health.* 1(3): 93–97.

Hansen, T. N., Cooper, T. R., & Weisman, L. E. (1998). *Contemporary diagnosis and management of neonatal respiratory diseases* (2nd ed.). Newton, PA: Handbooks in Health Care.

Hussey-Gardner, B. T., Wachtel, R. C., & Viscardi, R. M. (1998). Parent perceptions of an NICU follow-up clinic. *Neonatal Network, 17*(1), 33–39.

Juul, S. E. (1999). Erythropoietin in the neonate. *Current Problems in Pediatrics,* 29 pp. 133–149.

Kaplan, D. M., & Mason, E. A. (1974). Maternal reactions to premature birth viewed as an acute emotional disorder. In H. J. Parad (Ed.), *Crisis intervention.* New York: Family Services Association of America. Chap. 9. pp. 118–128.

Klaus, M. H., & Kennell, J. H. (1982). *Maternal-infant bonding* (2nd ed.). St. Louis: Mosby.

MacMahon, J. R., Stevenson, D. K., & Oski, F. A. (1998). Management of neonatal hyperbilirubinemia. In H. W. Taeusch & R. R. Ballard (Eds.), *Avery's diseases of the newborn* (7th ed.). Philadelphia: Saunders. Chap. 81, pp. 995–1002.

Maisels, M. J. (1999). Jaundice. In G. B. Avery, M. A. Fletcher, & M. G. MacDonald (Eds.), *Neonatology: Pathophysiology and management of the newborn* (5th ed.). Philadelphia: Lippincott Williams & Wilkins. Chap. 38, pp. 765–820.

Merenstein, G. B., & Gardner, S. L. (1998). *Handbook of neonatal intensive care* (4th ed.). St. Louis: Mosby.

Neonatal hypoglycemia. (2000). *NANN guidelines for practice* (pp. 1–16). Des Plaines, IL: NANN.

Neonatal thermoregulation. (1997). *NANN guidelines for practice* (pp. 1–15). Petaluma, CA: NICU Ink.

Ogata, E. S. (1999). Carbohydrate homeostasis. In G. B. Avery, M. A. Fletcher, & M. G. MacDonald (Eds.), *Neonatology: Pathophysiology and management of the newborn* (5th ed.). Philadelphia: Lippincott Williams & Wilkins. Chap. 35, pp. 699–714.

Payne, N. R., Schilling, C. G., & Steinberg, S. (1994). Selecting antibiotics for nosocomial bacterial infections in patients requiring neonatal intensive care. *Neonatal Network, 13*(3), 41–51.

Raines, D. A. (1998). Values of mothers of low birth weight infants in the NICU. *Neonatal Network, 17*(4), 41–46.

Schuchat, A. (1998). Epidemiology of group B streptococcal disease in the United States: Shifting paradigms. *Clinical Microbiology Reviews, 11*(3), 497–513.

Solnit, A., & Stark, M. (1961). Mourning and the birth of a defective child. *Psychoanalytic Study of the Child, 16,* 505.

Thureen, P. J., Deacon, J., O'Neill, P., & Hernandez, J. (1999). *Assessment and care of the well newborn.* Philadelphia: Saunders.

Whitsett, J. A., Pryhuber, G. S., Rice, W. R., Warner, B. B., & Wert, S. E. (1999). Acute respiratory disorders. In G. B. Avery, M. A. Fletcher, & M. G. MacDonald (Eds.), *Neonatology: Pathophysiology and management of the newborn* (5th ed.). Philadelphia: Lippincott Williams & Wilkins. Chap. 28. pp. 485–508.

Wiswell, T. E., Gannon, C. M., Jacob, J., Goldsmith, L., Szyld, E., Weiss, K., Schutzman, D., Cleary, G. M., Filipov, P., Kurlat, I., Caballero, C. L., Abassi, S., Sprague, D., Oltorf, C., & Padula, M. (2000). Delivery room management of the apparently vigorous meconium-stained neonate: Results of the multicenter, international collaborative trial. *Pediatrics, 105*(1), 1–7.

Wolach, B. (1997). Neonatal sepsis: Pathogenesis and supportive therapy. *Seminars in Perinatology, 21*(1), 28–38.

Young, T. E., & Mangum, O. B. (2000). *Neofax®: A manual of drugs used in neonatal care* (13th ed.). Raleigh, NC: Acorn Publishing.

## CONTEMPORARY MATERNAL-NEWBORN NURSING ON-LINE

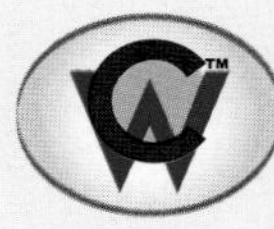

Additional interactive resources, including animations and video, for this chapter can be found on the Companion Website at http://www.prenhall.com/ladewig. Click on Chapter 26 and "Begin" to select the activities for this chapter.

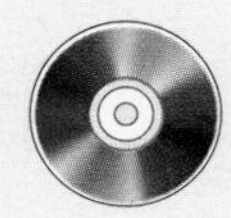

For NCLEX review questions and an audio glossary, access the accompanying CD-ROM in this book.

# Part Six

# Postpartum

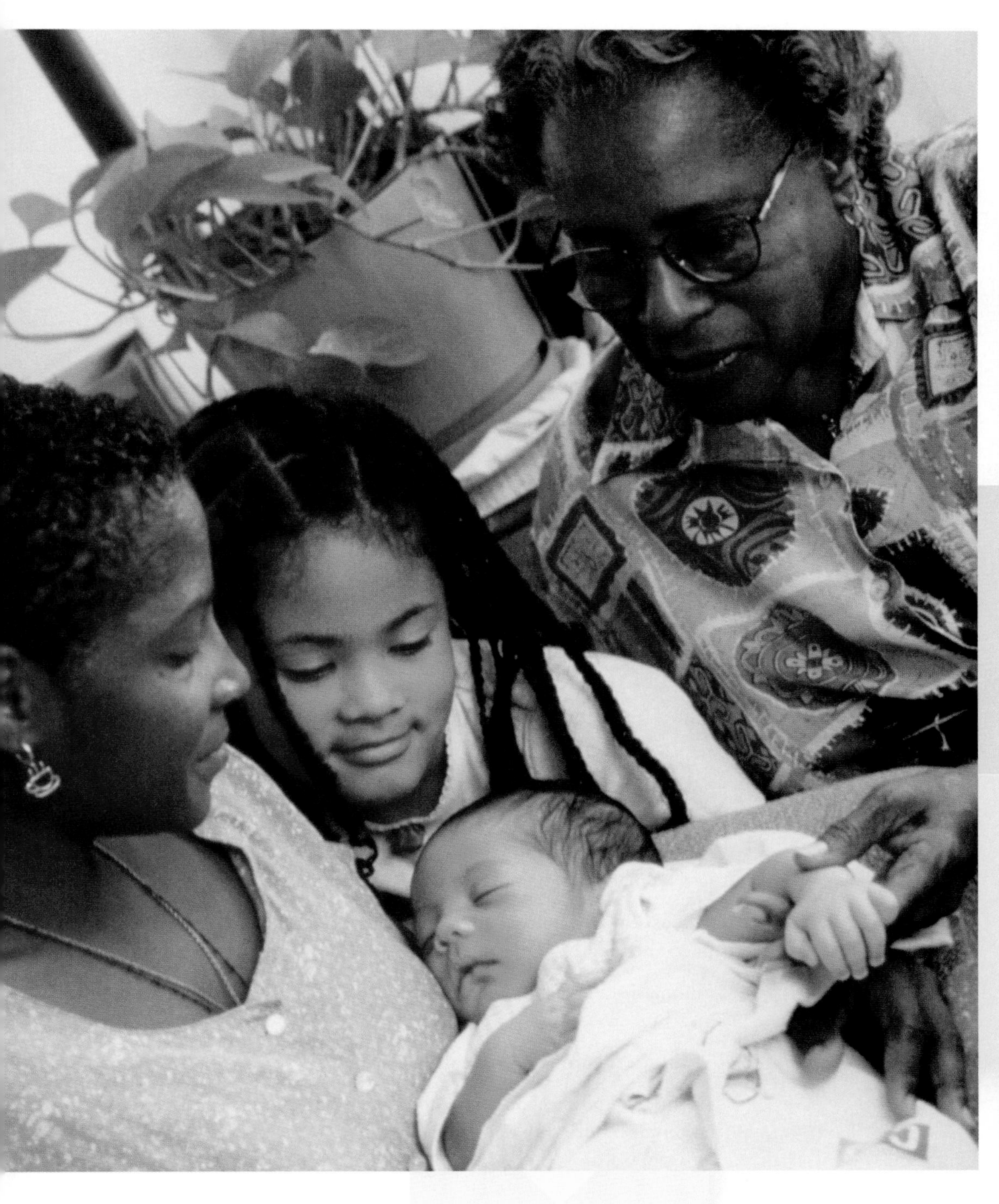

Chapter 27

# Postpartal Adaptation and Nursing Assessment

*My position as a mom-baby nurse involves helping the new family get to know one another. The real challenge is to balance the introduction of new skills and information with the time and space needed for the family to recover, both physically and mentally, from the birth experience. I want the families I care for to regard me as a resource, not an authority.*

—Postpartum Nurse

## KEY TERMS

| | |
|---|---|
| Afterpains | 732 |
| Boggy uterus | 729 |
| Diastasis recti abdominis | 731 |
| *En face* | 734 |
| Engrossment | 735 |
| Fundus | 729 |
| Involution | 729 |
| Lochia | 730 |
| Lochia alba | 730 |
| Lochia rubra | 730 |
| Lochia serosa | 730 |
| Postpartum blues | 734 |
| Puerperium | 729 |
| Reciprocity | 735 |

## OBJECTIVES

- Describe the basic physiologic changes that occur in the postpartal period as a woman's body returns to its prepregnant state.
- Discuss the psychologic adjustments that normally occur during the postpartal period.
- Summarize the factors that influence the development of parent-infant attachment.
- Delineate a normal postpartal assessment.
- Discuss the physical and developmental tasks that the mother must accomplish during the postpartal period.

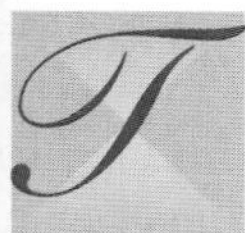

he **puerperium,** or postpartal period, is the period during which the woman adjusts, physically and psychologically, to the process of childbirth. It begins immediately after birth and continues for approximately 6 weeks, or until the body has returned to a near prepregnant state. This chapter describes the physiologic and psychologic changes that occur postpartally and the basic aspects of a thorough postpartal assessment.

# Postpartal Physical Adaptations

Comprehensive nursing assessment is based on a sound understanding of the normal anatomic and physiologic processes of the puerperium. These processes involve the reproductive organs and other major body systems.

## Reproductive System

### Involution of the Uterus

The term **involution** is used to describe the rapid reduction in size and the return of the uterus to a nonpregnant state. Following separation of the placenta, the decidua of the uterus is irregular, jagged, and varied in thickness. The spongy layer of the decidua is cast off as lochia, while the inner layer forms the basis for the development of new endometrium. Except at the placenta attachment site, this process takes about 3 weeks. Bleeding from the larger uterine vessels of the placenta site is controlled by compression of the retracted uterine muscle fibers. The clotted blood is gradually absorbed by the body. Some of these vessels are eventually obliterated and replaced by new vessels with smaller lumens.

Rather than forming a fibrous scar in the decidua, the placenta site heals by a process of exfoliation. In this process, the site is undermined by the growth of the endometrial tissue both from the margins of the site and from the fundi of the endometrial glands left in the basal layer of the site. The infarcted superficial tissue then becomes necrotic and is sloughed off (Resnik, 1999). Exfoliation is a very important aspect of involution. If healing of the placenta site left a fibrous scar, the area available for future implantation would be limited, as would the number of possible pregnancies.

The uterus gradually decreases in size as the cells grow smaller and the hyperplasia of pregnancy reverses. Protein material in the uterine wall is broken down and absorbed. Factors that slow uterine involution include prolonged labor, anesthesia or excessive analgesia, difficult birth, grand multiparity, a full bladder, and incomplete expulsion of all of the placenta or fragments of the membranes. Factors that enhance involution include an uncomplicated labor and birth, complete expulsion of the placenta or membranes, breastfeeding, and early ambulation.

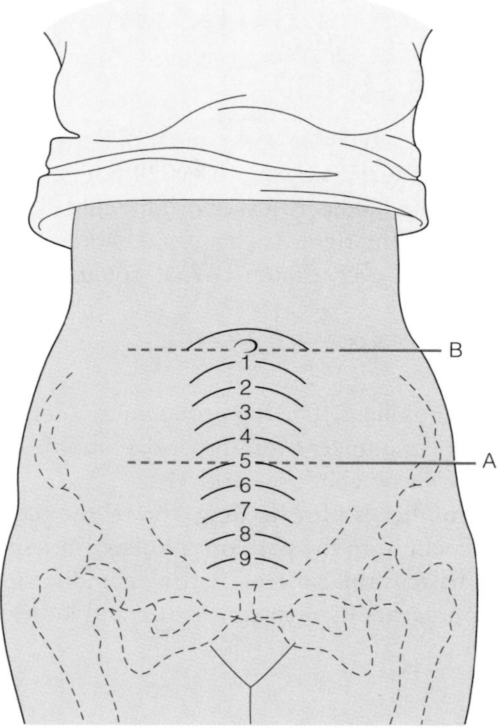


**FIGURE 27–1** ♦ Involution of the uterus. **A,** Immediately after delivery of the placenta, the top of the fundus is in the midline and approximately halfway between the symphysis pubis and the umbilicus. **B,** About 6 to 12 hours after birth, the fundus is at the level of the umbilicus. The height of the fundus then decreases about one finger breadth (approximately 1 cm) each day.

### Changes in Fundal Position

Immediately following the birth of the placenta, the uterus contracts to the size of a large grapefruit. The **fundus,** or top portion of the uterus, is situated in the midline midway between the symphysis pubis and the umbilicus (Figure 27–1♦). The walls of the contracted uterus are in close proximity, and the uterine blood vessels are firmly compressed by the myometrium. Within 6 to 12 hours after birth, the fundus of the uterus rises to the level of the umbilicus. A fundus that is above the umbilicus and is boggy (feels soft and spongy rather than firm and well contracted) is associated with excessive uterine bleeding. A **boggy uterus** results from collected blood and clot formation causing the fundus to rise and the interruption of uterine contractions. When the fundus is higher than expected on palpation and is not in the midline (usually deviated to the right), distension of the bladder should be suspected.

After birth the top of the fundus remains at the level of the umbilicus for about half a day. On the first postpartum day, the top of the fundus is located about 1 cm

## Critical Thinking in Practice

You have completed your assessment of Patty Clark, a 24-year-old, G2P2 woman who is 24 hours past childbirth. The fundus is just above the umbilicus and slightly to the right. Lochia rubra is present, and a pad is soaked every 2 hours. What would you do?

Answers can be found in Appendix I.

below the umbilicus. The top of the fundus descends approximately one finger breadth per day until it descends into the pelvis on about the 10th day.

If the mother is breastfeeding, the release of endogenous oxytocin from the posterior pituitary in response to suckling hastens this process. Barring complications, the uterus approaches its prepregnant size and location by 5 to 6 weeks.

### Lochia

The uterus rids itself of the debris remaining after birth through a discharge called **lochia,** which is classified according to its appearance and contents. **Lochia rubra** is dark red. It occurs for the first 2 to 3 days and contains epithelial cells, erythrocytes, leukocytes, shreds of decidua, and occasionally fetal meconium, lanugo, and vernix caseosa. Lochia should not contain large (plum-sized) clots; if it does the cause should be investigated without delay. Lochia serosa is a pinkish color. It follows from about the 3rd until the 10th day. **Lochia serosa** is composed of serous exudate (hence the name), shreds of degenerating decidua, erythrocytes, leukocytes, cervical mucus, and numerous microorganisms. Gradually the red blood cell component decreases, and **lochia alba,** a creamy or yellowish discharge, persists for an additional week or two. This final discharge is composed primarily of leukocytes, decidual cells, epithelial cells, fat, cervical mucus, cholesterol crystals, and bacteria. When the lochia flow stops, the cervix is considered closed, and chances of infection ascending from the vagina to the uterus decrease. Like menstrual discharge, lochia flow has a musty, stale odor that is not offensive. Foul-smelling lochia suggests infection and should be assessed promptly.

The total volume of lochia is about 240 to 270 mL, and the amount gradually declines with each passing day (Scoggin, 2000). The amount of discharge is greater in the morning due to pooling in the vagina and uterus while the mother lies sleeping. The amount of lochia may also be increased by exertion or breastfeeding.

Evaluation of lochia is necessary not only to determine the presence of hemorrhage but also to assess uterine involution. The type, amount, and consistency of lochia determine the stage of healing of the placenta site, and a progressive change from bright red at birth to dark red to pink to white or clear discharge should occur. Persistent discharge of lochia rubra or a return to lochia rubra indicates subinvolution or late postpartal hemorrhage (see Chapter 30).

### Cervical Changes

Following birth the cervix is flabby and formless and may appear bruised. The external os is markedly irregular and closes slowly. It admits two fingers for a few days following birth, but by the end of the first week it admits only a fingertip.

The shape of the external os is permanently changed by the first childbearing. The characteristic dimplelike os of the nullipara changes to the lateral slit (fish-mouth) os of the multipara. After significant cervical laceration or several lacerations, the cervix may appear lopsided.

### Vaginal Changes

Following birth the vagina appears edematous and may be bruised. Small superficial lacerations may be evident, and the rugae are obliterated. The apparent bruising is due to pelvic congestion and will quickly disappear. The hymen, torn and jagged, heals irregularly, leaving small tags called the *carunculae myrtiformes.*

The size of the vagina decreases and rugae return within 3 weeks, facilitating the gradual return to smaller, although not nulliparous, dimensions. By 6 weeks the nonlactating woman's vagina usually appears normal. The lactating woman is in a hypoestrogenic state because of ovarian suppression, and her vaginal mucosa may be pale and without rugae; the effects of the lowered estrogen level may lead to dyspareunia (painful intercourse). Tone and contractility of the vaginal orifice may be improved by perineal tightening exercises such as Kegel's (see Chapter 9). The labia majora and labia minora are more flaccid in the woman who has borne a child than in the nullipara.

### Perineal Changes

During the early postpartal period the soft tissue in and around the perineum may appear edematous, with some bruising (Figure 27–2♦). If an episiotomy is present, the edges should be drawn together. Occasionally ecchymosis occurs, which may delay healing.

### Recurrence of Ovulation and Menstruation

The return of ovulation and menstruation varies for each postpartal woman. Menstruation generally returns in 40% to 45% of nonnursing mothers between 6 and 8 weeks after birth; 50% of the first cycles are anovulatory.

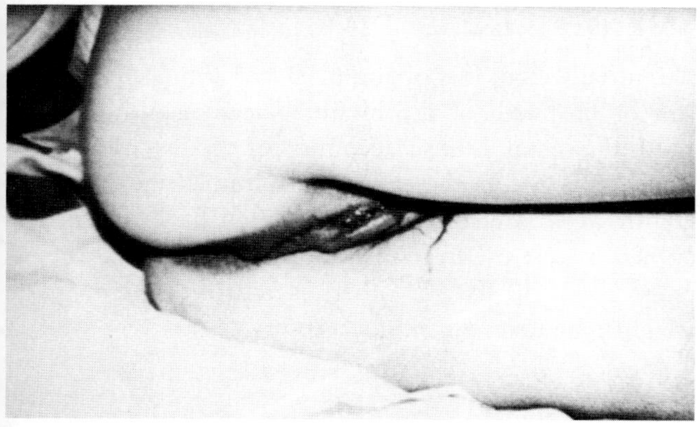

FIGURE 27–2 ♦ Bruising and edema of the vulva and perineum in a primipara 3 days after a forceps delivery. Source: Bennett, V. R., & Brown, L. K. (1989) *Myles Textbook for Midwives,* (11th ed.) (pp. 235). Edinburgh: Churchill Livingstone.

Overall 75% of nonnursing mothers resume menstruation by 12 weeks and the remaining 25% within 6 months following birth (Scoggin, 2000).

The return of ovulation and menstruation in nursing mothers is usually prolonged. It is associated with the length of time the woman breastfeeds and whether formula supplements are used. If a nursing mother breastfeeds for less than 1 month, the return of menstruation and ovulation is similar to that of the nonnursing mother. In women who exclusively breastfeed, menstruation is usually delayed for at least 3 months. However, since ovulation precedes menstruation, breastfeeding is not a reliable means of contraception (Farrington & Ward, 1999).

## Abdomen

Following birth the stretched abdominal wall appears loose and flabby, but it responds to exercise within 2 to 3 months. In the grand multipara, in the woman in whom overdistention of the abdomen has occurred, or in the woman with poor muscle tone before pregnancy, the abdomen may fail to regain good tone and will remain flabby. **Diastasis recti abdominis,** a separation of the abdominal muscle, may occur with pregnancy, especially in women with poor abdominal muscle tone. If diastasis occurs, part of the abdominal wall has no muscular support but is formed only by skin, subcutaneous fat, fascia, and peritoneum. If rectus muscle tone is not regained, support may be inadequate during future pregnancies. Inadequate support may result in a pendulous abdomen and increased maternal backache. Fortunately, diastasis responds well to exercise, and abdominal muscle tone can improve significantly.

Striae (stretch marks), which are caused by stretching and rupture of the elastic fibers of the skin, are red to purple at the time of birth. These marks gradually fade after a time but remain visible.

## Lactation

During pregnancy, breast development in preparation for lactation results from the influence of both estrogen and progesterone. After birth, the interplay of maternal hormones leads to milk production. (For further details, see the section on breastfeeding in Chapter 24.)

## Gastrointestinal System

Hunger following birth is common, and the mother may enjoy a light meal. She may also be quite thirsty and may drink large amounts of fluid. This helps replace fluids lost in labor, in the urine, and through perspiration.

The bowels tend to be sluggish following birth because of the lingering effects of progesterone and decreased abdominal muscle tone. Women who have had an episiotomy may tend to delay elimination for fear of increasing their pain or in the belief that their stitches will be torn if they bear down. In refusing or delaying the bowel movement, the woman may cause increased constipation and more pain when bowel elimination finally occurs.

The woman with a cesarean birth may receive clear liquids shortly after surgery; once bowel sounds are present, her diet is quickly advanced to solid food. The woman may experience some initial discomfort from flatulence; it is relieved by early ambulation and use of antiflatulent medications. It may take a few days for the bowel to regain its tone, especially if general anesthesia was used. The woman who has had a cesarean or a difficult birth may benefit from stool softeners.

## Urinary Tract

The postpartal woman has an increased bladder capacity, swelling and bruising of the tissue around the urethra, decreased sensitivity to fluid pressure, and a decreased sensation of bladder filling. Consequently, she is at risk for overdistention, incomplete bladder emptying, and a buildup of residual urine. Women who have had an anesthetic block have inhibited neural functioning of the bladder and are more susceptible to bladder distention, difficulty voiding, and bladder infections.

Puerperal diuresis causes rapid filling of the bladder. Thus adequate bladder elimination is an immediate concern. Urinary stasis increases the chances that a urinary tract infection will develop. A full bladder may also increase the tendency toward uterine relaxation by displacing the uterus and interfering with contractility, all of which may lead to hemorrhage. In the absence of infection, the dilated ureters and renal pelves return to prepregnant size by the end of the sixth week.

## Vital Signs

A maternal temperature of up to 38°C (100.4°F) may occur after childbirth as a result of the exertion and dehydration of labor. After the first 24 hours, the woman should be afebrile, and a temperature of 38°C (100.4°F) or greater suggests infection. (See discussion in Chapter 30.)

Blood pressure readings should remain stable after childbirth. A decrease may indicate physiologic readjustment to decreased intrapelvic pressure, or it may be related to uterine hemorrhage. Blood pressure elevations, especially when accompanied by headache, suggest pregnancy-induced hypertension (PIH), and the woman should be evaluated further.

Puerperal bradycardia with rates of 50 to 70 beats per minute commonly occurs during the first 6 to 10 days of the postpartal period. It may be related to decreased cardiac effort, the decreased blood volume following placental separation and contraction of the uterus, and increased stroke volume. Tachycardia occurs less frequently and is related to increased blood loss or difficult, prolonged labor and birth.

## HINTS FOR PRACTICE

During the first few hours after birth, the woman may have some orthostatic hypotension; it will cause her to have a lower blood pressure reading in a sitting position. For the most accurate reading, measure her BP with her in the same position each time, preferably lying on her back with her arm at her side.

## Blood Values

Blood values should return to the prepregnant state by the end of the postpartal period. Pregnancy-associated activation of coagulation factors may continue for variable amounts of time during the postpartal period. This condition, in conjunction with trauma, immobility, or sepsis, predisposes the woman to development of thromboembolism.

Leukocytosis often occurs, with white blood cell counts of 15,000 to 20,000/mL. Hemoglobin and hematocrit levels may be difficult to interpret in the first 2 days after birth because of the changing blood volume. In general, a decrease of two percentage points from the hematocrit at admission to the birthing unit indicates a blood loss of 500 mL (Varney, 1997).

Hemoglobin and hematocrit values should approximate or exceed prelabor values within 2 to 6 weeks as normal concentrations are reached. As extracellular fluid is excreted, hemoconcentration coincides with a rise in hematocrit.

## Weight Loss

An initial weight loss of about 10 to 12 lb occurs as a result of the birth of the infant, placenta, and amniotic fluid. Puerperal diuresis accounts for the loss of an additional 5 lb during the early puerperium. By the sixth to eighth week after birth, many women have returned to approximately prepregnant weight if they gained the average 25 to 30 lb. For others, a return to prepregnant weight may take longer.

## Postpartal Chill

Frequently the mother experiences a shaking chill immediately after birth, which is related to a nervous response or to vasomotor changes. If not followed by fever, this chill is of no clinical concern, but it is uncomfortable for the woman. The nurse can increase the woman's comfort by covering her with a warmed blanket and encouraging her to relax. Some women may also find a warm beverage helpful. Later in the puerperium, chill and fever indicate infection and require further evaluation.

## Postpartal Diaphoresis

The elimination of excess fluid and waste products via the skin during the puerperium produces greatly increased perspiration. Diaphoretic (sweating) episodes frequently occur at night, and the woman may awaken drenched with perspiration. This perspiration is not significant clinically, but the mother should be protected from chilling.

## Afterpains

**Afterpains** are more common in multiparas than in primiparas and are caused by intermittent uterine contractions. Although the uterus of the primipara usually remains consistently contracted, the lost tone of the multiparous uterus results in alternate contraction and relaxation. This phenomenon also occurs if the uterus has been markedly distended, as with a multiple-gestation pregnancy or hydramnios, or if clots or placental fragments were retained. These afterpains may cause the mother severe discomfort for 2 to 3 days after birth. The administration of oxytocic agents stimulates uterine contraction and increases the discomfort of the afterpains. Because endogenous oxytocin is released when the infant suckles, breastfeeding also increases the frequency and severity of the afterpains. The nursing mother may find it helpful to take a mild analgesic approximately 1 hour before feeding her infant. The nurse can assure the nursing mother that the prescribed analgesics are not harmful to the newborn and help improve the quality of the breastfeeding experience. An analgesic is also helpful at bedtime if the afterpains interfere with the mother's rest.

# Postpartal Psychologic Adaptations

## Maternal Role

The postpartal period is a time of readjustment and adaptation for the entire childbearing family, but especially for the mother. The woman experiences a variety of responses as she adjusts to a new family member, postpartum discomforts, changes in her body image, and the reality that she is no longer pregnant. During the first day or two after birth, the woman tends to be passive and somewhat dependent. She follows suggestions, hesitates to make decisions, and is still rather preoccupied with her needs. She may have a great need to talk about her perceptions of her labor and birth. Talking helps her work through the process, sort out the reality from her fantasized experience, and clarify anything that she did not understand. Food and sleep are major needs. In her early work, Rubin (1961) labeled this the *taking-in* period.

By the second or third day after birth, the new mother is ready to resume control over her life. She may be concerned about controlling her bodily functions such as elimination. If she is breastfeeding, she may worry about the quality of her milk and her ability to nurse her baby. If her baby spits up after a feeding, she may view it as a personal failure. She may also feel that the nurse handles her baby more proficiently than she does. She requires assurance that she is doing well as a mother. Rubin (1961) labeled this the *taking-hold* period. Today's mothers seem to be more independent and adjust more rapidly, exhibiting behaviors of "taking in" and "taking hold" in shorter time periods than those previously identified.

Postpartally the woman must adjust to a changed body image. Women often express dissatisfaction about their appearance and concern about the return of their weight and figure to normal. Multiparas tend to be more positive than primiparas. This difference may result because the multipara's previous experience has prepared her for the fact that the body does not immediately return to a prepregnant state.

The psychologic outcomes of the postpartal period are far more positive when the parents have access to a support network. Women and their partners may find that family relationships become increasingly important, but the increased family interaction can be a source of stress. The new parents may also have increasing contact with other parents of small children while contact with coworkers declines. Of great concern are women and their partners who have no family or friends to form a social network. Isolation at a time when the woman feels an increased need for support can result in tremendous stress and is often a contributing factor in situations of child neglect or abuse.

Maternal role attainment is the process by which a woman learns mothering behaviors and becomes comfortable with her identity as a mother. Formation of a maternal identity occurs with each child a woman bears. As the mother grows to know this child and forms a relationship, the mother's maternal identity gradually, systematically evolves and she "*binds in*" to the infant (Rubin, 1984).

Maternal role attainment often occurs in four stages (Mercer, 1995):

1. The *anticipatory stage* occurs during pregnancy. The woman looks to role models, especially her own mother, for examples of how to mother.
2. The *formal stage* begins when the child is born. The woman is still influenced by the guidance of others and tries to act as she believes others expect her to act.
3. The *informal stage* begins when the mother begins to make her own choices about mothering. The woman begins to develop her own style of mothering and finds ways of functioning that work well for her.
4. The *personal stage* is the final stage of maternal role attainment. When the woman reaches this stage, she is comfortable with the notion of herself as mother.

In most cases, maternal role attainment occurs within 3 to 10 months after birth. Social support, the woman's age and personality traits, the temperament of her infant, and the family's socioeconomic status all influence the woman's success in attaining the maternal role.

The postpartum woman faces a number of challenges as she adjusts to her new role:

- For many women, finding time for themselves is one of the greatest challenges. It is often difficult for the new mother to find time to read a book, talk to her partner, or even eat a meal without interruption.
- Women also report feelings of incompetence because they have not mastered all aspects of the mothering role. Often they are unsure of what to do in a given situation.
- The next greatest challenge involves fatigue resulting from sleep deprivation. The demands of nighttime care are tremendously draining, especially if the woman has other children.
- Another challenge faced by the new mother involves the feeling of responsibility that having a child brings. Women experience a sense of lost freedom, an awareness that they will never again be quite as carefree as they were before becoming mothers.

- Mothers sometimes cite the infant's behavior as a challenge, especially when the child is about 8 months old. Stranger anxiety develops, the infant begins crawling and getting into things, teething may cause fussiness, and the baby's tendency to put everything in his or her mouth requires constant vigilance by the parent.

All too often postpartum nurses are unaware of the long-term adjustments and stresses that the childbearing family faces as its members adjust to new and different roles. Nurses can help by providing anticipatory guidance about the realities of being a mother. Agencies should have literature available for reference at home. Ongoing parenting groups give parents an opportunity to discuss problems and become comfortable in new roles.

## Postpartum Blues

The **postpartum blues** consist of a transient period of depression that often occurs during the first few days of the puerperium. It may be manifested by tearfulness, anorexia, difficulty in sleeping, and a feeling of letdown. This depression frequently occurs while the woman is still hospitalized, but it may occur at home as well. Psychologic adjustments and hormonal factors are thought to be the main cause, although fatigue, discomfort, and overstimulation may play a part. The postpartum blues usually resolve naturally, but if persistent or worsening symptoms develop, the woman may need evaluation for postpartum depression (see Chapter 30).

## Development of Parent-Infant Attachment

A mother's first interaction with her infant is influenced by many factors, including her involvement with her family of origin, her relationships, the stability of her home environment, the communication patterns she developed, and the degree of nurturing she received as a child. These factors have shaped the person she has become. Certain personal characteristics are also important:

- *Level of trust.* What level of trust has this mother developed in response to her life experiences? What is her philosophy of childrearing? Will she be able to treat her infant as a unique individual with changing needs that should be met as much as possible?
- *Level of self-esteem.* How much does she value herself as a woman and as a mother? Does she feel generally able to cope with the adjustments of life?
- *Capacity for enjoying herself.* Is the mother able to find pleasure in everyday activities and human relationships?
- *Interest in and adequacy of knowledge about childbearing and childrearing.* What beliefs about the course of pregnancy, the capacities of newborns, and the nature of her emotions influence her behavior at first contact with her infant and later?
- *Her prevailing mood or usual feeling tone.* Is the woman predominantly content, angry, depressed, or anxious? Is she sensitive to her own feelings and those of others? Will she be able to accept her own needs and to obtain support in meeting them?
- *Reactions to the present pregnancy.* Was the pregnancy planned? Did it go smoothly? Were there ongoing life events that enhanced her pregnancy or depleted her reserves of energy?

By the time of birth each mother has developed an emotional orientation of some kind to the baby based on these factors.

### Initial Attachment Behavior

New mothers demonstrate a fairly regular pattern of maternal behaviors at first contact with a normal newborn. In a progression of touching activities, the mother proceeds from fingertip exploration of the newborn's extremities toward palmar contact with larger body areas and finally to enfolding the infant with the whole hand and arms. The time taken to accomplish these steps varies from minutes to days. The mother increases the proportion of time spent in the ***en face*** position (Figure 27–3♦). She arranges herself or the newborn so that she has direct face-to-face and eye-to-eye contact. There is an intense interest in having the infant's eyes open. When the infant's eyes are open, the mother characteristically greets the newborn and talks in high-pitched tones to him or her.

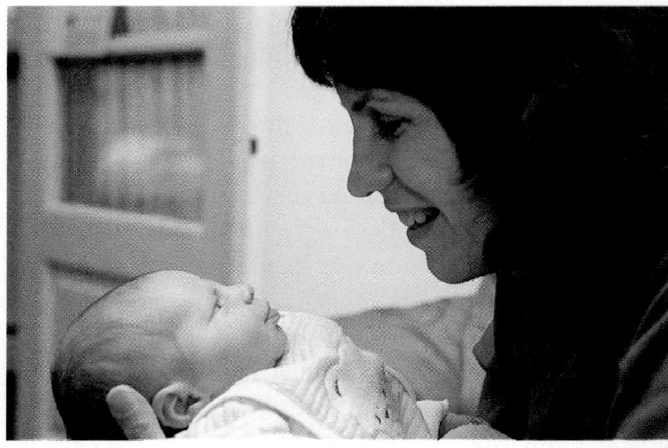

FIGURE 27–3 ♦ The mother has direct face-to-face and eye-to-eye contact in the *en face* position.

In most instances the mother relies heavily on her senses of sight, touch, and hearing in getting to know what her baby is really like. She tends also to respond verbally to any sounds emitted by the newborn, such as cries, coughs, sneezes, and grunts. The sense of smell may be involved as well.

In addition to interacting with the newborn, the mother is undergoing her own emotional reactions to the whole experience and, more specifically, to the baby as she perceives him or her. The frequency of the "I can't believe" reaction leads to speculation that human gains as well as losses may initially be met with a degree of shock, disbelief, and denial. A feeling of emotional distance from the newborn is quite common: "I feel like he is a stranger." On the other hand, feelings of connectedness between the newborn and the rest of the family can be expressed in positive or negative terms: "She's got your cute nose, Daddy" or "Oh, no! He looks just like the first one, and he was an impossible baby." A mother's facial expressions or the frequency and content of her questions may demonstrate concerns about the infant's general condition or normality, especially if her pregnancy was complicated or if a previously delivered baby was not healthy.

What are the characteristic behaviors of a newborn? Unless care is taken to effect a gentle birth, a number of harsh stimuli assault the senses of the newborn at birth. The newborn is probably suctioned, held with his or her head somewhat downward, exposed to bright lights and cool air, and in some way cleaned. The infant usually responds by crying. In fact, caregivers typically stimulate the newborn to cry to reassure themselves that the baby is well and normal. When newborns no longer need to concentrate most of their energy on physical and physiologic responses to the immediate crisis of birth, they are able to lie quietly with their eyes open, looking about, moving their limbs occasionally, making sucking motions, and possibly attempting to get their hand to their mouths. Placed in proximity to the mother, the newborn appears to focus briefly on her face and attend to her voice in the first moments of life.

During the first few days after her child's birth, the new mother applies herself to the task of getting to know her baby. This is termed the *acquaintance phase.* If the infant gives clear behavioral cues about needs, the infant's responses to mothering will be predictable, which will make the mother feel effective and competent. Other behaviors that make an infant more attractive to caretakers are smiling, grasping a finger, nursing eagerly, and being easy to console.

During this time the newborn is also becoming acquainted. Within a few days after birth, infants show signs of recognizing recurrent situations and responding to changes in routine. To the extent that their mother is their world, it can be said that they are actively acquainting themselves with her.

During the *phase of mutual regulation,* mother and infant seek to deal with the issue of the degree of control to be exerted by each partner in their relationship. In this phase of adjustment, a balance is sought between the needs of the mother and the needs of the infant. The most important consideration is that each should obtain a good measure of enjoyment from the interaction. During the mutual adjustment phase negative maternal feelings are likely to surface or intensify. Because "everyone knows that mothers love their babies," these negative feelings often go unexpressed and are allowed to build up. If they are expressed, the response of friends, relatives, or health care personnel is often to deny the feelings to the mother: "You don't mean that." Some negative feelings are normal in the first few days after birth, and the nurse should be supportive when the mother vocalizes these feelings.

When mutual regulation arrives at the point where both mother and infant primarily enjoy each other's company, reciprocity has been achieved. **Reciprocity** is an interactional cycle that occurs simultaneously between mother and infant. It involves mutual cuing behaviors, expectancy, rhythmicity, and synchrony. The mother develops a new relationship with an individual who has a unique character and evokes a response entirely different from the fantasy response of pregnancy. When reciprocity is synchronous, the interaction between mother and infant is mutually gratifying and is sought and initiated by both partners. They find pleasure and delight in each other's company and grow in mutual love.

### Father-Infant Interactions

Traditionally in Western cultures the primary role of the expectant father has been one of support for the pregnant woman. However, commitment to family-centered maternity care, has fostered interest in understanding the feelings and experiences of the new father. Evidence suggests that the father has a strong attraction to his newborn and that the feelings he experiences are similar to the mother's feelings of attachment (Figure 27–4♦). The characteristic sense of absorption, preoccupation, and interest in the infant demonstrated by fathers during early contact is termed **engrossment.**

### Siblings and Others

Infants are capable of maintaining a number of strong attachments without loss of quality. These attachments may include siblings, grandparents, aunts, and uncles. The social setting and personality of the individual seem to be significant factors in the development of multiple attachments. The advent of open visiting hours and

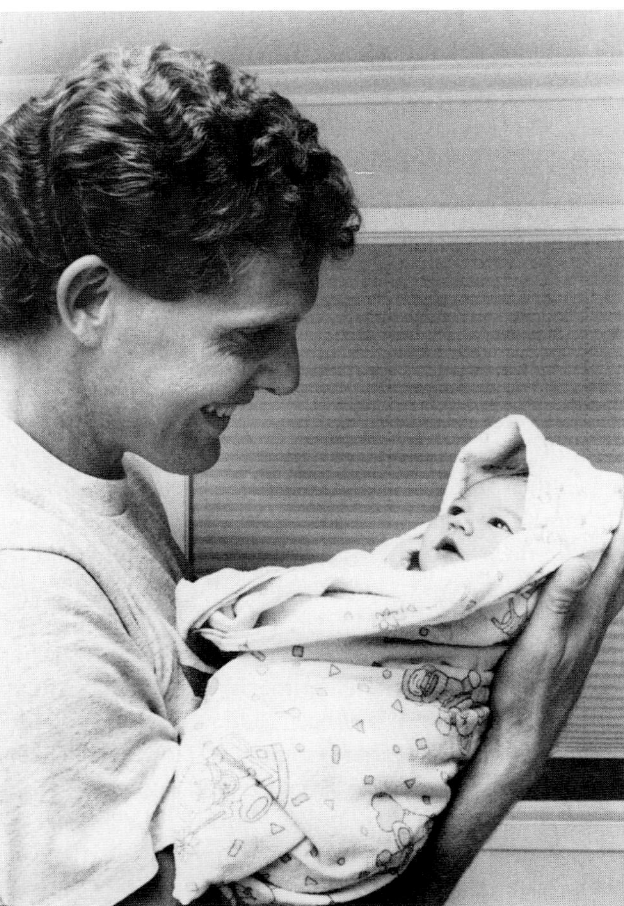

FIGURE 27–4 ♦ The father experiences strong feelings of attraction during engrossment.

rooming-in permits siblings and grandparents to participate in the attachment process.

## Cultural Influences in the Postpartal Period

The new mother's culture and personal values influence her beliefs about her postpartal care. Her expectations about food, fluids, rest, hygiene, medications and relief measures, support and counsel, and other aspects of her life are influenced by the beliefs and values of her family and cultural group. Sometimes, a new mother's wishes differ from what the physician or nurse expects.

Nurses belong to a particular personal culture and are also part of the health care cultural group. As part of the health care cultural group, nurses may take on some practices that support the general beliefs of that group, such as offering food in the recovery period after birth, providing iced fluids, expecting the woman to ambulate as soon as possible, and assuming the woman will want to shower and perhaps wash her hair soon after giving birth. It is important for nurses to recognize that they are approaching their client's care from their own perspective and that, to individualize care for each mother, they need to offer and support individual choices.

Although describing particular practices of differing cultural groups always involves some generalization, it is helpful for nurses to understand some of the possible differences in beliefs and practices. The woman of European heritage may expect to eat a full meal and have large amounts of iced fluids after the birth, in the belief that the food restores energy and the fluids help replace fluid lost during the labor. She may want to ambulate shortly after the birth and shower, wash her hair, and put on a fresh gown. She may expect a short stay in the hospital and may or may not be interested in educational classes.

Many cultures emphasize certain postpartal routines or rituals for mother and baby that are designed to restore the harmony, or the hot-cold balance, of the body (Howard & Berbiglia, 1997). Some women of Mexican, African, and Asian cultures may avoid cold after birth. This prohibition includes cold air, wind, and all water (even if heated). On the other hand, some traditional Mexican women may avoid eating "hot" foods such as pork just after the birth of a baby (considered a "hot" experience). It is important to note that individuals may define hot and cold conditions and foods differently. The nurse should ask each woman what she can eat and what foods she thinks would be helpful for healing (Chondhey, 1997). The nurse may encourage family members to bring preferred food and drink.

In many cultures, such as the Native Americans, the extended family plays an essential role during the puerperium. The grandmother is often the primary helper to the mother and newborn. She brings wisdom and experience, allowing the new mother time to rest and giving her ready access to someone who can help with problems and concerns as they arise. It is important to ensure access of all family members during the postpartal period. Visiting rules may be broadened to allow family members access to the mother and newborn. These practices show respect and foster a blending of old and new behaviors to meet the goals of all concerned (Cesario, 2001).

# Postpartal Nursing Assessment

Comprehensive care is based on a thorough assessment that identifies individual needs or potential problems. See the Assessment Guide: Postpartal—First 24 Hours after Birth.

## Risk Factors

Ongoing assessment and client education during the puerperium are designed to meet the needs of the childbearing

## ASSESSMENT GUIDE: POSTPARTAL—FIRST 24 HOURS AFTER BIRTH

| Physical Assessment/ Normal Findings | Alterations and Possible Causes* | Nursing Responses to Data† |
|---|---|---|
| **Vital Signs** | | |
| Blood pressure (BP): Should remain consistent with baseline BP during pregnancy | High BP (PIH, essential hypertension, renal disease, anxiety)<br>Drop in BP (may be normal; uterine hemorrhage) | Evaluate history of preexisting disorders and check for other signs of PIH (edema, proteinuria)<br>Assess for other signs of hemorrhage (↑ pulse, cool clammy skin) |
| Pulse: 50–90 bpm<br>May be bradycardia of 50–70 bpm | Tachycardia (difficult labor and birth, hemorrhage) | Evaluate for other signs of hemorrhage (↓ BP, cool clammy skin) |
| Respirations: 16–24/min | Marked tachypnea (respiratory disease) | Assess for other signs of respiratory disease |
| Temperature: 36.2–38°C (98–100.4°F) | After first 24 hours temperature of 28°C (100.4°F) or above suggests infection | Assess for other signs of infection; notify physician or certified nurse-midwife |
| **Breasts** | | |
| General appearance: Smooth, even pigmentation, changes of pregnancy still apparent; one may appear larger | Reddened area (mastitis) | Assess further for signs of infection |
| Palpation: Depending on postpartal day, may be soft, filling, full, or engorged | Palpable mass (caked breast, mastitis)<br>Engorgement (venous stasis)<br>Tenderness, heat, edema (engorgement, caked breast, mastitis) | Assess for other signs of infection: If blocked duct, consider heat, massage, position change for breastfeeding<br>Assess for further signs<br>Report mastitis to physician or certified nurse-midwife |
| Nipples: Supple, pigmented, intact; become erect when stimulated | Fissures, cracks, soreness (problems with breastfeeding), not erectile with stimulation (inverted nipples) | Reassess technique; recommend appropriate interventions |
| **Abdomen** | | |
| Musculature: Abdomen may be soft, have a "doughy" texture; rectus muscle intact | Separation in musculature (diastasis recti abdominis) | Evaluate size of diastasis; teach appropriate exercises for decreasing the separation |
| Fundus: Firm, midline; following expected process of involution | Boggy (full bladder, uterine bleeding) | Massage until firm; assess bladder and have woman void if needed; attempt to express clots when firm<br>If bogginess remains or recurs, report to physician or certified nurse-midwife |
| May be tender when palpated | Constant tenderness (infection) | Assess for evidence of endometritis |
| **Lochia** | | |
| Scant to moderate amount, earthy odor; no clots | Large amount, clots (hemorrhage)<br>Foul-smelling lochia (infection) | Assess for firmness, express additional clots; begin peripad count<br>Assess for other signs of infection; report to physician or certified nurse-midwife |
| Normal progression:<br>First 1–3 days: rubra<br>Following rubra:<br>Days 3–10: serosa (alba seldom seen in hospital) | Failure to progress normally or return to rubra from serosa (subinvolution) | Report to physician or certified nurse-midwife |

*Possible causes of alterations are placed in parentheses.

†This column provides guidelines for further assessment and initial nursing actions.

| Physical Assessment/ Normal Findings | Alterations and Possible Causes* | Nursing Responses to Data† |
|---|---|---|
| **Perineum** | | |
| Slight edema and bruising in intact perineum | Marked fullness, bruising, pain (vulvar hematoma) | Assess size; apply ice glove or ice pack; report to physician or certified nurse-midwife |
| Episiotomy: No redness, edema, ecchymosis, or discharge; edges well approximated | Redness, edema, ecchymosis, discharge, or gaping stitches (infection) | Encourage sitz baths; review perineal care, appropriate wiping techniques |
| Hemorrhoids: None present; if present, should be small and nontender | Full, tender, inflamed hemorrhoids | Encourage sitz baths, side-lying position; Tucks pads, anesthetic ointments, manual replacement of hemorrhoids, stool softeners, increased fluid intake |
| **Costovertebral Angle (CVA) Tenderness** | | |
| None | Present (kidney infection) | Assess for other symptoms of urinary tract infection (UTI); obtain clean-catch urine sample; report to physician or certified nurse-midwife |
| **Lower Extremities** | | |
| No pain with palpation; negative Homans' sign | Positive findings (thrombophlebitis) | Report to physician or certified nurse-midwife |
| **Elimination** | | |
| Urinary output: Voiding in sufficient quantities at least every 4–6 hours; bladder not palpable | Inability to void (urinary retention)<br>Symptoms of urgency, frequency, dysuria (UTI) | Employ nursing interventions to promote voiding; if not successful, obtain order for catheterization<br>Report symptoms of UTI to physician or certified nurse-midwife |
| Bowel elimination: Should have normal bowel movement by second or third day after birth | Inability to pass feces (constipation due to fear of pain from episiotomy, hemorrhoids, perineal trauma) | Encourage fluids, ambulation, roughage in diet; sitz baths to promote healing of perineum; obtain order for stool softener |

| Cultural Assessment‡ | Variations to Consider | Nursing Responses to Data† |
|---|---|---|
| Determine customs and practices regarding postpartum care<br>Ask the mother whether she would like fluids and ask what temperature she prefers | Individual preference may include<br>• Room-temperature or warmed fluids rather than iced drinks | Provide for specific request if possible<br>If woman is unable to provide specific information, the nurse may draw from general information regarding cultural variation |
| Ask the mother what foods or fluids she would like | • Special foods or fluids to hasten healing after childbirth | Mexican women may want food and fluids that restore hot-cold balance to the body<br>Women of European background may ask for iced fluids |
| Ask the mother whether she would prefer to be alone during breastfeeding | Some women may be hesitant to have someone with them when their breast is exposed | Provide privacy as desired by mother |

‡These are only a few suggestions. It is not our intent to imply this is a comprehensive cultural assessment.

*Possible causes of alterations are placed in parentheses.

†This column provides guidelines for further assessment and initial nursing actions.

## POSTPARTAL—FIRST 24 HOURS AFTER BIRTH *continued*

| Psychosocial Assessment/ Normal Findings | Variations to Consider | Nursing Responses to Data† |
|---|---|---|
| **Psychologic Adaptation** | | |
| During first 24 hours: Passive; preoccupied with own needs; may talk about her labor and birth experience; may be talkative, elated, or very quiet | Very quiet and passive; sleeps frequently (fatigue from long labor; feelings of disappointment about some aspect of the experience; may be following cultural expectation) | Provide opportunities for adequate rest; provide nutritious meals and snacks that are consistent with what the woman desires to eat and drink; provide opportunities to discuss birth experience in nonjudgmental atmosphere if the woman desires to do so |
| By 12 hours: Beginning to assume responsibility; some women eager to learn; easily feels overwhelmed | Excessive weepiness, mood swings, pronounced irritability (postpartum blues; feelings of inadequacy; culturally prescribed behavior) | Explain postpartum blues; provide supportive atmosphere; determine support available for mother; consider referral for evidence of profound depression |
| **Attachment** | | |
| *En face* position; holds baby close; cuddles and soothes; calls by name; identifies characteristics of family members in infant; may be awkward in providing care | Continued expressions of disappointment in sex, appearance of infant; refusal to care for infant; derogatory comments; lack of bonding behaviors (difficulty in attachment, following expectations of cultural/ethnic group) | Provide reinforcement and support for infant caretaking behaviors; maintain nonjudgmental approach and gather more information if caretaking behaviors are not evident |
| Initially may express disappointment over sex or appearance of infant but within 1–2 days demonstrates attachment behaviors | | |
| **Client Education** | | |
| Has basic understanding of self-care activities and infant care needs; can identify signs of complications that should be reported | Unable to demonstrate basic self-care and infant care activities (knowledge deficit; postpartum blues; following prescribed cultural behavior and will be cared for by grandmother or other family member) | Determine whether woman understands English and provide interpreter if needed; provide reinforcement of information through conversation and through written material (remember that some women and their families may not be able to understand written materials because of language difficulties or inability to read); provide information regarding infant care skills that are culturally consistent; give woman opportunity to express her feelings; consider social service home referral for women who have no family or other support, are unable to take in information about self-care and infant care, and demonstrate no caretaking activities |

‡These are only a few suggestions. It is not our intent to imply this is a comprehensive cultural assessment.

†This column provides guidelines for further assessment and initial nursing actions.

family and to detect and treat possible complications. Table 27–1, on page 736, identifies factors that may place the new mother at risk during the postpartal period. The nurse uses this knowledge during the assessment and is particularly alert for possible complications associated with identified risk factors.

## Physical Assessment

The nurse should remember several principles in preparing for and completing the assessment of the postpartal woman:

- Select a time that will provide the most accurate data. Palpating the fundus when the woman has

**TABLE 27–1 Postpartal High-Risk Factors**

| Factor | Maternal Implication |
|---|---|
| PIH | ↑ Blood pressure<br>↑ CNS irritability<br>↑ Need for bed rest → ↑ risk thrombophlebitis |
| Diabetes | Need for insulin regulation<br>Episodes of hypoglycemia or hyperglycemia<br>↓ Healing |
| Cardiac disease | ↑ Maternal exhaustion |
| Cesarean birth | ↑ Healing needs<br>↑ Pain from incision<br>↑ Risk of infection<br>↑ Length of hospitalization |
| Overdistension of uterus (multiple gestation, hydramnios) | ↑ Risk of hemorrhage<br>↑ Risk of anemia<br>↑ Stretching of abdominal muscles<br>↑ Incidence and severity of afterpains |
| Abruptio placentae, placenta previa | Hemorrhage → anemia<br>↓ Uterine contractility after birth → ↑ infection risk |
| Precipitous labor (<3 hours) | ↑ Risk of lacerations to birth canal → hemorrhage |
| Prolonged labor (>24 hours) | Exhaustion<br>↑ Risk of hemorrhage<br>Nutritional and fluid depletion<br>↑ Bladder atony and/or trauma |
| Difficult birth | Exhaustion<br>↑ Risk of perineal lacerations<br>↑ Risk of hematomas<br>↑ Risk of hemorrhage → anemia |
| Extended period of time in stirrups at birth | ↑ Risk of thrombophlebitis |
| Retained placenta | ↑ Risk of hemorrhage<br>↑ Risk of infection |

a full bladder, for example, may give false information about the progress of involution.

- Record the findings as clearly as possible.
- Perform the procedures as gently as possible to avoid unnecessary discomfort.
- Explain the purpose of regular assessment.

While performing the physical assessment, the nurse should also be teaching the woman. For example, when assessing the breasts of a nursing woman, the nurse can discuss breast milk production, the letdown reflex, and breast self-examination. A new mother may be very receptive to instruction on postpartal abdominal tightening exercises when the nurse assesses the woman's fundal height and diastasis. The assessment also provides an excellent time to provide information about the body's postpartal physical and anatomic changes as well as danger signs to report. (See Key Facts to Remember: Common Postpartal Concerns.) Because the time new mothers spend in the postpartum unit is often limited, nurses need to use every available opportunity for client education about self-care. One of the best opportunities comes during the normal postpartal assessment. To assist nurses in recognizing these opportunities, examples of client teaching during the assessment are provided throughout the following discussion.

**KEY FACTS TO REMEMBER**

### *Common Postpartal Concerns*

Several postpartal occurrences cause special concern for mothers. The nurse will frequently be asked about the following events:

| *Source of Concern* | *Explanation* |
|---|---|
| Gush of blood that sometimes occurs when she first arises | Due to normal pooling of blood in vagina when the woman lies down to rest or sleep; gravity causes blood to flow out when she stands. |
| Night sweats | Normal physiologic occurrence that results as body attempts to eliminate excess fluids that were present during pregnancy; may be aggravated by plastic mattress pad |
| Afterpains | More common in multiparas; due to contractions |

## Vital Signs

The nurse may choose to organize the physical assessment in a variety of ways. Many nurses begin by assessing vital signs because the findings are more accurate when they are obtained with the woman at rest. In addition, establishing whether the vital signs are within the expected normal range will assist the nurse in determining if other assessments are needed. For instance, if the temperature is elevated, the nurse considers the time since birth and gathers information to determine whether the woman is dehydrated or an infection is present.

Temperature elevations (less than 38°C [100.4°F]) due to normal processes should last for only 24 hours. The nurse evaluates any elevation of temperature in light of associated signs and symptoms and carefully reviews the woman's history to identify other factors, such as premature rupture of membranes (PROM) or prolonged labor, that might increase the incidence of infection in the genital tract.

Alterations in vital signs may indicate complications, so the nurse assesses them at regular intervals. The blood pressure should remain stable, but the pulse often shows a characteristic slowness that is no cause for alarm. Pulse rates return to prepregnant norms very quickly unless complications arise.

The nurse informs the woman of the results of the vital signs assessment and provides information about the normal changes in blood pressure and pulse. This may be an opportunity to determine whether the mother knows how to assess her own and her infant's temperature and how to read a thermometer.

### Auscultation of Lungs

The breath sounds should be clear. Women who have been treated for preterm labor or PIH are at higher risk for pulmonary edema (see Chapter 13 for further discussion).

### Breasts

The nurse can first assess the fit and support provided by the bra and offer information about how to select a supportive bra. A properly fitting bra supports the breasts and helps maintain breast shape by limiting stretching of supporting ligaments and connective tissue. If the mother is breastfeeding, the straps of the bra should be cloth, not elastic, and easily adjustable. The back should be wide and have at least three rows of hooks to adjust for fit. Traditional nursing bras have a fixed inner cup and a separate half cup that can be unhooked for breastfeeding while the cup continues to support the breast. Purchasing a nursing bra one size too large during pregnancy will usually result in a good fit because the breasts increase in size with milk production.

The nurse can then ask the woman to remove her bra so the breasts can be examined. The nurse notes the size and shape of the breasts and any abnormalities, reddened areas, or engorgement. The breasts are also lightly palpated for softness, slight firmness associated with filling, firmness associated with engorgement, warmth, and tenderness. The nipples are assessed for fissures, cracks, soreness, and inversion. The nurse teaches the woman the characteristics of the breast and explains how to recognize problems such as fissures and cracks.

The nonnursing mother is assessed for evidence of breast discomfort, and relief measures are instituted if necessary. (See discussion of lactation suppression in the nonnursing mother in Chapter 28.) Breast assessment findings for a nursing woman may be recorded as follows: breasts soft, filling, no evidence of nipple tenderness or cracking.

### Abdomen and Fundus

Before examination of the abdomen, the woman should void. This practice ensures that a full bladder is not displacing the uterus or causing any uterine atony; if atony is present, other causes must be investigated.

The nurse determines the relationship of the fundus to the umbilicus and also assesses the firmness of the fundus. She or he notes whether the fundus is in the midline or displaced to either side of the abdomen. Because the most common cause of displacement is a full bladder, this finding requires further assessment. The nurse should then record the results of the assessment (see Procedure 27–1).

While completing the assessment, the nurse teaches the woman about fundal position. The mother can be assisted in gently massaging her fundus to determine firmness.

In the woman who has had a cesarean birth, the abdominal incision is exquisitely tender. The fundus is therefore palpated with extreme care. The nurse also inspects the abdominal incision for any signs of infection, including drainage, foul odor, or redness. During the assessment, the nurse teaches the woman about her incision. Characteristics of normal healing may be reviewed and signs of infection discussed.

### Lochia

The nurse then evaluates the lochia, including character, amount, odor, and the presence of clots. Disposable gloves must be worn when assessing the perineum and lochia. Nurses may put on the gloves before beginning the assessment, just before assessing the abdomen and fundus, or when they are ready to assess the perineum and lochia. During the first 1 to 3 days the lochia should be rubra. A few small clots are normal and occur as a result of blood pooling in the vagina. However, the passage of numerous or large clots is abnormal, and the cause should be investigated immediately. After 2 to 3 days, the lochia flow becomes serosa.

Lochia should never exceed a moderate amount, such as four to eight partially saturated perineal pads daily, with an average of six. However, because this number is influenced by an individual woman's pad-changing practices, as well as the absorbency of the pad, the nurse needs to question her about the length of time the current pad has been in use, whether the amount is normal, and whether any clots were passed before this examination, such as during voiding. If heavy bleeding is reported but not seen, the nurse asks the woman to put on a clean perineal pad and then reassess the woman's pad in 1 hour (Figure 27–6♦). When a

# Procedure 27-1 Assessing the Fundus Following Vaginal Birth

| *Nursing Action* | *Rationale* |
|---|---|
| **OBJECTIVE: PREPARE THE WOMAN.** | |
| • Explain the procedure. | *Explanation decreases anxiety and increases cooperation.* |
| • Ask the woman to void. | *A full bladder will cause uterine atony.* |
| • Position the woman flat in bed with her head comfortably on a pillow. If the procedure is uncomfortable, the woman may flex her legs. | *The supine position prevents falsely high assessment of fundal height.* *Flexing the legs relaxes the abdominal muscles.* |
| **OBJECTIVE: DETERMINE UTERINE FIRMNESS.** | |
| • Gently place one hand on the lower segment of the uterus. Using the side of the other hand, palpate the abdomen until you locate the top of the fundus. | *This position provides support for the uterus and a larger surface for palpation.* |
| • Determine whether the fundus is firm. If it is not firm, massage the abdomen lightly until the fundus is firm. | *A firm fundus indicates that the muscles are contracted and bleeding will not occur.* |
| **OBJECTIVE: DETERMINE THE HEIGHT OF THE FUNDUS.** | |
| Measure the top of the fundus in finger breadths above, below, or at the umbilicus (Figure 27–5♦). | *Fundal height gives information about the progress of involution.* |

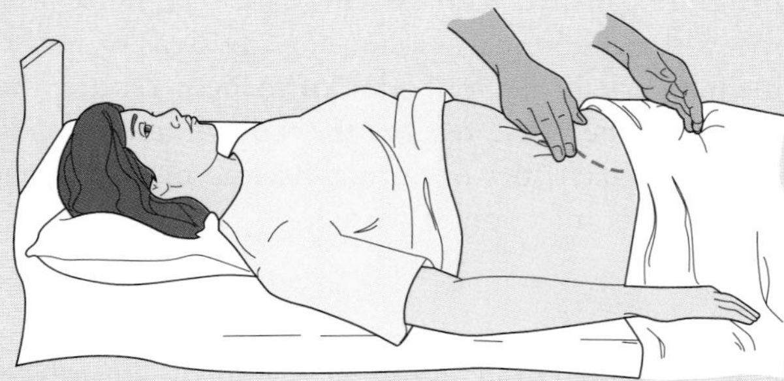

FIGURE 27–5 ♦ Measurement of descent of fundus for the woman with vaginal birth. The fundus is located two finger breadths below the umbilicus.

| *Nursing Action* | *Rationale* |
|---|---|
| **OBJECTIVE: ASCERTAIN THE POSITION OF THE FUNDUS.** | |
| • Determine whether the fundus has deviated from the midline. If it is not in the midline, locate the position. Evaluate the bladder for distention. | *The fundus may be deviated when the bladder is full.* |
| • Measure urine output for the next few hours until normal elimination status is established. | |
| **OBJECTIVE: CORRELATE THE UTERINE STATUS WITH LOCHIA.** | |
| Observe the amount, color, and odor of the lochia and the presence of clots. | *As normal involution occurs, the lochia decreases and changes from rubra to serosa. Increased amounts of lochia may be associated with uterine relaxation; failure to progress to the next type of lochia may indicate uterine relaxation or infection.* |
| **OBJECTIVE: RECORD THE FINDINGS.** | |
| • Fundal height is recorded in finger breadths (e.g., "2 FB ↓ U; 1 FB ↑ U"). | *Provides a permanent record.* |
| • If massage was necessary: "Uterus: Boggy → firm c̄ light massage." | |

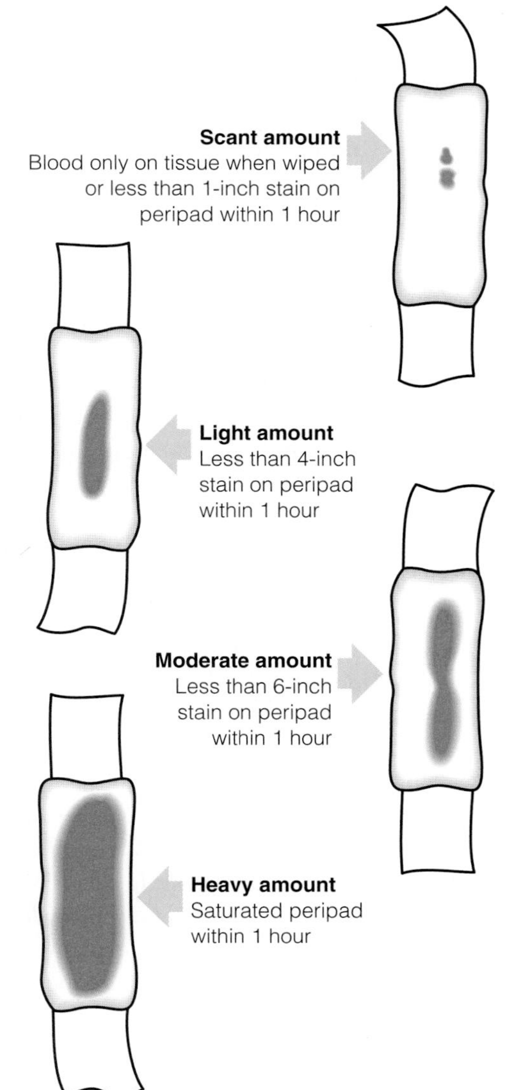
Scant amount
Blood only on tissue when wiped or less than 1-inch stain on peripad within 1 hour
Light amount
Less than 4-inch stain on peripad within 1 hour
Moderate amount
Less than 6-inch stain on peripad within 1 hour
Heavy amount
Saturated peripad within 1 hour

FIGURE 27–6 ♦ Suggested guideline for assessing lochia volume.
*Source:* Jacobson, H. (1985, May–June). A standard for assessing lochia volume. *Maternal-Child Nursing.*

more accurate assessment of blood loss is needed, the perineal pads can be weighed, with 1g considered the approximate equivalent of 1mL of blood. Clots and heavy bleeding may be caused by uterine relaxation (atony) or retained placental fragments and may require further assessment. Because of the evacuation of the uterine cavity during cesarean birth, women with such surgery usually have less lochia after the first 24 hours than mothers who give birth vaginally. If the woman is at increased risk for bleeding, or is actually experiencing heavy flow of lochia rubra, the physician may also order methylergonovine maleate (Methergine). (See Drug Guide: Methylergonovine Maleate [Methergine], in Chapter 28.)

The odor of the lochia is nonoffensive and never foul. If a foul odor is present, so is an infection. The amount of lochia is charted first, followed by character. For example:

- Lochia: moderate rubra
- Lochia: small rubra/serosa

Client teaching during assessment of the lochia may center on normal changes that can be expected in the amount and color of the flow. The nurse can review hygienic measures if appropriate. The nurse should approach the teaching of hygienic practices delicately and with the goals of promoting comfort, enhancing tissue healing, and preventing infection and avoid value-laden statements about the need for cleanliness or control of body odor.

## Perineum

The perineum is inspected with the woman lying in a Sims' position. The nurse lifts the buttock to expose the perineum and anus.

If an episiotomy was done or a laceration required suturing, the nurse assesses the wound and evaluates the state of healing by observing for ecchymosis and approximation. After 24 hours some edema may still be present, but the skin edges should be "glued" together (well approximated) so that gentle pressure does not separate them. Gentle palpation should elicit minimal tenderness, and there should be no hard areas suggesting infection. Ecchymosis interferes with normal healing, as does infection.

Foul odors associated with drainage indicate infection. The incision should be further observed for warmth, redness, tenderness, edema, and separation. The nurse next assesses whether hemorrhoids are present around the anus. If present, they are assessed for size, number, and pain or tenderness.

During the assessment, the nurse talks with the woman to determine the effectiveness of comfort measures that have been used. The nurse provides teaching about the episiotomy. Some women do not thoroughly understand what and where an episiotomy is, and they may believe that the stitches must be removed as with other types of surgery. Frequently, when women fear that the stitches must be removed manually, they are afraid to ask about them. While explaining the findings of the assessment, the nurse provides information about the episiotomy, its location, and the signs that are being assessed. In addition, the nurse can casually add that the sutures are special and will dissolve slowly over the next few weeks as the tissues heal. By the time the sutures are dissolved the tissues are strong and the incision edges will not separate. This is also an opportunity to teach comfort measures (see Chapter 29).

An example of charting a perineal assessment might be: Midline episiotomy; no edema, tenderness, or ecchymosis present. Skin edges well approximated. Woman reports pain relief measures are controlling discomfort.

### Lower Extremities

If thrombophlebitis occurs, the most likely site is in the woman's legs. To assess for it, her legs should be stretched out straight and relaxed with the knees flexed. The nurse grasps the woman's foot and sharply dorsiflexes it. No discomfort or pain should be present. The second leg is assessed in the same way. If pain is elicited, the nurse notifies the certified nurse-midwife or physician that the woman has a positive Homans' sign (Figure 27–7♦). The pain is caused by inflammation of the vessel. The nurse also evaluates the legs for edema by comparing both legs, since usually only one leg is involved. Any areas of redness, tenderness, and increased skin temperature are also noted.

Early ambulation is an important aspect in the prevention of thrombophlebitis. Most women are able to be up shortly after birth. The cesarean birth client requires range of motion exercises until she is ambulating more freely.

Client teaching associated with assessment of the lower extremities focuses on the signs and symptoms of thrombophlebitis. In addition, the nurse may review self-care measures to promote circulation and measures to prevent thrombophlebitis, such as ambulation and avoiding pressure behind the knees, using the knee gatch on the bed, and crossing the legs.

### Elimination

During the hours after birth the nurse carefully monitors a new mother's bladder status. A boggy uterus, a displaced uterus, or a palpable bladder are signs of bladder distention and require nursing intervention.

The postpartal woman should be encouraged to void every 4 to 6 hours. The nurse should assess the bladder for distention until the woman demonstrates complete emptying of the bladder with each voiding. The nurse may employ techniques to facilitate voiding, such as helping the woman out of bed to void or pouring warm water on the perineum. Catheterization is required when the bladder is distended and the woman cannot void or when no voiding has occurred in 8 hours. The cesarean birth mother may have an indwelling catheter inserted prophylactically. The same assessments should be made in evaluating bladder emptying once the catheter is removed.

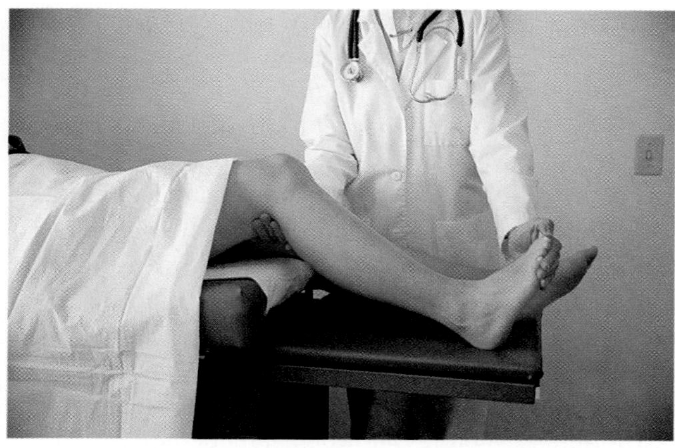

FIGURE 27–7 ♦ Homans' sign: with the woman's knee flexed, the nurse dorsiflexes the foot. Pain in the foot or leg is a positive Homans' sign.

During the physical assessment, the nurse elicits information from the woman about the adequacy of her fluid intake, whether she feels she is emptying her bladder completely when she voids, and any signs of urinary tract infection (UTI) she may be experiencing.

In the same way, the nurse obtains information about the new mother's intestinal elimination and any concerns she may have about it. Many mothers fear that the first bowel movement will be painful and possibly even damaging if an episiotomy has been done. Stool softeners may be ordered to increase bulk and moisture in the fecal material and to allow more comfortable and complete evacuation. Constipation is avoided to prevent pressure on sutures, which may increase discomfort. To enhance bowel elimination and help the woman reestablish her normal bowel pattern, the nurse can encourage ambulation, increased fluid intake (up to 2000 mL/day or more), and additional fresh fruits and roughage in her diet.

During the assessment, the nurse may provide information about postpartum diuresis and explain why the woman may be emptying her bladder so frequently. The need for additional fluid intake with suggestions of specific amounts may be helpful. The woman should drink at least eight 8-oz glasses of water or juice per day in addition to other fluids. The nurse discusses signs of urinary retention and overflow voiding and may review symptoms of UTI if it seems an appropriate moment for teaching. The nurse can also review methods of assisting bowel elimination and provide opportunities for the woman to ask questions.

### Rest and Sleep Status

As part of the postpartal assessment, the nurse evaluates the amount of rest a new mother is getting. If the woman reports difficulty sleeping at night, the nurse should try to determine the cause. If it is simply the strange environment, a warm drink and backrub may prove helpful. Appropriate nursing measures are indicated if the woman is bothered by normal postpartal discomforts such as afterpains, diaphoresis, or episiotomy or hemorrhoidal pain.

The nurse should encourage a daily rest period and schedule hospital activities to allow time for napping. The nurse can also provide information about the fatigue new mothers experience and the impact it can have on a woman's emotions and sense of control.

### Nutritional Status

Determination of postpartal nutritional status is based primarily on information provided by the mother and on direct assessment. During pregnancy the daily recommended dietary allowances call for increases in calories, protein, and most vitamins and minerals. After birth, the nonnursing mother's dietary requirements return to prepregnancy levels.

Visiting the mother during mealtime provides an opportunity for unobtrusive nutritional assessment and counseling. The nonnursing mother should be advised about the need to reduce her caloric intake by about 300 kcal and to return to prepregnancy levels for other nutrients. The nursing mother, on the other hand, should increase her caloric intake by about 200 kcal over the pregnancy requirements, or a total of 500 kcal over the nonpregnant requirement. Basic discussion often proves helpful, followed by referral as needed. In all cases, literature on nutrition should be provided, so that the woman will have a source of information after discharge.

The dietitian should be informed of any mother who is a vegetarian or whose cultural or religious beliefs require specific foods. Appropriate meals can then be prepared for her. Many women, especially those who gained excessive weight, are interested in losing weight after birth. The dietitian can design weight-reduction diets to meet nutritional needs and food preferences. The nurse may also refer women with unusual eating habits or numerous questions about good nutrition to the dietitian.

New mothers are advised that it is common practice to prescribe iron supplements for 4 to 6 weeks after birth. The hematocrit is then checked at the postpartal visit to detect any anemia.

## Psychologic Assessment

Adequate assessment of the mother's psychologic adjustment is an integral part of postpartal evaluation. This assessment focuses on the mother's general attitude, feelings of competence, available support systems, and caregiving skills. It also evaluates her fatigue level, sense of satisfaction, and ability to accomplish her developmental tasks.

Fatigue is often a highly significant factor in a new mother's apparent disinterest in her newborn. Frequently the woman is so tired from a long labor and birth that everything seems to be an effort. To avoid inadvertently classifying a very tired mother as one with a potential attachment problem, the nurse should do a psychologic assessment on more than one occasion. After a nap the new mother is often far more receptive to her baby and her surroundings.

Some new mothers have little or no experience with newborns and may feel totally overwhelmed. They may show these feelings by asking questions and reading all available material or by becoming passive and quiet because they simply cannot deal with their feelings of inadequacy. Unless a nurse questions the woman about her plans and previous experience in a supportive, nonjudgmental way, the nurse might conclude that the woman is disinterested, withdrawn, or depressed.

Problem clues might include excessive continued fatigue, marked depression, excessive preoccupation with physical status or discomfort, evidence of low self-esteem, lack of support systems, marital problems, inability to care for or nurture the newborn, and current family crises (illness, unemployment, and so on). These characteristics frequently indicate a potential for maladaptive parenting, which may lead to child abuse or neglect (physical, emotional, intellectual) and cannot be ignored. Referrals to public health nurses or other available community resources may provide greatly needed assistance and alleviate potentially dangerous situations.

## Assessment of Early Attachment

A nurse in any of the various postpartal settings can periodically observe and note progress toward attachment. The following questions can be addressed in the course of nurse-client interaction:

- Is the mother attracted to her newborn? To what extent does she seek face-to-face contact and eye contact? Has she progressed from fingertip touch, to palmar contact, to enfolding the infant close to her own body? Is attraction increasing or decreasing? If the mother does not exhibit increasing attraction, why not? Do the reasons lie primarily within her, in the baby, or in the environment?
- Is the mother inclined to nurture her infant? Is she progressing in her interactions with her infant?
- Does the mother act consistently? If not, is the source of unpredictability within her or her infant?
- Is her mothering consistently carried out? Does she seek information and evaluate it objectively? Does she develop solutions based on adequate knowledge of valid data? Does she evaluate the effectiveness of her maternal care and adjust appropriately?
- Is she sensitive to the newborn's needs as they arise? How quickly does she interpret her infant's behavior and react to cues? Does she seem happy and satisfied with the infant's responses to her efforts? Is she pleased with feeding behaviors? How much of this ability and willingness to respond is related to the baby's nature and how much to her own?

- Does she seem pleased with her baby's appearance and sex? Is she experiencing pleasure in interaction with her infant? What interferes with the enjoyment? Does she speak to the baby frequently and affectionately? Does she call him or her by name? Does she point out family traits or characteristics she sees in the newborn?
- Are there any cultural factors that might modify the mother's response? For instance, is it customary for the grandmother to assume most of the child care responsibilities while the mother recovers from childbirth?

When the nurse has addressed these questions and assembled the facts, the nurse's intuition and knowledge should combine to answer three more questions: Is there a problem in attachment? What is the problem? What is its source? The nurse can then devise a creative approach to the problem as it presents itself in the context of a unique, developing mother-infant relationship.

## Assessment of Physical and Developmental Tasks

During the first several postpartal weeks, the woman must accomplish certain physical and developmental tasks:

- Restoring physical condition
- Developing competence in caring for and meeting the needs of her infant
- Establishing a relationship with her new child
- Adapting to altered lifestyles and family structure resulting from the addition of a new member

The new mother may have an inadequate or incorrect understanding of what to expect during the early postpartal weeks. She may be concerned with restoring her figure and be surprised by continuing physical discomfort from sore breasts, episiotomy, or hemorrhoids. Fatigue is perhaps her greatest yet most underestimated problem during the early weeks. It may be aggravated if she has no extended family support or there are other young children at home.

Developing skill and confidence in caring for an infant may be especially anxiety provoking for a new mother. As she struggles to establish a mutually acceptable pattern with her baby, small unanticipated concerns may seem monumental. The woman may begin to feel inadequate and, if she lacks support systems, isolated.

Nurses have been in the forefront of health care providers in attempting to improve the care currently provided during the postpartal period. Many obstetricians and nurse practitioners now routinely see all postpartal women 1 to 2 weeks after birth in addition to the routine 6-week checkup. This extra visit provides an opportunity for physical assessment as well as evaluation of the mother's psychologic and informational needs.

### Postdischarge Care

Postdischarge care for the postpartal woman may be accomplished by home visits or follow-up phone calls. A home visit 1 to 3 days after discharge provides opportunities for further assessment and teaching. (See discussion of postpartum home care in Chapter 29.)

The follow-up telephone call is usually initiated by a nurse from the postpartal unit of the agency where the mother gave birth. It is made soon after discharge and is designed to provide assessment and care if necessary, to reinforce knowledge and provide additional teaching, and to make referrals if indicated.

In ideal situations a family approach involving the father, infant, other siblings, and grandparents permits a total evaluation and provides an opportunity for all family members to ask questions and express concerns. Such an approach also promotes diagnosis and treatment of disturbed family patterns to prevent future problems of neglect or abuse.

# Chapter Review

## CHAPTER HIGHLIGHTS

- The uterus involutes rapidly, primarily through a reduction in cell size.
- Involution is assessed by measuring fundal height. The fundus is at the level of the umbilicus within a few hours after childbirth and should decrease by approximately one finger breadth per day.
- The placental site heals by a process of exfoliation, so no scar formation occurs.
- Lochia flow progresses from rubra to serosa to alba and is assessed in terms of type, quantity, and characteristics.
- The abdomen may be flabby initially. Diastasis recti should be measured.
- Constipation may develop postpartally because of decreased tone, limited diet, and denial of the urge to defecate due to fear of pain.
- Decreased bladder sensitivity, increased capacity, and postpartal diuresis may lead to problems with bladder elimination. Frequent assessment and prompt intervention are indicated. A fundus that is boggy but does not respond to massage, is higher than expected, or deviates to the side usually indicates a full bladder.
- Postpartally a healthy woman should be normotensive and afebrile. Bradycardia is common.
- Postpartally the white blood cell count (WBC) is often elevated. Activation of clotting factors predisposes the woman to thrombus formation.
- Psychologic adaptations include maternal role attainment and attachment to the newborn.
- In consideration of the client's background, the nurse should recognize and respect cultural variations and individual preferences.
- Postpartal assessment should be completed in a systematic way, usually cephalocaudally. It provides a tremendous opportunity for informal teaching.
- In the weeks following birth, the woman's physical condition returns to a nonpregnant state and she gains competence and confidence in herself as a parent.

## CHAPTER REFERENCES


Cesario, S. K. (2001). Car of the native american woman: strategies for practice, education, and research. *Journal of Obstetric, Gynecologic and Neonatal Nursing, 30*(1), 13–18.

Chondhey, U. K. (1997). Traditional practices of women from India: Pregnancy, childbirth, and newborn care. *Journal of Obstetric, Gynecologic, and Neonatal Nursing, 26*(5), 533–539.

Farrington, P. F., & Ward, K. (1999). Normal labor, delivery, and puerperium. In J. R. Scott, P. J. DiSaia, C. B. Hammond, & W. N. Spellacy (Eds.), *Danforth's obstetrics and gynecology* (8th ed., pp. 91–109). Philadelphia: Lippincott, Williams & Wilkins.

Howard, J. Y., & Berbiglia, V. A. (1997). Caring for childbearing Korean women. *Journal of Obstetric, Gynecologic, and Neonatal Nursing, 26*(6), 665–671.

Mercer, R. T. (1995). *Becoming a mother.* New York: Springer.

Resnik, R. (1999). The puerperium. In R. K. Creasy & R. Resnik (Eds.), *Maternal-fetal medicine* (4th ed., pp. 102–105). Philadelphia: Saunders.

Rubin, R. (1961). Puerperal change. *Nursing Outlook, 9,* 753.

Rubin, R. (1984). *Maternal identity and the maternal experience.* New York: Springer.

Scoggin, J. (2000). Physical and psychological changes. In S. Mattson & J. Smith (Eds.), *AWHONN: Core curriculum for maternal-newborn nursing* (2nd ed., pp. 302–316). Philadelphia: Saunders.

Varney, H. (1997). *Varney's midwifery* (3rd ed.). Sudbury, MA: Jones & Bartlett.

## CONTEMPORARY MATERNAL-NEWBORN NURSING ON-LINE

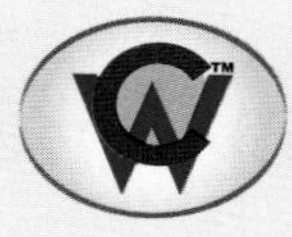

Additional interactive resources, including animations and video, for this chapter can be found on the Companion Website at http://www.prenhall.com/ladewig. Click on Chapter 27 and "Begin" to select the activities for this chapter.

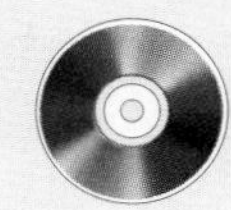

For NCLEX review questions and an audio glossary, access the accompanying CD-ROM in this book.

Chapter 28

# The Postpartal Family: Needs and Care

*I truly believe I have the best job there is in the nursing profession. I look forward to work each day, and I return home feeling satisfied that I have given my best. I'm using my nursing education to the fullest, as a hands-on caregiver, an educator, and a client advocate. There are plenty of challenges to keep me on my toes and plenty of new directions to explore. I know it may sound corny, but I love what I do!*

—Postpartum Staff Nurse

## OBJECTIVES

- Relate the use of nursing diagnoses to the findings of the "normal" postpartum assessment and analysis.
- Delineate nursing responsibilities for client teaching during the early postpartum period.
- Discuss appropriate nursing interventions to meet identified nursing goals for the childbearing family.
- Explore the nursing needs of the woman and family who experience a cesarean birth.
- Summarize the nursing needs of the childbearing adolescent during the postpartum period.
- Discuss the nursing needs of a woman with an unwanted pregnancy.
- Describe possible approaches to follow-up nursing care for the childbearing family.

## KEY TERMS

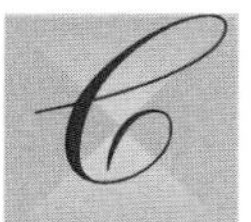

Certain premises form the basis of effective nursing care during the postpartal period:

- The best postpartal care is family centered; incorporates the family's needs, desires, and values as much as possible; and disrupts the family unit as little as possible. This approach uses the family's resources to support an early and smooth adjustment to the newborn by all family members.
- Knowledge of the range of normal physiologic and psychologic adaptations occurring during the postpartal period allows the nurse to recognize alterations and initiate interventions early. Communicating information about postpartal adaptations to the family members facilitates their adjustment to their situation.
- Nursing care aimed at accomplishing specific goals that are intended to meet individual and family needs. These goals are formulated after careful assessment, consultation with the woman and her family, and consideration of factors that could influence the outcome of care.

Chapter 27 provides a thorough discussion of postpartal assessment. This chapter describes how the nurse can use the remaining steps of the nursing process effectively to plan and provide care. Specific nursing responses to the mother's physical needs and the family's psychosocial needs are described at length. The Critical Pathway for the Postpartal Period begins on page 751.

## Community-Based Nursing Care

Various services are available to meet the needs of the childbearing family during the postpartal period and beyond. These services range from educational, such as classes on nutrition, exercise, infant care, and parenting, to specific health care programs, such as well-baby checks, family planning services, and more. Some are offered by private caregivers, whereas others are the domain of city, county, state, or federal agencies. In all cases, the goal is to help ensure that the mother, infant, and all family members have the opportunity to meet their health care needs, regardless of their resources.

### Home Health Care

Home health care is one of the most important forms of community-based nursing care offered to postpartal families. Home care visits and phone contacts help ensure that new parents have the necessary skills and resources to adequately care for their new infant and any other family members. (Home Care is discussed in depth in Chapter 29.)

# Nursing Care Management during the Early Postpartal Period

## Nursing Diagnosis

For most postpartal women, physical recovery goes smoothly and is considered a healthy process. Because of this perception, caregivers too often assume that the woman and her family have no real needs and that no care plan is needed. Nothing could be further from the truth. Every member of the family has needs, although the needs may not be obvious, especially if they are psychologic or educational.

The postpartal family's needs, which should be identified during assessment, are the basis for developing nursing diagnoses. Many nurses have suggested that nursing diagnoses are difficult to make in a wellness setting because of their emphasis on "problems." Nurses involved in the effort to formulate standardized diagnoses recognize this difficulty and continue working to develop nursing diagnoses that are more congruent with wellness settings.

Many agencies that use nursing diagnoses prefer to use only the NANDA list. Consequently, physiologic alterations form the basis of many postpartal diagnoses. Examples of such diagnoses include

- Altered patterns of urinary elimination related to dysuria
- Constipation related to fear of tearing stitches or pain
- Pain related to perineal edema or episiotomy from birth

Diagnoses related to family coping or instructional needs are also used frequently. Examples of these diagnoses include

- Health-seeking behaviors: information about infant care related to an expressed desire to improve parenting skills.
- Family coping: potential for growth related to successful adjustment to new baby

After completing the assessment and diagnosis steps of the nursing process, the nurse identifies expected outcomes and selects nursing interventions that will help the family meet the expected outcomes.

## Nursing Plan and Implementation

Nursing care management is individualized to meet the needs of each postpartal woman and her newborn. The plan of care needs to consider the newborn's schedule, as

Text continues on page 753.

# CRITICAL PATHWAY: *For the Postpartal Period*

| Category | First 4 Hours | 4–8 Hours Past Birth | 8–24 Hours Past Birth |
|---|---|---|---|
| **Referral** | **VB:** Report from labor nurse if applicable<br>**CB:** Report from OR Recovery nurse | Lactation consultation as needed<br>**CB:** Respiratory therapist as needed | Home nursing, WIC referral if indicated<br>**Expected Outcomes**<br>Referrals made |
| **Assessments** | **VB:** PP assess. q15 min × 4, q30 min × 2, q1h × 2, then q4h. Includes<br>• Fundus firm, midline, at or below umbilicus<br>• Lochia rubra <1 pad/hr; no free flow or passage of clots with massage<br>• Bladder: voids large amounts of urine; bladder not palpable following voiding<br>• Perineum: sutures intact; no bulging or marked swelling; no c/o severe pain. Minimal bruising may be present. If hemorrhoids present, no tenseness or marked engorgement; <2 cm diameter<br>• Breasts: soft, colostrum present<br>Vital Signs:<br>• BP WNL; no hypotension; not >30 mm Hg systolic or 15 mm Hg diastolic over baseline<br>• Temperature: <38°C (100.4°F)<br>• Pulse: bradycardia normal, consistent with baseline<br>• Respirations: 12–20/min; quiet, easy<br>Comfort level: <3 on scale of 1–10<br>**CB:** PP cesarean assess. q15min × 4, q30min × 4, q1 h per protocol; all assessment parameters for VB included, as well as<br>• Surgical dressing over incision clean and dry or with minimal drainage<br>• Foley catheter in place, urine color and amount noted<br>• IV: no swelling, pain, or redness at insertion site; infusing at prescribed rate<br>• Bowel sounds: present, decreased, or minimal<br>• LOC: alert and oriented, easily aroused if dozing<br>• LOS: sensation WNL for anesthesia or analgesia type administered<br>• Pulse ox: WNL<br>• Input and output: WNL | **VB:** Continue PP assess. q4h × 2, then q8h<br>Breast: evaluate nipple status; should be no evidence of cracks or bruising<br>Observe feeding technique with newborn<br>VS assess. q8h; all WNL; report temp > 38°C (100.4°F)<br>Assess Homans' sign q8h<br>Continue assess. of comfort level<br>**CB:** Continue cesarean assess. per protocol, including all assess. covered in VB; as well as<br>• Determine if woman passing flatus<br>• Determine if bowel sounds present | Continue PP assess. per protocol<br>Breasts: nipples should remain free of cracks, fissures, bruising<br>Feeding technique with newborn: should be good or improving<br>VS assess. q8h; all WNL; report temp >38°C (100.4°F)<br>Continue assessment of comfort level<br>**Expected Outcomes**<br>VS medically acceptable, voids qs, PP assessment WNL; comfort level <3 on a 1–10 scale, involution of uterus in process, demonstrates and verbalizes appropriate newborn feeding techniques |
| **Teaching/ psychosocial** | Explain PP assessments<br>Teach self-massage of fundus and expected findings; rationale for fundal massage<br>Instruct to call for assist. 1st time OOB and prn<br>Demonstrate peri-care, surgigator, sitz bath prn<br>Explain comfort measures<br>Begin newborn teaching; bulb suctioning, positioning, feeding, diaper change, cord care | Discuss psychologic changes of PP period; facilitate transition through tasks of taking on maternal role<br>Discuss peri-care/hygiene; encourage use of supportive brassiere for breast- or bottle-feeding<br>Stress need for frequent rest periods<br>Continue newborn teaching: soothing/ comfort techniques, swaddling; return demo indicates woman's understanding<br>Provide opportunities for questions and review, reinforce previous teaching | Reinforce previous teaching, complete teaching evaluation<br>Discuss involution; anticipated physical changes in first 2 weeks PP; PP exercises; need to limit visitors<br>Discuss PP nutrition; balanced diet<br>Breastfeeding:<br>• Increase calories by 500 kcal over nonpregnant state (200 kcal over pregnant intake)<br>• Explain milk production, letdown reflex, use of supplements, breast pumping, and milk storage |

Information is included for both vaginal birth (**VB**) and cesarean birth (**CB**). However, since many of the nursing care interventions are the same for either, specific interventions or suggestions related to vaginal birth are designated VB, and those specific to cesarean are designated CB.

ADL, activities of daily living; BP, blood pressure; CB, cesarean birth; CNM, certified nurse-midwife; DC, discontinue; LDR, labor, delivery, and recovery; OOB, out of bed; OR, operating room; PCA, patient-controlled analgesia; PRN, as needed; VB, vaginal birth; WNL, within normal limits; PP, postpartum; qs, quantity sufficient; VS, vital signs; c/o, complaints of; LOS, level of sensation; LOC, level of conscienceness; TC & DOB, turn-cough and deep breathe; D/C, discharge; s/s, signs and symptoms.

| Category | First 4 Hours | 4–8 Hours Past Birth | 8–24 Hours Past Birth |
|---|---|---|---|
| **Teaching/ psychosocial *continued*** | Orient to room if transferred from LDR room<br>Provide info. on early PP period<br>Assess mother-infant attachment<br>**CB:** Teach TC & DB exercise<br>Explain importance of moving around in bed and moving legs up and down<br>Demonstrate splinting of abdomen for ↑ comfort with movement<br>Discuss plan of care related to cesarean recovery; activity and ambulation recommendations, advancement of diet, incision care, schedule for IV and Foley catheter removal<br>Provide inform about PCA, pain meds, and alternate measures for pain management | Breastfeeding: nipple care: air-drying, lanolin; proper latch-on technique; tea bags<br>Bottle-feeding: supportive bra, ice bags, breast binder<br>Assess mother-infant attachment<br>Stress need for movement and ambulation<br>Discuss incision healing<br>Explain benefit of a regular schedule of medications for pain to optimize comfort | Bottle-feeding:<br>• Return to nonpregnant caloric intake<br>• Explain formula preparation and storage<br>Discuss birth control options, sexuality<br>Discuss sibling rivalry and plan for supporting siblings at home<br>Discuss pets; suggestions for improving acceptance of infant by pets<br>**Expected Outcomes**<br>Mother verbalizes teaching comprehension<br>Positive bonding and emotional behaviors observed |
| **Nursing care management and reports** | **VB:** Ice pack to perineum to ↓ swelling and ↑ comfort<br>Straight cath prn × 1 if distended or voiding small amounts<br>If continues unable to void or avoid small amounts, insert Foley catheter and notify CNM or physician<br>**CB:** Implement i/o regime<br>Maintain IV as ordered<br>Medicate for pain<br>Begin providing ice chips when bowel sounds are present | Sitz baths prn<br>If woman Rh negative and infant Rh positive, Rh-immune globulin workup; obtain consent; complete teaching<br>Determine rubella status<br>Obtain consent for rubella vaccine if indicated; explain purpose, procedure, implications of vaccine<br>**CB:** Advance diet as ordered and tolerated<br>Assist with perineal care and ADLs<br>Obtain hematocrit and hemaglobin<br>Discontinue Foley catheter when woman can ambulate to BR<br>Discontinue of heplock IV when woman can tolerate oral fluids, or as ordered<br>Maintain incision care as ordered | Continue sitz baths prn<br>May shower if ambulating without difficulty<br>DC buffalo cap (heplock) if present<br>Administer rubella vaccine as indicated<br>**Expected Outcomes**<br>Using sitz bath; voids qs; lab work WNL; performs ADL without sequelae |
| **Activity** | **VB:** Assistance when OOB first time, then prn<br>Ambulate ad lib<br>Rests comfortably between assessments<br>**CB:** Assistance with movement in bed, to include leg exercises and sitting upright | Encourage rest periods<br>Ambulate ad lib; may leave birthing unit after notifying staff of plan to ambulate off unit<br>**CB:** Advance movement to include hanging legs over edge of bed and brief standing | Up ad lib<br>**CB:** Assist woman to ambulate as soon as possible<br>**Expected Outcomes**<br>Ambulates ad lib |
| **Comfort** | Institute comfort measures:<br>• Perineal discomfort: peri-care; sitz baths, topical analgesics<br>• Hemorrhoids: sitz baths, topical analgesics, digital replacement of external hemorrhoids; side-lying or prone position<br>• Afterpains: prone with small pillow under abdomen; warm shower or sitz baths;<br>• Administer pain medication _____<br>**CB:** Implement PCA or pain med. as ordered | Continue with pain management techniques<br>Offer alternative pain management options: distraction with music, television, visitors; massage; warmed blankets or towels to affected area; using breathing techniques when infant latches on to breast and/or during cramping until medication's action is felt | Continue with pain management techniques<br>**Expected Outcomes**<br>Comfort level <3 on 1–10 scale<br>Verbalizes alternative pain management options |
| **Nutrition** | **VB:** Regular diet<br>Fluid ≥ 2000 mL/day<br>**CB:** Begin sips and chips when bowel sounds present or per protocol | Continue diet and fluids<br>**CB:** Advance diet to clear liquids as tolerated or per protocol | Continue diet and fluids<br>**CB:** Advance diet as tolerated<br>**Expected Outcomes**<br>Regular diet/fluids tolerated |

| Category | First 4 Hours | 4–8 Hours Past Birth | 8–24 Hours Past Birth |
|---|---|---|---|
| **Elimination** | Voiding large amounts straw-colored urine<br>**CB:** A min of 30 cc qh clear urine output in Foley catheter | Voiding large quantities<br>May have bowel movement<br>**CB:** A min of 30 cc qh clear urine output in Foley catheter | Same<br>**Expected Outcomes**<br>Voiding qs; passing flatus or bowel movement |
| **Medications** | Pain medications as ordered<br>Methergine 0.2 mg q4h po if ordered<br>Stool softener _____<br>Tucks pad prn, perineal analgesic spray | Continue meds<br>Lanolin to nipples prn; tea bags to nipples if tender; flush to buffalo cap/heplock (if present) q8h or as ordered<br>May take own prenatal vitamins | Continue medications<br>RhoGAM and rubella vaccine PRN<br>**Expected Outcomes**<br>Vaccines administered; pain controlled |
| **Discharge planning/ home care** | Evaluate knowledge of normal PP and newborn care<br>Evaluate support systems | Discuss typical newborn schedule; plan for periods of rest<br>Birth certificate paperwork completed<br>Evaluate plans for transporting newborn; car seat available<br>**CB:** Evaluate for physical help at home | Review D/C instruction sheet/checklist<br>Describe PP warning signs and when to call CNM or physician<br>Provide prescriptions; gift packs given appropriate for bottle- or breastfeeding<br>Arrangements for baby pictures as desired<br>Postpartum and newborn visits scheduled<br>**Expected Outcomes**<br>Discharged home; mother verbalizes PP warning s/s, follow-up appointments |
| **Family involvement** | Identify available support persons<br>Assess family perceptions of birth experience<br>Parenting: demonstrates culturally expected early parenting behaviors | Involve support persons in care, teaching; answer questions<br>Evidence of parental bonding behaviors present | Continue to involve support persons in teaching, involve siblings as appropriate.<br>Plans made for providing support to mother following D/C<br>**Expected Outcomes**<br>Evidence of parental bonding behavior; support persons verbalize understanding of woman's need for rest, good nutrition, fluids, and emotional support |
| **Date** | | | |

well as the physical and psychological well-being of each family member. An important component of nursing care is client teaching, which must be individualized to the learning capability and readiness of the parent(s). As part of the teaching role, the nurse discusses desired outcomes and goals with the mother and family members as soon as possible following the birth. Interventions can then be designed to achieve optimal health promotion.

## Promotion of Maternal Physical Well-Being

The nurse can promote and restore maternal physical well-being by monitoring uterine status, vital signs, cardiovascular status, elimination patterns, nutritional needs, sleep and rest, and support and educational needs. In addition, the postpartal woman may need medications to promote comfort, treat anemia, provide immunity to rubella, and prevent development of antigens (in the nonsensitized Rh-negative woman).

### Monitoring Uterine Status

The nurse completes an assessment of the uterus as discussed in Chapter 27. The assessment interval is usually every 15 minutes for the first hour after childbirth, every 30 minutes for the next hour, and then hourly for approximately 2 hours. After that, the nurse monitors uterine status every 8 hours or more frequently if problems arise such as bogginess, positioning out of midline, heavy lochia flow, or the presence of clots. (See Key Facts to Remember: Monitoring Postpartum Uterine Status.) Occasionally medications are needed to promote uterine contractions. (See Drug Guide: Oxytocin [Pitocin], in Chapter 20, and Drug Guide: Methylergonovine Maleate [Methergine], on page 755). The nurse monitors

## KEY FACTS TO REMEMBER

### *Monitoring Postpartal Uterine Status*

**Position of the Uterine Fundus Following Birth**

Immediately after birth: The top of the fundus is in the midline about midway between the symphysis-pubis and umbilicus.

Six to twelve hours after birth: The top of the fundus is in the midline and at the level of the umbilicus.

One day after birth: The top of the fundus is in the midline and one finger breadth below the umbilicus.

Second day after birth and thereafter: The top of the fundus remains in the midline and descends about one finger breadth per day.

**Normal Characteristics of Lochia**

Lochia rubra is red and is present for the first 2–3 days.

Lochia serosa is pinkish red and is present from day 3 to day 10.

Lochia alba is creamy white and is present from day 11 to about day 21.

amount, consistency, color, and odor of the lochia on an ongoing basis (see Table 28–1).

## Promotion of Comfort and Relief of Pain

The postpartal woman may experience varying degrees of discomfort. Potential sources of discomfort include an edematous perineum; an episiotomy, perineal laceration, or extension; vaginal hematoma; engorged hemorrhoids; or engorged breasts with sore nipples.

### Relief of Perineal Discomfort

There are many nursing interventions for the relief of perineal discomfort. Before selecting a method, the nurse needs to assess the perineum to determine the degree of edema and so on. It is also important to ask the woman if she believes any special measures will be particularly effective and to offer her choices when possible. The nurse uses disposable gloves while applying all relief measures and completes handwashing before and after using the gloves. At all times it is essential for the nurse to remember hygienic practices, such as moving from the front (area of the symphysis pubis) to the back (area around the anus) of the perineum. Avoiding contamination between the anal area and the urethral/vaginal area is vital to the prevention of infection.

## HINTS FOR PRACTICE

You may be surprised by how quickly the postpartal woman shows signs of bladder distention, possibly as soon as 1 to 2 hours after childbirth. It results because of normal postpartal diuresis. You can help prevent overdistention by palpating the woman's bladder frequently and encouraging her to void. When attempting to void for the first time after vaginal birth, some mothers may feel the urge to urinate but are unable to begin the flow of urine. Possible interventions include letting her hear running water by turning water on in the sink or tub, running warm water in the sink and having her place one hand in the water, and/or placing her feet in a basin of warm water.

#### Ice Pack

If an episiotomy is done at the time of birth, an ice pack is generally applied to the perineum to reduce edema and provide numbing of the tissues, which promotes comfort. In some agencies, chemical ice bags are used, these are usually activated by folding both ends toward the middle. The nurse can create inexpensive ice bags by filling a disposable glove with ice chips or crushed ice and then taping the top of the glove. To protect the perineum from burns caused by contact with such an ice pack, the glove needs to be rinsed under running water to remove any powder and then wrapped in an absorbent towel or washcloth before placing it against the perineum. To attain the maximum effect of this cold treatment, a pattern of applying the ice pack for approximately 20 minutes and then removing it for about 10 minutes should be followed. Usually ice packs are needed for the first 24 hours. The nurse provides information about the purpose of the ice pack, as well as anticipated effects, benefits, and possible problems, and explains how to prepare an ice pack for home use if edema is present and early discharge is planned.

#### Sitz Bath

The warmth of the water in the sitz bath provides comfort, decreases pain, and promotes circulation to the tissues, which promotes healing and reduces the incidence

# DRUG GUIDE

## METHYLERGONOVINE MALEATE (METHERGINE)

### *Overview of Action*

Methylergonovine maleate (Methergine) is an ergot alkaloid that stimulates smooth muscle tissue. Because the uterus is especially sensitive to this drug, it is used postpartally to stimulate the uterus to contract in order to decrease blood loss by clamping off uterine blood vessels and to promote involution. In addition, the drug has a vasoconstrictive effect on all blood vessels, especially the larger arteries. This may result in hypertension, particularly in a woman whose blood pressure is already elevated.

### *Route, Dosage, Frequency*

Methergine has a rapid onset of action and may be given orally or intramuscularly.

Usual IM dose: 0.2 mg following delivery of the placenta. The dose may be repeated every 2–4 hours if necessary.

Usual oral dose: 0.2 mg every 4 hours (six doses).

### *Maternal Contraindications*

Pregnancy, hepatic or renal disease, cardiac disease, and hypertension or pregnancy-induced hypertension contraindicate use of this drug. Methylergonovine maleate must be used with caution during lactation (Karch, 2001).

### *Maternal Side Effects*

Hypertension, nausea, vomiting, headache, bradycardia, dizziness, tinnitus, abdominal cramps, palpitations, dyspnea, chest pain, and allergic reactions may be noted.

### *Effects on Fetus or Neonate*

Because Methergine has a long duration (3 hours [Karch, 2000]) and action and can thus produce tetanic contractions, it **should never be used during pregnancy or in labor,** when it may result in a sustained uterine contraction that may cause amniotic fluid embolism (increased pressure in uterus may allow entry of amniotic fluid under the edge of the placenta and thus entry into the maternal venous system), uterine rupture, cervical and perineal lacerations (resulting from tetanic contractions and rapid birth of the baby), and hypoxia and intracranial hemorrhage in the baby (because of tetanic contractions, which severely decrease the maternal-placental-fetal blood flow, or uterine rupture, which causes cessation of blood flow to the unborn baby) (PDR Nurse's Handbook, 2001).

### *Nursing Considerations*

- Monitor fundal height and consistency and the amount and character of the lochia.
- Assess the blood pressure before and routinely throughout drug administration.
- Observe for adverse effects or symptoms of ergot toxicity (ergotism) such as nausea and vomiting, headache, muscle pain, cold or numb fingers and toes, chest pain, and general weakness (PDR Nurse's Handbook, 2001).
- Provide client and family teaching regarding importance of not smoking during Methergine administration (nicotine from cigarettes leads to constricted vessels and may lead to hypertension), signs of toxicity.

TABLE 28–1 Changes in Lochia That Cause Concern

| *Change* | *Possible Problem* | *Nursing Action* |
|---|---|---|
| Presence of clots | Inadequate uterine contractions that allow bleeding from vessels at the placental site. | Assess location and firmness of fundus.<br>Assess voiding pattern.<br>Record and report findings. |
| Persistent lochia rubra | Inadequate uterine contractions; retained placental fragments; infection | Assess location and firmness of fundus.<br>Assess activity pattern.<br>Assess for signs of infection.<br>Record and report findings. |

## EVIDENCE-BASED PRACTICE

### Postpartum Pain Management

You have been interviewed by a surveyor from the Joint Commission on Accreditation of Hospitals (JCAHO). As a first-year registered nurse on the mother-baby unit, you have never participated in an organizational review. When you were asked to describe how the "fifth vital sign" is assessed and monitored for your patients, you felt ill prepared to respond.

Some senior nurses on your unit explain to you that the JCAHO has incorporated pain management into its review for accreditation (JCAHO, 2000) to emphasize the importance of this aspect of care. They tell you that, in 1992, the Agency for Health Care Policy and Research published the first evidence-based guidelines, in this area titled *Acute Pain Management.* Despite the availability of this guideline, separate studies have shown that pain is underassessed and patients are regularly undermedicated (White, 1999; Zalon 1999).

"The patient's self report is the single most reliable indicator for pain," according to the National Institutes of Health (Zalon, 1999, p. 135). All women in labor should receive information about pain and pain relief measures. In addition, nurses must provide a baseline assessment of pain by using a pain intensity scale, evaluate the pain management regimen according to ongoing patient monitoring, and work with the client to optimize her comfort (JCAHO, 2000).

Your discussion with your colleagues prompts you to question whether there is a tendency to see pain as less significant for postpartum clients than for clients experiencing surgery or illness. You suggest this issue to your unit manager as a topic worthy of further nursing research.

#### References


Joint Commission on Accreditation of Hospitals. (2000). Pain management standards. *Comprehensive accreditation manual for hospitals [On-line]. Available: www.jacho.org*

White, C. (1999). Changing pain management and impacting on patient outcomes. *Clinical Nurse Specialist, 13*(4), 166–172.

Zalon, M. (1999). Comparison of pain measures in surgical patients. *Journal of Nursiing Management, 7*(2), 135–152.


of infection. Sitz baths may be ordered three times a day (TID) and as needed (prn). The nurse prepares the sitz bath by cleaning the sitz bath equipment and adding water at 102 to 105°F. The woman is encouraged to remain in the sitz bath for about 20 minutes. It is important for the woman to have a clean, unused towel to pat dry her perineum after the sitz bath and to have a clean perineal pad to apply. Care needs to be taken during the first sitz bath because the warm, moist heat and warm environment may cause the woman to faint. The nurse places a call bell well within reach and checks on the woman at frequent intervals to maintain safety. The nurse needs to observe the woman at frequent intervals for signs that she may faint, such as expressed feelings of dizziness, a floaty or spacy feeling, or difficulty hearing.

Cool sitz baths have gained popularity because they are effective in reducing perineal edema. Until research supports one temperature (warm or cold) as more effective, it may be best to offer the woman a choice. The nurse provides information about the purpose and use of the sitz bath; anticipated effects, benefits, and possible problems; and safety measures to prevent injury from fainting, slipping, or excessive water temperature. Home use of sitz baths may be recommended for the woman with an extensive episiotomy, and the woman may use a portable sitz bath or her bathtub. It is important for the nurse to emphasize that in using a bathtub, the woman draws only 4 to 6 in of water, assesses the temperature, and uses the water only for the sitz and not for bathing. If the woman takes a tub bath, she should release the water, have a helper clean the tub, and draw new water prior to the sitz bath to prevent infection.

#### Topical Agents

Topical anesthetics such as Dermoplast aerosol spray and Americain spray may be used to relieve perineal discomfort. The woman is advised to apply the anesthetic after a sitz bath or perineal care. Witch hazel compresses may be used to relieve perineal discomfort and edema. Nupercainal ointment or Tucks may be ordered for relief of hemorrhoidal pain. It is important for the nurse to emphasize the need for the woman to wash her hands before and after using the topical treatments.

The nurse provides information about the anesthetic spray or topical agent. The woman needs to understand the purpose, use, anticipated effects and benefits, and possible problems associated with the product. The nurse can combine a demonstration of application with teaching. A return demonstration is a useful method of evaluating the woman's understanding.

#### Perineal Care

Perineal care after each elimination cleanses the perineum and helps promote comfort. Many agencies provide "peri bottles" that the woman can use to squirt warm tap water over her perineum following elimination. To cleanse her perineum, the woman should use moist antiseptic towelettes or toilet paper in a blotting (patting) motion and should be taught to start at the front (area just under the symphysis pubis) and proceed toward the back (area around the anus), to prevent contamination from the anal area. In addition, to prevent contamination the perineal pad should be applied from front to back (place the front portion against the perineum first).

The nurse demonstrates how to cleanse the perineum and assists the woman as necessary. Many women have never used perineal pads and will need additional assistance in using them during the postpartal period. The pad needs to be placed snugly against the perineum but should not produce pressure. If the pad is worn too loosely, it may rub back and forth, irritating perineal tissues and causing contamination between the anal and vaginal areas. (For information regarding the care of the perineum following an episiotomy see the Teaching Guide: Episiotomy Care, on page 754 and for additional postpartum information see Teaching Cards.

### Relief of Hemorrhoidal Discomfort

Some mothers experience hemorrhoidal pain after giving birth. Relief measures include the use of sitz baths, topical anesthetic ointments, rectal suppositories, or witch hazel pads applied directly to the anal area. The woman may be taught to digitally replace external hemorrhoids in her rectum. She may also find it helpful to maintain a side-lying position when possible and to avoid prolonged sitting. The mother is encouraged to maintain an adequate fluid intake, and stool softeners are administered to ensure greater comfort with bowel movements. The hemorrhoids usually disappear a few weeks after birth if the woman did not have them before her pregnancy.

### Relief of Afterpains

Afterpains are the result of intermittent uterine contractions. A primipara may not experience afterpains because her uterus is able to maintain a contracted state. Multiparous women and those who have had a multiple-gestation pregnancy or hydramnios frequently experience discomfort from afterpains as the uterus contracts intermittently. Breastfeeding women are also more likely to experience afterpains than bottle-feeding women because of the release of oxytocin when the infant suckles. The nurse can suggest that the woman lie prone, with a small pillow under her lower abdomen, and explain that the discomfort may feel intensified for about 5 minutes but then diminishes greatly if not completely. The prone position applies pressure to the uterus and therefore stimulates contractions. When the uterus maintains a constant contraction, the afterpains cease. Additional nursing interventions include a sitz bath (for warmth), positioning, ambulation, or administration of an analgesic agent. For breastfeeding mothers, an analgesic administered an hour before nursing helps promote comfort and enhances maternal-infant interaction (Table 28–2).

The nurse provides information about the cause of afterpains and methods to decrease discomfort. She or he explains any medications that are ordered, including their expected effect, benefits, and possible side effects, and any special considerations such as the possibility of dizziness or sleepiness with particular medications.

### Discomfort from Immobility

Discomfort may be caused by immobility. The woman who has been in stirrups for any length of time may experience muscular aches from such extreme positioning. It is not unusual for women to experience joint pains and muscular pain in both arms and legs, depending on the effort they exerted during the second stage of labor.

Early ambulation is encouraged to help reduce the incidence of complications such as constipation and thrombophlebitis. It also helps promote a feeling of general well-being. The nurse provides information about ambulation and the importance of monitoring any signs of dizziness or weakness.

The nurse assists the woman the first few times she gets up during the postpartal period. Fatigue, effects of medications, loss of blood, and lack of food intake may cause feelings of dizziness or faintness when the woman stands up. Because this may be a problem during the woman's first shower, the nurse should remain in the room, check the woman frequently, and have a chair close by in case she becomes faint. During this first shower the nurse instructs the woman in the use of the emergency call button in the bathroom; if she becomes faint during a future shower, she is advised to sit down and can call for assistance.

## TEACHING GUIDE *Episiotomy Care*

### Assessment

During the time following labor and birth, assess the woman's understanding of the purpose of the episiotomy, the factors that contribute to wound healing, and the comfort measures available if needed. The woman's level of knowledge may be influenced by several factors, including for example, childbirth preparation activities and previous childbirth experience.

### Nursing Diagnosis

The key nursing diagnosis will probably be health-seeking behaviors regarding information about measures to promote episiotomy healing related to an expressed desire to take action to increase personal comfort.

### Client Goals

At the completion of teaching, the woman will be able to

- Identify the factors that both promote and interfere with wound healing.
- Summarize self-care activities to promote healing and increase personal comfort.
- Demonstrate the appropriate techniques used to keep the perineum clean.
- Demonstrate the correct procedure for taking a sitz bath.
- Discuss the judicious use of prescribed analgesics as needed.

### *Teaching Plan*

| CONTENT | TEACHING METHOD |
|---|---|
| • Describe the process of wound healing. Discuss the risk of contamination of the episiotomy by bacteria from the anal area.<br>• Explain techniques that are used to keep the episiotomy clean and promote healing:<br>  • Sitz bath<br>  • Use of peribottle following each voiding or defecation<br>  • Pad change following each elimination and at regular intervals | Many women do not consider the episiotomy a surgical incision. Discussion helps them understand the importance of good wound care.<br>Focus on open discussion. Demonstrate the peribottle or sitz bath. |
| • Describe comfort measures:<br>  • Ice pack or glove immediately following birth<br>  • Sitz bath<br>  • Judicious use of analgesics or topical anesthetics<br>  • Tightening buttocks before sitting | Focus on discussion and provide an opportunity for questions. |
| • Identify signs of episiotomy infection. Advise the woman to contact her caregiver if infection develops. | Encourage discussion and provide printed handouts. Some of this content may also be covered during a small postpartum class. |

### Evaluation

Evaluate the learning by asking the woman to explain the principles of wound healing and episiotomy care and/or demonstrate self-care measures, if necessary.

### Postpartal Diaphoresis

Postpartal diaphoresis (excessive perspiration) may cause discomfort for new mothers. The nurse can offer a fresh, dry gown and change bed linens to enhance comfort. Some women may feel refreshed by a shower. It is necessary to consider cultural practices and realize that some women of Hispanic or Asian cultural background may prefer not to shower in the first few days following birth. Because diaphoresis may also increase thirst, the nurse can offer fluids as the woman desires. Again, the nurse needs to consider cultural practices. Women of western European background may prefer iced water, whereas Asian women may prefer water at room temperature. It is important to ascertain the woman's wishes rather than operate solely from one's own value or cultural belief system. The nurse provides information about the normalcy of diaphoresis and methods to increase comfort.

## Suppression of Lactation in the Nonnursing Mother

For the woman who chooses not to breastfeed, lactation may be suppressed by mechanical inhibition. Although signs of engorgement do not usually appear until the second or third postpartum day, prevention of engorgement is best accomplished when the nurse encourages the woman to begin mechanical inhibition of lactation as soon as possible after birth. Ideally prevention involves having the woman begin wearing a supportive, well-fitting bra within 6 hours after birth. The bra is worn continuously until lactation is suppressed (usually about

## TABLE 28–2 Essential Information for Common Postpartum Drugs

### EMPIRIN #3 (325 MG ASPIRIN AND 30 MG CODEINE)

Drug class: Narcotic analgesic.

**Dose/Route:** Usual adult dose: 1–2 tablets PO every 4 hours prn.

**Indication:** For relief of mild to moderate pain.

**Adverse Effects:** Aspirin: Nausea, dyspepsia, epigastric discomfort, dizziness.
Codeine: Respiratory depression, apnea, light-headedness, dizziness, nausea, sweating, dry mouth, constipation, facial flushing, suppression of cough reflex, ureteral spasm, urinary retention, pruritus.

**Nursing Implications:** Determine whether woman is sensitive to ASA or codeine; has hs of impaired hepatic or renal function. Monitor bowel sounds, respiration, urine output.
Administer with food or after meals if GI upset occurs; encourage woman to drink one full glass (240mL) with the tablet to reduce the risk of the tablet lodging in the esophagus.

**Client Teaching:** Inform client about name of drug, expected action, possible side effects, that it is secreted in breast milk (*Note:* Some physicians and certified nurse-midwives may avoid ordering this medication for nursing mothers), and review safety measures (assess for dizziness, use side rails, call for assistance when getting out of bed and ambulating, report to nurse any signs of adverse effects); ask if she has any questions.

**Nursing Diagnosis Related to Drug Therapy:** ***Knowledge Deficit*** related to lack of information regarding the drug therapy.

***Risk for injury*** related to dizziness secondary to effect of drug.

### PERCOSET (325 MG ACETAMINOPHEN AND 5 MG OXYCODONE)

Drug Class: Narcotic analgesic.

**Drug/Route:** 1–2 tablets PO every 4 hours prn.

**Indication:** For moderate to moderately severe pain. Can be used in aspirin-sensitive women.

**Adverse Effects:** Acetaminophen: Hepatotoxicity, headache, rash, hypoglycemia.
Oxycodone: Respiratory depression, apnea, circulatory depression, euphoria, facial flushing, constipation, suppression of cough reflex, ureteral spasm, urinary retention.

**Nursing Implications:** Determine whether woman is sensitive to acetaminophen or codeine; has bronchial asthma, respiratory depression, convulsive disorder.
Observe woman carefully for respiratory depression if given with barbiturates or sedative/hypnotics. Consider that women who have undergone cesarean may have depressed cough reflex, so teaching and encouragement to TC & DB are needed. Monitor bowel sounds, urine and bowel elimination.

**Client Teaching:** Teaching should include name of drug, expected effect, possible adverse effects, that drug is secreted in the breast milk, encouragement to report any signs of adverse effects immediately.

**Nursing Diagnoses Related to Drug Therapy:** ***Ineffective Breathing Pattern*** related to depression.

***Constipation*** related to slowed gastrointestinal activity.

### RUBELLA VIRUS VACCINE, LIVE (MERUVAX 2)

**Dose/Route:** Single dose vial, inject subcutaneously in outer aspect of the upper arm.

**Indication:** Stimulate active immunity against rubella virus.

**Adverse Effects:** Burning or stinging at the injection site; about 2–4 weeks later may have rash, malaise, sore throat, or headache.

**Nursing Implications:** Determine whether woman has sensitivity to neomycin (vaccine contains neomycin); is immunosuppressed, or has received blood transfusions (not to be administered within 3 months of blood transfusion, plasma transfusion, or serum immune globulin).
*Note:* If a woman is to receive both RhoGAM and rubella, there is a possibility that the formation of antibodies to rubella may be suppressed by the RhoGAM injection. Most physicians will go ahead and order both injections and retest for maternal rubella immune status in about 3 months (Varney, 1997).

**Client Teaching:** Name of drug, expected effect, possible adverse effects, possible comfort measures to use if adverse effects occur; rubella titer will be assessed in about 3 months. Instruct woman to *avoid pregnancy for 3 months* following vaccination. Provide information regarding contraceptives and their use.

**Nursing Diagnosis Related to Drug Therapy:** ***Knowledge Deficit*** regarding drug therapy. ***Knowledge Deficit*** regarding types and use of contraceptives.
***Pain*** related to rash and malaise.

## TABLE 28–2 Essential Information for Common Postpartum Drugs *continued*

### RHOGAM (RH IMMUNE GLOBULIN SPECIFIC FOR D ANTIGEN)

**Dose/Route:** Postpartum: One vial IM within 72 hours of birth. Antepartal: One vial microdose RhoGAM IM at 28 weeks in Rh-negative women; after amniocentesis, spontaneous or therapeutic abortion, or ectopic pregnancy.

***Indication:*** Prevention of sensitization to the Rh factor in Rh-negative women and to prevent hemolytic disease in the newborn in subsequent pregnancies. Mother must be Rh negative, not previously sensitized to Rh factor. Infant must be Rh positive, direct antiglobulin negative.

**Adverse Effects:** Soreness at injection site.

**Nursing Implications:** Confirm that criteria for administration are present. Ensure correct vial is used for the client (each vial is cross-matched to the specific woman.
Inject entire contents of vial.

**Client Teaching:** Name of drug, expected action, possible side effects; report soreness at injection site to nurse; woman should carry information regarding Rh status and dates of RhoGAM injections with her at all times; explain use of RhoGAM with subsequent pregnancies.

**Nursing Diagnoses Related to Drug Therapy: *Knowledge Deficit*** related to the need for the RhoGAM and future implications.
***Pain*** related to soreness at injection site.

### SECONAL SODIUM (SECOBARBITAL SODIUM)

Drug Class: Sedative, short-acting barbiturate

**Dose/Route:** 100 mg PO at bedtime.

**Indication:** Promote sleep.

**Adverse Effects:** Somnolence, confusion, ataxia, vertigo, nightmares, hypoventilation, bradycardia, hypotension, nausea, vomiting, rashes.

**Nursing Implications:** Determine whether woman has sensitivity to barbiturates, or respiratory distress. Monitor respirations, blood pressure, pulse. Modify environment to increase relaxation and promote sleep. Monitor for drug interaction if woman also is taking tranquilizers or TACE.

**Client Teaching:** Name of drug, expected effect, possible adverse effects, safety measures (side rails, use call bell, ask for assistance when out of bed); medication is secreted in breast milk.

**Nursing Diagnoses Related to Drug Therapy: *Risk for Injury*** related to possible ataxia or vertigo.

***Altered Thought Processes*** related to drug-induced confusion.
***Knowledge Deficit*** related to lack of information regarding drug therapy.

5 to 7 days) and is removed only for showers. The bra provides support and eases the discomfort that can occur with tension on the breasts because of fullness. Ice packs should be applied over the axillary area of each breast for 20 minutes four times daily. This practice, too, should begin soon after birth. Ice is also useful in relieving discomfort if engorgement occurs. Breast engorgement may be a source of pain for the postpartal woman.

The mother is advised to avoid any stimulation of her breasts by her baby, herself, breast pumps, or her sexual partner until the sensation of fullness has passed (usually about 5 to 7 days). Such stimulation increases milk production and delays the suppression process. Heat is avoided for the same reason, and the mother is encouraged to let shower water flow over her back rather than her breasts.

## Promotion of Rest and Graded Activity

Following childbirth some women feel exhausted and in need of rest. Other women may be euphoric and full of psychic energy, ready to relive and recount the experience of birth repeatedly. The nurse can provide a period for airing of feelings and then encourage a period of rest.

Physical fatigue often affects other adjustments and functions of the new mother. For example, fatigue can reduce milk flow, thereby increasing problems with establishing breastfeeding. Energy is also needed to make the psychologic adjustments to a new infant and to assume new roles. Nurses can encourage rest by organizing their activities to avoid frequent interruptions for the woman. It is helpful for the new mother to know that fatigue may persist for several weeks or even months. Persistent fatigue is compounded by physical, psychological, situational, and environmental factors (Parks, Lenz, Milligan, et al., 1999).

Although most mothers feel tired, if they have perceived the pregnancy and birth as a natural process, they tend to view themselves as healthy and well. However, some mothers view the postpartal period as a time of sickness. For instance, some Korean women and their families view the new mother as sick and in need of care by the mother-in-law and the baby's father. A Korean mother may take on some activity, but for the most part it will be activities such as picking up the baby from the nursery rather than activity directed toward herself (Schneiderman, 1996).

### Postpartal Exercises

The woman should be encouraged to begin simple exercises while in the birthing unit and to continue them at home. She is advised that increased lochia or pain means she should reevaluate her activity and make necessary alterations. Most agencies provide a booklet describing suggested postpartal activities. (Exercise routines vary for women undergoing cesarean birth or tubal ligation after childbirth.) (See Figure 28–1♦ for a description of some commonly used exercises.)

Sampselle, Seng, Yeo, and coworkers (1999) report that exercise during the prenatal period is associated with positive views of the childbirth experience. The postpartal woman is more likely to have positive views of her well-being and less fatigue if she continues to do stretching and her own pattern of exercise after she is home.

### Resumption of Activities

Ambulation and activity may gradually increase after birth. The new mother should avoid heavy lifting, excessive stair climbing, and strenuous activity. One or two daily naps are essential and are most easily achieved if the mother sleeps when her baby does.

By the second week at home, the woman may resume light housekeeping. Although it is customary to delay returning to work for 6 weeks, most women are physically able to resume practically all activities by 4 to 5 weeks. Delaying the return to work until after the final postpartal examination minimizes the possibility of problems.

## Pharmacologic Interventions

### Rubella Vaccine

Women who have a rubella titer of less than 1:10, or test antibody negative on the enzyme-linked immunosorbent assay (ELISA), are usually given rubella vaccine in the postpartal period (Cunningham, MacDonald, Grant, et al., 1997) (see Table 28–2). The nurse needs to ensure that the woman understands the purpose of the vaccine and that she must avoid becoming pregnant in the next 3 months. To ensure that the woman understands, an informed consent is obtained before administration. Because the avoidance of pregnancy is so important, counseling regarding contraception is suggested.

### Rh Immune Globulin

All Rh-negative women who meet specific criteria should receive Rh immune globulin (RhoGAM) within 72 hours after childbirth to prevent sensitization from the fetomaternal transfusion of Rh-positive fetal red blood cells. (See discussion of criteria in Procedure 13–2.)

The Rh-negative woman needs to understand the implications of her Rh-negative status in future pregnancies. The nurse provides opportunities for questions.

## Promotion of Maternal Psychologic Well-Being

The birth of a child, with the changes in role and the increased responsibilities it produces, is a time of emotional stress for the new mother. During the early postpartum period the mother may be emotionally labile, and mood swings and tearfulness are common. Initially the mother may repeatedly discuss her experiences of labor and birth. This allows the mother to integrate her experiences (Banks-Wallace, 1999). If she believes that she did not cope well with labor, she may have feelings of inadequacy and may benefit from reassurance that she did well. Some women feel that they did not have any perception of time during the labor and birth and want to know how long it really lasted, or they may not remember the entire experience. In this case, it is helpful for the nurse to talk with the woman and provide information that she is missing and desires.

During this time the new mother must also adjust to the loss of her fantasized child and accept the child she has borne. This task may be more difficult if the child is not of the desired sex or if he or she has birth defects (see Chapter 26).

Immediately after the birth (the taking-in period) the mother is focused on bodily concerns and may not be fully ready to learn about personal and infant care. Following the initial dependent period, the mother becomes very concerned about her ability to be a successful parent (the taking-hold period). During this time the mother requires reassurance that she is effective. She also tends to be receptive to teaching and demonstration designed to assist her in mothering successfully. The depression, weepiness, and "let-down feeling" that characterize the postpartum blues are often a surprise for the new mother. She requires reassurance that these feelings are normal, an explanation about why they occur, and a supportive environment that permits her to cry without feeling guilty.

## Promotion of Effective Parent Education

Meeting the educational needs of the new mother and her family is one of the primary challenges facing the postpartum nurse. Each woman's educational needs vary based on her age, background, experience, and expectations. In addition, the brief period that the mother is in the postpartal area makes it even more difficult to address all individual characteristics and informational needs.

The nurse first assesses the learning needs of the new mother through observation and tactfully phrased questions. For example, "What plans have you made for handling things when you get home?" may elicit a response of several words and may provide the opportunity for some information sharing and guidance. Some agencies

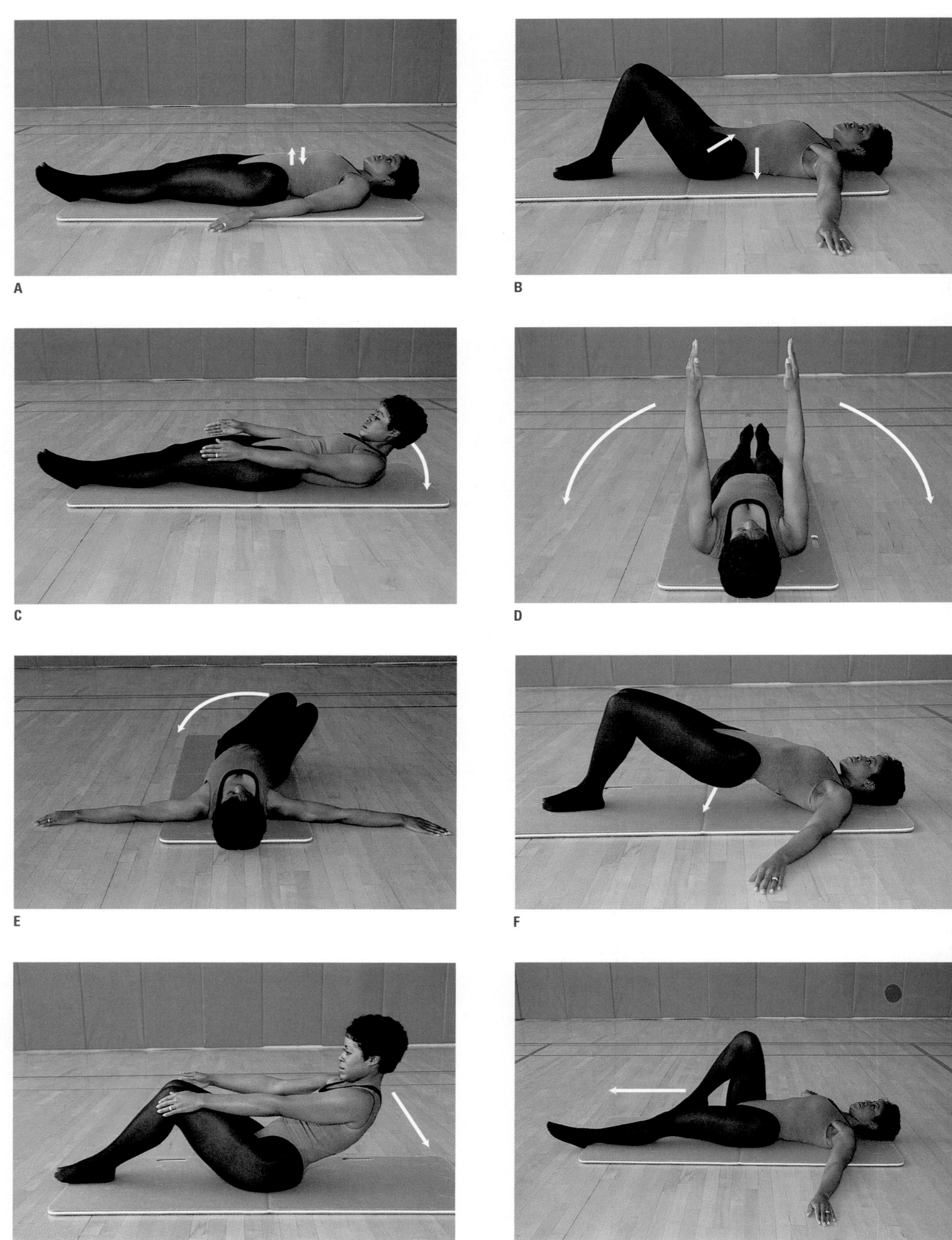
A
B
C
D
E
F
G
H

FIGURE 28–1 (at left) ♦ Postpartal exercises. Begin with 5 repetitions two or three times daily and gradually increase to 10 repetitions. First day: **A**, Abdominal breathing. Lying supine, inhale deeply using the abdominal muscles. The abdomen should expand. Then exhale slowly through pursed lips, tightening the abdominal muscles. **B**, Pelvic rocking. Lying supine with arms at sides, knees bent, and feet flat, tighten abdomen and buttocks and attempt to flatten back onto floor. Hold for a count of 10, then arch the back, causing the pelvis to "rock." On second day add the following: **C**, Chin to chest. Lying supine with no pillow, legs straight, raise head and attempt to touch chin to chest. Slowly lower head. **D**, Arm raises. Lying supine, arms extended perpendicular to the body, raise arms until hands touch. Lower slowly. On fourth day add the following: **E**, Knee rolls. Lying supine with knees bent, feet flat, arms extended to the side, roll knees slowly to one side, keeping shoulders flat. Return to original position and roll to opposite side. **F**, Buttocks lift. Lying supine, arms at sides, knees bent, feet flat, slowly raise the buttocks and arch the back. Return slowly to starting position. On sixth day add the following: **G**, Abdominal tighteners. Lying supine, knees bent, feet flat, slowly raise the head toward the knees. Arms should extend along either side of the legs. Return slowly to original position. **H**, Knee to abdomen. Lying supine, arms at sides, bend one knee and thigh until foot touches buttocks. Straighten leg and lower it slowly. Repeat with other leg. After 2 to 3 weeks, more strenuous exercises such as side leg raises may be added as tolerated. Kegel exercises, begun antepartally, should be done many times daily during postpartum to restore vaginal and perineal tone.

also use checklists of common concerns for new mothers. The woman can check the concerns that are of interest to her.

The nurse then plans and implements teaching in a logical, nonthreatening way based on knowledge and respect of the family's cultural values and beliefs. Unless the nurse believes an activity would be harmful, most cultural customs can be supported and encouraged. Postpartal units use a variety of approaches, including handouts, formal classes, videotapes, and individual interaction.

Regardless of the teaching technique, timing is important. The new mother becomes more receptive to teaching after the first 24 to 48 hours, when she is ready to assume responsibility for her own care and that of her newborn (Lamp & Howard, 1999). Unfortunately, many women are discharged during the first 48 hours after birth. Consequently, many units provide printed material for new mothers to consult if questions arise at home. Timing is also important for new fathers, who are more likely to attend teaching sessions if they are scheduled in the late afternoon or early evening.

Teaching should include information on role change and psychologic adjustments as well as skills. Anticipatory guidance can help prepare new parents for the many changes they will experience with a new family member.

Information is also essential for women with specialized educational needs such as the mother who has had a cesarean birth, the parents of twins, the parents of an infant with congenital anomalies, and so on (Koniak-Griffin, Mathenge, Anderson, et al., 1999). Nurses who are attuned to these individual problems can begin providing guidance as soon as possible.

Evaluation may take several forms: return demonstrations, question-and-answer sessions, and even formal evaluation tools. Follow-up phone calls after discharge provide additional evaluative information and continue the helping process for the family.

## Promotion of Family Wellness

The promotion of family wellness involves several considerations, including a satisfactory maternity experience, the need for follow-up care for mother and infant, and birth control. The new or expanding family may also need information about adjustment of siblings and resuming sexual relations.

Today most facilities support family-centered care that is focused on keeping the mother and baby together as much as the mother desires. This type of care is called **mother-baby care,** or **couplet care,** and provides increased opportunities for parent-child interaction because the newborn shares the mother's unit and they are cared for together. Mother-baby care enables the mother to have time to bond with her baby and learn to care for her or him in a supportive environment. It is especially conducive to a hunger-demand feeding schedule for both breast- and bottle-feeding babies. It also allows the father, siblings, and friends to participate in the care of the new baby.

Mother-baby unit policies must be flexible enough to permit the mother to return the baby to the nursery if she finds it necessary because of fatigue or physical discomfort. Some mother-baby units also return the newborns to a central nursery at night so the mothers can get more rest. Mother-baby care provides excellent opportunities for family bonds to grow because the father, mother, newborn, and often siblings can begin functioning as a family unit immediately.

### Reactions of Siblings

Sibling visitation helps meet the needs of both the siblings and their mother. A visit to the mother-baby unit reassures children that their mother is well and still loves them. It also provides an opportunity for the children to become familiar with the new baby. For the mother the pangs of separation are lessened as she interacts with her children and introduces them to the newest family member (Figure 28–2♦).

Although the parents have prepared their children for the presence of a new brother or sister, the actual arrival of the infant in the home requires some adjustments. If small children are waiting at home, it is helpful if the father carries the baby inside. This practice keeps the

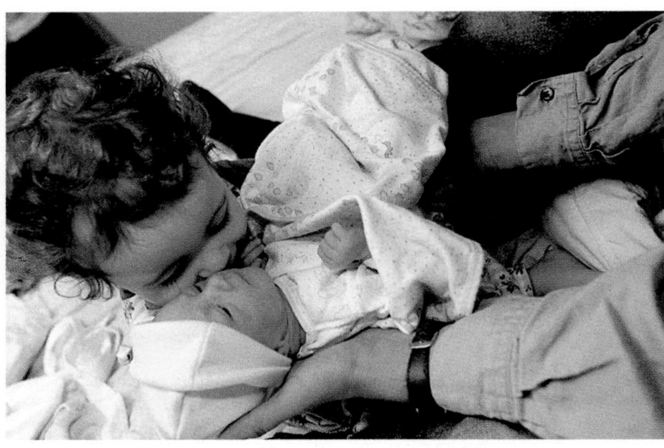

FIGURE 28–2 ♦ The sister of this newborn becomes acquainted with the new family member during a nursing assessment.

mother's arms free to hug and touch her older children. Many mothers bring a doll home with them for an older child. Caring for the doll alongside the mother or father helps the child to identify with the parents. This identification helps decrease anger and the need to regress for attention.

Parents may also provide supervised times when older children can hold the new baby and perhaps even help with a bottle-feeding. The older children feel a sense of accomplishment and learn tenderness and caring—qualities appropriate for both males and females. The nurse can help the parents come up with ways to show the other children that they, too, are valued and have their own places in the family.

### Sexual Activity and Contraception

Previously couples were discouraged from engaging in sexual intercourse until 6 weeks postpartum. Currently couples are advised to abstain from intercourse until the episiotomy has healed and the lochial flow has stopped (usually by the end of the third week). (For a more detailed discussion on resumption of sexual activity see Chapter 29.)

Because many couples resume sexual activity before the scheduled postpartal exam, family-planning information should be made available before discharge (Barrett, Pendry, Peacock, et al., 2000). Unfortunately, because of in-hospital time restraints, this subject is often overlooked. (Specific contraceptive methods are discussed in detail in Chapter 4.)

## Promotion of Parent-Infant Attachment

Nursing interventions to enhance the quality of parent-infant attachment should be designed to promote feelings of well-being, comfort, and satisfaction. Following are some suggestions for ways of promoting this:

- Determine the childbearing and childrearing goals of the infant's mother and father and adopt them wherever possible in planning nursing care for the family. This includes giving the parents choices about their labor and birth experience and their initial time with their new infant.
- Postpone eye prophylaxis for 1 hour after birth to facilitate eye contact between parents and their newborn (eye ointment further clouds the newborn's vision and makes eye contact difficult for the baby).
- Provide time in the first hour after birth for the new family to become acquainted, with as much privacy as possible.
- Arrange the health care setting so that the individual nurse-client relationship can be developed. A primary nurse can develop rapport and assess the mother's strengths and needs.
- Encourage the parents to involve the siblings in integrating the infant into the family by bringing them to the birthing center for visits.
- Use anticipatory guidance from conception through the postpartal period to prepare the parents for expected problems of adjustment.
- Include parents in any nursing intervention, planning, and evaluation. Give choices whenever possible.
- Initiate and support measures to alleviate fatigue in the parents.
- Help parents identify, understand, and accept both positive and negative feelings related to the overall parenting experience.
- Support and assist parents in determining the personality and unique needs of their infant.

Whenever possible, mother-baby care should be available. This practice gives the mother a chance to learn her newborn's normal patterns and develop confidence in caring for him or her. It also allows the father more uninterrupted time with his infant in the first days of life. If mother and baby are doing well, if help is available for the mother at home, and if the family and certified nurse-midwife or physician agree, early discharge may be advantageous.

The beginnings of parent-newborn attachment may be observed in the first few hours after birth. Continued assessments may occur in home visits after discharge. As the nurse assesses attachment, it is important to remember that cultural values, beliefs, and practices will direct the child care activities and self-care practices. For example, some Mexican-American women treat the umbilical

## TABLE 28–3 Parent Attachment Behaviors

| *Assessment Area* | *Attachment* | *Behavior Requiring Assessment and Information* |
|---|---|---|
| Caretaking | Talks with baby<br>Demonstrates and seeks eye-to-eye contact<br>Touches and holds baby<br>Changes diapers when needed<br>Baby is clean<br>Clothing is appropriate for room temperature<br>Feeds baby as needed and baby is gaining weight<br>Positions baby comfortably and checks on baby | Does not refer to baby<br>Completes activities without addressing the baby or looking at the baby<br>Lack of interaction<br>Does not recognize need for or demonstrate concern for baby's comfort or needs<br>Feeding occurs intermittently<br>Baby does not gain weight<br>Waits for baby to cry and then hesitates to respond |
| Perception of the baby | Has knowledge of expected child development<br>Understands that the baby is dependent and cannot meet parent's needs<br>Accepts sex and characteristics of child | Has unrealistic expectations of the baby's abilities and behaviors<br>Expects love and interaction from the baby<br>Believes that the baby will fulfill parent's needs<br>Is strongly distressed over sex of baby or feels that some aspect of the baby is unacceptable |
| Support | Has friends who are available for support<br>Seems to be comfortable with being a parent<br>Has realistic beliefs of parent role | Is alone or isolated<br>Is on edge, tense, anxious, and hesitant with the baby<br>Demonstrates difficulty incorporating parenting with own wants and needs |

*Please note:* These are a few of the behaviors that may be associated with attachment. It is vitally important for the nurse to observe the parents on more than one occasion and to take into consideration individual characteristics, values, beliefs, and customs.

stump by placing a coin or belly band over it. Some Mexican-American women or women from Southeast Asia may want to shield the baby from compliments and any extra attention because of their belief that they may attract the unwanted attention of evil spirits. (See Table 28–3 for behaviors related to infant attachment.)

# Nursing Care Management after Cesarean Birth

After a cesarean birth the new mother has postpartal needs similar to those of women who have given birth vaginally. Because she has undergone major abdominal surgery, the woman's nursing care needs are also similar to those of other surgical clients.

## Promotion of Maternal Physical Well-Being

The chances of pulmonary infection are increased because of immobility after the use of narcotics and sedatives and because of the altered immune response in postoperative clients. Therefore, the woman is encouraged to cough and deep breathe every 2 to 4 hours while awake until she is ambulating frequently.

Leg exercises are also encouraged every 2 hours until the woman is ambulating. These exercises increase circulation, help prevent thrombophlebitis, and also aid intestinal motility by tightening abdominal muscles.

The nurse monitors and manages the woman's pain experience during the postpartum period. Sources of pain include incisional pain, gas pain, referred shoulder pain, periodic uterine contractions (afterbirth pains), and pain from voiding, defecation, or constipation.

Nursing interventions are oriented toward preventing or alleviating pain or helping the woman cope with pain. The nurse should undertake the following measures:

- Administer analgesics as needed, especially during the first 24 to 72 hours after childbirth. Use of analgesics relieves the woman's pain and enables her to be more mobile and active.
- Promote comfort through proper positioning, back rubs, oral care, and the reduction of noxious stimuli such as noise and unpleasant odors.
- Encourage visits by significant others, including the newborn. These visits distract the woman from the painful sensations and help reduce her fear and anxiety.
- Encourage the use of breathing, relaxation, and distraction (eg, stimulation of cutaneous tissue) techniques taught in childbirth preparation class.

Epidural analgesia administered just after the cesarean birth is an effective method of pain relief for most women

## Critical Thinking in Practice

You walk in and find Dana Sullivan, a 29-year-old G2P2, crying 48 hours after a repeat cesarean birth. She states, "I'm not ready to go home. With my first baby they made me go home after 2 days. Can they make me again?"

Answers can be found in Appendix I.

in the first 24 hours following birth (see Drug Guide: Postpartum Epidural Morphine).

The physician may order **patient-controlled analgesia (PCA).** With this approach the woman is given a bolus of analgesia, usually morphine or meperidine, at the beginning of therapy. Using a special intravenous (IV) pump system, the woman presses a button to self-administer small doses of the medication as needed. For safety, the pump is preset with a time lockout so that the woman cannot deliver another dose until a specified period of time has elapsed. The use of a PCA helps women feel a greater sense of control and less dependence on nursing staff. The frequent, smaller doses help the woman experience rapid pain relief without grogginess and a drugged feeling and also avoid the discomfort associated with injections.

If a general anesthetic was used, abdominal distension may produce marked discomfort for the woman during the first few postpartal days. Measures to prevent or minimize abdominal distension include leg exercises, abdominal tightening, ambulation, avoiding carbonated or very hot or cold beverages, avoiding the use of straws, and providing a high-protein, liquid diet for the first 24 to 48 hours, until bowel sounds return. Medical intervention for gas pain includes using rectal suppositories and enemas to stimulate passage of flatus and stool and encouraging the woman to lie on her left side. Lying on the left side allows the gas to rise from the descending colon to the sigmoid colon so that it can be expelled more readily.

The nurse can minimize discomfort and promote satisfaction as the mother assumes the activities of her new role. Instruction and assistance in assuming comfortable positions when holding or breastfeeding the infant will do much to increase the mother's sense of competence and comfort.

The cesarean birth mother usually does extremely well postoperatively. Most women are ambulating by the day after the surgery. Usually by the second postpartal day the incision can be covered with plastic wrap so the woman can shower, which seems to provide a mental as well as physical lift. Most women are discharged by the third day after birth.

## Promotion of Parent-Infant Interaction after Cesarean Birth

Many factors associated with cesarean birth may hinder successful and frequent maternal-infant interaction. These factors include the physical condition of the mother and newborn and maternal reactions to stress, anesthesia, and medications. The mother and her infant may be separated after birth because of birthing unit routines, prematurity, or neonatal complications. A healthy infant born by uncomplicated cesarean is no more fragile than one born vaginally. However, some agencies automatically place cesarean birth infants in the high-risk nursery for a time. This practice may cause anxiety for the parents and interfere with early parent-infant interaction.

Signs of depression, anger, or withdrawal may indicate a grief response to the loss of the fantasized birth experience. Fathers as well as mothers may experience feelings of "missing out," guilt, or even jealousy toward another couple who had a vaginal birth. The cesarean birth couple may need the opportunity to tell their story repeatedly to work through these feelings. The nurse can provide factual information about their situation and support the couple's effective coping behaviors.

By the second or third day the cesarean birth mother moves into the "taking-hold period" and is usually receptive to learning how to care for herself and her infant. Special emphasis should be given to home management. The nurse can encourage the mother to let others assume responsibility for housekeeping and cooking. Fatigue not only prolongs recovery but also interferes with breastfeeding and mother-infant interaction.

The presence of the father or significant other during the birth process positively influences the woman's perception of the birth event. His or her presence reduces the woman's fears, enhances her sense of control, and enables the couple to share feelings and respond to one another with touch and eye contact. Later, they have the opportunity to relive the experience and fill in any gaps or missing pieces. The presence of the father or significant other is especially valuable if the mother has had general anesthesia. He or she can take pictures, hold the baby, and foster the discovery process by directing the mother's attention to the details of the newborn.

The perception of and reactions to a cesarean birth experience depend on how the woman defines that experience. Her reality is what she perceives it to be. If the

# DRUG GUIDE

## POSTPARTUM EPIDURAL MORPHINE

### *Overview of Obstetric Action*

Epidural morphine is used to provide relief of pain associated with cesarean birth, extensive episiotomies (mediolaterals), or third- and fourth-degree lacerations. Pain relief results directly from its effect on the opiate receptors in the spinal cord (it depresses pain impulse transmission). Morphine binds opiate receptors, thereby altering both the perception of and emotional response to pain. Women experience little or no discomfort during recovery and for up to 24 hours afterward. There is no motor or sympathetic block or associated hypotension. Onset of analgesia is slower, but duration is longer.

### *Route, Dosage, Frequency*

Morphine (5–7.5 mg) is injected through a catheter into the epidural space, providing pain relief for about 24 hours (Karch, 2001).

### *Maternal Contraindications*

Allergy to morphine, narcotic addiction, chronic debilitating respiratory disease, infection at the injection site, or administration of parenteral corticosteriods in past 14 days.

### *Maternal Side Effects*

Late-onset respiratory depression (rare but may occur 8–12 hours after administration), nausea and vomiting (occurring between 4 and 7 hours after injection), itching (begins within 3 hours and lasts up to 10 hours), urinary retention, and, rarely, somnolence. Side effects can be managed with naloxone.

### *Neonatal Effects*

No adverse effects since med is injected after birth of baby.

### *Nursing Considerations*

- Obtain history: sensitivity (allergy) to morphine, presence of any contraindications.
- Assess orientation, reflexes, skin color, texture, breath sounds, presence of lesions or infection over area of lumbar spine, voiding pattern, urinary output within normal limits (Karch, 2001).
- Monitor and evaluate analgesic effect. Ask client about comfort level and notify anesthesiologist of inadequate pain relief.
- Check catheter for obvious knots, breaks, and leakage at insertion site and catheter hub.
- Assess for pruritus (scratching and rubbing, especially around face and neck).
- Administer comfort measures for narcotic-induced pruritus, such as lotion, back rubs, cool/warm packs, or diversional activities. If the itching can be tolerated, naloxone should be avoided, especially since it counteracts the pain relief.
- If allergic reaction (urticaria, edema, or respiratory difficulties) occurs, administer naloxone or diphenhydramine per physician order.
- Provide comfort measures for nausea and vomiting, such as frequent oral hygiene or gradual increase of activity; administer naloxone, trimethobenzamide (Tigan), or metoclopramide HCl per physician order.
- Assess postural blood pressure and heart rate before ambulation.
- Assist client with her first ambulation and then as needed.
- Assess respiratory function every hour for 24 hours, then q2–8 h as needed. Also assess level of consciousness and mucous membrane color. May need to monitor client via apnea monitor for 24 hours.
- Monitor urinary output and assess bladder for distention. Assist client to void.

woman's attitude is more positive than negative, successful resolution of subsequent stressful events is more likely. Because the definition of events is transitory, change and growth are possible. Often the mothering role is perceived as an extension of the childbearing role. Inability to fulfill expected childbearing behavior (vaginal birth) may lead to parental feelings of role failure and frustration. The nurse can help families alter their negative definitions of cesarean birth and bolster and encourage positive perceptions.

## Nursing Care Management for the Postpartal Adolescent

The adolescent mother has special postpartal needs, depending on her level of maturity, support system, and cultural background. The nurse needs to assess maternal-infant interaction, roles of support people, plans for discharge, knowledge of childrearing, and plans for follow-up care. It is imperative that a community health service contact the adolescent shortly after discharge.

Contraception counseling is an important part of teaching. The incidence of repeat pregnancies during adolescence is high. The younger the adolescent, the more likely she is to become pregnant again. (See Chapter 10 on adolescent pregnancy.)

The nurse has many opportunities for teaching the adolescent about her newborn in the postpartal unit. Because the nurse is a role model, the manner in which she handles the newborn greatly influences the young mother. The father should be included in as much of the teaching as possible.

A newborn examination done at the bedside gives the adolescent information about her baby's health and shows her possible positions for handling a baby. The nurse can also use this time to provide information about newborn and infant behavior. Parents who have some idea of what to expect from their infant are less frustrated with the newborn's behavior.

The adolescent mother appreciates positive feedback about her newborn and her developing maternal responses. Praise and encouragement will increase her confidence and self-esteem.

Group classes for adolescent mothers should include information about infant care skills, taking the baby's temperature, clearing the nose and mouth, growth and development, infant feeding, well-baby care, and danger signals in the ill newborn.

Ideally, teenage mothers should visit adolescent clinics, for assessment of the mother and newborn, for several years after birth. In this way, the adolescent's enrollment in classes on parenting, need for vocational guidance, and school attendance can be supported and followed closely. School systems offering classes for young mothers are an excellent way of helping adolescents finish school and learn how to parent at the same time.

## Nursing Care Management for the Woman Who Is Relinquishing Her Baby

Sometimes a woman is unable to keep her baby. The woman may be single, an adolescent, or economically restricted, or the pregnancy may be the result of incest or rape. She may feel that she is not emotionally ready for the responsibilities of parenthood. Her partner may strongly disapprove of the pregnancy. These and many other reasons may cause the woman to continue to reject the idea of her pregnancy. An emotional crisis arises as she attempts to resolve the problem. She may choose to have an abortion, to carry the fetus to term and keep the baby, or to have the baby and relinquish it for adoption.

The decision of a mother to relinquish her infant is an extremely difficult one. There are social pressures against giving up one's child. Some women may want to prove to themselves that they can manage on their own by keeping their baby.

The mother who chooses to let her child be adopted usually experiences intense ambivalence. These feelings may heighten just before birth and upon seeing her baby. After childbirth, the mother needs to complete a grieving process to work through her loss.

The mother who decides to relinquish the child has usually made considerable adjustments in her lifestyle to give birth to this child. She may not have told friends and relatives about the pregnancy and so may lack an extended support system. During the prenatal period, the nurse can help the woman by encouraging her and providing opportunities to express her grief, loneliness, guilt, and other feelings.

When the relinquishing mother is admitted to the birthing unit, the nurse should be informed about the mother's decision to relinquish the baby. The nurse needs to respect any special requests for the birth and encourage the woman to express her emotions. After the birth the mother should have access to the baby; she will decide whether she wants to see the newborn. Seeing the newborn often aids the grieving process. When the mother sees her baby, she may feel strong attachment and love. The nurse needs to assure the woman that these feelings do not mean that her decision to relinquish the child is a wrong one; relinquishment is often a painful act of love (Arms, 1990). Postpartal nursing care also includes arranging ongoing care for the relinquishing mother.

If a woman decides to keep an unwanted child, the nurse should be aware of the potential for parenting problems. Families with unwanted children are more crisis prone than others, although in many cases, parents grow to love their child after attachment occurs. The nurse should be ready to initiate crisis strategies or make appropriate referrals as the need arises.

## Discharge Information

Ideally, preparation for discharge begins the moment a woman enters the birthing unit to give birth. Nursing efforts should be directed toward assessing the parents' knowledge, expectations, and beliefs and then providing anticipatory guidance and teaching accordingly. Since teaching is one of the primary responsibilities of the postpartum nurse, many agencies have elaborate teaching programs and videos. Before the actual discharge the nurse should spend time with the parents to determine if they have any last-minute questions. In general, discharge teaching includes at least the following information:

1. The signs of possible complications (see Key Facts to Remember: Signs of Postpartal Complications) and encouragement for the woman to contact her caregiver if she develops any of them.
2. Review of literature the woman has received that explains recommended postpartum exercises, the need for adequate rest, the need to avoid overexertion initially, and the recommendation to abstain from sexual intercourse until lochia has ceased. The woman may take either a tub bath or shower and may continue sitz baths at home. If the family desires information about birth control methods, the nurse can provide such information at this time.
3. The phone number of the mother-baby unit and encouragement to call if she has any questions or concerns.
4. Information on local agencies and/or support groups, such as La Leche League and Mothers of Twins, that might be of particular assistance to the new mother.
5. Information geared to the specific nutritional needs of breastfeeding or bottle-feeding mothers. If the mother has been receiving vitamins and/or iron supplements, the nurse encourages her to continue until the first postpartal examination.

**KEY FACTS TO REMEMBER**

*Signs of Postpartal Complications*

After discharge, a woman should contact her physician or certified nurse-midwife if any of the following develop:

- Sudden, persistent or spiking fever
- Change in the character of the lochia—foul smell, return to bright-red bleeding, excessive amount, passage of large clots
- Evidence of mastitis, such as breast tenderness, reddened areas, malaise
- Evidence of thrombophlebitis, such as calf pain, tenderness, redness
- Evidence of urinary tract infection, such as urgency, frequency, burning on urination
- Continued severe or incapacitating postpartal depression

6. When to schedule the first appointment for her postpartal examination and for her newborn's first well-baby examination.
7. The procedure for obtaining copies of her infant's birth certificate.
8. How to provide basic care for the infant; when to anticipate that the cord will fall off; when the infant can have a tub bath; when the infant will need her or his first immunizations; and so on. Parents should also be comfortable feeding and handling the baby, and should be aware of basic safety considerations, including the need to use a car seat whenever the infant is in a car.
9. The signs and symptoms that indicate possible problems in the infant and who the parents should contact about them.
10. Plans for home care visits so that the parents know when to expect the visit and what it entails (see Chapter 29).

The nurse can also use this final opportunity to reassure the couple of their ability to be successful parents. The nurse can stress the infant's need to feel loved and secure and urge parents to talk to each other and work together to solve any problems that arise.

The ideal teaching situation is a family approach involving the mother, the father, the infant, and possibly other siblings. This approach permits a total evaluation and provides opportunities for all family members to ask questions and express concerns. It also promotes diagnosis and treatment of disturbed family patterns to prevent future problems of neglect or abuse. A sample discharge teaching checklist (Table 28–4) is included on page 766.

## Evaluation

Anticipated outcomes of comprehensive nursing care of the postpartal family include the following:

- The mother is reasonably comfortable and has learned pain relief measures.
- The mother is rested and understands how to add more activity over the next few days and weeks.
- The mother's physiologic and psychologic well-being have been supported.
- The mother verbalizes her understanding of self-care measures.
- The new parents demonstrate how to care for their baby.
- The new parents have had opportunities to form attachment with their baby.
- The cesarean birth mother has been supported and has received safe care.

## TABLE 28–4 Areas to Include in Postpartal Teaching

| KNOWLEDGE AND SKILLS TO BE TAUGHT | TEACHING METHOD | | | |
|---|---|---|---|---|
| | *Video* | *Verbal Only* | *Verbally Reinforced* | *Demonstration* |
| **CARE OF THE MOTHER** | | | | |
| Breast care | | | | |
| Breastfeeding or lactation suppression | | | | |
| Possible problems and care | | | | |
| Involutional changes | | | | |
| Position of fundus | | | | |
| Aftercontractions | | | | |
| Changes in lochia | | | | |
| Signs of possible problems | | | | |
| Bladder function | | | | |
| Fluid needs | | | | |
| Signs of possible problems | | | | |
| Bowel function | | | | |
| Normal patterns | | | | |
| Dietary assistance | | | | |
| Perineal care | | | | |
| Expected healing changes in episiotomy | | | | |
| Comfort measures (rinsing with warm water, use of analgesic/anesthetic spray, sitz bath), home care | | | | |
| Signs of possible problems | | | | |
| Rest and activity | | | | |
| Scheduling rest periods, handling fatigue | | | | |
| Ambulation | | | | |
| Watching for circulatory problems in legs | | | | |
| Emotional changes | | | | |
| Changes in mood, crying, depression | | | | |
| **CARE OF THE FATHER OR PARTNER** | | | | |
| Emotional changes | | | | |
| Emotional changes and challenges that may occur | | | | |
| Encouragement to seek support as needed | | | | |
| Physiologic and psychologic changes that may occur in the mother and newborn | | | | |
| Infant care concerns | | | | |
| Possible supportive measures for the new family | | | | |
| **CARE OF THE BABY** | | | | |
| Observing the baby | | | | |
| General appearance | | | | |
| Senses | | | | |
| Visual | | | | |
| Hearing | | | | |
| Touch | | | | |
| Smell | | | | |
| Taste | | | | |
| Vital signs | | | | |
| Normal parameters | | | | |
| How to take a temperature | | | | |
| Skin | | | | |
| Coloring | | | | |
| Normal rashes | | | | |
| Diaper care | | | | |
| Cord care | | | | |
| Stool cycle | | | | |
| Normal characteristics | | | | |
| Signs of diarrhea and treatment | | | | |

## TABLE 28–4 Areas to Include in Postpartal Teaching *continued*

| KNOWLEDGE AND SKILLS TO BE TAUGHT | TEACHING METHOD | | | |
|---|---|---|---|---|
| | *Video* | *Verbal Only* | *Verbally Reinforced* | *Demonstration* |
| **CARE OF THE BABY** *continued* | | | | |
| Observing the baby *continued* | | | | |
|   Signs of constipation and treatment | | | | |
| Emotional and comforting needs | | | | |
| Protective reflexes | | | | |
|   Blinking | | | | |
|   Sneezing | | | | |
|   Swallowing | | | | |
| Normal reflexes | | | | |
|   Moro | | | | |
|   Fencing | | | | |
|   Head lag | | | | |
|   Stepping | | | | |
| Feeding the baby | | | | |
|   Breastfeeding | | | | |
|     Positioning, initiating, and ending feeding | | | | |
|     Infant cues for feeding (on demand) | | | | |
|     Identifying problem areas and possible solutions | | | | |
|     Breast care | | | | |
|   Bottle-feeding | | | | |
|     Positioning | | | | |
|     Preparation of bottles and formula | | | | |
|   Burping or bubbling the baby | | | | |
|   Holding, wrapping, and diapering the baby | | | | |
|     Various holds (cradle, football) | | | | |
|     Securing baby in blanket to provide warmth | | | | |
|     Diapering | | | | |
|       Comparison of reusable (cloth) and single use (paper) | | | | |
|       Methods of diapering and care of soiled diapers | | | | |
|     Perineal skin care | | | | |
|   Positioning the baby for sleep | | | | |
| Bathing the baby | | | | |
|   Supplies | | | | |
|   Method | | | | |
| Safety | | | | |
|   Use of bulb syringe and care if choking | | | | |
|   Positioning | | | | |
|   Car seat | | | | |
| Health promotion | | | | |
|   When to call health care provider | | | | |
|     Temperature | | | | |
|     Diarrhea | | | | |
|     Eating problems | | | | |
|     Malaise | | | | |
|   Protecting baby from infections | | | | |
|   Immunization schedule | | | | |
| **ASPECTS OF PARENTING** | | | | |
|   Interaction with newborn | | | | |
|     Newborn cues and capacity for interaction | | | | |
|     Parenting needs | | | | |
|     Acquaintance with individual characteristics of their newborn and possible techniques to use | | | | |
|     Resources available | | | | |

# Chapter Review

## CHAPTER HIGHLIGHTS

- Nursing diagnoses can be used effectively in caring for women postpartally.
- Postpartum discomfort may be due to a variety of factors, including engorged breasts, an edematous perineum, an episiotomy or extension, engorged hemorrhoids, or hematoma formation. Various self-care approaches are helpful in promoting comfort.
- Lactation suppression may be accomplished by mechanical techniques.
- The new mother requires opportunities to discuss her childbirth experience with an empathetic listener.
- In the first day or two after birth maternal behaviors are dependent and comfort oriented. Then the woman becomes more independent and ready to assume responsibility.
- Mother-baby care provides the childbearing family with opportunities to interact with their new member during the first hours and days of life. It enables the family to develop some confidence and skill in a safe environment.
- Sexual intercourse may resume once the episiotomy has healed and lochia has ceased.
- After a cesarean birth, the woman has the nursing care needs of an abdominal surgical client in addition to her needs as a postpartum client. She may also require assistance in working through her feelings if the cesarean birth was unexpected.
- Postpartally the nurse evaluates the adolescent mother in terms of her level of maturity, available support systems, cultural background, and existing knowledge and then plans care accordingly.
- The mother who decides to relinquish her baby needs emotional support. She should be able to decide whether to see and hold her baby, and any special requests regarding the birth should be honored.
- Prior to discharge the couple should be given any information necessary for the woman to provide appropriate self-care. Parents should have a beginning skill in caring for their newborn and should be familiar with warning signs of possible complications for mother or baby. Printed information is valuable in helping couples deal with questions that may arise at home.
- Because of the trend toward early discharge, follow-up care is more important than ever. Many approaches are used, especially home visits and telephone follow-up.

## CHAPTER REFERENCES


Arms, S. (1990). *Adoption: A handbook of hope.* Berkeley, CA: Celestial Arts.

Banks-Wallace, J. (1999). Storytelling as a tool for providing holistic care to women. *American Journal of Maternal-Child Nursing, 24,* 20–24.

Barrett, G., Pendry, E., Peacock, J., Victor, C., Thakar, R., & Manyonda, I. (2000). Women's sexual health after childbirth. *British Journal of Obstetrics and Gynecology, 107* (20), 186–195.

Cunningham, F. G., MacDonald, P. C., Gant, N. F., Leveno, K. J., Gilstrap, L. C., III, Hankins, G. D. V., & Clark, S. L. (Eds.). (1997). *Williams obstetrics* (20th ed.). Stamford, CT: Appleton & Lange.

Karch, A. M. (2001). *Lippincott's nursing drug guide.* Philadelphia, PA: Lippincott.

Koniak-Griffin, D., Mathenge, C., Anderson, N. L., & Verzemnieks, I. (1999). An early intervention program for adolescent mothers: A nursing demonstration project. *Journal of Obstetric, Gynecologic, and Neonatal Nursing, 28,* 51–59.

Lamp, J. M., & Howard, P. A. (1999). Guiding parents' use of the Internet for newborn education. *American Journal of Maternal-Child Nursing, 24,* 33–36.

Parks, P. L., Lenz, E. R., Milligan, R. A., & Han, H. R. (1999). What happens when fatigue lingers for 18 months after delivery? *Journal of Obstetric, Gynecologic, and Neonatal Nursing, 28,* 87–93.

*PDR nurse's handbook* (2001). Montvale, NJ: Demar Publishers.

Sampselle, C. M., Seng, J., Yeo, S., Killian, C., & Oakley, D. (1999). Physical activity and postpartum wellbeing. *Journal of Obstetric, Gynecologic, and Neonatal Nursing, 28,* 41–49.

Schneiderman, J. U. (1996). Postpartum nursing for Korean mothers. *American Journal of Maternal-Child Nursing, 21*(3), 155–158.

Varney, H. (1997). *Varney's Midwifery,* (3rd ed.). Sudbury, MA: Jones and Bartlett.

## CONTEMPORARY MATERNAL-NEWBORN NURSING ON-LINE

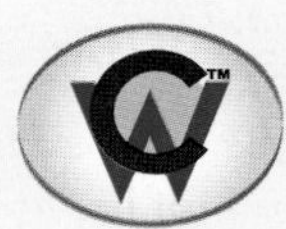

Additional interactive resources, including animations and video, for this chapter can be found on the Companion Website at http://www.prenhall.com/ladewig. Click on Chapter 28 and "Begin" to select the activities for this chapter.

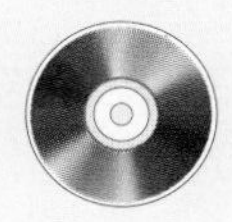

For NCLEX review questions and an audio glossary, access the accompanying CD-ROM in this book.

# Chapter 29

# Home Care of the Postpartal Family

*When I first became a nurse I thought I would always practice maternity nursing in a hospital. I loved the pace, the excitement! I began making home visits at the request of my supervisor when our unit partnered with the local midwives and obstetricians to provide postpartum follow-up services. Now I can't imagine doing anything else. Each day is different as I am challenged to improvise and help families deal with issues that arise. I value the independence of this role and the feeling that I am making a difference.*

—A Home Care Nurse Working with Postpartum Families

## KEY TERMS



## OBJECTIVES

- **Discuss the components of postpartal home care.**
- **Identify the main purposes of home visits during the postpartum period.**
- **Summarize actions a nurse should take to ensure personal safety during a home visit.**
- **Delineate aspects of fostering a caring relationship in the home.**
- **Describe assessment and care of the newborn and reinforcement of parent teaching in the home.**
- **Discuss maternal and family assessment and anticipated progress after birth.**

Home care has become essential because the length of stay in the birth setting has steadily decreased over the past few years. The length of time in the hospital or birthing center after birth has been referred to as *short stay;* however, there is no agreement about how long this period should be. The short stay has been fueled by efforts to contain health care costs rather than by well-developed research studies that validate the efficacy and safety of this practice (Bravemen, Egerter, Pearl, et al., 1995) or by cooperative decision making among health care professionals and families (American Academy of Pediatrics [AAP], Committee on Fetus and Newborn, 1995).

As the length of stay has declined, a number of new issues have been identified. New mothers who are discharged in 48 hours or less following childbirth must adjust to motherhood without the benefit of the assessment and teaching that are possible with a longer stay (Fishbein & Burggraf, 1998). The shortened stay (less than 48 hours) raises issues for the newborn because many conditions, such as jaundice, ductal-dependent cardiac lesions, and gastrointestinal obstructions, may take longer than 2 days to develop, and identification of these problems depends on a skilled, experienced professional (AAP, Committee on Fetus and Newborn, 1995). As a result, in one study, 1% to 4% of term infants with a less than 48-hour stay were readmitted, most often for jaundice (Catz, Hanson, Simpson, et al., 1995). However, research also suggests that there is no increase in the incidence of neonatal readmission when early discharge is combined with a structured program of postpartum home visits (Bragg, Rosenn, Khoury, et al., 1997).

Short stays also have implications for the mother. The stability of her health, availability of support systems, and opportunities to become comfortable with her new baby may be compromised, and less than 48 hours is too little time to establish breastfeeding (AAP, Committee on Fetus and Newborn, 1995). Furthermore, in the first 24 hours after childbirth, the mother is in the taking-in phase, which is not conducive to learning (Soskolne, Schumacher, Fyock, et al., 1996). The AAP Committee on Fetus and Newborn (1995) has developed minimum criteria to guide the timing of early discharge in order to enhance excellence in maternal-newborn care (Table 29–1).

In 1998 the U.S. federal government passed legislation that guaranteed a minimum stay of up to 48 hours following vaginal birth and up to 96 hours following cesarean birth at the discretion of the mother and her care provider. It does not require follow-up visits for women who leave earlier than the mandated time. Currently more than half the states have passed legislation strengthening the federal legislation by mandating coverage for home care follow-up (Carpenter, 1998).

## TABLE 29–1 Minimal Criteria for Discharge of Newborns

1. Uncomplicated prenatal, intrapartal, and postpartal course and vaginal birth.
2. A single baby who is term, 38–42 weeks, and average weight for gestational age (AGA).
3. The newborn's vital signs are within normal limits and have been stable for the 12 hours preceding discharge (respirations less than <60/min; apical pulse 100–160 beats per minute; axillary temperature of 36.1–37°C in an open crib with appropriate clothing).
4. The newborn has passed at least one stool and has urinated.
5. At least two feedings have been successfully completed, and the baby's ability to coordinate sucking, swallowing, and breathing has been observed and documented.
6. No physical abnormalities have been found that require continued hospitalization.
7. If a circumcision has been done, no excessive bleeding has been evident for at least 2 hours before discharge.
8. There has been no significant jaundice in the first 24 hours of life.
9. The mother has received education about breast-or bottle-feeding; the newborn's expected stool and urinary patterns; care of circumcision; cord, skin, and genital care; ways to recognize signs of illness or distress and common infant problems; signs of jaundice and who to contact if develops; infant safety, including positioning of baby after feeding and for sleep; and use of a car seat.
10. Review of pertinent laboratory data including maternal syphilis and hepatitis B surface antigen status; cord or infant blood type.
11. Completion of screening tests (eg; PKU).
12. First hepatitis B vaccine has been administered or appointment for administration has been scheduled within the first week.
13. Method and schedule for continuing care has been ascertained and planned, and the family is aware of the plan.
14. Family assessment has been completed for social and environmental risk factors such as history of previous child abuse or neglect; spousal or partner abuse either preceding or beginning during the pregnancy; parental substance abuse; lack of support within the family or community; lack of funds, shelter, or food; mental illness of one of the parents that impairs ability to care for self and newborn; single first-time mother without social support.

*Source:* Committee on Fetus and Newborn. (1995). Hospital stay for healthy term newborns. *Pediatrics, 96*(4), 788.

As the length of stay decreases, nursing professionals in the birthing center are pressed to complete essential assessments, ensure holistic care (physiologic, psychologic, and spiritual), and provide opportunities for education about maternal self-care and newborn care. The new family, eager to learn about important aspects of care, also needs to rest and spend time with the newborn. The needs of the family and the goals of the health care provider can be addressed through the provision of postpartal home care.

Home care for the postpartal family is focused more on assessment, teaching, and counseling than on physical care. Postpartal home care provides opportunities for enhancing information and self- and infant care techniques initially presented in the birth setting. In addition, the home setting provides an opportunity for the nurse and family to interact in a more relaxed environment in which the family has control of the setting. In some instances, the challenges of assessing and enhancing self-care and infant care may be unique in the home, and the nurse will have many opportunities to exercise critical thinking to develop creative options with the family.

## Considerations for the Home Visit

In planning a home visit the nurse should clearly understand the purpose of the visit and the content to be addressed. Other important considerations include ways of creating and fostering relationships with families, techniques for preplanning and executing the visit while maintaining safety, documentation of the visit, and telephone follow-up.

The postpartal home visit differs from community health visits in that only one or two home visits are typically planned, and long-term follow-up by the postpartal nurse is not anticipated. Although the postpartal home visit is comprehensive, it focuses specifically on the postpartal family's needs and care.

The established guidelines for discharge of the mother and baby (see Table 29–1) mean the nurse can expect certain levels of health and wellness. However, because the status of the mother and newborn can change, the nurse should stay alert for deviations from the norm.

### Purpose of the Home Visit

The postpartal home visit usually occurs within 24 to 48 hours of discharge and is conducted by a registered nurse who is experienced in postpartal maternal and newborn care. Prior to the home visit, the nurse prepares by identifying the purpose of the home visit and gathering anticipated materials and equipment. A personal contact while the woman is still in the birth setting or a previsit telephone call is used to arrange the appointment with the woman and her family. During the previsit contact, it is important for the nurse to identify clearly the purpose and goals of the visit and to begin establishing rapport.

The postpartal home visit has many purposes. It provides an opportunity to assess the status of the mother and infant after birth for signs of any complications, to complete follow-up blood work if needed, to ascertain current informational needs, and to offer additional information as needed. The home visit also provides time to cover additional information in a more relaxed setting. In addition, the nurse assesses adaptation of the family to the new baby and adjustment of any siblings, answers questions about breastfeeding, provides support and encouragement, and addresses the need for referrals (Lowdermilk, 1995).

### Fostering a Caring Relationship with the Family

Although the nurse in the birthing center strives to enhance family autonomy and control, the inherent atmosphere of the institutional environment may cause the new mother and family to feel unempowered. It is important for the professional nurse to recognize that the parameters of the home visit are different in many ways from those of the hospital or birthing center environment. In the home, the family members have control of their environment and the nurse is an invited visitor. The nurse can rely on the same characteristics of a caring relationship that have been integral to hospital-based practice—regard for clients, genuineness, empathy, and establishment of trust and rapport—but the relationship may take on new elements as the nurse moves into the home setting for the first time (see Key Facts to Remember: Fostering a Caring Relationship).

### Maintaining Safety

In the past, nurses were perceived as a mainstay of communities and could move in most settings without fear or concern for safety. However, today some communities are not safe for visiting nurses. It is important for the nurse to follow some basic safety rules when conducting a home visit. Obviously, the nurse needs to know the specific address and ask for directions during the previsit contact. If the area is not familiar, the nurse should trace out the route on a map before leaving for the visit and take the map along. It is also wise for the nurse to wear a name tag and sensible shoes. The nurse should avoid wearing expensive jewelry or pins of a religious or political nature that might be seen as offensive. A cellular phone or pager provides a means of contact and is advisable for any community visitor, as is a working flashlight, especially for night visits. In addition, the nurse should carry sufficient change to call from a pay phone if necessary. The nurse can also notify an instructor or supervisor when leaving for a visit and check in as soon as the visit is completed.

Many agencies that provide home care services have established violence prevention programs to help ensure safety. Nurses in the community need to be aware of their environment and alert to environmental cues, whether

## KEY FACTS TO REMEMBER

### *Fostering a Caring Relationship*

Evidence of genuineness and empathy, coupled with the establishment of trust and rapport, form the foundation for a caring relationship.

| Demonstrated Goal | Approaches to Achieve Goal |
|---|---|
| Regard | Introduce yourself to the family. Call the family members by their surnames until you have been invited to use the given or a less formal name.<br>Ask to be introduced to other members of the family who are present. Allow the mother or spokesperson to assume this role.<br>Use active listening. Maintain objectiveness.<br>Ask permission before sitting. |
| Genuineness | Mean what you say. Make sure that your verbal and nonverbal messages are congruent.<br>Be nonjudgmental. Do not make assumptions about individuals or settings.<br>Always strive to demonstrate caring behaviors.<br>Be prepared for the visit, honestly answer questions and provide information, and be truthful. If you do not know the answer to a question, tell the client you will find the information and report back. |
| Empathy | Listen to the mother and family where "they are" without judgment.<br>Be attentive to what the birthing experience is for them so that you will understand from their perspective.<br>Remember that empathy denotes understanding, not sympathy. |
| Trust and rapport | Do what you say you will do.<br>Be prepared for the visit and be on time.<br>Follow-up on any areas that are needed. |

overt or subtle. In addition, the following recommendations are important: (Durkin & Wilson, 1999):

- Invest time in personal safety by driving around a neighborhood before making an initial visit to identify potential cues to violence. Avoid walking through a crowd or staying in an elevator with others if it makes you uneasy.
- Lock personal belongings in the trunk of the car, out of sight.
- Pay attention to the body language of anyone present during the visit, not just the client.
- Be alert for signs that a person is becoming enraged (reddened neck and/or face, clenched fists, pacing).
- Be aware of personal body language and how it might be interpreted. (For example, avoid crossing arms or shoving hands in pockets, which may suggest hostility; remain calm and convey a sense of respect at all times.)
- Leave the home immediately if a gun is visible and the client or family member refuses requests to put it away.
- If a situation arises that feels unsafe, terminate the visit.

If the visit is in an area that seems very unsafe, it may be wise for two nurses to go together. Nurses should avoid entering areas where violence is in progress. In such cases, they should return to the car and contact the appropriate facility, such as 911.

Most people are more comfortable in familiar settings and have some hesitation in entering other residential areas. It is always important to be aware of one's surroundings and the people who are nearby. First home visits may feel uncomfortable because they are unfamiliar, but with experience comfort increases (Figure 29–1♦).

## Carrying Out the Home Visit

When the door is answered, the nurse should introduce herself or himself and confirm that the location is correct. If a place to sit is not indicated, the nurse may inquire "Where is the best place to sit so that we can talk for a while?" In some homes, the mother or family may offer refreshments, and this may be an important aspect of welcoming a visitor. In this case, it is beneficial to the relationship to accept the refreshment graciously.

The nurse completes planned assessments, provides direct care as necessary, carries out family and client teaching, makes necessary referrals to community agencies, and schedules additional home visits or telephone contact. The nurse should report significant medical concerns to the certified nurse-midwife or physician immediately and

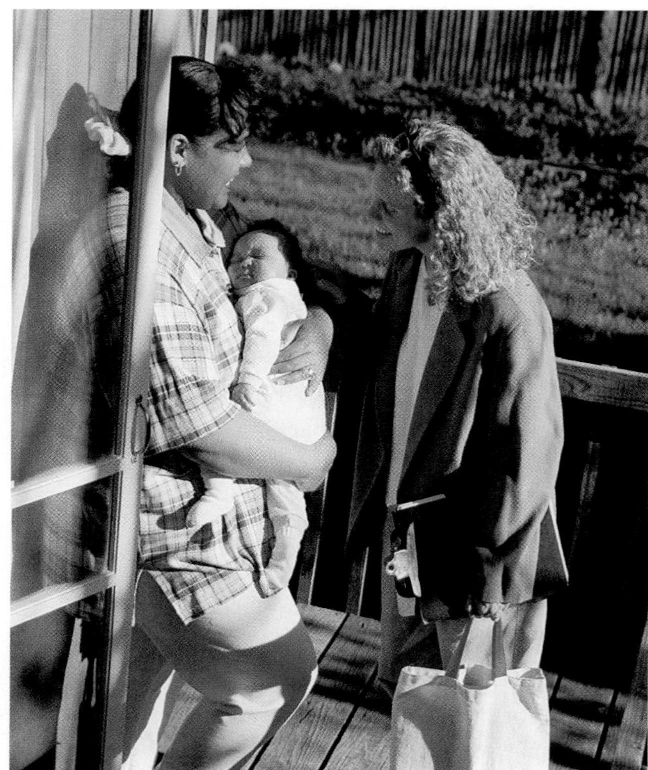

FIGURE 29–1 ♦ Nurse arriving for a home visit.

plan for appropriate follow-up (Carpenter, 1998). The aspects assessed and addressed during the home visit are discussed in the following sections.

# Home Care: The Newborn

## Positioning and Handling

The nurse demonstrates methods of positioning and handling the newborn as needed. As the family members provide care, the nurse can instill confidence by giving them positive feedback. If a family member encounters problems, the nurse can suggest alternatives and serve as a role model.

After the newborn is out of the crib, one of the following holds can be used (Figure 29–2♦). The *cradle hold* is frequently used during feeding. It provides a sense of warmth and closeness, permits eye contact, frees one of the adult's hands, and provides security because the cradling protects the newborn's body. Extra security is provided by gripping the baby's thigh with the hand while the arm supports the newborn's body. The *upright position* provides security and a sense of closeness and is ideal for burping. One hand should support the neck and shoulders, while the other hand holds the buttocks or is placed between the newborn's legs. The newborn may also be held upright in a cloth sling carrier that gently holds the baby against the parent's chest and frees the hands for other tasks. The *football hold* frees one of the caregiver's hands and permits eye contact. This hold is ideal for shampooing, carrying, or breastfeeding. It frees the caregiver to talk on the telephone, answer the door, or do the myriad tasks that await attention at this busy time.

The newborn is most frequently positioned on his or her side, with a rolled blanket or diaper behind the back for support and to prevent rolling (Figure 29–3♦). The side-lying position aids drainage of mucus and allows air to circulate around the cord. It is also more comfortable for the newly circumcised male. After feeding, the newborn is placed on the right side to aid digestion and to prevent aspiration of regurgitated feedings; this position makes it easier to expel air bubbles from the stomach.

A firm, flat mattress without pillows should be provided for the newborn. Research has shown an increased incidence of sudden infant death syndrome (SIDS) in infants who sleep on their stomachs. There is no evidence that sleeping on the back or side is harmful to healthy infants. Certain infants may need to be placed on their stomachs, including premature infants with respiratory distress (severe breathing problems), infants with symptoms of gastroesophageal reflux (severe spitting up), and infants with certain upper airway abnormalities. There may be other valid reasons for infants to be placed on their stomachs for sleep. Parents should discuss their individual circumstances with their care provider.

The infant's position should be changed periodically during the early months of life, because skull bones are soft, and permanently flattened areas may develop if the newborn consistently lies in one position. A newborn in the first days of life should not be left in a supine position when unattended, because of the danger of aspiration.

## Newborn Feeding

Newborn feeding is discussed in detail in Chapter 24. Problems a breastfeeding mother may face at home are discussed later in this chapter. Regardless of feeding method, it is important for the nurse to assess the newborn's fluid and nutritional intake. As part of the physical assessment the newborn's nude weight is determined. If the weight loss since birth is 10% or more, the nurse assesses the baby for signs of dehydration such as loose skin with decreased skin turgor, dry mucous membranes, sunken anterior fontanel, and decreased frequency and amount of voiding and stooling. Newborns who are postterm, small for gestational age, and one of a multiple gestation are at high risk for breastfeeding difficulty (Locklin & Jansson, 1999).

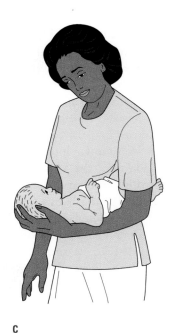

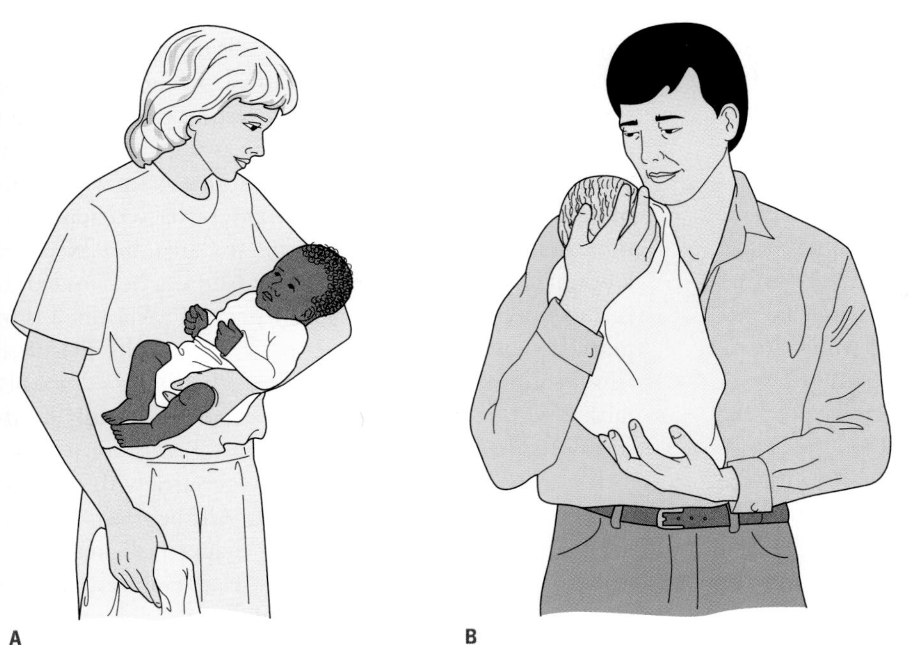


FIGURE 29–2 ♦ Various positions for holding an infant. **A,** Cradle hold. **B,** Upright position. **C,** Football hold.

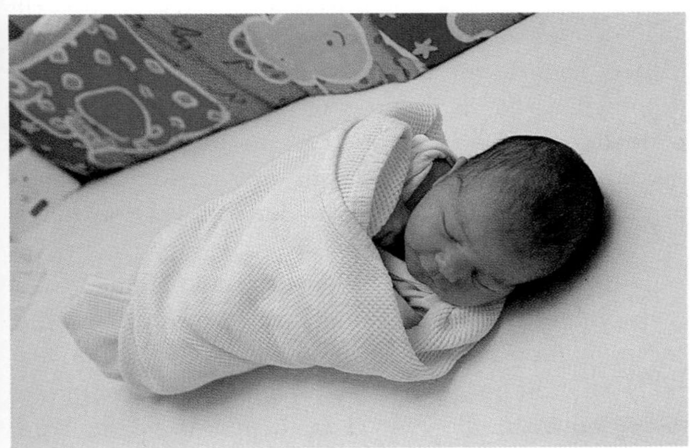

FIGURE 29–3 ♦ The most common sleeping position of the newborn is on the side. A rolled blanket may be placed behind the back to provide additional support.

## BATHING

An actual bath demonstration is the best way for the nurse to provide information to parents. Because excess bathing and the use of soap remove natural skin oils and dry out the newborn's sensitive skin, bathing should be done every other day or twice a week. Sponge baths are recommended for the first 2 weeks or until the umbilical cord completely falls off and the umbilicus has healed. Some agencies use a tub bath for the bath demonstration.

Supplies can be kept in a plastic bag or some type of container to eliminate the necessity of hunting for them each time. At home, the family may want to use a small plastic tub, a clean kitchen or bathroom sink, or a large bowl as the baby's tub. Expensive baby tubs are not necessary, but some prefer to purchase them.

Before starting, if no one else is at home, the parent may want to take the phone off the hook and put a sign on the door to prevent being disturbed. Having someone home during the first few baths will be helpful, because that person can get forgotten items, attend to interruptions, and provide moral support. The room should be warm and free of drafts.

### SPONGE BATHS

After the supplies are gathered, the tub (or any of the containers mentioned) is filled with water that is warm to the touch. Even though the newborn will not be placed in the tub, the bath giver carefully tests the water temperature with an elbow or forearm. Families may also choose to purchase a thermometer to help them determine when the bath water is at approximately 37.8°C (100°F) and safe to use. An unperfumed, mild soap such as Castile or Neutrogena should be used and kept on a soap dish or paper towel, not added to the water. The newborn should be wrapped in a blanket, with a T-shirt and diaper on, to keep her or him warm and secure.

To start the bath, the adult wraps a washcloth once around the index finger and wets it with water. Soap is not used on the face. Each eye is gently wiped from inner to outer corner. This direction prevents the potential for clogging the tear duct at the inner corner, where the eye naturally drains. A different portion of the washcloth is used for each eye to prevent cross contamination. Cotton balls can also be used for this purpose, a new one for each eye. Some swelling and drainage may be present the first few days after birth because of eye prophylaxis.

The bath giver washes the ears next by wrapping the washcloth once around an index finger and gently cleaning the external ear and behind the ear. Cotton swabs are never used in the ear canal because it is possible to put the swab too far into the ear and damage the ear drum. In addition, the swab may back any discharge farther down into the ear canal. The caregiver then wipes the remainder of the baby's face. Many babies start to cry at this point. The face should be washed every day and the mouth and chin wiped off after each feeding.

The neck is washed carefully but thoroughly with the washcloth. Soap may now be used. Formula or breast milk and lint collect in the skin folds of the neck, so it may be helpful to sit the newborn up, supporting the neck and shoulders with one hand while washing the neck with the other hand.

Next the bath giver unwraps the blanket, removes the T-shirt, and wets the chest, back, and arms with the washcloth. The bath giver may then lather the hands with soap and wash the baby's chest, back, and arms. Wetting the cord is avoided, if possible, because it delays drying. Soap is rinsed off with the wet washcloth, and the upper part of the body is dried with a towel or blanket. The newborn's upper body is then wrapped with a clean, dry blanket to prevent a chill.

The bath giver then unwraps the newborn's legs, wets them with the washcloth, and lathers, rinses, and dries them well. If the newborn has dry skin, a small amount of unscented lotion or ointment (petroleum jelly or A + D ointment) may be used. Ointments are thought to be better than lotions for dry, cracked feet and hands. Baby oil is not recommended, because it clogs skin pores. Powders are not currently recommended. Families should be warned that baby powder can cause serious respiratory problems if inhaled. If parents want to use powder, they should be advised to use one that is talc free. The powder should be shaken into the hand and then placed on the newborn rather than shaken directly onto the baby.

The genital area is cleansed with soap and water daily and with water after each wet or dirty diaper. Females are washed from the front of the genital area toward the rectum to prevent fecal contamination of the urethra and thus the bladder. Newborn females often have a thick, white mucus discharge or a slight bloody discharge from the vaginal area. This discharge is normal for the first 1 to 2 weeks after birth and should be wiped off with a damp cloth during diaper changes.

Parents of uncircumcised males should cleanse the penis daily. Even minimal retraction of the foreskin is not advised (see in-depth discussion of care of uncircumcised male babies in Chapter 23). Males who have been circumcised also need daily gentle cleansing. A very wet washcloth is rubbed over a bar of soap. The washcloth is squeezed above the baby's penis, letting the soapy water run over the circumcision site. The area is rinsed off with plain warm water and lightly patted dry. A small amount of petroleum jelly, A + D ointment, or bactericidal ointment may be put on the circumcised area, but excessive amounts may block the meatus and should be avoided. It is important to avoid using ointments if a Plastibell is in place because use of ointments may cause the Plastibell ring to slip off the penis too early. The Plastibell usually falls off within 5 to 8 days. If it does not, the family needs to call the health care provider.

It is important to cleanse the diaper area with each diaper change to prevent diaper rash. Although this cleansing is done on a routine basis, a diaper rash may occasionally occur. Baby powder or cornstarch is not recommended for diaper rash. Baby powder may cake with urine and irritate the perineal area; cornstarch may promote fungal infection. Ointments that provide a barrier, such as zinc oxide, A + D ointment, and petroleum jelly, are more effective for diaper rash. If the ointment does not help the rash, families using single-use (disposable) diapers should try another brand. If they use cloth diapers, a different detergent or fabric softener, more thorough rinsing, and hanging them in the sun to dry may alleviate the problem. If the rash persists, parents should discuss the problem with their nurse practitioner or physician, because it may be due to a yeast or fungal infection.

The umbilical cord should be kept clean and dry. The close proximity of the umbilical vessels makes the cord a common entry area for infection. The cord stump generally falls off in 7 to 14 days. The diaper should be folded down to allow air to circulate around the cord. The parents should consult their health care provider if redness, bright-red bleeding, or puslike drainage with foul odor appears around the umbilicus or if the area remains unhealed 2 to 3 days after the cord stump has sloughed off.

The last step in bathing is washing the hair (a step some suggest doing first). The newborn is swaddled in a dry blanket, leaving only the head exposed, and held in the football hold with the head tilted slightly downward to prevent water from running in the eyes. Water should be brought to the head by a cupped hand. The hair is moistened and lathered with a small amount of mild shampoo. A very soft brush may be used to massage the shampoo over the entire head, including the soft spots. The hair is then rinsed and toweled dry. Oils or lotions are not used on the newborn's head unless there is evidence of cradle cap. Moistening the scaly area with lotion or mineral oil half an hour or more before shampooing

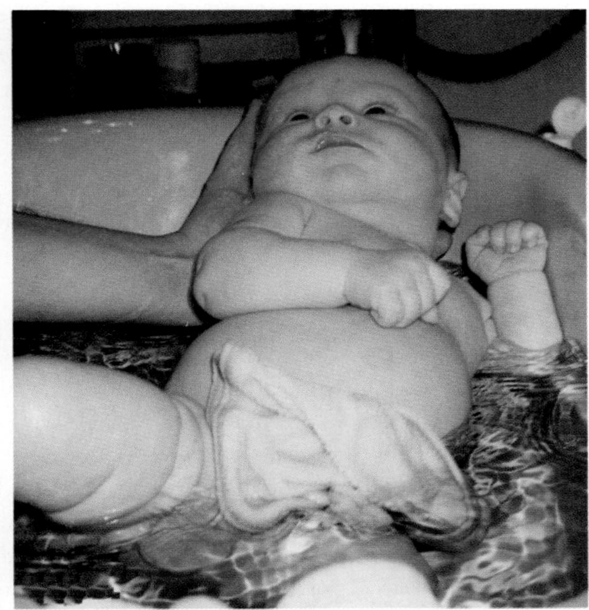

**FIGURE 29–4** ♦ When bathing the newborn, it is important to support the head. Wet babies are very slippery.

softens the crusts or scales and makes it easier to remove them with a soft brush during the shampoo.

### Tub Baths

The baby may be put in a small tub after the cord has fallen off and the circumcision site is healed (approximately 2 weeks) (Figure 29–4♦). Newborns usually enjoy a tub bath more than a sponge bath, although some cry during either type.

Only 3 or 4 in. of water is needed in the tub. To prevent slipping, a washcloth is placed in the bottom of the tub or sink. Some parents choose to bring the newborn into the tub with them.

The baby's face is washed in the same manner as for a sponge bath. The parent then places the newborn in the tub using the cradle hold and grasping the distal thigh. The neck is supported by the parent's elbow in the cradle position. An alternative hold is to support the newborn's head and neck with the forearm while grasping the distal shoulder and arm.

Because wet newborns are slippery, some parents pull a cotton sock (with holes cut out for the fingers) over the supporting arm to provide a "nonskid" surface. The newborn's body may be washed with a soapy washcloth or hand. To wash the back, the bath giver places his or her noncradling hand on the newborn's chest with the thumb under the newborn's arm closest to the adult. Gently tipping the newborn forward onto the supporting hand frees the cradling arm to wash the back. After the bath, the newborn is lifted out of the tub in the cradle position, dried well, and wrapped in a dry blanket. The hair is then washed in the same way as for a sponge bath.

## Nail Care

The nails of the newborn are seldom cut in the birthing center. During the first days of life, the nails may adhere to the skin of the fingers, and cutting is contraindicated. Within a week the nails separate from the skin and frequently break off. If the nails are long or if the newborn is scratching his or her face, the nails may be trimmed. Trimming is most easily done while the infant is asleep. Nails should be cut straight across using adult cuticle scissors or blunt-ended infant cuticle scissors.

## Dressing the Newborn

Newborns need to wear a T-shirt, diaper (diaper cover or plastic pants if using cloth diapers), and a sleeper. On a fairly cool day, they should be wrapped in a light blanket while being fed. Newborns should be covered with a blanket in air-conditioned buildings. The blanket should be unwrapped or removed when inside a warm building. At home, the amount of clothing the newborn wears is determined by the temperature. Families who maintain their home at 60 to 65°F should dress the infant more warmly than those who maintain a temperature of 70 to 75°F.

Newborns should wear head coverings outdoors to protect their sensitive ears from drafts. A blanket can be wrapped around the baby, leaving one corner free to place over the head while outdoors or in crowds for added protection. The nurse must advise families about the ease with which a newborn's skin can burn when exposed to the sun. To prevent sunburn, the newborn should remain shaded, wear a light layer of clothing, or be protected with sunscreen.

Diaper shapes vary and are subject to personal preference (Figure 29–5♦). Prefolded and disposable diapers are usually rectangular. Cloth diapers may also be triangular or kite folded. Extra material is placed in front for males and toward the back for females to increase absorbency.

Baby clothing should be laundered separately with a mild soap or detergent. Diapers may be presoaked before washing. All clothing should be rinsed twice to remove soap and residue and to decrease the possibility of rash. Some newborns may not tolerate clothing treated with fabric softeners added to the washer or dryer.

## Temperature Assessment

As the nurse prepares to teach parents about taking their baby's temperature, it is important to provide opportunities for discussion and demonstration. Families often need a review of how to take the baby's temperature and when to call their primary health care provider.

The nurse discusses the different types of thermometers available for home use. It is important that parents understand the differences and how to select the appropriate one. Although tympanic (ear) thermometers are

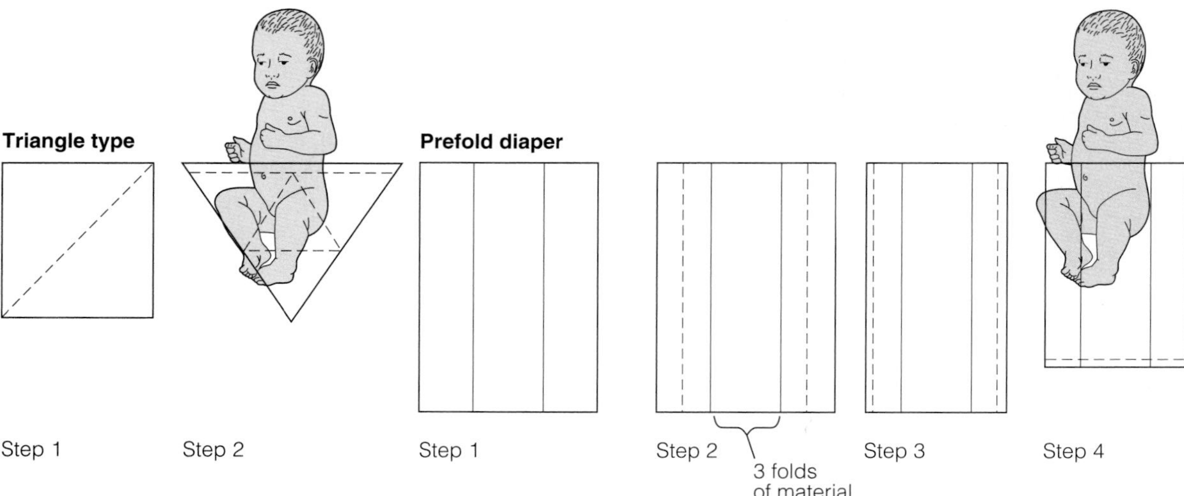


**FIGURE 29–5** ♦ Two basic cloth diaper shapes. Dotted lines indicate folds.

more expensive, many parents choose them because they are fast and easy to use. Other parents elect to use a digital thermometer. The nurse reviews the correct procedure for using the chosen thermometer.

## HINTS FOR PRACTICE

Health care facilities no longer use glass thermometers because of the risks associated with the resulting mercury spillage should one break. While some parents still have glass thermometers, they are used much less often than in the past. Before teaching families about temperature taking, you might find it helpful to visit a local pharmacy and review the types of thermometers available, the costs of the most commonly used methods, and the instructions provided. This will enable you to answer questions accurately when you work with parents or care givers.

Parents need to take the newborn's temperature only when the signs of illness are present. They should call their physician or pediatric nurse practitioner immediately if any signs of illness are present. (See Key Facts to Remember: When Parents Should Call Their Health Care Provider, in Chapter 23.) Parents should also check with their clinician for advice about over-the-counter medications to be kept in the medicine cabinet.

When parents find their newborn has a fever, they may expect to give an antipyretic such as Tylenol (acetaminophen). They should not give any form of aspirin for an illness that may be viral; use of aspirin in viral illnesses has been linked to Reye syndrome in children. Parents should discuss management of flu, colds, teething, constipation, diarrhea, and other common ailments with their clinician before they occur. When analgesic or antipyretic medication is needed, clinicians frequently recommend acetaminophen drops.

### STOOLS AND URINE

The appearance and frequency of a newborn's stools can cause concern for parents. The nurse prepares them by discussing and showing pictures of meconium stools and transitional stools and by describing the difference between breast milk and formula stools. Although each baby develops his or her own stooling patterns, parents can get an idea of what to expect (see Figure 21–8♦).

- Breastfed newborns may have 6 to 10 small, semiliquid, yellow stools per day by the third or fourth day, when milk production is established, unless the mother is having problems with her milk supply. Once breastfeeding is well established, usually by 1 month, the newborn may have only 1 stool every few days because of the increased digestibility of breast milk or still may have several daily. Constipation is unlikely to occur in newborns receiving only breast milk. Infrequent stooling in the first few weeks may indicate inadequate milk intake.
- Formula-fed babies may have only one or two stools a day; they are more formed and yellow or yellow-brown.

The parents may also be shown pictures of a constipated stool (small, pelletlike) and diarrhea (loose, green, or perhaps blood tinged). Families should understand that a green color is common in transitional stools, so that transitional stools are not confused with diarrhea during the first week of a newborn's life. Constipation may indicate that the newborn needs additional fluid intake. Parents may try offering additional water in an attempt to reverse the constipation.

Babies normally void (urinate) five to eight times per day. Fewer than six to eight wet diapers a day may indicate that the newborn needs more fluids. Frequency of voiding is easy to assess with cloth diapers. Parents who use superabsorbent single-use disposable diapers may have difficulty determining voiding patterns because the surface of the diaper feels dry. The liquid is pooling inside the filling of the diaper.

## Sleep and Activity

The newborn demonstrates several different sleep-wake states after the initial periods of reactivity described in Chapter 21. It is not uncommon for a newborn to sleep almost continuously for the first 2 to 3 days following birth, awakening only for feedings every 3 to 4 hours. Some newborns bypass this stage of deep sleep and require only 12 to 16 hours of sleep. The parents need to know that this pattern is normal.

**Quiet sleep** is characterized by regular breathing and no movement except for sudden body jerks. During this sleep state, normal household noise will not awaken the infant. In the active sleep state, the newborn has irregular breathing and fine muscular twitching. The newborn may cry out during sleep, but this does not mean he or she is uncomfortable or awake. Unusual household noise may awaken the newborn more easily in this state; however, he or she will quickly go back to sleep.

**Quiet alert state** is a state in which newborns are quietly involved with the environment. They watch a moving mobile, smile, and, as they age, discover and play with their hands and feet. When newborns become uncomfortable due to wet diapers, hunger, or cold, they enter the **active awake state** and **crying state.** In these states, parents should identify and eliminate the cause of the crying. Sometimes families are frustrated as they try to identify the external or internal stimuli that are causing the angry, hurt crying. Parents need to be told that the state may be changed from crying to quiet alert by moving the newborn toward an upright position where scanning and exploration are possible. (See Table 29–2 for the characteristics of the various states.)

## Crying

For the newborn, crying is the only means of expressing needs vocally. Families learn to distinguish different tones and qualities of the newborn's cry. The amount of crying is highly individual. Some cry as little as 15 to 30 minutes in 24 hours, and others cry as long as 2 hours every 24 hours. When crying continues after causes such as discomfort and hunger are eliminated, the newborn may be comforted by swaddling or by rocking and other reassuring activities. There is some indication that newborns who are held more tend to be calmer and cry less when not being held. Some parents are afraid that holding may "spoil" the newborn and need reassurance that this is not the case. Picking babies up when they cry teaches them that adults try to meet their needs and are responsive to them. This helps build a sense of trust in humankind. Excessive crying should be noted and assessed, taking other factors into consideration. After the first 2 or 3 days, newborns settle into individual patterns.

## Safety Considerations

Newborns should not have pillows or stuffed animals in the crib while they sleep; these items could cause suffocation. Mattresses should fit snugly in a crib to prevent entrapment and suffocation, and the crib should be inspected regularly to determine whether it is in safe working order. Crib slats should be no more than 2 3/8 in. apart. Parents can be encouraged to attend infant cardiopulmonary resuscitation (CPR) classes, especially if there is a family history of SIDS or the infant requires special care. See Evidence-Based Practice: Teaching Parents about Sudden Infant Death Syndrome.

## Newborn Screening and Immunization Program

Before the newborn and mother are discharged from the hospital, parents are informed about the normal screening tests for newborns and told when to return for further tests if needed. Newborn screening tests detect disorders that cause mental retardation, physical handicaps, or death if left undiscovered. Inborn errors of metabolism that can usually be detected from a drop of blood obtained by a heel stick on the second or third day include phenylketonuria (PKU) and congenital hypothyroidism (mandatory screening in all states in the United States), as well as sickle cell disease, galactosemia, and homocystinuria. Parents should be instructed that a second blood specimen will be required from the newborn after 7 to 14 days; in some states, the second blood specimen is not recommended if the first specimen is obtained 48 hours or longer after birth. Nurses should stress that an abnormal test result is not diagnostic. More definitive tests must be performed to verify the results. It is important to follow protocols that incorporate state laws about newborn testing.

If additional tests are positive, treatment is initiated. These conditions may be treated by dietary means or by administration of missing hormones. The inborn conditions

## TABLE 29–2 Infant State* Chart (Sleep and Awake States)

| Sleep States | *Characteristics of State* Body Activity | Eye Movement | Facial Movement | Breathing Pattern | Level of Response | Implications for Caregiving |
|---|---|---|---|---|---|---|
| Deep sleep | Nearly still except for occasional startle or twitch | None | Without facial movements, except for occasional sucking movement at regular intervals | Smooth and regular | Only very intense and disturbing stimuli will arouse infants. | Caregivers trying to feed infant in deep sleep will probably find the experience frustrating. Infants will be unresponsive, even if caregivers use disturbing stimuli (flicking feet) to arouse infants. Infants may arouse only briefly and then become unresponsive as they return to deep sleep. If caregivers wait until infants move to a higher, more responsive state, feeding or caregiving will be much more pleasant. |
| Light sleep | Some body movements | Rapid eye movement (REM): fluttering of eyes beneath closed eyelids | May smile and make brief fussy or crying sounds | Irregular | Infants are more responsive to internal and external stimuli. When these stimuli occur, infants may remain in light sleep or move to drowsy state. | Light sleep makes up the highest proportion of newborn sleep and usually precedes awakening. Caregivers who are not aware that the brief fussy or crying sounds made during this state occur normally may think it is time for feeding and may try to feed infants before they are ready to eat. |
| Drowsy | Activity level variable, with mild startles interspersed from time to time; movements usually smooth | Eyes open and close occasionally; are heavy lidded, with dull glazed appearance | May have some facial movements; often there are none and the face appears still | Irregular | Infants react to sensory stimuli, although responses are delayed. State change after stimulation is frequently noted. | From the drowsy state infants may return to sleep or awaken further. To wake them, caregivers can provide something for infants to see, hear, or suck. This may arouse them to a quite alert state, a more responsive state. Infants left alone without stimuli may return to a sleep state. |
| Quiet alert | Minimal | Brightening and widening of eyes | Faces have bright, shining, sparkling looks | Regular | Infants attend most to environment, focusing attention on any stimuli that are present. | Infants in this state provide much pleasure and positive feedback for caregivers. Providing something for infants to see, hear, or suck will often maintain a quiet alert state in the first few hours after birth. Most newborns commonly experience a period of intense alertness before going into a long sleeping period. |
| Active alert | Much body activity; may have periods of fussiness | Eyes open, with less brightening | Much facial movement; faces not as bright as in alert state | Irregular | Infants are increasingly sensitive to disturbing stimuli (hunger, fatigue, noise, excessive handling). | Caregivers may intervene at this stage to console and to bring infants to a lower state. |
| Crying | Increased motor activity, with color changes | Eyes may be tightly closed or open | Grimaces | More irregular | Infants are extremely responsive to unpleasant external or internal stimuli. | Crying is the infant's communication signal. If is a response to unpleasant stimuli from the environment or from within infants (fatigue, hunger, discomfort). Crying tells us infants have been reached. Sometimes infants can console themselves and return to lower states. At other times they need help from caregivers. |

**State* is a group of characteristics that regularly occur together: body activity, eye movements, facial movements, breathing pattern, and level of response to external stimuli (eg, handling) and internal stimuli (eg, hunger).

*Source:* Blackburn, S., & Kang, R. (1991). Early parent-infant relationships (2nd ed, module 3, series 1). In *The first six hours after birth.* White Plains, NY: March of Dimes Birth Defects Foundation. Reprinted with permission of the copyright holder.

## EVIDENCE-BASED PRACTICE

### Teaching Parents about Sudden Infant Death Syndrome

After 3 years of inpatient nursing, you decided to return to school and wanted to experience community-based nursing. So, you transferred from the inpatient mother-baby unit to the hospital's home care agency.

Providing care in the client's home is a new experience, one that makes you appreciate the value of your client-teaching skills. In particular, your agency is stressing parent teaching on reducing risk factors for sudden infant death syndrome (SIDS).

SIDS is the third leading cause of infant death in the United States; prematurity and congenital anomalies are the first and second (Huffman, Smok-Pearsall, Silvestri, et al., 1999). Although the cause of SIDS is still unknown, some risk factors should alert the caregiver to the need for more detailed assessment and education with the family. The American Academy of Pediatrics (AAP) created recommendations aimed at eliminating three of the risk factors for SIDS in 1992 (see AAP, Task Force on Infant Sleep Positioning and Sudden Infant Death Syndrome, 1992). These three risk factors are prone positioning, overbundling, and sleeping on soft bedding. However, studies show that parents are getting this information not from their caregivers but from the lay media (Huffman et al., 1999).

During your home visits you will therefore screen for maternal and infant risk factors for SIDS. You will also assess the infant's sleeping environment and position and make recommendations on your findings that reflect the AAP position (AAP, 2000).

#### References


American Academy of Pediatrics. (2000). Changing concepts of sudden infant death syndrome: Implications for infant sleeping environment and sleep position (RE 9946). *Pediatrics, 105*(5), 650–656. Available: http://www.aap.org/policy/re9946.html

American Academy of Pediatrics, Task Force on Infant Sleep Positioning and Sudden Infant Death Syndrome. (1992). *Pediatrics, 89*, 1120–1126.

Huffman, A., Smok-Pearsall, S., Silvestri, J., & Weese-Mayer, D. (1999). SIDS risk factor awareness: Assessment among nursing students. *Journal of Obstetric, Gynecologic and Neonatal Nursing, 28*(1), 68–73.


cannot be cured, but they can be treated. They are not contagious, but they may be inherited.

## Follow-up Care

Routine well-baby visits should be scheduled with the clinic, pediatric nurse practitioner, or physician. It is helpful if these appointments are scheduled before the woman leaves the birthing center or hospital.

To help parents care for their newborn at home, some physicians encourage prenatal pediatric visits to establish this contact before the birth. Public health nurses have long been involved as guides in newborn care and parent education. Birthing units are now expanding their support for the new family to include one home visit by the nurse who cared for the family in the birthing unit.

The family should be taught all necessary caregiving methods before discharge. A checklist may be helpful to determine whether the teaching has been completed. The mother should have the phone number, address, and any specific instructions from the certified nurse-midwife, nurse practitioner, or physician and the lactation consultant. Having the nursery phone number is also reassuring to a new family. Parents are encouraged to call with questions.

Nurses engaged in telephone triage must consider several important strategies to provide optimum care and avoid legal pitfalls. These strategies include the following (Cady, 1999):

1. Develop and follow triage protocols for the most commonly occurring calls.
2. Document all triage calls carefully and accurately.
3. Initiate timely follow-up contacts. (This may include instructions to the client to call back after a specific period or if the condition does not improve; it may also involve calls from the nurse to the client as a follow-up.)

# Home Care: The Mother and Family

During the first few days and weeks postpartally many changes are occurring. The family adjusts to a new family member, and siblings become familiar with new roles and responsibilities. During this period the woman must accomplish a variety of physical and developmental tasks, including

- Restoring physical condition
- Developing competence in caring for and meeting the needs of her infant
- Establishing a relationship with her new child
- Adapting to altered lifestyles and family structure resulting from the addition of a new member

The nurse can interact with the family following discharge by telephone follow-up, home visit, or a combination. The approach used depends on the mother's needs and preferences and established practices in the community.

## Assessment of the Mother and Family

During the first home visit, the nurse completes a physical and psychologic assessment. Before completing the assessment the nurse should ensure privacy. The physical assessment focuses on maternal physical adaptation, which is assessed by focusing on vital signs, breasts, abdominal musculature, elimination patterns, reproductive tract, and laboratory values. The nurse also talks with the mother about her diet, fatigue level, ability to rest and sleep, pain management, and signs of postpartal complications. In addition, for breastfeeding mothers, the nurse assesses the woman's feeding technique and presents information about possible problems that may occur.

The psychologic assessment focuses on attachment, adjustment to the parental role, sibling adjustment, and educational needs. When appropriate, the nurse mentions available community resources, including public health department follow-up visits. If not already discussed, teaching about family planning is appropriate at this time, and the nurse provides information about birth control methods. In ideal situations a family approach involving the presence of the father and any siblings provides an opportunity to observe family interactions and opportunities for all family members to ask questions and express concerns. In addition, any questionable family interaction pattern such as one suggestive of abuse or neglect may be evident and further referral could be considered if needed. (See Assessment Guide: Postpartal—First Home Visit and Anticipated Progress at 6 Weeks.)

In addition, the nurse continues to provide teaching to the mother and her family as needed, including descriptions of relevant self-care measures. The nurse discusses infant care and answers any questions the family may have. Generally the new mother has a final postpartum examination with her caregiver about 6 weeks after childbirth. However, if the nurse's assessment indicates a need, the nurse refers the woman to her health care provider for further care prior to the 6-week check.

## Breastfeeding Issues Following Discharge

Because mothers are discharged from the birthing unit before breastfeeding is well established, they are frequently alone when they encounter changes in the breastfeeding process. Many women stop nursing if the situations they encounter seem problematic. The nurse can offer anticipatory guidance regarding common breastfeeding phenomena and provide resources for the woman's use after discharge. Table 29–3 on page 791 summarizes self-care measures the nurse can suggest to a woman with a breastfeeding problem.

### Nipple Soreness

Some discomfort often occurs initially with breastfeeding; it peaks between the third and sixth days and then recedes (Riordan & Auerbach, 1999). However, the mother should not switch to bottle-feeding or delay feedings because these measures cause engorgement and more soreness. Discomfort that lasts throughout the feeding or past the first week demands attention.

The baby's position at the breast is a critical factor in nipple soreness. The mother's hand should be off the areola, and the baby should be facing the mother's chest, with ear, shoulder, and hip aligned (see Figure 24–5♦). Because the area of greatest stress to the nipple is in line with the newborn's chin and nose, nipple soreness may be decreased by encouraging the mother to rotate positions when feeding the infant. Changing positions alters the focus of greatest stress and promotes more complete breast emptying.

Nipple soreness may also develop if the infant has faulty sucking habits. Nipples may have injured tips that are bruised, scabbed, or blistered from the nipple entering the baby's mouth at an upward angle and rubbing against the roof of the mouth (Riordan & Auerbach, 1999). Soreness may also result from continuous negative pressure if the infant falls asleep with the breast in his or her mouth.

Chewed nipples, which result from improper positioning, are cracked or tender at or near the base. In these cases, the baby's jaws close only on the nipple instead of on the areola, the baby's mouth is not opened wide

Text continues on page 792.

## ASSESSMENT GUIDE: POSTPARTAL—FIRST HOME VISIT AND ANTICIPATED PROGRESS AT 6 WEEKS

| Physical Assessment/ Normal Findings | Alterations and Possible Causes* | Nursing Responses to Data† |
|---|---|---|
| **Vital Signs** | | |
| Blood pressure: Return to normal prepregnant level. | Elevated blood pressure (anxiety, essential hypertension, renal disease). | Review history, evaluate normal baseline; refer to physician or CNM is necessary. |
| Pulse: 60–90 beats/minute (or prepregnant normal rate). | Increased pulse rate (excitement, anxiety, cardiac disorders). | Count pulse for full minute and note irregularities; marked tachycardia or beat irregularities require additional assessment and possible physician or CNM referral. |
| Respirations: 16–24/minute. | Marked tachypnea or abnormal patterns (respiratory disorders). | Evaluate for respiratory disease; refer to physician or CNM if necessary. |
| Temperature: 36.2–37.6°C (98–99.6°F). | Increased temperature (infection). | Assess for signs and symptoms of infection or disease state. |
| **Weight** | | |
| 2 days: Possible weight loss of 12–20+ lb. | Minimal weight loss (fluid retention, pregnancy-induced hypertension [PIH]. | Evaluate for fluid retention, edema, deep tendon reflexes, and blood pressure elevation. |
| 6 weeks: Returning to normal prepregnant weight. | Retained weight (excessive caloric intake). | Determine amount of daily exercise. Provide dietary teaching. Refer to dietitian if necessary for additional dietary counseling. |
| | Extreme weight loss (excessive dieting, inadequate caloric intake). | Discuss appropriate diets; refer to dietitian for additional counseling if necessary. |
| **Breasts** | | |
| *Nonnursing*<br>2 days: May have mild tenderness; small amount of milk may be expressed.<br>6 weeks: Soft, with no tenderness; return to prepregnant size. | Some engorgement (incomplete suppression of lactation).<br>Redness; marked tenderness (mastitis).<br>Palpable mass (tumor). | Engorgement may be seen in nonnursing mothers. Advise client to wear a supportive, well-fitted bra, avoid very warm showers, use ice packs for comfort; evaluate for signs and symptoms of mastitis (rare in nonnursing mothers). |
| *Nursing*<br>Full with prominent nipples; lactation established. | Cracked, fissured nipples (feeding problems).<br>Redness, marked tenderness, or even abscess formation (mastitis).<br>Palpable mass (full milk duct, tumor) | Counsel about nipple care.<br>Evaluate client condition, evidence of fever; refer to physician or certified nurse midwife for initiation of antibiotic therapy, if indicated.<br>Opinion varies as to value of breast examination for nursing mothers; some feel a nursing mother should examine her breasts monthly, after feeding, when breasts are empty; if palpable mass is felt, refer to physician for further evaluation. |

*Possible causes of alterations are placed in parentheses.

†This column provides guidelines for further assessment and initial nursing interventions.

## POSTPARTAL—FIRST HOME VISIT AND ANTICIPATED PROGRESS AT 6 WEEKS *continued*

| Physical Assessment/ Normal Findings | Alterations and Possible Causes* | Nursing Responses to Data† |
|---|---|---|
| **Breasts** *continued* | | |
| | | For breast inflammation instruct the mother to<br>**1.**. Keep breast empty by frequent feeding.<br>**2.**. Rest when possible.<br>**3.**. Take prescribed pain relief med.<br>**4.**. Force fluids.<br>If symptoms persist for more than 24 hours, instruct her to call her physician or CNM. |
| **Abdominal Musculature** | | |
| 2 days: Improved firmness, although "bread-dough" consistency is not unusual, especially in multipara.<br>Striae pink and obvious. | Marked relaxation of muscles. | Evaluate exercise level; provide information on appropriate exercise program. |
| Cesarean incision healing. | Drainage, redness, tenderness, pain, edema (infection). | Evaluate for infection; refer to physician or CNM if necessary. |
| 6 weeks: Muscle tone continues to improve; striae may be beginning to fade, may not achieve a silvery appearance for several more weeks; linea nigra fading. | | |
| **Elimination Pattern** | | |
| *Urinary Tract* | | |
| Return to prepregnant urinary elimination routine. | Urinary incontinence, especially with lifting, coughing, laughing, and so on (urethral trauma, cystocele). | Assess for cystocele; instruct in appropriate muscle tightening exercises; refer to physician or CNM. |
| | Pain or burning when voiding, urgency and/or frequency, pus or white blood cells (WBC) in urine, pathogenic organisms in culture (urinary tract infection). | Evaluate for urinary tract infection; obtain clean-catch urine sample; refer to physician or certified nurse-midwife for treatment if indicated. |
| Routine urinalysis within normal limits (proteinuria disappeared). | Sugar or ketone in urine—may be some lactose present in urine of breastfeeding mothers (diabetes). | Evaluate diet; assess for signs and symptoms of diabetes; refer to physician or CNM. |
| *Bowel Habits* | | |
| 2 days: May be some discomfort with defecation, especially if client had severe hemorrhoids or third-or fourth-degree extension. | Severe constipation or pain when defecating (trauma or hemorrhoids). | Discuss dietary patterns; encourage fluid, adequate roughage.<br>Continue use of stool softener if necessary to prevent pain associated with straining; continue sitz baths, periods of rest for severe hemorrhoids; assess healing of episiotomy and/or lacerations; severe constipation may require administration of laxatives, stool softeners, and an enema. |
| | ***Possible causes of alterations are placed in parentheses.** | **†This column provides guidelines for further assessment and initial nursing intervention.** |

## POSTPARTAL—FIRST HOME VISIT AND ANTICIPATED PROGRESS AT 6 WEEKS *continued*

| Physical Assessment/ Normal Findings | Alterations and Possible Causes* | Nursing Responses to Data† |
|---|---|---|
| Bowel Habits *continued* | | |
| 6 weeks: Return to normal prepregnancy bowel elimination patterns. | Marked constipation. | See previous page. |
| | Fecal incontinence or constipation (rectocele). | Assess for evidence of rectocele; instruct in muscle-tightening exercises; refer to physician or CNM. |
| **Reproductive Tract** | | |
| *Lochia* | | |
| 2 days: Lochia rubra or lochia serosa, scant amounts, fleshy odor. | Excessive amounts (nonfirm uterus), foul odor (infection). | Assess for evidence of infection and/or failure of the uterus to decrease in size; refer to physician or CNM. |
| 6 weeks: No lochia, or return to normal menstruation pattern. | See above. | See above. |
| *Fundus and Perineum* | | |
| 2 days: Fundus is at least two finger breadths below the umbilicus; uterine muscles still somewhat lax; introitus of vagina lacks tone—gapes when intraabdominal pressure is increased by coughing or straining. | Uterus not decreasing in size appropriately (infection). | Assess fundus for firmness and/or signs of infection; refer to physician or CNM if indicated. |
| Episiotomy and/or lacerations healing; no signs of infection. | Evidence of redness, tenderness, poor tissue approximation in episiotomy and/or laceration (wound infection). | |
| 6 weeks: Uterus almost returned to prepregnant size, with almost completely restored muscle tone. | Continued flow of lochia, failure to decrease appropriately in size (subinvolution). | Assess for evidence of subinvolution and/or infection; refer to physician for further evaluation and for dilatation and curettage if necessary. |
| **Hemoglobin and Hematocrit Levels** | | |
| 6 weeks: Hb 12g/dL.<br>Hct 37% plus or minus 5% | HB less than 12 g/dL.<br>Hct 32% (anemia). | Assess nutritional status, begin (or continue) supplemental iron; for marked anemia (Hb less than or equal to 9g/dL) additional assessment and/or physician or CNM referral may be necessary. |
| **Attachment** | | |
| Bonding process demonstrated by soothing, cuddling, and talking to infant; appropriate feeding techniques; eye-to-eye contact; calling infant by name. | Failure to bond demonstrated by lack of behaviors associated with bonding process, calling infant by nickname that promotes ridicule, inadequate infant weight gain, infant is dirty, hygienic measures are not being maintained, severe diaper rash, failure to obtain adequate supplies to provide infant care (malattachment). | Provide counseling; talk with the woman about her feelings regarding the infant; provide support for the caretaking activities that are being performed; refer to public health nurse for continued home visits. |

***Possible causes of alterations are placed in parentheses.**

**†This column provides guidelines for further assessment and initial nursing interventions.**

## POSTPARTAL—FIRST HOME VISIT AND ANTICIPATED PROGRESS AT 6 WEEKS *continued*

| Psychosocial Assessment/ Normal Findings | Alterations and Possible Causes* | Nursing Responses to Data† |
|---|---|---|
| **Attachment** *continued* | | |
| Parent interacts with infant and provides soothing, caretaking activities. | Parent is unable to respond to infant needs (inability to recognize needs, inadequate education and support, fear, family stress). | Provide support for caretaking activities observed; provide information regarding caretaking activities, such as responding to infant cry; methods of wrapping infant; methods of soothing the infant such as swaddling, rocking, increasing stimuli by singing to the infant or decreasing stimuli by putting infant to rest in quiet room; methods of holding the infant; differences in the cry. Identify support system such as friends, neighbors; provide information regarding community resources and support groups. |
| Parents express feelings of comfort and success with the parent role. | Evidence of stress and anxiety (difficulty moving into or dealing with the parent role). | Provide support and encouragement; provide information regarding progression into parent role and assist parents in talking through their feelings; refer to community resources and support groups. |
| Woman is in the informal or personal stage of maternal role attainment. | Woman is still greatly influenced by others, has not developed an image or style of her own (woman remains in the anticipatory stage). | Provide role modeling for the woman in working through problem solving with the infant; provide encouragement as she thinks through decisions and develops her sense of problem solving; encourage her to make decisions regarding infant care. |
| **Adjustment to Parental Role** | | |
| Parents are coping with new roles in terms of division of labor, financial status, communication, readjustment of sexual relations, and adjusting to new daily tasks. | Inability to adjust to new roles (immaturity, inadequate education and preparation, ineffective communication patterns, inadequate support, current family crisis). | Provide counseling; refer to parent groups. |
| **Education** | | |
| Mother understands self-care measures. | Inadequate knowledge of self-care (inadequate education). | Provide education and counseling. |
| Parents are knowledgeable regarding infant care. | Inadequate knowledge of infant care (inadequate education). | |
| Siblings are adjusting to new baby. | Excessive sibling rivalry. | |
| Parents have a method of contraception. | Birth control method not chosen. | |

*Possible causes of alterations are placed in parentheses.

†This column provides guidelines for further assessment and initial nursing interventions.

## TABLE 29–3 Breastfeeding Problems and Remedies

### NIPPLES NOT GRASPABLE

Flat or inverted nipples

- Use Hoffman technique to break adhesions.
- Wear milk cups to encourage nipples to protrude.
- Use nipple tug and roll to increase protractility.
- Form the nipple prior to nursing by hand shaping, ice, wearing milk cups a half-hour before feeding.
- As a last resort, use nipple shield for first few minutes of feeding to draw out nipple; then place baby on breast.

Engorged breasts

Treat engorgement by relieving fullness with hand expression of milk prior to nursing and instituting frequent feeding so nipple is more prominent.

Large breasts

- Support breast with opposite hand or use rolled towel under breast to bring nipple to the level of baby's mouth.
- Use C-hold to make nipple accessible to baby.

### ENGORGEMENT

Missed or infrequent feedings

- Nurse frequently (every 1 1/2 hours).
- Massage and hand express or pump to empty breasts completely when feedings are missed or when a full feeling develops in breasts and baby is not available or willing to nurse.

Breasts not emptied at feedings

- Nurse long enough to empty breasts (10–15 minutes on each side at each feeding).
- If baby will not nurse long enough to empty breasts, hand express or pump after feeding.

Inadequate letdown

- Use relaxation techniques, massage, and warm or cool compresses before nursing.
- Relax in warm shower with water running from back over shoulders and breasts, hand expressing to relieve fullness.
- If due to anxiety, try to eliminate the source of tension.

Baby sleepy or not eager to nurse

- Use rousing techniques (eg. hold baby upright, unwrap blanket, change diaper).
- Preexpress milk onto nipple or baby's lips to entice baby.
- Avoid use of bottles of water or formula; these will decrease baby's willingness to suckle.

### INADEQUATE LETDOWN

Letdown not well established

- Give the baby ample time at the breast (at least 15 minutes per side) to allow for letdown and complete emptying.
- Nurse in a quiet spot away from distractions.
- Massage breasts before nursing.
- Drink juice, water, tea (no caffeine) before and during nursing.
- Condition letdown by setting up a routine for beginning feedings.
- Use relaxation and breathing techniques.
- Stimulate the nipple manually before nursing.
- Concentrate thought on the baby and milk flow; turn on a faucet so that the sound of running water helps stimulate letdown.
- Use synthetic oxytocin nasal spray several times during a feeding (This should condition letdown within 24 hours. Then it is no longer needed. Spray must be prescribed by a doctor.)

Mother overtired or overextended

- Nap or rest when the baby rests.
- Lie down to nurse.
- Nurse the baby in bed at night.
- Simplify daily chores; set priorities.

Mother tense, pressured

- Identify the causes of tensions and eliminate or minimize them.
- Decrease fatigue.

Mother caught in cycle of little milk, worry, less milk

- Try all the actions mentioned earlier.
- Develop confidence in mothering skills. (A home visit by a counselor may help.)

### CRACKED NIPPLES

All causes of sore nipples carried to extreme

- Refer to all actions for sore nipples.
- Consult doctor about using aspirin, acetaminophen (Tylenol), or other painkiller.
- Improve nutritional status, increasing protein, vitamin C, zinc.

Local infection (baby with staph or other organism may have infected mother's nipples)

Refer to physician.

### PLUGGED DUCTS

Poor positioning

Try a variety of positions for complete emptying.

Incomplete emptying of breast

- Nurse at least 10 minutes per side after letdown.
- Alternate nursing positions.
- If baby does not empty breasts, pump or express milk after feedings.

External pressure on breast

- Use larger size bras, insert bra extender, or go braless.
- Use nursing bra instead of pulling up conventional bra to nurse to avoid pressure on ducts.
- Avoid bunching up sweater or nightgown under arm during nursing.

## TABLE 29–3 Breastfeeding Problems and Remedies continued

### SORE NIPPLES

Poor positioning

- Alternate nursing positions throughout the day.
- Bring the baby close to nurse so the baby does not pull on the breast.
- Place the nipple and some of the areola in the baby's mouth.
- Check to ensure the baby is put on and off the breast properly.
- Check to ensure the nipple is back far enough in the baby's mouth.
- Hold the baby closely during nursing so the nipple is not constantly being pulled.

Baby chewing or nuzzling onto nipple

- Form the nipple for the baby.
- Set up a pattern of getting the baby onto the breast using the rooting reflex.

Baby nursing on end of nipple

- Ensure the nipple is way back in the baby's mouth by getting the baby properly onto the breast.
- Check for an inverted nipple.
- Check for engorgement.

Baby chewing his or her way off the nipple (nipple being pulled out of baby's mouth at end of feeding)

- Remove the baby from the breast by placing a finger between the baby's gums to ensure suction is broken.
- End feeding when the baby's suckling slows, before he or she has a chance to chew on the nipple.

Baby overly eager to nurse

- Nurse more often.
- Preexpress milk to hasten letdown, avoiding vigorous suckling.

Dry colostrum or milk causing nipple to stick to bra or breast pads

Moisten bra or pads before taking off so as not to remove keratin.

Nipples not allowed to dry

- Remove plastic liners from milk pads.
- Air dry breasts completely after nursing.
- Change milk pads frequently.

Improper use of breast shield

- Use shield only to draw out nipple; then have the baby nurse on the breast.
- Cut tip of shield back bit by bit and eventually discard.

Nipple skin not resistant to stress

- Improve diet, especially adding fresh fruits and vegetables and vitamin supplements.
- Eliminate or decrease use of sugary foods, alcohol, caffeine, cigarettes.
- Check use of cleansing or drying agents.

Natural oils removed or keratin layers broken down by drying agents (soap, alcohol, shampoo, deodorant)

- Eliminate irritants.
- Wash breasts with water only.

*Source:* Adapted from Lauwers, J., & Woessner, C. (1990). *Counseling the nursing mother: A reference handbook for health care providers and lay counselors* (2nd ed., pp.385–397). Garden City Park, NY: Avery.

enough, or the infant's mouth has slipped down to the nipple from the areola as a result of engorgement. Soreness on the underside of the nipple is caused by the infant nursing with her or his bottom lip tucked in rather than out, causing a friction burn. In such cases, even vigorous sucking produces little milk because the milk sinuses under the areola are not compressed. This situation results in a frustrated infant and marked soreness for the mother. The problem is overcome by positioning the infant with as much areola as possible in his or her mouth and rotating the baby's positions at the breast.

Nipple soreness is especially pronounced during the first few minutes of a feeding. If the mother is not expecting this discomfort, she may become discouraged and quickly stop. The letdown reflex may take a few minutes to activate, and it may not occur if the mother stops nursing too quickly. The infant is unsatisfied, and the possibility of breast engorgement increases.

Nipple soreness can result from the vigorous feeding of an overeager infant. Thus the mother may find it helpful to nurse more frequently. The woman can also apply ice to her nipples and areola for a few minutes before feeding to promote nipple erectness and numb the tissue initially. To prevent skin breakdown, after feeding the mother can wash her nipples and areolae with water and allow them to dry well. To promote dryness, the mother may leave her bra flaps down for a few minutes after feeding or expose her nipples to sunlight or ultraviolet light for 30 seconds at first, gradually increasing to 3 minutes. Drying the nipples with a hair dryer on a low heat setting also facilitates drying and promotes healing (Riordan & Auerbach, 1999).

The use of petroleum-based products such as Vaseline, A + D, cocoa butter, and baby oil to lubricate the nipples is discouraged because the petroleum interferes with skin respiration and may prolong soreness. Because of the risk of allergic reactions, products such as Massé cream (risk of peanut allergy) and lubricants containing lanolin (risk of wool allergy) are also discouraged. In addition, products that are washed off before breastfeeding are avoided because of the irritation that washing produces (Lauwers & Shinskie, 2000).

Currently research as to the effectiveness of nipple lubricants is inconclusive. Thus many lactation experts recommend that the mother's own milk be applied to the nipples and allowed to air dry. Breast milk is high in fat, fights infection, and will not irritate the nipples. Moreover, it is readily available at no cost to the mother. In cases of very dry or severely sore nipples, hypoallergenic medical-grade anhydrous lanolin may be helpful. This product poses a low risk of allergy because the alcohols that contribute to the allergic response have been removed (Lauwers & Shinskie, 2000).

If the woman finds that her bra or clothing rubs against her nipples and adds to her discomfort, she may insert shields into her bra. Both Medela Shells and Woolrich Shields relieve friction and promote air circulation. If a woman uses breast pads inside her bra to keep milk from leaking onto her clothes, she should change the pads frequently so the nipples remain dry.

Older remedies for nipple soreness are receiving renewed acceptance. For instance, tea bags may be moistened in warm water and applied to the nipples. The tannic acid seems to help toughen the nipples, and the warmth is soothing and promotes healing. However, tannic acid can cause drying and cracking and is not appropriate in all situations (Lawrence, 1994).

Nipple dermatitis, which causes swollen, reddened, burning nipples, is most commonly caused by thrush or by allergic response to breast cream preparations. If the nipple soreness has a sudden onset and is accompanied by burning or itching, shooting pains through the breast, and a deep pink coloration of the nipple, it may be caused by a thrush infection transmitted from the infant to the mother. White patches or streaks in the infant's mouth indicate a need for treatment of the mouth and nipple infection. The disease can be treated with a variety of antifungal preparations and does not preclude breastfeeding.

### Cracked Nipples

Nipple soreness is often coupled with cracked nipples. When a breastfeeding mother complains of soreness, the nurse carefully examines the nipples for fissures or cracks and observes the mother during breastfeeding to see whether the infant is correctly positioned at the breast. If the positioning is correct and cracks exist, interventions are necessary. All the interventions described for sore nipples may be used. It may also help the mother to begin nursing on the breast that is less sore. This approach allows the letdown reflex to occur in the affected breast and permits the infant to do more vigorous sucking on the less tender breast, which decreases trauma to the cracked nipple. With severe cases, the temporary use of a nipple shield for nursing may be appropriate. For the mother's comfort, analgesics may be taken after nursing.

## Critical Thinking in Practice

Ann calls you from home in tears on her third postpartum day. She states that, although breastfeeding was going well in the hospital, her breasts are now swollen, hard, and very painful, and her baby is refusing to suckle. Ann expresses extreme disappointment that "the breastfeeding didn't work' because she truly believes that breast milk is best for babies and she had enjoyed her breastfeeding experience in the hospital, especially nursing the baby immediately after delivery. But she also states she has not been able to stop crying all day and can no longer tolerate her painful breasts. In addition she says that the baby "seems happier" with the bottle. What would you do?

Answers can be found in Appendix H.

### Breast Engorgement

A distinction exists between breast fullness and engorgement. All lactating women experience a transition fullness at first, initially due to venous congestion and later due to accumulating milk. However, this fullness generally lasts only 24 hours, the breasts remain soft enough for the newborn to suckle, and there is no pain. Engorged breasts are hard, painful, and warm and appear taut and shiny.

The infant should suckle for an average of 15 minutes per feeding and should feed at least eight times in 24 hours (Riordan & Auerbach, 1999). If the baby is unable to nurse more frequently, the mother may express some milk manually or with a pump, taking care to avoid traumatizing the breast tissue. Warm or cool compresses before nursing stimulate letdown and soften the breast so that the infant can grasp the areola more easily. The mother should wear a well-fitting nursing bra 24 hours a day to support the breasts and prevent discomfort from tension.

The use of fresh green cabbage leaves placed inside the bra to treat engorgement is a long-recognized home remedy that has sparked renewed interest. Although the exact action of the cabbage is not understood, it appears to reduce the edema of engorgement. The amount of relief women experience varies. Some women report relief in as little as 30 minutes, whereas other women require more continuous use to perceive an effect. It should be noted that prolonged use of cabbage can cause the milk to dry up, which may be helpful if sudden weaning is necessary (Lauwers & Shinskie, 2000). Analgesics such as acetaminophen and aspirin, alone or in combination with codeine, are appropriate, especially if taken just before nursing. The pain will be relieved, but the medication will not reach the milk for at least 30 minutes (Lawrence, 1994).

### Plugged Ducts

Some mothers experience plugging of one or more ducts, especially in conjunction with or following engorgement. This condition is often referred to as "caked breasts." Manifested as an area of tenderness or lumpiness in an otherwise well woman, plugging may be relieved by the use of heat and massage. The nurse can encourage the mother to massage her breasts from her chest wall forward to the nipple while standing in a warm shower or following the application of moist heat to the breast (Riordan & Auerbach, 1999). The mother should then nurse her infant, starting on the unaffected breast if the plugged breast is tender. Frequent nursing and the use of a variety of positions to ensure complete emptying helps prevent the problem.

### Breastfeeding and the Working Mother

The best preparation for maintaining lactation after return to work is frequent, unlimited breastfeeding. Even when well planned, the first day back to work may be fraught with emotional and physical distress. Anticipatory guidance from the nurse may facilitate the transition from maternity leave to work. The earlier the breastfeeding mother returns to work, the more often she will need to pump her breasts to express the breast milk. Because milk production follows the principle of supply and demand, if breasts are not pumped, the milk supply will decrease.

An electric breast pump and double collection system are considered the optimal means of milk expression. However, this is not the only method; mechanical means may not suit some women. Sometimes a mother has a flexible schedule and can return home or have the baby brought to her to nurse at lunch time. If this is not possible, the infant may be fed expressed milk. (For proper storage of breast milk, see the section on "Storing Breast Milk" in Chapter 24.) When the mother is absent, the infant can be bottle-fed or spoon-fed. If the baby is 3 months or older, cup feeding is an option. The mother should wait until lactation is well established before introducing the bottle. Most babies adjust to the bottle within 7 to 10 days.

To maintain a milk supply, the working mother must pay special attention to her fluid intake. She can ensure adequate intake by drinking extra fluid at each break and whenever possible during the day. It is also helpful to nurse more on weekends, nurse during the night, eat a nutritionally sound diet, and continue manual expression or pumping when not nursing (Bocar, 1997).

Night nursing presents a dilemma: it may help a working mother maintain her milk supply, but it may also contribute to fatigue. Some women choose to have the infant sleep with them so that breastfeeding is more easily accomplished; other women find it difficult to sleep soundly when the infant is in the same bed. For the mother who works long hours or has a rigid work schedule, the best alternative may be to limit breastfeeding to morning and evening feedings, with supplemental feedings at other times. This choice allows her to maintain a close relationship with the infant and provides some of the unique benefits of breast milk.

### Weaning

The decision to *wean* the baby from the breast may be made for a variety of reasons, including family or cultural pressures, changes in the home situation, pressure from the woman's partner, or a personal opinion about when weaning should occur. For the woman who is comfortable with breastfeeding and well informed about the process, the appropriate time to wean her infant will become evident if she is sensitive to the child's cues. Often weaning falls between periods of great developmental activity for the child. Thus weaning commonly occurs at 8 to 9 months, 12 to 14 months, 18 months, 2 years, and 3 years of age. The infant who is weaned before 12 months should be given iron-fortified infant formula, not cows' milk (American College of Obstetricians and Gynecologists, 2000).

If weaning is timed to respond to the child's cues, and if the mother is comfortable with the timing, it can be accomplished with less difficulty than if the process begins before mother and child are ready emotionally. Nevertheless, weaning is a time of emotional separation for mother and baby; it may be difficult for them to give up the closeness of their nursing sessions. The nurse who is understanding about this possibility can help the mother see that her infant is growing up and plan other comforting, consoling, and play activities to replace breastfeeding. A gradual approach is the easiest and most comforting way to wean the child from breastfeedings.

During weaning, the mother should substitute one cup feeding or bottle-feeding for one breastfeeding session over a few days to a week so that her breasts gradually produce less milk. Eliminating the breastfeedings associated with meals first facilitates the mother's ability to wean the infant, because satiation with food lessens the desire for milk. Over a period of several weeks she can substitute more cup feedings or bottle-feedings for breastfeedings. The slow method of weaning prevents breast engorgement, allows infants to alter their eating methods at their own rates, and provides time for psychologic adjustment.

## Resumption of Sexual Activity

Typically, postpartum couples resume sexual intercourse once the episiotomy is healed and the lochial flow has stopped. Because this usually occurs by the end of the third week, prior to the 6-week check, it is important that the woman and her partner have information about what to expect. The nurse may inform the couple that, because the vaginal vault is "dry" (hormone poor), some form of lubrication such as K-Y jelly may be necessary during intercourse. The female-superior and side-lying coital positions may be preferable because they allow the woman to control the depth of penile penetration.

Breastfeeding couples should be forewarned that during orgasm milk may spurt from the nipples due to the release of oxytocin. Some couples find this spurt pleasurable or amusing, but others choose to have the woman wear a bra during sexual activity. Nursing the baby before lovemaking may reduce the chance of milk release.

Other factors may inhibit satisfactory sexual experiences: the baby's crying may "spoil the mood," the woman's changed body may seem unattractive to her or her partner, maternal sleep deprivation may interfere with a mutually satisfying experience, and the woman's physiologic response to sexual stimulation may be altered due to hormonal changes. By 3 months postpartum, sexual interest and activity are generally regular in frequency. However, a return to prepregnant levels of sexual activity varies by couple and may take from a few weeks to a year after childbirth (Alteneder & Hartzell, 1997).

With anticipatory guidance during the prenatal and postpartal periods, the couple can be forewarned of potential temporary problems. Anticipatory guidance is enhanced if the couple can discuss their feelings and reactions as they are experienced. (See Teaching Guide: Resumption of Sexual Activity after Childbirth.)

### Contraception

Information on contraception is often provided as part of discharge teaching. However, the nurse can also be an important resource for the woman and her partner during postpartum follow-up. Couples typically choose to use contraception to control the number of children they will have or to determine the spacing of future children. In choosing a specific method, consistency of use is essential. The nurse needs to identify the advantages, disadvantages, risks, and contraindications of the various methods to help the couple, or the single mother, make an informed choice about the most practical and compatible method. (For a more detailed discussion of contraceptive methods, see Chapter 4.)

## Additional Community Resources

### Telephone Follow-up

Telephone follow-up is offered to families prior to discharge, and a mutually agreed upon time is set for the call. Typically the call is made within 3 days after discharge or earlier if desired. To perform effective telephone assessment, the nurse must be able to listen skillfully, ask open-ended questions, and project an attitude of caring. The plan of care developed and implemented during a telephone conversation is limited to supportive counseling, teaching, and referral.

It is also fairly common for a home care nurse to make a telephone follow-up call to a family a few days after a home visit to provide additional information, address questions or areas of confusion, and make referrals if indicated.

### Return Visits

If the mother, family, and physician or certified nurse-midwife have chosen discharge earlier than 48 hours after vaginal birth, in some states, the mother may request a total of three visits. In such cases the nurse would schedule the first visit about 24 hours after discharge and then space out the other two visits over the next week. In other instances the nurse may schedule additional home visits based on the findings of the first home visit and the follow-up phone call.

### Help Lines for Parents

Many communities have established 24-hour help lines for new parents to call when they have questions or need support. In areas where help lines are not available, parents may be directed to call the birthing center. In either case, the nurse may provide the number so that it is readily accessible for the family.

### Postpartal Classes and Support Groups

Postpartal classes are becoming more common as caregivers recognize the continuing needs of the childbearing family. In many instances, classes are prepared to meet the specific needs of a variety of families so that, for example, single mothers and adolescent mothers can attend class with peers. A series of structured classes may focus on topics such as parenting, postpartal exercise, or nutrition, or there may be loosely structured group sessions that address mothers' concerns as they arise. Such classes offer

# TEACHING GUIDE *Resumption of Sexual Activity after Childbirth*

## Assessment

The nurse recognizes that couples, especially if they have become parents for the first time, may have questions about resuming sexual activity. Although the woman may initiate this discussion, often the nurse can best assess the woman's (and her partner's) understanding by providing some general information followed by some tactful questions.

## Nursing Diagnosis

The key nursing diagnosis will probably be health-seeking behaviors: information on sexuality related to expressed desire to learn more about changes in sexual functioning and about family planning following childbirth.

## Nursing Plan and Implementation

For the teaching plan to be effective the nurse first establishes rapport with the couple and promotes an environment that is conducive to teaching and discussion. It is helpful to provide privacy during the session so that the couple feels free to ask questions without fear of interruption. The format is generally a question-and-answer or discussion approach.

## Client Goals

At the completion of the teaching the couple will be able to

1. Discuss the changes in the woman's body that affect sexual activity.
2. Formulate alternative approaches to sexual activity based on an understanding of these changes.
3. Identify the length of time it is advisable to wait before resuming sexual activity.
4. Discuss information needed to make contraceptive choices.

## *Teaching Plan*

| CONTENT | TEACHING METHOD |
|---|---|
| Present information about changes that may affect sexual activity, including the following:<br>• Tenderness of the vagina and perineum<br>• Presence of lochia and the healing process<br>• Dryness of the vagina<br>• Breast engorgement and tenderness<br>• Escape of milk during sexual activity | Discussion is a logical approach. It may be useful to make a universal statement and link it with a question to determine a couple's initial level of knowledge. For example, "Many women experience vaginal dryness when they resume intercourse for the first several weeks after childbirth. Are you familiar with this change and the cause for it?"<br>Use the information gained during this discussion to determine the depth to which to cover the material. Avoid a patronizing tone. |
| Discuss healing at the placental site; stress that the presence of lochia indicates that healing is not yet complete. Point out that because the vagina is "hormone-poor" postpartally, vaginal dryness may be problematic. Dryness can be avoided by using a water-soluble lubricant. Escape of milk during sexual activity can be minimized by having the breastfeeding mother nurse immediately beforehand. | Provide printed information to clarify content and serve as a resource for the couple following discharge. |
| Discuss the importance of contraception even during the early postpartal period. Provide information on the advantages and disadvantages of different methods. The woman's body needs adequate time to heal and recover from the stress of pregnancy and childbirth. Couples who are opposed to contraception may choose abstinence at this time. | Have samples of different types of contraceptives available. Provide literature on specific contraceptive methods. |
| Discuss impact of fatigue and the new baby's schedule on the woman's feelings of desire. Refer the couple to physician or certified nurse-midwife for additional information if needed. | Many couples are unprepared for the impact of fatigue and the baby on lovemaking. Information enables the couple to anticipate this impact. Allow sufficient time for questions. |

## Evaluation

Evaluate the couple's learning by providing time for discussion and questions. If the couple indicates that they plan to use a particular contraceptive method, ask them about aspects of the method to ascertain that they have correct and complete information.

chances for the new mother to socialize, share her concerns, and receive encouragement. Because baby-sitting arrangements may be difficult or expensive, it is desirable to provide child care for newborns and siblings; in some instances infants may remain with mothers in the class.

Many parents today look to the Internet for information and advice. Criteria that suggest that Internet information is reliable and of high quality include affiliation with a university medical or nursing school; inclusion of authors' credentials, education, board certification, and affiliations; referencing of information; currency of information; similarity of information when compared with other sources, and easy accessibility (Lamp & Howard, 1999).

# Chapter Review

## CHAPTER HIGHLIGHTS

- The overall goal of postpartal home visits is to enhance opportunities for smooth transition of the new family. The home visit provides opportunities for assessment, teaching, and fostering a caring relationship with new families.
- Professional nursing has a role in establishing and maintaining excellence in care for the new family after discharge from the birthing center.
- Nurses need to act proactively to maintain their safety when making home visits by exercising reasonable caution and remaining alert to environmental cues.
- Nursing goals during home visits include reinforcement of daily newborn care, maintenance of neutral thermal environment, promotion of adequate hydration and nutrition, prevention of complications, promotion of safety, and enhancement of attachment and family knowledge of child care.
- Essential care during a home visit includes assessments of the vital signs, weight, overall color, intake and output, umbilical cord and circumcision, newborn nutrition, parent education, and attachment.
- The physician or pediatric nurse practitioner should be notified if there is evidence of redness around the umbilicus, bright-red bleeding or puslike drainage near the cord stump, or the umbilicus remains unhealed.
- Following a circumcision, the newborn must be observed closely for inability to void and signs of infection.
- Signs of illness in newborns include temperature above 38.4°C (101°F) or below 36.1°C (97°F), more than one episode of forceful vomiting, refusal of two feedings in a row, lethargy, cyanosis with or without a feeding, and absence of breathing for longer than 15 seconds.
- Screening for galactosemia, hemocystinuria, hypothyroidism, phenylketonuria, and sickle cell anemia is done on all newborns in the first 1 to 3 days, with a second blood specimen drawn after 7 to 14 days.
- Signs of illness in mothers include mastitis, excessive or foul-smelling lochia, failure of fundus to descend at anticipated rate, temperature of 100.4°F (38°C) or above, elevation of blood pressure, and tenderness, redness, or pain in the legs.
- To prevent sore nipples the nurse can encourage the breastfeeding mother to nurse frequently, to change the infant's position regularly, and to allow her nipples to air dry after breastfeeding.
- Sexual intercourse may resume once the episiotomy is healed and lochial flow has stopped. Couples should be forewarned of possible changes. For example, the vagina may be "dry," fatigue may inhibit desire, or the woman's breasts may leak during orgasm.

## CHAPTER REFERENCES


Alteneder, R. R., & Hartzell, D. (1997). Addressing couples sexuality concerns during the childbearing period: Use of the PLISSIT Model. *Journal of Obstetric, Gynecologic, and Neonatal Nursing, 26*(6), 651–8.

American Academy of Pediatrics, Committee on Fetus and Newborn. (1995). Hospital stay for healthy term newborns. *Pediatrics, 96*(4, Pt. 1), 788–790.

American College of Obstetricians and Gynecologists. (2000). *Breastfeeding: Maternal and infant aspects* (ACOG Educational Bulletin No. 258). Washington, DC: Author.

Bocar, D. L. (1997). Combining breastfeeding and employment: Increasing success. *Journal of Perinatal and Neonatal Nursing, 11* (2), 23–43.

Bragg, E. J., Rosenn, B. M., Khoury, J. C., Miodovnik, M., & Siddiqi, T. A. (1997). The effect of early discharge after vaginal delivery on neonatal readmission rates. *Obstetrics and Gynecology, 89*(6), 930–933.

Braveman, P., Egerter, S., Pearl, M., Marchi, K., & Miller, C. (1995). Problems associated with early discharge of newborn infants. Early discharge of newborns and mothers: A critical review of the literature. *Pediatrics, 96*(4, Pt. 1), 716–726.

Cady, R. (1999). Telephone triage: Avoiding the pitfalls. *Maternal-Child Nursing, 24*(4), 209.

Carpenter, J. A. (1998). Shortening the short stay. *AWHONN Lifelines, 2*(1), 29–34.

Catz, C., Hanson, J. W., Simpson, L., & Yaffe, S. J. (1995). Summary of workshop: Early discharge and neonatal hyperbilirubinemia. *Pediatrics, 96*(4, Pt. 1), 743–745.

Durkin, N., & Wilson, C. (1999). Simple steps to keep yourself safe. *Home Healthcare Nurse, 17*(7), 430–435.

Fishbein, E. G., & Burggraf, E. (1998). Early postpartum discharge: How are mothers managing? *Journal of Obstetric, Gynecologic, and Neonatal Nursing, 27*(2), 142–150.

Lamp, J. M., & Howard, P. A. (1999). Guiding parents' use of the Internet for newborn education. *American Journal of Maternal-Child Nursing, 24,* 33–36.

Lauwers, J., & Shinskie, D. (2000). *Counseling the nursing mother: A lactation consultant's guide* (3rd ed.). Boston: Jones & Bartlett.

Lawrence, R. A. (1994). *Breastfeeding: A guide for the medical profession* (4th ed.). St. Louis: Mosby.

Locklin, M. P., & Jansson, M. J. (1999). Home visits: Strategies to protect the breastfeeding newborn at risk. *Journal of Obstetric, Gynecologic, and Neonatal Nursing, 28,* 33–40.

Lowdermilk, D. (1995, December 14–15). *AWHONN perinatal home care guidelines: An overview.* Paper presented at the perinatal home care conference. New Orleans, LA.

Riordan, J., & Auerbach, K. (1999). *Breastfeeding and human lactation.* (2nd ed.). Boston: Jones & Bartlett.

Soskolne, E. I., Schumacher, R., Fyock, C., Young, M. L., & Schork, A. (1996). The effect of early discharge and other factors on readmission rates of newborns. *Archives of pediatric and adolescent medicine* 150, 373–78.


## CONTEMPORARY MATERNAL-NEWBORN NURSING ON-LINE

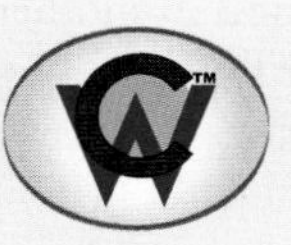

Additional interactive resources, including animations and video, for this chapter can be found on the Companion Website at http://www.prenhall.com/ladewig. Click on Chapter 29 and "Begin" to select the activities for this chapter.

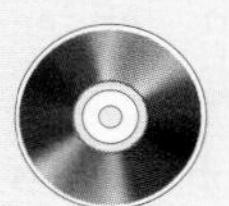

For NCLEX review questions and an audio glossary, access the accompanying CD-ROM in this book.

Chapter 30

# The Postpartal Family at Risk

*With hospital stays lasting only a couple of days, and most of that time being used to recover from labor and birth, many new parents arrive home needing lots of information and support. Our childbirth education classes have cut out the parenting information that they used to teach, and our birthing units all discontinued the newborn care class they sponsored, so there is a big gap in the "what do I do with this newborn?" area. Fortunately, in my community, the home care agency provides nurses like me to fill that gap. My clients receive a minimum of two postpartum well-baby visits, and more if a specific problem is identified. At the end of my day I always wonder about the new moms, dads, and babies that don't have this type of follow-up care. It is so needed.*

—Home Care/Postpartum Nurse

## OBJECTIVES

- Describe assessment of the postpartum woman for predisposing factors, signs, and symptoms of various postpartum complications.
- Summarize the preventive measures for various complications of the postpartum period that should be incorporated into nursing care of the postpartum woman.
- List the causes of and appropriate nursing interventions for hemorrhage during the postpartal period.
- Develop a nursing care plan that reflects a knowledge of etiology, pathophysiology, and current medical management for the woman experiencing postpartum hemorrhage, reproductive tract infection, urinary tract infection, mastitis, thromboembolic disease, or a postpartal psychiatric disorder.
- Evaluate the woman's knowledge of self-care measures, signs of complications to be reported to the primary care provider, and measures to prevent recurrence of complications.
- Describe the role of telephone follow-up and home visits in the extended care of postpartum families at risk.

## KEY TERMS

| | |
|---|---|
| Early postpartal hemorrhage | 800 |
| Endometritis or metritis | 806 |
| Late postpartal hemorrhage | 800 |
| Mastitis | 813 |
| Pelvic cellulitis (parametritis) | 806 |
| Peritonitis | 806 |
| Puerperal infection | 805 |
| Puerperal morbidity | 806 |
| Subinvolution | 803 |
| Thrombophlebitis | 816 |
| Uterine atony | 800 |

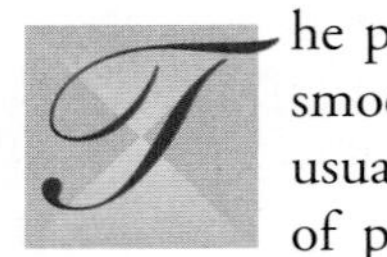

The postpartal period is typically viewed as a smooth, uneventful transition time—and it usually is. However, the nurse must be aware of problems that may develop postpartally and their implications for the childbearing family.

# Nursing Care Management of the Postpartal Family at Risk

## Hospital-Based Care

Ongoing comprehensive nursing assessment of postpartal clients is an important aspect of care. Systematic data collection allows the nurse to note the normality of findings and identify early signs of complications that might necessitate a longer hospital stay. Data collected before hospital discharge provide baseline findings against which subsequent data, collected by telephone or home visits, can be evaluated.

Signs and symptoms of many postpartal complications (late hemorrhage, mastitis, thromboembolic disease, major depression) typically occur only after the woman has returned home; they may appear even though she met criteria for early discharge. Consequently, it is critical that predischarge teaching for the woman and her partner (or her support person) include signs of postpartal complications; findings to report to her physician or certified nurse-midwife; and preventive measures, if available. Written instructions to supplement any discussion will be of great value in the early weeks at home with a newborn, when life can be chaotic and instructions may be forgotten. The family should have telephone numbers for postpartum follow-up services and other resources to answer questions. By communicating an attitude of willingness to answer questions and listen to concerns, the nurse enhances the parents' comfort in making calls later for what they might otherwise perceive as issues too trivial to bother someone about.

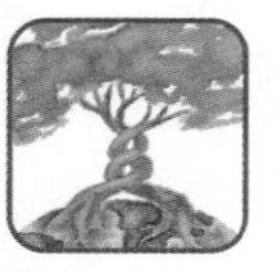

## Community-Based Nursing Care

Telephone or home visit follow-up may facilitate earlier recognition of, and thus earlier medical intervention for, such complications than might otherwise be possible. (See Chapter 29 for a more detailed discussion of home care for the postpartum family.)

# Care of the Woman with Postpartal Hemorrhage

Hemorrhage in the postpartal period is described as either early (immediate) or late (delayed) postpartal hemorrhage. **Early postpartal hemorrhage** occurs in the first 24 hours after childbirth. **Late postpartal hemorrhage** occurs from 24 hours to 6 weeks after birth. The traditional definition of postpartal hemorrhage has been a blood loss of greater than 500 mL of blood following childbirth. That definition is currently being questioned, however, because careful quantification indicates that the average blood loss in a vaginal birth is actually greater than 500 mL, and the average blood loss after cesarean childbirth exceeds 1000 mL. Some clinicians believe that postpartal hemorrhage can be objectively and reliably defined as either a decrease in the hematocrit of 10 points between the time of admission and the time postbirth or the need for fluid replacement following childbirth (American College of Obstetricians and Gynecologist [ACOG], 1998). Clinical estimation of blood loss at childbirth is difficult because blood mixes with amniotic fluid and is obscured as it oozes onto sterile drapes or is sponged away; without vigilance, it may be difficult over the next hours to appreciate the significance of slow, steady blood loss.

### HINTS FOR PRACTICE

Women who are natural redheads tend to experience heavier bleeding after childbirth.

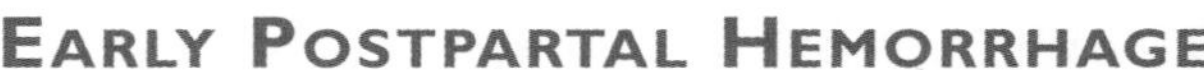

## Early Postpartal Hemorrhage

The normal mechanism for hemostasis after delivery of the placenta is contraction of the interlacing uterine muscles to occlude the open sinuses that previously brought blood into the placenta. Absence of prompt and sustained uterine contractions (uterine atony) can result in significant blood loss. Other causes of postpartal hemorrhage include laceration of the genital tract; episiotomy; retained placental fragments; vulvar, vaginal, or subperitoneal hematomas; uterine inversion; and coagulation disorders.

### Uterine Atony

**Uterine atony** (relaxation of the uterus) accounts for 80% to 90% of early postpartal hemorrhage (Gonik, 1999). Although uterine atony can occur after any childbirth, its contributing factors include the following:

- Overdistension of the uterus due to multiple gestation, hydramnios, or a large infant (macrosomia)
- Rapid or prolonged labor, which indicates that the uterus is contracting abnormally
- Oxytocin augmentation or induction of labor
- Grand multiparity, because stretched uterine musculature contracts less vigorously
- Use of anesthesia or other drugs, such as magnesium sulfate and terbutaline, that cause the uterus to relax
- Intra-amniotic infection
- Pregnancy-induced hypertension (PIH)
- Asian or Hispanic heritage

Hemorrhage from uterine atony may be slow and steady rather than sudden and massive. The blood may escape the vagina or collect in the uterus, evident as large clots. Because of the increased blood volume associated with pregnancy, changes in maternal blood pressure and pulse may not occur until blood loss has been significant. The woman with PIH is an exception to this finding because she does not have the normal hypervolemia of pregnancy and cannot tolerate even normal postchildbirth blood loss.

Ideally, postpartal hemorrhage is prevented, beginning with adequate prenatal care, good nutrition, avoidance of traumatic procedures, risk assessment, early recognition, and management of complications as they arise. Any woman at risk should be typed and cross matched for blood and have intravenous lines in place with needles suitable for blood transfusion (18-gauge minimum).

After expulsion of the placenta, the fundus is palpated to ensure that it is firmly contracted. If it is not firm (if it is boggy), fundal massage is performed until the uterus contracts. Fundal massage is painful for the woman who has not received regional anesthesia; consequently, she will need explanation for why this uncomfortable procedure is necessary and support as massage is initiated. If bleeding is excessive, the clinician will likely order intravenous oxytocin at a rapid infusion rate and may elect to do a bimanual massage (Figure 30–1A♦). Other uterine stimulants may be necessary to manage postpartal uterine atony. Table 30–1 summarizes critical nursing information about

Text continues on page 803.

## HINTS FOR PRACTICE

As you know, bogginess indicates that the uterus is not contracting well, which results in increased uterine bleeding. This blood may remain in the uterus and form clots or may result in increased flow. In assessing the amount of blood loss, you must first massage the uterus until it is firm and then express clots. Do not be misled by the firmness of a woman's uterus. Significant bleeding can have causes other than uterine atony. To accurately determine the amount of blood loss, it is not sufficient to assess only the perineal pad. You should also ask the woman to turn on her side so you can assess underneath her for pooling of blood.

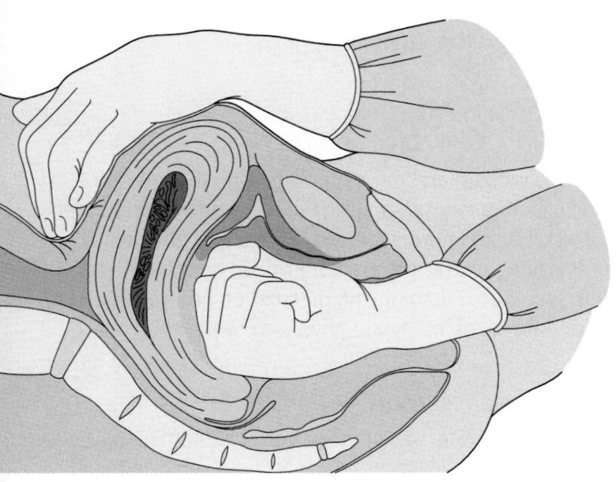

A

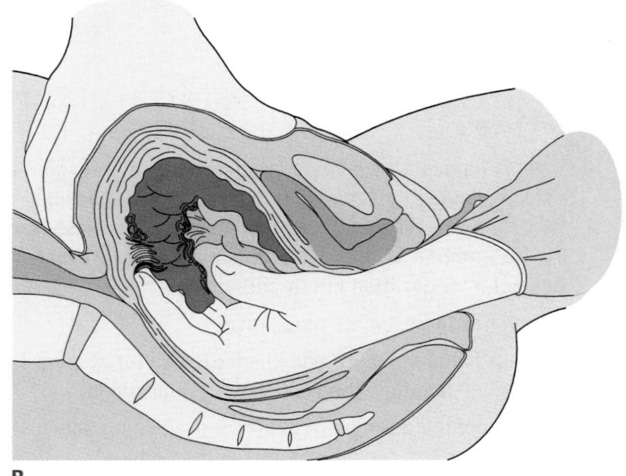

B

**FIGURE 30–1** ♦ **A,** Manual compression of the uterus and massage with the abdominal hand usually will effectively control hemorrhage from uterine atony. **B,** Manual removal of placenta. The fingers are alternately abducted, adducted, and advanced until the placenta is completely detached. Both procedures are performed only by the medical clinician. *Source:* Adapted from Cunningham, F. G., MacDonald, P. C., & Gant, N. F. [Eds.] (1989). *Williams obstetrics* (18th ed., pp. 417–418). Norwalk, CT: Appleton & Lange.

**TABLE 30–1 Uterine Stimulants Used to Prevent and Manage Uterine Atony**

| Drug | Dosing Information | Contraindications | Expected Effects | Side Effects |
|---|---|---|---|---|
| Oxytocin (Pitocin, Syntocinon) | IV use: 10–40 units in 500–1000 mL crystalloid fluid @ 50 mU/min administration rate. Onset: immediate. Duration: 1 h. **IV bolus administration not recommended.** | | Rhythmic uterine contractions that help to prevent or reverse pospartal hemorrhage caused by uterine atony. | Uterine hyperstimulation, mild transient hypertension, water intoxication rare in postpartum use. |
| Methylergonovine malaeate (Methergine) | IM use: 10–20 units. Onset: 3–5 min. Duration: 2–3 hours. IM use: 0.2 mg q2–4h. Onset: 2–5 min. Duration: 3 h (× 5 dose maximum). PO use: 0.2 mg q6–12h. Onset: 7–15 min. Duration: 3 h (× 1 week). **IV administration not recommended.** | Women with labile or high blood pressure or known sensitivity to drug. | Sustained uterine contractions that help to prevent or reverse pospartal hemorrhage caused by uterine atony; management of postpartal subinvolution. | Hypertension, dizziness, headache, flushing/hot flashes, tinnitus, nausea and vomiting, palpitations, chest pain. Overdose or hypersensitivity is recognized by seizures; tingling and numbness of fingers and toes from vasconstrictive effect, leading rarely to gangrene; hypertension; weak pulse; chest pain. |
| Ergonovine maleate (Ergotrate Maleate) | IM use: 0.2 mg q2–4h. Onset: 7 min. Duration: 3 h (5 dose maximum). PO use: 0.2 mg q6–12h. Onset: 15 min. Duration: 3 h (× 2–7 days). **IV administration not recommended.** | Women with labile or high blood pressure or known sensitivity to drug. | Sustained uterine contractions that help to prevent or reverse postpartal hemorrhage caused by uterine atony; management of postpartal subinvolution. | Hypertension, dizziness, headache, nausea and vomiting, chest pain. Hypersensitivity is noted on systemic vasoconstrictive effects: seizure, chest pain, and tingling and numbness of fingers and toes that lead rarely to gangrene. |
| Prostaglandin ($PGF_{2a}$, Hemabate, Prostin/15M) | IM use: 0.25 mg repeated up to maximum 5 doses; may be repeated q15–90min. Physician may elect to administer by direct intramyometrial injection. | Women with active cardiovascular, renal, liver disease, or asthma or with known hypersensitivity to drug. | Control of refractory cases of postpartal hemorrhage caused by uterine atony; generally used after failed attempts at control of hemorrhage with oxytoxic agents. | Nausea, vomiting, diarrhea, headache, flushing, bradycardia, bronchospasm, wheezing, cough, chills, fever. |

## IMPLICATIONS FOR NURSING MANAGEMENT OF THE POSTPARTAL WOMAN RECEIVING UTERINE STIMULANTS

- Assess fundus for evidence of contraction and amount of uterine bleeding at least q10–15min × 1–2 h after administration, then q30–60min until stable. **More frequent assessments are determined by the woman's condition or by orders of the physician or certified nurse-midwife.**
- Weigh pads to estimate blood loss.
- Monitor blood pressure and pulse q15 min for at least 1 h after administration, then q30–60 min until stable.
- Note expected duration of action of drug being administered and take care to recheck fundus at that time.
- When the drug is ineffective, the fundus remains atonic (boggy or uncontracted), and bleeding continues, massage the fundus. If massage fails to cause sustained contraction, notify the physician or certified nurse-midwife immediately.
- Monitor woman for signs of known side effects of the drug; report to physician or certified nurse-midwife if side effects occur.
- Remind the woman and her support person that uterine cramping is an expected result of these drugs and that medication is available for discomfort. Administer analgesic medications as needed for pain relief. Provide nonpharmacologic comfort measures. If analgesic medication ordered is insufficient for pain relief, notify the physician or certified nurse-midwife.

*When Prostaglandin Is Used*

- Check temperature q1–2h and/or after chill. Administer antipyretic medication as ordered for prostaglandin-induced fever.
- Auscultate breath sounds frequently for signs of adverse respiratory effects.
- Assess for nausea, vomiting, and diarrhea. Administer antiemetic and antidiarrheal medications as ordered. (In some settings, women are premedicated with these drugs.)

the use of uterine stimulants. The need for intravenous fluid replacement and blood transfusion is determined on the basis of hemoglobin and hematocrit results.

Vessel ligation may be used to slow blood loss and allow normal clotting mechanisms to occur (ACOG, 1998; Bowes, 1999). Arterial embolization may be used when the bleeding is not immediately life threatening. In severe, uncontrolled hemorrhage, surgical management may be the only alternative.

## Lacerations of the Reproductive Tract

Early postpartum hemorrhage is associated with lacerations of the perineum, vagina, or cervix. Several factors predispose women to higher risk of reproductive tract lacerations:

- Nulliparity
- Epidural anesthesia
- Precipitous childbirth
- Forceps- or vacuum-assisted birth
- Macrosomia

Thorough inspection of the reproductive tract by the birth attendant facilitates recognition and timely repair of most lacerations. Genital tract lacerations should be suspected when vaginal bleeding persists in the presence of a firmly contracted uterus. The nurse who suspects a laceration should notify the clinician so that the laceration can be immediately sutured to control the hemorrhage and restore the integrity of the reproductive tract. Episiotomies can be a source of postpartal blood loss. Episiotomy is an often underappreciated source of blood loss because of slow, steady bleeding. The risk for bleeding is increased with mediolateral episiotomies. (See discussion in Chapter 20.)

## Retained Placental Fragments

Retained placental fragments and a retained placental lobe may both cause immediate postpartal hemorrhage and are the most common causes of delayed hemorrhage. The most common cause of partial separation of the placenta with retention of fragments is massage of the fundus prior to placental separation, so this practice should be avoided.

Following birth, the placenta should always be inspected for intactness and for evidence of missing fragments or cotyledons on the maternal side and for vessels that transverse to the edge of the placenta outward along the membranes of the fetal side, which may indicate succenturiate placenta and a retained lobe. Based on the findings, uterine exploration may be required to remove missing fragments. This cause should be immediately suspected if bleeding persists and no lacerations are noted (Figure 30–1B♦).

## Vulvar, Vaginal, and Pelvic Hematomas

Hematomas occur as a result of injury to a blood vessel from birth trauma, often without noticeable trauma to the superficial tissue, or from inadequate hemostasis at the site of repair of an incision or laceration. The soft tissue in the area offers no resistance, and hematomas containing 250 to 500 mL of blood may develop rapidly. Signs and symptoms vary somewhat with the type of hematoma. Hematomas may be vulvar, vaginal (especially in the area of the ischial spines), or subperitoneal. The most frequently observed hematomas are of the vagina and vulva. Risk factors for hematomas include PIH, use of pudendal anesthesia, first full-term birth, precipitous labor, prolonged second stage of labor, macrosomia, forceps- or vacuum-assisted births, and history of vulvar varicosities.

Nonexpanding hematomas less than 5 cm in size are managed with the application of ice packs and analgesia. They usually resolve over several days. For larger hematomas and those that expand, surgical management is usually required; the hematoma is evacuated, the bleeding vessel ligated, and the wound closed, with or without vaginal packing. An indwelling urinary catheter may be necessary for 24 hours because voiding may be impossible with a vaginal pack in place (Cunningham, MacDonald, Gant, et al., 1997).

The hematoma site is an ideal medium for the growth of flora normally present in the genital tract. Consequently, broad-spectrum antibiotics are usually ordered to prevent infection or abscess.

## Late Postpartal Hemorrhage

Although early postpartal hemorrhage usually occurs within hours after birth, delayed hemorrhage generally occurs within 1 to 2 weeks after childbirth, most frequently as a result of subinvolution of the placental site due to retained placental fragments. Blood loss at this time may be excessive but rarely poses the same risk as that from immediate postpartal hemorrhage.

With **subinvolution,** the postpartum fundal height is greater than expected. In addition, lochial flow often fails to progress from rubra to serosa to alba normally. Lochia rubra that persists longer than 2 weeks postpartum is highly suggestive of subinvolution (Cunningham et al., 1997). Some women report scant brown lochia or irregular heavy bleeding. Leukorrhea, backache, and foul lochia may occur if infection is a cause. There may be a history of heavy early postpartal bleeding or difficulty in delivery of the placenta.

Subinvolution is most commonly diagnosed during the routine postpartal examination at 4 to 6 weeks. The woman may relate a history of irregular or excessive bleeding or describe the symptoms listed previously. An enlarged, softer-than-normal uterus palpated bimanually is an objective indication of subinvolution. Treatment includes oral administration of methylergonovine maleate 0.2 mg orally every 4 hours for 24 to 48 hours (see Drug Guide: Methylergonovine Maleate [Methergine], in Chapter 28). When uterine infection is present, antibiotics are also administered and the uterus is reevaluated in 2 weeks. If retained placenta is suspected or other treatment is ineffective, curettage may be indicated.

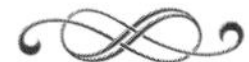

# Nursing Care Management

## Nursing Assessment and Diagnosis

The nurse carefully evaluates the woman's prenatal history and the results of ongoing assessment during labor and birth to identify factors that put the woman at risk for postpartal hemorrhage. Following birth, periodic assessment for evidence of vaginal bleeding is a major nursing responsibility. Regular and frequent assessment of fundal height and evidence of uterine tone or contractility will alert the nurse to the possible development or recurrence of hemorrhage. The nurse observes and documents vaginal bleeding to determine whether further medical intervention is needed. This assessment can be done visually, by pad counts, or by weighing the perineal pads.

When regional anesthesia is used, frequent assessment of the woman's perineum is important. Once the effects of anesthesia have subsided, vaginal and vulvar hematomas are generally associated with perineal pain. The pain is often intense, out of proportion or excessive, and usually from the woman's "stitches." If the hematoma is localized in the posterior vaginal area, rectal pressure may also be a presenting complaint. Hematomas that develop in the upper vagina may cause difficulty voiding because of pressure against the urinary meatus or urethra. Rather than automatically attributing complaints of perineal pain to the presence of an episiotomy, the nurse should examine the perineal area for signs of hematomas: ecchymosis; edema; tenseness of tissue overlying the hematomas; fluctuant, bulging mass at the introitus; and extreme tenderness to palpation. Estimating the size of the hematoma on first assessment of the perineum enables the nurse to better identify increases in size and the potential blood loss. The nurse notifies the physician or certified nurse-midwife if a hematoma is suspected.

Nursing diagnoses that may apply to a woman experiencing postpartal hemorrhage include the following:

- ***Knowledge deficit*** related to lack of information about signs of delayed postpartal hemorrhage
- ***Fluid volume deficit*** related to blood loss secondary to uterine atony, lacerations, or retained placental fragments

## Nursing Plan and Implementation

If the nurse detects a soft, boggy uterus, it is massaged until firm. If the uterus is not contracting well and appears larger than anticipated, the nurse may express clots during fundal massage. Once clots are removed, the uterus tends to contract more effectively.

If the woman seems to have a slow, steady, free flow of blood, the nurse begins to weigh the perineal pads (500 mL fluid weighs approximately 1 lb [454 g]) and monitors the woman's vital signs every 15 minutes, or more frequently if indicated. If the fundus is displaced upward or to one side because of a full bladder, the nurse encourages the woman to empty her bladder—or catheterizes her if she is unable to void—to allow for efficient uterine contractions.

During the initial postpartum period, the nurse maintains the vascular access started during labor in case additional fluid or blood is necessary. When physicians and certified nurse-midwives write orders that specify "discontinue IV after present bottle," the astute postpartum nurse will assess the consistency of the fundus and the presence of normal versus excessive lochia prior to discontinuing the infusion. If the assessments are not reassuring, the nurse continues the intravenous (IV) infusion and notifies the physician or certified nurse-midwife.

The nurse assesses the woman for signs of anemia, such as fatigue, pallor, headache, thirst, and orthostatic changes in pulse or blood pressure and reviews the results of all hematocrit determinations. All medical interventions, intravenous infusions, blood transfusions, oxygen therapy, and medications such as uterine stimulants are monitored as necessary and evaluated for effectiveness. The nurse also monitors urinary output to determine adequacy of fluid replacement and renal perfusion and reports amounts less than 30 mL/h to the physician. The nurse also helps the woman plan activities so that adequate rest is possible.

The woman who is experiencing anemia and fatigue related to hemorrhage may need assistance with self-care and progressive ambulation for several days. When she is able to be out of bed to shower, use of a shower chair permits independence while providing a measure of safety in case the woman experiences weakness or dizziness. The emergency call light should be easily accessible.

The mother may find it difficult to care for her baby because of the fatique associated with blood loss. The nurse can often find ways to promote maternal-infant attachment while accommodating the health needs of the mother. The mother may require additional assistance in caring for her infant. The nurse can work with the woman's partner and family to find ways to help the mother cope.

The nurse can decrease the risk of vulvar or vaginal hematoma by applying an ice pack to the woman's perineum during the first hour after birth and intermittently thereafter for the next 8 to 12 hours. If a hematoma develops despite preventive measures, a sitz bath after the first 12 hours will aid fluid absorption once the bleeding has stopped and will promote comfort, as will the judicious use of analgesics.

The women and her family or other support persons should receive clear, preferably written, explanations of the normal postpartum course, including changes in the lochia and fundus and signs of abnormal bleeding. Instructions for the prevention of bleeding should include fundal massage, ways to assess the fundal height and consistency, and inspection of any episiotomy and lacerations, if possible. The woman and her family are advised to contact her caregiver if any of the signs of postpartal hemorrhage occur. (See Key Facts to Remember: Signs of Postpartal Hemorrhage.) If iron supplementation is ordered, instructions for proper dosage should be provided to enhance absorption and avoid constipation and stomach upset.

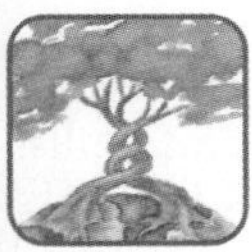

## Community-Based Nursing Care

The woman may continue to need help with self-care for a time. She should be advised to rise slowly to minimize the likelihood of orthostatic hypotension. Until she regains strength, she should be seated when holding the newborn.

The support person who assumes responsibility for grocery shopping and meal preparation needs advice about the importance of including foods high in iron in the daily menus. Having the woman indicate her preferences from a list of such foods will promote cooperation with the diet. The nurse also explains the rationale for continuing medications containing iron.

The woman should continue to count perineal pads for several days so that she can recognize any recurring problems with excessive blood loss. The debilitated condition and anemia associated with hemorrhage increase the woman's risk of puerperal infection. She and her caregivers should use good handwashing and minimize exposure to infection in the home. The nurse should give the woman's caregiver a list of the signs of infection and ensure that she or he understands the importance of alerting the physician immediately if signs occur.

A sense of emergency often accompanies late postpartal hemorrhage. Because it commonly occurs 1 to 2 weeks after birth, the couple is generally at home, involved in the day-to-day activities demanded by their new roles, when the unexpected, excessive bleeding begins. Quick decisions about child care arrangements must often be made so that the mother can return to the hospital. Both mother and father are likely to be alarmed by the excessive bleeding and concerned about her prognosis. There may be additional worries about separation from the newborn, especially when the mother is breastfeeding. The father may find himself torn between the needs of the mother and those of the newborn. Ideally, arrangements can be made to minimize separation of the family members.

**KEY FACTS TO REMEMBER**

***Signs of Postpartal Hemorrhage***

Excessive or bright-red bleeding

A boggy fundus that does not respond to massage

Abnormal clots

Any unusual pelvic discomfort or backache

Persistent bleeding in the presence of a firmly contracted uterus

Rise in the level of the fundus of the uterus

Increased pulse or decreased BP

Hematoma formation or bulging/shiny skin in the perineal area

Decreased level of consciousness

### Evaluation

Expected outcomes of nursing care include the following:

- Signs of postpartal hemorrhage are detected quickly and managed effectively.
- Maternal-infant attachment is maintained successfully.
- The woman is able to identify abnormal changes that might occur following discharge and understands the importance of notifying her caregiver if they develop.

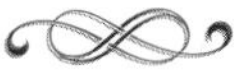

# Care of the Woman with a Reproductive Tract Infection or Wound

**Puerperal infection** is an infection of the reproductive tract associated with childbirth that occurs any time up to 6 weeks postpartum. The most common infection is metritis (endometritis), which is limited to the uterus. However, infection can spread by way of the lymphatic system to become a progressive disease resulting in parametrial cellulitis and peritonitis.

The standard definition of **puerperal morbidity,** established in the 1930s by the Joint Committee on Maternal Welfare, is a temperature of 38°C (100.4°F) or higher, with the temperature occurring on any 2 of the first 10 postpartum days, exclusive of the first 24 hours, and when taken by mouth by standard technique at least four times a day. However, serious infections can occur in the first 24 hours or may cause only persistent low-grade temperatures. Therefore, careful assessment of all postpartum women with elevated temperatures is essential.

Antibiotic therapy alone has not caused the decrease in postpartal morbidity and mortality seen today. Aseptic technique, fewer traumatic operative births, a better understanding of labor dystocia, improved surgical intervention, and a population generally at less risk from malnutrition and chronic debilitative disease have also contributed to this reduction.

The vagina and cervix of approximately 70% of all healthy pregnant women contain pathogenic bacteria that, alone or in combination, are sufficiently virulent to cause excessive infection. However, other factors must be present for infection to occur. Uterine infections are relatively uncommon following uncomplicated vaginal births, but they continue to be a major source of morbidity for women who give birth by cesarean, occurring in 12% to 51% of cases (Gibbs & Sweet, 1999).

## Postpartal Uterine Infection

Postpartal uterine infection is known variously as metritis, endometritis, endomyometritis, and endoparametritis. Risk factors for postpartal uterine infection include the following:

- Cesarean birth, which is the single most significant risk
- Prolonged rupture of the amniotic membranes
- Multiple vaginal examinations during labor
- Compromised health status (due to low socioeconomic status, anemia, obesity, cigarette smoking, use of illicit drugs or alcohol)
- Use of fetal scalp electrode or intrauterine pressure catheter for internal monitoring during labor
- Obstetric trauma (including episiotomy and lacerations of perineum, vagina, or cervix)
- Chorioamnionitis
- Preexisting bacterial vaginosis or *Chlamydia trachomatis* infection
- Instrument-assisted childbirth (vacuum or forceps)
- Manual removal of the placenta
- Lapses in aseptic technique by surgical staff

## Endometritis (Metritis)

**Endometritis** or **metritis,** an inflammation of the endometrium, may occur postpartally. After expulsion of the placenta, the placental site provides an excellent culture medium for bacterial growth. The remaining portion of the decidua is also susceptible to pathogenic bacteria because of its thinness (approximately 2 mm) and its large blood supply. The cervix may also be a bacterial breeding ground because of the multiple small lacerations attending normal labor and spontaneous birth. Both aerobic and anerobic organisms cause postpartal uterine infections. Late-onset postpartal endometritis or metritis is most commonly associated with genital mycoplasmas and *Chlamydia trachomatis. C. trachomatis* has a longer replication time and latency period than other bacteria and are not consistently eradicated by antibiotics used for early postpartal infections.

In mild cases of endometritis the woman generally has discharge that is either scant or profuse, bloody, and foul smelling. In more severe cases, she also has uterine tenderness; sawtooth temperature spikes, usually between 38.3 and 40°C (101 and 104°F); tachycardia; and chills. Foul-smelling lochia is cited as a classic sign of endometritis, but in the case of infection with β-hemolytic streptococcus, the lochia may be scant and odorless (Gibbs & Sweet, 1999).

## Pelvic Cellulitis (Parametritis) and Peritonitis

**Pelvic cellulitis (parametritis)** is infection involving the connective tissue of the broad ligament or, in more severe forms, the connective tissue of all the pelvic structures. The infection generally ascends upward in the pelvis by way of the lymphatics in the uterine wall but may also occur if pathogenic organisms invade a cervical laceration that extends upward into the connective tissue of the broad ligament—a direct pathway into the pelvis.

A pelvic abscess may form in the case of postpartal **peritonitis** (infection involving the peritoneal cavity) and is most commonly found in the uterine ligaments, the cul-de-sac of Douglas, and the subdiaphragmatic space. Pelvic cellulitis may be a secondary result of pelvic vein thrombophlebitis. This condition occurs when the clot, usually in the right ovarian vein, becomes infected and the wall of the vein breaks down from necrosis, spilling the infection into the connective tissues of the pelvis.

A woman with parametritis may demonstrate a variety of symptoms, including marked high temperature (38.9 to 40°C [102 to 104°F], chills, malaise, lethargy, abdominal pain, subinvolution of the uterus, tachycardia, and

## EVIDENCE-BASED PRACTICE

### Postpartum Infection

Yolanda had a cesarean birth 2 days ago. Her incision is clean, with staples intact, but she is complaining of deep pain and is very tender to your palpation of the fundus; when her temperature spikes to 102.5°F, you contact her physician.

The physician diagnoses endometritis and orders gentamicin and clindamycin administered intravenously. You check for drug allergies and administer the medications as ordered. During the pharmacist's rounds later in the shift, you ask why these two drugs were ordered. In other words, is there any evidence to indicate that these drugs are more effective than another combination of antibiotics?

The pharmacist explains that there are convincing data from 41 trials reviewed by the Cochrane Collaborative (French & Smaill, 2000) that combining gentamicin and clindamycin is effective treatment of endrometritis. This systematic review also showed that there was no difference in the incidence of allergic reactions among the various antibiotics studied; no treatment form has fewer side effects.

Finally, you learn that there is no evidence to support oral antibiotic therapy following completion of the intravenous therapy if the woman has uncomplicated endometritis. You will raise this issue with Yolanda's physician as you coordinate the plan for her discharge. If the physician prescribes oral antibiotic therapy, how will you respond? Are there cases in which a woman who has received the prescribed treatment receive additional medication that the evidence says is unnecessary? How does this affect the broader issue of antibiotic resistance? And what is the professional's responsibility to use resources wisely?

#### Reference

French, L. M., & Smaill, F. M. (2000). Antibiotic regimens for endometritis after delivery. *Cochrane Library*, 2. Oxford: Update Software.

local and referred rebound tenderness. If peritonitis develops, the woman becomes acutely ill, with severe pain, marked anxiety, high fever, rapid and shallow respirations, pronounced tachycardia, excessive thirst, abdominal distension, nausea, and vomiting.

## Perineal Wound Infections

Given the degree of bacterial contamination that occurs with normal vaginal birth, it is surprising that more women do not have infections of the episiotomy or repaired lacerations of the perineum, vagina, or vulva. When perineal wound infection occcurs, it is recognized by the classic signs: redness, warmth, edema, purulent drainage, and, later, gaping of the wound that had previously been well approximated. Local pain may be severe. Infected perineal wounds, like other infected wounds, are treated by draining purulent material. Sutures are removed, and the wound is left open. A regimen of broad-spectrum antibiotics is used. When the surface of the wound is free of infectious exudate and tissue granulation is evident, the mother returns for secondary closure of the wound under regional anesthesia (Cunningham et al., 1997).

## Cesarean Wound Infection

The infection rate following cesarean births is 4% to 12%, with the highest rate occurring after emergency cesarean because there is more traumatization of the tissue (Gibbs & Sweet, 1999). Signs of an abdominal wound infection, which may not be evident until after discharge, include erythema; warmth; skin discoloration; edema; tenderness; purulent drainage, sometimes mixed with sanguineous liquid; and gaping of the wound edges. Fever, pain, malodorous lochia, and other systemic signs are also common. Culture of the wound drainage commonly reveals mixed pathogens.

## Clinical Therapy

The infection site and causative organism are diagnosed by careful history and complete physical examination, blood tests, aerobic and anaerobic endometrial cultures (although cultures may be of limited value because multiple organisms are usually present), and urinalysis to rule out urinary tract infection. When a localized infection develops, it is treated with antibiotics, sitz baths, and analgesics as necessary for pain relief. If an abscess has developed or a stitch site is infected, the suture is removed and the area is allowed to drain. Packing the wound with saline gauze twice to three times daily, using aseptic technique, allows removal of necrotic debris when packing is removed. Broad-spectrum antibiotic coverage is used to treat postpartal wound infections (Gibbs & Sweet, 1999).

Endometritis (metritis) is treated by aggressive administration of antibiotics. With appropriate antibiotic coverage, improvement should occur within a few days. Antibiotics are generally continued until the woman is afebrile for 24 to 48 hours. The route and dosage are determined by the severity of the infection. Careful monitoring is also necessary to prevent the development of a more serious infection.

Parametritis and peritonitis are treated with intravenous antibiotics. Broad-spectrum antibiotics effective against the most commonly occurring causative organisms are chosen initially, until the results of culture and sensitivity reports are available. If multiple organisms are present, the approach to antibiotic therapy is continued unless no improvement is observed; then the antibiotic is changed.

An abscess is frequently manifested by the development of a palpable mass and may be confirmed with ultrasound. It usually requires incision and drainage to prevent rupture into the peritoneal cavity and the possible development of peritonitis. After drainage of the abscess, the cavity may be packed with iodoform gauze to promote drainage and facilitate healing.

The woman with a severe systemic infection is acutely ill and may require care in an intensive care unit. Supportive therapy includes maintenance of adequate hydration with intravenous fluids, analgesic medications, ongoing assessment of the infection, and possibly continuous nasogastric suctioning if paralytic ileus develops.

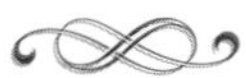

# Nursing Care Management

## Nursing Assessment and Diagnosis

The nurse should inspect the woman's perineum every 8 to 12 hours for signs of early infection. The REEDA scale helps the nurse remember to consider redness, edema, ecchymosis, discharge, and approximation. The nurse immediately reports any degree of induration (hardening) to the clinician. The nurse notes and reports the presence of fever, malaise, abdominal pain, foul-smelling lochia, tachycardia, and other signs of infection so that treatment can be instituted.

Nursing diagnoses that may apply to the women with a puerperal infection include the following:

- ***Risk for injury*** related to the spread of infection
- ***Pain*** related to the presence of infection
- ***Risk for altered parenting*** related to delayed parent-infant attachment secondary to woman's malaise and other symptoms of infection

## Nursing Plan and Implementation

### *Hospital-Based Nursing Care*

The nurse caring for a woman during the postpartal period is responsible for teaching the woman self-care measures that are helpful in preventing infection. The woman should understand the importance of perineal care, good hygiene practices to prevent contamination of the perineum (including wiping from front to back, changing perineal pads after voiding), and thorough handwashing. Once edema and perineal pain are under control, the nurse can also encourage sitz baths, which are cleansing and promote healing. Adequate fluid intake and a diet high in protein and vitamin C, which are necessary for wound healing, also help prevent infection.

If the woman is seriously ill, ongoing assessment of urine specific gravity and intake and output is necessary. The nurse also carefully administers antibiotics as ordered and regulates the intravenous fluid rate. Ongoing assessment of the woman's condition is vital to detect subtle changes in her health status. The nurse also addresses the woman's comfort needs related to hygiene, positioning, oral hygiene, and pain relief.

Promoting maternal-infant attachment can be difficult with the acutely ill woman. The nurse may provide pictures of the infant and keep the mother informed of the infant's well-being. See the Critical Pathway for the Woman with a Puerperal Infection, for specific nursing care measures.

## Community-Based Nursing Care

The woman with a puerperal infection needs assistance when she is discharged from the hospital. If the family cannot provide this home assistance, a referral to home care services is needed. Home care services should be contacted as soon as puerperal infection is diagnosed so that the nurse can meet with the woman for a family and home assessment and development of a home care plan.

The family needs instruction in the care of a newborn, including feeding, bathing, cord care, immunizations, and

Text continues on page 811.

## CRITICAL PATHWAY: *For the Woman with a Puerperal Infection*

| Category | 1–4 Hours Postpartum | 4–8 Hours Postpartum | 8–24 Hours Postpartum |
|---|---|---|---|
| **Referral** | Report from labor nurse if not continuing in an LDR room | Lactation consultation if needed | Home nursing referral if indicated<br>**Expected Outcomes**<br>Appropriate resources identified and utilized |
| **Assessment** | Postpartum assessment q ½ × 2, q1h × 2, then q4h, includes:<br>• Fundus firm, in midline, at or below umbilicus<br>• Lochia rubra <1 pad/hr: no free flow or passage of clots with massage<br>• Bladder: voids large amounts of urine spontaneously; bladder not palpable following voiding<br>• Perineum: sutures intact, no bulging or marked swelling, no c/o severe pain; minimal bruising may be present; if hemorrhoids present, no tenseness or marked engorgement; <2 cm diameter<br>• Breasts: soft, colostrum present<br>Vital signs:<br>• BP WNL; no hypotension; not >30 mm Hg systolic or 15 mm Hg diastolic over baseline<br>• Temperature: <38°C (100.4°F)<br>• Pulse: bradycardia normal; consistent with baseline<br>• Respirations: 12–20/min; quiet; easy<br>Comfort level: <3 on scale of 1 to 10 | Continue postpartum assessment q4h ×2, then q8h<br>• Assess for bowel sounds<br>• Assess lochia for color, odor, amount<br>Breasts: evaluate nipple status; should be no evidence of cracks or bruising<br>Observe feeding technique with newborn<br>Assess VS q8h; all WNL; report temp >38°C (100.4°F)<br>Continue assessment of comfort level q3–4h | Continue postpartum assessment q8h<br>Breasts: nipples should remain free of cracks, fissures, bruising<br>Feeding technique with newborn should be good or improving<br>Assess VS q4h; report temp >38°C (100.4°F)<br>Continue assessment of comfort level q3–4h<br>Continue s/s of infection (ie, episiotomy, endometritis, pelvic cellulitis, or peurperal peritonitis)<br>Inspect incision/episiotomy for redness, approximation, and drainage<br>Assess for signs of progressive infection (ie, uterine subinvolution, foul-smelling lochia, uterine tenderness, severe lower abdominal pain, fever, elevated WBC, malaise, chills, lethargy, tachycardia, nausea and vomiting, abdominal rigidity)<br>**Expected Outcomes**<br>Findings indicate infection identified, treated, and reduced or eliminated in timely manner<br>No additional complications found |
| **Comfort** | Institute comfort measures:<br>• Perineal discomfort peri-care, sitz baths, topical analgesics<br>• Hemorrhoids: sitz baths, topical analgesics, digital replacement of external hemorrhoids, side-lying or prone position<br>• Afterpains: prone with small pillow under abdomen; warm shower or sitz baths; ambulation<br>Administer pain medication _____ | Continue with pain management techniques | Continue with pain management techniques<br>Promote comfort by<br>• Ensuring adequate periods of rest<br>• Minimizing disturbing environmental stimuli<br>• Judicious use of analgesics and antipyretics<br>• Providing emotional support<br>• Using supportive nursing measures (ie, back rubs, instruction in relaxation techniques, maintenance of cleanliness, provision of diversional activities) |
| **Teaching/ psychosocial** | Explain postpartum assessments<br>Teach self-massage of fundus and expected findings<br>Instruct to call for assistance first time OOB and prn<br>Demonstrate peri-care, surgigator, sitz baths prn<br>Explain comfort measures<br>Begin newborn teaching (bulb suctioning, positioning, feeding, diaper change, cord care)<br>Orient to room if transferred from LDR room<br>Provide information on early postpartum period<br>If breastfeeding mother is unable to nurse, assist her in pumping her breasts to maintain adequate milk supply | Discuss psychologic changes of postpartum period<br>Stress need for frequent rest periods<br>Continue newborn teaching: soothing/comforting techniques, swaddling; return demonstrations indicate woman's understanding<br>Provide opportunities for questions and review; reinforce previous teaching<br>Breastfeeding: nipple care; air drying, lanolin; tea bags; proper latch-on technique<br>Bottle-feeding: supportive bra; ice bags, breast binder<br>**Expected Outcomes**<br>Client verbalizes/demonstrates understanding of teaching and related plan of care<br>Client incorporates teaching into self-care | Reinforce previous teaching: answer questions<br>Discuss need to take antibiotics until course completed<br>Discuss involution; anticipated physical changes in first 2 weeks postpartum; postpartum exercises; need to limit visitors<br>Breastfeeding/bottle-feeding:<br>• Explain milk production, letdown reflex, use of supplements, breast pumping, and milk storage<br>• If cannot breastfeed, assist mother with pumping her breasts<br>• Explain formula preparation and storage<br>Discuss sibling rivalry; mother should have plan for supporting siblings at home<br>Teaching evaluation completed |

ad lib, as desired; BSI, body substance isolation; CNM, certified nurse-midwife; dr, doctor; hep-lock, intravenous catheter that allows intermittent access; I/O, intake and output; IV, intravenous; LDR, labor, delivery, and recovery; meds, medications; OOB, out of bed; peri-care, perineal care; prn, as desired; s/s, signs and symptoms; vit C, vitamin C; VS, vital signs; WBC, white blood count; WNL, within normal limits.

| Category | 1–4 Hours Postpartum | 4–8 Hours Postpartum | 8–24 Hours Postpartum |
|---|---|---|---|
| **Therapeutic nursing interventions and reports** | Ice pack to perineum to decrease swelling and increase comfort<br>Straight cath prn × 1 if distended or voiding small amounts<br>If continues unable to void or voiding small amounts, insert Foley catheter and notify CNM or physician | Sitz baths prn<br>If woman Rh negative and infant Rh positive, RhoGAM workup; obtain consent; complete teaching<br>Obtain consent for rubella vaccine if indicated; explain purpose, procedure, implications<br>Obtain hematocrit<br>Determine rubella status<br>**Expected Outcomes**<br>Labs and cultures indicate infection reduced/resolved<br>Complications have been minimized | Continue sitz baths two to three times daily or surgigator<br>May shower if ambulating without difficulty<br>Obtain blood cultures per dr order if temp elevated<br>Obtain wound culture and assist with wound drainage and packing<br>Use principles of BSI<br>Promote normal wound healing by peri-care, wiping from front to back after each voiding, frequent changing of pads |
| **Activity** | Assistance when OOB first time, then prn<br>Ambulate ad lib<br>Rests comfortably between checks | Encourage rest periods<br>Ambulate ad lib; may leave birthing unit | Up ad lib<br>**Expected Outcomes**<br>Optimal comfort and activity maintained |
| **Nutrition** | Regular diet, high in vit C and protein<br>Fluid intake ≥2000 mL/day | Continue diet and fluids<br>**Expected Outcomes**<br>Nutritional needs met with emphasis on calories needed for healing | Continue diet and fluids<br>Increase calories by 500 kcal over non-pregnant state (200 kcal over pregnant intake) if breastfeeding<br>Return to normal caloric intake for non-pregnant state if bottle-feeding |
| **Elimination** | Voiding large amounts straw-colored urine | Voiding large quantities<br>May have bowel movement, assess bowel sounds | Monitor I/O, urine specific gravity, and level of hydration<br>**Expected Outcomes**<br>Intake and output WNL |
| **Medications** | Methergine 0.2 mg q4h prn if ordered<br>Stool softener _____<br>Tucks pads prn | Continue meds<br>Lanolin to nipples prn; tea bags to nipples if tender; heparin flush to hep-lock (if present) q8h or as ordered | IV antibiotics<br>Continue meds<br>May take own prenatal vitamins<br>RhoGAM administered if indicated<br>Rubella vaccine administered if indicated<br>**Expected Outcomes**<br>Infection successfully treated<br>Medications utilized to further support health |
| **Discharge planning/ home care** | Evaluate knowledge of normal postpartum, newborn care<br>Evaluate support systems | Discuss typical newborn schedule; plan for periods of rest<br>Birth certificate paperwork completed<br>Evaluate plans for transporting newborn; car seat used | Provide information regarding predisposing factors, s/s, and treatment<br>Discuss the value of a nutritious diet in promoting healing<br>Review hygiene practice (ie, correct wiping after voiding, and handwashing, to prevent the spread of infection)<br>Discuss home care routines to be used following postpartal infection<br>Review discharge instruction sheet and checklist<br>Describe postpartum and infection warning signs and when to call CNM or physician<br>Provide prescriptions; gift pack given to woman<br>Arrangements made for baby pictures if desired<br>Postpartum visit scheduled<br>Newborn check scheduled<br>**Expected Outcomes**<br>Woman participates in self-care and continued medication therapy<br>Discharge teaching complete with emphasis on follow-up care, adequate rest, and infant attachment |

| :ategory | 1–4 Hours Postpartum | 4–8 Hours Postpartum | 8–24 Hours Postpartum |
|---|---|---|---|
| **amily involvement** | Identify available support persons<br>Assess family perceptions of birth experience<br>Parenting: demonstrates culturally expected early parenting behaviors | Involve support persons in care, teaching; answer questions<br>Evidence of parental bonding behaviors apparent<br>Provide and maintain mother-infant interaction:<br>• Provide opportunities for the mother to see and hold her infant<br>• Encourage partner or support person to discuss infant with woman and to become involved in infant's care if the woman is not able to care for the infant | Continue to involve support persons in teaching<br>Evidence of parental bonding behaviors continued<br>Plans made for providing support to mother following discharge; support persons verbalize understanding of need for woman to rest, eat nutritionally, recover<br>**Expected Outcomes**<br>Family demonstrates understanding of resources<br>Support network identified<br>Family development unimpaired |
| **ate** | | | |

ignificant observations that should be reported. A well-›aby appointment should be scheduled. Breastfeeding nothers receiving antibiotics should be instructed to in-pect the infant's mouth for signs of thrush and to report he finding to their physician.

The mother should be instructed regarding activity, est, medications, diet, and signs and symptoms of com-›lications, and she should be scheduled for a return med-cal visit. She needs to know the importance of taking the entire course of prescribed antibiotics even though she nay begin to feel better before the bottle is empty. She also needs to be informed about the importance of pelvic est; that is, she should not use tampons or douches or nave intercourse until she has been examined by the ›hysician and told it is safe to resume those activities.

### Evaluation

Expected outcomes of nursing care include the following:

- The infection is quickly identified and treated successfully, without further complications.
- The woman understands the infection and the purpose of therapy; she cooperates with ongoing antibiotic therapy after discharge.
- Maternal-infant attachment is maintained.

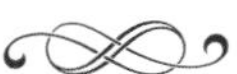

## Care of the Woman with a Urinary Tract Infection

The postpartal woman is at increased risk of developing urinary tract problems due to the normal postpartal diuresis, increased bladder capacity, decreased bladder sensitivity from stretching or trauma, and possible inhibited neural control of the bladder following the use of general or regional anesthesia and contamination from catheterization.

Emptying the bladder is vital. Women who have not sufficiently recovered from the effects of anesthesia cannot void spontaneously, and catheterization is necessary. Retention of residual urine, bacteria introduced at the time of catheterization, and a bladder traumatized by birth combine to provide an excellent environment for the development of cystitis.

### Overdistension of the Bladder

Overdistension occurs postpartally when the woman is unable to empty her bladder as a result of the predisposing factors previously identified. After the effects of regional anesthesia have worn off, postpartal urinary retention is highly indicative of urinary tract infection (UTI).

### Clinical Therapy

Overdistension in the early postpartal period is often managed by draining the bladder with a straight catheter as a onetime measure. If the overdistension recurs or is diagnosed later in the postpartal period, an indwelling catheter is generally ordered for 24 hours.

# Nursing Care Management

## Nursing Assessment and Diagnosis

The overdistended bladder appears as a large mass, reaching sometimes to the umbilicus and displacing the uterine fundus upward. Increased vaginal bleeding occurs, the fundus is boggy, and the woman may complain of cramping as the uterus attempts to contract. Some women also experience backache and restlessness.

Nursing diagnoses that may apply when a woman has difficulties with overdistension of the bladder include the following:

- ***Risk for infection*** related to urinary stasis secondary to overdistension
- ***Urinary retention*** related to decreased bladder sensitivity and normal postpartal diuresis

## Nursing Plan and Implementation

Diligent monitoring of the bladder during the recovery period and preventive health measures greatly reduce the chances for overdistension of the bladder. Encouraging the mother to void spontaneously and helping her use the toilet, if possible, or the bedpan, if she has received conductive anesthesia, prevents overdistension in most cases. The nurse assists the woman to a normal position for voiding (ie, sitting with the legs and feet lower than the trunk) and provides privacy to encourage voiding. The woman should receive medication for whatever pain she may be having before she attempts to void because pain may cause a reflex spasm of the urethra. Applying perineal ice packs after childbirth helps minimize edema, which may interfere with voiding. Pouring warm water over the perineum or having the woman void in the sitz bath may also be effective.

If catheterization becomes necessary, careful, meticulous aseptic technique is employed during catheter insertion. The vagina and vulva are traumatized to some degree by vaginal birth, and edema is common. Because this edema may obscure the urinary meatus, the nurse needs to be extremely careful in cleansing the vulva and inserting the catheter. It is imperative to discard a catheter that has inadvertently been introduced into the vagina and thus contaminated. Because catheterization is an uncomfortable procedure due to the postpartal trauma and edema of the tissue, the nurse should be careful and gentle not only in inserting the catheter but also in handling and cleaning the perineal area.

The catheter is clamped after draining the desired amount of urine and taped firmly to the woman's leg. The nurse takes the woman's vital signs before and after the procedure and notes the women's responses. The nurse then carefully documents the procedure and assessment findings. After an hour, the catheter may be unclamped and placed on gravity drainage. This technique protects the bladder and prevents rapid intra-abdominal decompression. When the indwelling catheter is removed, a urine specimen is often sent to the laboratory. The tip of the catheter may also be removed and sent for culture.

## Evaluation

Expected outcomes of nursing care include the following:

- The woman voids adequately.
- The woman does not develop infection due to stasis of urine.
- The woman actively incorporates self-care measures to decrease bladder overdistension.

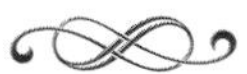

# Cystitis (Lower Urinary Tract Infection)

*Escherichia coli* has been demonstrated to be the causative agent in most cases of postpartal cystitis and pyelonephritis (in both lower and upper UTI). Generally, the infection ascends the urinary tract from the urethra to the bladder and then to the kidneys because vesiculoureteral reflux (backward flow of urine) forces contaminated urine into the renal pelvis.

# Clinical Therapy

When cystitis is suspected, a clean-catch midstream urine sample is obtained for microscopic examination, culture, and sensitivity tests. The specimen may require collection by the nurse with the woman on a bedpan because few postpartal women can collect a true midstream, clean-catch specimen without contaminating the specimen with lochia. A catheterized specimen is avoided when possible because of the increased risk of infection. When the bacterial concentration is greater than 100,000 colonies of the same organism per milliliter of fresh urine, infection is generally present. Counts between 10,000 and 100,000 suggest infection, particularly if clinical symptoms are noted.

In the clinical setting, antibiotic therapy is often initiated before culture and sensitivity reports are available.

Frequently used antibiotics include a preparation of trimethoprim and sulfamethoxazole (Bactrim, Septra), one of the short-acting sulfonamides, nitrofurantoin (Macrodantin), and, in the case of sulfa allergy, ampicillin. The antibiotic is changed later if indicated by the results of the sensitivity report. Antispasmodics or urinary analgesic agents, such as phenazopyridine hydrochloride (Pyridium), may be given to relieve discomfort.

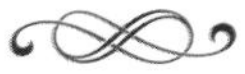

# Nursing Care Management

## Nursing Assessment and Diagnosis

Symptoms of cystitis often appear 2 to 3 days after childbirth. The initial symptoms of cystitis may include frequency, urgency, dysuria, and nocturia. Hematuria and suprapubic pain may also be present. A slightly elevated temperature may occur, but systemic symptoms are often absent.

When a UTI progresses to pyelonephritis, systemic symptoms usually occur, and the woman becomes acutely ill. Symptoms include chills, high fever, flank pain (unilateral or bilateral), nausea, and vomiting, in addition to all the signs of lower UTI. Costovertebral angle tenderness on palpation and pain may or may not be present. The nurse obtains a urine culture so that sensitivity can identify the causative organism.

Nursing diagnoses that may apply if a woman develops a UTI postpartally include the following:

- ***Pain*** with voiding related to dysuria secondary to infection
- ***Knowledge deficit*** related to lack of information about self-care measures to prevent UTI

## Nursing Plan and Implementation

Screening for asymptomatic bacteriuria in pregnancy should be routine. The nurse needs to encourage frequent emptying of the bladder during labor and postpartum to prevent overdistension and trauma to the bladder. Catheterization technique and nursing actions to prevent overdistension (previously discussed) also apply. The woman with pyelonephritis must understand the importance of follow-up care after discharge to prevent recurrence or further complications.

The nurse should advise the postpartal woman to continue good perineal hygiene after discharge, to maintain a good fluid intake (at least 8 to 10 8-oz glasses daily), especially of water, and to empty her bladder whenever she feels the urge to void, but at least every 2 to 4 hours while awake. Once sexual intercourse is resumed, the new mother should void before (to prevent bladder trauma) and following intercourse (to wash contaminents from the vicinity of the urinary meatus). Wearing underwear with a cotton crotch to facilitate air circulation also reduces the risk of UTI.

Acidification of the urine is thought to aid in preventing and managing UTI. The nurse thus advises the woman to avoid carbonated beverages, which increase the alkalinity of urine, and to drink unsweetened cranberry, plum, apricot, and prune juices, which increase the acidity of urine.

## Evaluation

Expected outcomes of nursing care include the following:

- Signs of UTI are detected quickly and the condition is treated successfully.
- The woman incorporates self-care measures to prevent the recurrence of UTI as part of her personal hygiene routine.
- The woman cooperates with any long-term therapy or follow-up.
- Maternal-infant attachment is maintained and the woman is able to care for her newborn effectively.

# Care of the Woman with Mastitis

**Mastitis** is an infection of the breast connective tissue that occurs primarily in lactating women. The usual causative organisms are *Staphylococcus aureus, Haemophilus parainfluenzae, H. influenzae,* and *Streptococcus* species. (Gibbs & Sweet, 1999). Because symptoms seldom occur before the second to fourth week postpartum, birthing unit nurses often are not fully aware of how uncomfortable and acutely ill the woman can be; they must ensure that all breastfeeding women are taught preventive techniques and ways of recognizing this condition if it develops.

The infection usually begins when bacteria invade the breast tissue. Often the tissue has been traumatized in some way (fissured or cracked nipples, overdistension, manipulation, milk stasis) and is especially susceptible to pathogenic invasion. The most common sources of these organisms are the infant's nose and throat, but other sources include the hands of the mother or birthing unit personnel and the woman's circulating blood.

Poor drainage of milk, lowered maternal defenses due to fatigue or stress, and poor hygiene practices make the

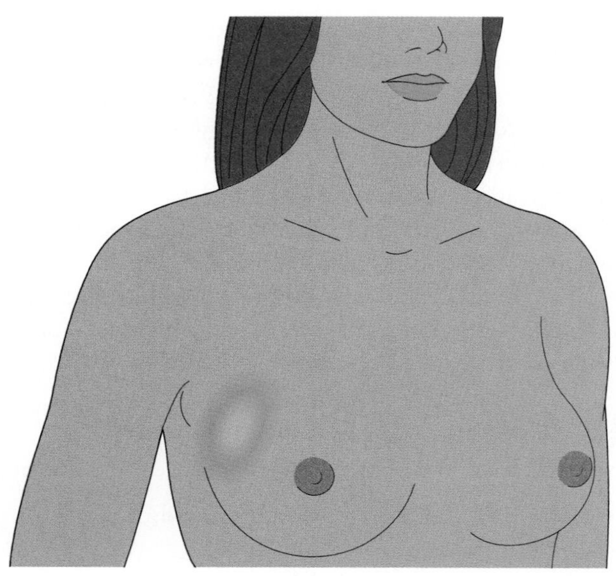

FIGURE 30–2 ♦ Mastitis. Erythema and swelling are present in the upper outer quadrant of the breast. Axillary lymph nodes are enlarged and tender.

woman susceptible to mastitis (Lauwers & Shinskie, 2000). Tight clothing, missed feedings, poor support of pendulous breasts, lack of regular breast pumping when away from the baby, and a baby who suddenly begins to sleep through the night can result in milk stasis, which is a milder inflammatory condition.

Infectious mastitis is a more serious infection, with fever, headache, flulike symptoms, and a warm, reddened, painful area of the breast, often wedge shaped because of the connective tissue septal divisions of the breast (Figure 30–2♦).

In other cases *Candida albicans* is the causative organism of mastitis, entering the breast through a small fissure or abrasion on the nipple. Signs include late-onset nipple pain, followed by shooting pain during and between feedings. Eventually, the skin of the affected breast becomes pink, flaking, and pruritic.

## Clinical Therapy

Diagnosis is usually based on history and physical examination; a culture and sensitivity may be done. A culture and sensitivity assessment of breast milk allows susceptibility-directed antibiotic therapy; a leukocyte count of 1 million/mL and bacterial colony count of greater than 10,000/mL is diagnostic (Gibbs & Sweet, 1999). Treatment involves bed rest (may be needed for the first several days), use of a supportive bra, frequent breastfeeding, local application of warm, moist-heat compresses, and analgesics (such as acetaminophen) as needed for discomfort. Nonsteroidal antiinflammatory agents are recommended to treat both fever and inflammation. Also, a 10-day course of antibiotics (usually a penicillinase-resistant penicillin) is completed (Johnson & Riddick, 2000). Improved outcome, decreased duration of symptoms, and decreased incidence of breast abscess result if the breasts continue to be emptied by either nursing or pumping. Thus continued breastfeeding is recommended in the presence of mastitis. The woman should be contacted within 24 hours of initiation of treatment to ensure that symptoms are subsiding (Lauwers & Shinskie, 2000). Early treatment may prevent the progression of milk stasis and noninfectious inflammation to mastitis; 10% of all mastitis cases result in abscess formation requiring aspiration (if small) or, more commonly but still rare, incision and drainage (Vogel, Hutchison, & Mitchell, 1999).

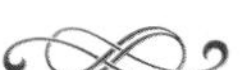

# Nursing Care Management

### Nursing Assessment and Diagnosis

Daily the nurse assesses breast consistency, skin color, surface temperature, nipple condition, and presence of pain to detect early signs of problems that may predispose a woman to mastitis. The nurse also observes the mother nursing her baby to ensure proper technique.

If an infection develops, the nurse assesses for contributing factors such as cracked nipples, poor hygiene, engorgement, supplemental feedings, change in routine or infant feeding pattern, abrupt weaning, and lack of proper breast support so that these factors can be corrected as part of the treatment plan.

Nursing diagnoses that may apply to the woman with mastitis include the following:

- ***Health seeking behaviors*** related to lack of information about appropriate breastfeeding practices
- ***Ineffective breastfeeding*** related to pain secondary to development of mastitis

### Nursing Plan and Implementation

Preventing mastitis is far simpler than treating it. Ideally mothers are instructed in proper breastfeeding technique prenatally. The nurse assists the mother to breastfeed soon after childbirth and reviews correct technique. Comanagement of breastfeeding between the nurse and a certified lactation specialist is often possible. Nurses need to encourage new mothers, even those not breastfeeding, to wear a good supportive bra at all times to prevent milk stasis, especially in the lower lobes.

Meticulous handwashing by the breastfeeding mother and all personnel is the primary measure in preventing epidemic nursery infections and subsequent maternal mastitis. Prompt attention to mothers who have blocked milk ducts eliminates stagnant milk as a growth medium for bacteria. If the mother finds that one area of her breast feels distended, she can rotate the position of her infant for nursing, manually express milk remaining in the breast after nursing (usually necessary only if the infant is not sucking well), or massage the caked area toward the nipple as the infant nurses. Mothers who develop mastitis can apply warm, moist compresses to the affected area before and during breastfeeding. The nurse encourages the mother to breastfeed frequently, starting with the unaffected breast until letdown occurs in the affected breast, then feeds from the affected breast until it is emptied completely (Lauwers & Shinskie, 2000). While feeding on the affected breast, the baby's chin is pointed toward the inflamed area. After nursing, the mother can leave a small amount of milk on each nipple to prevent cracking and allow nipples to air dry. Early identification of and intervention for sore nipples are also essential.

### *Teaching for Self-Care*

The nurse stresses to the breastfeeding woman the importance of adequate breast and nipple care to prevent the development of cracks and fissures, a common portal for bacterial entry. (For a detailed discussion of breastfeeding, see Chapter 24.)

The woman should be aware of the importance of regular, complete emptying of the breasts to prevent engorgement and stasis. She should also understand the role of letdown in successful breastfeeding, correct positioning of the infant on the nipple, proper latch-on, and the principle of supply and demand. If the mother is taking antibiotics, she needs to understand the importance of completing the full course of antibiotics, even if the infection seems to clear quickly. Breastfeeding mothers who are returning to work outside the home need information on how to do so successfully. Because mastitis tends to develop after discharge, it is important to include information about signs and symptoms in the discharge teaching and printed materials (Table 30–2). All flulike symptoms should be considered a sign of mastitis until proven otherwise. If symptoms develop, the woman should contact her caregiver immediately because prompt treatment helps to prevent abscess formation.

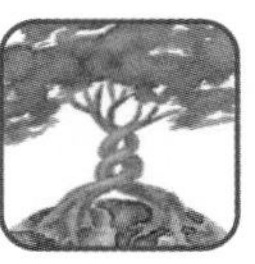

## Community-Based Nursing Care

The home care nurse who suspects mastitis on the basis of assessment findings refers the woman to the physician. The nurse may be asked to obtain a sample of breast milk to be cultured for the causative organism.

If the mother feels too ill to breastfeed or develops an abscess that prevents nursing, the home care nurse can help the mother obtain a breast pump to help her maintain lactation and can provide opportunities for demonstration and return demonstration of pumping. Referral to a lactation consultant or to La Leche League can be invaluable to the woman's physical and emotional adjustment to mastitis.

### Evaluation

Expected outcomes of nursing care include the following:

- The woman is aware of the signs and symptoms of mastitis.
- The woman's mastitis is detected early and treated successfully.
- The woman can continue breastfeeding if she chooses.
- The woman understands self-care measures she can employ to prevent the recurrence of the mastitis.

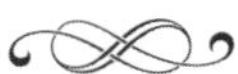

**TABLE 30–2 Comparison of Findings of Engorgement, Plugged Duct, and Mastitis**

| *Characteristics* | *Engorgement* | *Plugged Duct* | *Mastitis* |
|---|---|---|---|
| Onset | Gradual, immediately postpartum | Gradual, after feedings | Sudden, after 10 days |
| Site | Bilateral | Unilateral | Usually unilateral |
| Swelling and heat | Generalized | May shift, little or no heat | Localized, red, hot, and swollen |
| Pain | Generalized | Mild but localized | Intense but localized |
| Body temperature | <38.4°C (101.1°F) | <38.4°C (101.1°F) | >38.4°C (101.1°F) |
| Systemic symptoms | Feels well | Feels well | Flulike symptoms |

*Source:* Lawrence, R. A. (1994). *Breastfeeding: A guide for the medical profession* (p. 261). St. Louis: Mosby.

## Care of the Woman with Postpartal Thromboembolic Disease

Thromboembolic disease may occur antepartally, but it is generally considered a postpartal complication. Venous thrombosis refers to thrombus formation in a superficial or deep vein, with the accompanying risk that a portion of the clot might break off and result in pulmonary embolism. When the thrombus is formed in response to inflammation in the vein wall, it is termed **thrombophlebitis.** In this type of thrombosis, the clot tends to be more firmly attached and therefore is less likely to result in embolism. In noninflammatory venous thrombosis (also called phlebothrombosis) the clot, caused by venous stasis, tends to be more loosely attached and the risk of embolism is greater.

Factors contributing directly to the development of thromboembolic disease postpartally include (1) increased amounts of certain blood-clotting factors; (2) postpartal thrombocytosis (increased quantity of circulating platelets and their increased adhesiveness); (3) release of thromboplastin substances from the tissue of the decidua, placenta, and fetal membranes; and (4) increased amounts of fibrinolysis inhibitors. Predisposing factors include (1) obesity, increased maternal age, and high parity; (2) anesthesia and surgery, with possible vessel trauma and venous stasis due to prolonged inactivity; (3) previous history of venous thrombosis; (4) maternal anemia, hypothermia, or heart disease; (5) endometritis (metritis); and (6) varicosities. Thromboembolic disease is more likely to occur after cesarean birth than after vaginal birth (Laros, 1999).

### Superficial Vein Leg Disease

Superficial thrombophlebitis is far more common postpartally than during pregnancy. Often the clot involves one of the saphenous veins. This disorder is more common in women with preexisting varices (enlarged veins), although it is not limited to these women. Symptoms—including tenderness in a portion of the vein, some local heat and redness, normal temperature or low-grade fever, and occasionally slight elevation of the pulse—usually become apparent about the third or fourth postpartal day. Treatment involves application of local heat, elevation of the affected limb, bed rest, analgesics, and the use of elastic support hose. Anticoagulants are usually not necessary unless complications develop. Pulmonary embolism is extremely rare. Occasionally the involved veins have incompetent valves, and, as a result, the problem may spread to the deeper leg veins, such as the femoral vein.

### Deep Vein Thrombosis

Deep vein thrombosis (DVT) is more frequently seen in women with a history of thrombosis. Certain obstetric complications, such as hydramnios, PIH, and operative birth, are associated with an increased incidence.

Clinical manifestations may include edema of the ankle and leg and an initial low-grade fever often followed by high temperature and chills. Depending on the vein involved, the woman may complain of pain in the popliteal and lateral tibial areas (popliteal vein), pain in the entire lower leg and foot (anterior and posterior tibial veins), inguinal tenderness (femoral vein), or pain in the lower abdomen (iliofemoral vein). The Homans' sign (refer to Figure 27–7♦) may or may not be positive, but pain often results from calf pressure. Because of reflex arterial spasm, sometimes the limb is pale and cool to the touch—the so-called *milk leg* or *phlegmasia alba dolens*—and peripheral pulses may be decreased.

### Septic Pelvic Thrombophlebitis

Septic pelvic thrombophlebitis is a complication that develops in conjunction with infections of the reproductive tract and is more common in women who have had a cesarean birth. The diagnosis is suspected when infection is unresponsive to antibiotics. Abdominal pain, flank pain, or both, sometimes accompanied by guarding, occurs on the second or third day postpartum, along with fever and tachycardia. Bimanual examination may reveal a parametrial mass. On occasion, paralytic ileus develops. Treatment consists of anticoagulation and antibiotic therapy. Although most women show significant clinical improvement with antibiotics, a sawtooth fever spike and chills may persist (Laros, 1999).

### Clinical Therapy

Because cases of thromboembolic disease are seldom clear-cut, diagnosis involves a variety of approaches, such as client history and physical examination, occlusive cuff impedence plethysmography (IPG), Doppler ultrasonography, and contrast venography (increased circumference of affected extremity). In questionable cases, venography provides the most accurate diagnosis of DVT; unfortunately, however, it is not practical for multiple examinations or prospective screening and may itself induce phlebitis (Laros, 1999).

Treatment involves the administration of intravenous heparin, using an infusion pump to permit continuous, accurate infusion of medication. Strict bed rest and elevation of the leg are required; analgesics are given as necessary to relieve discomfort. If fever is present, deep thrombophlebitis is suspected, and the woman is also given antibiotics. In most cases thrombectomy (surgical removal of the clot) is not necessary.

## Critical Thinking in Practice

Lei Chang, GIPI, had a cesarean birth after a prolonged labor and failure to progress. As she is walking in the hallway with her husband, you notice that Lei is limping slightly, and you comment on that observation. Lei responds that she is having pain in her right lower leg. She says, "Maybe I pulled a muscle during labor." What would you do?

Answers can be found in Appendix I.

Once the symptoms have subsided (usually in several days), the woman may begin ambulation while wearing elastic support stockings. Intravenous heparin is continued until prothrombin time reaches 1.5 to 1.7, and treatment with sodium warfarin (Coumadin) is begun. The woman continues taking Coumadin for 2 to 6 months at home. While taking warfarin, prothrombin times are assessed periodically to maintain correct dosage levels.

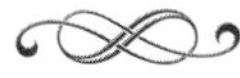

## Nursing Care Management

### Nursing Assessment and Diagnosis

The nurse carefully assesses the woman's history for factors predisposing her to development of thrombosis or thrombophlebitis. In addition, the nurse is alert to any complaints of pain in the legs, inguinal area, or lower abdomen because such pain may indicate DVT. The nurse also assesses the woman's legs for evidence of edema, temperature change, or pain with palpation.

Nursing diagnoses that may apply to a postpartal woman with a thrombolic disease include the following:

- ***Altered tissue perfusion*** in periphery related to obstructed venous return
- ***Pain*** related to tissue hypoxia and edema secondary to vascular obstruction
- ***Risk for altered parenting*** related to decreased maternal-infant interaction secondary to bed rest and intravenous lines

### Nursing Plan and Implementation

The need for support hose for women with varicosities is evaluated during labor and the postpartum period. Adequate fluid intake is necessary during labor to prevent dehydration. Because trauma is often a factor in the development of thrombophlebitis, the nurse avoids keeping the woman's legs elevated in stirrups for prolonged periods. If stirrups are used, they should be comfortably padded and adjusted to provide correct support and prevent pressure on popliteal vessels. In addition, early ambulation is encouraged following birth, and the knee gatch on the bed should be avoided. Women confined to bed following a cesarean birth are encouraged to perform regular leg exercises to promote venous return.

Once DVT is diagnosed, the nurse maintains the heparin therapy, provides appropriate comfort measures, and monitors the woman closely for signs of pulmonary embolism. The nurse also assesses for evidence of bleeding related to heparin and keeps the antagonist for heparin, protamine sulfate, readily available.

The nurse instructs the woman to avoid prolonged standing or sitting because these positions contribute to venous stasis. The nurse also advises the woman to avoid crossing her legs because of the pressure it causes. The nurse recommends that the woman take frequent breaks during car trips and while working if she sits most of the day. Walking is acceptable because it promotes venous return. The woman is reminded to mention her history of thrombosis or thrombophlebitis to her physician during subsequent pregnancies so that preventive measures can be instituted early.

Women who are discharged while taking warfarin must understand the purpose of the medication and be alert for signs of bleeding such as bleeding gums, epistaxis, petechiae or ecchymosis, and evidence of blood in the urine or stool. Because careful monitoring is important, the woman should clearly understand the need to keep scheduled appointments for prothrombin time assessment. Certain medications such as aspirin and other nonsteroidal antiinflammatory drugs increase anticoagulant activity and should be avoided; when she is taking warfarin the woman should check for possible medication interaction before taking *any* other medication. The nurse encourages the woman to carry a MedicAlert card in case of emergency, inform all health care providers, including dentists, that she is taking anticoagulants, and have vitamin K available in case of bleeding (Shaver, 1999).

Warfarin is excreted in the breast milk and thus may present problems for infants of breastfeeding mothers. Women who wish to continue nursing may be maintained at home on low doses of subcutaneous heparin, because heparin is not excreted in breast milk. (See the Critical Pathway for the Woman with Thromboembolic Disease on pages 814 to 817 for specific nursing care measures.)

Text continues on page 821.

# CRITICAL PATHWAY: *For the Woman with Thromboembolic Disease**

| Category | Antepartal Management | Intrapartal Management | Postpartal Management |
|---|---|---|---|
| **Referral** | Perinatologist<br>Internist<br>Social worker<br>Psychiatric clinical nurse practitioner<br>Dietary/nutritionist<br>Infectious disease consult | Obtain prenatal record | Home nursing referral if indicated<br>**Expected Outcomes**<br>Appropriate resources identified and utilized |
| **Assessment** | Obtain hx of present pregnancy<br>Assess estimated gestational age<br>Assess any sensitivity to medications<br>Obtain complete physical examination to include<br>• Fetal size, fetal status (FHR), and fetal maturity<br>• Signs of fatigue, weakness, recurrent diarrhea, pallor, night sweats<br>• Present weight and amount of weight gain or weight loss<br>Obtain diagnostic studies:<br>• Ultrasound<br>• Fetal maturity studies (L/S ratio, PG, creatine)<br>• Hemoglobin, hematocrit, platelet count<br>• WBC and differential<br>• HIV<br>• CD4 + T lymphocyte count<br>• ESR | | Monitor daily Hct<br>Continue normal postpartum assessment q8h<br>Feeding technique with newborn: should be good or improving<br>TPR assessment: q8h; all WNL; report temperature >38°C (100.4°F)<br>Continue assessment of comfort level<br>Assess for superficial thrombophlebitis:<br>• Tenderness along involved vein<br>• Areas of palpable thrombosis<br>• Warmth and redness in the involved area<br>Deep venous thrombosis (DVT):<br>• Positive Homans' sign (pain occurs when foot is dorsiflexed while leg is extended)<br>• Tenderness and pain in affected area<br>• Fever (initially low, followed by high fever and chills)<br>• Edema in affected extremity<br>• Pallor and coolness in affected limb<br>• Diminished peripheral pulses<br>• Increased potential for pulmonary embolus<br>Immediately report the development of any signs of pulmonary embolism, including the following:<br>• Sudden onset of severe chest pain, often located substernally<br>• Apprehension and sense of impending catastrophe<br>• Cough (may be accompanied by hemoptysis)<br>• Tachycardia<br>• Fever<br>• Hypotension<br>• Diaphoresis, pallor, weakness<br>• Shortness of breath<br>• Neck engorgement<br>• Friction rub and evidence of atelectasis upon auscultation<br>**Expected Outcomes**<br>Findings indicate complications of thrombosis minimized, and condition stable or improved |
| **Comfort** | | | Continue with pain management techniques<br>No aspirin or ibuprofen; acetaminophen may be ordered<br>Provide supportive nursing comfort measures such as back rubs, provision of quiet time for sleep, diversional activities<br>Maintain warm, moist soaks as ordered, with legs elevated |

*All of the interventions for a normal labor and birth and postpartal client may be found in those appropriate critical pathways.

CNM, certified nurse-midwife; DC, discharge; Het, hematocrit; ICN, intensive care nursing; IV, intravenous; heparin lock, intravenous catheter that allows intermittent access; hx, history; prn, as needed; PT, prothromfin time; s/s, signs and symptoms; TPR, temperature, pulse, and respiration; WNL, within normal limits.

## CRITICAL PATHWAY *Continued*

| Category | Antepartal Management | Intrapartal Management | Postpartal Management |
|---|---|---|---|
| **Teaching/ psychosocial** | Room orientation<br>Explain s/s of labor<br>Increase client awareness of fetal monitoring<br>Evaluation of client teaching | Tour of ICN<br>Discuss with woman:<br>• Mode of childbirth<br>• Postpartum expectation | Implement normal postpartum teaching and psychosocial support (see Chapter 28)<br>Maintain mother-infant attachment; when mother is on bed rest provide frequent contacts for mother and infant; modified rooming-in is possible if the crib is placed close to the mother's bed and nurse checks often to help mother lift or move infant<br>**Expected Outcomes**<br>Woman demonstrates/verbalizes understanding of plan of care and teaching<br>Infant-maternal bonding unimpaired |
| **Nursing care management and reports** | Assess emotional response so that support and teaching can be planned accordingly<br>Weigh woman<br>Obtain food history<br>Establish rapport<br>Provide opportunities to talk without interruption<br>Monitor for signs of infection<br>Maintain appropriate isolation precautions | Ongoing monitoring of blood pressure<br>Electronic fetal monitoring in place<br>Try to have same nurses caring for woman during her hospitalization<br>Monitor for signs of infections<br>**Expected Outcomes**<br>Maternal/fetal circulation optimized | Continue sitz baths prn<br>May shower if ambulating without difficulty<br>DC buffalo cap (heparin lock) if present<br>Monitor for signs of infection<br>For DVT obtain prothrombin time (PT) and review prior to beginning warfarin; repeat periodically per physician order<br>**Expected Outcomes**<br>Thromoembolic disease treated successfully, without related complications |
| **Activity and comfort** | Decreased stimulation in room including visitors | | Maintain bed rest and limb in elevated position<br>Initiate progressive ambulation following the acute phase; provide properly fitting elastic stockings prior to ambulation for management of superficial thrombophlebitis and DVT<br>**Expected Outcomes**<br>Activity initiated as appropriate<br>Optimal comfort maintained |
| **Nutrition** | Plan high-protein, high-calorie diet | | Continue diet and fluids<br>**Expected Outcomes**<br>Nutritional needs met |
| **Elimination** | | | |
| **Medications** | | Continuous IV infusion | May take own prenatal vitamins<br>RhoGAM administered if indicated<br>Rubella vaccine administered if indicated<br>For DVT administer intravenous heparin as ordered by continuous intravenous drip, heparin lock, or subcutaneously, including<br>• Monitor IV or heparin lock site for signs of infiltration<br>• Obtain Lee-White clotting times or partial thromboplastin time (PTT) per physician order and review prior to administering heparin<br>• Observe for signs of anticoagulant overdose with resultant bleeding, including the following: hematuria, epistaxis, ecchymosis, and bleeding gums<br>• Provide protamine sulfate per physician order to combat bleeding problems related to heparin overdose<br>**Expected Outcomes**<br>Thrombosis resolved and control of related bleeding problems achieved<br>Minimized complications and side effects |

| Category | Antepartal Management | Intrapartal Management | Postpartal Management |
|---|---|---|---|
| **Discharge planning/ home care** | Assess home care needs<br>Provide support and counseling | | Discuss ways of avoiding circulatory stasis such as avoiding prolonged standing, sitting, and crossing legs<br>Review need to wear support stockings and to plan for rest periods with legs elevated<br>In the presence of DVT, discuss the following:<br>• The use of warfarin, its side effects, possible interactions with other medications, and need to have dosage assessed through periodic checks of the prothrombin time<br>• Signs of bleeding, which may be associated with warfarin sodium and which need to be reported immediately, including the following: hematuria, epistaxis, ecchymosis, bleeding gums, and rectal bleeding<br>• Monitor menstrual flow: bleeding may be heavier<br>• Review need for woman to eat a consistent amount of leafy green vegetables (lettuce, cabbage, brussels sprouts, broccoli) every day (high in vit K also affects dose of warfarin and PT balance)<br>• Instruct the woman to report any bleeding that continues more than 10 minutes<br>Instruct the woman to do the following:<br>• Routinely inspect the body for bruising<br>• Carry MedicAlert card indicating she is on anticoagulant therapy<br>• Use electric razor to avoid scratching skin<br>• Use soft-bristle toothbrush<br>• Avoid alcohol intake or keep intake at a minimum<br>• Avoid taking any other drugs without checking with the physician<br>• Note that stools may change color to pink, red, or black as result of anticoagulant use<br>• Advise all health providers, including dentists, that she is taking anticoagulants<br>Review discharge instructions and checklist<br>Provide list or make appropriate referrals to available community resources<br>Describe postpartum warning signs and when to call CNM or physician<br>Provide prescriptions; gift pack given to woman<br>Arrangements made for baby pictures if desired<br>Postpartum visit scheduled<br>Newborn check scheduled<br>**Expected Outcomes**<br>Client discharge teaching done with emphasis on follow-up care, continued therapy needs, and precautions<br>Support network identified |

| Category | Antepartal Management | Intrapartal Management | Postpartal Management |
|---|---|---|---|
| **Family involvement** | Assess support systems | Encourage family member to stay with the woman as long as possible throughout labor and childbirth | Involve support persons in teaching<br>Plans made for providing support to mother following discharge; support persons verbalize understanding of need for woman to rest, eat nutritionally, recover<br>Encourage woman to express her concerns to her partner; assist couple in planning ways to manage while woman is hospitalized and after her discharge<br>Encourage partner or support person to bring other children to hospital to visit mother and meet new sibling<br>Encourage partner or support person to bring in family pictures; encourage phone calls<br>Contact social services if indicated to obtain additional assistance for family if needed<br>**Expected Outcomes**<br>Family demonstrates resource availability and utilization<br>Family bonding and development unimpaired |
| **Date** | | | |

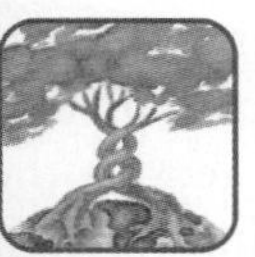

## Community-Based Nursing Care

Because the mother with postpartal thromboembolic disease will depend on others for much of her initial home care, it is helpful for the father of the newborn to be involved in preparations for discharge. The nurse should provide ample time to answer questions and clarify instructions, verbally and in writing. The nurse will evaluate the extent to which both the mother and father have understood instructions regarding the plan of care. It is especially important to assess the couple's plans to ensure complete bed rest for the mother. They might explore ways for her to maintain bed rest and still spend quality time with her newborn and any other children. For example, young children can sit on the bed for storytelling or play quiet games, and the newborn's crib can be placed next to the mother's bed.

Many concerns will not surface until the couple actually returns home and fully comprehends the reality of their situation. For that reason, it is valuable to provide them with an accessible resource person and to plan telephone or home visit follw-up care.

Signs of postpartum thrombophlebitis may not occur until after discharge from the birthing unit. Consequently all couples must be taught to recognize its signs and symptoms and appreciate the importance of reporting them immediately and of not massaging the affected leg. If signs and symptoms occur after discharge, a short readmission may be required. In that case every effort is made to allow mother, father, and newborn to remain together.

### Evaluation

Expected outcomes of nursing care include the following:

- If thrombophlebitis develops, it is detected quickly and managed successfully, without further complications.
- At discharge the woman is able to explain the purpose, dosage regimen, and necessary precautions associated with any prescribed medications such as anticoagulants.

- The woman can discuss the self-care measures and ongoing therapies (such as the use of elastic stockings) indicated.
- The woman has bonded successfully with her newborn and is able to care for her baby effectively.

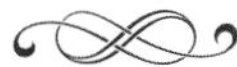

## Care of the Woman with a Postpartum Psychiatric Disorder

Many types of psychiatric problems may occur in the postpartum period. The classification of postpartum psychiatric disorders is a subject of some controversy. The *Diagnostic and Statistical Manual of Mental Disorders,* 4th edition (DSM-IV), (American Psychiatric Association, 1994), has added a postpartum onset specifier to the mood disorder diagnostic category of psychiatric disorders. It is proposed that postpartum psychiatric disorders be considered one diagnosable syndrome with three subclasses: (1) adjustment reaction with depressed mood, (2) postpartum psychosis, and (3) postpartum major mood disorder. The incidence, etiology, symptoms, treatment, and prognosis vary with each subclass.

*Adjustment reaction with depressed mood* is also known as postpartum, maternal, or "baby blues." It is characterized by mild depression interspersed with happier feelings. Postpartum blues typically occur within a few days after the baby's birth and are self-limiting, lasting from a few hours to several days (O'Hara, 1999). The depression is more severe in primiparas than in multiparas and seems related to the rapid alteration of estrogen, progesterone, and prolactin levels after birth. New mothers experiencing postpartum blues commonly report feeling overwhelmed, unable to cope, fatigued, anxious, irritable, and oversensitive. A key feature is episodic tearfulness, often without an identifiable reason.

Validating the existence of this phenomenon, labeling it as a real but normal adjustment reaction, and providing reassurance can offer a measure of relief. Assistance with self- and infant care, information, and family support aids recovery. The partner should be encouraged to watch for and report signs that the new mother is not returning to a more normal mood but slipping into a deeper depression.

*Postpartum psychosis,* which has an incidence of 1 to 2 per 1000, usually becomes evident within the first 3 months postpartum. Symptoms include agitation, hyperactivity, insomnia, mood lability, confusion, irrationality, difficulty remembering or concentrating, poor judgment, delusions, and hallucinations. Improvement is seen in 95% of women in 2 to 3 months (O'Hara, 1999). Treatment may include hospitalization, antipsychotics, sedatives, electroconvulsive therapy, removal of the infant, social support, and psychotherapy.

*Postpartum major mood disorder,* also known as postpartum depression, develops in about 7% to 16% of all postpartum women in North America (O'Hara, 1999). Although it may occur at any time during the first postpartum year, the periods of greatest risk occur around the fourth week, just before the initiation of menses, and upon weaning. Surprisingly, it is not associated with depression during pregnancy.

Risk factors for postpartum depression include the following:

- Primiparity
- Ambivalence about maintaining the pregnancy
- History of postpartum depression or bipolar illness
- Lack of social support
- Lack of a stable and supportive relationship with parents or partner
- The woman's dissatisfaction with herself, including body image problems and eating disorders

### Clinical Therapy

Medication, individual or group psychotherapy, and practical assistance with child care and other demands of daily life are common treatment measures. Support groups have proved to be successful adjuncts to such treatment. Within a support group of postpartal women and their partners, a couple may feel consolation that they are not alone in their experience. Moreover, the group provides a forum for exchanging information about postpartum depression, learning stress-reduction measures, and experiencing renewed self-esteem and support. If a support group is not available locally, the woman and her family may be encouraged to contact Depression after Delivery (DAD), a national support network that provides literature and volunteers (PO Box 1282, Morrisville, PA 19067, or 800-944-4773).

## Nursing Care Management

### Nursing Assessment and Diagnosis

Assessment for factors predisposing a client to postpartal depression or psychosis should begin prenatally. Questions designed to detect problems can be included as part of the routine prenatal history interview or questionnaire. Beck (1995) developed a practical and simple screening checklist to use during routine care with all postpartum women to identify those who might be experiencing postpartum depression so that early management might be initiated (Table 30–3). Willingness to listen as the mother shares her experiences of postpartum depression not only enables the nurse to recognize symptoms and initiate timely management but also conveys to the mother a sense of caring (Beck, 1999). The nurse recognizes that depressive symptomatology frequently occurs among first-time mothers of low socioeconomic status. Chronic stressors and inadequate social support are significant factors associated with postpartum depression (Seguin, Potvin, St-Denis, et al., 1999).

In providing daily care, the nurse observes the woman for objective signs of depression—anxiety, irritability, poor concentration, forgetfulness, sleep difficulties, appetite change, fatigue, and tearfulness—and listens for statements indicating feelings of failure and self-accusation. Severity and duration of symptoms should be noted. Behavior and verbalizations that are bizarre or seem to indicate a potential for violence against herself or others, including the infant, are reported as soon as possible for further evaluation.

The nurse needs to be aware that many normal physiologic changes of the puerperium are similar to symptoms of depression (lack of sexual interest, appetite change, fatigue). It is essential that observations be as specific and as objective as possible and that they be carefully documented.

### TABLE 30–3 Suggested Questions to Elicit Responses from the Postpartum Depression Checklist (PDC)*

**LACK OF CONCENTRATION**
Are you experiencing difficulty concentrating?
Does your mind seem to be filled with cobwebs?
Does it seem at times like fogginess sets in?

**LOSS OF INTERESTS**
Do you feel your life is empty of your previous interests and goals?
Have you lost interest in your hobbies that used to bring you pleasure and enjoyment?

**LONELINESS**
Are you experiencing feelings of loneliness?
Do you feel as though no one really understands what you are experiencing?
Do you feel uncomfortable around other people?
Have you been isolating yourself from other people?

**INSECURITY**
Have you been feeling insecure, fragile, or vulnerable?
Does the responsibility of motherhood seem overwhelming?

**OBSESSIVE THINKING**
Is your mind constantly filled with obsessive thinking such as, "What's wrong with me?" "Am I going crazy?" "Why can't I enjoy being with my baby?"
When trying to fall asleep at night, is your mind still racing with repetitive thoughts?

**LACK OF POSITIVE EMOTIONS**
Are you experiencing feelings of emptiness?
Do you feel like a robot just going through the motions?
When caring for your infant/child, do you feel any joy or love?

**LOSS OF SELF**
Do you feel as though you are not the same person you used to be?
Are you afraid that your life will never be normal again?

**ANXIETY ATTACKS**
Are you experiencing uncontrollable anxiety attacks?
Are you experiencing periods of palpitations, chest pains, sweating, or tingling hands?
When going through an anxiety attack, do you feel as though you're losing your mind?

**LOSS OF CONTROL**
Do you feel you are in control of your emotions and thoughts?
Are you experiencing loss of control in any aspects of your life?

**GUILT**
Are you feeling guilty because you believe you are not giving your infant/child the love and attention he/she needs?
Are you experiencing guilt over thoughts of harming your infant/child?
Do you feel you are a good mother?

**CONTEMPLATING DEATH**
Have you experienced thoughts of harming yourself?
Have you been feeling so low that the thought of leaving this world was appealing to you?

*Bold print reflects areas of concern expressed by depressed women in Beck's qualitative studies. Questions answered "Yes" by women during screening with this checklist can be followed with further dialogue between nurse and client.

*Source:* Beck, C. T. (1995). Screening methods for postpartum depression. *Journal of Obstetric, Gynecologic, and Neonatal Nursing, 24*(4), 113. Used with permission of Lippincott-Raven Publishers.

Possible nursing diagnoses that may apply to a woman with a postpartum psychiatric disorder include the following:

- ***Ineffective individual coping*** related to postpartum depression
- ***Risk*** for altered parenting related to postpartal mental illness

## Nursing Plan and Implementation

Nurses working in antepartal settings or teaching childbirth classes play independsable roles in helping prospective parents appreciate the lifestyle changes and role demands associated with parenthood. Offering realistic information and anticipatory guidance and debunking myths about the perfect mother or perfect newborn may help prevent postpartum depression. Social support teaching guides are available for nurses to help postpartum women explore their needs for postpartum support (Logsdon, Birkimer, & Usui, 2000). The nurse should alert the mother, spouse, and other family members to the possibility of postpartum blues in the early days after birth and reassure them of the short-term nature of the condition. Symptoms of postpartum depression should be described and the mother encouraged to call her health care provider if symptoms become severe, if they fail to subside quickly, or if at any time she feels she is unable to function. Encouraging the mother to plan how she will manage at home and providing concrete suggestions on how to cope aid in her adjustment to motherhood.

## Community-Based Nursing Care

Home visits, especially for early-discharge families, are essential to fostering positive adjustments for the new family constellation. Telephone follow-up at 3 weeks postpartum to ask whether the mother is experiencing difficulties is also helpful.

Women with a history of depression or postpartum psychosis should be referred to a mental health professional for counseling and biweekly visits between the second and sixth week postpartum for evaluation of depression. Medication, social support, and assistance with child care may also be necessary.

In all women the presence of three symptoms or one symptom of depression for 3 days may signal serious depression and requires immediate referral to a mental health professional. Immediate referral should also be made if rejection of the infant or threatened or actual aggression against the infant has occurred. In such cases the newborn is never left unattended with the mother.

A diagnosis of postpartum depression or other psychiatric disorder poses major problems for the family, especially the father (Meighan, Davis, Thomas, et al., 1999). The symptoms of these disorders are difficult to witness and may be harder to understand than physical problems such as hemorrhage and infection. The father may feel hurt by his partner's hostility, worry that she is becoming insane, or be baffled by her mood swings and lack of concern about herself, the newborn, or household responsibilities. Very real practical matters—running the household; managing the children, including the totally dependent newborn; and caring for the mother—may be added to his usual routines and work responsibilities.

Information, emotional support, and assistance in providing or obtaining care for the infant may be needed. The nurse can assist family members by identifying community resources and making referrals to public health nursing services and social services. Postpartum follow-up and visits from a psychiatric home health nurse are especially important.

## Evaluation

Expected outcomes of nursing care include the following:

- Signs of potential postpartal disorders are detected quickly and therapy is implemented.
- The newborn is cared for effectively by the father or another support person until the mother is able to do her share.

# Chapter Review

## CHAPTER HIGHLIGHTS

- The main causes of early postpartal hemorrhage are uterine atony, lacerations of the vagina and cervix, and retained placental fragments.
- The most common postpartal infection is endometritis, which is limited to the uterine cavity.
- A postpartal woman is at increased risk for developing urinary tract problems due to normal postpartal diuresis, increased bladder capacity, decreased bladder sensitivity from stretching or trauma, and, possibly, inhibited neural control of the bladder following the use of anesthetic agents.
- Mastitis is an inflammation of the breast caused by a variety of organisms and is primarily seen in breastfeeding women. Symptoms seldom occur before the second to fourth week after birth.
- Thromboembolic disease originating in the veins of the leg, thigh, or pelvis may occur in the antepartum or postpartum periods and carries with it the potential for creating a pulmonary embolus.
- Although many different types of psychiatric problems may be encountered in the postpartal period, depression is the most common. Episodes occur frequently in the week after childbirth and are typically transient.
- Telephone calls and home visits are effective measures for extending comprehensive care into the home setting of the postpartum family at risk.

## CHAPTER REFERENCES


American College of Obstetricians and Gynecologists. (1998). *Postpartum hemorrhage* (ACOG Educational Bulletin No. 243). Washington, DC: Author.

American Psychiatric Association. (1994). *Diagnostic and statistical manual of mental disorders: DSM-IV* (4th ed.). Washington DC: Author.

Beck, C. T. (1995). Perceptions of nurses' caring by mothers experiencing postpartum depression. *Journal of Obstetric, Gynecologic, and Neonatal Nursing, 24*(9), 819–825.

Beck, C. T. (1999). Maternal depression and child behaviour problems: A meta-analysis. *Journal of Advanced Nursing, 29*(3), 623–629.

Bowes, W. (1999). Clinical aspects of normal and abnormal labor. In R. K. Creasy & R. Resnik (Eds.), *Maternal-fetal medicine* (4th ed.). Philadelphia: Saunders. Chap. 34 pp. 541–568.

Cunningham, F. G., MacDonald, P. C., Gant, N. F., Leveno, K. J., Gilstrap, L. C., III, Hankins, G. D. V., & Clark, S. L. (1997). *Williams obstetrics* (20th ed.). Stamford, CT: Appleton & Lange.

Gibbs, R. S., & Sweet, R. L. (1999). Maternal and fetal infectious disorders. In R. K. Creasy & R. Resnik (Eds.), *Maternal-fetal medicine* (4th ed.). Philadelphia: Saunders. Chap. 41 pp. 659–724.

Gonik, B. (1999). Intensive care monitoring of the critically ill pregnant patient. In R. K. Creasy & R. Resnik (Eds.), *Maternal-fetal medicine* (4th ed.). Philadelphia: Saunders. Chap. 50 pp. 895–920.

Johnson, J. V., & Riddick, D. H. (2000). The nonlactating human breast. In J. J. Sciarri & T. J. Watkins (Eds.), *Gynecology and obstetrics* (Vol. 5, pp. 1–19). Philadelphia, PA: Lippincott Williams & Wilkins.

Laros, R. K. (1999). Thromboembolic disease. In R. K. Creasy & R. Resnik (Eds.), *Maternal-fetal medicine* (4th ed.). Philadelphia: Saunders. Chap. 47 pp. 821–832.

Lauwers, J., & Shinskie, D. (2000). *Counseling the nursing mother: The lactation consultant's reference* (3rd ed.). Boston: Jones & Bartlett.

Logsdon, M. C., Birkimer, J. C., & Usui, W. M. (2000). The link of social support and postpartum depressive symptoms in African-American women with low incomes. *Journal of Maternal-Child Nursing, 25*(5), 262–266.

Meighan, M., Davis, M. W., Thomas, S. P., & Droppleman, P. G. (1999). Living with postpartum depression: The father's experience. *Journal of Maternal-Child Nursing, 24*(4), 202–208.

O'Hara, M. W. (1999). Postpartum mental disorders. In J. J. Sciarri & T. J. Watkins (Eds.), *Gynecology and obstetrics* (Vol. 6, pp. 1–19). Philadelphia, PA: Lippincott Williams & Wilkins.

Seguin, L., Potvin, L., St-Denis, M., & Loiselle, J. (1999). Depressive symptoms in the late postpartum among low socioeconomic status women. *Birth, 26*(3), 157–163.

Shaver, D. C. (1999). Thromboembolic disease. In J. J. Sciarri & T. J. Watkins (Eds.), *Gynecology and obstetrics* (Vol. 2, pp. 1–11). Philadelphia, PA: Lippincott Williams & Wilkins.

Vogel, A., Hutchison, B. L., & Mitchell, E. A. (1999). Mastitis in the first year postpartum. *Birth, 26*(4), 218–225.

## CONTEMPORARY MATERNAL-NEWBORN NURSING ON-LINE

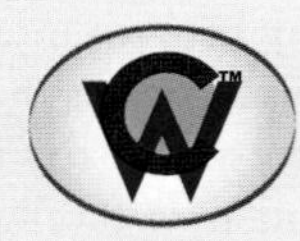

Additional interactive resources, including animations and video, for this chapter can be found on the Companion Website at http://www.prenhall.com/ladewig. Click on Chapter 30 and "Begin" to select the activities for this chapter.

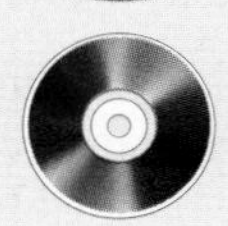

For NCLEX review questions and an audio glossary, access the accompanying CD-ROM in this book.

# Appendices

# Appendix A

## Common Abbreviations in Maternal-Newborn and Women's Health Nursing

| | |
|---|---|
| **AC** | Abdominal circumference |
| **accel** | Acceleration of fetal heart rate |
| **AFAFP** | Amniotic fluid alpha-fetoprotein |
| **AFP** | Alpha-fetoprotein |
| **AFV** | Amniotic fluid volume |
| **AGA** | Average for gestational age |
| **AID or AIH** | Artificial insemination donor (*H* designates mate is donor) |
| **AMOL** | Active management of labor |
| **ARBOW** | Artificial rupture of bag of waters |
| **AROM** | Artificial rupture of membranes |
| **BAT** | Brown adipose tissue (brown fat) |
| **BBT** | Basal body temperature |
| **BL** | Baseline (fetal heart rate baseline) |
| **BOW** | Bag of waters |
| **BPD** | Biparietal diameter *or* Bronchopulmonary dysplasia |
| **BPP** | Biophysical profile |
| **BSE** | Breast self-examination |
| **BSST** | Breast self-stimulation test |
| **CC** | Chest circumference *or* Cord compression |
| **C–H** | Crown-to-heel length |
| **CID** | Cytomegalic inclusion disease |
| **CMV** | Cytomegalovirus |
| **CNM** | Certified nurse-midwife |
| **CNS** | Clinical nurse specialist |
| **CPAP** | Continuous positive airway pressure |
| **CPD** | Cephalopelvic disproportion *or* Citrate-phosphate-dextrose |
| **CRL** | Crown-rump length |
| **C/S** | Cesarean section (or C-section) |
| **CST** | Contraction stress test |
| **CVA** | Costovertebral angle |
| **CVS** | Chorionic villus sampling |
| **D&C** | Dilatation and curettage |
| **decels** | Deceleration of fetal heart rate |
| **DFMR** | Daily fetal movement response |
| **dil** | Dilatation |
| **DRG** | Diagnostic related groups |
| **DTR** | Deep tendon reflexes |
| **ECMO** | Extracorporal membrane oxygenator |
| **EDB** | Estimated date of birth |
| **EDC** | Estimated date of confinement |
| **EDD** | Estimated date of delivery |
| **EFM** | Electronic fetal monitoring |
| **EFW** | Estimated fetal weight |
| **EIA** | Enzyme immunoassay |
| **ELF** | Elective low forceps |
| **ELISA** | Enzyme-linked immunosorbent assay |
| **epis** | Episiotomy |
| **ERT** | Estrogen replacement therapy |
| **FAD** | Fetal activity diary |
| **FAE** | Fetal alcohol effects |
| **FAS** | Fetal alcohol syndrome |
| **FBD** | Fibrocystic breast disease |
| **FBM** | Fetal breathing movements |
| **FBS** | Fetal blood sample *or* Fasting blood sugar test |
| **FECG** | Fetal electrocardiogram |
| **FHR** | Fetal heart rate |
| **FHT** | Fetal heart tones |
| **FL** | Femur length |
| **FM** | Fetal movement |
| **FPG** | Fasting plasma glucose test |
| **FSH** | Follicle-stimulating hormone |
| **FSHRH** | Follicle-stimulating hormone–releasing hormone |
| **G or grav** | Gravida |
| **GDM** | Gestational diabetes mellitus |
| **GIFT** | Gamete intrafallopian transfer |
| **GnRF** | Gonadotropin-releasing factor |
| **GnRH** | Gonadotropin-releasing hormone |
| **GTD** | Gestational trophoblastic disease |
| **GTPAL** | Gravida, term, preterm, abortion, living children; a system of recording maternity history |
| **HA** | Head-abdominal ratio |
| **HAI** | Hemagglutination-inhibition test |
| **HC** | Head compression |
| **hCG** | Human chorionic gonadotropin |
| **hCS** | Human chorionic somatomammotropin (same as hPL) |
| **HMD** | Hyaline membrane disease |
| **hMG** | Human menopausal gonadotropin |
| **hPL** | Human placental lactogen |
| **HPV** | Human papilloma virus |
| **HVH** | Herpesvirus hominis |
| **IDM** | Infant of a diabetic mother |
| **IPG** | Impedance phlebography |
| **IU** | International units |
| **IUD** | Intrauterine device |
| **IUFD** | Intrauterine fetal death |
| **IUGR** | Intrauterine growth restriction |
| **IVF** | In vitro fertilization |
| **LADA** | Left-acromion-dorsal-anterior |
| **LADP** | Left-acromion-dorsal-posterior |
| **LBW** | Low birth weight |
| **LDR** | Labor, delivery, and recovery room |
| **LGA** | Large for gestational age |
| **LH** | Luteinizing hormone |
| **LHRH** | Luteinizing hormone–releasing hormone |
| **LMA** | Left-mentum-anterior |
| **LML** | Left mediolateral (episiotomy) |
| **LMP** | Last menstrual period *or* Left-mentum-posterior |
| **LMT** | Left-mentum-transverse |
| **LOA** | Left-occiput-anterior |

# APPENDIX A

## Common Abbreviations in Maternal-Newborn and Women's Health Nursing

| | |
|---|---|
| **LOF** | Low outlet forceps |
| **LOP** | Left-occiput-posterior |
| **LOT** | Left-occiput-transverse |
| **L/S** | Lecithin/sphingomyelin ratio |
| **LSA** | Left-sacrum-anterior |
| **LSP** | Left-sacrum-posterior |
| **LST** | Left-sacrum-transverse |
| **MAS** | Meconium aspiration syndrome |
| **mec** | Meconium |
| **mec** st | Meconium stain |
| **ML** | Midline (episiotomy) |
| **MSAFP** | Maternal serum alpha-fetoprotein |
| **MUGB** | 4-methylumbelliferyl quanidinobenzoate |
| **multip** | Multipara |
| **NEC** | Necrotizing enterocolitis |
| **NGU** | Nongonococcal urethritis |
| **NP** | Nurse practitioner |
| **NSCST** | Nipple stimulation contraction stress test |
| **NST** | Nonstress test *or* Nonshivering thermogenesis |
| **NSVD** | Normal sterile vaginal delivery |
| **NTD** | Neural tube defects |
| **OA** | Occiput anterior |
| **OC** | Oral contraceptives |
| **OCT** | Oxytocin challenge test |
| **OF** | Occipitofrontal diameter of fetal head |
| **OFC** | Occipitofrontal circumference |
| **OGTT** | Oral glucose tolerance test |
| **OM** | Occipitomental (diameter) |
| **OP** | Occiput posterior |
| **p** | Para |
| **Pap smear** | Papanicolaou smear |
| **PDA** | Patent ductus arteriosus |
| **PEEP** | Positive end-expiratory pressure |
| **PG** | Phosphatidylglycerol *or* Prostaglandin |
| **PI** | Phosphatidylinositol |
| **PID** | Pelvic inflammatory disease |
| **PIH** | Pregnancy-induced hypertension |
| **Pit** | Pitocin |
| **PKU** | Phenylketonuria |
| **PMS** | Premenstrual syndrome |
| **PPHN** | Persistent pulmonary hypertension |
| **Premie** | Premature infant |
| **primip** | Primipara |
| **PROM** | Premature rupture of membranes |
| **PSI** | Prostaglandin synthesis inhibitor |
| **PUBS** | Percutaneous umbilical blood sampling |
| **RADA** | Right-acromion-dorsal-anterior |
| **RADP** | Right-acromion-dorsal-posterior |
| **RDS** | Respiratory distress syndrome |
| **REM** | Rapid eye movements |
| **RIA** | Radioimmunoassay |
| **RLF** | Retrolental fibroplasia |
| **RMA** | Right-mentum-anterior |
| **RMP** | Right-mentum-posterior |
| **RMT** | Right-mentum-transverse |
| **ROA** | Right-occiput-anterior |
| **ROM** | Rupture of membranes |
| **ROP** | Right-occiput-posterior *or* Retinopathy of prematurity |
| **ROT** | Right-occiput-transverse |
| **RRA** | Radioreceptor assay |
| **RSA** | Right-sacrum-anterior |
| **RSP** | Right-sacrum-posterior |
| **RST** | Right-sacrum-transverse |
| **SET** | Surrogate embryo transfer |
| **SGA** | Small for gestational age |
| **SIDS** | Sudden infant death syndrome |
| **SMB** | Submentobregmatic diameter |
| **SOB** | Suboccipitobregmatic diameter |
| **SPA** | Sperm penetration assay |
| **SRBOW** | Spontaneous rupture of bag of waters |
| **SROM** | Spontaneous rupture of membranes |
| **STH** | Somatotropic hormone |
| **STI** | Sexually transmitted infection |
| **STS** | Serologic test for syphilis |
| **SVE** | Sterile vaginal exam |
| **TC** | Thoracic circumference |
| **TCM** | Transcutaneous monitoring |
| **TDI** | Therapeutic donor insemination |
| **TNZ** | Thermal neutral zone |
| **TOL** | Trail of labor |
| **TORCH** | Toxoplasmosis, rubella, cytomegalovirus, herpesvirus hominis type 2 |
| **TSS** | Toxic shock syndrome |
| **ū** | Umbilicus |
| **UA** | Uterine activity |
| **UAC** | Umbilical artery catheter |
| **UAU** | Uterine activity units |
| **UC** | Uterine contraction |
| **UPI** | Uteroplacental insufficiency |
| **US** | Ultrasound |
| **VBAC** | Vaginal birth after cesarean |
| **VDRL** | Venereal Disease Research Laboratories |
| **VLBW** | Very low birth weight |
| **WIC** | Supplemental food program for Women, Infants, and Children |
| **ZIFT** | Zygote intrafallopian transfer |

# Appendix B

## Conversions and Equivalents

### Temperature Conversion

(Fahrenheit temperature − 32) × 5/9 = Centigrade temperature
(Centigrade temperature − 9/5) + 32 = Fahrenheit temperature

### Selected Conversion to Metric Measures

| *Known Value* | *Multiply by* | *To find* |
|---|---|---|
| inches | 2.54 | centimeters |
| ounces | 28 | grams |
| pounds | 454 | grams |
| pounds | 0.45 | kilogram |

### Selected Conversion from Metric Measures

| *Known Value* | *Multiply by* | *To find* |
|---|---|---|
| centimeters | 0.4 | inches |
| grams | 0.035 | ounces |
| grams | 0.0022 | pounds |
| kilograms | 2.2 | pounds |

### Conversion of Pounds and Ounces to Grams

| | *Ounces* | | | | | | | | | | | | | | | |
|---|---|---|---|---|---|---|---|---|---|---|---|---|---|---|---|---|
| S (*Pounds*) | 0 | 1 | 2 | 3 | 4 | 5 | 6 | 7 | 8 | 9 | 10 | 11 | 12 | 13 | 14 | 15 |
| 0 | — | 28 | 57 | 85 | 113 | 142 | 170 | 198 | 227 | 255 | 283 | 312 | 340 | 369 | 397 | 425 |
| 1 | 454 | 482 | 510 | 539 | 567 | 595 | 624 | 652 | 680 | 709 | 737 | 765 | 794 | 822 | 850 | 879 |
| 2 | 907 | 936 | 964 | 992 | 1021 | 1049 | 1077 | 1106 | 1134 | 1162 | 1191 | 1219 | 1247 | 1276 | 1304 | 1332 |
| 3 | 1361 | 1389 | 1417 | 1446 | 1474 | 1503 | 1531 | 1559 | 1588 | 1616 | 1644 | 1673 | 1701 | 1729 | 1758 | 1786 |
| 4 | 1814 | 1843 | 1871 | 1899 | 1928 | 1956 | 1984 | 2013 | 2041 | 2070 | 2098 | 2126 | 2155 | 2183 | 2211 | 2240 |
| 5 | 2268 | 2296 | 2325 | 2353 | 2381 | 2410 | 2438 | 2466 | 2495 | 2523 | 2551 | 2580 | 2608 | 2637 | 2665 | 2693 |
| 6 | 2722 | 2750 | 2778 | 2807 | 2835 | 2863 | 2892 | 2920 | 2948 | 2977 | 3005 | 3033 | 3062 | 3090 | 3118 | 3147 |
| 7 | 3175 | 3203 | 3232 | 3260 | 3289 | 3317 | 3345 | 3374 | 3402 | 3430 | 3459 | 3487 | 3515 | 3544 | 3572 | 3600 |
| 8 | 3629 | 3657 | 3685 | 3714 | 3742 | 3770 | 3799 | 3827 | 3856 | 3884 | 3912 | 3941 | 3969 | 3997 | 4026 | 4054 |
| 9 | 4082 | 4111 | 4139 | 4167 | 4196 | 4224 | 4252 | 4281 | 4309 | 4337 | 4366 | 4394 | 4423 | 4451 | 4479 | 4508 |
| 10 | 4536 | 4564 | 4593 | 4621 | 4649 | 4678 | 4706 | 4734 | 4763 | 4791 | 4819 | 4848 | 4876 | 4904 | 4933 | 4961 |
| 11 | 4990 | 5018 | 5046 | 5075 | 5103 | 5131 | 5160 | 5188 | 5216 | 5245 | 5273 | 5301 | 5330 | 5358 | 5386 | 5415 |
| 12 | 5443 | 5471 | 5500 | 5528 | 5557 | 5585 | 5613 | 5642 | 5670 | 5698 | 5727 | 5755 | 5783 | 5812 | 5840 | 5868 |
| 13 | 5897 | 5925 | 5953 | 5982 | 6010 | 6038 | 6067 | 6095 | 6123 | 6152 | 6180 | 6209 | 6237 | 6265 | 6294 | 6322 |
| 14 | 6350 | 6379 | 6407 | 6435 | 6464 | 6492 | 6520 | 6549 | 6577 | 6605 | 6634 | 6662 | 6690 | 6719 | 6747 | 6776 |
| 15 | 6804 | 6832 | 6860 | 6889 | 6917 | 6945 | 6973 | 7002 | 7030 | 7059 | 7087 | 7115 | 7144 | 7172 | 7201 | 7228 |
| 16 | 7257 | 7286 | 7313 | 7342 | 7371 | 7399 | 7427 | 7456 | 7484 | 7512 | 7541 | 7569 | 7597 | 7626 | 7654 | 7682 |
| 17 | 7711 | 7739 | 7768 | 7796 | 7824 | 7853 | 7881 | 7909 | 7938 | 7966 | 7994 | 8023 | 8051 | 8079 | 8108 | 8136 |
| 18 | 8165 | 8192 | 8221 | 8249 | 8278 | 8306 | 8335 | 8363 | 8391 | 8420 | 8448 | 8476 | 8504 | 8533 | 8561 | 8590 |
| 19 | 8618 | 8646 | 8675 | 8703 | 8731 | 8760 | 8788 | 8816 | 8845 | 8873 | 8902 | 8930 | 8958 | 8987 | 9015 | 9043 |
| 20 | 9072 | 9100 | 9128 | 9157 | 9185 | 9213 | 9242 | 9270 | 9298 | 9327 | 9355 | 9383 | 9412 | 9440 | 9469 | 9497 |
| 21 | 9525 | 9554 | 9582 | 9610 | 9639 | 9667 | 9695 | 9724 | 9752 | 9780 | 9809 | 9837 | 9865 | 9894 | 9922 | 9950 |
| 22 | 9979 | 10007 | 10036 | 10064 | 10092 | 10120 | 10149 | 10177 | 10206 | 10234 | 10262 | 10291 | 10319 | 10347 | 10376 | 10404 |

# Spanish Translations of English Phrases*

This appendix includes phrases you might find helpful in working with families during pregnancy, labor and birth, and after the birth. There are many ways to phrase questions. We have chosen some statements we consider essential and have tried to phrase them in a straightforward way. The phrases are designed to help you in situations in which translation is not possible at the moment.

This list begins with introductory statements, which are presented in a logical conversational flow. The remaining phrases are arranged according to the phases of pregnancy and birth during which they are most applicable.

| **Essential Introductory Phrases** | **Frases Introductoras Esenciales** |
|---|---|
| Hello | Hola |
| I am a nurse. | Soy enferera (enfermero).† |
| I am a student nurse. | Soy estudiante de enfermería. |
| My name is ______________. | Mi nombre es ______________. |
| | Me llamo ______________. |
| What is your name? | ¿Cuál es su nombre? |
| | ¿Cómo se llama? |
| | ¿Cómo quiere que la llamemos? |
| What name should I call you? | ¿Cómo quiere ser llamada? |
| Thank you | Gracias |
| Please | Por favor |
| Is someone here with you? | ¿Hay alquien aquí con usted? |
| Does he (she) speak English? | ¿Habla él (ella) English? |
| Goodbye | Adiós. |

| **Phrases for the Antepartal Period** | **Frases para el Periodo Prenatal** |
|---|---|
| Are you taking any medications now? | ¿Está tomando algunas medicinas ahora? |
| Show me the medicine bottles please. | Por favor, muéstreme los frascos. |
| Have you ever had trouble with your blood pressure? | ¿Ha tenido problemas alguna vez con la presión arterial? |
| When was the first day of your last period? | ¿Cuál fue el primer día de su última regla? |
| | ¿Cuál fue el primer día de su última menstruación? |
| Have you had any spotting or bleeding since your last period? | ¿Ha sangrado o ha tenido manchas de sangre desde su última regla? |
| Have you been on birth control pills? | ¿Ha estado tomando píldoras anticonceptivas? |
| When did you stop taking them? | ¿Cuándo dejó de tomarlas? |

| **Phrases for the Antepartal Period** | **Frases para el Periodo Prenatal** |
|---|---|
| Do you have an intrauterine device (IUD)? | ¿Usa un aparato intrauterino? |
| How many times have you been pregnant? | ¿Cuántas veces ha estado usted embarazada? |
| Are you having any problems with your pregnancy? | ¿Tiene problemas con su embarazo? |
| Is there anything that is worrying you? | ¿Hay algo o alguna cosa que la preocupe? |

*Prepared by Elizabeth Medina, Ph.D. Associate Professor of Spanish, Regis University, Denver, Colorado.

†In Spanish, nouns that end in *a* indicate female gender; nouns that end in *o* indicate male gender.

# APPENDIX C

## Spanish Translations of English Phrases

| | |
|---|---|
| I would like to take your blood pressure. | Quisiera tomarle la presió arterial. |
| I would like to take your pulse. | Quisiera tomarle el pulso. |
| I would like to take your temperature. | Quisiera tomarle la temperatura. |
| I would like to listen to your heart and lungs. | Quisiera escucharle el corazon y los pulmones. |
| I would like to check your uterus. | Quisiera examinarle el útero. |
| Please urinate in this cup and leave it in the bathroom? | Puede orinar en este vaso y dejarlo en el baño. |
| Please stand up. | Por favor, levántese. |
| Please sit down. | Por favor, sie'ntese. |
| Please lie down. | Por favor, acuéstese. |
| **Phrases Related to Client Safety** | **Frases Relacionadas con la Seguridad del Cliente** |
| I would like to talk to you alone. | Quisiera hablar a solas con usted. |
| Are you safe at home? | ¿Sufre de peligros en casa? |
| Are you afraid of your partner? | ¿Le tiene miedo a su compañero? |
| During your pregnancy has your partner hit, slapped, kicked, or punched you? | Durante su embarazo,<br>¿la ha golpeado?<br>¿la ha abofeteado?<br>¿la ha pateado? o<br>¿le ha dado puñetazos? |
| How many times? | ¿Cuántas veces? |
| Do you have someone for support? | ¿Cuénta con alguien que la pueda ayudar? |
| **Questions the Mother or Father May Ask** | **Posibles Preguntas que Madres o Padres Hacen** |
| How big is my baby? | ¿De qué tamaño es el (la) bebé? |
| How much does the baby weigh now? | ¿Cuánto pesa el bebé ahora? |
| When will I feel my baby move? | ¿Cuándo lo (la) voy a sentir moverse? |
| **Phrases for the Intrapartal Period** | **Frases Durante el Parto** |
| *Note:* Review the essential introductory phrases for beginning a conversation. | *Nota:* Repase las frases introductoras para comenzar una conversación. |
| Are you having labor pains? | ¿Tiene dolores de parto? |
| Are you having contractions? | ¿Tiene contracciones? |
| Are you having pain? | ¿Tiene dolores? |
| Do you need medicine for pain? | ¿Necesita medicina para el dolor? |
| Do you need to urinate? | ¿Necesita orinar? |
| This is a bedpan to urinate in. | Aquí tiene el bacín (la chata) (el pato) para orinar. |
| Can I help you to the bathroom? | ¿La ayudo a ir al baño? |
| Do you need to have a bowel movement? | ¿Necesita mover el vientre (obrar)? Necesita "Hacer caca"—coloquial |

# Appendix C

## Spanish Translations of English Phrases

| | |
| --- | --- |
| Has your bag of water broken? | ¿Se le ha roto la bolsa de agua(s)? |
| Have you had any bright-red bleeding during your pregnancy? | ¿Ha tenido algún sangramiento de color rojo durante su embarazo? |
| **Phrases for the Intrapartal Period** | **Frases Durante el Parto** |
| How many births have you had? | ¿Cuántos niños le han nacido? |
| I need to do a vaginal examination. | Necesito hacerle un examen vaginal. |
| I will help you. | La voy a ayudar. |
| I will stay with you. | Me quedaré con usted. |
| Please pant. I will show you how. | Por favor, jadee. Le voy a mostrar cómo. |
| Do not push now. | No puje ahora. |
| Push now. | Puje ahora. |
| Stop pushing. | Pare de pujar.<br>No puje más. |
| The doctor needs to do a cesarean birth. | El doctor le va a hacer una operación cesárea. |
| This is medicine for your pain. You will feel better soon. | Esta medicina es para el dolor. Va a sentirse mejor pronto. |
| When is your baby supposed to be born? | ¿Cuando está supuesto a nacer el bebé? |

| | | | |
| --- | --- | --- | --- |
| January | February | enero | febrero |
| March | April | marzo | abril |
| May | June | mayo | junio |
| July | August | julio | agosto |
| September | October | septiembre | octubre |
| November | December | noviembre | diciembre |

| | |
| --- | --- |
| What is your doctor's name? | ¿Cuál es el nombre de su doctor? |
| What is your midwife's name? | ¿Cuál is el nombre de su comadrona (partera)? |
| Your baby is having some trouble now. | El bebé está pasando por algunos problemas.<br>El bebé está sufriendo algunas dificultades. |
| I need to put this oxygen mask on you. It will help your baby. It may smell funny, but it is OK. | Le voy a poner esta máscara de oxígeno. Va a ayudar al bebé. Huele extraño, pero no hay problemas. |
| Please turn on your left side. | Por favor voltéese al lado izquierdo. |
| Please turn on your right side. | Por favor voltéese al lado derecho. |
| Your baby is OK. | El bebé está bien. |
| **Phrases for the Postpartal Period and the Newborn Area** | **Frases para el Periodo Despues del Parto y el Area del Recien Nacido** |
| *Note:* Review the essential introductory phrases for beginning a conversation. | *Nota:* Repase las frases introductoras para comenzar una conversación. |
| Are you hungry? | ¿Tiene hambre? |
| Are you thirsty? | ¿Tiene sed? |
| Are you cold? | ¿Tiene frío? |

# Appendix C

## Spanish Translations of English Phrases

| | |
|---|---|
| Are you tired? | ¿Está cansada? |
| I am going to put antibiotic ointment in the baby's eyes. It will help protect your baby from some infections. | Le voy a poner al bebé un ungüento antibiótico alrededor de los ojos. Lo (la) va a proteger contra al gunos infecciones. |
| I am going to take some blood from your baby's foot to check the blood sugar and hemocrit. | Le voy a sacar sangre del pie al bebé para determinar el azúcar del la sangre ye el hematocrítico. |
| If your baby begins to spit up, please turn him (her) on his (her) side. | Si el bebé comienza a vomitar, colóquelo (colóquela) de costado. |
| It may help to position your baby like this. | Lo (la) ayudará—si lo coloca así.<br>Lo (la) ayudaría—si lo colocara así. |
| I would like to suggest that you clean your nipples this way before you breastfeed your baby. | Es bueno que se lave los pezones de esta manera antes de darle el pecho al bebé. |

| **Phrases for the Postpartal Period and the Newborn Area** | **Frases para el Periodo Despues del Parto y el Area del Recien Nacido** |
|---|---|
| It is better that you clean your baby's cord this way. | Es mejor para el bebé que le lave el ombligo de esta manera. |
| It is better that you bathe your baby this way. | Es mejor que lo (la) bañe de esta manera. |
| It is better that you clean your baby's penis this way. | Es mejor que le limpie el pene así. |
| I would like to suggest that you fold the diaper this way. | Le sugiero que doble el pañal así. |
| I would like to suggest that you fasten the diaper this way. | Le sugiero que asegure el pañal así. |
| Take the baby's temperature this way. | Tómele la temperature así. |
| I need to check [your breasts, your uterus, your flow, your stitches, your legs and feet]. | Necesito examinarle [los pechos, el útero, el flujo, los puntos, las pierns y los pies]. |
| I need to feel your uterus. | Necesito examinarle el útero. |
| I need to massage your uterus. | Necesito darle un masaje en la región del útero. |
| Place your baby on its side. | Coloque al bebé de costado. |
| Place the baby's used diapers here. | Coloque aquí los pañales usados. |
| Please rub your uterus every half hour to keep it firm. I will show you how. | Necesita darse un masaje en la región del útero cada media hora para mantenerlo firme. Le voy a mostrar cómo. |
| Would you like to see your baby now? | ¿Quiere ver a su bebé ahora? |
| Would you like me to help you feed your baby? | ¿Quiere que le ayude a alimentarlo (la)? |
| Your baby needs a car seat to go home in. | El (la) bebé necesita un asiento para bebé en el automóvil. |

| **Special Neonatal Needs** | **Necesidades del Recien Nacido** |
|---|---|
| We are giving your baby oxygen. | Le vamos a dar oxígeno al (a la) bebé. |
| Your baby is having problems breathing. | El (la) bebé tiene problemas al respirar. |
| Your baby needs extra help. | El (la) bebé necesita ayuda especial. |
| Your baby needs to go to a special care nursery. | El (la) bebé necesita ir a la sala de cuidados especiales para bebés. |

# Guidelines for Working with Deaf Clients and Interpreters

1. First, remember that it requires trust on the part of the client to allow nonsigning caregivers and an interpreter into her life.
2. It is important to use a registered interpreter. Medical interpreters are registered with the Registry of Interpreters for the Deaf. Although family members and friends may offer to interpret, it is best to use registered medical interpreters because they are required to translate the clients' and nurses' words accurately without adding in any other opinion.
3. Greet the client and family with a handshake and body posture that indicates welcome. You may point to your name tag and use the American Sign Language (ASL) alphabet cards to spell out your name. The client may wish to select cards to indicate her name. It is especially important as you work together to make the effort to provide a greeting as you would with speaking clients; greetings help develop rapport.
4. Once the interpreter is present, continue to look at the client and speak directly to her. There will be a temptation to look at the interpreter, and it will help to remember that you are speaking to the client.
5. Avoid phrasing your words as if you are talking to the interpreter (eg, "Can you tell her . . . ?"). Instead, phrase your questions as you do with speaking clients (eg, "I'm going to ask you some questions now.").
6. Depend on the deaf client to ask questions.
7. Look at the client's face for signs of difficulty in understanding. Deaf clients have a behavior of "gesturing" that involves shaking their heads as if to indicate "yes" even when they do not understand. If the client is nodding "yes," ask her to repeat the directions you have just given.
8. Be as direct as possible. Keep to what you want to know or what you want to convey. Speak in short sentences, using nontechnical words. Avoid colloquial or slang words. Be sure to explain what you want to do before you do it. For instance, tell her you want to start an IV and explain the equipment. Then, with her permission, start the IV.
9. Be aware that deaf clients may have difficulty understanding when to take medications. It will be helpful to associate taking medications or completing some treatment or activity with meals. (For instance, while showing her the two capsules she is to take when she goes home, tell her to take the two capsules at breakfast and another two capsules at bedtime.) Avoid saying "take two capsules at 8:00 A.M., 2:00 P.M., and 12:00 A.M."
10. The difference in interpreting time may also affect obtaining a history. It is best to begin with a specific event in the past and work forward.

**What to Do Until the Interpreter Arrives**

1. Role-play as much as possible.
2. Demonstrate what you want the client to do or what you want to do.
3. Be resourceful.
4. Remember that some deaf clients can read lips. Some may read written language, but use care in assuming the client understands.

**What to Do to Prepare for Working with a Deaf Client**

1. Contact local agencies that work with deaf clients to see what resources are available. Ask about classes in ASL. Being able to use some basic signs will be very helpful while waiting for an interpreter to arrive.
2. Read to learn more about the deaf culture. Contact your local agency or the National Information Center on Deafness, Silver Springs, Maryland, to get suggestions on books you might read.
3. Investigate your health facility. What is available to assist you? Look for videos used for teaching in the maternal-child unit and note if they have captions. Remember that many deaf clients do not read written language, so it will be important to review the content of the video with an interpreter present.

Prepared with the kind assistance of Mr. Gerald Dement, Interpreter Coordinator, Pikes Peak Center on Deafness, Colorado Springs, Colorado.

# APPENDIX E

## Sign Language for Health Care Professionals

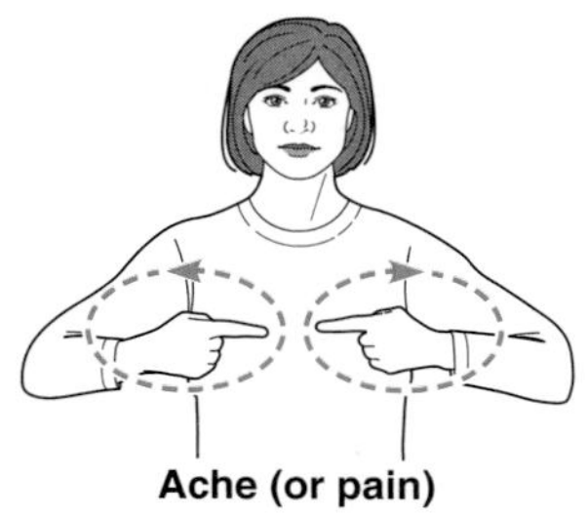
Ache (or pain)

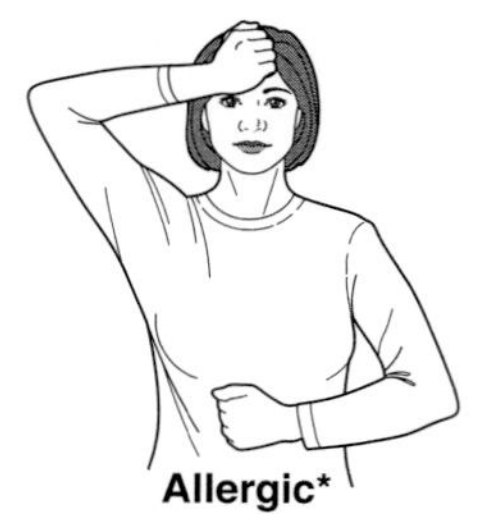
Allergic*

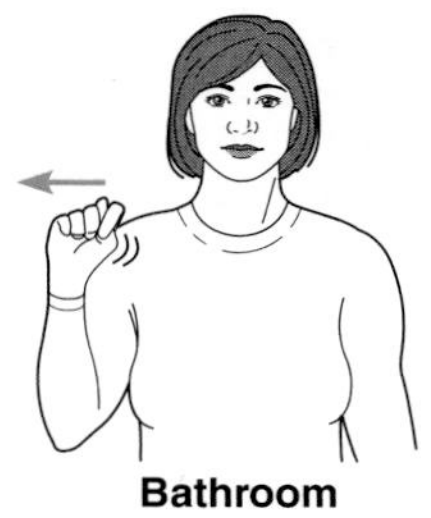
Bathroom

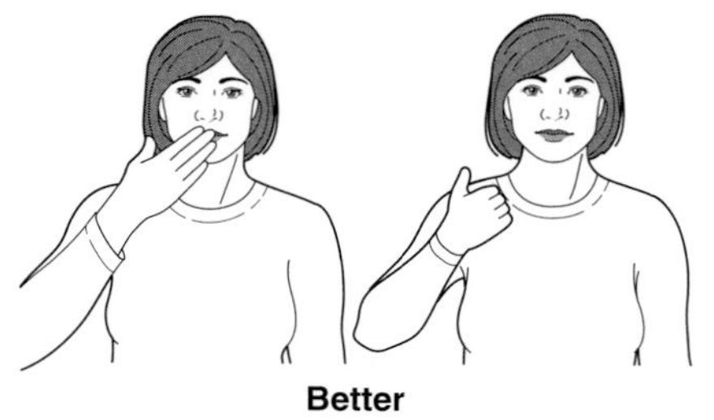
Better

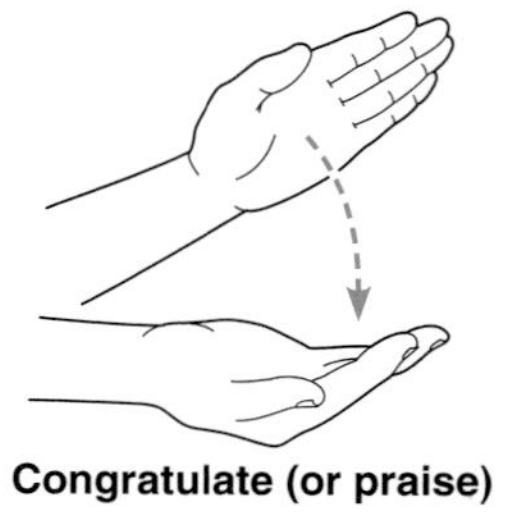
Congratulate (or praise)

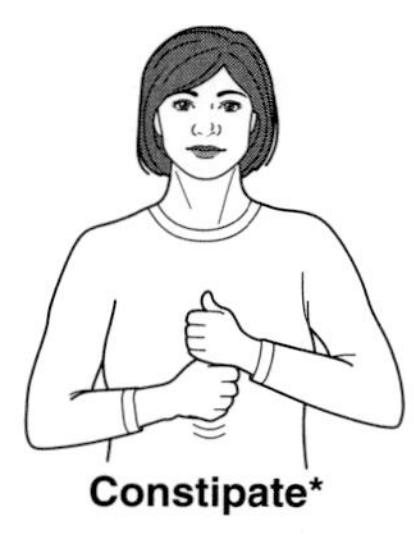
Constipate*

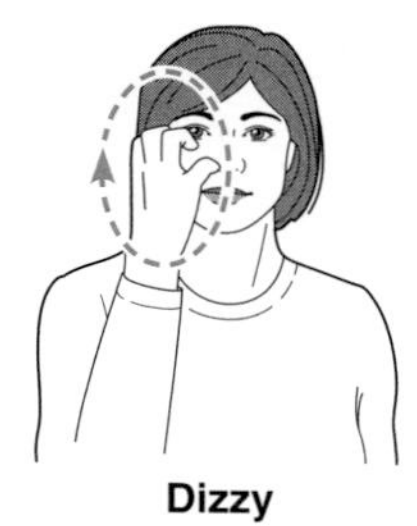
Dizzy

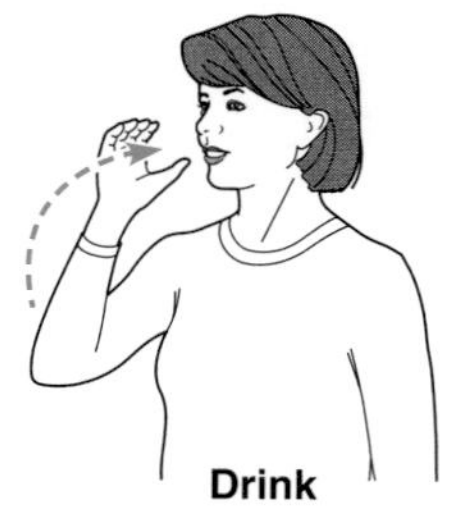
Drink

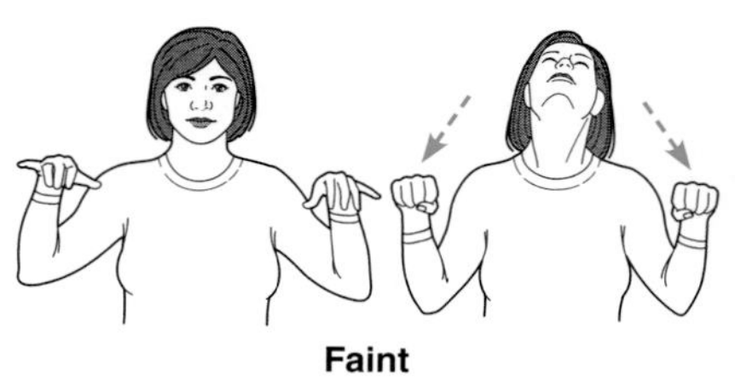
Faint

*Indicates signs that are in manually signed English. Those without an asterisk are in American Sign Language.

# Sign Language for Health Care Professionals

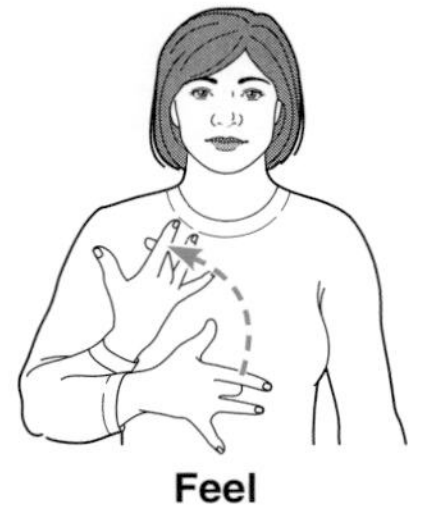
Feel

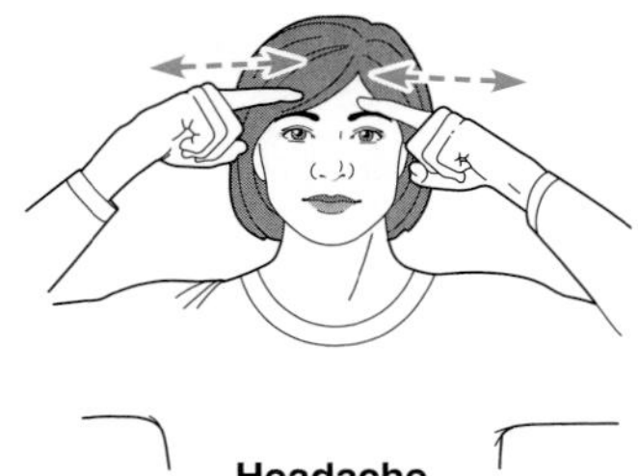
Headache

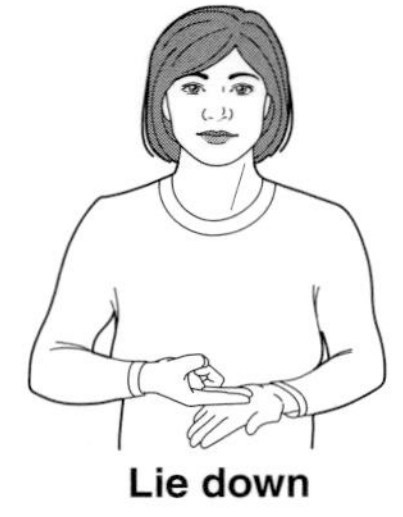
Lie down

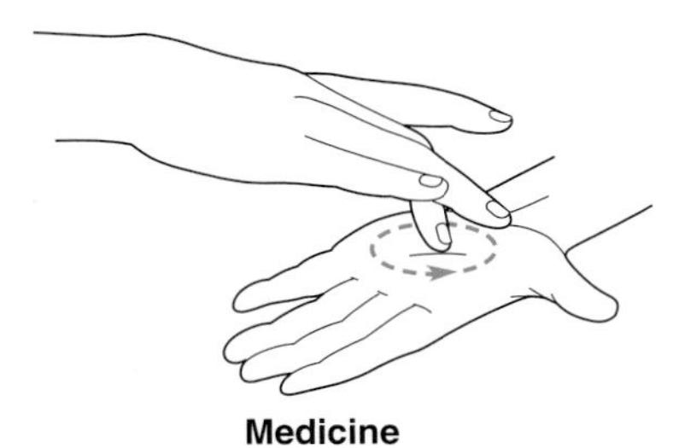
Medicine

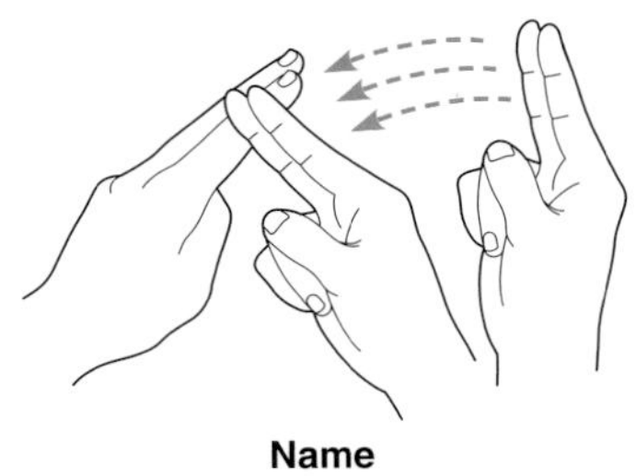
Name

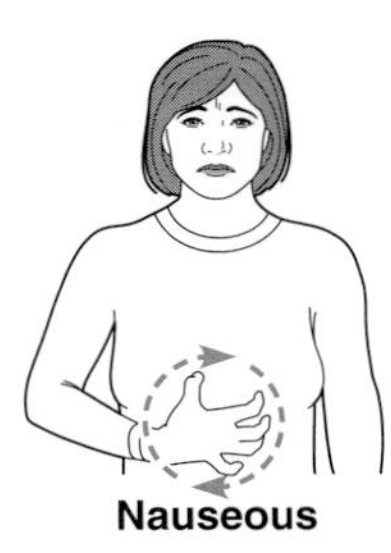
Nauseous

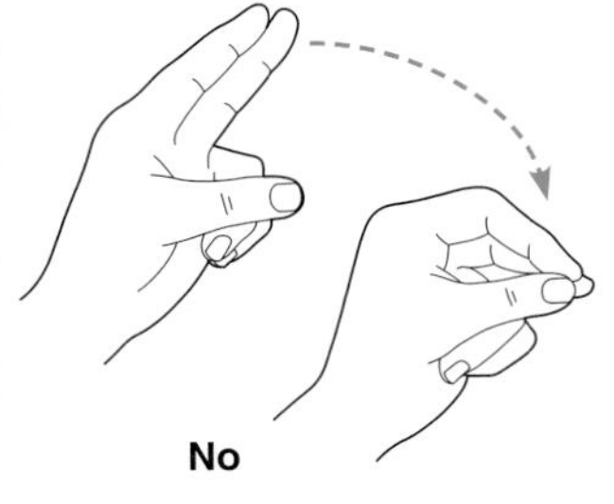
No

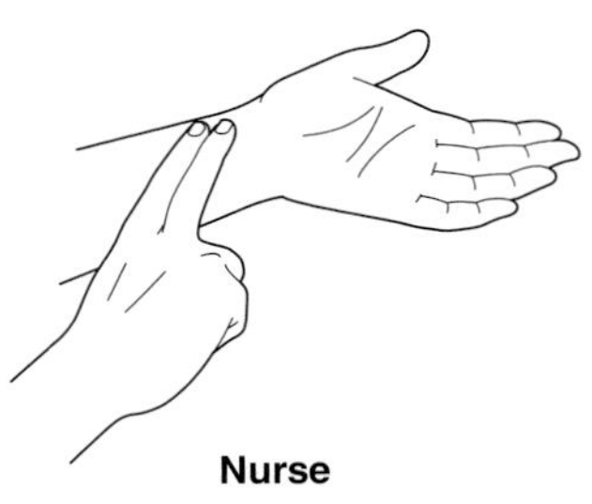
Nurse

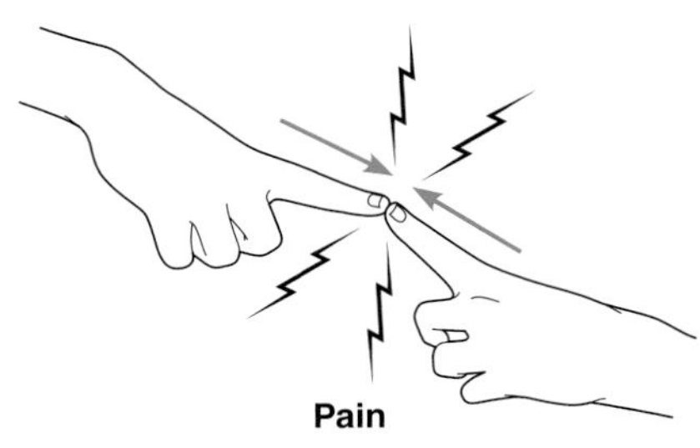
Pain

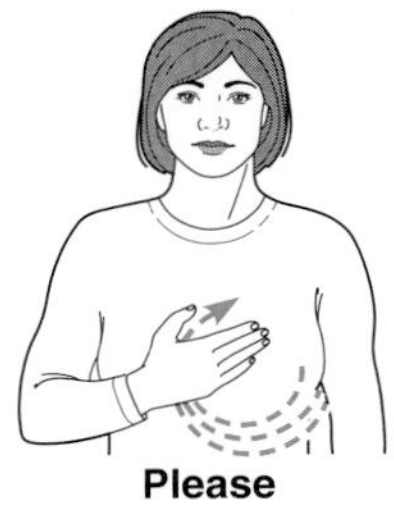
Please

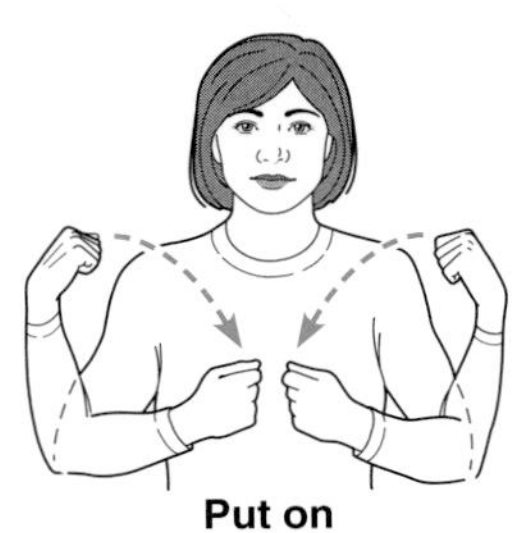
Put on

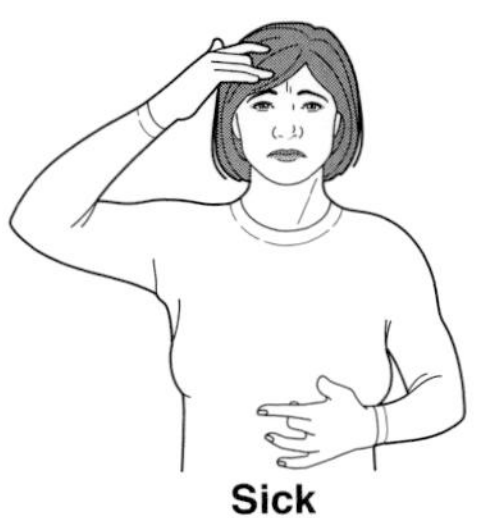
Sick

# Sign Language for Health Care Professionals

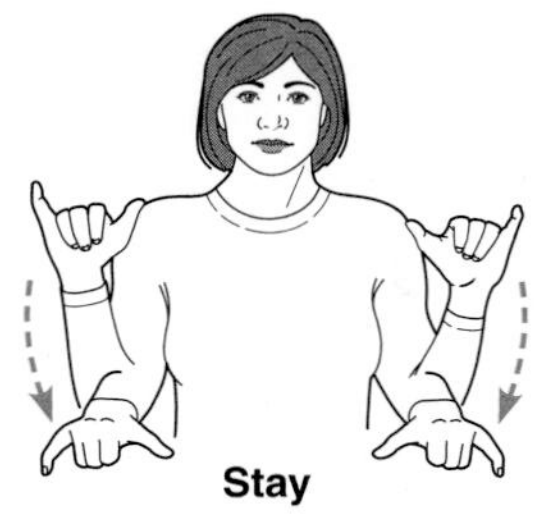
Stay

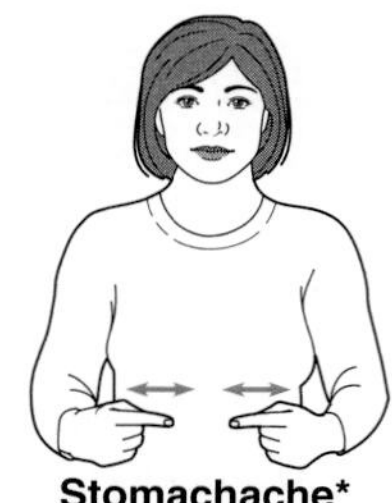
Stomachache*

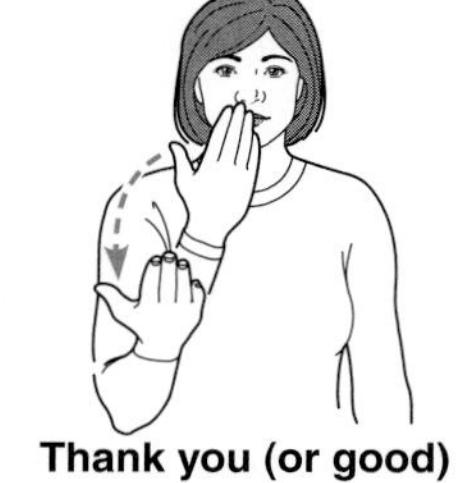
Thank you (or good)

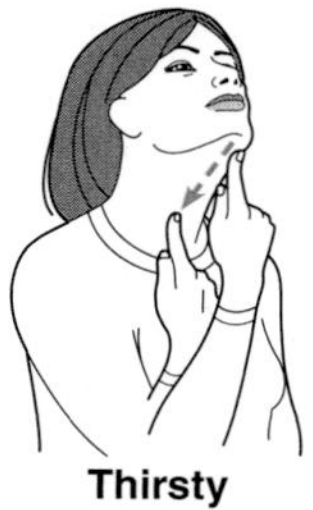
Thirsty

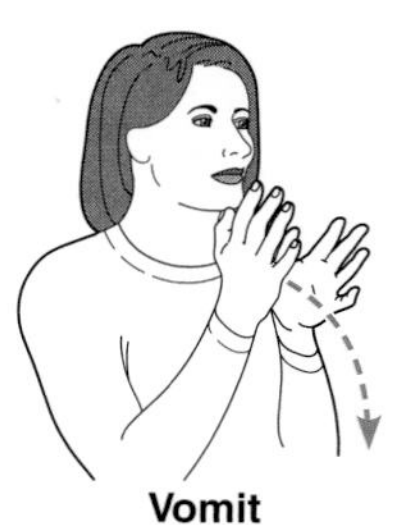
Vomit

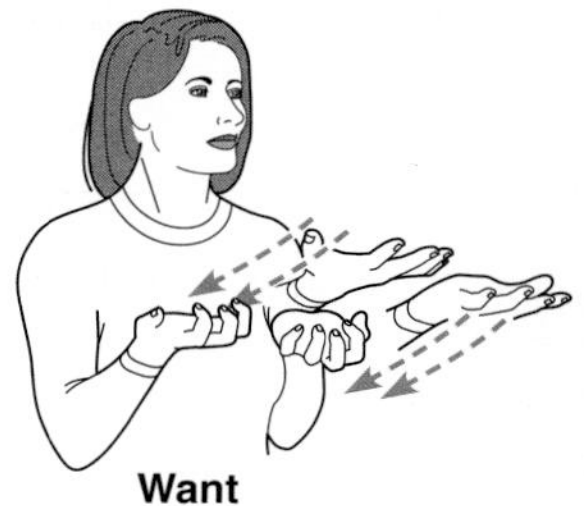
Want

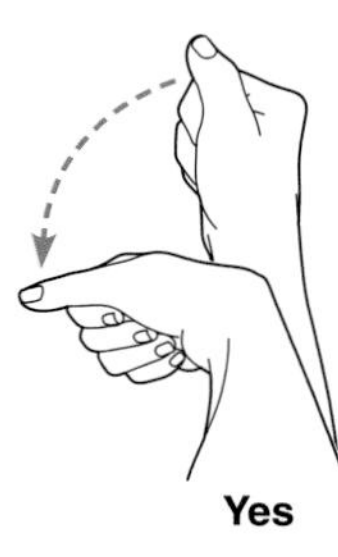
Yes

*Indicates signs that are in manually signed English. Those without an asterisk are in American Sign Language.

# Clinical Estimation of Gestational Age

## Examination First Hours

## CLINICAL ESTIMATION OF GESTATIONAL AGE

An Approximation Based on Published Data*

WEEKS GESTATION: 20 21 22 23 24 25 26 27 28 29 30 31 32 33 34 35 36 37 38 39 40 41 42 43 44 45 46 47 48

| PHYSICAL FINDINGS | | | | | | | | | |
|---|---|---|---|---|---|---|---|---|---|
| VERNIX | | APPEARS | COVERS BODY, THICK LAYER | ON BACK, SCALP, IN CREASES | SCANT, IN CREASES | NO VERNIX | | | |
| BREAST TISSUE AND AREOLA | | AREOLA & NIPPLE BARELY VISIBLE NO PALPABLE BREAST TISSUE | AREOLA RAISED | 1-2 MM NODULE | 3-5 MM | 5-6 MM | 7-10 MM | ?12 MM | |
| EAR | FORM | FLAT, SHAPELESS | BEGINNING INCURVING SUPERIOR | INCURVING UPPER 2/3 PINNAE | WELL-DEFINED INCURVING TO LOBE | | | | |
| | CARTILAGE | PINNA SOFT, STAYS FOLDED | CARTILAGE SCANT RETURNS SLOWLY FROM FOLDING | THIN CARTILAGE SPRINGS BACK FROM FOLDING | PINNA FIRM, REMAINS ERECT FROM HEAD | | | | |
| SOLE CREASES | | SMOOTH SOLES T CREASES | 1-2 ANTERIOR CREASES | 2-3 ANTERIOR CREASES | CREASES ANTERIOR 2/3 SOLE | CREASES INVOLVING HEEL | DEEPER CREASES OVER ENTIRE SOLE | | |
| SKIN | THICKNESS & APPEARANCE | THIN, TRANSLUCENT SKIN, PLETHORIC, VENULES OVER ABDOMEN EDEMA | SMOOTH THICKER NO EDEMA | PINK | FEW VESSELS | SOME DESQUAMATION PALE PINK | THICK, PALE, DESQUAMATION OVER ENTIRE BODY | | |
| | NAIL PLATES | APPEAR | | NAILS TO FINGER TIPS | NAILS EXTEND WELL BEYOND FINGER TIPS | | | | |
| HAIR | | APPEARS ON HEAD | EYE BROWS & LASHES | FINE, WOOLLY, BUNCHES OUT FROM HEAD | SILKY, SINGLE STRANDS LAYS FLAT | ?RECEDING HAIRLINE OR LOSS OF BABY HAIR SHORT, FINE UNDERNEATH | | | |
| LANUGO | | APPEARS | COVERS ENTIRE BODY | VANISHES FROM FACE | PRESENT ON SHOULDERS | NO LANUGO | | | |
| GENITALIA | TESTES | | TESTES PALPABLE IN INGUINAL CANAL | IN UPPER SCROTUM | IN LOWER SCROTUM | | | | |
| | SCROTUM | | FEW RUGAE | RUGAE, ANTERIOR PORTION | RUGAE COVER | PENDULOUS | | | |
| | LABIA & CLITORIS | | PROMINENT CLITORIS LABIA MAJORA SMALL WIDELY SEPARATED | LABIA MAJORA LARGER NEARLY COVERED CLITORIS | LABIA MINORA & CLITORIS COVERED | | | | |
| SKULL FIRMNESS | | BONES ARE SOFT | SOFT TO 1" FROM ANTERIOR FONTANELLE | SPONGY AT EDGES OF FONTANELLE CENTER FIRM | BONES HARD SUTURES EASILY DISPLACED | BONES HARD, CANNOT BE DISPLACED | | | |
| POSTURE | RESTING | HYPOTONIC LATERAL DECUBITUS | HYPOTONIC | BEGINNING FLEXION THIGH | STRONGER HIP FLEXION | FROG-LIKE | FLEXION ALL LIMBS | HYPERTONIC | VERY HYPERTONIC |
| | RECOIL - LEG | NO RECOIL | PARTIAL RECOIL | PROMPT RECOIL | | | | | |
| | ARM | NO RECOIL | BEGIN FLEXION NO RECOIL | PROMPT RECOIL MAY BE INHIBITED | PROMPT RECOIL AFTER 30" INHIBITION | | | | |

WEEKS GESTATION: 20 21 22 23 24 25 26 27 28 29 30 31 32 33 34 35 36 37 38 39 40 41 42 43 44 45 46 47 48

*Brazie, J. V., & Lubchenco, L. O. (1974). The estimation of gestational age chart. In Kempe, Silver, & O'Brien (Eds.), *Current pediatric diagnosis and treatment* (3rd ed., chap. 4). Los Altos, CA: Lange Medical Publications. Form courtesy of Mead Johnson Laboratories, Evansville, IN.

# Appendix G

## Actions and Effects of Selected Drugs during Breastfeeding*

### Anticoagulants

*Coumarin derivatives (warfarin, dicumarol):* Relatively safe to use; only small amount in breast milk; check PTT

*Heparin:* Does not cross into breast milk; check PTT

*Phenindione (Hedulin):* Passes easily into breast milk; neonate may have increased prothrombin time and PTT

### Anticonvulsants

*Phenytoin (Dilantin), phenobarbital:* Generally considered safe; if high doses of phenobarbital are ingested, may cause drowsiness; short-acting phenobarbiturates (secobarbital) preferred, because they appear in lower concentration in milk

*Magnesium sulfate:* Lactogenesis may be delayed

### Antihistamines

*Diphenhydramine (Benadryl), pheniramine (Dimetane), Claritin, Allegra:* May cause decreased milk supply; infant may become drowsy or irritable

**Antimetabolites** Unknown, probably long-term anti-DNA effect on the infant; potentially very toxic

### Antimicrobials

*Aminoglycosides:* May cause ototoxicity or nephrotoxicity if given for more than 2 weeks

*Ampicillin:* Skin rash, candidiasis; diarrhea

*Chloramphenicol:* Possible bone marrow suppression; too low a dose for Gray syndrome; refusal of breast

*Methacycline:* Possible inhibition of bone growth; may cause discoloration of the teeth; use should be avoided

*Metronidazole (Flagyl):* Possible neurologic disorders or blood dyscrasias; delay breastfeeding for 12 hours after dose

*Penicillin:* Possible allergic response; candidiasis

*Quinolones (synthetic antibiotics):* Can cause arthropathies

*Sulfonamides:* May cause hyperbilirubinemia; use contraindicated until infant over 1 week old

*Tetracycline:* Long-term use and large doses should be avoided; may cause tooth staining or inhibition of bone growth

### Antithyroids

*Thiouracil:* Contraindicated during lactation; may cause goiter or agranulocytosis

### Barbiturates

*Propylthiouracil:* Safe; monitor infant thyroid function

*Phenothiazines:* May produce sedation

### Bronchodilators

*Aminophylline:* May cause insomnia or irritability in the infant

*Ephedrine, cromolyn (Intal):* Relatively safe

**Caffeine** Excessive consumption may cause jitteriness or wakefulness

### Cardiovascular

*Methyldopa:* Increase in milk volume

*Propranolol (Inderal):* May cause hypoglycemia; possibility of other blocking effects, especially if infant has renal or liver dysfunction

*Quinidine:* May cause arrhythmias in infant

*Reserpine (Serpasil):* Nasal stuffiness, lethargy, or diarrhea in infant

**Corticosteroids** Adrenal suppression may occur with long-term administration of doses greater than 10 mg/day

### Diuretics

*Furosemide (Lasix):* Not excreted in breast milk

*Thiazide diuretics (Esidrix, Hydrodiuril, Oretic):* Safe but can cause dehydration, reduce milk production

### Heavy metals

*Gold:* Potentially toxic; gold salts—compatible with nursing

*Mercury:* Excreted in the milk and hazardous to infant

### Hormones

*Androgens:* Suppress lactation

*Thyroid hormones:* May mask hypothyroidism

### Laxatives

*Peri-Colaces Ducolax:* Relatively safe

*Milk of magnesia, metamucil:* Relatively safe

### Narcotic analgesics

*Codeine:* Accumulation may lead to neonatal depression

*Meperidine:* May lead to neonatal depression

*Morphine:* Long-term use may cause newborn addiction

*Based on data from Riordan, J., & Auerbach, K. J. (1999). *Breastfeeding and human lactation* (2nd ed., pp. 163–220). Boston: Jones & Bartlett. Briggs, G. G., Freeman, R. K., & Yaffe, S. J. (1998). *Drugs in pregnancy and lactation* (5th ed.). Baltimore: Williams & Wilkins. Committee on Drugs, American Academy of Pediatrics. (1994). The transfer of drugs and other chemicals into human milk. *Pediatrics,* 93, 137–150. Taeusch, H., & Ballard, R. A. (1998). *Avery's diseases of the newborn* (7th ed., pp. 1348–1352). Philadelphia: Saunders.

# Actions and Effects of Selected Drugs during Breastfeeding

## Nonnarcotic analgesics, NSAIDs

*Acetaminophen (Tylenol):* Relatively safe for short-term analgesia

*Ibuprofen (Motrin):* Safe

*Propoxyphene (Darvon):* May cause sleepiness and poor nursing in infant

*Salicylates (aspirin):* Safe after first week of life; monitor protime

## Oral contraceptives

*Combined estrogen/progestin pills:* Significantly decrease milk supply; may alter milk composition; may cause gynecomastia in male infants

*Progestin only (DMPA, Norplant):* Safe if started after lactation is established

## Radioactive materials for testing

*Gallium citrate ($^{67}G$):* Insignificant amount excreted in breast milk; no nursing for 2 weeks

*Iodine:* Contraindicated; may affect infant's thyroid gland

*$^{125}I$:* Discontinue nursing for 48 hours

*$^{131}I$:* Nursing should be discontinued until excretion is no longer significant; nursing may be resumed after 10 days

*Technetium-99m:* Discontinue nursing for 3 days (half-life = 6 hours)

## Sedatives/tranquilizers

*Diazepam (Valium):* May accumulate to high levels; may increase neonatal jaundice; may cause lethargy and weight loss

*Lithium:* Contraindicated; may cause neonatal flaccidity and hypotonia

## Substance abuse

*Alcohol:* Potential motor developmental delay; mild sedative effect

*Amphetamines:* Controversial; may cause irritability, poor sleeping pattern

*Cocaine, crack:* Extreme irritability, tachycardia, vomiting, apnea

*Marijuana:* Drowsiness

*Heroin:* Tremors, restlessness, vomiting, poor feeding

*Nicotine (smoking):* Shock, vomiting, diarrhea, decreased milk production

# APPENDIX H

## Selected Maternal-Newborn Laboratory Values

### Normal Maternal Laboratory Values

| Test | Nonpregnant Values | Pregnant Values |
|---|---|---|
| Hematocrit | 37%–47% | 32%–42% |
| Hemoglobin | 12–16 g/dL* | 10–14 g/dL* |
| Platelets | 150,000–350,000/mm$^3$ | Significant increase 3–5 days after birth (predisposes to thrombosis) |
| Partial thromboplastin time (PTT) | 12–14 seconds | Slight decrease in pregnancy and again in labor (placental site clotting) |
| Fibrinogen | 250 mg/dL | 400 mg/dL |
| Serum glucose | | |
| Fasting | 70–80 mg/dL | 65 mg/dL |
| 2-hour postprandial | 60–110 mg/dL | Less than 140 mg/dL |
| Total protein | 6.7–8.3 g/dL | 5.5–7.5 g/dL |
| White blood cell total | 4500–10,000/mm$^3$ | 5000–15,000/mm$^3$ |
| Polymorphonuclear cells | 54%–62% | 60%–85% |
| Lymphocytes | 38%–46% | 15%–40% |

### Normal Neonatal Laboratory Values

| Test | Normal Values |
|---|---|
| Hematocrit | 51%–56% |
| Hemoglobin | 16.5 g/dL (cord blood) |
| Platelets | 150,000–400,000/mm$^3$ |
| White blood cell total | 18,000/mm$^3$ |
| White blood cell differential | |
| Bands | 1600/mm$^3$ (9%) |
| Polymorphonuclear (segs) | 9400/mm$^3$ (52%) |
| Eosinophils | 400/mm$^3$ (2.2%) |
| Basophils | 100/mm$^3$ (0.6%) |
| Lymphocytes | 5500/mm$^3$ (31%) |
| Monocytes | 1050/mm$^3$ (5.8%) |
| Serum glucose | 40–80 mg/dL |
| Serum electrolytes | |
| Sodium | 135–147 mEq/L |
| Potassium | 4–6 mEq/L |
| Chloride | 90–114 mEq/L |
| Carbon dioxide | 15–25 mEq/L |
| Bicarbonate | 18–23 mEq/L |
| Calcium | 7–10 mg/dL |

*At sea level.

# Suggested Answers to Critical Thinking in Practice Questions

## Chapter 4

Rita has described a normal menstrual cycle. Although it is variable in frequency, it is not outside the range of what is acceptable in a teenager. The flow that she thinks is heavy is really quite normal, and her cramps indicate that she is having ovulatory cycles.

It is important to reassure Rita that there is nothing wrong with her menstrual cycle. It would be appropriate to suggest an antiprostaglandin such as ibuprofen for the relief of dysmenorrhea. Of utmost importance is to follow up on her request for birth control pills. She may be considering becoming sexually active and may need contraception. Sometimes teenagers have a difficult time asking for what they really want, and this is an ideal situation in which to bring up issues of sexuality with a young woman.

## Chapter 7

Elena's height and prepregnancy weight are normal. Her weight gain during pregnancy has been appropriate but not excessive. Research indicates that assessment of fundal height is more accurate between 22–24 and 34 weeks' gestation. At 33 weeks Elena's baby was growing normally. Thus this finding is not abnormal by itself and may simply be a reflection of decreased accuracy of the procedure late in pregnancy. It may also reflect variations in growth of the baby. To make your best assessment you need further information about the results of this week's examination. If during her examination there are no indicators of problems, such as decreased fetal activity, maternal urinary tract infection, maternal hypertension, and so forth, you can reassure Elena that this finding is probably a normal variation.

## Chapter 8

Certainly Karen should continue with her exercising, including light weight lifting. She also can continue to use the heated pool. However, current recommendations suggest that hot tubs not be used during pregnancy. There is a potential for hot tub (and sauna) hyperthermia in early pregnancy to induce fetal damage.

## Chapter 9

Competing in the marathon is not recommended. Even though Constance is in excellent shape, we do not know what impact prolonged participation in such a strenuous event might have on her fetus. The normal fetus seems able to withstand decreased uterine blood flow during exercise as blood is shunted to the muscles. We do not know, however, whether this decreased blood flow to the fetus interferes with the fetus's ability to dissipate heat, especially since the fetus is not able to decrease temperature via perspiration or respiration. With this in mind, during pregnancy, competitive athletes avoid competition, and all women should avoid reaching their maximal physical effort by maintaining their pulse at 140 beats per minute or less.

## Chapter 10

Cindy has only recently turned 15. She may not be aware of good nutrition and probably has minimal knowledge about how her nutritional habits impact the growing fetus. The nurse can begin by showing Cindy and her boyfriend pictures of the uterus, placenta, and umbilical cord and discussing how the fetus is nourished. She or he then needs to help Cindy understand good nutritional habits and which of her favorite foods in the different food groups will also be healthy for her fetus. The use of audiovisual aids is important in teaching young teenagers. The nurse needs to determine food practices in Cindy's home. Who is cooking and preparing the food? How much control does Cindy have? If the mother prepares the food, the nurse and Cindy can discuss ways of sharing information about good nutrition with Cindy's mother. Evaluation of nutritional habits and reinforcement for positive changes throughout her pregnancy will be important. Since this was a planned pregnancy with a supportive boyfriend, compliance in health behaviors to produce a healthy baby is likely.

Expected weight gain in pregnancy also needs to be discussed. Body image is a concern in the teen years. Knowing that a specific amount of weight needs to be gained each trimester for normal growth of a healthy fetus, and that this weight will be lost after pregnancy, will be important for both Cindy and her boyfriend.

## Chapter 11

Although Diane's intake is supporting an appropriate weight gain, her diet is not nutritionally adequate. Comparing her diet to the Food Guide Pyramid shows that she lacks servings from the grain and dairy groups and that she has a high intake from the meat group.

**Grain group** Diane should not restrict her intake from this group. Breads, pasta, and other grain products will not cause weight gain unless they are prepared with large amounts of fat or eaten in excessive quantities.

# Appendix I

## Suggested Answers to Critical Thinking in Practice Questions

**Meat group** The number of servings from this group exceeds the recommended intake. This contributes to Diane's fat and calorie intake even though she may be selecting lean cuts of meat. The number of servings should be decreased and each portion size should be about 2–3 ounces.

**Dairy group** A restricted dairy intake has decreased Diane's calcium intake. The items she consumes from this group tend to have a high fat content. She could use dairy products that have a reduced fat content in order to limit her calorie intake but maintain the calcium level in her diet.

**Vegetable group** Broccoli and green leafy vegetables such as beet greens, collards, and kale will provide calcium to the diet but must be consumed in amounts greater than usual serving sizes for Diane to obtain adequate calcium. Most salad greens contain very little calcium.

**Beverages** The total amount of fluid consumed is adequate. The consumption of soda should be limited because it would increase the calorie intake without contributing to the nutrient content of the diet.

### Chapter 12

It is not unusual for women to be upset and frustrated with news that they may have newly diagnosed glucose intolerance during pregnancy. It has been described that women with gestational diabetes approach the new diagnosis as a crisis or anxiety-provoking situation. These women may experience more difficulty with coping and learning than do women with chronic diabetes who become pregnant.

It is important for the nurse to first assess the woman's knowledge about gestational diabetes before attempting to provide any teaching. The woman will benefit most from discussions that build on her current knowledge level. It will usually take several sessions to ensure that the new information is accurately understood and retained.

The nurse can reassure Mrs. Chang that the baby should be fine and can stress the importance of keeping her glucose levels in a normal range. Women with gestational diabetes may require treatment with diet therapy alone, or they may need insulin administration to control hyperglycemia.

It is believed that gestational diabetes does not cause birth defects because it occurs later in pregnancy, after the baby's organs are formed. The two most common risks to the baby are macrosomia, potentially causing a problem in labor and birth, and hypoglycemia.

### Chapter 13

About 30% to 40% of pregnant women with bacteriuria develop cystitis or pyelonephritis unless their bladder infection is treated (Lentz, 2000). This is related to the anatomic and physiologic changes of pregnancy, including decreased ureteral peristalsis, ureteral dilation, and increased bladder capacity. Since Rachel is 6 months pregnant, she is probably being seen monthly for prenatal care. Because prompt treatment is essential, you should urge her to call her caregiver and discuss her symptoms.

### Chapter 18

We hope you would encourage her to take medication if she felt she needed it. Many types of analgesic agents and many types of regional blocks can help her if she decides she needs them. Sometimes, giving permission for someone to ask relieves her anxiety and decreases the need for intervention.

### Chapter 19

Decreased amniotic fluid contributes to fetal head compression, which may result in the early FHR decelerations described. This type of deceleration is considered benign; no action is required. (However, the lower volume of fluid may also result in cord compression and cause variable decelerations. Variable decelerations require careful nursing assessment.)

### Chapter 20

Once uterine contractions reach the desired characteristics (frequency of every 2–3 minutes, duration of 40–60 seconds, and moderate to strong intensity), and cervical dilatation is 5–6 cm, the infusion rate can be decreased by increments similar to those by which it was increased. In this case you should decrease the rate to the step it was just prior to 6 mU/min (36 mL/hr).

### Chapter 22

The unique behavioral and temperamental characteristics of newborn infants should be discussed. Additionally, aspects of the Brazelton exam may be helpful to show Mrs. Reyes how her

# Suggested Answers to Critical Thinking in Practice Questions

infant changes state with different stimuli and intervention. Teaching her how to console her newborn may also be helpful.

## Chapter 23

Reassure the mother that you will help her baby as you carry out the following activities:

- Position the infant with her head lowered and to the side.
- Bulb suction the nares and mouth repeatedly until the airway is cleared.
- Hold and comfort the infant when normal respirations are restored.
- Reassure the mother and review this procedure with her.

*Note:* If bulb suctioning alone does not clear the airway, use DeLee wall suction and administer oxygen as needed to restore normal respirations.

## Chapter 23

We hope you would first examine the infant's genitalia and wipe between the labia to verify the source of bleeding. If there were no external lacerations, you would explain to the mother that a small amount of bleeding, called pseudomenstruation, sometimes occurs in newborn girls because of maternal hormone levels. This is considered normal and generally resolves in a few days. The tissue she observes is a vaginal skin tag, also a normal finding. It usually disappears in a few weeks.

## Chapter 25

We hope that you would tell her that nurses always wear gloves during the initial assessment of a newborn, during all admission procedures until the newborn has its first bath, and sometimes during diaper changes. You should also tell her that her baby will not be isolated from the other babies when in the nursery and that her baby can remain with her if she wishes. It is important to recognize the concern that Mrs. Corrigan may have about people knowing that her baby may have HIV and to assess her own feelings of social isolation.

## Chapter 26

It is important to give this mother clear, factual information regarding the type, cause, and usual course of the baby's respiratory problem. You see that Linn's laboratory tests, chest x-ray, and clinical course so far are indicative of transient tachypnea of the newborn. Respiratory distress syndrome is probably not the problem since Linn is not premature and did not have any asphyxia at birth. You recognize that prior experience with a premature newborn with respiratory distress and prolonged hospitalization will add to this mother's fear and anxiety regarding her new baby. Therefore, in addition to giving factual information regarding the baby's condition, it is important for you to see whether the mother can be brought to the nursery to see her baby or to have the mother receive a picture of the baby for reassurance. Before the mother visits the baby, clearly describe the oxygen and monitoring equipment that is helping Linn so that the mother will not be alarmed upon seeing her daughter.

## Chapter 27

These findings are not within the normal range. At 24 hours past birth the fundus should be approximately one finger breadth below the umbilicus and located in the midline. A uterus that is deviated to the right may indicate that the bladder is full and the woman needs to urinate. You should determine whether she is having difficulty urinating and emptying her bladder; if so, you can try some nursing measures to help her void. The lochia will still be rubra, but the amount is excessive and may be related to a boggy uterus.

## Chapter 28

Your best response would be, "You can only be discharged if both you and your physician feel you are ready. Federal law now states that you can stay in the hospital for up to 4 days (96 hours) when you have had a cesarean section."

## Chapter 29

Acknowledge Ann's frustration and pain. Tell her you are glad she called and ask how you may be of help. Let her ventilate about how she feels. Explain that her breasts are engorged, which is a problem that many women encounter. It is not unusual for infants to refuse to nurse when the breast is hard and the nipple difficult to grasp.

Identify methods to relieve the engorgement.

**a.** Warm or cool soaks, whichever she prefers, for comfort and to stimulate let-down.

**b.** Express a small amount of milk.

**c.** Put the baby to breast after stimulating let-down and expressing a little milk. (The breast will be softer and it will be easier to grasp the nipple.)

**d.** Use analgesics. (If taken immediately before nursing, less medication will go to the baby.)

# Suggested Answers to Critical Thinking in Practice Questions

Explain to Ann that her emotional upheaval is probably the "baby blues" or "postpartum blues" and that they usually subside in 24–72 hours. Instruct her to call her physician if the blues do not subside, or if she develops symptoms of depression.

Ask why she started supplemental feedings. Upon questioning, Ann tells you that she had started supplementing her baby with formula after each feeding because her mother-in-law told her that the baby was nursing too frequently (every 1–3 hours, sometimes clustering 3–4 feedings in one 2–3 hour period). She told Ann that the baby was obviously not getting enough breast milk. After receiving supplemental feedings, the baby began feeding once every 3–5 hours.

Tactfully explain that although Ann's mother-in-law meant well, her comments indicate a lack of information about breastfeeding; that is,

**a.** Breast milk digests faster than formula, so breastfeeding babies feed more frequently.

**b.** On average, babies nurse 8–12 times in 24 hours.

**c.** After lactation is well established, the baby will nurse less frequently. During growth spurts, however, all babies nurse more frequently for a few days.

Explain that Ann may still breastfeed successfully, and if she desires to continue breastfeeding, she should stop supplementing with formula.

## Chapter 30

You should have Lei return to her room via wheelchair. Assess her leg for warmth, edema, redness, tenderness, and Homan's sign. Discuss with Lei that she should not massage her leg or get out of bed until you consult with the primary provider concerning your findings. Notify her primary health care provider and document your assessment findings.

**Abdominal effleurage** Gentle stroking used in massage.

**Abortion** Loss of pregnancy before the fetus is viable outside the uterus; miscarriage.

**Abruptio placentae** (ab-rŭp′shē-ō plasen′tē) Partial or total premature separation of a normally implanted placenta.

**Abstinence** Refraining voluntarily, especially from indulgence in food, alcoholic beverages, or sexual intercourse.

**Acceleration** Periodic increase in the baseline fetal heart rate.

**Acini cells** Secretory cells in the human breast that create milk from nutrients in the bloodstream.

**Acme** Peak or highest point; time of greatest intensity (of a uterine contraction).

**Acrocyanosis** Cyanosis of the extremities.

**Acrosomal reaction** Breakdown of the hyaluronic acid in the corona radiata by enzymes from the heads of sperm; allows one spermatozoon to penetrate the ovum zona pellucida.

**Active acquired immunity** Formation of antibodies by the pregnant woman in response to illness or immunization

**Active management of labor** Medical protocol for augmentation of labor that includes (1) a strict criterion for labor admission, (2) early amniotomy, (3) high-dose oxytocin infusion for inefficient labor contractions, and (4) a commitment to provision of continuous nursing care.

**Adnexa** Adjoining or accessory parts of a structure, such as the uterine adnexa: the ovaries and fallopian tubes.

**Adolescence** Period of human development initiated by puberty and ending with the attainment of young adulthood.

**Afterbirth** Placenta and membranes expelled after the birth of the infant, during the third stage of labor. Also called secundines.

**Afterpains** Cramplike pains due to contractions of the uterus that occur after childbirth. They are more common in multiparas, tend to be most severe during nursing, and last 2 to 3 days.

**AIDS (acquired immune deficiency syndrome)** A sexually transmitted viral disease that so far has proved fatal in 100% of cases.

**Alveoli** Small units of the breast tissue in which milk is synthesized by the alveolar secretory epithelium.

**Amenorrhea** Suppression or absence of menstruation.

**Amniocentesis** Removal of amniotic fluid by insertion of a needle into the amniotic sac; amniotic fluid is used to assess fetal health or maturity.

**Amnioinfusion** Procedure used to infuse a sterile fluid (such as normal saline) through an intrauterine catheter into the uterus in an attempt to increase the fluid around the umbilical cord to decrease or prevent cord compression during labor contractions; also used to dilute thick meconium-stained amniotic fluid.

**Amnion** The inner of the two membranes that form the sac containing the fetus and the amniotic fluid.

**Amnionitis** Infection of the amniotic fluid.

**Amniotic fluid** The liquid surrounding the fetus in utero. It absorbs shocks, permits fetal movement, and prevents heat loss.

**Amniotic fluid embolism** Amniotic fluid that has leaked into the chorionic plate and entered the maternal circulation.

**Amniotomy** (am-nē-ot′ō-mē) The artificial rupturing of the amniotic membrane.

**Ampulla** The outer two-thirds of the fallopian tube; fertilization of the ovum by a spermatozoon usually occurs here.

**Androgen** Substance producing male characteristics, such as the male hormone testosterone.

**Android pelvis** Male-type pelvis.

**Antepartum** Time between conception and the onset of labor; usually used to describe the period during which a woman is pregnant.

**Anterior fontanelle** Diamond-shaped area between the two frontal and two parietal bones just above the newborn's forehead.

**Anthropoid pelvis** Pelvis in which the anteroposterior diameter is equal to or greater than the transverse diameter.

**Apgar score** A scoring system used to evaluate newborns at 1 minute and 5 minutes after birth. The total score is achieved by assessing five signs: heart rate, respiratory effort, muscle tone, reflex irritability, and color. Each of the signs is assigned a score of 0, 1, or 2. The highest possible score is 10.

**Apnea** A condition that occurs when respirations cease for more than 20 seconds, with generalized cyanosis.

**Areola** Pigmented ring surrounding the nipple of the breast.

**Artificial insemination** Introduction of viable semen into the vagina by artificial means for the purpose of impregnation.

**Artificial rupture of membranes (AROM)** Use of a device such as an amnihook or allis forceps to rupture the amniotic membranes.

**Assisted reproductive technology (ART)** Term used to describe the highly technologic approaches used to produce pregnancy.

**Attachment** Enduring bonds or relationship of affection between persons.

**Attitude** Attitude of the fetus refers to the relationship of the fetal parts to each other.

**Autosome** A chromosome that is not a sex chromosome.

**Babinski reflex** Reflex found normally in infants under 6 months of age in which the great toe dorsiflexes when the sole of the foot is stimulated.

**Bacterial vaginosis** A bacterial infection of the vagina, formerly called *Gardnerella vaginalis* or *Hemophilus vaginalis,* characterized by a foul-smelling, grayish vaginal discharge that exhibits a characteristic fishy odor when 10% potassium hydroxide (KOH) is added. Microscopic examination of a vaginal wet prep reveals the presence of "clue cells" (vaginal epithelial cells coated with gram-negative organisms).

**Bag of waters (BOW)** The membrane containing the amniotic fluid and the fetus.

**Ballottement** (bal-ot-maw′) A technique of palpation to detect or examine a floating object in the body. In obstetrics, the fetus, when pushed, floats away and then returns to touch the examiner's fingers.

**Barr body** Deeply staining chromatin mass located against the inner surface of the cell nucleus. It is found only in normal females. Also called sex chromatin.

**Basal body temperature (BBT)** The lowest waking temperature.

**Baseline rate** The average fetal heart rate observed during a 10-minute period of monitoring.

**Baseline variability** Changes in the fetal heart rate that result from the interplay between the sympathetic and the parasympathetic nervous systems.

**Battledore placenta** Placenta in which the umbilical cord is inserted on the periphery rather than centrally.

**Bimanual palpation** Examination of the pelvic organs by placing one hand on the abdomen and one or two fingers of the other hand into the vagina.

**Biophysical profile (BPP)** Assessment of five variables in the fetus that help to evaluate fetal risk: breathing movement, body movement, tone, amniotic fluid volume, and fetal heart rate reactivity.

**Birth center** A setting for labor and birth that emphasizes a family-centered approach rather than obstetric technology and treatment.

**Birthing room** A room for labor and birth with a relaxed atmosphere.

**Birth preference plan** Decisions made by the expectant couple about aspects of the childbearing experience that are most important to them.

**Birth rate** Number of live births per 1000 population.

**Bishop score** A prelabor scoring system to assist in predicting whether an induction of labor may be successful. The total score is achieved by assessing five components: cervical dilatation, cervical effacement, cervical consistency, cervical position, and fetal station. Each of the components is assigned a score of 0 to 3, and the highest possible score is 13.

**Blastocyst** The inner solid mass of cells within the morula.

**Bloody show** Pink-tinged mucous secretions resulting from rupture of small capillaries as the cervix effaces and dilates.

**Body stalk** Future umbilical cord; structure that attaches the embryo to the yolk sac and contains blood vessels that extend into the chorionic villi.

**Boggy uterus** A term used to describe the uterine fundus when it is not firmly contracted after the birth of the baby and in the early postpartum period; excessive bleeding occurs from the placental site, and maternal hemorrhage may occur.

**Bonding** Process of parent-infant attachment occurring at or soon after birth.

**Brachial palsy** Partial or complete paralysis of portions of the arm resulting from trauma to the brachial plexus during a difficult birth.

**Braxton Hicks contractions** Intermittent painless contractions of the uterus that may occur every 10 to 20 minutes. They occur more frequently toward the end of pregnancy and are sometimes mistaken for true labor signs.

**Brazleton's neonatal behavioral assessment** A brief examination used to identify the infant's behavioral states and responses.

**Breasts** Mammary glands.

**Breast self-examination** Recommended monthly procedure by which women may detect changes or abnormalities in their breasts.

**Breech presentation** A birth in which the buttocks and/or feet are presented instead of the head.

**Broad ligament** The ligament extending from the lateral margins of the uterus to the pelvic wall; keeps the uterus centrally placed and provides stability within the pelvic cavity.

**Bronchopulmonary dysplasia (BPD)** Chronic pulmonary disease of multifactorial etiology characterized initially by alveolar and bronchial necrosis, which results in bronchial metaplasia and interstitial fibrosis. Appears in x-ray films as generalized small, radiolucent cysts within the lungs.

**Brown adipose tissue (BAT)** Fat deposits in neonates that provide greater heat-generating activity than ordinary fat. Found around the kidneys, adrenals, and neck; between the scapulas; and behind the sternum. Also called brown fat.

**Calorie** Amount of heat required to raise the temperature of 1 kg of water 1 degree centigrade.

**Capacitation** Removal of the plasma membrane overlying the spermatozoa's acrosomal area with the loss of seminal plasma proteins and the glycoprotein coat. If the glycoprotein coat is not removed, the sperm will not be able to penetrate the ovum.

**Caput succedaneum** (kap′ut suk″sĕ-da′ne-um) Swelling or edema occurring in or under the fetal scalp during labor.

**Cardinal ligaments** The chief uterine supports, suspending the uterus from the side walls of the true pelvis.

**Cardinal movements of labor** The positional changes of the fetus as it moves through the birth canal during labor and birth. The positional changes are descent, flexion, internal rotation, extension, restitution, and external rotation.

**Cardiopulmonary adaptation** Adaptation of the neonate's cardiovascular and respiratory systems to life outside the womb.

**Cephalhematoma** (sef′ăl-hē-mă-tō′mă) Subcutaneous swelling containing blood found on the head of an infant several days after birth; it usually disappears within a few weeks to 2 months.

**Cephalic presentation** Birth in which the fetal head is presenting against the cervix.

**Cephalopelvic disproportion (CPD)** A condition in which the fetal head is of such a shape or size, or in such a position, that it cannot pass through the maternal pelvis.

**Certified nurse-midwife (CNM)** An RN who has received special training and education in the care of the family during childbearing and the prenatal, labor and birth, and postpartal periods. After a period of formal education, the nurse-midwife takes a certification test to become a CNM.

**Cervical cap** A cup-shaped device placed over the cervix to prevent pregnancy.

**Cervical dilatation** Process in which the cervical os and the cervical canal widen from less than a centimeter to approximately 10 cm, allowing birth of the fetus.

**Cervical ripening** Softening of the cervix; occurs normally as a physiologic process prior to labor or is stimulated to occur through the process of induction of labor.

**Cervix** The "neck" between the external os and the body of the uterus. The lower end of the cervix extends into the vagina.

**Cesarean birth** Birth of the fetus by means of an incision into the abdominal wall and the uterus.

**Chadwick's sign** Violet bluish color of the vaginal mucous membrane caused by increased vascularity; visible from about the fourth week of pregnancy.

**Chemical conjunctivitis** Irritation of the mucous membrane lining of the eyelid; may be due to instillation of silver nitrate ophthalmic drops.

**Child abuse** Nonaccidental physical or threatened harm, including mental or emotional injury, sexual abuse, and sexual exploitation.

**Child neglect** Failure by parents or other custodians to meet the medical, emotional, physical, or supervisory needs of a child.

**Chloasma** (klō-az′mă) Brownish pigmentation over the bridge of the nose and the cheeks during pregnancy and in some women who are taking oral contraceptives. Also called mask of pregnancy.

**Chorioamnionitis** (kō′rē-ō-am′nē-ō-nī′tis) An inflammation of the amniotic membranes stimulated by organisms in the amniotic fluid, which then becomes infiltrated with polymorphonuclear leukocytes.

**Chorion** The fetal membrane closest to the intrauterine wall that gives rise to the placenta and continues as the outer membrane surrounding the amnion.

**Chorionic villus sampling** Procedure in which a specimen of the chorionic villi is obtained from the edge of the developing placenta at about 8 weeks' gestation. The sample can be used for chromosomal, enzyme, and DNA tests.

**Chromosomes** The threadlike structures within the nucleus of a cell that carry the genes.

**Circumcision** Surgical removal of the prepuce (foreskin) of the penis.

**Circumoral cyanosis** Bluish appearance around the mouth.

**Circumvallate** (ser-kŭm-val′āt) **placenta** A placenta with a thick, white fibrous ring around the edge.

**Cleavage** Rapid mitotic division of the zygote; cells produced are called blastomeres.

**Client advocacy** An approach to client care in which the nurse educates and supports the client and protects the client's rights.

**Climacteric** The period of time that marks the cessation of a woman's reproductive function; the "change of life," or menopause.

**Clitoris** Female organ homologous to the male penis; a small oval body of erectile tissue situated at the anterior junction of the vulva.

**Coitus interruptus** Method of contraception in which the male withdraws his penis from the vagina prior to ejaculation.

**Cold stress** Excessive heat loss resulting in compensatory mechanisms (increased respirations and nonshivering thermogenesis) to maintain core body temperature.

**Colostrum** (kō-los′trŭm) Secretion from the breast before the onset of true lactation; contains mainly serum and white blood corpuscles. It has a high protein content, provides some immune properties, and cleanses the neonate's intestinal tract of mucus and meconium.

**Colposcopy** The use of an instrument inserted into the vagina to examine the cervical and vaginal tissues by means of a magnifying lens.

**Conception** Union of male sperm and female ovum; fertilization.

**Conceptional age** The number of complete weeks since the moment of conception. Because the moment of conception is almost impossible to determine, conceptional age is estimated at 2 weeks less than gestational age.

**Condom** A rubber sheath that covers the penis to prevent conception or disease.

**Conduction** Loss of heat to a cooler surface by direct skin contact.

**Condyloma** (kon-di-lō′mă) Wartlike growth of skin, usually seen on the external genitals or anus. There are two types, a pointed variety and a broad, flat form usually found with syphilis.

**Conjugate** Important diameter of the pelvis, measured from the center of the promontory of the sacrum to the back of the symphysis pubis. The diagonal conjugate is measured and the true conjugate is estimated.

**Conjugate vera** The true conjugate, which extends from the middle of the sacral promontory to the middle of the pubic crest.

**Contraception** The prevention of conception or impregnation.

**Contraction** Tightening and shortening of the uterine muscles during labor, causing effacement and dilatation of the cervix; contributes to the downward and outward descent of the fetus.

**Contraction stress test** A method of assessing the reaction of the fetus to the stress of uterine contractions. This test may be utilized when contractions are occurring spontaneously or when contractions are artificially induced by oxytocin challenge test (OCT) or breast self-stimulation test (BSST).

**Convection** Loss of heat from the warm body surface to cooler air currents.

**Coombs' test** (kōōmz) A test for antiglobulins in the red cells. The indirect test determines the presence of Rh-positive antibodies in maternal blood; the direct test determines the presence of maternal Rh-positive antibodies in fetal cord blood.

**Cornua** The elongated portions of the uterus where the fallopian tubes open.

**Corpus** The upper two-thirds of the uterus.

**Corpus luteum** A small yellow body that develops within a ruptured ovarian follicle; it secretes progesterone in the second half of the menstrual cycle and atrophies about 3 days before the beginning of menstrual flow. If pregnancy occurs, the corpus luteum continues to produce progesterone until the placenta takes over this function.

**Cotyledon** (kot-i-lē′don) One of the rounded portions into which the placenta's uterine surface is divided, consisting of a mass of villi, fetal vessels, and an intervillous space.

**Couvade** (kū-vahd′) In some cultures, the male's observance of certain rituals and taboos to signify the transition to fatherhood.

# GLOSSARY

**Crack** A form of freebase cocaine that is smoked.

**Crisis intervention** Actions taken by the nurse to help the client deal with an impending, potentially overwhelming crisis; regain his or her equilibrium, grow from the experience; and improve coping skills.

**Critical thinking** Intellectual processes that include separating fact from opinion, identifying prejudices and stereotypes that may influence interpretation of information, exploring differing ideas and views, and arriving at conclusions or insights.

**Crowning** Appearance of the presenting fetal part at the vaginal orifice during labor.

**Deceleration** Periodic decrease in the baseline fetal heart rate.

**Decidua** (dē-sid′yū-ă) Endometrium or mucous membrane lining of the uterus in pregnancy that is shed after childbirth.

**Decidua basalis** The part of the decidua that unites with the chorion to form the placenta. It is shed in lochial discharge after childbirth.

**Decidua capsularis** The part of the decidua surrounding the chorionic sac.

**Decidua vera (parietalis)** Nonplacental decidua lining the uterus.

**Decrement** Decrease or stage of decline, as of a contraction.

**Depo-Provera** A long-acting, injectable progestin contraceptive.

**Descriptive statistics** Statistics that describe or summarize a set of data.

**Desquamation** (des-kwă-mā′shŭn) Shedding of the epithelial cells of the epidermis.

**Diagonal conjugate** Distance from the lower posterior border of the symphysis pubis to the sacral promontory; may be obtained by manual measurement.

**Diaphragm** A flexible disk that covers the cervix to prevent pregnancy.

**Diastasis** (dī-as′tă-sis) **recti** (rek-ti′) **abdominis** Separation of the recti abdominis muscles along the median line. In women, it is seen with repeated childbirths or multiple gestations. In the newborn, it is usually caused by incomplete development.

**Dilatation and curettage (D&C)** Stretching of the cervical canal to permit passage of a curette, which is used to scrape the endometrium to empty the uterine contents or to obtain tissue for examination.

**Dilatation of the cervix** Expansion of the external os from an opening a few millimeters in size to an opening large enough to allow the passage of the infant.

**Diploid number of chromosomes** Containing a set of maternal and a set of paternal chromosomes; in humans, the diploid number of chromosomes is 46.

**Dissociation relaxation** A pattern of active relaxation in which the woman learns to tighten one area of the body and then relax other areas simultaneously. This relaxation pattern is very effective for some women during labor.

**Doula** A supportive companion who accompanies a laboring woman to provide emotional, physical, and informational support and acts as an advocate for the woman and her family.

**Down syndrome** An abnormality resulting from the presence of an extra chromosome number 21 (trisomy 21); characteristics include mental retardation and altered physical appearance. Formerly called mongolism.

**Drug-dependent infant** The newborn of an alcoholic or drug-addicted woman.

**Ductus arteriosus** A communication channel between the main pulmonary artery and the aorta of the fetus. It is obliterated after birth by rising $PO_2$ and changes in intravascular pressure in the presence of normal pulmonary functioning. It normally becomes a ligament after birth but sometimes remains patent (patent ductus arteriosus, a treatable condition).

**Ductus venosus** A fetal blood vessel that carries oxygenated blood between the umbilical vein and the inferior vena cava, bypassing the liver; it becomes a ligament after birth.

**Duncan's mechanism** Occurs when the maternal surface of the placenta rather than the shiny fetal surface presents upon delivery.

**Duration** The time length of each contraction, measured from the beginning of the increment to the completion of the decrement.

**Dysmenorrhea** Painful menstruation.

**Dyspareunia** Painful intercourse.

**Dystocia** (dis-tō′sē-ă) Difficult labor due to mechanical factors produced by the fetus or the maternal pelvis or due to inadequate uterine or other muscular activity.

**Early decelerations** Periodic change in fetal heart rate pattern caused by head compression; deceleration has a uniform appearance and early onset in relation to maternal contraction.

**Early postpartal hemorrhage** See *Postpartal hemorrhage.*

**Eclampsia** (ek-lamp′sē-ă) A major complication of pregnancy. Its cause is unknown; it occurs more often in the primigravida and is accompanied by elevated blood pressure, albuminuria, oliguria, tonic and clonic convulsions, and coma. It may occur during pregnancy (usually after the 20th week of gestation) or within 48 hours after childbirth.

**Ectoderm** Outer layer of cells in the developing embryo that gives rise to the skin, nails, and hair.

**Ectopic pregnancy** Implantation of the fertilized ovum outside the uterine cavity; common sites are the abdomen, fallopian tubes, and ovaries. Also called oocyesis.

**Effacement** Thinning and shortening of the cervix that occurs late in pregnancy or during labor.

**Effleurage** (e-fler-ahz′) A light stroking movement of the fingertips over the abdominal area during labor; used to provide distraction during labor contractions.

**Ejaculation** Expulsion of the seminal fluids from the penis.

**Embryo** The early stage of development of the young of any organism. In humans the embryonic period is from about 2 to 8 weeks' gestation and is characterized by cellular differentiation and predominantly hyperplastic growth.

**Embryonic membranes** The amnion and chorion.

**Endoderm** The inner layer of cells in the developing embryo that give rise to internal organs such as the intestines.

**Endometriosis** Ectopic endometrium located outside the uterus in the pelvic cavity. Symptoms may include pelvic pain or pressure, dysmenorrhea, dyspareunia, abnormal bleeding from the uterus or rectum, and sterility.

**Endometritis** Infection of the endometrium.

**Endometrium** (en′dō-mē′trē-ŭm) The mucous membrane that lines the inner surface of the uterus.

***En face*** An assumed position in which one person looks at another and maintains his or her face in the same vertical plane as that of the other.

**Engagement** The entrance of the fetal presenting part into the superior pelvic strait and the beginning of the descent through the pelvic canal.

**Engorgement** Vascular congestion or distention. In obstetrics, the swelling of breast tissue brought about by an increase in blood and lymph supply to the breast, preceding true lactation.

**Engrossment** Characteristic sense of absorption, preoccupation, and interest in the infant demonstrated by fathers during early contact with their infants.

**Entrainment** Phenomenon in which a newborn moves in rhythm to adult speech.

**Epidural block** Regional anesthesia effective through the first and second stages of labor.

**Episiotomy** (ĕ-piz″e-ot′o-me) Incision of the perineum to facilitate birth and to avoid laceration of the perineum.

**Epstein's** (ep′stīnz) **pearls** Small, white blebs found along the gum margins and at the junction of the hard and soft palates; commonly seen in the newborn as a normal manifestation.

**Erb-Duchenne palsy** Paralysis of the arm and chest wall as a result of a birth injury to the brachial plexus or a subsequent injury to the fifth and sixth cervical nerves.

**Erythema toxicum** Innocuous pink papular rash of unknown cause with superimposed vesicles; it appears within 24 to 48 hours after birth and resolves spontaneously within a few days.

**Erythroblastosis fetalis** Hemolytic disease of the newborn characterized by anemia, jaundice, enlargement of the liver and spleen, and generalized edema. Caused by isoimmunization due to Rh incompatibility or ABO incompatibility.

**Estimated date of birth (EDB)** During a pregnancy, the approximate date when childbirth will occur; the "due date."

**Estrogens** The hormones estradiol and estrone, produced by the ovary.

**Ethnocentrism** An individual's belief that the values and practices of his or her own culture are the best ones.

**Evaporation** Loss of heat incurred when water on the skin surface is converted to a vapor.

**Exchange transfusion** The replacement of 70% to 80% of circulating blood by withdrawing the recipient's blood and injecting a donor's blood in equal amounts, for the purpose of preventing the accumulation of bilirubin or other by-products of hemolysis in the blood.

**External (cephalic) version (ECV)** Procedure involving external manipulation of the maternal abdomen to change the presentation of the fetus from breech to cephalic.

**External os** The opening between the cervix and the vagina.

**Fallopian tubes** Tubes that extend from the lateral angle of the uterus and terminate near the ovary; they serve as a passageway for the ovum from the ovary to the uterus and for the spermatozoa from the uterus toward the ovary. Also called oviducts and uterine tubes.

**False labor** Contractions of the uterus, regular or irregular, that may be strong enough to be interpreted as true labor but that do not dilate the cervix.

**False pelvis** The portion of the pelvis above the linea terminalis; its primary function is to support the weight of the enlarged pregnant uterus.

**Family-centered care** An approach to health care based on the concept that a hospital can provide professional services to mothers, fathers, and infants in a homelike environment that would enhance the integrity of the family unit.

**Female condom** A thin, disposable polyurethane sheath with a flexible ring at each end that is placed inside the vagina and serves to prevent sperm from entering the cervix, thus preventing conception.

**Female reproductive cycle (FRC)** The monthly rhythmic changes in sexually mature women.

**Ferning** Formation of a palm-leaf pattern by the crystallization of cervical mucus as it dries at mid-menstrual cycle. Helpful in determining time of ovulation. Observed via microscopic examination of a thin layer of cervical mucus on a glass slide. This pattern is also observed when amniotic fluid is allowed to air dry on a slide and is a useful and quick test to determine whether amniotic membranes have ruptured.

**Fertility rate** Number of births per 1000 women aged 15 to 44 in a given population per year.

**Fertilization** Impregnation of an ovum by a spermatozoon; conception.

**Fetal acoustic stimulation test (FAST)** A fetal assessment test that uses sound from a speaker, bell, or artificial larynx to stimulate acceleration of the fetal heart; may be used in conjunction with the nonstress test.

**Fetal activity diary (FAD)** A method for tracking fetal activity taught to pregnant women.

**Fetal alcohol effects (FAE)** The less severe fetal manifestations of maternal alcohol ingestion, including mild to moderate cognitive problems and physical growth retardation.

**Fetal alcohol syndrome (FAS)** Syndrome caused by maternal alcohol ingestion and characterized by microcephaly, intrauterine growth restriction, short palpebral fissures, and maxillary hypoplasia.

**Fetal attitude** Relationship of the fetal parts to one another. Normal fetal attitude is one of moderate flexion of the arms onto the chest and flexion of the legs onto the abdomen.

**Fetal blood sampling** Blood sample drawn from the fetal scalp (or from the fetus in breech position) to evaluate the acid-base status of the fetus.

**Fetal bradycardia** A fetal heart rate less than 120 beats per minute during a 10-minute period of continuous monitoring.

**Fetal death** Death of the developing fetus after 20 weeks' gestation. Also called fetal demise.

**Fetal distress** Evidence that the fetus is in jeopardy, such as a change in fetal activity or heart rate.

**Fetal heart rate (FHR)** The number of times the fetal heart beats per minute; normal range is 120 to 160.

**Fetal lie** Relationship of the cephalocaudal axis (spinal column) of the fetus to the cephalocaudal axis (spinal column) of the woman. The fetus may be in a longitudinal or transverse lie.

**Fetal movement record** See *Fetal activity diary (FAD).*

**Fetal position** Relationship of the landmark on the presenting fetal part to the front, sides, or back of the maternal pelvis.

**Fetal presentation** The fetal body part that enters the maternal pelvis first. The three possible presentations are cephalic, shoulder, and breech.

**Fetal tachycardia** A fetal heart rate of 160 beats per minute or more during a 10-minute period of continuous monitoring.

**Fetoscope** An adaptation of a stethoscope that facilitates auscultation of the fetal heart rate.

**Fetoscopy** A technique for directly observing the fetus and obtaining a sample of fetal blood or skin.

**Fetus** The child in utero from about the seventh to ninth week of gestation until birth.

**Fibrocystic breast disease** Benign breast disorder characterized by a thickening of normal breast tissue and the formation of cysts.

**Fimbria** Any structure resembling a fringe; the fringelike extremity of the fallopian tubes.

**Folic acid** An important vitamin directly related to the outcome of pregnancy and to maternal and fetal health.

**Follicle-stimulating hormone (FSH)** Hormone produced by the anterior pituitary during the first half of the menstrual cycle, stimulating development of the graafian follicle.

**Fontanelle** (fon′tă-nel′) In the fetus, an unossified space, or soft spot, consisting of a strong band of connective tissue lying between the cranial bones of the skull.

**Foramen ovale** Special opening between the atria of the fetal heart. Normally, the opening closes shortly after birth; if it remains open, it can be repaired surgically.

**Forceps** Obstetric instrument occasionally used to aid in childbirth.

**Foremilk** Breast milk obtained at the beginning of the breastfeeding episode.

**Fourth trimester** First several postpartal weeks during which the woman returns to an essentially prepregnant state and becomes competent in caring for her newborn.

**Frequency** The time between the beginning of one contraction and the beginning of the next contraction.

**Fundus** The upper portion of the uterus between the fallopian tubes.

**Galactorrhea** Nipple discharge.

**Gamete** (gam′ēt) Female or male germ cell; contains a haploid number of chromosomes.

**Gamete intrafallopian transfer (GIFT)** Retrieval of oocytes by laparoscopy; immediately combining oocytes with washed, motile sperm in a catheter; and placement of the gametes into the fimbriated end of the fallopian tube.

**Gametogenesis** The process by which germ cells are produced.

**Genotype** The genetic composition of an individual.

**Gestation** (jes-tā′shŭn) Period of intrauterine development from conception through birth; pregnancy.

**Gestational age** The number of complete weeks of fetal development, calculated from the first day of the last normal menstrual cycle.

**Gestational age assessment tools** Systems used to evaluate the newborn's external physical characteristics and neurologic and/or neuromuscular development to accurately determine gestational age. These replace or supplement the traditional calculation from the woman's last menstrual period.

**Gestational diabetes mellitus** A form of diabetes of variable severity with onset or first recognition during pregnancy.

**Gestational trophoblastic disease (GTD)** Disorder classified into two types: benign (hydatidiform mole) and malignant.

**Gonadotropin-releasing hormone (GnRH)** A hormone secreted by the hypothalamus that stimulates the anterior pituitary to secrete FSH and LH.

**Goodell's sign** Softening of the cervix that occurs during the second month of pregnancy.

**Graafian follicle** The ovarian cyst containing the ripe ovum; it secretes estrogens.

**Grasping reflex** Normal newborn reflex elicited by stimulating the palm with a finger or object, resulting in newborn firmly holding on to the finger or object.

**Gravida** (grav′i-dă) A pregnant woman.

**Grief work** The inner process of working through or managing the bereavement.

**Gynecoid pelvis** Typical female pelvis in which the inlet is round instead of oval.

**Habituation** (ha-bit-chū-ā′shŭn) Infant's ability to diminish innate responses to specific repeated stimuli.

**Haploid number of chromosomes** Half the diploid number of chromosomes. In humans there are 23 chromosomes, the haploid number, in each germ cell.

**Harlequin sign** A rare color change that occurs between the longitudinal halves of the newborn's body, such that the dependent half is noticeably pinker than the superior half when the newborn is placed on one side; it is of no pathologic significance.

**Hegar's sign** A softening of the lower uterine segment found upon palpation in the second or third month of pregnancy.

**HELLP syndrome** A cluster of changes including *h*emolysis, *e*levated *l*iver enzymes, and *l*ow *p*latelet count; sometimes associated with severe preeclampsia.

**Hemolytic disease of the newborn** *Hyperbilirubinemia* secondary to Rh incompatibility.

**Heterozygous** A genotypic situation in which two different alleles occur at a given locus on a pair of homologous chromosomes.

**Hindmilk** Breast milk released after initial letdown reflex; high in fat content.

**Homozygous** A genotypic situation in which two similar genes occur at a given locus on homologous chromosomes.

**Hormone replacement therapy (HRT)** Administration of hormones, usually estrogen and a progestin, to alleviate the symptoms of menopause.

**Huhner test** Postcoital examination to evaluate sperm and cervical mucus.

**Human chorionic gonadotropin (hCG)** A hormone produced by the chorionic villi and found in the urine of pregnant women. Also called prolan.

**Human placental lactogen (hPL)** A hormone synthesized by the syncytiotrophoblast that functions as an insulin antagonist and promotes lipolysis to increase the amounts of circulating free fatty acids available for maternal metabolic use.

**Hydatidiform** (hī-da-tid′i-form) **mole** Degenerative process in chorionic villi, giving rise to multiple cysts and rapid growth of the uterus, with hemorrhage.

**Hydramnios** (hī-dram′-nē-os) An excess of amniotic fluid, leading to overdistension of the uterus. Frequently seen in diabetic pregnant women, even if there is no coexisting fetal anomaly. Also called polyhydramnios.

**Hydrops fetalis** See *Erythroblastosis fetalis.*

**Hyperbilirubinemia** (hī′per-bil′i-rū-bi-nē′mē-ă) Excessive amount of bilirubin in the blood; indicative of hemolytic processes due to blood incompatibility, intrauterine infection, septicemia, neonatal renal infection, and other disorders.

**Hyperemesis gravidarum** Excessive vomiting during pregnancy, leading to dehydration and starvation.

**Hypoglycemia** Abnormally low level of sugar in the blood.

**Hysterectomy** Surgical removal of the uterus.

**Hysterosalpingogram** Result of testing by instillation of radiopaque substance into the uterine cavity to visualize the uterus and fallopian tubes.

**Hysteroscopy** Use of a special endoscope to examine the uterus.

**Inborn error of metabolism** A hereditary deficiency of a specific enzyme needed for normal metabolism of specific chemicals.

**Incompetent cervix** The premature dilatation of the cervix, usually in the second trimester of pregnancy.

**Increment** Increase or addition; to build up, as of a contraction.

**Induction of labor** The process of causing or initiating labor by use of medication or surgical rupture of membranes.

**Infant** A child under 1 year of age.

**Infant mortality rate** Number of deaths of infants under 1 year of age per 1000 live births in a given population per year.

**Infant of a diabetic mother (IDM)** At-risk infant born to a woman previously diagnosed as diabetic or who develops symptoms of diabetes during pregnancy.

**Inferential statistics** Statistics that allow an investigator to draw conclusions about what is happening between two or more variables in a population and to suggest or refute casual relationships between them.

**Infertility** Diminished ability to conceive.

**Informed consent** A legal concept that protects a person's rights to autonomy and self-determination by specifying that no action may be taken without that person's prior understanding and freely given consent.

**Infundibulopelvic ligament** Ligament that suspends and supports the ovaries.

**Intensity** The strength of a uterine contraction during acme.

**Internal os** An inside mouth or opening; the opening between the cervix and the uterus.

**Internal version** Procedure used to vaginally deliver a second twin. The obstetrician inserts a hand into the uterus, grasps the feet of the fetus, and changes the fetus from a transverse to a breech presentation.

**Intrapartum** The time from the onset of true labor until the birth of the infant and delivery of the placenta.

**Intrauterine device (IUD)** Small metal or plastic form that is placed in the uterus to prevent implantation of a fertilized ovum.

**Intrauterine fetal surgery** Surgery performed on a fetus to correct anatomic lesions that are not compatible with life if left untreated.

**Intrauterine growth restriction (IUGR)** Fetal undergrowth due to any etiology, such as intrauterine infection, deficient nutrient supply, or congenital malformation. Formerly called intrauterine growth retardation.

**Intrauterine pressure catheter (IUPC)** A catheter that can be placed through the cervix into the uterus to measure uterine pressure during labor. Some types of catheters may be inserted for the purpose of infusing warmed saline to add additional intrauterine fluid when oligohydramnios is present.

**Intrauterine resuscitation** Interventions initiated when nonreassuring fetal heart rate patterns are noted; they are directed at improving intrauterine blood flow.

**Introitus** Opening or entrance into a cavity or canal such as the vagina.

**In vitro fertilization (IVF)** Procedure during which oocytes are removed from the ovary, mixed with spermatozoa, fertilized, and incubated in a glass petri dish; then up to four viable embryos are placed in the woman's uterus.

**Involution** Rolling or turning inward; the reduction in size of the uterus following childbirth.

**Ischial spines** Prominences that arise near the junction of the ilium and ischium and jut into the pelvic cavity; used as a reference point during labor to evaluate the descent of the fetal head into the birth canal.

**Isthmus** The straight, narrow part of the fallopian tube with a thick muscular wall and an opening (lumen) 2–3 mm in diameter; the site of tubal ligation. Also, a constriction in the uterus that is located above the cervix and below the corpus.

**Jaundice** Yellow pigmentation of body tissues caused by the presence of bile pigments. See also *Physiologic jaundice.*

**Karyotype** The set of chromosomes arranged in a standard order.

**Kegel's exercises** Perineal muscle tightening that strengthens the pubococcygeus muscle and increases its tone.

**Kernicterus** (ker-nik′ter-ŭs) An encephalopathy caused by deposition of unconjugated bilirubin in brain cells; may result in impaired brain function or death.

**Kilocalorie (kcal)** Equivalent to 1000 calories, it is the unit used to express the energy value of food.

**Klinefelter syndrome** A chromosomal abnormality caused by the presence of an extra X chromosome in the male. Characteristics include tall stature; sparse pubic and facial hair; gynecomastia; small, firm testes; and absence of spermatogenesis.

**Labor** The process by which the fetus is expelled from the maternal uterus. Also called childbirth, confinement, or parturition.

**Lactation** The process of producing and supplying breast milk.

**Lacto-ovovegetarians** Vegetarians who include milk, dairy products, and eggs in their diets and occasionally fish, poultry, and liver.

**Lactose intolerance** A condition in which an individual has difficulty digesting milk and milk products.

**Lactovegetarians** Vegetarians who include dairy products but no eggs in their diets.

**La Leche League** Organization that provides information on and assistance with breastfeeding.

**Lamaze method** A method of childbirth preparation.

**Lanugo** (lă-nū′gō) Fine, downy hair found on all body parts of the fetus, with the exception of the palms of the hands and the soles of the feet, after 20 weeks' gestation.

**Laparoscopy** Procedure that enables direct visualization of pelvic organs.

**Large for gestational age (LGA)** Excessive growth of a fetus in relation to the gestational time period.

**Last menstrual period (LMP)** The last normal menstrual period experienced by the woman prior to pregnancy; sometimes used to calculate the infant's gestational age.

**Late decelerations** Periodic change in fetal heart rate pattern caused by uteroplacental insufficiency; deceleration has a uniform shape and late onset in relation to maternal contraction.

**Late postpartal hemorrhage** See *Postpartal hemorrhage.*

**Lecithin-sphingomyelin** (les′i-thin sfing′gō-mī′ĕ-lin) **(L/S) ratio** Lecithin and sphingomyelin are phospholipid components of surfactant; their ratio changes during gestation. When the L/S ratio reaches 2:1, the fetal lungs are thought to be mature and the fetus will have a low risk of respiratory distress syndrome (RDS) if born at that time.

**Leiomyoma** A benign tumor of the uterus, composed primarily of smooth muscle and connective tissue. Also referred to as a myoma or a fibroid.

**Leopold's maneuvers** A series of four maneuvers designed to provide a systematic approach whereby the examiner may determine fetal presentation and position.

**Letdown reflex** Pattern of stimulation, hormone release, and resulting muscle contraction that forces milk into the lactiferous ducts, making it available to the infant. Also called milk ejection reflex.

**Leukorrhea** Mucous discharge from the vagina or cervical canal that may be normal or pathologic, as in the presence of infection.

**Lie** Relationship of the long axis of the fetus and the long axis of the pregnant woman. The fetal lie may be longitudinal, transverse, or oblique.

**Lightening** Moving of the fetus and uterus downward into the pelvic cavity.

**Linea nigra** (lin′ē-ă ni′gră) The line of darker pigmentation extending from the umbilicus to the pubis noted in some women during the later months of pregnancy.

**Local anesthesia** Injection of an anesthetic agent into the subcutaneous tissue in a fanlike pattern.

**Lochia** (lō′kē-ă) Maternal discharge of blood, mucus, and tissue from the uterus; may last for several weeks after birth.

**Lochia alba** White vaginal discharge that follows lochia serosa and that lasts from about the 10th to the 21st day after birth.

**Lochia rubra** Red, blood-tinged vaginal discharge that occurs following birth and lasts 2 to 4 days.

**Lochia serosa** Pink, serous, and blood-tinged vaginal discharge that follows lochia rubra and lasts until the 7th to 10th day after birth.

**Long-term variability (LTV)** Large rhythmic fluctuations of the FHR that occur from two to six times per minute.

**Luteinizing hormone (LH)** Anterior pituitary hormone responsible for stimulating ovulation and for development of the corpus luteum.

**Macrosomia** (mak-rō-sō′mē-ă) A condition seen in neonates of large body size and high birth weight, as those born of prediabetic and diabetic mothers.

**Malposition** An abnormal position of the fetus in the birth canal.

**Malpresentation** A presentation of the fetus into the birth canal that is not "normal"—that is, brow, face, shoulder, or breech presentation.

**Mammogram** A soft tissue radiograph of the breast without the injection of a contrast medium.

**Mastitis** Inflammation of the breast.

**Maternal mortality rate** The number of maternal deaths from any cause during the pregnancy cycle per 100,000 live births.

**Mature milk** Breast milk that contains 10% solids for energy and growth.

**McDonald's sign** A probable sign of pregnancy characterized by an ease in flexing the body of the uterus against the cervix.

**Meconium** Dark green or black material present in the large intestine of a full-term infant; the first stools passed by the newborn.

**Meconium aspiration syndrome (MAS)** Respiratory disease of term, postterm, and SGA newborns caused by inhalation of meconium or meconium-stained amniotic fluid into the lungs; characterized by mild to severe respiratory distress, hyperexpansion of the chest, hyperinflated alveoli, and secondary atelectasis.

**Meiosis** The process of cell division that occurs in the maturation of sperm and ova that decreases their number of chromosomes by one-half.

**Menarche** (me-nar′kē) Beginning of menstrual and reproductive function in the female.

**Mendelian inheritance** A major category of inheritance whereby a trait is determined by a pair of genes on homologous chromosomes. Also called single gene inheritance.

**Menopause** The permanent cessation of menses.

**Menorrhagia** Excessive or profuse menstrual flow.

**Menstrual cycle** Cyclic buildup of the uterine lining, ovulation, and sloughing of the lining occurring approximately every 28 days in nonpregnant females.

**Mentum** The chin.

**Mesoderm** The intermediate layer of germ cells in the embryo that gives rise to connective tissue, bone marrow, muscles, blood, lymphoid tissue, and epithelial tissue.

**Metrorrhagia** Abnormal uterine bleeding occurring at irregular intervals.

**Milia** (mil′ē-ă) Tiny white papules appearing on the face of a neonate as a result of unopened sebaceous glands; they disappear spontaneously within a few weeks.

**Miscarriage** See *Spontaneous abortion.*

**Mitosis** Process of cell division whereby both daughter cells have the same number and pattern of chromosomes as the original cell.

**Molding** Shaping of the fetal head by overlapping of the cranial bones to facilitate movement through the birth canal during labor.

**Mongolian spot** Dark, flat pigmentation of the lower back and buttocks noted at birth in some infants; usually disappears by the time the child reaches school age.

**Moniliasis** Yeastlike fungal infection caused by *Candida albicans.*

**Mons pubis** (monz pu′bis) Mound of subcutaneous fatty tissue covering the anterior portion of the symphysis pubis.

**Moro reflex** Flexion of the newborn's thighs and knees accompanied by fingers that fan, then clench, as the arms are simultaneously thrown out and then brought together, as though embracing something. This reflex can be elicited by startling the newborn with a sudden noise or movement. Also called the startle reflex.

**Morula** Developmental stage of the fertilized ovum in which there is a solid mass of cells.

**Mosaicism** Condition of an individual who has at least two cell lines with differing karyotypes.

**Mottling** (mot′ling) Discoloration of the skin in irregular areas; may be seen with chilling, poor perfusion, or hypoxia.

**Mucous plug** A collection of thick mucus that blocks the cervical canal during pregnancy. Also called operculum.

**Multigravida** (mŭl-tē-grav′i-dă) Woman who has been pregnant more than once.

**Multipara** (mŭl-tip′ă-ră) Woman who has had more than one pregnancy in which the fetus was viable.

**Multiple pregnancy** More than one fetus in the uterus at the same time.

**Myometrium** Uterine muscular structure.

**Nägele's rule** A method of determining the estimated date of birth (EDB): after obtaining the first day of the last menstrual period, subtract 3 months and add 7 days.

**Neonatal mortality rate** Number of deaths of infants in the first 28 days of life per 1000 live births.

**Neonatal mortality risk** The chance of death within the newborn period.

**Neonatal transition** The first few hours of life, in which the newborn stabilizes its respiratory and circulatory functions.

**Neonate** Infant from birth through the first 28 days of life.

**Neonatology** The specialty that focuses on the management at-risk conditions of the newborn.

**Neutral thermal environment (NTE)** An environment that provides for minimal heat loss or expenditure.

**Nevus** (nē′vŭs) **flammeus** (flaem′iŭs) Large port-wine stain.

**Nevus vasculosus** "Strawberry mark": raised, clearly delineated, dark-red, rough-surfaced birthmark commonly found in the head region.

**Newborn screening tests** Tests that detect inborn errors of metabolism that, if left untreated, cause mental retardation and physical handicaps.

**Nidation** Implantation of a fertilized ovum in the endometrium.

**Nipple** A protrusion about 0.5 to 1.3 cm in diameter in the center of each mature breast.

**Nipple preparation** Prenatal activities designed to toughen the nipple in preparation for breastfeeding.

**Non-Mendelian (multifactorial) inheritance** The occurrence of congenital disorders that result from an interaction of multiple genetic and environmental factors.

**Nonstress test (NST)** An assessment method by which the reaction (or response) of the fetal heart rate to fetal movement is evaluated.

**Norplant** A subdermal progestin contraceptive that is implanted in a woman's arm and provides contraceptive protection for up to 5 years.

**Nuchal cord** Term used to describe the umbilical cord when it is wrapped around the neck of the fetus.

**Nulligravida** (nŭl-i-grav′i-dă) A woman who has never been pregnant.

**Nullipara** A woman who has not delivered a viable fetus.

**Obstetric conjugate** Distance from the middle of the sacral promontory to an area approximately 1 cm below the pubic crest.

**Oligohydramnios** (ol′i-gō-hī-dram′nē-os) Decreased amount of amniotic fluid, which may indicate a fetal urinary tract defect.

**Oocyte** Early primitive ovum before it has completely developed.

**Oogenesis** Process during fetal life whereby the ovary produces oogenia, cells that become primitive ovarian eggs.

**Oophoritis** Infection of the ovaries.

**Ophthalmia** (of-thal′mē-ă) **neonatorum** Purulent infection of the eyes or conjunctiva of the newborn, usually caused by gonococci.

**Oral contraceptives** Birth control pills that work by inhibiting the release of an ovum and by maintaining a type of mucus that is hostile to sperm.

**Orientation** Infant's ability to respond to auditory and visual stimuli in the environment.

**Ortolani's maneuver** A manual procedure performed to rule out the possibility of developmental dysplastic hip.

**Ovarian ligaments** Ligaments that anchor the lower pole of the ovary to the cornua of the uterus.

**Ovary** Female sex gland in which the ova are formed and in which estrogen and progesterone are produced. Normally there are two ovaries, located in the lower abdomen on each side of the uterus.

**Ovulation** Normal process of discharging a mature ovum from an ovary approximately 14 days prior to the onset of menses.

**Ovum** Female reproductive cell; egg.

**Oxygen toxicity** Excessive levels of oxygen therapy that result in pathologic changes in tissue.

**Oxytocin** Hormone normally produced by the posterior pituitary, responsible for stimulation of uterine contractions and the release of milk into the lactiferous ducts.

**Oxytocin challenge test (OCT)** See *Contraction stress test.*

**Papanicolaou (Pap) smear** Procedure to detect the presence of cancer of the uterus by microscopic examination of cells gently scraped from the cervix.

**Para** (par′ă) A woman who has borne offspring who reached the age of viability.

**Parametritis** Inflammation of the parametrial layer of the uterus.

**Parent-newborn attachment** Close affectional ties that develop between parent and child. See also *Attachment.*

**Passive acquired immunity** Transfer of antibodies (IgG) from the mother to the fetus in utero.

**Pedigree** Graphic representation of a family tree.

**Pelvic cavity** Bony portion of the birth passages; a curved canal with a longer posterior than anterior wall.

**Pelvic cellulitis** Infection involving the connective tissue of the broad ligament or, in severe cases, the connective tissue of all the pelvic structures.

**Pelvic diaphragm** Part of the pelvic floor composed of deep fascia and the levator ani and the coccygeal muscles.

**Pelvic floor** Muscles and tissue that act as a buttress to the pelvic outlet.

**Pelvic inflammatory disease (PID)** An infection of the fallopian tubes that may or may not be accompanied by a pelvic abscess; may cause infertility secondary to tubal damage.

**Pelvic inlet** Upper border of the true pelvis.

**Pelvic outlet** Lower border of the true pelvis.

**Pelvic tilt** Also called pelvic rocking; exercise designed to reduce back strain and strengthen abdominal muscle tone.

**Penis** The male organ of copulation and reproduction.

**Percutaneous umbilical blood sampling (PUBS)** A technique used to obtain pure fetal blood from the umbilical cord while the fetus is in utero. Also called cordocentesis.

**Perimetrium** The outermost layer of the corpus of the uterus. Also known as the serosal layer.

**Perinatal mortality rate** The number of neonatal and fetal deaths per 1000 live births.

**Perinatology** The medical specialty concerned with the diagnosis and treatment of high-risk conditions of the pregnant woman and her fetus.

**Perineal** (per′i-nē′ăl) **body** Wedge-shaped mass of fibromuscular tissue found between the lower part of the vagina and the anal canal.

**Perineum** (per′i-nē′ŭm) The area of tissue between the anus and scrotum in a man or between the anus and vagina in a woman.

**Periodic breathing** Sporadic episodes of apnea, not associated with cyanosis, that last for about 10 seconds and commonly occur in preterm infants.

**Periods of reactivity** Predictable patterns of neonate behavior during the first several hours after birth.

**Persistent occiput posterior position** Malposition of the fetus in which the fetal occiput is posterior in the maternal pelvis.

**Persistent pulmonary hypertension of the newborn (PPHN)** Respiratory disease resulting from right-to-left shunting of blood away from the lungs and through the ductus arteriosus and patent foramen ovale.

**Phenotype** The whole physical, biochemical, and physiologic makeup of an individual as determined both genetically and environmentally.

**Phenylketonuria** (fen′il-kē′tō-nū′rē-ă) A common metabolic disease caused by an inborn error in the metabolism of the amino acid phenylalanine.

**Phosphatidylglycerol (PG)** (fos-fă-tī′dĭl-glis′er-ol) A phospholipid present in fetal surfactant after about 35 weeks' gestation.

**Phototherapy** The treatment of jaundice by exposure to light.

**Physiologic anemia of infancy** A harmless condition in which the hemoglobin level drops in the first 6 to 12 weeks after birth, then reverts to normal levels.

**Physiologic anemia of pregnancy** Apparent anemia that results because during pregnancy the plasma volume increases more than the erythrocytes increase.

**Physiologic jaundice** A harmless condition caused by the normal reduction of red blood cells, occurring 48 or more hours after birth, peaking at the 5th to 7th day, and disappearing between the 7th and 10th day.

**Pica** The eating of substances not ordinarily considered edible or to have nutritive value.

**Placenta** (plă-sen′tă) Specialized disk-shaped organ that connects the fetus to the uterine wall for gas and nutrient exchange. Also called afterbirth.

**Placenta accreta** Partial or complete absence of the decidua basalis and abnormal adherence of the placenta to the uterine wall.

**Placenta previa** Abnormal implantation of the placenta in the lower uterine segment. Classification of type is based on proximity to the cervical os: *total*—completely covers the os; *partial*—covers a portion of the os; *marginal*—is in close proximity to the os.

**Platypelloid pelvis** An unusually wide pelvis, having a flattened oval transverse shape and a shortened anteroposterior diameter.

**Polar body** A small cell resulting from the meiotic division of the mature oocyte.

**Polycythemia** An abnormal increase in the number of total red blood cells in the body's circulation.

**Polydactyly** (pol-ē-dak′ti-lē) A developmental anomaly characterized by more than five digits on the hands or feet.

**Positive signs of pregnancy** Indications that confirm the presence of pregnancy.

**Postconception age periods** Period of time in embryonic/fetal development calculated from the time of fertilization of the ovum.

**Postmature newborn** See *Postterm newborn.*

**Postpartal hemorrhage** A loss of blood of greater than 500 mL following birth. The hemorrhage is classified as *early* if it occurs within the first 24 hours and *late* if it occurs after the first 24 hours.

**Postpartum** After childbirth or delivery.

**Postpartum blues** A maternal adjustment reaction occurring in the first few postpartal days, characterized by mild depression, tearfulness, anxiety, headache, and irritability.

**Postterm labor** Labor that occurs after 42 weeks' gestation.

**Postterm newborn** Any infant born after 42 weeks' gestation.

**Postterm pregnancy** Pregnancy that lasts beyond 42 weeks' gestation.

**Precipitous birth** (1) Unduly rapid progression of labor. (2) A birth in which no physician is in attendance.

**Precipitous labor** Labor lasting less than 3 hours.

**Preeclampsia** (prē-ē-klamp′sē-ă) Toxemia of pregnancy, characterized by hypertension, albuminuria, and edema. See also *Eclampsia.*

**Pregnancy-induced hypertension (PIH)** A hypertensive disorder including preeclampsia and eclampsia as conditions, characterized by the three cardinal signs of hypertension, edema, and proteinuria.

**Premature infant** See *Preterm infant.*

**Premature rupture of the membranes (PROM)** See *Rupture of membranes (ROM).*

**Premenstrual syndrome (PMS)** Cluster of symptoms experienced by some women, typically occurring from a few days up to 2 weeks prior to the onset of menses.

**Prenatal education** Programs offered to expectant families, adolescents, women, or partners to provide education regarding the pregnancy, labor, and birth experience.

**Prep** Shaving of the pubic area.

**Presentation** The fetal body part that enters the maternal pelvis first. The three possible presentations are cephalic, shoulder, and breech.

**Presenting part** The fetal part present in or on the cervical os.

**Presumptive signs of pregnancy** Symptoms that suggest but do not confirm pregnancy, such as cessation of menses, quickening, Chadwick's sign, and morning sickness.

**Preterm infant** Any infant born before 38 weeks' gestation.

**Preterm labor** Labor occurring between 20 and 38 weeks of pregnancy. Also called premature labor.

**Primigravida** (prī-mi-grav′i-dă) A woman who is pregnant for the first time.

**Primipara** (prī-mip′ă-ră) A woman who has given birth to her first child (past the point of viability),whether or not that child is living or was alive at birth.

**Probable signs of pregnancy** Manifestations that strongly suggest the likelihood of pregnancy, such as a positive pregnancy test, enlarging abdomen, and positive Goodell's, Hegar's, and Braxton Hicks signs.

**Progesterone** A hormone produced by the corpus luteum, adrenal cortex, and placenta whose function is to stimulate proliferation of the endometrium to facilitate growth of the embryo.

**Progressive relaxation** A relaxation technique that involves relaxing first one portion of the body and then another portion, until total body relaxation is achieved; may be used during labor.

**Prolactin** A hormone secreted by the anterior pituitary that stimulates and sustains lactation in mammals.

**Prolapsed cord** Umbilical cord that becomes trapped in the vagina before the fetus is born.

**Prolonged labor** Labor lasting more than 24 hours.

**Prostaglandins** Complex lipid compounds synthesized by many cells in the body.

**Pseudomenstruation** Blood-tinged mucus from the vagina in the newborn female infant; caused by withdrawal of maternal hormones that were present during pregnancy.

**Ptyalism** Excessive salivation.

**Pubic** Pertaining to the pubes or pubis.

**Pudendal** (pyū-den′dăl) **block** Injection of an anesthetizing agent at the pudendal nerve to produce numbness of the external genitals and the lower one-third of the vagina, to facilitate childbirth and permit episiotomy if necessary.

**Puerperal morbidity** A maternal temperature of 38°C (100.4°F) or higher on any 2 of the first 10 postpartal days, excluding the first 24 hours. The temperature is to be taken by mouth at least four times per day.

**Puerperium** (pyū-er-pēr′ē-ŭm) The period after completion of the third stage of labor until involution of the uterus is complete, usually 6 weeks.

**Quickening** The first fetal movements felt by the pregnant woman, usually between 16 and 18 weeks' gestation.

**Radiation** Heat loss incurred when heat transfers to cooler surfaces and objects not in direct contact with the body.

**Rape** Sexual activity, often intercourse, against the will of the victim.

**Reciprocal inhibition** The principle that it is impossible to feel relaxed and tense at the same time; the basis for relaxation techniques.

**Recommended dietary allowances (RDA)** Government recommended allowances of various vitamins, minerals, and other nutrients.

**Regional anesthesia** Injection of local anesthetic agents so that they come into direct contact with nervous tissue.

**Relaxin** A water-soluble protein secreted by the corpus luteum that causes relaxation of the symphysis and cervical dilatation.

**Respiratory distress syndrome (RDS)** Respiratory disease of the newborn characterized by interference with ventilation at the alveolar level, thought to be caused by the presence of fibrinoid deposits lining the alveolar ducts. Formerly called hyaline membrane disease.

**Retinopathy** (ret-i-nop′ă-thē) **of prematurity (ROP)** Formation of fibrotic tissue behind the lens; associated with retinal detachment and arrested eye growth, seen with hypoxemia in preterm infants.

**Rh factor** Antigens present on the surface of blood cells that make the blood cell incompatible with blood cells that do not have the antigen.

**RhoGAM** An anti-Rh (*D*) gamma globulin given after delivery to an Rh-negative mother of an Rh-positive fetus or child. Prevents the development of permanent active immunity to the Rh antigen.

**Rhythm method** The timing of sexual intercourse to avoid the fertile time associated with ovulation.

**Risk factors** Any findings that suggest the pregnancy may have a negative outcome, for either the woman or her unborn child.

**Rooting reflex** An infant's tendency to turn the head and open the lips to suck when one side of the mouth or cheek is touched.

**Round ligaments** Ligaments that arise from the side of the uterus near the fallopian tube insertion to help the broad ligament keep the uterus in place.

**Rugae** (rū′gē) Transverse ridges of mucous membranes lining the vagina that allow the vagina to stretch during the descent of the fetal head.

**Rupture of membranes (ROM)** Rupture may be PROM (premature), SROM (spontaneous), or AROM (artificial). Some clinicians may use the abbreviation RBOW (rupture of bag of waters).

**Sacral promontory** A projection into the pelvic cavity on the anterior upper portion of the sacrum; serves as an obstetric guide in determining pelvic measurements.

**Salpingitis** Infection of the fallopian tubes.

**Saltatory pattern** A fetal heart rate pattern of marked or excessive variability.

**Scalp stimulation test (SST)** A test used during labor to assess fetal well-being by pressing a fingertip on the fetal scalp. A fetus not under excessive stress will respond to the digital stimulation with heart rate accelerations.

**Scarf sign** The position of the elbow when the hand of a supine infant is drawn across to the other shoulder until it meets resistance.

**Schultze's mechanism** Delivery of the placenta with the shiny, or fetal, surface presenting first.

**Self-quieting activity** Infant's ability to use personal resources to quiet and console him- or herself.

**Semen** Thick whitish fluid ejaculated by the male during orgasm and containing the spermatozoa and their nutrients.

**Sepsis neonatorum** Infections experienced by a neonate during the first month of life.

**Sex chromosomes** The X and Y chromosomes, which are responsible for sex determination.

**Sexually transmitted infection (STI)** Refers to infections ordinarily transmitted by direct sexual contact with an infected individual. Also called sexually transmitted disease.

**Short-term variability (STV)** Refers to the differences between successive heart beats as measured by the R–R wave interval of the QRS cardiac cycle. Measured only by internal electronic fetal monitoring.

**Show** A pinkish mucous discharge from the vagina that may occur a few hours to a few days prior to the onset of labor.

**Simian line** A single palmar crease frequently found in children with Down syndrome.

**Sinusoidal pattern** A waveform of fetal heart rate in which long-term variability is present but there is no short-term variability.

**Situational contraceptives** Contraceptive methods that involve no prior preparation (eg, abstinence or coitus interruptus).

**Skin turgor** Elasticity of skin; provides information on hydration status.

**Small for gestational age (SGA)** Inadequate weight or growth for gestational age; birth weight below the 10th percentile.

**Spermatogenesis** The process by which mature spermatozoa are formed, during which the number of chromosomes is halved.

**Spermatozoa** Mature sperm cells of the male animal, produced by the testes.

**Spermicides** A variety of creams, foams, jellies, and suppositories that, when inserted into the vagina prior to intercourse, destroy sperm or neutralize any vaginal secretions and thereby immobilize sperm.

**Spinal block** Injection of a local anesthetic agent directly into the spinal fluid in the spinal canal to provide anesthesia for vaginal and cesarean births.

**Spinnbarkheit** The elasticity of the cervical mucus that is present at ovulation.

**Spontaneous abortion** Abortion that occurs naturally. Also called miscarriage.

**Station** Relationship of the presenting fetal part to an imaginary line drawn between the pelvic ischial spines.

**Stillbirth** The delivery of a dead infant.

**Striae** (strī′ă) **gravidarum** Stretch marks; shiny reddish lines that appear on the abdomen, breasts, thighs, and buttocks of pregnant women as a result of stretching the skin.

**Subconjunctival hemorrhage** (sŭb′kon-jŭnk-tī′văl hem′ŏ-rij) Hemorrhage on the sclera of a newborn's eye, usually caused by changes in vascular tension during birth.

**Subdermal implants** See *Norplant.*

**Subinvolution** (sŭb-in-vō-lū′shŭn) Failure of a part to return to its normal size after functional enlargement, such as failure of the uterus to return to normal size after pregnancy.

**Sucking reflex** Normal newborn reflex elicited by inserting a finger or nipple in the newborn's mouth, resulting in forceful, rhythmic sucking.

**Surfactant** (ser-fak′tănt) A surface-active mixture of lipoproteins secreted in the alveoli and air passages that reduces surface tension of pulmonary fluids and contributes to the elasticity of pulmonary tissue.

**Suture** Fibrous connection of opposed joint surfaces, as in the skull.

**Symphysis pubis** Fibrocartilaginous joint between the pelvic bones in the midline.

**Syndactyly** (sin-dak′ti-lē) Malformation of the fingers or toes in which there may be webbing or complete fusion of two or more digits.

**Telangiectatic nevi** (tel-an′jē-ek-tat′ik nē′vī) **(stork bites)** Small clusters of pink-red spots appearing on the nape of the neck and around the eyes of infants; localized areas of capillary dilatation.

**Teratogens** Nongenetic factors that can produce malformations of the fetus.

**Term** The normal duration of pregnancy.

**Testes** The male gonads, in which sperm and testosterone are produced.

**Testosterone** The male hormone; responsible for the development of secondary male characteristics.

**Therapeutic abortion** Medically induced termination of pregnancy when a malformed fetus is suspected or when the woman's health is in jeopardy.

**Thrombophlebitis** Inflammation of a vein wall, resulting in thrombus.

**Thrush** A fungal infection of the oral mucous membranes caused by *Candida albicans.* Most often seen in infants; characterized by white plaques in the mouth.

**Tocolysis** Use of medications to arrest preterm labor.

**Tonic neck reflex** Postural reflex seen in the newborn. When the supine infant's head is turned to one side, the arm and leg on that side extend while the extremities on the opposite side flex. Also called the fencing position.

**TORCH** An acronym used to describe a group of infections that represent potentially severe problems during pregnancy. TO, toxoplasmosis; R, rubella; C, cytomegalovirus;, H, herpesvirus.

**Total serum bilirubin** Sum of conjugated (direct) and unconjugated (indirect) bilirubin.

**Touch relaxation** A relaxation technique that involves relaxing an area of one's body as another person provides a "touch" cue to that specific area. Touch relaxation is very effective during labor contractions.

**Toxic shock syndrome** Infection caused by *Staphylococcus aureus,* found primarily in women of reproductive age.

**Transitional milk** Breast milk produced from the end of colostrum production until about 2 weeks postpartum.

**Transverse diameter** The largest diameter of the pelvic inlet; helps determine the shape of the inlet.

**Transverse lie** A lie in which the fetus is positioned crosswise in the uterus.

***Trichomonas vaginalis*** A parasitic protozoan that may cause inflammation of the vagina, characterized by itching and burning of vulvar tissue and by white, frothy discharge.

**Trimester** Three months, or one-third of the gestational time for pregnancy.

**Trisomy** The presence of three homologous chromosomes rather than the normal two.

**Trophoblast** The outer layer of the blastoderm that will eventually establish the nutrient relationship with the uterine endometrium.

**True pelvis** The portion that lies below the linea terminalis, made up of the inlet, cavity, and outlet.

**Tubal ligation** Sterilization of a woman accomplished by transecting or occluding the fallopian tubes.

**Turner syndrome** A number of anomalies that occur when a woman has only one X chromosome. Characteristics include short stature; little sexual differentiation; webbing of the neck, with a low posterior hairline; and congenital cardiac anomalies.

**Ultrasound** High-frequency sound waves that may be directed, through the use of a transducer, into the maternal abdomen. The ultrasonic sound waves reflected by the underlying structures of varying densities allow identification of various maternal and fetal tissues, bones, and fluids.

**Umbilical cord** (ŭm-bil′i-kăl kōrd) The structure connecting the placenta to the umbilicus of the fetus and through which nutrients from the woman are exchanged for wastes from the fetus.

**Uterine atony** Relaxation of uterine muscle tone following birth.

**Uterine inversion** Prolapse of the uterine fundus through the cervix into the vagina; may occur just prior to or during delivery of the placenta; associated with massive hemorrhage, requiring emergency treatment.

**Uterosacral ligaments** Ligaments that provide support for the uterus and cervix at the level of the ischial spines.

**Uterus** The hollow muscular organ in which the fertilized ovum is implanted and in which the developing fetus is nourished until birth.

**Vagina** The musculomembranous tube or passageway located between the external genitals and the uterus of a woman.

**Vaginal birth after cesarean (VBAC)** Practice of permitting a trial of labor and possible vaginal birth for women following a previous cesarean birth for nonrecurring causes such as fetal distress or placenta previa.

**Variable deceleration** Periodic change in fetal heart rate caused by umbilical cord compression; decelerations vary in onset, occurrence, and waveform.

**Vasectomy** Surgical removal of a portion of the vas deferens (ductus deferens) to produce infertility.

**Vegan** A "pure" vegetarian; one who consumes no food from animal sources.

**Vena caval syndrome** Symptoms of dizziness, pallor, and clamminess that result from lowered blood pressure when a pregnant woman lies supine and the enlarged uterus presses on the vena cava. Also known as supine hypotensive syndrome.

**Vernix caseosa** (ver′niks kā′sē-ōs) A protective, cheeselike, whitish substance made up of sebum and desquamated epithelial cells that is present on the fetal skin.

**Version** Turning of the fetus in utero.

**Vertex** The top or crown of the head.

**Vulva** The external structure of the female genitals, lying below the mons veneris.

**Weaning** The process of discontinuing breastfeeding and accustoming an infant to another feeding method.

**Wharton's** (hwar′tunz) **jelly** Yellow-white gelatinous material surrounding the vessels of the umbilical cord.

**Zona pellucida** Transparent inner layer surrounding an ovum.

**Zygote** A fertilized egg.

**Zygote intrafallopian transfer (ZIFT)** Retrieval of oocytes under ultrasound guidance, followed by in vitro fertilization and laparoscopic replacement of fertilized eggs into the fimbriated end of the fallopian tube.

## Art Credits

**Chapter 2** 2-1: Barbara Cousins. 2-2: Wendy Hiller Gee/Biomed Arts Associates. 2-3A-B: Kristin Mount. 2-4: Wendy Hiller Gee/Biomed Arts Associates. 2-5A-B: Precision Graphics. 2-6: Wendy Hiller Gee/Biomed Arts Associates. 2-7: Wendy Hiller Gee/Biomed Arts Associates. 2-8: Kristin Mount. 2-9: Kristin Mount. 2-10A-B: Precision Graphics. 2-11: Kristin Mount. 2-12: Wendy Hiller Gee/Biomed Arts Associates. 2-13: Nea Hanscomb. 2-14: Kristin Mount. 2-15: Barbara Cousins. 2-16: Kristin Mount.

**Chapter 3** 3:1: Nea Hanscomb. 3-2A: Kristin Mount. 3-3A-B: Precision Graphics. 3-4: Kristin Mount. 3-5A-C: Kristin Mount. 3-6: Kristin Mount. 3-7: Kristin Mount. 3-10: Kristin Mount. 3-11: Kristin Mount. 3-12: Precision Graphics.

**Chapter 4** 4-1: Nea Hanscomb. 4-2B: Precision Graphics. 4-3B-D: Precision Graphics. 4-4A-D: Precision Graphics. 4-6: Nea Hanscomb. 4-8: Precision Graphics. 4-9: Precision Graphics.

**Chapter 5** 5-1: Nea Hanscomb. 5-2A-B: The Left Coast Group. 5-3A: Precision Graphics. 5-4: Nea Hanscomb. 5-12: Precision Graphics. 5-13: Precision Graphics. 5-14: Precision Graphics. 5-15: Kristin Mount. 5-16A-B: Precision Graphics. 5-17: Precision Graphics.

**Chapter 6** 6-1: The Left Coast Group. 6-3: Precision Graphics.

**Chapter 7** 7-1: Kristin Mount. 7-3A-B: Kristin Mount. 7-4: Kristin Mount. 7-5: Kristin Mount. 7-6: Kristin Mount. 7-7: Kristin Mount. 7-8: Kristin Mount.

**Chapter 8** 8-1: Nea Hanscomb. 8-3: Kristin Mount. 8-5A-D: Kristin Mount. 8-6: Kristin Mount.

**Chapter 9** 9-5: The Left Coast Group. 9-9: Kristin Mount.

**Chapter 10** 10-1: Shirley Bortoli.

**Chapter 11** 11-1: Robert Voights/Nea Hanscomb. 11-2: Shirley Bortoli. 11-4: The Left Coast Group.

**Chapter 13** 13-1A-C: Precision Graphics. 13-2: Kristin Mount. 13-5A-E: Kristin Mount.

**Chapter 14** 14-5: Nea Hanscomb. 14-6: Nea Hanscomb. 14-7: Kristin Mount. 14-8: Nea Hanscomb. 14-9: Kristin Mount.

**Chapter 15** 15-1: Kristin Mount. 15-2: Kristin Mount. 15-3: Kristin Mount. 15-4A-B: Kristin Mount. 15-5: Precision Graphics. 15-6A-D: Precision Graphics. 15-7A-C: Precision Graphics. 15-8: Precision Graphics. 15-9: Precision Graphics. 15-10: Nea Hanscomb. 15-11A-D: Precision Graphics. 15-13A-E: Kristin Mount. 15-14A-B: Kristin Mount. 15-15: Precision Graphics. 15-16: Precision Graphics. 15-17A-C: Precision Graphics.

**Chapter 16** 16-2: Kristin Mount. 16-3A-D: Precision Graphics. 16-4: Precision Graphics. 16-5: Kristin Mount. 16-6: Precision Graphics. 16-10: Nea Hanscomb. 16-11A-D: Nea Hanscomb. 16-12: Nea Hanscomb. 16-13: Nea Hanscomb.

**Chapter 17** 17-7A-C: Precision Graphics. 17-9: Precision Graphics.

**Chapter 18** 18-1A-C: Precision Graphics. 18-2: Kristin Mount. 18-3A-D: Kristin Mount. 18-4: Kristin Mount. 18-5A-B: Kristin Mount. 18-6: Kristin Mount. 18-7 Precision Graphics.

**Chapter 19** 19-1A-B: The Left Coast Group. 19-2A-B: Precision Graphics. 19-3A-D: Nea Hanscomb. 19-4A-B: Precision Graphics. 19-5: Precision Graphics. 19-6A-B: Precision Graphics. 19-7A-D: Precision Graphics. 19-8A-B: Precision Graphics. 19-10: Nea Hanscomb. 19-11A-C: Precision Graphics. 19-12A-C: Precision Graphics. 19-14: Nea Hanscomb. 19-15: Precision Graphics. 19-9A-F: Precision Graphics.

**Chapter 20** 20-1: Precision Graphics. 20-2A-B: Wendy Hiller Gee/Biomed Arts Associates. 20-3A-C: Precision Graphics. 20-4A-C: Precision Graphics. 20-5A-C: Nea Hanscomb.

**Chapter 21** 21-1: Nea Hanscomb. 21-2: Nea Hanscomb. 21-3: Kristin Mount. 21-4: Nea Hanscomb. 21-5A-D: Precision Graphics. 21-6: Precision Graphics. 21-7: Nea Hanscomb.

**Chapter 22** 22-1: The Left Coast Group. 22-11: Nea Hanscomb. 22-12: The Left Coast Group. 22-14A-B: Precision Graphics. 22-15: Precision Graphics. 22-24: Kristin Mount. 22-25: Kristin Mount. 22-34A-C: Kristin Mount.

**Chapter 23** 23-3: Kristin Mount. 23-5A-B: Precision Graphics. 23-6: Precision Graphics. 23-7: The Left Coast Group. 23-10: Precision Graphics. 23-10: Precision Graphics. 23-11: Precision Graphics. 23-12: The Left Coast Group.

**Chapter 24** 24-2A-D: Precision Graphics. 24-5: Precision Graphics. 24-6: Shirley Bortoli.

**Chapter 25** 25-1: Nea Hanscomb. 25-2: Nea Hanscomb. 25-8: Precision Graphics. 25-9: Precision Graphics.

**Chapter 26** 26-2A-B: Precision Graphics. 26-3: Nea Hanscomb. 26-6: Nea Hanscomb. 26-8: Nea Hanscomb. 26-10: Nea Hanscomb. 26-13: Nea Hanscomb. 26-14: Nea Hanscomb.

**Chapter 27** 27-1: Kristin Mount. 27-5: Precision Graphics. 27-6: Nea Hanscomb.

**Chapter 29** 29-2: Precision Graphics. 29-5: Precision Graphics.

**Chapter 30** 30-1A-B: Kristin Mount. 30-2: Kristin Mount.

## Photography Credits

**Chapter 1** 1-1: © Richard Tauber/Addison Wesley Longman.

**Chapter 3** 3-2B: © Lennart Nillson/Albert Bonniers Forlag AB: *A Child is Born,* Dell, 1990. 3-8: Courtesy of Marcia London, RNC, MSN, NNP. 3-9: Courtesy of Marcia London, RNC, MSN, NNP. 3-13: © Petit Format/Nestle/Science Source/Photo Researchers, Inc. 3-14: © Petit Format/Nestle/Science Source/Photo Researchers, Inc. 3-15: © Lennart Nillson/Albert Bonniers Forlag AB: *A Child is Born,* Dell, 1990. 3-16: © Lennart Nillson/Albert Bonniers Forlag AB: *A Child is Born,* Dell, 1990. 3-17: © Lennart Nillson/Albert Bonniers Forlag AB: *A Child is Born,* Dell, 1990.

**Chapter 4** 4-2A: © Kathleen Cameron/Addison Wesley Longman. 4-3A: © Kathleen Cameron/Addison Wesley Longman. 4-5: © Kathleen Cameron/Addison Wesley Longman. 4-7 (left): © Kathleen Cameron/Addison Wesley Longman. 4-7 (right): © Alain McLaughlin/Addison Wesley Longman. 4-10: Courtesy of Centers for Disease Control and Prevention. 4-11: Courtesy of Centers for Disease Control and Prevention. 4-12: © D.M. Phillips/Visuals Unlimited. 4-13: © Kenneth Greer/Visuals Unlimited.

**Chapter 5** 5-3B: Courtesy of Lovena L. Porter. 5-3C: Speroff, L., et al.: *Clinical Gynecologic Endocrinology and Infertility,* 5th ed. 5-5: Courtesy of David Peakman, Reproductive Genetics Center, Denver, CO. 5-6: Courtesy of David Peakman, Reproductive Genetics Center, Denver, CO. 5-7: Courtesy Dr. Arthur Robinson, National Jewish Hospital and Research Center, Denver, CO. 5-8: From Jones, K. L.: *Smith's Recognizable Patterns of Human Malformations,* 4th ed.. Philadelphia: Saunders, 1988. 5-9: From Jones, K. L.: *Smith's Recognizable Patterns of Human Malformations,* 4th ed.. Philadelphia: Saunders, 1988. 5-10: From Jones, K. L.: *Smith's Recognizable Patterns of Human Malformations,* 4th ed.. Philadelphia: Saunders, 1988. 5-11: From Lemli, L., Smith, D. W. (1963). The XO syndrome: A study of the different phenotype in 25 patients. *Journal of Pediatrics, 63,* 577.

**Chapter 6** 6-2: The Left Coast Group

**Chapter 7** 7-2: © Annie Dowie/Addison Wesley Longman. 7-5: Unknown.

**Chapter 8** 8-2: © Elena Dorfman/Addison Wesley Longman. 8-4: © Elena Dorfman/ Addison Wesley Longman.

**Chapter 9** 9-1: Photos courtesy of Birthways Childbirth Resource Center, Inc. 9-2: © Richard Tauber/Addison Wesley Longman. 9-3: © Jenny Thomas Photography/Addison Wesley Longman. 9-5: © Elena Dorfman/Addison Wesley Longman. 9-6: © Elena Dorfman/ Addison Wesley Longman. 9-7A-D: © Elena Dorfman/Addison Wesley Longman. 9-9: © Elena Dorfman/Addison Wesley Longman.

**Chapter 10** 10-2: © Elena Dorfman/ Addison Wesley Longman. 10-3: © Jenny Thomas Photography/Addison Wesley Longman.

**Chapter 11** 11-3: © Elena Dorfman/ Addison Wesley Longman.

**Chapter 12** 12-1: © Jenny Thomas Photography/Addison Wesley Longman.

**Chapter 13** 13-3: © Elena Dorfman/ Addison Wesley Longman. 13-4: © Elena Dorfman/Addison Wesley Longman.

**Chapter 14** 14-1: © Elena Dorfman/ Addison Wesley Longman. 14-2: © Elena Dorfman/Addison Wesley Longman. 14-3: From Cundiff, J. L., Haybrich, K. L., Hinzman, N. G. (1990, Nov./Dec.). Umbilical artery Doppler flow studies during pregnancy. *JOGNN, 19*(6), 475, fig. 3. 14-4: From Cundiff, J. L., Haybrich, K. L., Hinzman, N. G. (1990, Nov./Dec.). Umbilical artery Doppler flow studies during pregnancy. *JOGNN, 19*(6), 475, fig. 4.

**Chapter 15** 15-12: © Stella Johnson/ Addison Wesley Longman.

**Chapter 16** 16-1: © Stella Johnson/Addison Wesley Longman. 16-7A-B: © Elena Dorfman/Addison Wesley Longman. 16-7C: © Stella Johnson/Addison Wesley Longman.

**Chapter 17** 17-1: © Elena Dorfman/ Addison Wesley Longman. 17-2: © Elena Dorfman/Addison Wesley Longman. 17-3: © Elena Dorfman/Addison Wesley Longman. 17-4: © Suzanne Arms/Addison Wesley Longman. 17-5A: © Elena Dorfman/Addison Wesley Longman. 17-5B: © Stella Johnson/ Addison Wesley Longman. 17-6: © Stella Johnson/Addison Wesley Longman. 17-8: © Elena Dorfman/Addison Wesley Longman. 17-10: © Suzanne Arms/Addison Wesley Longman.

**Chapter 19** 19-13: Courtesy of Dr. Dan Farine, University of Toronto.

**Chapter 21** 21-9: © Beth Elkin/Addison Wesley Longman. 21-10: © Elena Dorfman/Addison Wesley Longman.

**Chapter 22** 22-2A-C: Reprinted by permission of V. Dubowitz, M.D., Hammersmith Hospital, London, England. 22-3A: Courtesy of Barbara Carey, RNC, MSN, NNP. 22-3B-C: Reprinted by permission of V. Dubowitz, M.D., Hammersmith Hospital, London, England. 22-4A-B: Reprinted by permission of V. Dubowitz, M.D., Hammersmith Hospital, London, England. 22-4C: © Suzanne Arms/ Addison Wesley Longman. 22-5A-B: Reprinted by permission of V. Dubowitz, M.D., Hammersmith Hospital, London, England. 22-5C: © Suzanne Arms/Addison Wesley Longman. 22-6A: Reprinted by permission of V. Dubowitz, M.D., Hammersmith Hospital, London, England. 22-6B: © Suzanne Arms/Addison Wesley Longman. 22-7A-C: Reprinted by permission of V. Dubowitz, M.D., Hammersmith Hospital, London, England. 22-8A-C: Reprinted by permission of V. Dubowitz, M.D., Hammersmith Hospital, London, England. 22-9A-C: Reprinted by permission of V. Dubowitz, M.D., Hammersmith Hospital, London, England. 22-10A-B: Reprinted by permission of V. Dubowitz, M.D., Hammersmith Hospital, London, England. 22-13: © Elena Dorfman/Addison Wesley Longman. 22-16: © Elena Dorfman/ Addison Wesley Longman. 22-23: From Korones, S. B. (1986). *High-Risk newborn infants* (4th ed.). St. Louis: Mosby. 22-24: Photo reproduced with permission from Potter, E. L., & Craig, J. M. (1975). *Pathology of the fetus and infant* (3rd ed.). Chicago: Year Book Medical Publishers. 22-25: Photo courtesy of Mead Johnson Laboratories, Evansville, IN. 22-26: Courtesy of Dr. Ralph Platow from Potter, E. L., & Craig, J. M. (1975). *Pathology of the fetus and infant* (3rd ed.). Chicago: Year Book Medical Publishers. 22-27: Courtesy of Mead Johnson Laboratories, Evansville, IN. 22-28: © Stella Johnson/ Addison Wesley Longman. 22-29A-B: Courtesy of Mead Johnson Laboratories, Evansville, IN. 22-30: : From Korones, S. B. (1986). *High-Risk newborn infants* (4th ed.). St. Louis: Mosby. 22-31A-B: © Elena Dorfman/Addison Wesley Longman. 22-32: © Elena Dorfman/ Addison Wesley Longman. 22-33: Reproduced with permission from Potter, E. L., & Craig, J. M. (1975). *Pathology of the fetus and infant* (3rd ed.). Chicago: Year Book Medical Publishers. 22-35A: Provided courtesy Mead Johnson Nutritionals. 22-35B: © Stella Johnson/Addison Wesley Longman. 22-36: © Stella Johnson/ Addison Wesley Longman. 22-37: © Stella Johnson/Addison Wesley Longman. 22-38: © Stella Johnson/Addison Wesley Longman. 22-39: © Stella Johnson/Addison Wesley Longman. 22-40: © Elena Dorfman/Addison Wesley Longman.

**Chapter 23** 23-1: © Stella Johnson/Addison Wesley Longman. 23-2: © Elena Dorfman/ Addison Wesley Longman. 23-4: Courtesy of Ruth Likler RNC, BSN. 23-8: © Stella Johnson/Addison Wesley Longman. 23-9: © Stella Johnson/Addison Wesley Longman.

**Chapter 24** 24-1: © Stella Johnson/Addison Wesley Longman. 24-3: © Stella Johnson/ Addison Wesley Longman. 24-4B: © Stella Johnson/Addison Wesley Longman. 24-7: © Stella Johnson/Addison Wesley Longman. 24-8: © Jenny Thomas Photography/Addison Wesley Longman.

**Chapter 25** 25-3: Courtesy of Carol Harrigan, RNC, MSN, NNP. 25-4: © Stella Johnson/Addison Wesley Longman. 25-5: From Dubowitz, L., & Dubowitz, V. (1977). *The gestational age of the newborn.* Menlo Park, CA: Addison-Wesley. Reprinted by permission of V. Dubowitz, MD, Hammersmith Hospital, London, England. 25-6: Courtesy of Carol Harrigan, RNC, MSN, NNP. 25-7: Courtesy of Carol Harrigan, RNC, MSN, NNP. 25-10: Courtesy of Kadlac Medical Center Kangaroo Care Study and Carol Thompson, MSN, NNP. 25-11: Courtesy of Carol Harrigan, RNC, MSN, NNP. 25-12: Courtesy of Theresa Kledzik, RN. Table 25-3 (photo): Newborn with lumbar myelomeningocele photo courtesy of Dr. Paul Winchester.

**Chapter 26** 26-1: © Stella Johnson/Addison Wesley Longman. 26-4: Courtesy of Carol Harrigan, RNC, MSN, NNP. 26-5: Courtesy of Carol Harrigan, RNC, MSN, NNP. 26-7: © Stella Johnson/Addison Wesley Longman. 26-9: © Elena Dorfman/Addison Wesley Longman. 26-11: © Stella Johnson/Addison Wesley Longman. 26-12: © Stella Johnson/Addison Wesley Longman. 26-15: © Stella Johnson/ Addison Wesley Longman.

**Chapter 27** 27-2: Reprinted from *Myles textbook for midwives 11/e,* Bennett R., p. 235, F 16.2, 1989, by permission of the publisher Churchill Livingstone. 27-3: © Stella Johnson/Addison Wesley Longman. 27-4: © Beth Elkin/Addison Wesley Longman. 27-7: © Elena Dorfman/Addison Wesley Longman.

**Chapter 28** 28-1: © Stella Johnson/Addison Wesley Longman. 28-2A-H: © Anne Dowie/Addison Wesley Longman.

**Chapter 29** 29-1: © Kathy Kieliszewski/ Addison Wesley Longman. 29-3: © Stella Johnson/Addison Wesley Longman. 29-4: © Kathy Kieliszewski/Addison Wesley Longman.

# INDEX

# INDEX

# Special Features

## Assessment Guides



## Critical Pathways



## Critical Thinking in Practice



## Drug Guides



## Evidence-Based Practice



## Key Facts to Remember